CHURCHILL LIVINGSTONE

# MEDICAL
# DICTIONARY

*For Elsevier:*

*Commissioning Editor:* Mairi McCubbin
*Development Editor:* Ailsa Laing/Ewan Halley
*Project Manager:* Rory MacDonald
*Designer:* Erik Bigland
*Illustrations Manager:* Gillian Richards/Kirsteen Wright

CHURCHILL LIVINGSTONE

# MEDICAL DICTIONARY

Edited by

## Chris Brooker BSc MSc RGN SCM RNT

Author and Editor, Norfolk, UK

SIXTEENTH EDITION

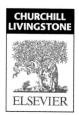

EDINBURGH LONDON NEW YORK OXFORD PHILADELPHIA ST LOUIS SYDNEY
TORONTO 2008

# CHURCHILL LIVINGSTONE
## ELSEVIER

An imprint of Elsevier Limited
© E. & S. Livingstone Limited 1963, 1966, 1969
© Longman Group Limited 1974, 1978
© Longman Group UK Limited 1987
© Pearson Professional Limited 1995
© Harcourt Brace and Company Limited 1998
© Elsevier Limited 2003
© 2008, Elsevier Limited. All rights reserved.

The right of Chris Brooker to be identified as editor of this work has been asserted by her in accordance with the Copyright, Designs and Patents Act 1988.

| First edition 1933 | Ninth edition 1961 |
| Second edition 1935 | Tenth edition 1966 |
| Third edition 1938 | Eleventh edition 1969 |
| Fourth edition 1940 | Twelfth edition 1974 |
| Fifth edition 1941 | Thirteenth edition 1976 |
| Sixth edition 1943 | Fourteenth edition 1987 |
| Seventh edition 1946 | Fifteenth edition 2003 |
| Eighth edition 1949 | Sixteenth edition 2008 |

Standard Edition ISBN 978-0-443-10412-1

International Edition of Fourteenth Edition 1987
International Edition of Fifteenth Edition 2003
International Edition of Sixteenth Edition 2008

International Edition ISBN 978-0-443-10410-7

**British Library Cataloguing in Publication Data**
A catalogue record for this book is available from the British Library

**Library of Congress Cataloging in Publication Data**
A catalog record for this book is available from the Library of Congress

**Notice**
Neither the Publisher nor the Author assumes any responsibility for any loss or injury and/or damage to persons or property arising out of or related to any use of the material contained in this book. It is the responsibility of the treating practitioner, relying on independent expertise and knowledge of the patient, to determine the best treatment and method of application for the patient.
*The Publisher*

**ELSEVIER**

your source for books, journals and multimedia in the health sciences

**www.elsevierhealth.com**

Working together to grow libraries in developing countries

www.elsevier.com | www.bookaid.org | www.sabre.org

ELSEVIER | BOOK AID International | Sabre Foundation

The publisher's policy is to use paper manufactured from sustainable forests

Printed in China

# Contents

# Preface

Health care and medical practice continue to change at a rapid pace, with exciting developments leading to many new interventions. Thus all those concerned need easy access to up-to-date information from many medical specialties and other health care disciplines. The 16th edition of the *Churchill Livingstone Medical Dictionary* aims to meet the needs of a broad group that includes medical students, practising doctors, students and practitioners of the allied health professions, others working in the medical/health fields, such as medical secretaries and receptionists, and members of the public.

This well-established dictionary has been extensively enlarged—over 3500 new words/terms have been added and it now has over 11 000 main entries. Existing entries have been revised and updated.

New features for this edition include the introduction of 150 informative two-colour illustrations and photographs. An icon included in some main entries/appendices alerts readers to further material on the DVD that accompanies the dictionary. This contains the following features:

- Basic life support (BLS) algorithms from the *2005 Resuscitation Guidelines* (Resuscitation Council, UK)
- Colour photographs of a selection of disorders
- Reference values for hormones in the blood
- Links to several professional, evidence-based practice and information websites
- Spell checker
- The full image bank for the dictionary.

Many subject areas that were introduced in the 15th edition have been expanded, including: critical care, complementary medicine, epidemiology, ethics, nutrition, occupational medicine, oncology, podiatry, public health and health promotion, quality issues, research and sports medicine. The entries relating to nutrition, occupational therapy, physiotherapy, radiography, and speech and language therapy have been expanded to reflect the increasingly multiprofessional and interprofessional approaches to health care. The pharmacological entries are mostly general and most relate to pharmacological terms and drug groups, rather than specific drug names. However, further drug information is provided in Appendix 5.

The eight appendices have been revised and updated:

- **Appendix 1** contains full-page, full-colour line illustrations of the major body systems. At the appropriate anatomical term in the dictionary, the reader is directed to the relevant illustration.
- **Appendix 2** explains about SI units and the metric system and provides useful conversion scales for certain chemical pathology tests and common units of measurement.

- **Appendix 3** details normal values for blood, cerebrospinal fluid, faeces and urine.
- **Appendix 4** provides an overview of the nutrients required for health and well-being.
- **Appendix 5** introduces the wide-ranging topic of drugs. An overview of drugs and the relevant legislation is provided. Essential information about the measurement of drugs follows. A further feature is information about the drug groups in common use, with subgroups, drug examples and clinical indications provided in a table for easy reference.
- **Appendix 6** lists abbreviations of commonly used medical terms and related organizations.
- **Appendix 7** lists useful websites, helping you to access the very latest information.
- **Appendix 8** provides some common chemical symbols and formulae.

It is 75 years since the publication of the first edition of this dictionary and I hope that the 16th edition will continue to be a valuable resource for students, registered practitioners and all those with an interest in health and health care.

Chris Brooker
Norfolk 2008

# Acknowledgements

The editor would like to thank Mairi McCubbin, Ailsa Laing and Rory MacDonald at Elsevier; Jennifer Kelly, who revised Appendix 5, and the advisers for the 15th edition.

The following figures have been reproduced or adapted with permission from the following publications:

Bale S, Jones V 1997 Wound Care Nursing. A Patient-Centred Approach. Baillière Tindall, London: Figure V.1.

Boon N, Colledge N, Walker B, Hunter J (eds) 2006 Davidson's Principles and Practice of Medicine, 20th edn. Churchill Livingstone, Edinburgh: Figures B.2, C.12, N.5, P.13, S.3, S.9, V.3 and Table G.1.

Brooker C 1998 Human Structure and Function. Nursing Applications in Clinical Practice, 2nd edn. Mosby, London: Figure P.6.

Brooker C (ed) 2002 Mosby Nurse's Pocket Dictionary, 32nd edn. Mosby, Edinburgh: Figure A.7.

Brooker C (ed) 2006A Mosby Nurse's Pocket Dictionary, 33rd edn. Mosby, Edinburgh: Figures A.6, B.1, B.6, C.3, C.4, C.9, F.3, I.3, M.7, O.3, O.4, P.10, P.11, R.3, S.1, S.7, T.2.

Brooker C (ed) 2006B Churchill Livingstone's Dictionary of Nursing, 19th edn. Churchill Livingstone, Edinburgh: Figure C.2.

Brooker C, Nicol M (eds) 2003 Nursing Adults. The Practice of Caring. Mosby, Edinburgh: Figures A.2, A.10, A.11, A.12, A.13, B.4, B.5, C.14, C.16, D.3, D.4, E.3, E.4, I.2, L.2, M.4, N.4, O.1, P.1, P.12, R.2, S.6, T.5, V.2, W.1 and Table B.1.

Brooker C, Waugh A (eds) 2007 Foundations of Nursing Practice. Fundamentals of Holistic Care. Mosby, Edinburgh: Figures A.8, C.7, C.10, E.5, M.5, N.2, R.4, R.5, R.7, S.5, V.4.

Downie G, Mackenzie J, Williams A 2003 Pharmacology and Medicines Management for Nurses, 3rd edn. Churchill Livingstone, Edinburgh: Figure Z.1.

Fraser D, Cooper M (eds) 2003 Myles Textbook for Midwives, 14th edn. Churchill Livingstone, Edinburgh: Figures B.8, C.6, E.1, M.9, P.8, S.4, U.2 and Table A.1.

Gangar E (ed) 2001 Gynaecological Nursing. A Practical Guide. Churchill Livingstone, Edinburgh: Figure U.1.

Gunn C 2001 Using Maths in Health Sciences. Churchill Livingstone, Edinburgh: Figures C.5, H.7, N.6.

Hinchliff S, Montague S, Watson R (eds) 1996 Physiology for Nursing Practice, 2nd edn. Baillière Tindall, London: Figures D.1, F.4, K.1, M.2, M.3, M.6, M.11, P.9, T.6.

Huband S, Trigg E (eds) 2000 Practices in Children's Nursing. Guidelines for Hospital and Community. Churchill Livingstone, Edinburgh: Figures H.3, P.4.

Jamieson E, McCall J, Whyte L 2002 Clinical Nursing Practices, 4th edn. Churchill Livingstone, Edinburgh: Figure S.8.

Kanski J 1999 Clinical Ophthalmology. A Systematic Approach, 4th edn. Butterworth-Heinemann, Oxford: Figure F.5.

Mallik M, Hall C, Howard D (eds) 1998 Nursing Knowledge and Practice. A Decision-Making Approach. Baillière Tindall, London: Figures H.2, J.1.

Nicol M, Bavin C, Bedford-Turner S, Cronin P, Rawlings-Anderson K 2004

Essential Nursing Skills, 2nd edn. Mosby, Edinburgh: Figures A.5, C.1, E.2, H.9, N.1, P.3, P.14, R.1.

Parsons M, Johnson M 2001 Diagnosis in Colour: Neurology. Mosby, Edinburgh: Figure E.8.

Peattie P, Walker S (eds) 1995 Understanding Nursing Care, 4th edn. Churchill Livingstone, Edinburgh: Figure H.4.

Porter S 2005 Dictionary of Physiotherapy. Butterworth-Heinemann, Edinburgh: Figures A.9, B.7, C.11, C.13, D.2, G.1, I.1, M.1, M.10, N.1, O.2, S.2, S.10, W.2 and Table M.1.

Pudner R (ed) 2000 Nursing the Surgical Patient. Baillière Tindall, Edinburgh: Figure S.11.

Rodeck C, Whittle M (eds) 1999 Fetal Medicine. Basic Science and Clinical Practice. Churchill Livingstone, Edinburgh: Figure C.8.

Rutishauser S 1994 Physiology and Anatomy. A Basis for Nursing and Health Care. Churchill Livingstone, Edinburgh: Figure F.2.

Walsh M (ed) 2002 Watson's Clinical Nursing and Related Sciences, 6th edn. Baillière Tindall, Edinburgh: Figure L.4.

Watson R 2000 Anatomy and Physiology for Nurses, 11th edn. Baillière Tindall, Edinburgh: Figures E.6, E.7, G.2, G.4, H.6, L.1, L.3, M.8, P.5, P.7, R.6, T.3.

Waugh A, Grant A 2006 Ross and Wilson Anatomy and Physiology in Health and Illness, 10th edn. Churchill Livingstone, Edinburgh: Figures A.1, A.4, C.15, F.1, H.1, H.5, H.8, N.3, N.7, P.2, S.12, T.1, T.4.

Westwood O 1999 The Scientific Basis for Health Care. Mosby, London: Figure G.3.

Wilson J 1995 Infection Control in Clinical Practice. Baillière Tindall, London: Figure B.3.

Zhu H 2005 Running a Safe and Successful Acupuncture Clinic. Churchill Livingstone, Edinburgh: Figure A.3.

# Panel of advisers

**For the 16th edition**

**Jennifer Kelly** BA(Hons) MSc RGN DipN DipNEd
Lecturer, University of East Anglia, King's Lynn, UK

**For the 15th edition**

**David Assheton** MB ChB MRC
Specialist Registrar, Merseyside Hospital, Royal Liverpool University Hospital, Prescott St, Liverpool, UK

**Anne Ballinger** MD FRCP
Senior Lecturer and Honorary Consultant Physician, Department of Adult and Paediatric Gastroenterology, Barts and the London Queen Mary's School of Medicine and Dentistry, London, UK

**Helen Barker** BSc SRD MPH PGCE
Senior Lecturer in Dietetics, School of Health and Social Sciences, Coventry University, Coventry, UK

**Roger Barker** BA MBBS MRCP PhD
University Lecturer and Honorary Consultant in Neurology, Cambridge Centre for Brain Repair and Addenbrooke's Hospital, Cambridge, UK

**Mark Batterbury** BSc MBBS DO FRCS FRCOphth
Consultant Ophthalmologist and Director of Clinical Studies, St Paul's Eye Unit, Royal Liverpool University Hospital, Liverpool, UK

**Philip Benington** BDS MSc MOrthRCS FDS(Orth)RCS FDSRCPS
Consultant Orthodontist, Glasgow Dental Hospital and School, Glasgow, UK

**Ewen Cameron** MA MB BChir MRCP
Specialist Registrar, Department of Gastroenterology, Ipswich Hospital, Ipswich, UK

**Andrew Currie** BM DCH MRCP(UK) FRCPCH
Consultant Neonatologist, Leicester Royal Infirmary, Leicester, UK

**David Gawkrodger** MD FRCP FRCPE
Consultant Dermatologist and Honorary Senior Clinical Lecturer, Department of Dermatology, Royal Hallamshire Hospital, Sheffield, UK

**Paddy Gibson** BSc MB ChB MRCP
Consultant Nephrologist, Department of Renal Medicine, Royal Infirmary of Edinburgh, Edinburgh, UK

**Peter Hammond** BM BCh MA MD FRCP
Consultant Physician, Department of Medicine, Harrogate District Hospital, Harrogate, UK

**Paul Hateley** MPH BSc(Hons) DMS RGN RMN OND
Head of Nursing, Pathology and Patient Services, Barts and the London NHS Trust, London, UK

**Ariane Herrick** MD FRCP
Senior Lecturer in Rheumatology, University of Manchester Rheumatic Diseases Centre, Hope Hospital, Salford, UK

**Philip Hopley** MB BS(Dist) MRCPsych
Consultant Forensic Psychiatrist, West London Mental Health NHS Trust, London, UK

**Diana Hulbert** BSc(Hons) MBBS FRCS FFAEM
Consultant, Emergency Department, Southampton General Hospital, Southampton, UK

**Susan Ingamells** BSc(Hons) PhD BM MRCOG
Subspeciality Registrar in Reproductive Medicine, Department of Obstetrics and Gynaecology, The Princess Anne Hospital, Southampton, UK

**Greg Kelly** DipCOT BSc(Hons) Psychology
Lecturer in Occupational Therapy, School of Rehabilitation Sciences, University of Ulster at Jordanstown, Newtownabbey, Co Antrim, UK

**Donald L Lorimer** BEd(Hons) MChS DPodM SRCh
Former Head of Durham School of Podiatric Medicine, Past Chairman of Council, Society of Chiropodists and Podiatrists, Baldock, UK

**Islay M McEwan** MSc BSc(Hons) GradDipPhys SRP MCSP
Senior Lecturer in Sports Physiotherapy and Programme Leader MSc Science of Sports Injury, Manchester Metropolitan University, Manchester, UK

**Gerald W McGarry** MB ChB MD FRCS (Ed. Glas) FRCS ORLHNS
Consultant Otorhinolaryngologist, Department of ENT, Glasgow Royal Infirmary, Glasgow, UK

**Alexander McMillan** MD FRCP FRCP (Ed)
Consultant Physician, Department of Genitourinary Medicine, Royal Infirmary of Edinburgh, Edinburgh, UK

**J Kilian Mellon** MD FRCS(Urol)
Professor of Urology, Leicester Warwick Medical School, Leicester General Hospital, Leicester, UK

**Cathy Meredith** MPH BA DCRt TQFF Cert CT
Senior Lecturer, Division of Radiography, School of Health and Social Care, Glasgow Caledonian University, Glasgow, UK

**Jeannette Naish** MBBS MSc FRCGP
Senior Lecturer, Department of General Practice and Primary Care, Barts and The London Queen Mary's School of Medicine and Dentistry, University of London, UK

**Andrew Nicol** BSc MBBS FRCA
Consultant Anaesthetist, Department of Anaesthesia, Barnet Hospital, Barnet, Herts, UK

**Marianne Nicolson** BSc MD FRCP(Ed)
Consultant Medical Oncologist, Aberdeen Royal Infirmary, Aberdeen, UK

**Rowan Parks** MD FRCSI FRCS(Ed)
Senior Lecturer in Surgery, Department of Clinical and Surgical Sciences, Royal Infirmary of Edinburgh, Edinburgh, UK

**Anne Parry** PhD MCSP DipTP
Professor of Physiotherapy and Senior Research Fellow, Professions Allied to Medicine, School of Health and Social Care, Sheffield Hallam University, Sheffield, UK

**Helen Richmond** MA PGDipE MSc DPSM RM SRN
Senior Lecturer in Midwifery, Anglia Polytechnic University, Chelmsford, Essex, UK

**Jillian Riley** MSc BA(Hons) RGN RM
Senior Lecturer, Cardio-respiratory Nursing, Thames Valley University, Royal Brompton Hospital, London, UK

**Carrock Sewell** MB PhD MRCP MRCPath
Consultant Immunologist, Path Links Immunology, Lincolnshire, UK

**Anne Shields** BA(Hons) RGN OHND
Occupational Health Nurse,
Occupational Health Unit, University
of Hull, Hull, UK

**Christina H Smith** BSc MSc PhD
Lecturer, Department of Human
Communication Science, University
College London, London, UK

**Mike Smith** MSc PGDipEd RN
Postgraduate Orthopaedic Nursing
Course, Nursing Professional
Development Unit, Royal Perth
Hospital, and Lecturer (adjunct),
Faculty of Nursing, Edith Cowan
University, Perth, Australia

**David Soutar** MB ChB ChM FRCS(Ed)
FRCS(Glas)
Consultant Plastic Surgeon, Plastic
Surgery Unit, Canniesburn Hospital,
Glasgow, UK

**Andrew Stewart** BA MB ChB MRCP
MRCPath
Consultant Haematologist, Monklands
and Hairmyres Hospitals, Lanarkshire,
UK

**Quintin van Wyk** MB ChB
Specialist Registrar in Histopathology,
Department of Histopathology, Royal
Hallamshire Hospital, Sheffield, UK

**Roger Watson** BSc PhD RGN CBiol
FIBiol ILTM FRSA
Professor of Nursing, School of
Nursing, Social Work and Applied
Health Studies, University of Hull, Hull,
UK

**Jessica White** MB BChir MRCP(UK)
Clinical Research Fellow, Department
of Medicine, Addenbrooke's Hospital,
Cambridge, UK

**Simon M Whiteley** MBBS FRCA
Consultant in Anaesthesia and
Intensive Care, Anaesthetic
Department, St James's University
Hospital, Leeds, UK

# How to use this dictionary

**Main entries**
These are listed in alphabetical order and appear in **bold** type. Derivative forms of the main entry also appear in **bold** type and along with their parts of speech are to be found at the end of the definition. For example:

**amoebicide** *n* an agent that kills amoebae, such as metronidazole—**amoebicidal** *adj*.

**Separate meanings of main entry**
Different meanings of the same word are separated by means of an Arabic numeral before each meaning. For example:

**articulation 1.** the junction of two or more bones; a joint. **2.** enunciation of speech—**articular** *adj*.

**Subentries**
Subentries relating to the defined main entry are listed in alphabetical order and appear in *italic* type, following the main definition. For example:

**alkalosis** *n* process leading to low levels of acid (excess of alkali) in the body. *metabolic alkalosis* due to loss of body acids (e.g. vomiting of gastric acid) or excess administration of alkali. *respiratory alkalosis* due to hyperventilation and lowering of carbon dioxide level.

**Parts of speech and other abbreviations**
The parts of speech follow single-word main entries and derivative forms of the main entry, and appear in *italic* type. The parts of speech and other

abbreviations used in the dictionary are:

| | |
|---|---|
| *abbr* | abbreviation |
| *acron* | acronym |
| *adj* | adjective |
| *adv* | adverb |
| *Am* | American |
| e.g. | for example |
| i.e. | that is |
| *n* | noun |
| *npl* | noun, plural |
| *opp* | opposite |
| *pl* | plural |
| *sing* | singular |
| *syn* | synonym |
| *v* | verb |
| *vi* | intransitive verb |
| *vt* | transitive verb |

**Cross-references**
Cross-references alert you to related words and additional information elsewhere in the dictionary. A single symbol has been used for this purpose—an arrow ⇒. Either within or at the end of the definition, the arrow indicates the word(s) you can then look up for related subject matter. For example:

**achalasia** *n* loss of oesophageal peristalsis and failure of lower oesophageal sphincter relaxation. ⇒ cardiomyotomy.

Most drug entries relate to drug groups rather than specific drug names and the cross-reference will be to Appendix 5 for more information. For example:

**anthelmintic** *adj* describes a drug for the destruction or elimination of parasitic worms, e.g. mebendazole. ⇒ Appendix 5.

Many anatomical terms are cross-referenced to the appropriate figure(s) in Appendix 1 to show the term's position in the body. For example:

**clavicle** *n* the collar bone (⇒ Appendix 1, Figure 2)—**clavicular** *adj*.

# Prefixes

Prefixes which can be used as combining forms in compounded words

| Prefix | Meaning |
|---|---|
| a- | without, not |
| ab- | away from |
| abdo-<br>abdomino- | abdominal |
| acro- | extremity |
| ad- | towards |
| adeno- | glandular |
| aer- | air |
| amb<br>ambi- | both, on both sides |
| amido- | NH$_2$ group united to an acid radical |
| amino- | NH$_2$ group united to a radical other than an acid radical |
| amphi- | on both sides, around |
| amyl- | starch |
| an- | not, without |
| ana- | up |
| andro- | male |
| angi- | vessel (blood) |
| aniso- | unequal |
| ant-<br>anti- | against, counteracting |
| ante-<br>antero- | before |
| antro- | antrum |
| aorto | aorta |
| app- | away, from |
| arachn- | spider |
| arthro- | joint |
| auto- | self |
| bi- | twice, two |
| bili- | bile |
| bio- | life |
| blenno- | mucus |
| bleph- | eyelid |
| brachio- | arm |
| brachy- | short |
| brady- | slow |
| broncho- | bronchi |
| calc- | chalk |
| carcin- | cancer |
| cardio- | heart |
| carpo- | wrist |
| cata- | down |
| cav- | hollow |
| centi- | a hundredth |
| cephal- | head |
| cerebro- | brain |
| cervic- | neck |
| cheil- | lip |
| cheir- | hand |
| chemo- | chemical |
| chlor- | green |
| chol- | bile |
| cholecysto- | gallbladder |
| choledocho- | common bile duct |
| chondro- | cartilage |
| chrom- | colour |
| cine- | film, motion |
| circum- | around |
| co-<br>col-<br>com-<br>con- | together |
| coli- | bowel |
| colpo- | vagina |
| contra- | against |
| costo- | rib |
| cox- | hip |
| crani-<br>cranio- | skull |
| cryo- | cold |
| crypt- | hidden, concealed |

| | | | |
|---|---|---|---|
| cyan- | blue | ger- | old age |
| cysto- | bladder | glosso- | tongue |
| cyto- | cell | glyco- | sugar |
| | | gnatho- | jaw |
| dacryo- | tear | gynae- | female |
| dactyl- | finger | | |
| de- | away, from, reversing | haema- ⎫ | |
| deca- | ten | haemo- ⎭ | blood |
| deci- | tenth | hemi- | half |
| demi- | half | hepa- ⎫ | |
| dent- | tooth | hepatico- ⎬ | liver |
| derma- ⎫ | skin | hepato- ⎭ | |
| dermat- ⎭ | | hetero- | unlikeness, dissimilarity |
| dextro- | to the right | | |
| di-/dip- | twos, double | hexa- | six |
| dia- | through | histo- | tissue |
| dis- | separation, against | homeo- | like |
| dorso- | dorsal | homo- | same |
| dys- | difficult, painful, abnormal | hydro- | water |
| | | hygro- | moisture |
| ecto- | outside, without, external | hyper- | above |
| | | hypno- | sleep |
| electro- | electricity | hypo- | below |
| em- | in | hystero- | uterus |
| en- ⎫ | | | |
| end- ⎬ | in, into, within | iatro- | physician |
| endo- ⎭ | | idio- | peculiar to the individual |
| ent- | within | | |
| entero- | intestine | ileo- | ileum |
| epi- | on, above, upon | ilio- | ilium |
| ery- | red | immuno- | immunity |
| eu- | well, normal | in- | not, in, into, within |
| ex- ⎫ | away from, out, out of | infra- | below |
| exo- ⎭ | | inter- | between |
| extra- | outside | intra- | within |
| | | intro- | inward |
| faci- | face | ischio- | ischium |
| ferri- ⎫ | iron | iso- | equal |
| ferro- ⎭ | | | |
| feto- | fetus | karyo- | nucleus |
| fibro- | fibre, fibrous tissue | kerato- | horn, skin, cornea |
| flav- | yellow | kypho- | rounded, humped |
| fore- | before, in front of | | |
| | | lact- | milk |
| gala- | milk | laparo- | flank |
| gastro- | stomach | laryngo- | larynx |
| genito- | genitals, reproductive | | |

| | | | |
|---|---|---|---|
| lepto- | thin, soft | orchido- | testis |
| leuco- ⎫ | white | oro- | mouth |
| leuko- ⎭ | | ortho- | straight |
| lympho- | lymphatic | os- | bone, mouth |
| | | osteo- | bone |
| macro- | large | oto- | ear |
| mal- | abnormal, poor | ova- | egg |
| mamm- ⎫ | breast | ovari- | ovary |
| mast- ⎭ | | | |
| medi- | middle | pachy- | thick |
| mega- | large | paed- | child |
| melano- | pigment, dark | pan- | all |
| meso- | middle | para- | beside |
| meta- | between | patho- | disease |
| metro- | uterus | ped- | child, foot |
| micro- | small | penta- ⎫ | five |
| milli- | a thousandth | pento- ⎭ | |
| mio- | smaller | per- | by, through |
| mono- | one, single | peri- | around |
| muco- | mucus | perineo- | perineum |
| multi- | many | pharma- | drug |
| myc- | fungus | pharyngo- | pharynx |
| myelo- | spinal cord, bone marrow | phlebo- | vein |
| | | phono- | voice |
| myo- | muscle | photo- | light |
| | | phren- | diaphragm, mind |
| narco- | stupor | physio- | form, nature |
| naso- | nose | pleuro- | pleura |
| necro- | corpse, dead | pluri- | many |
| neo- | new | pneumo- | lung |
| nephro- | kidney | podo- | foot |
| neuro- | nerve | polio- | grey |
| noct- | night | poly- | many, much |
| normo- | normal | post- | after |
| nucleo- | nucleus | pre- ⎫ | before |
| nyc- | night | pro- ⎭ | |
| | | proct- | anus |
| oculo- | eye | proto- | first |
| odonto- | tooth | pseudo- | false |
| oligo- | deficiency, diminution | psycho- | mind |
| onc- | mass | pyelo- | pelvis of the kidney |
| onycho- | nail | pyo- | pus |
| oo- | egg, ovum | pyr- | fever |
| oophor- | ovary | | |
| ophthalmo- | eye | quadri- | four |
| opisth- | backward | quint- | five |

| | | | |
|---|---|---|---|
| radi- | ray | teno- | tendon |
| radio- | radiation | tetra- | four |
| re- | again, back | thermo- | heat |
| ren- | kidney | thoraco- | thorax |
| retro- | backward | thrombo- | blood clot |
| rhin- | nose | thyro- | thyroid gland |
| rub- | red | tibio- | tibia |
| | | tox- | poison |
| racchar- sacchar- | sugar | tracheo- | trachea |
| sacro- | sacrum | trans- | across, through |
| salpingo- | uterine (fallopian) tube | tri- | three |
| sapro- | dead, decaying | trich- | hair |
| sarco- | flesh | tropho- | nourishment |
| sclero- | hard | ultra- | beyond |
| scota- | darkness | uni- | one |
| semi- | half | uretero- | ureter |
| sept- | seven | urethro- | urethra |
| sero- | serum | uri- | urine |
| socio- | sociology | uro- | urine, urinary organs |
| sphygm- | pulse | utero- | uterus |
| spleno- | spleen | | |
| spondy- | vertebra | vaso- | vessel |
| steato- | fat | veno- | vein |
| sterno- | sternum | vesico- | bladder |
| sub- | below | | |
| supra- | above | xanth- | yellow |
| syn- | together, union, with | xero- | dry |
| | | xiphi- ⎫ | ensiform cartilage of |
| tabo- | tabes | xipho- ⎭ | sternum |
| tachy- | fast | | |
| tarso- | foot, edge of eyelid | zoo- | animal |

# Suffixes

Suffixes which can be used as combining forms in compounded words

| Suffix | Meaning |
|---|---|
| -able | able to, capable of |
| -aemia | blood |
| -aesthesia | sensibility, sense perception |
| -agra | attack, severe pain |
| -al | characterized by, pertaining to |
| -algia | pain |
| -an | belonging to, pertaining to |
| -ase | catalyst, enzyme |
| -asis | state of |
| -blast | cell |
| -caval | pertaining to venae cavae |
| -cele | tumour, swelling |
| -centesis | to puncture |
| -cide | destructive, killing |
| -clysis | infusion, injection |
| -coccus | spherical cell |
| -cule | little |
| -cyte | cell |
| -derm | skin |
| -desis | to bind together |
| -dynia | pain |
| -ectasis | dilation, extension |
| -ectomy | removal of |
| -facient | making |
| -form | having the form of |
| -fuge | expelling |
| -genesis ⎫ -genetic ⎬ | formation, origin |
| -genic | capable of causing |
| -gogue | increasing flow |
| -gram | a tracing |
| -graph | instrument for writing or recording |
| -iasis | condition of, state |
| -iatric | practice of healing |
| -itis | inflammation of |
| -kinesis ⎫ -kinetic ⎬ | motion |
| -lith | calculus, stone |
| -lithiasis | presence of stones |
| -logy | science of, study of |
| -lysis ⎫ -lytic ⎬ | breaking down, disintegration |
| -malacia | softening |
| -megaly | enlargement |
| -meter | measure |
| -morph | form |
| -odynia | pain |
| -ogen | precursor |
| -oid | likeness, resemblance |
| -ol | alcohol |
| -ology | the study of |
| -oma | tumour |
| -opia | eye |
| -opsy | looking |
| -ose | sugar |
| -osis | condition, disease, excess |
| -ostomy | to form an opening or outlet |
| -otomy | incision of |
| -ous | like, having the nature of |
| -pathy | disease |
| -penia | lack of |
| -pexy | fixation |
| -phage | ingesting |
| -phagia | swallowing |
| -phasia | speech |

| | | | |
|---|---|---|---|
| -philia | affinity for, loving | -somatic | pertaining to the body |
| -phobia | fear | -somy | pertaining to chromosomes |
| -phylaxis | protection | | |
| -plasty | reconstructive surgery | -sonic | sound |
| -plegia | paralysis | -stasis | stagnation, cessation of movement |
| -pnoea | breathing | | |
| -poiesis | making | -sthenia | strength |
| -ptosis | falling | -stomy | to form an opening or outlet |
| -rhage | to burst forth | | |
| -rhaphy | suturing | -taxia | |
| -rhoea | excessive discharge | -taxis | arrangement, co-ordination, order |
| -rhythmia | rhythm | -taxy | |
| | | -tome | cutting instrument |
| -saccharide | basic carbohydrate molecule | -tomy | incision of |
| | | -trophy | nourishment |
| -scope | instrument for visual examination | -trophy | turning |
| -scopy | to examine visually | -uria | urine |

# A

**A band** the dark constrictions formed in muscle myofibrils when the actin and myosin filaments overlap. They are visible on electron microscopy.

**AA** *abbr* Alcoholics Anonymous.

**AAA** *abbr* abdominal aortic aneurysm.

**AAMI** *abbr* age-associated memory impairment.

**abacterial** *adj* without bacteria. A condition, such as inflammation, that is not caused by bacteria.

**Abbreviated Injury Scale (AIS)** a scoring system (1 to 6) used to provide a ranking of the severity of injuries and the threat to life. ⇒ advanced trauma life support (ATLS).

**ABCs of proprioception** agility, balance and co-ordination. ⇒ proprioception.

**abdomen** *n* the largest body cavity.

**abdominal** *adj* pertaining to the abdomen.

**abdominal aorta** *n* that part of the aorta within the abdomen. Smaller arteries branch from it to supply oxygenated blood to abdominal structures, for example, the renal arteries supply the kidneys. ⇒ Appendix 1, Figures 9 and 19. *abdominal aortic aneurysm (AAA)* a swelling in the abdominal aorta. ⇒ aneurysm.

**abdominal breathing** more than usual use of the diaphragm and abdominal muscles to increase the input of air to and output from the lungs. It can occur in disease as a compensatory mechanism for inadequate oxygenation.

**abdominal excision of the rectum** an operation sometimes performed for rectal cancer. The rectum is mobilized via an abdominal approach. The bowel is divided well proximal to the cancer. The proximal end is brought out as a permanent colostomy. Excision of the distal bowel, containing the cancer and the anal canal, is completed through a perineal incision.

**abdominal reflex** a superficial reflex where the abdominal muscles contract when the skin is lightly stroked.

**abdominal regions** where the surface anatomy is divided into nine regions used to describe the location of organs or symptoms, such as pain. ⇒ Appendix 1, Figure 18A.

**abdominal thrust** a first-aid measure for choking. ⇒ Heimlich's manoeuvre.

**abdominocentesis** *n* paracentesis (aspiration) of the peritoneal cavity. ⇒ amniocentesis, colpocentesis, thoracentesis.

**abdominopelvic** *adj* pertaining to the abdomen and pelvis or pelvic cavity.

**abdominoperineal** *adj* pertaining to the abdomen and perineum.

**abdominoplasty** *n* plastic surgical procedure used to tighten the abdominal muscles and remove surplus skin. It may be performed following a large reduction in weight that has resulted in a pendulous abdomen with the anterior abdominal wall hanging down over the pubis. It is also undertaken for cosmetic reasons. Known colloquially as a 'tummy tuck'.

**abducens nerve** the sixth pair of cranial nerves. They control the lateral rectus muscle of the eyeball, which turns the eyeball outwards.

**abduct** *vt* to draw away from the median line of the body ⇒ adduct *opp*.

**abduction** *n* the act of moving (or abducting) away from the midline ⇒ adduction *opp*.

**abductor** *n* a muscle which, on contraction, draws a part away from the median line of the body. ⇒ adductor *opp*.

**aberrant** *adj* abnormal; usually applied to a blood vessel or nerve which does not follow the normal course.

**aberration** *n* a deviation from normal—**aberrant** *adj*. *chromosomal aberration* loss, gain or exchange of genetic material in the chromosomes of a cell resulting in deletion, duplication, inversion or translocation of genes. ⇒ amniocentesis. *optical aberration* imperfect focus of light rays by a lens.

**ABGs** *abbr* arterial blood gases.

**ability** *n* the physical and cognitive capacity to perform a task.

**ablation** *n* removal. In surgery, the word means excision or eradication (destruction)—**ablative** *adj*.

**ablepharia** *n* absence or partial absence of the eyelids.

**ABO blood group system** comprises four main blood groups – A, B, AB and O. Discovered in 1901 by Nobel laureate Karl Landsteiner (1868–1943). ⇒ anti-D, blood groups, Rhesus incompatibility.

**abort** *vt, vi* to terminate before full development.

**abortifacient** *adj* causing abortion, such as the drug mifepristone.

**abortion** *n* **1.** abrupt termination of a process. **2.** the induced expulsion from the uterus of the product of conception before viability by medical or surgical means. N.B.: The preferred term for unintentional loss of the product of conception prior to 24 weeks' gestation is miscarriage. *criminal abortion* intentional evacuation of the uterus by other than trained licensed personnel, or where abortion is prohibited by a country's law.

**ABPI** *abbr* ankle–brachial pressure index.

**abrasion** *n* **1.** superficial injury to skin or mucous membrane from scraping or rubbing; excoriation. **2.** can be used therapeutically for removal of scar tissue (dermabrasion).

**abscess** *n* localized collection of pus produced by pyogenic organisms. May be acute or chronic. *alveolar abscess* ⇒ dentoalveolar abscess. *Brodie's abscess* chronic osteomyelitis occurring without previous acute phase. *cold abscess* one occurring in the course of such chronic inflammation as may be due to *Mycobacterium tuberculosis*. *psoas abscess* ⇒ psoas.

*Absidia* *n* a genus of fungus. Some species cause lung and ear infections in humans.

**absolute risk reduction** in a comparative study the difference in the event rate between the control group and the group having the treatment.

**absorption rate constant** a value describing the amount of a drug absorbed in a unit of time.

**absorptive state** the metabolic state immediately after a meal and continuing for about 4 hours. Absorbed nutrients are used as energy or to build up other substances through anabolic processes, such as glycogenesis. ⇒ postabsorptive state.

**abstract** *n* a clear and concise summary of a research paper. It details the study design, results and implications for practice.

**abulia (aboulia)** *n* inability or reduced capacity to make decisions or to show initiative.

**abuse** *n* **1.** deliberate injury to another person. It may be physical, sexual, psychological or through neglect, such as failure to feed or keep clean. The term can apply to any group of individuals, especially those most vulnerable, such as children, older people and those with mental health problems or learning disabilities. ⇒ child abuse, elder abuse. **2.** misuse of equipment, drugs and other substances, power and position.

**abutment** *n* a structure, such as a root, tooth or implant that functions to support and retain a removable or fixed prosthesis.

**acalculia** *n* inability to do simple arithmetic.

*Acanthamoeba* *n* a genus of amoebae typically present in water and soil. May cause local infections or infections of the respiratory, nervous or genitourinary system.

**acanthamoebiasis** *n* meningoencephalitis caused by *Acanthamoeba*. Cleaning contact lenses in water containing *Acanthamoeba* can cause keratitis and serious corneal ulceration.

**acanthosis** *n* diffuse proliferation of the cells in the prickle layer of the epidermis, associated with skin conditions, such as eczema. *acanthosis nigricans* hyperpigmentation and velvety thickening of the skin, especially in the axilla and groin. It is related to the insulin resistance accompanying diabetes, obesity and syndrome X.

**acapnia** *n* ⇒ hypocapnia.

**acardia** *n* absence of the heart. Can occur in conjoined twins where one twin has the heart which circulates blood to both twins.

**acariasis** *n* a condition caused by an acarid (mite), e.g. scrub typhus, which is transmitted by mites.

**acarid** *n* a mite belonging to the order Acarina.

**acatalasia (Takahara's disease)** *n* a rare genetic condition caused by the lack of catalase activity. It is usually asymptomatic but can cause mouth ulceration.

**ACBT** *abbr* active cycle of breathing technique.

**acceleration** *n* the rate of change of velocity.

**acceptable daily intake (ADI)** the quantity of a food additive that could be ingested daily for the entire lifespan without appreciable risk.

**Access to Health Records Act (1990)** allows access to both paper and computerized health records made after 1991, with certain exceptions, such as where they may cause serious physical or mental harm to a person.

**accessory motion** sliding, gliding or rolling motion that occurs within and between joint surfaces during active or passive joint movement.

**accessory nerve** *n* sometimes referred to as the spinal accessory nerve. The 11th pair of cranial nerves. They supply the muscles of the larynx and pharynx and the muscles of the neck and shoulder to control movement of the head and shoulders.

**acclimation** *n* the chronic adaptation caused by artificially imposed stress, which mimics the natural environmental stress.

**acclimatization** *n* the body's ability to adapt physiologically to environmental stress, such as variation in climate or altitude.

**accommodating resistance** muscle activity during which the resistance provided changes as the muscle moves through its range of motion. Also known as isokinetic activity.

**accommodation** *n* **1.** ability of the lens of the eye to increase its refractive power in order to focus on near objects. **2.** decreased sensitivity to stimuli demonstrated by neurons that have been exposed to subthreshold stimuli for long periods of time.

**accommodation reflex** *n* constriction of the pupils and convergence of the eyes for near vision.

**accouchement** *n* delivery in childbirth. Confinement.

**accountability** *n* health professionals have a duty to care according to law. In some countries the statutory body, and/or the professional organization, develops a code of conduct via which each practitioner can accept responsibility and accountability for the professional service delivered to each patient/client. ⇒ duty of care, malpractice, negligence.

**accretion** *n* an increase of substance or deposit round a central object—**accrete** *adj, vt, vi*, **accretive** *adj*.

**ACE inhibitor** *acron* **a**ngiotensin-**c**onverting **e**nzyme inhibitor.

**acentric** *adj* **1.** (in genetics) describes a chromosome fragment without a centromere. **2.** without a centre.

**acephalous** *adj* without a head.

**acetabuloplasty** *n* an operation to improve the depth and shape of the hip socket (acetabulum); necessary in such conditions as developmental dysplasia of the hip and osteoarthritis of the hip.

**acetabulum** *n* a cup-like socket on the external lateral surface of the pelvis into which the head of the femur fits and articulates to form the hip joint—**acetabula** *pl*.

**acetate** *n* a salt of acetic acid.

**acetic acid** an organic acid present in vinegar.

**acetoacetate** *n* an acidic ketone produced during an intermediate stage of fat oxidation in the body. Some can be utilized as a fuel by tissues, such as the kidney. In situations where carbohydrate molecules are not available for metabolism, such as in diabetes mellitus or starvation, excess is produced and the high levels in the blood result in ketoacidosis with severe disturbances of pH, fluid and electrolytes.

**acetonaemia** *n* ⇒ ketonaemia.

**acetone** *n* inflammable liquid with odour of 'pear drops'; used as a solvent. *acetone bodies* ⇒ ketones.

**acetonuria** *n* acetone and other ketones in the urine. ⇒ ketonuria—**acetonuric** *adj*.

**acetyl coenzyme A** (*syn* acetyl CoA) coenzyme A linked with an acetyl group. An important metabolic molecule involved in many biochemical reactions, such as glycolysis.

**acetylcholine (ACh)** *n* a chemical neurotransmitter released from nerve endings to allow the transmission of a nerve impulse at the neuromuscular junction in voluntary (skeletal) muscle, in preganglionic sympathetic neurons and across all synapses in parasympathetic neurons. The nerve fibres releasing this chemical are described as 'cholinergic'. Acetylcholine is broken down into choline and acetate by the enzyme acetylcholinesterase. ⇒ myasthenia gravis.

**acetylcholinesterase** *n* enzyme that inactivates acetylcholine following the transmission of a nerve impulse across the synapse.

**ACh** *abbr* acetylcholine.

**ACH index** arm, chest, hip index.

**achalasia** *n* loss of oesophageal peristalsis and failure of lower oesophageal sphincter relaxation. ⇒ cardiomyotomy.

**Achilles tendinitis** inflammation of the Achilles tendon.

**Achilles tendon** the tendinous termination of the soleus and gastrocnemius muscles inserted into the heel bone (os calcis or calcaneus) (Figure A.1).

**achlorhydria** *n* the absence of gastric acid (hydrochloric). Found in pernicious anaemia and gastric cancer—**achlorhydric** *adj*.

**acholia** *n* the absence of bile—**acholic** *adj*.

**acholuria** *n* the absence of bile pigments from the urine. ⇒ jaundice—**acholuric** *adj*.

**achondroplasia** *n* an inherited condition characterized by arrested growth of the long bones resulting in short-limbed dwarfism with a large head. The intellect is not impaired. Inheritance is dominant—**achondroplastic** *adj*.

**achromatopsia** *n* inability to see colours.

**acid** *n* any substance that has an excess of hydrogen ions over hydroxyl ions, e.g. hydrochloric acid. They have a pH below 7 and turn blue litmus red. They react with alkalis to form salts plus water.

**acid etching** (in dentistry) the application of substances, usually phosphoric acid, to the tooth enamel in order to provide retention of orthodontic brackets, sealant or restorative material.

**acid foods, basic (alkaline) foods** describes the residue of the metabolism of different foods. Foods containing phosphorus, sulphur and chlorine are acid-forming whereas those containing sodium, potassium, calcium and magnesium are base-forming. The predominant foods in the diet determine the nature of the residue: meat, cheese, eggs and cereals

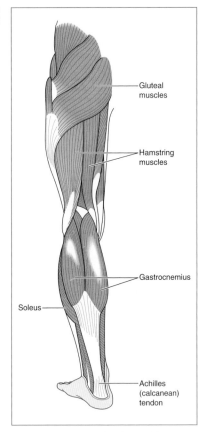

Gluteal muscles

Hamstring muscles

Gastrocnemius

Soleus

Achilles (calcanean) tendon

**Figure A.1** Achilles tendon *(adapted from Waugh & Grant 2006 with permission)*.

produce an acidic residue, whereas milk, vegetables and some fruits leave a basic (alkaline) residue.

**acid phosphatase** *n* an enzyme which synthesizes phosphate esters of carbohydrates in an acid medium. An increase of this enzyme in the blood may be indicative of cancer of the prostate gland.

**acidaemia** *n* a high level of acid (hydrogen ions) in the blood resulting in a below-normal blood pH <7.35 (hydrogen ion concentration >44 mmol/L). ⇒ acidosis—**acidaemic** *adj*.

**acid-alcohol-fast** *adj* in microbiology, describes a micro-organism which, when stained, is resistant to decolorization by alcohol as well as acid, e.g. *Mycobacterium tuberculosis*. ⇒ Ziehl–Neelsen technique.

**acid–base balance** equilibrium between the acid and base elements of the blood and body fluids. The net rate at which acids or bases are produced in the body is equal to the net rate at which acids and bases are excreted.

**acid-fast** *adj* in microbiology, describes a micro-organism which, when stained, does not become decolorized when washed with dilute acids. *acid-fast bacilli (AFB)* a type of bacteria identified using acid-fast techniques.

**acidity** *n* the state of being acid or sour. The degree of acidity can be measured on the pH scale where a pH below 7 is acid and pH 6 denotes a weak acid and pH 1 a strong acid.

**acidosis** *n* process leading to the accumulation of excess acid in the body. *respiratory acidosis* due to hypoventilation and the accumulation of waste carbon dioxide. *metabolic acidosis* due to the generation of excess acid (lactic acidosis) or depletion of alkali (e.g. due to diarrhoea). ⇒ acidaemia, ketoacidosis, ketosis—**acidotic** *adj*.

**aciduria** *n* excretion of an acid urine. It can be caused by the intake of acid-forming foods, inborn errors of metabolism and certain medications.

*Acinetobacter n* a genus of aerobic bacteria of the family Neisseriaceae. They cause infections that include wound infection, pneumonia and meningitis. The micro-organism has developed antibiotic resistance and is a particular danger to critically ill patients who require intensive or high-dependency care.

**acini** *npl* minute saccules or alveoli, lined or filled with secreting cells. Several acini combine to form a lobule—**acinus** *sing*, **acinous**, **acinar** *adj*.

**acme** *n* **1.** the highest point. **2.** crisis or critical point of a disease.

**acne, acne vulgaris** *n* a condition in which the pilosebaceous units are overstimulated by circulating androgens and the excessive sebum is trapped by a plug of keratin, one of the protein constituents of human skin. Skin bacteria then colonize the glands and convert the trapped sebum into irritant fatty acids responsible for the swelling and inflammation (pustules) which follow. Treatment options include topical benzoyl peroxide, topical or oral antibiotics, topical azelaic acid, topical or oral retinoids or antiandrogen hormone therapy (for young women).

**acneiform** *adj* resembling acne.

**acoustic** *adj* pertaining to sound or the sense of hearing.

**acoustic neuroma** a benign tumour (schwannoma) affecting the eighth cranial nerve (vestibulocochlear nerve) as it passes through the skull into the brainstem, causing problems in hearing and with balance.

**acquired immune deficiency syndrome (AIDS)** a term used to denote a particular stage of infection with human immunodeficiency virus (HIV). The Centers for Disease Control and Prevention (CDC) define AIDS as the development of an AIDS-defining illness in a patient with HIV infection. A low CD4+ T-cell count of less than 200 per μL (or less than 14% of lymphocytes) in an HIV-positive person is also regarded as AIDS-defining, regardless of symptoms or opportunistic infections.

**acrocentric** *adj* describes a chromosome that has the centromere at or close to one end.

**acrocephalia; acrocephaly** *n* a congenital malformation whereby the top of the head is pointed and the eyes protrude, due to premature closure of sagittal and coronal skull sutures—**acrocephalic, acrocephalous** *adj.*

**acrocephalosyndactyly** *n* a congenital malformation consisting of a pointed top of head, with fusion of fingers and/or toes. ⇒ Apert's syndrome.

**acrocyanosis** *n* coldness and blueness of the extremities due to circulatory disorder—**acrocyanotic** *adj.*

**acrodermatitis enteropathica** *n* an inherited disorder of zinc malabsorption. The zinc deficiency leads to vesicles and bullae affecting the skin and mucosae, poor growth, chronic diarrhoea and alopecia. Treatment is with zinc supplements.

**acrodynia** *n* acute, painful reddening of the extremities, such as occurs in erythroedema polyneuropathy.

**acromegaly** *n* enlargement of the hands, face and feet, occurring due to excess growth hormone in an adult, almost always from a pituitary adenoma. Treatment may be with drugs, radiation or surgery—**acromegalic** *adj.*

**acromicria** *n* smallness of the hands, face and feet.

**acromioclavicular** *adj* pertaining to the acromion process (of scapula) and the clavicle.

**acromion** *n* the point or summit of the shoulder: the triangular process at the extreme outer end of the spine of the scapula—**acromial** *adj.*

**acrophobia** *n* morbid fear of being at a height.

**acrosome** *n* structure surrounding the nucleus of a spermatozoon. It contains lytic enzymes, which when released by many spermatozoa (during the acrosome reaction) facilitate the penetration of an oocyte by a single spermatozoon.

**acrylamide** *n* chemical formed when starchy foods, such as crisps and chips, are cooked at high temperatures.

**ACTH** *abbr* adrenocorticotrophic hormone.

**actin** *n* one of the contractile proteins in a muscle myofibril; it reacts with myosin to cause contraction.

**acting out** reducing distress by the release of disturbed or violent behaviour, which is unconsciously determined and reflects previous unresolved conflicts and attitudes.

**actinic dermatoses** skin conditions in which the integument is abnormally sensitive to ultraviolet radiation.

**actinism** *n* the chemical action of radiant energy, especially in the ultraviolet spectrum—**actinic** *adj.*

**actinobiology** *n* study of the effects of radiation on living organisms.

**Actinomyces** *n* a genus of branching microorganisms. *Actinomyces israelii* causes disease in humans. ⇒ actinomycosis.

**actinomycosis** *n* a disease caused by *Actinomyces israelii*, the sites most affected being the face, neck, lung and abdomen. There is pus containing yellow 'sulphur granules', abscess formation with sinuses and necrosis—**actinomycotic** *adj.*

**actinotherapy** *n* treatment by use of infrared or ultraviolet radiation.

**action** *n* the activity or function of any part of the body. *specific action* that brought about by certain remedial agents in a particular disease, e.g. antibiotics in infection.

**action potential** change in electrical potential and charge that occurs across excitable cell membranes during nerve impulse conduction or when muscles contract (Figure A.2). ⇒ nerve impulse.

**action research** a type of social research involving a systematic and planned implementation of a cycle of social interventions and an evaluation of the change within the environment/situation being researched. The aims are to solve practical problems within the environment/situation and augment knowledge.

**activated partial thromboplastin time (APTT)** a test of blood coagulation ability.

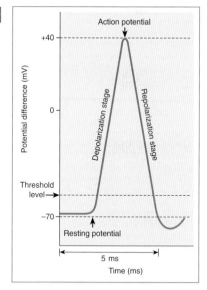

Figure A.2 Action potential *(reproduced from Brooker & Nicol 2003 with permission).*

**activator** *n* a substance which renders something else active, e.g. the hormone secretin, the enzyme enterokinase—**activate** *v*.

**active** *adj* energetic. ⇒ passive *opp.* active *hyperaemia* ⇒ hyperaemia. *active immunity* ⇒ immunity.

**active assisted exercise** exercise that involves the person's own efforts combined with assistance from the therapist or the use of equipment.

**active cycle of breathing technique (ACBT)** techniques used to clear excessive pulmonary secretions in people with dyspnoea. The techniques include control of breathing, chest expansion exercises and 'huffing' out through the mouth. Great care is needed in patients prone to bronchospasm because strenuous huffing and insufficient relaxation between techniques can lead to bronchospasm. Care should also be taken postoperatively as patients tire easily

**active principle** an ingredient which gives a complex drug its chief therapeutic value, e.g. atropine is the active principle in belladonna.

**active range of motion (AROM)** the movement of a joint without assistance through a range of motion. Those produced by patients using their own neuromuscular mechanisms.

**active transport** movement of substances across cell membranes that requires the use of energy, usually adenosine triphosphate (ATP). For example, moving substances against a concentration gradient. Substances transported by active transport include nutrients and ions, e.g. the sodium–potassium pump in cell membranes. ⇒ diffusion, filtration, osmosis.

**activities of daily living (ADLs)** tasks focusing on the occupational performance areas of self-care, work and play that enable individuals to perform their occupational roles in society consistently and competently. ⇒ DADL, IADL, PADL. *ADL assessment and training* a technique whereby formal and informal evaluation of a person's ability to perform ADLs is followed by a treatment programme designed to maintain or improve function.

**activity** *n* the execution of a series of linked, purposeful, productive, playful or creative tasks by an individual with the specific goal of changing objective reality or subjective experience. These may include physical and mental tasks at various levels of complexity.

**activity analysis** a cognitive process used to reduce an activity into its component tasks in order to understand the skills required for consistent and competent performance of activities of daily living (ADLs) in a specific environment.

**activity diaries** a collaboration between a patient/client and the occupational therapist. The diary outlines agreed activities for a period (e.g. a week) and records the patient's/client's success in accomplishing the goals set.

**activity limitations** inability of an individual to perform activities of daily living as expected by his or her cultural and social environment.

**activity theory** a psychosocial theory of ageing. It supports the view that older people who develop different roles and are socially active into old age gain benefit and satisfaction. ⇒ disengagement theory.

**actomyosin** *n* the protein complex of actin and myosin formed during muscle fibre contraction.

**acuity** *n* clearness, sharpness, keenness. ⇒ auditory acuity, visual acuity.

**acupuncture** *n* a technique that involves the insertion of fine needles into specific parts of the body (Figure A.3). There are approximately 365 points along meridians (channels

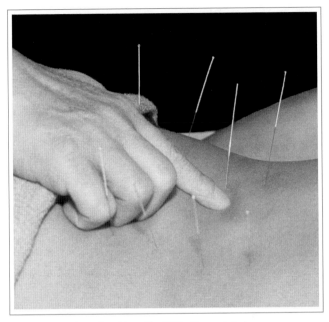

**Figure A.3** Acupuncture *(reproduced from Zhu 2005 with permission).*

through which energy known as *Qi* flows) at which needles can be inserted into the body to stimulate or depress the energy flow. Sometimes the herb moxa is also used to warm and stimulate certain points. This is known as moxibustion. Used for the treatment of disease, relief of pain or production of anaesthesia.

**acute** *adj* short and severe; not long-drawn-out or chronic.

**acute abdomen** a pathological condition within the abdomen requiring immediate surgical intervention. Causes include a perforated viscera, acute appendicitis, diverticulitis or intestinal obstruction.

**acute confusional state** sudden-onset confusion with loss of awareness and disorientation due to a physical or metabolic disturbance affecting brain function. It may be misdiagnosed as dementia when it occurs in older people. Often there is an acute medical cause, such as stroke, urinary tract or chest infection, but may be caused by medications or recent loss or bereavement.

**acute coronary syndromes** describes the spectrum of events ranging from chest pain, the partial occlusion of a coronary artery resulting in unstable angina, a minor heart attack to a major heart attack. ⇒ myocardial infarction.

**acute defibrination syndrome** ⇒ hypofibrinogenaemia.

**acute dilatation of the stomach** sudden enlargement of this organ due to paralysis of the muscular wall ⇒ gastrectasia, paralytic ileus.

**acute heart failure** cessation or impairment of heart action, in previously undiagnosed heart disease, or in the course of another disease.

**acute injury** an injury that presents with a rapid onset and has a short duration, due to a traumatic episode. Term used to describe the first 24–48 hours after onset of an injury, such as that sustained during a sporting activity.

**acute leukaemia** ⇒ leukaemia.

**acute necrotizing ulcerative gingivitis (ANUG)** a recurrent periodontal condition characterized by ulceration and necrosis affecting the interdental tissues.

**acute pain** pain of brief duration usually associated with tissue injury (nociceptive pain) which reduces as healing occurs. ⇒ chronic pain, nociceptive pain.

**acute suppurative otitis media (ASOM)** an acute infection of the middle ear, often due to bacterial infection.

**acute tubular necrosis (ATN)** rapid-onset necrosis of the renal tubules. It is usually caused by renal ischaemia due to shock, but may be due to the nephrotoxic effects of bacterial toxins or chemical toxins. ⇒ renal failure.

**acute wound** usually describes a surgical incision or uncomplicated trauma. The wound usually heals quickly. ⇒ chronic wound, wound healing.

**acute yellow atrophy** acute diffuse necrosis of the liver; icterus gravis; malignant jaundice.

**acute/adult respiratory distress syndrome (ARDS)** characterized by difficulty breathing, poor oxygenation, stiff lungs and typical changes on a chest X-ray, following a recognized cause of acute lung injury. Analysis of arterial blood gases reveals a fall in $PaO_2$ and eventually an increased $PaCO_2$ and a fall in pH.

**acute-phase proteins** a class of proteins produced by the liver. They include C-reactive protein, etc., and are produced in response to inflammation and trauma and with malignancy.

**acyanosis** n without cyanosis.

**acyanotic** adj without cyanosis; a word used to differentiate congenital cardiovascular defects.

**acyesis** n absence of pregnancy—**acyetic** adj.

**acystia** n congenital absence of the bladder—**acystic** adj.

**Adam's apple** the laryngeal prominence in the anterior part of the neck, especially in the adult male, formed by the junction of the two wings of the thyroid cartilage.

**adaptability** n the ability to adjust mentally and physically to circumstances in a flexible way.

**adaptation** n **1.** a positive change in the function of an individual in order to meet the demands of the environment. **2.** an alteration made to the environment in order to improve an individual's ability to perform activities of daily living consistently and competently. **3.** in sports medicine describes the long-term physical changes that occur from the training effects produced as a result of overload. ⇒ aerobic adaptations, anaerobic adaptations.

**adaptive behaviour** advantageous or appropriate behaviour that follows a change.

**addiction** n craving for chemical substances, such as a drug, alcohol and tobacco, which the addicted person finds difficult to control.

**Addison's disease** (T Addison, British physician, 1793–1860) deficient secretion of cortisol and aldosterone due to primary failure of the adrenal cortex, causing electrolyte imbalance, diminished blood volume, hypotension, weight loss, hypoglycaemia, muscular weakness, gastrointestinal upsets and pigmentation of skin.

**addisonian crisis** ⇒ adrenal crisis.

**additive** n a substance not usually considered to be or used as a food which is added to foods to assist processing/manufacture, or to enhance flavour, texture, colour, keeping properties, appearance or stability of the food, or as a convenience to the consumer. Nutrients, such as vitamins and minerals, added to enhance the nutritional value of food are not included as additives. Other substances that include spices, salt, herbs, yeast, air and water are also usually excluded.

**adduct** vt to draw towards the midline of the body. ⇒ abduct opp.

**adduction** n the act of adducting, drawing towards the midline of the body. ⇒ abduction opp.

**adductor** n any muscle which moves a part toward the median axis of the body. ⇒ abductor opp. *adductor longus* ⇒ Appendix 1, Figure 4. *adductor magnus* ⇒ Appendix 1, Figures 4 and 5.

**adenectomy** n surgical removal of a gland.

**adenine** n a nitrogenous base derived from purine. With other bases, one or more phosphate groups and a sugar it is part of the nucleic acids DNA and RNA. ⇒ deoxyribonucleic acid, ribonucleic acid.

**adenitis** n inflammation of a gland, or lymph node. *hilar adenitis* inflammation of bronchial lymph nodes.

**adenocarcinoma** n a malignant, epithelial cell tumour of glandular tissue—**adenocarcinomata** pl, **adenocarcinomatous** adj.

**adenofibroma** n ⇒ fibroadenoma.

**adenohypophysis** n the glandular anterior lobe of the pituitary gland. It develops from the ectoderm of the mouth/pharynx in the embryo. ⇒ pituitary gland.

**adenoid** adj resembling a gland. ⇒ adenoids.

**adenoidectomy** n surgical removal from the nasopharynx of enlarged pharyngeal tonsil (adenoid tissue).

**adenoids** *npl* abnormally enlarged pharyngeal tonsils. Lymphoid tissue situated in the nasopharynx which can obstruct breathing and impede hearing.

**adenoma** *n* a benign tumour of glandular epithelial tissue—**adenomata** *pl*, **adenomatous** *adj*.

**adenomyoma** *n* a benign tumour composed of muscle and glandular elements, usually applied to benign growths of the uterus—**adenomyomata** *pl*, **adenomyomatous** *adj*.

**adenopathy** *n* any disease of a gland—**adenopathic** *adj*.

**adenosine** *n* a nucleoside formed from the sugar ribose and adenine. With the addition of one, two or three phosphate groups forms the three nucleotides: *adenosine monophosphate, adenosine diphosphate* and *adenosine triphosphate*.

**adenosine deaminase** the enzyme that facilitates the conversion of adenosine to the nucleoside inosine. *adenosine deaminase deficiency* a genetic condition that affects lymphocyte function and can lead to severe combined immunodeficiency syndrome.

**adenosine diphosphate (ADP)** an important cellular metabolite involved in energy exchange within the cell. Chemical energy is conserved in the cell by the phosphorylation of ADP to adenosine triphosphate (ATP), primarily in the mitochondrion, as a high-energy phosphate bond.

**adenosine monophosphate (AMP)** an important cellular metabolite involved in energy release for cell use. ⇒ cyclic adenosine monophosphate (cAMP).

**adenosine triphosphate (ATP)** an intermediate high-energy compound which on hydrolysis to adenosine diphosphate (ADP) releases chemically useful energy. ATP is generated during catabolism and utilized during anabolism.

**adenosis** *n* a disease or enlargement of a gland or glandular tissue.

**adenotonsillectomy** *n* surgical removal of the pharyngeal tonsil (adenoid tissue) and palatine tonsils.

**adenovirus** *n* a group of DNA-containing viruses. They cause upper respiratory and gastrointestinal infections, cystitis and conjunctivitis.

**adequate intake** in situations where there is insufficient scientific evidence to confirm needs and reference intakes for a particular nutrient for which deficiency is rarely, if ever, seen. The observed intake levels are assumed to be greater than requirements, and thus give an approximation of intakes that are greater than adequate to meet needs.

**ADH** *abbr* antidiuretic hormone ⇒ antidiuretic hormone, vasopressin (or arginine vasopressin [AVP]).

**ADHD** *abbr* attention deficit hyperactivity disorder.

**adhesion** *n* abnormal union of two parts, occurring after inflammation; a band of fibrous tissue which joins such parts. In the abdomen such a band may cause intestinal obstruction; in joints it restricts movement; between two surfaces of pleura it prevents complete pneumothorax—**adherent** *adj*, **adherence** *n*, **adhere** *vi*.

**adhesion molecules** *npl* specific cell surface molecules that bind cells to each other within tissues.

**ADI** *abbr* acceptable daily intake.

**Adie's syndrome** (W Adie, British physician, 1886–1935) a condition characterized by one pupil reacting more slowly to light, convergence and accommodation than the other pupil. There is also a reduction in, or absent, tendon reflexes, such as the ankle reflexes.

**adipocyte** *n* a fat (adipose) cell (Figure A.4). Able to store fat as triglycerides (triacylglycerol).

**adiponectin** *n* a hormone produced by adipose tissue, which may be concerned with energy balance. Its effects include increased insulin sensitivity and glucose tolerance, and oxidation of fatty acids in muscle tissue.

**adipose** *n, adj* fat; of a fatty nature. White adipose tissue (or fat) is stored by the body, under the skin, within body cavities, e.g. in the

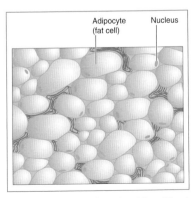

**Figure A.4** Adipocyte *(reproduced from Waugh & Grant 2006 with permission).*

abdominal cavity, and around organs. It contains cells that are able to synthesize and store fat, releasing it into blood to be used as an energy source in the fasted state. Brown fat is metabolically more active and is important for the production of heat needed for maintaining body temperature within the normal range.

**adiposity** *n* excessive accumulation of fat in the body.

**adiposogenital dystrophy** Fröhlich's syndrome. Affects males; it is characterized by obesity with female fat distribution, underdevelopment of the genitalia and female secondary sexual characteristics, somnolence, disturbance of temperature regulation and diabetes insipidus due to damage of the pituitary and hypothalamus.

**adipsia** *n* absence of thirst.

**aditus** *n* in anatomy, an entrance or opening.

**adjustment** *n* **1.** stability within an individual and an acceptable relationship between the individual and his or her environment. **2.** the mechanism used in focusing a microscope.

**adjuvant** *n* a substance included in a prescription to assist the action of other drugs, e.g. a preservative. *adjuvant therapy* additional treatment, such as a drug, that acts synergistically to assist or increase the action of other drugs or therapies. Especially used to describe the use of drugs, such as antidepressants, e.g. amitriptyline, given with an analgesic for pain relief. It is also applied to the treatment of cancer where cytotoxic drugs are used after removal of the tumour by surgery or radiotherapy. The purpose of treatment is to enhance the chance of cure and prevent recurrence. ⇒ neoadjuvant therapy.

**ADLs** *abbr* activities of daily living.

**adnexa** *npl* structures that are in close proximity to a part—**adnexal** *adj. adnexa oculi* the lacrimal apparatus. *adnexa uteri* the ovaries and uterine (fallopian) tubes.

**adolescence** *n* the period between the onset of puberty and full maturity; youth—**adolescent** *adj, n.*

**adoption** *n* the acquisition of legal responsibility for a child who is not a natural offspring of the adopter.

**ADP** *abbr* adenosine diphosphate.

**adrenal** *adj* near the kidney.

**adrenal crisis (addisonian crisis)** acute life-threatening situation occurring in patients with adrenal cortex (adrenocortical) insufficiency. It may present as shock in previously undiagnosed Addison's disease, or in a patient who is having insufficient corticosteroid replacement therapy during a concurrent illness. There is low blood pressure with weakness and commonly fever and abdominal tenderness.

**adrenal function tests** tests to identify adrenocortical hypofunction or hyperfunction; random cortisol may identify gross abnormalities in function, but for the vast majority dynamic testing of the hypothalamo–pituitary–adrenal axis is needed. ⇒ dexamethasone suppression tests, glucagon stimulation test, insulin tolerance test, tetracosactide (Synacthen) test.

**adrenal glands** endocrine glands, one situated on the upper pole of each kidney. (⇒ Appendix 1, Figure 19). The *adrenal cortex* secretes glucocorticoids, mineralocorticoids and sex hormones which control metabolism, the chemical constitution of body fluids and secondary sexual characteristics. Under the control of the pituitary gland via the secretion of adrenocorticotrophic hormone (ACTH). The *adrenal medulla* secretes the catecholamines noradrenaline (norepinephrine) and adrenaline (epinephrine).

**adrenalectomy** *n* removal of an adrenal gland, usually for tumour. If both adrenal glands are removed, replacement administration of cortical hormones is required.

**adrenaline (epinephrine)** *n* a catecholamine hormone, produced by the adrenal medulla. It enhances the effects of the sympathetic nervous system during times of physiological stress by preparing the body for 'fight or flight' responses. These include increased heart rate, bronchodilation and increased respiratory rate and glucose release. Adrenaline (epinephrine) is used therapeutically as a sympathomimetic in situations that include acute allergic reactions, and in local anaesthetic to prolong the anaesthetic effects. ⇒ alpha (α)-adrenoceptor agonist, alpha (α)-adrenoceptor antagonist, beta (β)-adrenoceptor agonist, beta (β)-adrenoceptor antagonist, monoamine, noradrenaline (norepinephrine).

**adrenarche** *n* increased adrenal cortex activity occurring at around 6–8 years of age. Hormone secretion is increased, especially androgens.

**adrenergic** *adj* describes nerves which liberate the catecholamine noradrenaline (norepinephrine) from their terminations. Most postganglionic sympathetic neurons release noradrenaline as the neurotransmitter at the tissue or organ supplied. The exceptions to this are the postganglionic sympathetic neurons that supply the skin, sweat glands and the blood vessels in skeletal voluntary muscle (structures having no parasympathetic supply); these generally use acetylcholine ⇒ cholinergic *opp*.

**adrenoceptor** *n* (*syn* adrenergic receptor) receptor sites on the effector structures innervated by sympathetic nerves. There are two main types: alpha (α) and beta (β). Both receptor types, which respond differently to neurotransmitters, have further subdivisions.

**adrenocorticotrophic hormone (ACTH)** (*syn* corticotrophin) secreted by the anterior lobe of the pituitary gland, it stimulates the production of hormones by the adrenal cortex.

**adrenogenital syndrome** an endocrine disorder, usually congenital, resulting from abnormal activity of the adrenal cortex. A female child will show enlarged clitoris and possibly labial fusion, perhaps being confused with a male. The male child may show pubic hair and enlarged penis. In both male and female there is rapid growth, muscularity and advanced bone age.

**adrenoleucodystrophy (ALD)** a group of neurodegenerative disorders associated with adrenocortical insufficiency. X-linked inheritance. ⇒ Schilder's disease.

**adrenolytic** *adj* describes a substance that inhibits the function of adrenergic nerves.

**ADRs** *abbr* adverse drug reactions.

**adsorbents** *npl* solids that bind dissolved substances or gases on their surfaces. Charcoal can be used to adsorb gases to act as a deodorant, such as in certain wound-dressing products. Bacterial and other toxins are adsorbed by kaolin, which may be used in the treatment of food poisoning.

**adsorption** *n* the property of a substance to attract and to hold to its surface a gas, liquid or solid in solution or suspension—**adsorptive** *adj*, **adsorb** *vt*.

**adult basic life support** the basic resuscitation measures used in people who have reached puberty. ⊙DVD

**adult polycystic kidney diseases (APKD)** ⇒ polycystic kidney disease.

**adulteration** *n* the addition of cheaper substances to foods etc. in order to increase the bulk and reduce the cost, with intent to mislead and defraud the customer.

**advance directive** referred to as an advance decision to refuse treatment in the Mental Capacity Act 2005 but also known colloquially as a 'living will'. It is a written declaration made by a mentally competent adult before they lose the capacity to make decisions about medical treatment. An advance directive is legally binding if it is in the form of an advanced refusal and the adult is competent at the time of making it. An advance directive allows a competent adult to specify which medical interventions they wish to refuse and the situations/circumstances where the refusal would apply. There must be a clear refusal to have a specified treatment and if there is any doubt about the validity a declaration may be sought or treatment is given that is in the best interests of the person.

**advanced life support (ALS)** the use of drugs, artificial aids and advanced skills to save or preserve life during resuscitation procedures, including tracheal intubation, intravenous drugs, etc. ⇒ cardiopulmonary resuscitation. *paediatric advanced life support (PALS)* the special techniques, drug doses and equipment appropriate to the body weight and surface area of the child being resuscitated.

**advanced trauma life support (ATLS)** a simple systematic method of managing patients with major trauma, such as following a road traffic accident, explosions, gunshot, etc., and dealing with the most life-threatening injury. Specialist courses prepare doctors, nurses and paramedics to use the approach.

**advancement** *n* surgical detachment of a tendon or muscle followed by reattachment at an advanced point.

**adventitia** *n* the external coat, especially of an artery or vein—**adventitious** *adj*.

**adventitious** *adj* **1.** occurring outside the usual location, in an inappropriate place. **2.** relating to an accidental condition. **3.** acquired, not hereditary.

**adverse drug reactions (ADRs)** *npl* a term describing any unwanted effects of a drug. They range from very minor through to extremely unpleasant or life-threatening. They are usually classified into five types: A–E. Type A or augmented effects are adverse effects that occur as a result of the drug's pharmacology, i.e. they are pharmacologically predictable. They are sometimes referred to as side-effects, for example, the dry mouth and constipation caused by morphine. Type B or bizarre effects are unpredictable adverse effects that are not dose-related, for example, hypersensitivity reactions to penicillin. Although the occurrence of type B ADRs is relatively uncommon, they do have a high morbidity and mortality rate. Type C or chronic effects occur after prolonged drug usage, for example, tardive dyskinesia, that occurs with typical antipsychotic drugs (neuroleptics) and the phenothiazines used to manage symptoms in serious mental health problems. Type D or delayed effects occur years after the original drug therapy, for example, cancers caused by the use of cytotoxic drugs for childhood leukaemia. In some cases, the adverse effect may affect the offspring of the original recipient, as in the case of a rare vaginal cancer occurring in the daughters of women who took diethylstilbestrol (a sex hormone) during pregnancy. Type E or ending-of-use effects are adverse effects that occur when the drug is stopped suddenly, i.e. withdrawal effects, illustrated by delirium tremens which occurs when a person stops misusing alcohol. ⇒ Commission on Human Medicines, side-effects, yellow card reporting.

**advocacy** *n* process by which a person supports or argues for the needs of another. Health care professionals may act as advocate for their patients or clients, or assist individuals to develop the skills needed for self-advocacy by, for instance, providing sufficient information for the person to make an informed decision.

**AED** *abbr* automated external defibrillator.

***Aedes*** *n* a genus of mosquitoes which includes *Aedes aegypti*, an important vector of dengue and yellow fever.

**aerobe** *n* a micro-organism that requires oxygen to maintain life—**aerobic** *adj*. ⇒ anaerobe, aerobic micro-organisms.

**aerobic** *adj* requiring free oxygen or air to support life or a specific process.

**aerobic adaptations** long-term physical changes that result from aerobic exercise. They increase the body's ability to deal with endurance exercise. ⇒ anaerobic adaptations.

**aerobic energy** the production of adenosine triphosphate (ATP) by oxidative phosphorylation. ⇒ anaerobic energy.

**aerobic exercise** physical activity that requires the heart and lungs to work harder in order to obtain and supply increased oxygen to strenuously contracting skeletal muscles. ⇒ anaerobic exercise.

**aerobic fitness** the capacity to deliver oxygen to the strenuously contracting muscles and to use it to produce energy during exercise.

**aerobic micro-organisms (aerobes)** *npl* micro-organisms that require oxygen for growth. *facultative aerobes* micro-organisms

that can grow within an anaerobic environment but grow more quickly if aerobic conditions prevail. *obligate aerobes* micro-organisms that are unable to grow in the absence of oxygen, e.g. *Mycobacterium tuberculosis*.

**aerodontalgia** *n* ⇒ barodontalgia.

**aerogenous** *adj* gas-producing.

**aerophagia, aerophagy** *n* excessive air swallowing.

**aerosol** *n* small particles finely dispersed in a gas phase. May be used: to deliver inhalation drug therapy, such as bronchodilators, in insect control and for skin application. Aerosols produced during sneezing and coughing can be responsible for the spread of infection.

**aetiology** *n* (etiology) the science of the causation of disease—**aetiological** *adj*, **aetiologically** *adv*.

**AFB** *abbr* acid-fast bacillus.

**afebrile** *adj* without fever.

**affect** *n* emotion or mood.

**affection** *n* the feeling or emotional aspects of mind; one of the three aspects. ⇒ cognition, conation.

**affective** *adj* pertaining to emotions or moods. *affective psychosis* a mental health problem characterized by mood disturbance together with psychotic symptoms. ⇒ mood, psychosis.

**afferent** *adj* conducting inward to a part or organ; used to describe nerves, blood and lymphatic vessels ⇒ efferent *opp*. *afferent degeneration* that which spreads up sensory nerves.

**affiliation** *n* settling of the paternity of an illegitimate child on the putative father.

**affinity** *n* describes the chemical attraction between two substances, e.g. oxygen and haemoglobin.

**afibrinogenaemia** *n* a lack of fibrinogen resulting in a serious disorder of blood coagulation—**afibrinogenaemic** *adj*.

**aflatoxin** *n* carcinogenic metabolites of certain strains of *Aspergillus flavus* that can affect peanuts and carbohydrate foods stored in warm humid climates. Hepatic enzymes produce the metabolites of aflatoxins which predispose to liver cancer.

**AFP** *abbr* alphafetoprotein.

**afterbirth** *n* the placenta, cord and membranes which are expelled from the uterus after childbirth.

**aftercare** *n* a word denoting the care given during convalescence and rehabilitation. It may be within the remit of health professionals, including therapists or nurses, or may be provided by social care staff or family members.

**aftereffect** *n* a response occurring after the initial effect of a stimulus.

**afterimage** *n* a visual impression of an object persisting after the object has been removed. May be 'positive' when the image is seen in its natural bright colours or 'negative' if the dark parts are light and the bright parts become dark.

**afterload** *n* the pressure of blood in aorta and vessel constriction that forms the resistance or load that left ventricular contraction must overcome to pump blood into the circulation. ⇒ preload.

**afterpains** *n* the pains felt after childbirth, due to contraction and retraction of the uterine muscle fibres.

**agalactia** *n* non-secretion or imperfect secretion of milk after childbirth—**agalactic** *adj.*

**agammaglobulinaemia** *n* absence of gammaglobulin in the blood, with consequent inability to produce immunity to infection—**agammaglobulinaemic** *adj.* ⇒ Bruton's agammaglobulinaemia, ⇒ dysgammaglobulinaemia.

**aganglionosis** *n* absence of ganglia. For example, the parasympathetic ganglion cells of the distal bowel. ⇒ Hirschsprung's disease, megacolon.

**agar** *n* a gelatinous substance obtained from certain seaweeds. It is used as a bulk-increasing laxative and for solidifying bacterial culture media.

**age** *n* ⇒ mental age.

**age-associated memory impairment (AAMI)** an abnormal decline in memory (greater than one standard deviation from the normal) with age where there is no premorbid problem with IQ or the presence of dementia.

**ageism** *n* stereotyping people according to chronological age: overemphasizing negative aspects to the disadvantage of more positive points. Discriminatory attitudes in society disadvantage older people on the basis of age alone. Ageism is also interpreted to be stigmatizing and to separate the older person from others who are younger. Ageist behaviours are often demonstrated in the choice of terms or labels used. For example, 'elderly', 'seniors', 'senile' and 'geriatric'. The media often reinforce this negative stereotyping. Furthermore, ageist views can impact on people of any age. For example, a group of teenagers chatting on a street corner may be perceived, by others, as a potential threat.

**agenesis** *n* incomplete and imperfect development—**agenetic** *adj.*

**age-related macular degeneration (AMD)** degenerative changes of the retina in the macular region which may lead to loss of central vision. There are problems with reading and distinguishing fine features. It is a leading cause of blindness in people aged over 50. AMD may be 'dry' or atrophic, when Bruch's membrane accumulates debris known as drusen, or 'wet', which involves the growth of new, abnormal blood vessels in Bruch's membrane.

**ageusia** *n* loss or impairment of the sensation of taste.

**agglutination** *n* the clumping of bacteria, red blood cells or antigen-coated particles by antibodies called agglutinins, developed in the blood serum of a previously infected or sensitized person or animal. Agglutination forms the basis of many laboratory tests—**agglutinable**, **agglutinative**, *adj.* **agglutinate** *vt, vi.*

**agglutinins** *npl* antibodies that agglutinate or clump organisms or particles.

**agility** *n* the ability to control the direction of the body or body part during rapid movement.

**aglossia** *n* absence of the tongue—**aglossic** *adj.*

**aglutition** *n* dysphagia.

**agnathia** *n* absence or incomplete development of the jaw.

**agnosia** *n* inability to perceive the nature of sensory impressions. People and things are not recognized; usually classified by the sense or senses affected—**agnosic** *adj.* *spatial agnosia* loss of spatial appreciation.

**agonal** *adj* relating to the events occurring just before death. ⇒ Cheyne–Stokes respiration. *agonal rhythm* the terminal arrhythmia recorded just prior to death. Usually there is broad-based bradycardia without a cardiac output.

**agonist** *n* a muscle that shortens to perform a movement. Also describes a drug or other chemical that imitates the response of the ligand (natural chemical) at a receptor site. ⇒ antagonist *opp.*

**agoraphobia** *n* morbid fear of being alone in large open places—**agoraphobic** *adj.*

**agranulocyte** *n* a non-granular leucocyte.

**agranulocytosis** *n* marked reduction in or complete absence of granulocytes (the polymorphonuclear leucocytes, neutrophils, eosinophils and basophils). Usually results from bone marrow depression caused by (a) hypersensitivity to drugs; (b) cytotoxic drugs; or (c) irradiation. Symptoms include fever and ulceration of the mouth and throat. There is an inability to fight infection and this can lead to overwhelming infection and ultimately to death. ⇒ neutropenia—**agranulocytic** *adj*.

**agraphia** *n* loss of language facility. *motor agraphia* inability to express thoughts in writing, usually due to left precentral cerebral lesions. *sensory agraphia* inability to interpret the written word, due to lesions in the posterior part of the left parieto-occipital region—**agraphic** *adj*.

**AHF/G** *abbr* antihaemophilic factor/globulin.

**AHI** *abbr* apnoea hypopnoea index.

**Aicardi syndrome** (J Aicardi, French paediatrician/neurologist, b. 1926) a rare genetic defect affecting females. There is abnormal brain development with the partial or total absence of the corpus callosum which normally connects the two hemispheres of the brain. Affected children have seizures, a learning disability and retinal abnormalities.

**AICD** *abbr* automatic implantable cardioverter defibrillator.

**AID** *abbr* artificial insemination of a female with donor semen.

**AIDS** *abbr* acquired immune deficiency syndrome.

**AIDS-defining illness** the US Centers for Disease Control and Prevention (CDC) criteria for acquired immune deficiency syndrome (AIDS) in a patient infected with human immunodeficiency virus (HIV) disease. Examples include candidiasis of bronchus, trachea, lungs or oesophagus, invasive cervical cancer, Kaposi's sarcoma, pulmonary tuberculosis or other mycobacterial infection, and *Pneumocystis jirovecii* (former name *Pneumocystis carinii*) pneumonia.

**AIH** *abbr* artificial insemination of a female with her husband's (partner's) semen.

**ainhum** *n* the spontaneous amputation of the fifth toe. It may be due to the formation of a constricting fibrous band. It may occur in Africa, in people who habitually walk barefoot.

**air** *n* the gaseous mixture which makes up the atmosphere surrounding the earth. It consists of approximately 78% nitrogen, 20% oxygen, 0.04% carbon dioxide, 1% argon, traces of ozone, neon, helium, etc. and a variable amount of water vapour.

**air embolism** obstruction to the flow of blood resulting from an air bubble entering the circulation. This may occur during surgery, during intravenous fluid infusion or injection, cardiac catheterization or trauma.

**air hunger** a deep indrawing of breath which characterizes the late stages of uncontrolled haemorrhage.

**air swallowing (aerophagia)** swallowing of excessive air particularly when eating: it may result in belching or the passage of flatus from the anus.

**airway** *n* used to describe the entry to the larynx from the pharynx. *Brook airway* oropharyngeal airway used in expired air resuscitation. *nasopharyngeal airway* a curved airway introduced into the pharynx via the nostril. It is located behind the tongue and so prevents a flaccid tongue from obstructing the airway in an unconscious patient. *oropharyngeal airway* a flexible oval tube, such as a Guedel airway (Figure A.5), which can be placed along the upper surface of the tongue to prevent a flaccid tongue from resting against the posterior pharyngeal wall, thereby obstructing the airway; it is commonly used during general anaesthesia. Also used during cardiopulmonary resuscitation.

**airway conductance** the ease in which air/gas flows through the airways. It is the reciprocal of airways resistance.

**airways resistance ($R_{aw}$)** the change in pressure between the mouth/nose and the alveoli divided by air flow. It is increased in conditions that reduce the diameter of the airways (bronchoconstriction) including bronchospasm in asthma and inflammation.

**AIS** *abbr* abbreviated injury scale.

**akathisia** *n* a subjective state of persistent motor restlessness: it can occur as a side-effect of antipsychotic (neuroleptic) drugs.

**akinesia** *n* impairment in initiation of movement or delay in reaction time—**akinetic** *adj*.

**ALA** *abbr* alpha (α)-linolenic acid.

**alactacid (alactic) anaerobic system** a series of chemical reactions occurring within the cells whereby adenosine triphosphate (ATP) for energy use is produced, without oxygen, from adenosine diphosphate (ADP) and creatine phosphate (CP) (phosphocreatine).

**alactacid oxygen debt component** the amount of oxygen required to replace the adenosine triphosphate (ATP) and creatine phosphate (phosphocreatine) stores in cells during the process of recovery from exercise.

**alactasia** *n* the deficiency (partial or total) of the intestinal enzyme lactase. The affected person is unable to digest lactose (sugar) in milk. ⇒ lactase deficiency.

**Alagille syndrome** a dominantly inherited autosomal condition. There is jaundice due

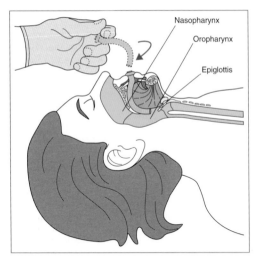

**Figure A.5** Airway *(reproduced from Nicol et al. 2004 with permission).*

to faulty development of the intrahepatic bile ducts. It may be associated with pulmonary stenosis and other heart defects, and abnormalities affecting the eyes and nervous system.

**alanine** *n* a non-essential (dispensable) amino acid.

**alanine aminotransferase (ALT)** an enzyme that facilitates the reversible transfer of amino groups during amino acid metabolism. ⇒ aminotransferases.

**Albers-Schönberg disease** (H Albers-Schönberg, German surgeon/radiologist, 1865–1921) ⇒ osteopetrosis.

**albinism** *n* a congenital hypopigmentation of the hair, skin and eyes. It is caused by a deficiency of melanin pigment in skin and/or the eye. Other associated eye and neurological defects can contribute to poor vision.

**albino** *n* a person affected with albinism— **albinotic** *adj.*

**Albright's syndrome** (F Albright, American physician, 1900–1969) a condition that includes fibrous dysplasia of bone, endocrine problems, such as precocious puberty in females, and brown macular areas on the skin. ⇒ fibrous dysplasia.

**albumin** *n* a protein found in animal and vegetable material. It is soluble in water and coagulates on heating. *serum albumin* the main

protein of blood plasma. ⇒ lactalbumin— **albuminous, albuminoid** *adj.*

**albuminuria** *n* the presence of albumin in the urine. The condition may be temporary and clear up completely, as in many febrile states. May be indicative of serious kidney disease— **albuminuric** *adj.* ⇒ microalbuminuria, orthostatic albuminuria, proteinuria.

**albumose** *n* an intermediate substance formed during protein digestion.

**alcohol** *n* a group of organic compounds. Absolute alcohol is occasionally used by injection for the relief of trigeminal neuralgia and other intractable pain. Ethyl alcohol (ethanol) is the intoxicating constituent of alcoholic drinks: wine, beer, cider and spirits. It potentiates the effects of hypnotics and tranquillizers. ⇒ alcohol dependence/misuse, Korsakoff's syndrome, Wernicke's encephalopathy.

**alcohol dependence/misuse** the morbid state of dependence upon an excessive intake of alcohol. A syndrome of physical, psychological and behavioural responses related to alcohol misuse. Characteristically there are withdrawal symptoms and drinking to relieve the same, tolerance to the effects of alcohol, compulsion to drink alcohol, narrowing of repertoire of drinking, etc. Poisoning resulting from alcoholic dependence may be acute or chronic. Chronic poisoning causes severe damage to most body systems, e.g. the liver, digestive organs with malnutrition, the heart and nervous system. Long-term alcohol misuse is associated with hepatitis, cirrhosis, hepatic portal hypertension, oesophageal varices and gastrointestinal haemorrhage, gastritis, iron overload, primary liver cancer, other cancers, e.g. head and neck, pancreatitis, arterial hypertension, coronary heart disease and neurological problems caused by alcohol toxicity or vitamin B deficiency. Misuse of alcohol by a woman during pregnancy can lead to the birth of an infant with fetal alcohol syndrome (FAS). Additionally, the chronic misuse of alcohol causes social, emotional and psychological problems, such as the breakdown of relationships, financial difficulties and debt, the loss of employment and homelessness.

**alcohol units** a useful way of estimating how much alcohol has been consumed, and in promoting safe intake. One unit of alcohol is defined as 10 mL of absolute alcohol.

**alcohol-fast** *adj* in bacteriology, describes a micro-organism which, when stained, is resistant to decolorization by alcohol.

**Alcoholics Anonymous (AA)** a fellowship of people who have had problems with alcohol dependence. Their aim is helping others with similar difficulties.

**ALD** *abbr* adrenoleucodystrophy.

**aldehydes** *npl* a group of organic compounds. Formed by the oxidation of an alcohol (e.g. acetaldehyde from ethyl alcohol).

**aldolase** *n* an enzyme present in muscle tissue. *aldolase test* increased levels of aldolase and other enzymes in the blood are indicative of some muscle diseases, e.g. severe muscular dystrophy.

**aldosterone** *n* mineralocorticoid hormone secreted by the adrenal cortex. Secretion is regulated by the action of renin and angiotensin. It enhances the reabsorption of sodium accompanied by water and the excretion of potassium by the renal tubules.

**aldosterone antagonist** a drug that acts as an aldosterone antagonist. ⇒ potassium-sparing diuretics, Appendix 5.

**aldosteronism** *n* ⇒ hyperaldosteronism.

**Aleppo boil** ⇒ leishmaniasis.

**Alexander technique** (F Alexander, Australian actor, 1869–1955) a series of techniques used to improve the functioning of mind and body in movement known as 'psychophysical' re-education. It is based on the belief that poor posture can lead to ill health, injury and chronic pain. The technique aims to promote postural improvement through self-awareness.

**alexia** *n* word blindness; an inability to interpret the significance of the printed or written word, but without loss of visual power. Can be due to a brain lesion or insufficient/inappropriate sensory experience during an *ab initio* stage of learning—**alexic** *adj*.

**ALG** *abbr* antilymphocyte globulin.

**algesia** *n* excessive sensitivity to pain.

**algesimeter** *n* an instrument that registers the degree of sensitivity to pain.

**alginates** *npl* seaweed derivatives used in some wound dressings. They have high absorbency and haemostatic properties and can be removed without damaging delicate tissues. They can be used for wounds with moderate to high exudate, for wet wound débridement and on infected wounds.

**algodystrophy** *n* ⇒ complex regional pain syndrome.

**algorithm** *n* **1.** a step-by-step protocol or guide for the management of a particular situation or health problem. **2.** a computer procedure for problem solving using logical or mathematical operations.

**alienation** *n* in psychology and sociology, estrangement from people.

**alimentary** *adj* pertaining to food.

**alimentary tract** *n* comprises the mouth, oesophagus, stomach, small intestine, ascending colon, transverse colon, descending colon, sigmoid colon, rectum and anal canal. ⇒ Appendix 1, Figure 18B.

**alimentation** *n* the act of nourishing with food; feeding.

**alkalaemia** *n* low level of acid (hydrogen ions) in the blood, resulting in an above normal pH >7.45 (hydrogen ion concentration <36 mmol/L). ⇒ alkalosis—**alkalaemic** *adj*.

**alkali** *n* also called a base. Substances that have an excess of hydroxyl ions over hydrogen ions, e.g. sodium bicarbonate, sodium hydroxide. They have a pH greater than 7 and turn red litmus blue. Alkalis react with acids to produce salts plus water, and with fats to form soaps.

**alkaline** *adj* **1.** relating to or possessing the properties of an alkali. **2.** containing an excess of hydroxyl over hydrogen ions.

**alkaline phosphatase** an enzyme present in several tissues, e.g. bone, liver and kidney. An increase of this enzyme in the blood is indicative of obstructive jaundice and increased osteoblast activity associated with some bone diseases.

**alkaline reserve** the amount of buffered alkali (normally bicarbonate) available in the blood for buffering acids (normally dissolved $CO_2$) formed in or introduced into the body and limiting pH changes in the blood.

**alkaline tide** describes the movement of basic bicarbonate (hydrogen carbonate) ($HCO_3^-$) ions from the parietal (oxyntic) cells of the stomach into the venous blood. The hydrogen carbonate ions are formed during the secretion of hydrochloric acid (HCl) by the oxyntic cells. This results in a small rise in blood pH.

**alkalinuria** *n* alkalinity of urine—**alkalinuric** *adj*.

**alkaloid** *n* similar to an alkali. Also describes a large group of organic bases present in plants and which have important pharmacological actions, e.g. morphine, atropine, quinine and caffeine. Also result from fungal action on cereal crops, such as ergot. They may also be present in animal foods, e.g. puffer fish contains tetrodotoxin—**alkaloidal** *adj*.

**alkalosis** *n* process leading to low levels of acid (excess of alkali) in the body. *metabolic alkalosis* due to loss of body acids (e.g. vomiting of acidic gastric contents) or excess administration of alkali. *respiratory alkalosis* due to hyperventilation and lowering of carbon dioxide level.

**alkaptonuria** *n* the presence of alkaptone (homogentisic acid) in the urine, resulting from only partial oxidation of the amino acids phenylalanine and tyrosine. The condition is usually noticed because urine turns black in the nappies, or when left to stand. Apart from this, and a tendency to arthritis in later life, there are no ill effects from alkaptonuria.

**alkylating agents** organic molecules that disrupt cell division by binding to the DNA in the nucleus, e.g. busulfan. ⇒ cytotoxic. ⇒ Appendix 5.

**ALL** *abbr* acute lymphoblastic leukaemia.

**allele** *n* allelomorph. Describes the alternative forms of a gene at the same chromosomal location (locus). Previously used to denote inherited characteristics that are alternative and contrasting, such as normal colour vision contrasting with colour blindness, or the different ABO blood groups.

**allelomorph** *n* ⇒ allele.

**allergen** *n* an antigen which produces an allergic, or immediate-type hypersensitivity response—**allergenic** *adj*, **allergenicity** *n*.

**allergy** *n* an immune response induced by exposure to an allergen causing a harmful hypersensitivity reaction on subsequent exposure—**allergic** *adj*. ⇒ anaphylaxis, sensitization.

**Allied and Complementary Medicine Database (AMED)** computerized database of literature relevant to a variety of professions allied to medicine, such as physiotherapy, podiatry, etc., palliative care and complementary medicine.

**allied health professions** a large and varied group of registered health profession practitioners distinct from medicine, dentistry and nursing. They work autonomously in multiprofessional and interagency teams. Professionals included as allied health vary from country to country but may include: art therapists, biomedical scientists, chiropodists/podiatrists, dental hygienists, dietitians, occupational therapists, operating department practitioners, paramedics, physiotherapists (physical therapists), radiographers (diagnostic and therapeutic), prosthetists/orthotists, speech and language therapists.

**allograft** *n* grafting or transplanting an organ or tissue from one person to another who does not share exactly the same transplantation antigens. Also known as a homograft.

**allopathy** *n* describes conventional medicine and health care—**allopathic** *adj*. ⇒ homoeopathy.

**all-or-none law/phenomenon** *n* relates to the conduction of action potentials in nerve or muscle fibres (excitable tissue). The action potential in a particular fibre is always the same size regardless of the intensity of the stimulus. The nerve or muscle fibre either responds in full or does not respond at all. There is no partial response to a reduced intensity stimulus.

**allotriophagy** *n* desire for extraordinary or abnormal foods. Also known as cissa, cittosis and pica.

**alopecia** *n* baldness, which can be congenital, premature or senile. *alopecia areata* a patchy baldness, usually of a temporary nature. Cause unknown, probably autoimmune, but stress is a common precipitating factor. Exclamation mark hairs are diagnostic. The broken stump found at the periphery of spreading bald patches in alopecia areata is called an exclamation mark hair, from the characteristic shape caused by atrophic thinning of the hair shaft. ⊙DVD *cicatricial alopecia* progressive alopecia of the scalp in which tufts of normal hair occur between scarred bald patches. Folliculitis decalvans is an alopecia of the scalp characterized by pustulation and scarring.

**alpha (α)-adrenoceptor agonists** (*syn* α-stimulants) a group of drugs that stimulate α-adrenoceptors, e.g. adrenaline (epinephrine). ⇒ Appendix 5.

**alpha (α)-adrenoceptor antagonists** (*syn* α-blockers) a group of drugs that block the stimulation of α-adrenoceptors, e.g. doxazosin. ⇒ Appendix 5.

**alpha (α)-glucosidase inhibitor** an oral hypoglycaemic drug that slows the digestion and absorption of complex carbohydrates and sucrose from the intestine, e.g. acarbose. ⇒ Appendix 5.

**alpha (α)-linolenic acid (ALA)** a polyunsaturated fatty acid. ⇒ linolenic acids.

**alpha (α)-redistribution phase** the point after an intravenous injection when the blood concentration of the drug begins to fall below the peak levels achieved.

**alpha$_1$ (α)-antitrypsin** a liver protein that normally opposes the proteolytic enzyme trypsin. Reduced blood levels are linked with a genetic predisposition to emphysema and liver disease.

**alphafetoprotein (AFP)** *n* a protein produced by the fetal gut and liver cells and by adult liver cancer cells. Raised levels are found in maternal serum and amniotic fluid in fetal abnormalities, including neural tube defects. May be used as a tumour marker for cancers, including those of the liver and the testes, affecting children and adults. It is also present in the serum in liver cirrhosis. ⇒ oncofetal antigens.

**alphaviruses** *npl* a group of very small togaviruses. They are transmitted by mosquito bites and cause diseases that include Ross river virus disease/fever. ⇒ arboviruses.

**Alport's syndrome** (A Alport, South African physician, 1880–1959) an inherited disorder characterized by glomerulonephritis and haematuria which, in males, usually progresses to end-stage renal failure. A kidney transplant and some form of dialysis may be successful. Affected females may be asymptomatic. Other problems include progressive sensorineural deafness and eye disorders, such as cataracts and lenticonus.

**ALS** *abbr* **1.** advanced life support. **2.** amyotrophic lateral sclerosis.

**ALT** *abbr* alanine aminotransferase. ⇒ aminotransferases.

**alternative medicine** ⇒ complementary and alternative medicine.

**altitude sickness (mountain sickness)** signs and symptoms including nausea, tachycardia, headache, dizziness, mood changes and dyspnoea, sometimes with pulmonary oedema caused by the reduced partial pressure of atmospheric oxygen at high altitudes. This is encountered during mountaineering or flights in unpressurized aircraft.

**altitude training** programme of exercise that aims to produce reversible physiological adaptations that increase a person's tolerance to reduced $PO_2$ at altitude.

**altitudinal** *adj* when describing a visual field defect implies loss of vision in superior or inferior half of field.

**alveolar ridge** the bony ridge of the mandible and maxillae; it contains the alveoli or sockets for the teeth.

**alveolitis** *n* inflammation of alveoli. When caused by inhalation of an allergen, such as microbial spores or animal proteins, it is termed *extrinsic allergic alveolitis*.

**alveolus** *n* **1.** an air sac of the lung. **2.** in dentistry, a bony tooth socket within the jaw bone. **3.** a gland follicle or acinus—**alveoli** *pl*, **alveolar** *adj*.

**Alzheimer's disease** (A Alzheimer, German neurologist, 1864–1915) a neurodegenerative disorder of the brain with distinct pathology causing a progressive loss of cognitive function (dementia). It is primarily a disease that occurs in older people for no obvious reason but can affect younger patients (i.e. <65 years of age), when it may be familial. Alzheimer's disease is the most common cause of dementia in people under 65 years of age and may be linked to the inheritance of a gene that codes for apolipoprotein E (a transport protein). The brains of people with Alzheimer's disease exhibit specific abnormalities, including: plaques containing amyloid (abnormal protein) in the cortex, loss of neurons, brain atrophy with shrinkage and the presence of neurofibrillary tangles. The onset is insidious and some changes may be put down to growing older. The disorder is characterized by progressive memory loss (particularly short-term or recent), failing intellectual ability, confusion, restlessness, speech problems, motor retardation, depression and personality changes. As the disease progresses the person becomes bed-bound and completely reliant upon family or carers for every need.

**AMA** *abbr* antimitochondrial antibody.

**amalgam** *n* any of a group of alloys containing mercury. ⇒ dental amalgam.

***Amanita*** *n* a genus of fungi, some of which are highly toxic. They include the death cap (*A. phalloides*) mushroom. Some hours after ingestion the toxins cause vomiting, diarrhoea, abdominal pain and acute liver necrosis and failure. Intensive care and support for specific organ failure are required. The mortality rate is high in the absence of treatment.

**amastia** *n* congenital absence of the breasts.

**amaurosis** *n* partial or total blindness. In particular, loss of vision associated with a systemic disorder, such as neurological diseases, diabetes, kidney disease, excessive misuse of alcohol and tobacco, rather than conditions directly affecting the eye. *amaurosis fugax* temporary loss of vision in an eye due to interruption of arterial blood supply to the retina.

**ambidextrous** *adj* able to use both hands equally well—**ambidexter** *adj*, **ambidexterity** *n*.

**ambivalence** *n* **1.** uncertainty that results from an inability to choose between opposites **2.** the situation where opposite conflicting feelings, drives, desires or attitudes towards the same object, person, or place coexist in a person. For example, love and hate or pain and pleasure.

**amblyopia** *n* defective vision. Usually refers to failure of normal visual development (may be strabismic, refractive, deprivation). *toxic amblyopia* damage to the optic nerve by a noxious agent, usually related to heavy smoking—**amblyopic** *adj*.

**amblyoscope** *n* an instrument used to assess the angle of strabismus (squint) and the manner in which both eyes are used together.

**ambulant** *adj* able to walk, i.e. not confined to bed or chair.

**ambulatory** *adj* mobile, walking about.

**ambulatory ECG** ⇒ electrocardiogram.

**ambulatory surgery (day surgery)** surgery carried out on the day of admission and, in the absence of problems, the person is discharged the same day to the care of the primary care team. Examples include hernia surgery, cataract removal, endoscopic examinations, and minor orthopaedic and gynaecological procedures.

**ambulatory treatment** interventions, such as blood product transfusion or chemotherapy, provided for patients as day care. ⇒ continuous ambulatory peritoneal dialysis.

**AMD** *abbr* age-related macular degeneration.

**AMED** *abbr* Allied and Complementary Medicine Database.

**amelia** *n* a congenital absence of a limb or limbs. *complete amelia* absence of both arms and legs.

**amelioration** *n* a reduction in the severity of symptoms.

**amelogenesis** *n* the formation of the tooth enamel. It is finished before the teeth erupt. *amelogenesis imperfecta* an inherited condition where there is a complete failure of tooth enamel production (agenesis) or severe hypoplasia. The condition, which is inherited as an autosomal-dominant character, gives rise to brown discoloration of the teeth.

**amelolast** *n* an epithelial cell which secretes tooth enamel during the period when the teeth are being formed.

**amenorrhoea** *n* absence of the menses. Amenorrhoea is normal before the menarche (the commencement of menstruation) occurring during puberty, during pregnancy and for varying periods during lactation and following the menopause (cessation of menstruation) occurring during the climacteric. When menstruation has not been established at the time when it should have been, it is termed *primary amenorrhoea.* Causes include eating disorders, Turner's syndrome, absence of the uterus or faulty hormone secretion; absence of the menses after they have once commenced is referred to as *secondary amenorrhoea.* Causes include hypothalamic disorders, hormonal disturbances, certain medications, emotional crisis, change in circumstances, eating disorders or some mental health problems—**amenorrhoeal** *adj*.

**Ames test** a method of in vitro testing for the ability of chemicals, such as potential food additives, to cause mutation in a strain of *Salmonella* bacteria (the mutagenic potential). Frequently used as a preliminary screening test to identify substances likely to be carcinogenic. Also known as the mutagenicity test.

**ametria** *n* congenital absence of the uterus.

**ametropia** *n* defective sight due to imperfect refractive power of the eye—**ametropic** *adj*, **ametrope** *n*. ⇒ astigmatism, hypermetropia, myopia.

**amines** *npl* group of organic compounds containing the functional group -NH$_2$. Many are important biochemical molecules, e.g. catecholamines, histamine, dopamine, etc. There are three potentially important amines present in protein foods containing amino acids: phenylethylamine (from the amino acid phenylalanine), tyramine (from the amino acid tyrosine) and tryptamine (from the amino acid tryptophan). These amines can stimulate the activity of the sympathetic nervous system and can cause an increase in blood pressure. In some people they are a possible dietary cause of migraine. The intake of foods high in these amines, (e.g. mature cheese, fermented soya bean foods and yeast extract) is contraindicated for people taking monoamine oxidase inhibitor (MAOI) antidepressant drugs, as a dangerous increase in blood pressure can occur.

**amino acids** organic acids in which one or more of the hydrogen atoms are replaced by a basic amino group (-NH$_2$); they also contain one or more acidic carboxyl groups (-COOH). They are the end-product of protein hydrolysis and from them the body synthesizes its own proteins. In this process individual amino acids are linked together by peptide bonds, in a dehydration reaction, to form new polypeptides or proteins. There are 20 common amino acids which are classified as either essential (indispensable) or non-essential (dispensable). Ten (eight in adults and a further two during childhood) cannot be synthesized in sufficient quantities in the body and are therefore essential (indispensable) in the diet—isoleucine, leucine, lysine, methionine, phenylalanine, threonine, tryptophan and valine. Arginine and histidine are the two amino acids that are essential during childhood. The remainder, which can be synthesized in the body if the diet contains sufficient amounts of the precursor amino acids, are designated non-essential (dispensable) amino acids. They are alanine, asparagine, aspartic acid (aspartate), cysteine, glutamic acid (glutamate), glutamine, glycine, proline, serine and tyrosine. However, some of these are conditionally essential and depend upon adequate amounts of their precursor being present in the diet. ⇒ essential amino acids.

**aminoacidopathy** *n* disease caused by imbalance of amino acids.

**aminoaciduria** *n* the abnormal presence of amino acids in the urine; it usually indicates an inborn error of metabolism as in cystinosis, tyrosinaemia and Fanconi syndrome—**aminoaciduric** *adj*.

**aminoglycosides** *npl* a group of bactericidal antibiotic drugs, e.g. gentamicin, with a wide range of activity. They have toxic effects on the kidney (nephrotoxicity) and on the ear (ototoxicity) and so are only prescribed if other, safer drugs would be ineffective. ⇒ Appendix 5.

**aminopeptidases** *npl* intestinal enzymes present in the outer membrane of the enterocytes (intestinal cells) that act upon the amine end (-NH$_2$) of the peptide chain during the digestion of protein. They break the peptide bond and release the terminal amino acid.

**aminotransferases** *npl* transaminases. A group of enzymes that catalyse the transfer of an α-amino group from an α-amino acid to an α-keto acid. The major site for these is the liver. *alanine aminotransferase (ALT)* formerly known as serum glutamic pyruvic transaminase (SGPT). *aspartate aminotransferase (AST)* formerly known as serum glutamic oxalacetic transaminase (SGOT). Aminotransferases are released by certain damaged cells and when blood levels are measured may be useful, along with other biochemical tests, in the diagnosis of liver disease (ALT, AST) and myocardial infarction (AST).

**amitosis** *n* division of a cell by direct fission—**amitotic** *adj*.

**AML** *abbr* acute myeloblastic leukaemia.

**ammonia** *n* (NH$_3$) a pungent gaseous compound of nitrogen and hydrogen.

**ammonium bicarbonate** sometimes used in expectorant cough mixtures but of doubtful value.

**ammonium ion (NH$_4^+$)** an ion formed from a reaction between ammonia and hydrogen. Ammonium ions are formed in the liver during amino acid metabolism. Several inherited errors of ammonia/ammonium metabolism can cause a learning disability, seizures and other neurological manifestations. ⇒ urea cycle.

**amnesia** *n* complete loss of memory; can be divided into organic (true) amnesia (e.g. delirium, dementia, postelectroconvulsive therapy [ECT]) and psychogenic amnesia (e.g. dissociative states, Ganser's syndrome). The term *anterograde amnesia* is used when there is impaired continuous recall for events following an accident or brain insult, and *retrograde amnesia* when the impairment is of events prior to the insult—**amnesic** *adj*.

**amnesic syndrome** chronic profound impairment of recent memory with preserved immediate recall. Often accompanied by disorientation for time and confabulation (the creation of false memory to fill the gaps in memory). Commonly caused by thiamin(e) deficiency, which can be secondary to chronic alcohol use, dietary deficiency, gastric cancer, etc. ⇒ Korsakoff's (Korsakov's) syndrome.

**amniocentesis** *n* a diagnostic procedure for detecting chromosomal, metabolic and haematological abnormalities of the fetus. It involves inserting a wide-bore needle under

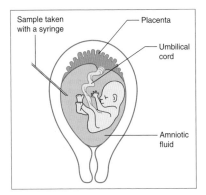

Sample taken with a syringe

Placenta

Umbilical cord

Amniotic fluid

**Figure A.6** Amniocentesis *(reproduced from Brooker 2006A with permission).*

ultrasound guidance through the abdominal wall into the amniotic sac to obtain a sample of amniotic fluid (Figure A.6). Many single-gene and chromosome abnormalities can be diagnosed from testing amniotic fluid and fetal cells shed into the amniotic fluid surrounding the fetus. The cells obtained from the fluid are grown and examined for chromosomal abnormalities, such as Down's syndrome. The amniotic fluid may contain chemical markers for a particular abnormality, e.g. the presence of alphafetoprotein (AFP) may indicate neural tube defects. Amniocentesis is usually performed after 15 weeks' gestation. Testing for genetic defects takes time and final results are usually available in about 10–14 days. There are, however, risks associated with amniocentesis, for example spontaneous miscarriage occurs in around 1% of women. ⇒ chorionic villus sampling.

**amniohook** *n* an instrument for rupturing the fetal membranes. Also called an amniotome. ⇒ amniotomy.

**amnion** *n* membrane of embryonic origin lining the cavity of the uterus during pregnancy containing amniotic fluid and the fetus—**amnionic, amniotic** *adj.* ⇒ chorion.

**amnionitis** *n* inflammation of the amnion. May result from premature rupture of the fetal membranes.

**amnioscopy** *n* an amnioscope passed through an incision in the abdominal wall and into the amniotic cavity enables direct viewing of the fetus and amniotic fluid. Clear, colourless fluid is normal; yellow or green staining is due to

meconium and occurs in cases of fetal hypoxia—**amnioscopic** *adj.* **amnioscopically** *adv. cervical amnioscopy* can be performed late in pregnancy. A different instrument is inserted via the vagina and uterine cervix for the same purposes.

**amniotic cavity** the fluid-filled cavity between the fetus and the amnion.

**amniotic fluid** fluid produced by the inner fetal membrane (amnion) and the fetus, which surrounds the fetus throughout pregnancy. About 1 litre of fluid is present at the 38th week of gestation. It protects the fetus from temperature variations and physical trauma, and permits fetal movement. It is secreted and reabsorbed by cells lining the amniotic cavity and is swallowed by the fetus and excreted as urine. ⇒ amniocentesis, amnioscopy, oligohydramnios, polyhydramnios. *amniotic fluid embolism* an embolus caused by amniotic fluid entering the maternal circulation. An extremely rare but very serious complication of pregnancy. ⇒ disseminated intravascular coagulation.

**amniotome** *n* ⇒ amniohook.

**amniotomy** *n* artificial rupture of the fetal membranes to induce or expedite labour.

**amoeba** *n* a unicellular (single-cell) protozoon. Strains that are human parasites include *Entamoeba histolytica*, which causes amoebic dysentery (intestinal amoebiasis). ⇒ protozoon—**amoebae** *pl.* **amoebic** *adj.*

**amoebiasis** *n* infestation of the large intestine by the protozoon *Entamoeba histolytica*, where it causes mucosal ulceration leading to pain, diarrhoea alternating with constipation, and blood and mucus passed rectally, hence the term 'amoebic dysentery'. Metronidazole or tinidazole is used to treat amoebic dysentery. If the amoebae enter the hepatic portal circulation they may cause a liver abscess. Hepatic involvement is treated with metronidazole or tinidazole followed by a course of diloxanide to destroy any amoebae in the intestine. Diagnosis is by isolating the amoeba in the stools. Cutaneous amoebiasis may cause perianal or genital ulceration in homosexual men.

**amoebicide** *n* an agent that kills amoebae, such as metronidazole—**amoebicidal** *adj.*

**amoeboid** *adj* resembling an amoeba in shape or in mode of movement, such as some leucocytes.

**amoeboma** *n* a tumour (swelling) in the caecum or rectum caused by *Entamoeba histolytica*. Fibrosis may occur and obstruct the bowel.

**A**

**amorph** *n* a gene that is inactive, i.e. does not express a trait.

**amorphous** *adj* not having a regular shape.

**AMP** *abbr* adenosine monophosphate.

**ampere (A)** *n* (A M Ampère, French physicist, 1775–1836) one of the seven base units of the International System of Units (SI). A measurement of electrical current. ⟹ Appendix 2.

**amphetamines** *npl* a group of sympathomimetic agents. A potent central nervous system (CNS) stimulant. This stimulant effect has led to the increased misuse of, and dependence on, individual drugs, such as amfetamine. Clinical use is extremely limited. *amfetamine poisoning* is indicated by signs and symptoms that include hallucinations, delerium, agitation, excessive activity, paranoia, tachycardia, hypertension, exhaustion, seizures, hyperthermia and altered consciousness.

**amphiarthrosis** *n* a cartilaginous, slightly movable joint. There are two types: synchondrosis and symphysis.

**amphipathic** *adj* describes a molecule that has parts with very different chemical properties. For example, possessing a non-polar (hydrophobic) end and a polar (hydrophilic) end.

**ampoule** *n* a hermetically sealed glass or plastic phial containing a single sterile dose of a drug.

**ampulla** *n* any flask-like dilatation, such as that in the uterine (fallopian) tube ⟹ Appendix 1, Figure 17—**ampullae** *pl,* **ampullar, ampullary, ampullate** *adj. ampulla of Vater* ⟹ hepatopancreatic ampulla.

**amputation** *n* removal of an appending part of the body, e.g. breast, or a limb or part of a limb. A limb may be amputated following severe trauma, to remove a cancer and in the case of gangrene in peripheral vascular disease. A limb may also be lost by traumatic amputation in an industrial accident, an explosion or a road traffic accident.

**amputee** *n* a person who has had amputation of one or more limbs.

**Amsler grid** a grid comprising black lines on a white background arranged horizontally and vertically to produce a checkerboard effect with a black or white dot in the centre. It is used to identify a central visual field defect, such as that which occurs with age-related macular degeneration. The person is asked to look at the grid wearing normal reading spectacles at normal reading distance, to cover one eye and stare at the central spot. This is repeated with the other eye. In order to detect the presence of a potential problem the person is asked to report if any of the lines are blurred, wavy, missing or a different colour, or crooked or bent, and whether any of the boxes are distorted in terms of shape or size.

**amygdala** *n* an almond-shaped nucleus (mass of grey matter) sited deep within the temporal lobe of the cerebrum. It is part of the limbic system and associated with emotional behaviour and the olfactory system, and may have a role in memory processing. It is closely connected to the caudate nucleus, one of the basal nuclei (also known as basal ganglia). ⟹ limbic system.

**amylase** *n* any enzyme that converts starches into sugars. Found in saliva and pancreatic juice; it converts starchy foods to maltose, a disaccharide. The amount of amylase in the blood is increased in disorders of the pancreas, such as pancreatitis, and in some gastrointestinal conditions, e.g. perforation of a peptic ulcer.

**amylin** *n* also called islet amyloid polypeptide. A polypeptide hormone produced by the beta (β) cells of the islets of the pancreas with insulin. It has a role in glycaemic control in conjunction with insulin and glucagon.

**amylodyspepsia** *n* a condition characterized by an inability to digest starchy foods.

**amyloid** *adj, n* **1.** resembling starch. **2.** describes the abnormal proteins associated with amyloidosis. It was previously thought to be a starch-like glycoprotein (a protein–carbohydrate complex). ⟹ amyloidosis.

**amyloidosis** *n* a group of diseases in which amyloid, an abnormal protein, is deposited in one or more organ systems, notably the liver, kidney, heart, gastrointestinal system and nervous system, leading to impaired organ function. Amyloidosis can be primary, secondary or familial. There are also other types that include the abnormal protein (β-amyloid protein) associated with Alzheimer's disease. *primary amyloidosis* affects the plasma cells (formed from B cells) and may be associated with multiple myeloma. *secondary amyloidosis* can occur in conditions where there is chronic inflammation or infection. These include rheumatoid arthritis, tuberculosis, osteomyelitis, bronchiectasis and leprosy. It also occurs in the genetic disease familial Mediterranean fever. *familial amyloidosis* occurs rarely and is caused by the production of an abnormal protein in the liver.

**amylolysis** *n* starch digestion—**amylolytic** *adj.*

**amylopectin** *n* a type of starch that forms a branched-chain structure. It forms about 75–80% of most starches.

**amylose** *n* a type of starch that forms a straight-chain structure. It forms about 20–25% of most starches.

**amyotrophic lateral sclerosis (ALS)** a form of motor neuron disease in which there is a loss of the upper motor neurons from the cortex to the brainstem and spinal cord, as well as the loss of the lower motor neurons from the brainstem and spinal cord to the muscles.

**ANA** *abbr* antinuclear antibody.

**anabolic hormones** natural or synthetic hormones that stimulate growth and the development of muscle tissue. They include insulin, insulin-like growth factors, growth hormone and the sex hormones oestrogen and testosterone. Compare with catabolic hormones.

**anabolic steroids** a group of androgens (e.g. nandrolone) that stimulate anabolic effects, such as the synthesis of body protein. They are used therapeutically for aplastic anaemia and are sometimes used to support patients who are very debilitated. They may be misused by body builders and athletes. Anabolic steroids can cause serious adverse effects, which include disordered liver function and liver cancer with long-term use, acne, oedema, masculinizing effects in women (e.g. voice changes, facial hair, amenorrhoea) and reduced sperm production. ⇒ Appendix 5.

**anabolism** *n* the series of chemical reactions in the living body requiring energy to change simple substances into complex ones. For example, the use of amino acids to form functional proteins such as protein hormones, enzymes, antibodies and plasma proteins—**anabolic** *adj.* ⇒ adenosine triphosphate, catabolism, metabolism.

**anacidity** *n* lack of normal acidity, especially in the gastric juice. ⇒ achlorhydria.

**anacrotic** *adj* a wave in the ascending opening of an arterial tracing, indicating the opening of the aortic valve (that between the left ventricle and the aorta). An abnormality of this occurs in aortic stenosis. ⇒ dicrotic.

**anaemia** *n* diminished oxygen-carrying capacity of the blood, due to a reduction in the haemoglobin content of the blood. This may be due to reduced amounts of haemoglobin in the red blood cells and/or a reduction in the number of red blood cells. Produces clinical manifestations arising from hypoxaemia, such as lassitude and breathlessness on exertion. There are very many possible causes. ⇒ haemolytic disease of the newborn, megaloblastic anaemia, sickle-cell disease, thalassaemia—**anaemic** *adj. anaemia of chronic disease* anaemia associated with chronic inflammatory diseases such as rheumatoid arthritis, infection or cancer. *anaemia of pregnancy* this is caused by a lower concentration of haemoglobin in the blood. It may be physiological because, during pregnancy, the blood is diluted. The plasma volume increases without a corresponding increase in red cell numbers. However, there are pathological causes that include insufficient intake of nutrients required for haemoglobin production, e.g. iron, loss of red cells through bleeding or damage. *aplastic anaemia* is the result of complete bone marrow failure. *haemolytic anaemia* is caused by the premature destruction of red blood cells, as with some drugs and toxins, autoimmune processes, or inherited red cell or haemoglobin disorders. *pernicious anaemia* results from the inability of the bone marrow to produce normal red cells because of the lack of a protein released by gastric cells, called the intrinsic factor, which is necessary for the absorption of vitamin $B_{12}$ from food in the ileum. An autoimmune mechanism may be responsible. ⇒ pernicious. *sickle-cell anaemia* ⇒ sickle-cell disease.

**anaerobe** *n* a micro-organism that is unable to grow in the presence of molecular oxygen. When this is strictly so, it is called an *obligatory anaerobe*. These include *Clostridium tetani, C. perfringens and C. botulinum*. Most pathogens are indifferent to atmospheric conditions and will grow whether oxygen is present or not and are therefore called *facultative anaerobes*. Some, however, will grow more vigorously if anaerobic conditions prevail—**anaerobic** *adj*.

**anaerobic** *adj* relating to the absence of oxygen. Describes processes that occur without oxygen, and certain micro-organisms that survive without free oxygen or air.

**anaerobic adaptations** long-term physical changes that result from anaerobic exercise. They increase the body's ability to deal with powerful dynamic exercise.

**anaerobic capacity** the capacity that decides a person's ability to continue high-intensity exercise associated with the finite capacity for anaerobic energy production.

**anaerobic endurance** ⇒ anaerobic capacity.

**anaerobic endurance training** also known as lactate tolerance training. Anaerobic endurance training aims to place maximum stress on the systems that produce energy when oxygen is in short supply, i.e. anaerobically (ATP-CP pathway, anaerobic glycolysis). The high intensity of training results in fatigue so the repetition of periods of maximal-intensity exercise are interspersed with rest periods with a variable exercise:rest ratio, such as 1:1 or 1:4. *long-duration anaerobic endurance training* is a regime with an exercise:rest ratio of around 1:4. It makes increased demands on the anaerobic glycolysis energy system. *short-duration anaerobic endurance training* involves very short bursts of maximal-intensity exercise bouts with an exercise:rest ratio of around 1:10. Short-duration endurance training improves the ATP-CP energy pathway and increases muscular power. ⇒ alactacid (alactic) anaerobic system, lactacid (lactic) anaerobic system.

**anaerobic energy** energy that is produced without using oxygen via two energy systems: alactacid and lactacid.

**anaerobic exercise** vigorous short-duration exercise where skeletal muscle oxygen supply is inadequate. Metabolic fuel molecules are broken down anaerobically to produce adenosine triphosphate (ATP).

**anaerobic fitness** the ability to perform maximal anaerobic exercise.

**anaerobic glycolysis** the anaerobic process comprising a series of enzyme-catalysed chemical reactions that break down stored muscle glycogen or glucose to provide energy for ATP resynthesis.

**anaerobic threshold ($T_{AN}$)** the level of exercise intensity at which the rate of oxygen available for muscle contraction is limiting and anaerobic energy pathways are utilized. The onset of a sustained increase in the concentration of lactate in the blood. ⇒ lactate threshold.

**anaesthesia** *n* loss of sensation. ⇒ caudal anaesthesia, epidural anaesthesia. *general anaesthesia* loss of sensation with loss of consciousness. In *local anaesthesia* injection of a drug, e.g. lidocaine, that inhibits peripheral nerve conduction so that painful stimuli fail to reach the brain. *spinal anaesthesia* loss of sensation by the injection of local anaesthetic into the cerebrospinal fluid, which is accessed by introducing the needle/cannula between the vertebrae, usually of the lower back, causing loss of sensation but no loss of consciousness. Also used to describe the loss of feeling produced by a spinal lesion.

**anaesthesiology** *n* the science dealing with anaesthetics, their administration and effect.

**anaesthetic** *n* **1.** *n* a drug that induces general or local anaesthesia. **2.** *adj* causing anaesthesia. **3.** *adj* insensible to stimuli—**anaesthetize** *vt*. *general anaesthetic* a drug that produces general anaesthesia by inhalation or injection. *local anaesthetic* a drug that when injected into the tissues or applied topically causes local insensibility to pain. *spinal anaesthetic* ⇒ spinal.

**anaesthetic assistant** a qualified health care professional who provides support for the anaesthetist. A role undertaken by anaesthetic nurses, operating department practitioners (ODP) or operating department assistants (ODA). ⇒ anaesthetic practitioner.

**anaesthetic practitioner (AP)** a new non-medically qualified role in anaesthesia care in the UK. Specially trained and qualified individuals will undertake certain parts of anaesthesia care without the direct supervision of an anaesthetist. The diploma course is open to existing health care staff and to science graduates.

**anaesthetist** *n* a doctor with specialist training to administer general anaesthesia.

**anaesthetize** *vt* to administer drugs or gases to produce general anaesthesia.

**anagen** *n* the active growth phase (lasting 2–3 years) in the hair development cycle. Most scalp hairs are in the anagen phase at any given time. ⇒ catagen, telogen. *anagen effluvium* loss of hair during the active growth phase due to a variety of causes that include chemotherapy drugs used to treat cancer, toxins and alopecia areata.

**anal** *adj* pertaining to the anus.

**anal canal** *n* the last portion of the large intestine. It is about 4 cm long in an adult and leads from the rectum to the exterior at the anus. It has the internal and external muscular sphincters, which are involved in the process of defecation. The anal canal is lined with stratified squamous epithelium: this is continuous with the rectal mucosa above and merges with the skin (perianal) outside the external sphincter.

**anal fissure** painful split or break in the anal mucosa or skin, associated with constipation. Also known as a fissure-in-ano.

**anal fistula** an abnormal opening on the cutaneous surface close to the anus. Also known as a fistula-in-ano. It is usually associated with local abscess formation and often occurs in Crohn's disease.

**anal reflex** a superficial reflex. Normally there is reflex contraction of the external anal sphincter when the perianal skin or mucosa is stroked. The reflex is absent if there is disease or damage affecting the relevant segments of the spinal cord.

**analeptic** *adj, n* restorative.

**analgesia** *n* loss of sensation of pain without loss of touch—**analgesic** *adj.* ⇒ patient-controlled analgesia.

**analgesic** *n* a drug used to produce analgesia, i.e. relieves pain. For example, paracetamol, codeine or morphine. ⇒ Appendix 5.

**analogous** *adj* similar in function but not in evolutionary origin.

**analogue** *n* a chemical, such as a drug, which is similar in structure or composition to other drugs but its action produces different effects. For example, an analogue drug may have enhanced potency or cause fewer adverse drug reactions.

**analysis** *n* in chemistry the determination of the component parts of a compound substance. ⇒ psychoanalysis—**analyses** *pl*, **analytic** *adj*, **analytically** *adv*.

**analysis by intention to treat** a method of analysis used in randomized controlled trials (RCT). The analysis is based on all participants who were randomly assigned to the groups, regardless of whether or not they withdrew from the study or received the treatment. Using 'intention to treat' rather than 'on treatment' analysis avoids biases.

**analysis of variance (ANOVA)** a statistical method of comparing sample means.

**anaphase** *n* the third stage of mitosis (see Figure M.6, p. 308) and in both divisions of meiosis (see Figure M.3, p, 296). During anaphase in mitosis and the second division of meiosis the double chromosomes split at the centromeres with each chromatid arranged in the equatorial region of the mitotic spindle. The fibres of the spindle contract and the chromatids move to opposite poles of the cell where they become complete chromosomes. During anaphase in the first division of meiosis, the 23 pairs (i.e. 46) of homologous chromosomes in humans separate from each other and 23 move intact to one pole and 23 to the other pole of the cell. ⇒ metaphase, prophase, telophase.

**anaphylactoid** *adj* a systemic reaction, resembling anaphylaxis but not immunoglobulin (Ig) E-mediated.

**anaphylaxis** *n* an exaggerated systemic reaction due to a type I, or immediate-type, hypersensitivity reaction caused by immunoglobulin E (IgE)-mediated release of inflammatory mediators, e.g. histamine, from mast cells on exposure to an allergen. The allergen that triggers the reaction may be a certain food, such as nuts, eggs or shellfish, drugs that include penicillin, foreign proteins including vaccines, or insect stings, especially bees and wasps. Characterized by urticaria, pruritus, angioedema, airway obstruction, bronchospasm, respiratory distress, vascular collapse, hypotension and shock. ⇒ allergy, sensitization—**anaphylactic** *adj*.

**anaplasia** *n* loss of the distinctive characteristics of a cell, associated with abnormal proliferative cellular activity as in cancer—**anaplastic** *adj*.

**anarthria** *n* a severe form of dysarthria. The affected person is unable to produce the motor movements required for speech. The muscle weakness is apparent in the phonatory, articulatory, respiratory and resonatory speech systems. ⇒ dysarthria.

**anasarca** *n* severe generalized oedema. It is associated with renal disease.

**anastomosis** *n* **1.** the anatomical intercommunication of the branches of two or more tubular structures, e.g. arteries or veins. **2.** in surgery, the establishment of an intercommunication between two hollow organs, ducts, vessels or nerves, such as the anastomosis between two segments of bowel following the resection of a diseased length of bowel. The types of anastomosis are end-to-end or side-to-side—**anastomoses** *pl*, **anastomotic** *adj*, **anastomose** *vt*.

**anatomical dead space** the area of the conducting airways containing the inspired air that takes no part in gaseous exchange. It has a volume of around 150 mL in an adult and comprises the nasal cavity, pharynx, larynx, trachea and bronchi.

**anatomical position** for the purpose of accurate description the anterior view is of the upright body facing forward, hands by the sides with palms facing forwards. The posterior view is of the back of the upright body in that position.

**anatomy** *n* the science which deals with the structure of the body—**anatomical** *adj*, **anatomically** *adv*.

**ANCA** *abbr* antineutrophil cytoplasmic antibody.

**anconeus** *n* a triangular superficial muscle of the arm. Its origin is on the lateral epicondyle of the humerus and it inserts on the olecranon process of the ulna. Contraction of the muscle extends the forearm and abducts the ulna during forearm pronation.

**A**

**Ancylostoma** *n* a genus of parasitic nematode hookworms that includes *Ancylostoma duodenale* that is mostly found in southern Europe and the Middle and Far East. It is usually only significant when infestation is moderate or heavy. The worm lives in the duodenum and upper jejunum; eggs are passed in faeces, hatch in moist soil and produce larvae that can penetrate bare feet and reinfest individuals. Infestation is prevented by wearing shoes and using latrines. ⇒ *Necator*.

**ancylostomiasis** *n* (*syn* hookworm disease, miners' anaemia) infestation of the human intestine with *Ancylostoma duodenale*, giving rise to malnutrition and severe anaemia.

**androblastoma** *n* (*syn* arrhenoblastoma) a tumour of the ovary; can produce male or female hormones and can cause masculinization in women or precocious puberty in girls.

**androgen insensitivity syndrome** a disorder where body tissues are unresponsive to androgen hormones. The affected individual has a male genotype (XY) but has a female phenotype (physical appearance). The relevant gene is inherited on the X chromosome; the disorder is therefore X-linked. The presentation is primary amenorrhoea and, although the person has breast development, there is no uterus.

**androgens** *npl* steroid hormones secreted by the testes (testosterone) and adrenal cortex in both sexes. They have widespread anabolic effects, produce the male secondary sex characteristics, e.g. male hair distribution, and stimulate spermatogenesis—**androgenic, androgenous** *adj*.

**andrology** *n* the medical/surgical specialties that deal with men's health. The focus is urological and reproductive problems. It covers diverse areas that include specific, targeted health promotion; diseases that include cancer or infections affecting the penis, testes and epididymis, prostate gland; family planning; infertility; and erectile dysfunction and rapid ejaculation.

**anencephaly** *n* absence of the brain. The condition is incompatible with life. It can be detected by raised levels of alphafetoprotein (AFP) in the amniotic fluid obtained by amniocentesis—**anencephalous, anencephalic** *adj*.

**aneuploidy** *n* a chromosome number that is not a multiple of the normal haploid number (23). Includes: (a) trisomy, e.g. Down's syndrome, Edward's syndrome, Patau's syndrome, etc. where the individual has 47 chromosomes; and (b) monosomy where there are 45 chromosomes, e.g. Turner's syndrome. ⇒ monosomy, polyploidy, trisomy.

**aneurysm** *n* a sac formed by localized dilatation of a blood vessel, usually an artery, due to a local fault in the wall through defect, disease or injury, producing a swelling, often pulsating, over which a murmur may be heard. They are common in the aorta but also occur elsewhere, e.g. in the popliteal artery, carotid artery and in the cerebral arteries (berry aneurysm). True aneurysms may be saccular, fusiform or dissecting, where the blood flows between the layers of the arterial wall (Figure A.7). An aneurysm can predispose to the formation of a thrombus which may enter the circulation as emboli to block a smaller distal vessel, or rupture causing catastrophic haemorrhage—**aneurysmal** *adj*.

**Angelman syndrome** an inherited condition that arises from mutations in the maternal chromosome 15 during formation of the gamete. Features include: a jerky 'puppet-like' gait and movements, a learning disability, brachycephaly (short, broad skull), hooked nose, tongue protrusion, inappropriate emotional outbursts and seizures. ⇒ Prader–Willi syndrome.

**angiectasis** *n* abnormal dilatation of blood vessels. ⇒ telangiectasis—**angiectatic** *adj*.

**angiitis** *n* inflammation of a blood or lymph vessel. ⇒ vasculitis—**angiitic** *adj*.

**angina** *n* sense of constriction—**anginal** *adj*.

**angina pectoris** a common condition in developed countries. It is caused by narrowing of the coronary arteries, usually by atherosclerosis, but it may be due to coronary artery spasm. The narrowing of the coronary arteries

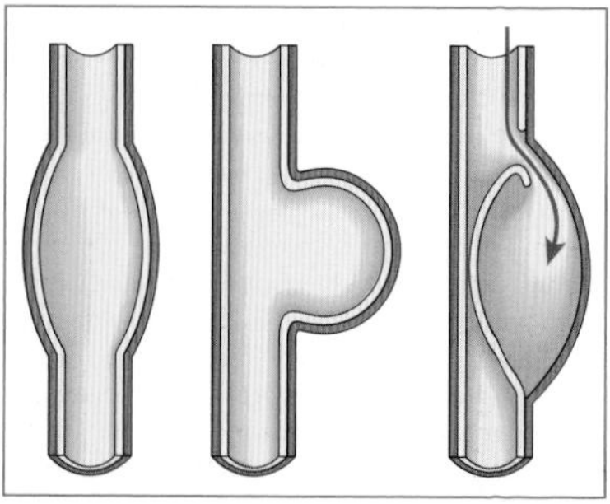

**Figure A.7** Aneurysms *(reproduced from Brooker 2002 with permission).*

reduces the blood supply and hence the amount of oxygen reaching the myocardium (myocardial ischaemia), which results in severe but transient chest pain that may radiate to the inner aspect of both arms but especially the left, throat, lower jaw, upper abdomen or the back. There may also be breathlessness. Often the attack is induced by exercise (angina of effort), emotional upsets, cold and windy weather and sometimes after eating a large meal. The pain is promptly relieved by rest and the use of coronary vaso-dilators, such as glyceryl trinitrate. ⇒ acute coronary syndrome, coronary heart disease, myocardial infarction.

**angiocardiography** *n* radiographic demonstration of the chambers of the heart and great vessels after injection of a contrast medium—**angiocardiographic** *adj*. **angiocardiogram** *n*, **angiocardiograph** *n*, **angiocardiographically** *adv*.

**angiodysplasia** *n* vascular malformation comprising a collection of small blood vessels initially involving the large bowel, which may cause lower gastrointestinal bleeding.

**angioedema** *n* (*syn* angioneurotic oedema) a severe form of urticaria which may involve the skin of the face, hands or genitalia and the mucous membrane of the mouth and throat: oedema of the glottis may be fatal. Immediately there is an abrupt local increase in vascular permeability, as a result of which fluid escapes from blood vessels into surrounding tissues. Swelling may be due to an allergic hypersensitivity reaction to drugs, pollens or other known allergens, but in many cases no cause can be found.

**angiogenesis** *n* the formation of new blood vessels (vascularization). Angiogenesis is a feature of wound healing, new blood vessels are formed during stage 2 (inflammation) and stage 3 (proliferation) in response to growth factors released by white blood cells (leucocytes). New blood vessels also develop, in response to growth factors, to supply the blood that supports the growth of cancers. Recent advances in cancer treatment include drugs that suppress angiogenesis, thus reducing the tumour's blood supply. One such drug is the monoclonal antibody bevacizumab, which inhibits vascular endothelial growth factor. It is used with cytotoxic drugs in the management of metastatic colorectal cancer.

**angiography** *n* demonstration of the blood vessels of the arterial system after injection of a contrast medium. *computed tomography (CT)* *angiography* contrast medium injected intravenously into an arm vein during CT scanning enhances the visualization of the relevant arterial system, e.g. the cerebral circulation. *fluorescein angiography* fluorescein is injected intravenously into a vein in the arm or hand to demonstrate the retinal blood vessels and any retinal pathology, the macula and optic disc and the presence of tumours of the choroid. Before the fluorescein is injected, the pupils of the eyes are dilated with a mydriatic drug, such as tropicamide, to allow the fundus to be examined and photographs taken. *indocyanine green angiography* demonstration of the choroidal and retinal vessels using indocyanine green in the same way as with fluorescein. It provides better information about the state of the choroidal circulation, in particular the presence of abnormal new blood vessels (neovascularization). *magnetic resonance angiography* the use of magnetic resonance technology to demonstrate blood vessels. It may be undertaken with or without a specific contrast medium—**angiographic** *adj*. **angiogram** *n*, **angiograph** *n*, **angiographically** *adv*. ⇒ digital subtraction angiography.

**angiokeratoma corporis diffusum** also known as Fabry's disease or Anderson–Fabry disease. A rare X-linked recessive familial disease in which the absence of an enzyme leads to the accumulation of a glycolipid in blood vessels, other tissues and organs, including the liver and kidneys.

**angiology** *n* the science dealing with blood and lymphatic vessels—**angiological** *adj*, **angiologically** *adv*.

**angioma** *n* a benign tumour affecting blood vessels; a haemangioma. Many angiomas are congenital. ⇒ haemangioma, lymphangioma.

**angioplasty** *n* surgical reconstruction of blood vessels—**angioplastic** *adj*. *percutaneous transluminal angioplasty* (PTA) a balloon is passed into a stenosed artery and inflated with contrast medium; it presses the atheroma against the vessel wall, thereby increasing the diameter of the lumen. The technique is commonly used to reopen coronary arteries, renal arteries, those in the leg and the carotid artery. A stent is often inserted at the same time in order to prevent the artery becoming occluded again.

**angiosarcoma** *n* a malignant tumour arising from blood vessels—**angiosarcomata** *pl*, **angiosarcomatous** *adj*.

**angiospasm** *n* spasm of blood vessels—**angiospastic** *adj*.

**angiotensin** *n* a polypeptide formed by the action of renin on the precursor protein angiotensinogen in the blood plasma. Renin is mainly released by the juxtaglomerular cells in the kidney. In the lungs angiotensin I is converted into angiotensin II, a highly active substance which constricts blood vessels and causes release of aldosterone from the adrenal cortex in the *angiotensin–aldosterone response* (also called *renin–angiotensin–aldosterone response*). ⇒ renin.

**angiotensin-converting enzyme (ACE) inhibitor** a group of drugs that inhibit the conversion of angiotensin I to angiotensin II and thereby reduce the angiotensin–aldosterone response, e.g. enalapril maleate. ⇒ Appendix 5.

**Angle's classification of malocclusion (modified)** (E Angle, American orthodontist, 1855–1930) a classification of various forms of malocclusion between the upper and lower teeth. The classification depends on the point at which contact is made between the buccal groove of the first molar in the mandible and the mesiobuccal cusp of the maxillary first molar. There are three classes, I, II and III, each with further subdivisions or types.

**angstrom (Å)** *n* (A J Angström, Swedish physicist, 1814–1874) a unit of measurement equal to 0.1 nanometre or $10^{-10}$ metre. It is not a SI unit but is sometimes used for wavelength.

**angular stomatitis** ⇒ stomatitis.

**anhedonia** *n* a total inability to take pleasure in life. The person is unable to feel happiness in response to events that are ordinarily enjoyable. Associated with severe depressive disorders and schizophrenia.

**anhidrosis** *n* deficient sweat secretion—**anhidrotic** *adj*.

**anhidrotic** *n* an agent that reduces perspiration.

**anhydraemia** *n* deficient fluid content of blood—**anhydraemic** *adj*.

**anhydrase** *n* an enzyme that catalyses the removal of water molecules. For example, carbonic andydrase, which catalyses the removal of water from carbonic acid in the reversible reactions that transport waste carbon dioxide from the cells, maintain normal blood pH and regulate the amount of carbon dioxide excreted by the lungs.

**anhydrous** *adj* entirely without water, dry.

**anicteric** *adj* without jaundice.

**anion** *n* a negatively charged ion, e.g. chloride ($Cl^-$). They move towards the positive electrode (anode) during electrolysis. ⇒ cation.

**anion exchange resin** one of several high-molecular-weight organic substances that exchange anions with other ions. ⇒ ion exchange resins.

**anion gap** the difference between the amount of anions and cations in the plasma. It is calculated by measuring the concentration of sodium and potassium ions and subtracting the concentration of bicarbonate (hydrogen carbonate) and chloride ions: $(Na^+ + K^+) - (HCO_3^- + Cl^-)$. It may also be determined by subtracting the concentration of bicarbonate and chloride from that of sodium: $(Na^+) - (HCO_3^- + Cl^-)$, Normally the gap is between 8 and 14 mmol/L plasma. It is useful in the diagnosis of metabolic acidosis.

**aniridia** *n* absence of the iris; usually congenital.

**aniseikonia** *n* an abnormal condition where each eye perceives the image of an object as being strikingly different.

**anisocoria** *n* inequality in diameter of the pupils.

**anisocytosis** *n* inequality in size of red blood cells. ⇒ macrocytosis, microcytosis, poikilocytosis.

**anisomelia** *n* unequal length of limbs—**anisomelous** *adj*.

**anisometropia** *n* a difference in the refractive power of the two eyes—**anisometropic** *adj*.

**ankle** *n* the joint formed between the talus, fibula and tibia.

**ankle clonus** a tendon reflex characterized by a series of rapid muscular contractions of the calf muscle when the foot is dorsiflexed by pressure upon the sole.

**ankle equinus** a congenital or acquired condition or deformity, which is characterized by deficient dorsiflexion at the ankle joint. During the stance phase of normal gait a minimum 10° of ankle joint dorsiflexion is needed for normal walking. ⇒ talipes.

**ankle foot orthosis** *n* a splint used to facilitate function in people with insufficient ankle dorsiflexion for walking, or those with unstable ankle and subtalar joints. It enables the person to walk without tripping. The increased stability often allows people to walk more quickly and safely, which in turn increases their confidence.

**ankle–brachial pressure index (ABPI)** also known as ankle–arm index. The ratio of ankle systolic blood pressure to systolic blood pressure in the arm. It is calculated by dividing

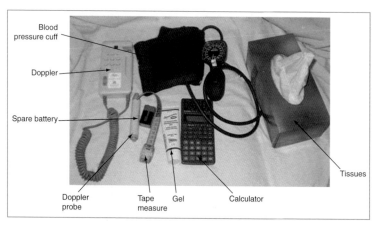

Blood pressure cuff

Doppler

Spare battery

Tissues

Doppler probe | Tape measure | Gel | Calculator

**Figure A.8** Ankle–brachial pressure equipment *(reproduced from Brooker & Waugh 2007 with permission).*

ankle blood pressure by arm blood pressure; this is calculated for both the right and left legs. Doppler ultrasound is used to assess the arterial blood flow to the lower limb (Figure A.8). An ABPI of 1 indicates that 100% of blood is reaching the lower leg, whereas an ABPI of 0.85 means that only 85% of blood reaches the lower leg and is indicative of arterial disease.

**ankyloblepharon** *n* adhesion of the eyelid margins, usually lateral, often secondary to chronic inflammation.

**ankylosing spondylitis** polyarthritis affecting mainly the spine. It is characterized by inflammation involving ligament and tendon attachments to bone. This results in painful stiffness of ligaments and joints, which in severe cases leads to a forward flexion of the spine ('bamboo' or 'poker' spine). It occurs more commonly in males—M:F ratio is 3:1—and generally affects young men under 30 years of age. ⇒ spondylitis.

**ankylosis** *n* stiffness or fixation of a joint. Fusion of a joint. ⇒ spondylitis—**ankylosed** *adj*, **ankylose** *vt, vi*.

**annular** *adj* ring-shaped. *annular ligaments* hold in proximity two long bones, as in the wrist and ankle joints.

**annulus** *n* any ring-shaped structure or circular aperture.

**annulus fibrosus** the ring-shaped outer part of the intervertebral disc. It is formed from sheets of collagen fibres arranged in marginally different orientations. The posterior part is the thinnest part of the annulus fibrosus, which makes it more likely to rupture.

**anodontiau** *n* the failure of the teeth to develop. It may be partial, where some teeth develop, or total, when all teeth are absent. ⇒ oligodontia.

**anodyne** *n* a drug, other substance or treatment that eases or relieves pain.

**anogenital** *adj* pertaining to the anus and the genital region.

**anomaly** *n* that which is unusual or differs from the normal—**anomalous** *adj*.

**anomia** *n* a difficulty in word finding that affects many people with aphasia. Most frequently demonstrated when the person is required to perform a naming task but may also be recognized by the use of circumlocutions in spontaneous speech samples.

**anomie** *n* sociological term that describes a circumstance where the norms that guide behaviour are absent. The normless state that results from weak social controls and moral obligations leads to derangement in social behaviour.

**anonychia** *n* absence of nails.

**anoperineal** *adj* pertaining to the anus and perineum.

***Anopheles*** *n* a genus of mosquito. The females of some species are the host of the malarial parasite, and their bite is the means of transmitting malaria to humans.

**anophthalmos** *n* congenital absence of an eye.

**anoplasty** *n* surgical repair or reconstruction of the anus—**anoplastic** *adj*.

**anorchism** *n* congenital absence of one or both testes—**anorchic** *adj*.

**anorectal** *adj* pertaining to the anus and rectum, e.g. a fissure. ⇒ anal fissure.

**anorectic** *adj* **1.** relating to anorexia. **2.** leading to loss or reduction in appetite, such as drugs that suppress appetite. **3.** lacking appetite.

**anorexia** *n* lack of appetite for food.

**anorexia nervosa** a psychological illness with a complex aetiology that may include poor self-esteem, fear of obesity, distorted body image and an obsession with being thin. It is most common in female adolescents but also affects males and adults. There is refusal to eat, excessive exercising, self-induced vomiting and misuse of laxatives. Can lead to severe emaciation, life-threatening metabolic consequences and death in severe cases—**anorexic, anorectic** *adj*. ⇒ eating disorders.

**anosmia** *n* absence of the sense of smell—**anosmic** *adj*.

**ANOVA** *abbr* analysis of variance.

**anovular** *adj* relating to absence of ovulation. *anovular bleeding* occurs in dysfunctional uterine bleeding associated with hormone disturbance. *anovular menstruation* is the result of taking oral contraceptives.

**anoxaemia** *n* literally, no oxygen in the blood. Usually used to indicate hypoxaemia—**anoxaemic** *adj*.

**anoxia** *n* literally, no oxygen in the tissues. Usually used to signify hypoxia—**anoxic** *adj*.

**ANP** *abbr* atrial natriuretic peptide.

**antacid** *n* a substance that neutralizes acidity. Often used in alkaline indigestion medicines, e.g. magnesium trisilicate. ⇒ Appendix 5.

**antagonist** *n* a muscle that reverses or opposes the action of an agonist muscle. Also describes a drug or chemical that blocks the action of another molecule at a cell receptor site, e.g. the narcotic antagonist naloxone reverses the action of opioid drugs. ⇒ agonist *opp*—**antagonism** *n*, **antagonistic** *adj*.

**antagonistic action** action performed by those muscles that limit the movement of an opposing group.

**antalgia** *n* literally away from pain, such as the adoption of a particular posture or gait in order to reduce pain.

**anteflexion** *n* the bending forward of an organ, commonly applied to the position of the uterus. ⇒ retroflexion *opp*.

**antemortem** *adj* before death. ⇒ postmortem *opp*.

**antenatal** *adj* prenatal. ⇒ postnatal *opp*—**antenatally** *adj*.

**antepartum** *adj* before birth. From 24 weeks' gestation to full term. *antepartum haemorrhage* (APH) any bleeding from the genital tract after the 24th week of gestation and before the commencement of labour. Causes include placenta praevia, placental abruption, trauma, cervicitis, genital cancers, etc. ⇒ postpartum *opp*.

**anterior** *adj* in front of; the front surface of; ventral. ⇒ posterior *opp*—**anteriorly** *adv*.

**anterior chamber of the eye** the space between the posterior surface of the cornea and the anterior surface of the iris. Contains aqueous fluid. ⇒ aqueous.

**anterior cruciate ligament** a major ligament within the knee joint (Figure A.9). It is important in stabilizing the knee by limiting the chance of hyperextending the tibia beyond the femur, and is also concerned with proprioception. A common sports injury where there is violent twisting combined with rapid deceleration, such as in soccer, rugby football, skiing or basketball.

**anterior tibial syndrome** severe pain and inflammation over anterior tibial muscle group, with inability to dorsiflex the foot.

**anterograde** *adj* proceeding forward. ⇒ retrograde *opp*, amnesia.

**anteversion** *n* the normal forward tilting, or displacement forward, of an organ or part. ⇒ retroversion *opp*—**anteverted** *adj*, **antevert** *vt*.

**anthelmintic** *adj* describes a drug for the destruction or elimination of parasitic worms, e.g. mebendazole. ⇒ Appendix 5.

**anthracosis** *n* coal miner's/worker's pneumoconiosis. Accumulation of carbon in the lungs due to inhalation of coal dust; may cause a fibrotic reaction. A form of pneumoconiosis—**anthracotic** *adj*.

**anthrax** *n* a contagious disease of domestic animals such as cattle, which may be transmitted to humans by inoculation, inhalation and ingestion, causing malignant pustule (skin lesion) with septicaemia, inhalation anthrax or woolsorter's disease (haemorrhagic

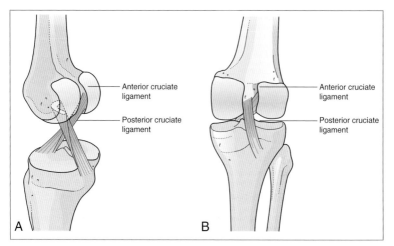

**Figure A.9** Cruciate ligaments: (A) oblique view showing twisting of fibres; (B) posterior view showing them crossing in space *(reproduced from Porter 2005 with permission).*

bronchopneumonia), meningitis and severe gastroenteritis. Causative organism is the bacterium *Bacillus anthracis.* Preventive measures include immunization of humans and animals, postexposure prophylaxis with antibiotics, e.g. ciprofloxacin, and proper disposal of infected animals. Occupations at high risk include veterinary surgeons, livestock farmers, butchers and those handling hides and wool.

**anthropoid** *adj* resembling man. The word is also used to describe a pelvis that is narrow from side to side, a form of contracted pelvis.

**anthropology** *n* the study of humankind. Subdivided into several specialties. ⇒ ethnology.

**anthropometry** *n* measurement of the human body and its parts for the purposes of comparison and establishing norms for gender, age, weight, race and so on. Used to assess development, nutritional status and as a non-invasive way of assessing body composition. Anthropometric measurements include weight for age; weight for height; height for age; skinfold thickness to assess subcutaneous fat; and mid-upper-arm circumference to assess muscle wastage—**anthropometric** *adj.*

**antianabolic** *adj* preventing the synthesis of body protein.

**antiandrogens** *npl* a group of drugs that block the activity of testosterone, e.g. finasteride. ⇒ Appendix 5.

**antiarrhythmic** *adj* describes drugs and treatments used to treat a variety of cardiac arrhythmias, e.g. verapamil. ⇒ Appendix 5.

**antibacterial** *adj* describes an agent that destroys bacteria or inhibits their growth. ⇒ antibiotics, antiseptics, bactericidal, bacteriostatic, disinfectants.

**antiberi-beri** *adj* against beri-beri, e.g. the thiamin(e) portion of vitamin B complex.

**antibilharzial** *adj* against *Bilharzia.* ⇒ *Schistosoma.*

**antibiosis** *n* an association between organisms that is harmful to one of them. ⇒ symbiosis *opp*—**antibiotic** *adj.*

**antibiotics** *npl* antibacterial substances derived from fungi and bacteria, exemplified by penicillin. However, the term is generally used for all drugs that act against bacteria. Some have a narrow spectrum of activity whereas others act against a wide range of bacteria (broad-spectrum). ⇒ aminoglycosides, antituberculosis drugs, bactericidal, bacteriostatic, β-lactam antibiotics, cephalosporins, glycylcyclines, glycopeptide antibiotics, macrolides, penicillins, fluoroquinolones, sulphonamides, tetracyclines. ⇒ Appendix 5.

**antibodies** *npl* (*syn* immunoglobulins) often used to indicate immunoglobulins with specific antigen-binding activity.

**anticholinergic** *adj* inhibitory to the action of a cholinergic nerve by interfering with the action of the neurotransmitter acetylcholine at synapses. ⇒ muscarinic antagonists (antimuscarinic).

**anticholinesterase** *n* any agent that inactivates cholinesterase.

**anticipatory postural adjustments** small postural adjustments made by postural muscles, (e.g. those in the trunk), in anticipation of movement or movement of a body part such as an arm. They form part of the many mechanisms that operate to maintain balance.

**anticoagulant** *n* an agent that reduces the propensity of blood to clot. Uses: (a) to obtain specimens suitable for pathological examination and chemical analyses where whole blood or plasma is required instead of serum; (b) during the collection of blood for transfusion, the anticoagulant usually being sodium citrate; (c) as therapy in the prophylaxis and treatment of thromboembolic conditions. ⇒ Appendix 5, coumarins, heparin.

**anticoagulation** *n* the process of suppressing or reducing blood coagulation.

**anticodon** *n* in genetics, the three bases (triplet) in transfer ribonucleic acid (tRNA) concerned with the synthesis of proteins (translation stage). ⇒ codon.

**anticonvulsant** *n* ⇒ antiepileptics—**anticonvulsive** *adj.*

**anti-D** *n* an antibody directed against the Rhesus D blood group antigen. It is formed when Rhesus-negative individuals are exposed to Rhesus-positive blood, such as being transfused with Rhesus-positive blood, or a Rhesus-negative woman who is pregnant with a Rhesus-positive fetus. *anti-D (Rh$_O$) immunoglobulin* is given to prevent the formation of anti-D antibody by Rhesus-negative women after the birth of the baby, or following an ectopic pregnancy, threatened miscarriage, spontaneous miscarriage or termination of pregnancy. It is also given after amniocentesis and other invasive procedures, abdominal trauma, antepartum haemorrhage and in cases of intrauterine death or stillbirth. Anti-D (Rh$_O$) immunoglobulin reduces the risk of isoimmunization and problems with subsequent pregnancies, including stillbirth or haemolytic disease of the newborn. ⇒ ABO blood group system, blood groups, Rhesus incompatibility.

**antidepressants** *npl* drugs used to manage depression. There are three main groups: monoamine oxidase inhibitors (MAOIs), e.g. phenelzine, selective serotonin reuptake inhibitors (SSRIs), e.g. fluoxetine and tricyclic antidepressants (TCA), e.g. amitriptyline. ⇒ Appendix 5.

**antidiabetic** *adj* literally 'against diabetes'. Used to describe therapeutic measures in people with diabetes mellitus to control blood glucose. ⇒ insulin, hypoglycaemic drugs.

**antidiarrhoeals** *npl* agents such as drugs used to reduce diarrhoea, e.g. loperamide. ⇒ Appendix 5.

**antidiscriminatory practice** professional codes of practice and policies of health care providers seek to eliminate discrimination experienced by patients/clients, employees and groups, particularly on the basis of their age, gender, sexual orientation, social class, health behaviours, religion, race, disability, political views or their illness. Specific legislation, such as the UK Sex Discrimination Act (1975), exists to safeguard the interests of people and can be used to challenge discriminatory practices.

**antidiuretic** *adj* reducing the volume of urine.

**antidiuretic hormone (ADH)** also called vasopressin, or arginine vasopressin (AVP). A hormone formed in the hypothalamus and stored in the posterior lobe of the pituitary gland. ADH increases the permeability of the renal tubule, thereby increasing water reabsorption into the blood stream. ADH is released in response to a reduction in blood volume or increased level of sodium in the blood. When the levels of ADH in the plasma are low, a large volume of dilute urine is excreted (diuresis) by the kidneys. In contrast, when plasma levels are high, a small volume of concentrated urine is excreted (antidiuresis). ⇒ vasopressin.

**antidote** *n* a remedy that opposes, counteracts or neutralizes the action of a poison. For example, protamine sulphate is used to counteract the effects of an overdose of heparin.

**antiembolic** *adj* against embolism.

**antiembolism hosiery/stockings** elastic hosiery (knee or full-length) that exerts linear graduated compression on the superficial veins of the legs. This increases venous return to the heart, thus preventing venous stasis, which predisposes to deep-vein thrombosis (DVT) following surgery and in other situations where patients are immobile. Also known as thromboembolic deterrents (TEDs) stockings.

**antiemetic** *adj* against emesis. Any agent such as a drug that prevents or treats nausea and vomiting. ⇒ cannabinoids, D$_2$-receptor antagonists, H$_1$-receptor antagonists, 5-HT$_3$-receptor antagonists, muscarinic antagonists (antimuscarinic), neurokinin receptor antagonist. ⇒ Appendix 5.

**antienzyme** *n* a substance that exerts a specific inhibiting action on an enzyme. Found in the digestive tract to prevent autodigestion of the mucosa, and in blood where they act as immunoglobulins.

**antiepileptic** *adj* (*syn* anticonvulsant) describes drugs which reduce the frequency of seizures, e.g. sodium valproate. ⇒ Appendix 5.

**antifebrile** *adj* describes any agent which reduces or allays fever.

**antifibrinolytic** *adj* describes any agent which prevents fibrinolysis.

**antifungal** *adj* describes any agent which destroys fungi, e.g. fluconazole. ⇒ Appendix 5.

**anti-GBM disease** disease caused by specific antibodies that target the glomerular basement membranes. It features rapidly progressive glomerulonephritis and pulmonary haemorrhage. Previously known as Goodpasture's disease.

**antigen** *n* substance inducing a specific immune response which interacts with the product of that immune response. This may be a specific immunoglobulin or T cells bearing T-cell receptors specific for that antigen—**antigenic** *adj*.

**antigenetic determinant** the site on an antigen molecule that binds with the corresponding site on the specific antibody or T-lymphocyte receptor. Also known as an epitope. ⇒ epitope, paratope.

**antigenic drift** the mutations occurring in a micro-organism over time that alter their antigenic characteristics. This leads to difficulties in the provision of effective vaccines and antimicrobial drugs. For example, the changes that occur in the influenza virus, which creates problems for vaccine production, as a new influenza vaccine is required each year.

**antigenicity** *n* the ability or power of micro-organisms and their products to stimulate the production of antibodies by immune cells, as in a vaccine.

**antigen-presenting cells (APC)** *npl* part of the immune response. They are cells of the monocyte–macrophage (reticuloendothelial) system that include macrophages, and dendritic cells that are present in the skin (called Langerhans cells) and in the gastrointestinal tract and respiratory tract. They process antigens so they can be presented to T-lymphocyte receptors. ⇒ macrophages.

**antigonococcal** *adj* describes any measures used against infections caused by *Neisseria gonorrhoeae*.

**antihaemophilic factor (AHF)** also called antihaemophilic globulin (AHG). Factor VIII in the blood coagulation cascade, present in plasma. It has two portions, a low-molecular-weight part and a high-molecular-weight part; they are involved at different stages of coagulation. A deficiency causes haemophilia A (classical).

**antihaemophilic factor B** ⇒ Christmas factor.

**antihaemorrhagic** *adj* describes any agent which prevents haemorrhage.

**antihelix** *n* a curved ridge in the auricle (pina) of the outer/external ear.

**antihistamines** *npl* drugs which suppress some of the effects of histamine released in the body, e.g. chlorphenamine. ⇒ Appendix 5.

**antihypertensive** *adj* describes any agent that reduces high blood pressure. ⇒ ($\alpha$)-adrenoceptor antagonists, angiotensin-converting enzyme inhibitors, ($\beta$)-adrenoceptor antagonists, calcium antagonists, diuretics. ⇒ Appendix 5.

**anti-infective** *adj* describes any agent which prevents infection.

**anti-inflammatory** *adj* tending to prevent or relieve inflammation. ⇒ non-steroidal anti-inflammatory drugs (NSAIDs). ⇒ Appendix 5.

**antileprotic** *adj* describing any agent which prevents or cures leprosy, e.g. rifampicin. ⇒ Appendix 5.

**antilipidaemic** *n* dietary modification, drug or other treatment used to manage hyperlipidaemia by lowering the level of blood lipids.

**antilymphocyte globulin (ALG)** an immunoglobulin which binds to antigens on T cells and inhibits T-cell-dependent immune responses; occasionally used in preventing graft rejection during organ transplantation.

**antimalarial** *adj* against malaria, e.g. mefloquine. ⇒ Appendix 5.

**antimetabolites** *npl* molecules that prevent cell division. They are sufficiently similar to essential cell metabolites to be incorporated into the metabolic pathways, thereby preventing their use by the cell, e.g. methotrexate. ⇒ cytotoxic. ⇒ Appendix 5.

**antimicrobial** *adj* against microbes.

**antimitochondrial antibody (AMA)** autoantibodies against mitochondrial components. Certain types are a marker for primary biliary cirrhosis.

**antimitotic** *adj* preventing cell replication by mitosis. ⇒ cytotoxic.

**antimutagen** *n* a substance that cancels out the action of a mutagen—**antimutagenic** *adj*.

**antimycotic** *adj* ⇒ antifungal.

**antineoplastic** *adj* describes any substance or procedure that kills or slows the growth of cancerous/neoplastic cells, such as cytotoxic chemotherapy, radiotherapy or hormonal or biological response modification therapy.

**antineuritic** *adj* describes any agent which prevents neuritis. Specially applied to vitamin B complex.

**antineutrophil cytoplasmic antibody (ANCA)** a group of autoantibodies directed against cytoplasmic components of neutrophils and associated with a range of pathological conditions such as polyarteritis.

**antinuclear antibody (ANA)** a family of many types of autoantibody directed against cell nuclei that are found in connective tissue diseases, particularly in systemic lupus erythematosus (SLE) and Sjögren syndrome. The many types recognized can be used to categorize rheumatological disorders.

**antioestrogens** *npl* antagonist drugs that block cell surface oestrogen receptors in various body sites, e.g. tamoxifen. ⇒ oestrogen receptors, selective (o)estrogen receptor modulators (SERMS). ⇒ Appendix 5.

**antioxidant** *n* a substance that delays the process of oxidation of fats in stored food. Many fats, and especially vegetable oils, contain natural antioxidants, such as vitamin E, which guard against rancidity for some time.

**antioxidant nutrients** *npl* a number of nutrients, notably carotene, vitamins C and E, and the mineral selenium contained in a balanced diet, function as antioxidants and help to minimize or prevent free radical oxidative damage to cells. Extremely reactive oxygen radicals are produced normally during metabolism and in response to other insults, such as some chemicals and infection. The free radicals disrupt the fatty acids in cell membranes, which eventually leads to damage to cell proteins and DNA. ⇒ reactive oxygen species.

**antiparasitic** *adj* describes agents that prevent or destroy parasites.

**antiparkinson(ism) drugs** drugs used in the management of parkinsonism, e.g. orphenadrine. ⇒ Appendix 5.

**antipellagra** *adj* against pellagra; a function of the nicotinic acid portion of vitamin B complex.

**antiperistalsis** *n* reversal of the normal peristaltic action—**antiperistaltic** *adj*.

**antiphospholipid antibody syndrome** *n* an autoimmune condition where the presence of antiphospholipid antibodies is linked to thromboembolism and pregnancy loss through miscarriage, fetal death and preterm birth with eclampsia or intrauterine growth restriction. Management with low-dose aspirin and low-molecular-weight heparin increases the chance of a successful pregnancy and reduces the risk of a thromboembolic condition.

**antiplatelet drugs** a group of drugs that reduce platelet aggregation, e.g. dipyridamole. ⇒ Appendix 5.

**antiprothrombin** *n* stops blood coagulation by preventing conversion of prothrombin into thrombin. Anticoagulant.

**antiprotozoal** *n* a drug used to prevent or cure a protozoal disease, e.g. metronidazole. ⇒ Appendix 5.

**antipruritic** *adj* describes any agent which relieves or prevents itching.

**antipsychotic drugs** *adj* also known as neuroleptics. Against psychosis, such as drugs used to treat psychotic episodes. Most are antagonists of dopamine receptors and other receptors. They can be divided into typical and atypical neuroleptics. ⇒ dibenzodiazepines, extrapyramidal, neuroleptic malignant syndrome, phenothiazines, tardive dyskinesia, Appendix 5.

**antipyretic** *adj* describes any agent which prevents or reduces fever, e.g. aspirin. ⇒ Appendix 5.

**antirachitic** *adj* describes any agent which prevents or cures rickets, a function of vitamin D.

**anti-Rhesus** ⇒ anti-D.

**antischistosomal** *adj* describes any agent which destroys *Schistosoma*.

**antiscorbutic** *adj* describes any agent which prevents or cures scurvy, a function of vitamin C.

**antisecretory drug** a drug that reduces the secretion of a specific body substance, such as proton pump inhibitors (e.g. esomeprazole), and reduces the amount of hydrochloric acid secreted by the gastric parietal (oxyntic) cells.

**antisepsis** *n* prevention of sepsis (tissue infection); introduced into surgical procedures in 1880 by Lord Lister—**antiseptic** *adj*.

**antiseptic** *n* chemical substances that destroy or inhibit the growth of micro-organisms. They can be applied to living tissues, e.g.

chlorhexidine, used for skin preparation before invasive procedures and for routine hand decontamination.

**antiserum** *n* serum prepared from the blood of an animal or human immunized by the requisite antigen, containing a high concentration of polyclonal antibodies against that antigen.

**antisocial** *adj* against society. Used to describe a person who does not accept the responsibilities and constraints placed on a community by its members—**antisocialism** *n.*

**antispasmodic** *adj* (*syn* spasmolytic) describes any measure or drugs used to relieve spasm in muscle, mebeverine hydrochloride. ⇒ Appendix 5.

**antistatic** *adj* preventing the accumulation of static electricity.

**antistreptolysin** *adj* against streptolysins. A raised antistreptolysin titre in the blood is indicative of recent streptococcal infection.

**antisyphilitic** *adj* describes any measures taken to combat syphilis.

**antithrombin III** *n* substance that inhibits blood coagulation. It is synthesized in the liver and is normally present in the blood, where it restricts coagulation to areas where it is needed. Deficiency is uncommon but is associated with an increased risk of thrombosis. ⇒ thrombin, thrombophilia.

**antithrombotic** *adj* describes any measures that prevent or cure thrombosis.

**antithyroid** *n* any agent used to decrease the activity of the thyroid gland, e.g. carbimazole. ⇒ Appendix 5.

**antitoxin** *n* an antibody which neutralizes a given toxin. Made in response to the invasion by toxin-producing bacteria, or the injection of toxoids—**antitoxic** *adj.*

**antitreponemal** *adj* describes any measures used against infections caused by *Treponema*.

**antituberculosis drugs** drugs used in the treatment of tuberculosis, e.g. ethambutol—**antitubercular** *adj.* ⇒ Appendix 5.

**antitumour antibiotics** cytotoxic antibiotics that act against tumour cells by disrupting cell membranes and DNA, e.g. doxorubicin. ⇒ cytotoxic. ⇒ Appendix 5.

**antitussive** *adj* describes any measures which suppress cough.

**antivenom** *n* a serum prepared from animals injected with the venom of snakes; used as an antidote in cases of poisoning by snakebite.

**antiviral** *adj* acting against viruses. *antiviral drugs*, e.g. aciclovir. ⇒ Appendix 5.

**antivitamin** *n* a substance interfering with the absorption or utilization of a vitamin, e.g. a large intake of avidin in raw egg white is associated with deficiency of biotin.

**antrectomy** *n* surgical excision of the antrum of the stomach.

**antro-oral** *adj* pertaining to the maxillary antrum and the mouth.

**antroscopy** *n* an endoscopic examination of the maxillary air sinus.

**antrostomy** *n* surgical opening from nasal cavity to antrum of Highmore (maxillary sinus).

**antrum** *n* **1.** a cavity, especially in bone—**antral** *adj. antrum of Highmore* an air sinus in the superior maxillary bone. **2.** the pyloric antrum, the lowest part of the stomach, continuous with the pylorus.

**ANUG** *abbr* acute necrotizing ulcerative gingivitis.

**anuria** *n* complete absence of urine output by the kidneys. ⇒ suppression—**anuric** *adj.*

**anus** *n* the end of the alimentary canal, at the extreme termination of the rectum and anal canal. The internal and external sphincter muscles relax to allow faecal matter to pass through the anus to the exterior—**anal** *adj. artificial anus* ⇒ colostomy. *imperforate anus* ⇒ imperforate. ⇒ anal canal.

**anxiety** *n* feelings of fear, apprehension and dread. *anxiety disorder* a mental health problem characterized by recurrent acute anxiety attacks (panic) or by chronic anxiety. The attacks consist of both physical and psychological anxiety signs and symptoms.

**anxiolytics** *npl* agents that reduce anxiety, e.g. diazepam. ⇒ Appendix 5.

**aorta** *n* the main artery arising out of the left ventricle of the heart. It comprises four parts: ascending aorta, aortic arch, thoracic descending part and the abdominal descending part. It carries oxygen-rich blood which it supplies to all organs, tissues and cells. Its first branch, the coronary arteries, supply oxygen and nutrients to the heart muscle (myocardium). ⇒ Appendix 1, Figures 8 and 9.

**aortic** *adj* pertaining to the aorta.

**aortic arch** a continuation of the ascending aorta that arches over the heart to become the thoracic part of the descending aorta. The left common carotid artery, left subclavian artery and the brachiocephalic artery branch from the aortic arch to supply oxygen-rich blood to the head, neck and upper limbs. ⇒ Appendix 1, Figures 8 and 9.

**aortic murmur** abnormal heart sound heard over aortic area: a systolic murmur alone is

**A**

the murmur of aortic stenosis; a diastolic murmur denotes aortic regurgitation.

**aortic regurgitation (incompetence)** regurgitation of blood from the aorta back into the left ventricle.

**aortic stenosis** narrowing of aortic valve. This is usually due to rheumatic heart disease or a congenital fusion of the valve which predisposes to the deposit of calcium.

**aortic valve** semilunar valve between the aorta and the left ventricle.

**aortitis** *n* inflammation of the aorta.

**aortography** *n* demonstration of the aorta after introduction of a contrast medium, either via a catheter passed along the femoral or brachial artery or by direct translumbar injection—**aortographic** *adj*, **aortogram** *n*, **aortograph** *n*, **aortographically** *adv*.

**AP** *abbr* anaesthesia practitioner.

**apathy** *n* **1.** abnormal listlessness and deficiency of activity. **2.** attitude of indifference—**apathetic** *adj*.

**APC** *abbr* antigen-presenting cell.

**APD** *abbr* **1.** auditory processing disorder. **2.** automated peritoneal dialysis.

**aperients** *npl* ⇒ laxatives.

**aperistalsis** *n* absence of peristaltic movement in the bowel. Characterizes the condition of paralytic ileus—**aperistaltic** *adj*.

**Apert's syndrome** (E Apert, French paediatrician, 1868–1940) congenital craniosynostosis accompanied by deformities of the hands. ⇒ acrocephalosyndactyly, syndactyly.

**apertognathia** *n* an occlusion where there is vertical separation between the upper (maxillary) and lower (mandibular) anterior teeth.

**apex** *n* the summit or top of anything which is cone-shaped, e.g. the tip of a lung. ⇒ Appendix 1, Figure 7—**apices** *pl*, **apical** *adj*. In a

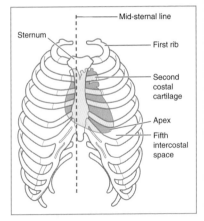

**Figure A.10** Apex beat *(reproduced from Brooker & Nicol 2003 with permission).*

heart of normal size the *apex beat* (systolic impulse) can be seen or felt in the fifth left intercostal space in the mid-clavicular line (Figure A.10). It is the lowest and most lateral point at which an impulse can be detected and provides a rough indication of the size of the heart.

**Apgar score** (V Apgar, American anaesthetist, 1909–1974) a measure used to evaluate the general condition of a newborn baby. A score of 0, 1 or 2 is given for the criteria of heart rate, respiratory effort, skin colour, muscle tone and response to stimulation (Table A.1). A score between 8 and 10 indicates a baby in good condition.

**Table A.1** The Apgar score. The score is assessed at 1 minute and 5 minutes after birth. Medical aid should be sought if the score is less than 7. 'Apgar minus colour' score omits the fifth sign. Medical aid should be sought if the score is less than 6

| Sign | Score | | |
| --- | --- | --- | --- |
| | 0 | 1 | 2 |
| Heart rate | Absent | Less than 100 beats/min | More than 100 beats/min |
| Respiratory effort | Absent | Slow, irregular | Good or crying |
| Muscle tone | Limp | Some flexion of limbs | Active |
| Reflex response to stimulus | None | Minimal grimace | Cough or sneeze |
| Colour | Blue, pale | Body pink, extremities blue | Completely pink |

Reproduced from Fraser & Cooper (2003) with permission.

**APH** *abbr* antepartum haemorrhage.

**aphagia** *n* inability to swallow—**aphagic** *adj*.

**aphagosis** *n* the lack of ability to eat.

**aphakia** *n* absence of the lens. Describes the eye after removal of a cataract without artificial lens implantation—**aphakic** *adj*.

**aphasia** *n* a language disorder that follows brain damage, due primarily to an impaired linguistic system. The term does not describe language disorders that involve problems with expression or comprehension caused by mental health problems, including psychoses, confusion and dementia, or muscle weakness, or problems with hearing. There are several classifications but generally aphasia is described as being *expressive (motor) aphasia* or *receptive (sensory) aphasia*. However, many people exhibit problems with both language expression and comprehension—**aphasic** *adj*. ⇒ dysarthria.

**apheresis** *n* a technique in which blood is transferred from a donor into a cell separator which collects the required components, e.g. red cells, plasma (plasmapheresis) platelets (platelet pheresis), or white cells (leucopheresis) and returns the remainder to the donor. Plasmapheresis may be used in the treatment of some diseases caused by antibodies or immune complexes circulating in the patient's plasma, e.g. myasthenia gravis. ⇒ plasmapheresis.

**aphonia** *n* inability to make sound due to neurological, behavioural, psychogenic or organic causes. ⇒ dysarthria—**aphonic** *adj*.

**aphrodisiac** *n* an agent that stimulates sexual arousal.

**aphthae** *npl* small ulcers of the gastrointestinal mucosa surrounded by a ring of erythema—**aphtha** *sing*, **aphthous** *adj*.

**aphthous stomatitis** ⇒ stomatitis.

**apical abscess** an abscess involving the apex of a tooth root. ⇒ periapical.

**apicectomy (apicoectomy)** *n* the removal of the apex or apical part of a tooth root.

**APKD** *abbr* adult polycystic kidney disease.

**aplasia** *n* incomplete development of tissue; absence of growth.

**aplastic** *adj* **1.** without structure or form. **2.** incapable of forming new tissue. *aplastic anaemia* ⇒ anaemia.

**Apley's test** a manoeuvre that tests for a torn meniscus of the knee ('grind test'); or a manoeuvre for testing the range of motion at both shoulders ('scratch test').

**apneustic breathing** abnormal gasping inspiratory breathing pattern seen after brain injury. It is characterized by a protracted inspiratory phase followed by expiration apnoea.

**apneustic centre** a respiratory control centre in the pons. Responsible for stimulating the inspiratory centre. It also has a minor role in ensuring a smooth respiratory rhythm. ⇒ pneumotaxic centre.

**apnoea** *n* a transitory cessation of breathing as seen in Cheyne–Stokes respiration. It is due to lack of the necessary $CO_2$ tension in the blood for stimulation of the respiratory centre—**apnoeic** *adj*. *apnoea of the newborn* ⇒ periodic breathing.

**apnoea hypopnoea index (AHI)** the frequency of periods of apnoea and hypopnoea that occur during sleep. The index is calculated on the number of apnoeic or hypopnoeic periods per hour of sleep. It is used in the diagnosis of various sleep apnoea syndromes and to ascertain its severity. ⇒ obstructive sleep apnoea (hypopnoea) syndrome, sleep apnoea syndrome.

**apnoea monitor** an electronic device that detects changes that indicate that breathing has stopped. The device has an alarm, which is activated when breathing stops for a given time period. Apnoea monitors are used for infants, especially preterm infants and those at risk of sudden infant death syndrome. The alarm may be a pad placed on the cot/bed, a nasal airflow sensor or an abdominal movement sensor.

**apocrine gland** a type of exocrine gland in which the apical portion of the secretory cell buds off and is lost when its secretion is released. ⇒ holocrine gland, merocrine (eccrine) gland.

**apocrine sweat glands** modified sweat glands, especially in axillae, genital and perineal regions. Responsible after puberty for body odour. ⇒ eccrine.

**apodia** *n* congenital absence of the feet.

**apoenzyme** *n* a protein part of an enzyme that needs the specific coenzyme or metal ion to become active.

**apolipoprotein** *n* the protein part of a lipoprotein.

**aponeurosis** *n* a broad glistening sheet of tendon-like tissue which serves to invest and attach muscles, e.g. abdominal muscles, to each other, and also to the parts that they move—**aponeuroses** *pl*, **aponeurotic** *adj*.

**aponeurositis** *n* inflammation of an aponeurosis.

**apophysis** *n* a projection, protuberance or outgrowth. Usually used in connection with bone.

**apoplexy** *n* historical term for cerebrovascular accident (stroke)—**apoplectic, apoplectiform** *adj*.

**apoprotein** *n* a protein before it binds to the prosthetic group required for biological activity.

**apoptosis** *n* programmed cell death.

**appendectomy** *n* ⇒ appendicectomy.

**appendicectomy** *n* excision of the appendix vermiformis.

**appendicitis** *n* inflammation of the appendix vermiformis.

**appendix** *n* an appendage. *appendix vermiformis* a worm-like appendage of the caecum about the thickness of a pencil and usually measuring from 2.5 to 15 cm in length. It contains lymphoid tissue and its position is variable. (⇒ Appendix 1, Figure 18B)—**appendices** *pl*, **appendicular** *adj*.

**apperception** *n* clear perception of a sensory stimulus, in particular where there is identification or recognition—**apperceptive** *adj*.

**appetite** *n* the desire for food, influenced by physical activity, metabolic, dietary, psychological and behavioural factors. It may be increased or decreased pharmacologically. Appetite is also influenced by health status. ⇒ anorexia, bulimia, eating disorders.

**applanation** *n* a way of flattening the cornea during contact tonometry to determine intraocular pressure. ⇒ Goldmann applanation tonometer, tonometry.

**applicator** *n* an instrument used for local application of remedies, e.g. vaginal medication applicator.

**apposition** *n* the approximation or bringing together of two surfaces or edges.

**appraisal** *n* making a valuation. *performance appraisal or review* a formal procedure whereby an appraiser (manager) systematically reviews the role performance of the appraisee and they jointly set goals for the future.

**approved name** the generic or non-proprietary name of a drug, such as salbutamol. Should be used in prescribing, except in the case of drugs where bioavailability differs between brands. ⇒ recommended International Non-proprietary Name (rINN).

**approved social worker (ASW)** in England and Wales a social worker appointed by the local health authority with statutory duties under the Mental Health Act 1983, including: (a) making applications for compulsory or emergency admission to hospital and conveyance of patients there; (b) applications concerning guardianship, the functions of the nearest relative, or

acting as a nearest relative if so appointed; (c) planning and providing aftercare of discharged mentally disordered patients.

**apraxia** *n* inability to perform a motor act or use an object normally, due typically to damage in the parietal lobe of the brain—**apraxic, apractic** *adj*. *constructional apraxia* inability to arrange objects to a plan.

**apronectomy** *n* ⇒ abdominoplasty.

**aptitude** *n* natural ability and facility in performing tasks, either physical or mental.

**APTT** *abbr* activated partial thromboplastin time.

**APUD cells** amine precursor uptake and decarboxylation cells. A large group of cells widespread throughout the body, especially in the hypothalamus, pituitary gland, thyroid gland, parathyroid glands, pancreas and the mucosa of gastrointestinal tract. They convert precursor substances to various hormones and physiologically active amines, such as dopamine, 5-hydroxytryptamine (serotonin), etc.

**apudoma** *n* a hormone- or amine-secreting tumour of APUD cells. ⇒ argentaffinoma, carcinoid syndrome.

**apyrexia** *n* absence of fever—**apyrexial** *adj*.

**aqueduct** *n* a canal. *aqueduct of Sylvius* the canal connecting the third and fourth ventricles of the brain; aqueductus cerebri.

**aqueous** *adj* watery. *aqueous humour* the fluid contained in the anterior and posterior chambers of the eye. ⇒ Appendix 1, Figure 15.

**arachidonic acid** a polyunsaturated fatty acid with four double bonds. Used in the body for the synthesis of important regulatory lipids that include: prostaglandins, prostacyclins and thromboxanes. A high concentration is found in brain and nervous tissue membranes. Arachidonic acid is important for brain development. The dietary intake of arachidonic acid is associated with birth weight, head circumference and placental weight. It can be synthesized from linoleic acid in the body, but may be considered to be an essential fatty acid (EFA) when linoleic acid is deficient in the diet.

**arachis oil** oil expressed from peanuts (groundnuts). Used for cooking, in the food industry and for some pharmaceutical products. Contains monounsaturated fatty acids. Should not be used by those with a peanut allergy.

**arachnodactyly** *n* congenital abnormality resulting in long, slender fingers. Said to resemble spider legs (hence 'spider fingers').

**arachnoid** *adj* resembling a spider's web. *arachnoid mater or membrane* a delicate membrane enveloping the brain and spinal cord, lying between the pia mater internally and the dura mater externally; the middle membrane of the meninges—**arachnoidal** *adj.*

**arborization** *n* an arrangement resembling the branching of a tree. Characterizes both ends of a neuron, i.e. the dendrites and the axon as it supplies each muscle fibre.

**arboviruses** *npl* abbreviation for arthropod-borne viruses. Include various RNA viruses transmitted by arthropods: mosquitoes, ticks, sandflies, etc. They cause diseases such as yellow fever, dengue, sandfly fever and several types of encephalitis.

**arc eye** a painful but usually temporary condition of the eyes following exposure to the light from arc welding equipment.

**arch of aorta** ⇒ aortic arch. Appendix 1, Figures 8 and 9.

**arcus** *n* an arch- or ring-shaped structure.

**arcus senilis** an opaque ring round the edge of the cornea, seen in older people.

**ARDS** *abbr* acute/adult respiratory distress syndrome.

**areola** *n* the pigmented area round the nipple of the breast. A *secondary areola* surrounds the primary areola in pregnancy—**areolar** *adj.* ⇒ Montgomery's glands.

**areolar tissue** a loose connective tissue comprising cells and fibres in a semisolid matrix.

**ARF** *abbr* **1.** acute renal failure. ⇒ renal failure. **2.** acute respiratory failure. ⇒ respiratory failure.

**argentaffin cells** *npl* cells found, for example, in the mucosa of the gastrointestinal tract. They take up stains containing silver and chromium.

**argentaffinoma (carcinoid)** *n* tumour affecting argentaffin cells in the gastrointestinal tract, or in those within the bronchi. ⇒ carcinoid syndrome.

**arginase** *n* an enzyme present in the liver, kidney and spleen. It converts arginine into ornithine and urea.

**arginine** *n* one of the essential amino acids during childhood, it is found in protein foods required for growth and recovery. It is hydrolysed by the enzyme arginase to urea and ornithine. Supplements have been shown to enhance immune function in high-risk surgical patients.

**argininosuccinuria** *n* the presence of arginine and succinic acid in urine. Associated with learning disability and seizures. Also called argininosuccinic aciduria.

**argon** *n* an inert gas. Forms less than 0.1% of atmospheric air.

**Argyll Robertson pupil** (D M Argyll Robertson, British ophthalmologist, 1837–1909) small, irregular pupil that responds to accommodation but not to light, associated with neurosyphilis and chronic alcohol misuse.

**argyria** *n* slate grey discoloration of the skin and conjunctivae resulting from chronic exposure to silver.

**ariboflavinosis** *n* a deficiency state caused by lack of riboflavin and other members of the vitamin B complex. Characterized by cheilosis, seborrhoea, angular stomatitis, glossitis and photophobia.

**ARM** *abbr* artificial rupture of the membranes. ⇒ amniotomy.

**arm, chest, hip index (ACH index)** a way of assessing nutritional status using measurements of the arm circumference, chest and hip size.

**Arnold–Chiari malformation** a group of disorders affecting the base of the brain. Commonly occurs in hydrocephalus associated with meningocele and myelomeningocele. There are degrees of severity but usually there is some 'kinking' or 'buckling' of the brainstem with cerebellar tissue herniating through the foramen magnum at the base of the skull.

**AROM** *abbr* active range of motion.

**aromatase inhibitors** *npl* a group of drugs, such as exemestane, used in the treatment of breast cancer in postmenopausal women.

**aromatherapy** *n* a complementary therapy that involves the use of fragrances derived from essential oils. These may be combined with a base oil, inhaled or massaged into intact skin.

**arousal** *n* the state of alertness and responsiveness to sensory stimuli.

**arrectores pilorum** *npl* internal, plain, involuntary muscles (⇒ Appendix 1, Figure 12) attached to hair follicles, which, by contraction, erect the hair follicles, causing 'gooseflesh' when the person is cold or aroused, as in fright—**arrector pili** *sing.* ⇒ pilomotor reflex.

**arrhythmia** *n* any deviation from the normal rhythm, usually referring to the heart beat. ⇒ asystole, extrasystole, fibrillation, heart block, Stokes–Adams syndrome, supraventricular tachycardia, Wolff–Parkinson–White syndrome.

**arsenic (As)** *n* a poisonous metallic element present in preparations such as herbicides and pesticides. Vegetables, fruit and other foods may contain small amounts. Toxic effects include malaise, gastrointestinal symptoms, pigmentation of the skin, anaemia and nervous symptoms.

**artefact** *n* any artificial product resulting from a physical or chemical agent; an unnatural change in a structure or tissue.

**arteralgia** *n* pain in an artery.

**arterial blood gases (ABGs)** measurement of the oxygen ($PaO_2$), carbon dioxide ($PaCO_2$) and acid–base (pH or hydrogen ion concentration) content of the arterial blood.

**arterial line** a cannula placed in an artery to sample blood for gas analysis and for continuous blood pressure monitoring. Usually only used in specialist units (intensive therapy unit, high-dependency unit and theatre) because of the potential risk of severe blood loss. They should always be attached to a pressure transducer and monitor, and have an alarm that indicates any disconnection. ⇒ arterial blood gases, blood pressure.

**arterial ulcer** a leg ulcer caused by a defect in arterial blood supply. They are found on the foot, usually between the toes or close to the ankle; the adjacent skin is discoloured, shiny and hairless; and the ulcer is small and deep with some exudate (Figure A.11). They are often associated with a history of cardiovascular disease or diabetes mellitus. ⇒ claudication.

**arteriectomy** *n* surgical excision of part of an artery.

**arteriography** *n* demonstration of the arterial system after injection of an opaque contrast medium—**arteriographic** *adj*, **arteriogram** *n*, **arteriograph** *n*, **arteriographically** *adv*.

**arteriole** *n* a small artery, joining an artery to a capillary network. They control the amount of blood entering the capillary network. They are able to constrict and dilate to change peripheral resistance, thereby influencing blood pressure.

**arteriopathy** *n* disease of any artery—**arteriopathic** *adj*.

**arterioplasty** *n* reconstructive surgery applied to an artery—**arterioplastic** *adj*.

**arteriosclerosis** *n* degenerative arterial change associated with advancing age. Primarily a thickening of the medial (middle) layer and usually associated with some degree of atheroma—**arteriosclerotic** *adj*.

**arteriotomy** *n* incision or needle puncture of an artery.

**arteriovenous** *adj* pertaining to an artery and a vein.

**arteriovenous fistula** the anastomosis of an artery to a vein to promote the enlargement of the latter, to facilitate the removal and replacement of blood during long-term haemodialysis.

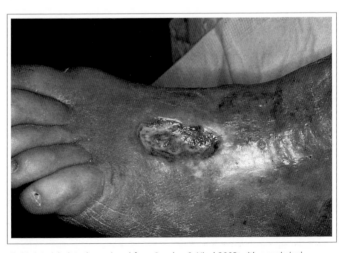

**Figure A.11** Arterial ulcer *(reproduced from Brooker & Nicol 2003 with permission)*.

**arteriovenous oxygen difference** the difference in oxygen content between the arterial and venous blood. It is the arterial oxygen content minus the oxygen content in the central veins.

**arteritis** *n* an inflammatory disease affecting layers of the arterial wall. It may be due to an infection such as syphilis or it may be part of a connective tissue (collagen) disease. The arteries may become swollen and tender and the blood may clot in them. ⇒ temporal arteritis—**arteritic** *adj.*

**artery** *n* a vessel carrying blood away from the heart to the various tissues. The internal endothelial lining provides a smooth surface to prevent intravascular clotting of blood. The middle layer of plain muscle and elastic fibres allows for distension as blood is pumped from the heart. The outer, mainly connective tissue layer prevents overdistension. The lumen is largest nearest to the heart; it gradually decreases in size—**arterial** *adj.* *artery forceps* forceps used to achieve haemostasis during surgery.

**arthralgia** *n* (*syn* articular neuralgia, arthrodynia) pain in a joint, used especially when there is no inflammation—**arthralgic** *adj.* *intermittent* or *periodic arthralgia* is the term used when there is pain, usually accompanied by swelling of the knee at regular intervals.

**arthrectomy** *n* surgical excision of a joint.

**arthritis** *n* inflammation of one or more joints which swell, become warm to touch, and are tender and painful on movement. There are many causes and the treatment varies according to the cause—**arthritic** *adj.* ⇒ arthropathy, gout, juvenile idiopathic arthritis, osteoarthritis, rheumatoid arthritis, Still's disease.

**arthrocentesis** *n* aspiration of fluid from a synovial joint using a needle and syringe. Synovial fluid samples may be obtained for diagnosis. Therapeutic removal of effusion fluid, pus or blood may be performed. Drugs may also be injected into the synovial cavity.

**arthroclasis** *n* breaking down of adhesions within the joint cavity to produce a wider range of movement.

**arthrodesis** *n* the stiffening or fusion of a joint by operative means. Sometimes performed to relieve pain by limiting movement at the joint, or to stabilize an unstable joint.

**arthrodynia** *n* ⇒ arthralgia—**arthrodynic** *adj.*

**arthrography** *n* a radiographic examination to determine the internal structure of a joint, outlined by contrast media—either a gas or a liquid contrast medium or both— **arthrographic** *adj,* **arthrogram** *n,* **arthrograph** *n,* **arthrographically** *adv.*

**arthrogryposis multiplex congenita** *n* a congenital condition characterized by fibrous stiffness of one or more joints. It is often accompanied by poor development of associated muscles and changes to the motor nerves that innervate the muscles.

**arthrology** *n* the science that studies the structure and function of joints, their diseases and treatment.

**arthropathy** *n* any joint disease—**arthropathies** *pl,* **arthropathic** *adj.* Arthropathy may be classified as: *enteropathic arthropathies* resulting from chronic diarrhoeal disease; *psoriatic arthropathies* accompanying psoriasis; *seronegative arthropathies* include all other instances of inflammatory arthritis other than rheumatoid arthritis; *seropositive arthropathies* include all instances of rheumatoid arthritis.

**arthroplasty** *n* surgical remodelling of a joint—**arthroplastic** *adj.* *cup arthroplasty* articular surface is reconstructed and covered with a vitallium cup. *excision arthroplasty* gap is filled with fibrous tissue as in Keller's operation for hallux valgus. *Girdlestone arthroplasty* excision arthroplasty of the hip. *replacement arthroplasty* insertion of an inert prosthesis of similar shape into a joint, such as the hip, knee, shoulder, etc. *total replacement arthroplasty* replacement of the head of femur and the acetabulum, both being cemented into the bone.

**arthroscope** *n* an endoscopic instrument used for the visualization of the interior of a joint cavity. Used to take tissue biopsies, and also for treatments such as removing loose bodies from the knee joint. ⇒ endoscope—**arthroscopic** *adj.*

**arthroscopy** *n* the act of visualizing the interior of a joint. Uses an intra-articular endoscopic camera to assess, repair or reconstruct various tissues within and around joints—**arthroscopic** *adj.*

**arthrosis** *n* degeneration in a joint.

**arthrostomy** *n* operative procedure to make an opening (temporary) in a joint cavity.

**arthrotomy** *n* incision into a joint.

**articular** *adj* pertaining to a joint or articulation. Applied to cartilage, surface, capsule, etc.

**articulation** *n* **1.** the junction of two or more bones; a joint. **2.** enunciation of speech—**articular** *adj.*

**artificial blood** a fluid able to transport $O_2$.

**artificial heart** ⇒ left ventricular assist device (LVAD).

**artificial insemination** ⇒ insemination.

**artificial kidney** ⇒ dialyser.

**artificial limb** ⇒ orthosis, prosthesis.

**artificial lung** ⇒ respirator.

**artificial pacemaker** cardiac pacemaker. ⇒ cardiac.

**artificial pneumothorax** ⇒ pneumothorax.

**artificial respiration** ⇒ cardiopulmonary resuscitation.

**asbestos** *n* a fibrous, mineral substance which does not conduct heat and is incombustible. It has many uses, including brake linings, asbestos textiles and asbestos-cement sheeting. Inhalation of asbestos fibres leads to pulmonary fibrous. Long-term contact with asbestos, such as during employment, can cause mesothelioma and lung cancer. ⇒ mesothelioma.

**asbestosis** *n* a form of pneumoconiosis from inhalation of asbestos dust and fibre. ⇒ mesothelioma.

**ascariasis** *n* infestation by nematodes (roundworms). The ova are ingested and hatch in the duodenum. The larvae pass to the lungs in the blood, from where they ascend to be swallowed and returned to the intestine. They may occasionally obstruct the intestine or the bile ducts.

**ascaricide** *n* a substance that kills ascarides, e.g. levamisole—**ascaricidal** *adj*.

*Ascaris* *npl* a genus of nematode worms of the family Ascaridae, e.g. the roundworm *Ascaris lumbricoides*. ⇒ ascariasis.

**ascending colon** ⇒ Appendix 1, Figure 18B.

**Aschoff's nodules** (K A Aschoff, German pathologist, 1866–1942) nodules present in the myocardium in myocarditis caused by rheumatic fever.

**ascites** *n* (*syn* hydroperitoneum) free fluid in the peritoneal cavity—**ascitic** *adj*.

**ascorbic acid** vitamin C. A water-soluble antioxidant vitamin which is necessary for healthy connective tissue, particularly the collagen fibres and cell membranes. Also enhances absorption of dietary iron and is necessary for functioning of the immune system. Deficiency causes scurvy. Used as nutritional supplement in anaemia and to promote wound healing.

**ASD** *abbr* atrial septal defect.

**asepsis** *n* the condition of being free from living pathogenic micro-organisms—**aseptic** *adj*.

**aseptic technique** describes procedures used to exclude pathogenic micro-organisms from an environment. It includes the use of sterile gloves and gowns in theatre, non-touch technique and the use of sterilized equipment. Used where there is a possibility of introducing micro-organisms into the patient's body.

**ash** *n* the residue of components in a food after all organic matter and water has been burnt off. It is all the non-organic matter in a food, a measure of the total content of minerals in a food.

**asialorrhoea** *n* diminished flow or lack of saliva.

**ASO** *abbr* antistreptolysin O.

**ASOM** *abbr* acute suppurative otitis media.

**asomatognosia** *n* loss of awareness of parts of the body (soma) and their position in space, a perceptual sequela of cerebrovascular accident (stroke) affecting the right parietal lobe of the cerebrum, which may lead to lack of awareness, even denial, of the presence of disability.

**asparaginase** *n* an enzyme derived from micro-organisms. In the form of crisantaspase, used pharmacologically to treat cancers, e.g. acute lymphoblastic leukaemia. ⇒ cytotoxic.

**asparagine** *n* a non-essential (dispensable) amino acid.

**aspartame** *n* an artificial sweetener. It is converted to phenylalanine in the body and consequently should not be used by people with phenylketonuria.

**aspartate aminotransferase (AST)** an enzyme that facilitates the reversible transfer of amino groups during amino acid metabolism. ⇒ aminotransferases.

**aspartic acid (aspartate)** *n* a non-essential (dispensable) amino acid. At physiological pH aspartic acid is negatively charged and is known as aspartate.

**Asperger's syndrome** (H Asperger, Austrian psychiatrist, 1906–1980) a pervasive developmental syndrome classified as part of the autistic spectrum of disorders. It is diagnosed during childhood and is associated with various problems with social interactions, communication and expressing emotion, but without delay in language or cognitive development. The problems with social interaction frequently continue into adult life.

**aspergillosis** *n* opportunist infection, most frequently of the lungs, caused by any species of *Aspergillus*. ⇒ bronchomycosis.

*Aspergillus* *n* a genus of fungi, found in soil, manure and on various grains. Some species are pathogenic.

**aspermia** *n* lack of secretion or expulsion of semen—**aspermic** *adj*.

**asphyxia** *n* lack of oxygen reaching the brain leading to unconsciousness and, in the absence of effective treatment, eventually death.

**aspiration** *n* (*syn* paracentesis, tapping) **1.** the removal of fluids from a body cavity by means of suction or siphonage such as fluid from the peritoneal cavity, postoperative gastric aspiration, etc. **2.** describes the entry of fluids or food into the airway. *aspiration pneumonia* inflammation of lung tissue from inhalation of a foreign body, most often food particles or fluids. ⇒ Heimlich's manoeuvre.

**aspirator** *n* a negative-pressure device used for withdrawing fluids from body cavities.

**aspirin** *n* ⇒ non-steroidal anti-inflammatory drugs. ⇒ Appendix 5.

**assault** *n* an attempt or offer of unlawful contact in which the person is put in fear of violence or unlawful force. Constitutes a trespass against the person. ⇒ battery.

**assay** *n* a quantitative test used to measure the amount of a substance present or its level of activity, e.g. hormones or drugs.

**assertiveness training** developing self-confidence in personal and professional relationships. It concentrates on the honest expression of feelings, both negative and positive: learning occurs through role playing in a therapeutic setting followed by practice in real-life situations.

**assessment** *n* the collection of information, including subjective and objective data which are relevant to formulating an individual plan of treatment, a specific therapy or care package.

**assimilation** *n* the process whereby digested foodstuffs are absorbed and used by the cells and tissues—**assimilable** *adj*, **assimilate** *vt*, *vi*.

**assisted conception** techniques used when the normal method of conception has failed. They include in vitro fertilization (IVF) and transcervical embryo transfer or gamete intra-fallopian tube transfer (GIFT), zygote intra-fallopian transfer (ZIFT), intracytoplasmic sperm injection (ICSI) and microsurgical epididymal sperm aspiration (MESA).

**assisted movements** movements aided by a therapist, or equipment, another health professional or carer. May be self-assisted (auto-assisted) when, for instance, a person moves an arm paralysed after a stroke using the unaffected arm.

**associated movements** described by some authorities as the normal movements that occur during considerable effort, such as when attempting a new activity. Other authorities use the term to include both normal and abnormal movements.

**associated reactions** the postural muscle reactions that happen when a muscle is freed from its usual nervous control. They are involuntary stereotyped movements that can occur when a person is having balance problems, or is putting a great deal of effort into a task.

**association** *n* a term used in psychology. *association of ideas* the principle by which ideas, emotions and movements are connected so that their succession in the mind occurs. *controlled association* ideas called up in consciousness in response to words spoken by the examiner. *free association* ideas arising spontaneously when censorship is removed: an important feature of psychoanalysis.

**AST** *abbr* aspartate aminotransferase. ⇒ aminotransferases.

**astereognosis** *n* inability to recognize objects by touch and manipulation, especially inability to perceive the shape, texture and size of objects.

**asteroid hyalosis** a degenerative condition, usually asymptomatic, in which the vitreous body (humour) of the eye contains numerous small opacities.

**asthenia** *n* lack of strength; weakness, debility—**asthenic** *adj*.

**asthenopia** *n* eye strain. Describes symptoms related to excessive effort of accommodation, e.g. headaches—**asthenopic** *adj*, **asthenope** *n*.

**asthma** *n* paroxysmal dyspnoea characterized by wheezing and difficulty in expiration because of muscular spasm in the bronchi (bronchospasm). Immunological studies have implicated mast cells, lymphocytes and cytokines in an inflammatory cascade leading to bronchial wall hyperactivity and narrowing in response to a stimulus. Inhaled or oral corticosteroids damp down the acute immune reaction, while inhaled $\beta_2$ receptor-agonists, e.g. salbutamol, relieve bronchial spasm. ⇒ Appendix 5. Newer leukotriene receptor antagonist drugs, e.g. zafirlukast, offer more targeted therapy. The monoclonal antibody omalizumab, which binds to immunoglobulin E (IgE), can be used for patients with severe IgE-mediated sensitivity to inhaled allergens who do not respond adequately to other therapies. ⇒ occupational asthma, severe acute asthma—**asthmatic** *adj*.

**astigmatism** *n* defective vision caused by refractive surfaces, usually corneal, focusing light on to more than one focal plane—**astigmatic, astigmic** *adj.*

**astringency** *n* the action of chemicals in foods, such as unripe fruits, on the tongue. They cause contraction of the epithelium of the tongue.

**astringent** *adj* describes an agent which contracts organic tissue, thus lessening secretion. May be used in the management of heavily exuding wounds—**astringency, astringent** *n.*

**astrocytes** *npl* part of the macroglia. Star-shaped neuroglial cells, which are the main supporting tissue in the central nervous system. They are sited close to blood vessel walls where they contribute to the blood–brain barrier.

**astrocytoma** *n* a slowly growing tumour of astrocytes (neuroglial tissue) of the brain.

**ASW** *abbr* approved social worker.

**asymmetric tonic neck reflex** also called tonic neck reflex. A reflex present in newborns. When an infant is lying on its back with the head turned to one side, the limbs on the side that the head is facing should be straight, while the limbs on the other side should bend. The reflex normally disappears around 6 months of age.

**asymmetry** *n* lack of similarity of the organs or parts on each side.

**asymptomatic** *adj* symptomless.

**asynclitism** *n* the lateral tilting of the fetal head so that the biparietal diameter can negotiate the narrowest anteroposterior diameter of the pelvic brim.

**asyndesis** *n* a disorder of thought with disruption of the association of ideas. Thought and speech are fragmented because the person cannot assemble related thoughts into a coherent notion.

**asystole** *n* absence of heart beat and output from the heart. One type of cardiac arrest.

**ataractic** *adj* describes drugs that tranquillize and relieve anxiety. ⇒ tranquillizers.

**atavism** *n* the reappearance of a hereditary characteristic that has missed one or more generations—**atavic, atavistic** *adj.*

**ataxia, ataxy** *n* ill-timed and incoordinate movements caused by hypotonia, dyssynergia and dysmetria—**ataxic** *adj.* ⇒ Friedreich's ataxia, gait.

**atelectasis** *n* numbers of pulmonary alveoli do not contain air due to failure of expansion (congenital atelectasis) or resorption of air from the alveoli (collapse)—**atelectatic** *adj.*

**ateliosis** *n* a form of dwarfism caused by lack of hormones from the anterior lobe of the pituitary gland. The person appears childlike and sexual development does not occur.

**atherogenic** *adj* capable of producing atheroma—**atherogenesis** *n.*

**atheroma** *n* plaques of fatty (lipid) material in the intimal (inner) layer of the arteries. Starts as fatty streaks on the intima, deposition of low-density lipoprotein and plaque formation (Figure A.12). Eventually the lumen of the artery is reduced and ischaemia results. A thrombus may form if a plaque ruptures, which leads to further occlusion of the artery. Of great importance in the coronary arteries in predisposing to coronary thrombosis and myocardial infarction—**atheromatous** *adj.*

**atherosclerosis** *n* coexisting atheroma and arteriosclerosis—**atherosclerotic** *adj.*

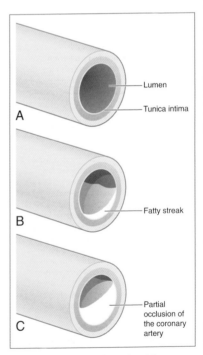

**Figure A.12** Atheroma *(reproduced from Brooker & Nicol 2003 with permission).*

**athetosis** *n* a largely obsolete word used to describe a slow writhing movement disorder typically in the context of cerebral palsy. Made worse by excitement and emotional stress—**athetoid, athetotic** *adj*.

**athlete's foot** tinea pedis. ⇒ tinea.

**athlete's heart** the cardiac adaptations to physical training. They include resting bradycardia, changes to the ECG trace, alteration in heart sounds and physical changes to heart muscle.

**athletic trainer** a term used in North America for an individual who is trained in the prevention, evaluation, treatment and rehabilitation of athletic injuries.

**atlas** *n* the first cervical vertebra.

**ATLS** *abbr* advanced trauma life support.

**ATN** *abbr* acute tubular necrosis.

**atom** *n* the smallest particle of an element capable of existing individually, or in combination with one or more atoms of the same or another element—**atomic** *adj*.

**atomic mass unit (amu) or dalton** a relative weight used to measure atoms and sub-atomic particles. Protons and neutrons have both been designated as being 1 amu.

**atomic number** the number of protons in the atomic nucleus or the number of electrons, for example, hydrogen which, with one of each, has the atomic number 1.

**atomic weight (mass)** or relative atomic mass. The relative average mass of an atom based on the mass of an atom of carbon-12.

**atomizer** *n* nebulizer.

**atonia** *n* total flaccidity or no muscle tone caused by complete loss of motor supply to a muscle—**atonic** *adj*.

**atonic bladder** a condition marked by over-filling of the urinary bladder and involuntary leakage of small volumes of urine. It arises from some interruption to the nerve pathways to the bladder, such as with diabetes, which leads to loss of the sensation of a full bladder and an inability to empty the bladder normally.

**atopic syndrome** a hereditary predisposition to develop hypersensitivity disorders, such as eczema, asthma, hayfever and allergic rhinitis. Associated with excess immunoglobulin E (IgE) production.

**ATP** *abbr* adenosine triphosphate.

**ATP–CP energy pathway** the energy pathway that produces energy from the skeletal muscle stores of the high-energy phosphates adenosine triphosphate (ATP) and creatine phosphate (CP). Important during short-duration, high-intensity physical activity.

**atresia** *n* imperforation or closure of a normal body opening, duct or canal such as the oesophagus, bowel, anus or bile duct—**atresic, atretic** *adj*.

**atrial fibrillation** a cardiac arrhythmia. Chaotic irregularity of atrial rhythm with an irregular ventricular response (Figure A.13). There is a risk of thrombi forming on the atrial wall. When sinus rhythm returns emboli may be dislodged and travel in the circulation to cause, for instance, a stroke. Commonly associated with mitral stenosis, hyperthyroidism (thyrotoxicosis) or heart failure.

**atrial flutter** a cardiac arrhythmia caused by an irritable focus in atrial muscle and usually associated with coronary heart disease. Speed of atrial beats is between 260 and 340 per minute. The ventricular response is slower and may respond to every four atrial beats.

**atrial natriuretic peptides (ANP)** peptides produced by cells in the cardiac atria. They are involved in the control of blood pressure by inhibiting the release of antidiuretic hormone and aldosterone when blood pressure rises.

**atrial septal defect (ASD)** a hole in the atrial septum. Most commonly due to a congenital defect. Types include: ostium secundum defect, which is most common and is situated around the site of the foramen ovale; and ostium primum defects, situated lower down on the atrial septum.

**atrioventricular (A-V)** *adj* pertaining to the atria and the ventricles of the heart. Applied to a node, tract and valves.

**atrioventricular bundle** also called the bundle of His. Part of the conducting system of the heart. Carries impulses from the atrioventricular node to the ventricles. Divides into right and left bundle branches that transmit the impulses to the apex of each ventricle.

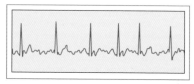

**Figure A.13** Atrial fibrillation *(reproduced from Brooker & Nicol 2003 with permission)*.

A

**atrioventricular node** part of the conducting system of the heart. Situated at the bottom of the right atrium, it transmits impulses from the sinus node (sinoatrial node) to the atrioventricular bundle.

**atrioventricular valves** valves between the atria and ventricles in the heart. ⇒ bicuspid, tricuspid.

**atrium** *n* cavity, entrance or passage. One of the two upper receiving chambers of the heart ⇒ Appendix 1, Figure 8—**atria** *pl*, **atrial** *adj*.

**atrophic rhinitis** (*syn* ozaena) chronic infective condition of the nasal mucous membrane with associated crusting and fetor.

**atrophy** *n* loss of substance of cells, tissues or organs. There is wasting and a decrease in size and function. The process may be physiological such as that occurring as part of normal ageing, or pathological, as in disuse atrophy when a limb is immobilized—**atrophied**, **atrophic** *adj*. *progressive muscular atrophy* ⇒ motor neuron disease.

**atropine** *n* the principal alkaloid of belladonna. ⇒ muscarinic antagonists.

**attachment** *n* in psychology a term describing the dependent relationship which one individual forms with another, emanating from the unique bonding between infant and parent figure.

**attention** *n* ability to select some stimuli for closer examination while discarding others considered less salient.

**attention deficit hyperactivity disorder (ADHD)** term used to describe children who have short attention spans and are easily distracted. They are frequently overactive, may be aggressive and often have learning difficulties. ⇒ hyperkinetic disorder/syndrome.

**attentional deficits** can involve different areas of attention. These include the ability to transfer the focus of attention and to change it between activities; the ability to avoid being distracted; being able to respond to multiple tasks simultaneously; the ability to sustain concentration; and the ability to be focused and recognize individual pieces of information.

**attenuation** *n* the process whereby pathogenic micro-organisms are induced to develop or show less virulent characteristics. They can then be used in the preparation of vaccines—**attenuant**, **attenuated** *adj*, **attenuate** *vt, vi*.

**atticotomy** *n* operation to remove cholesteatoma from the middle ear and mastoid process.

**attitudes** *npl* reactions to and evaluations of individuals, situations and objects. They may be positive or negative.

**attribution** *n* in psychology, the theory that deals with the inferences that individuals make regarding the causes of their own and other individuals' behaviour.

**attrition** *n* the normal wear of tooth surfaces caused by friction.

**atypical** *adj* not typical; unusual, irregular; not conforming to type, e.g. atypical pneumonia.

**atypical mole syndrome** dysplastic naevus syndrome. A syndrome characterized by the presence of multiple moles. The moles or naevi are pigmented and irregular in size. Occurs in individuals at risk of familial or non-familial malignant melanoma.

**audiogram** *n* a graph of the acuity of hearing tested with an audiometer.

**audiology** *n* the scientific study of hearing—**audiological** *adj*, **audiologically** *adv*.

**audiometer** *n* apparatus for the clinical testing of hearing. It generates pure tones over a wide range of pitch and intensity—**audiometric** *adj*, **audiometry** *n*.

**audiometrist** *n* a person qualified to carry out audiometry.

**audit** *n* investigative methods used to measure outcomes and review performance systematically. *audit trail* a way of working and record keeping that allows the processes to be transparent and clear. *medical audit* systematic and critical review of medical care, including diagnosis and treatment, outcomes and quality of life.

**Audit Commission** within the NHS the main role of the Audit Commission is to promote best practice in terms of economy, effectiveness and efficiency.

**auditory** *adj* pertaining to the sense of hearing. *auditory canal* ⇒ external auditory meatus/canal.

**auditory acuity** ability to hear clearly and distinctly. Tests include the use of tuning fork, whispered voice and audiometer. Hearing can be tested in infants by otoacoustic emission (OAE) testing and automated auditory brainstem response (AABR). ⇒ audiometer, automated auditory brainstem response, neonatal hearing screening, otoacoustic emission testing.

**auditory area** that portion of the temporal lobe of the cerebral cortex which interprets sound.

**auditory nerves** the eighth pair of cranial nerves. More usually called the vestibulocochlear nerve.

**auditory ossicles** three small bones—malleus, incus and stapes—located within the middle ear.

**auditory-processing disorder (APD)** previously known as central auditory processing disorder. A condition in which the brain does not perceive auditory information despite normal auditory pathways, i.e. there is no sensory impairment. There are several types and it may be genetic or acquired (e.g. following brain injury). It is characterized by difficulty with the localization of sounds, difficulty remembering spoken instructions, understanding speech in situations with background noise (e.g. television on, parties), etc.

**Auerbach's (myenteric) plexus** (L Auerbach, German anatomist, 1828–1897) ⇒ myenteric plexus.

**augmentation** *n* enlargement. Commonly applied to plastic surgical procedures that increase breast size.

**augmentation of labour** interventions that include amniotomy and/or the administration of oxytocin to rectify slow progress in labour.

**aura** *n* a premonition; a peculiar sensation or warning of an impending attack, such as occurs in epilepsy or migraine. They may include visual disturbances, abnormal sensations such as tingling, or strange tastes.

**aural** *adj* pertaining to the ear.

**auricle** *n* **1.** the pinna of the outer/external ear. ⇒ Appendix 1, Figure 13. **2.** an appendage to the cardiac atrium. **3.** obsolete term for cardiac atrium—**auricular** *adj*.

**auriculoventricular** *adj* obsolete term ⇒ atrioventricular.

**auriscope** *n* ⇒ otoscope.

**auscultation** *n* a method of listening to the body sounds, particularly the heart, lungs and fetal circulation for diagnostic purposes. It may be: (a) immediate, by placing the ear directly against the body; or (b) mediate, by the use of a stethoscope—**auscultatory** *adj*, **auscult, auscultate** *v*.

**autism** *n* a pervasive form of disordered child development characterized by difficulties with social interaction, communication and repetitive stereotyped behaviours. ⇒ Asperger's syndrome.

**autoagglutination** *n* the agglutination of red blood cells (erythrocytes) by the person's own antibodies, such as occurs in autoimmune haemolytic anaemia.

**autoantibody** *n* an antibody which binds self-antigen expressed in normal tissue.

**autoantigen** *n* a self-antigen, expressed in normal tissue, which is the target of autoantibodies or self-reactive T cells.

**autoclave** *n* **1.** an apparatus for high-pressure steam sterilization. **2.** *vt* sterilize in an autoclave.

**autocrine** *adj* describes the action of a hormone or growth factor upon the cells that secrete it. ⇒ endocrine, paracrine.

**autodigestion** *n* self-digestion of body tissue during life. ⇒ autolysis.

**autoeroticism** *n* self-gratification of the sex instinct. ⇒ masturbation—**autoerotic** *adj*.

**autofluorescence** *n* the fluorescence of structures in the eye, for example drusen in the retina. ⇒ angiography.

**autogenic** *adj* describes a process or condition that originates from within the organism.

**autogenic drainage** a breathing technique used to clear secretions from the airways. It improves ventilation and ensures optimal chest movements.

**autogenic facilitation** reflex activation of a muscle through activation of its own sensory receptors; self-generated excitation of muscle, e.g. the stretch reflex.

**autogenic inhibition** reflex inhibition of a muscle through activation of stretch receptors, the Golgi tendon organs, in its own tendons; self-generated relaxation of muscle that normally prevents build-up of too much, potentially injurious, tension in a muscle.

**autogenic therapy** a complementary therapy that employs a combination of self-hypnosis and relaxation.

**autograft** *n* tissue grafted from one part of the body to another.

**autoimmune disease** an illness caused by, or associated with, the development of an immune response to normal body tissues.

**autoinfection** *n* ⇒ infection.

**autointoxication** *n* poisoning from abnormal or excessive metabolic products produced in the body, some of which may originate from infected or necrotic tissue.

**autologous** *adj* when a patient acts as the source of cells or a graft.

**autologous bone marrow transplant** reinfusion of bone marrow cells originating from the recipient. May be performed for patients with leukaemia. Their bone marrow is harvested, stored and replaced after leukaemic cells have been destroyed with cytotoxic chemotherapy or radiotherapy.

**autologous transfusion** a patient donates blood or blood products prior to elective surgery to be transfused during surgery or postoperatively. Cross-matching and compatibility problems are avoided, as is the risk of bloodborne infections.

**autolysis** *n* autodigestion, which occurs if digestive enzymes escape into surrounding tissues. Occurs as a physiological process, e.g. of the uterus during the puerperium—**autolytic** *adj*.

**automated auditory brainstem response (AABR)** a way of testing hearing in newborns. It is performed by exposing the infant (usually when asleep) to clicking sounds via small headphones. Small sensors on the infant's head and neck convey responses to a computer, which analyses the responses to sounds beyond the cochlea of the inner ear. Specific brainstem response testing is being developed for premature infants in order to detect deafness resulting from hypoxia occurring during delivery.

**automated external defibrillator (AED)** a device that delivers electric shocks to victims of cardiac arrest in order to treat ventricular fibrillation. They are suitable for use by members of the public and health professionals, as they direct the operator with visual and voice prompts. AEDs may be semi-automatic or fully automatic but all devices analyse the casualty's cardiac rhythm in order to ascertain whether a shock is required and then deliver the shock if needed.

**automated lamellar keratectomy** an operative procedure whereby the cornea is reshaped for the correction of refractive errors.

**automated peritoneal dialysis (APD)** a type of peritoneal dialysis where the fluid exchanges are performed at night by the use of a mechanical device.

**automatic** *adj* occurring without the influence of the will; spontaneous; without volition; involuntary acts.

**automatic implantable cardioverter defibrillator (AICD)** used for patients who have recurrent life-threatening arrhythmias, such as ventricular tachycardia and ventricular fibrillation. Also used in the management of patients with some types of sudden adult/arrhythmic death syndrome (SADS). The device detects the arrhythmia and delivers a small electric shock to restore sinus rhythm.

**automatism** *n* organized behaviour which occurs without subsequent awareness of it. For example, somnambulism, hysterical and epileptic states.

**autonomic** *adj* independent; self-governing.

**autonomic dysreflexia** a serious condition that can affect people with spinal cord injuries above the level of the seventh thoracic vertebra. It results from a life-threatening sympathetic nervous system response to noxious harmful stimuli, such as bowel distension, constipation, full bladder, etc. It is characterized by tachycardia, hypertension, headache, sweating and flushing above the spinal lesion, seizures, exaggerated reflexes and distension of the bowel or bladder.

**autonomic nervous system (ANS)** is divided into parasympathetic and sympathetic portions. They are made up of nerve cells and fibres which cannot be controlled at will. They are concerned with the control of glandular secretion and involuntary muscle.

**autonomy** *n* the ability to function independently, such as in decision making.

**autopsy** *n* the examination of a dead body (cadaver) for diagnostic purposes.

**autosome** *n* in humans one of 44 (22 pairs) of non-sex chromosomes. The full chromosome complement of 46 (23 pairs) found in somatic cells comprises 44 autosomes and 2 sex chromosomes—**autosomal** *adj* relating to autosomes. *autosomal inheritance* is determined by the expression or not of genes on the autosomes. It may be dominant or recessive.

**autosuggestion** *n* self-suggestion; uncritical acceptance of ideas arising in the individual's own mind. Occurs in hysteria.

**autotransfusion** *n* ⇒ autologous transfusion.

**auxotrophe** *n* a mutant strain of microorganisms that needs specific nutrients for growth not needed by the parent microorganism. Used for microbiological assays of vitamins, etc.

**availability** *n* ⇒ bioavailability.

**avascular** *adj* bloodless; not vascular, i.e. without blood supply. *avascular necrosis* death of tissue due to complete depletion of its blood supply. Usually applied to that of bone tissue following injury or possibly through disease. Commonly seen with fractures of the femoral neck, leading to death of the femoral head. Also seen in scaphoid and head of humerus fractures. Often a precursor of osteoarthritis—**avascularity** n, **avascularize** vt, vi.

**aversion therapy** a method of treatment by deconditioning. Effective in some forms of dependence and abnormal behaviour.

**avian** adj relating to birds.

**avian influenza** 'bird flu'. An extremely contagious viral disease affecting wild birds and domestic poultry. Some strains are highly pathogenic (H5N1) and cause up to 100% mortality in affected birds. Infection and, in some cases, death has occurred in humans who had close contact with sick, dead or dying birds, or infected products, such as faeces. Of major concern to health authorities worldwide is the potential for the virus to mutate to a highly infectious form that is passed from person to person to cause an influenza pandemic.

**avian tuberculosis** is caused by *Mycobacterium avium* complex (MAC) or *M. avium intracellulare* (MAI), which also cause atypical tuberculosis in humans, especially in immunocompromised individuals.

**avidin** n a high-molecular-weight protein with an affinity for biotin which can interfere with the absorption of biotin. Found in raw egg white.

**avitaminosis** n any disease resulting from a deficiency of vitamins.

**Avogadro's number** ⇒ mole.

**AVP** abbr arginine vasopressin.

**AVPU scale** n a simplified tool used to assess level of consciousness. A, alert; V, voice responses present; P, pain response present; U, unresponsive. ⇒ Glasgow Coma Scale.

**avulsion** n a forcible wrenching away of a structure or part of the body.

**axilla** n the armpit.

**axillary** adj applied to nerves, blood and lymphatic vessels, of the axilla. *axillary artery* ⇒ Appendix 1, Figure 9. *axillary vein* ⇒ Appendix 1, Figure 10.

**axis** n **1.** the second cervical vertebra. **2.** an imaginary line passing through the centre; the median line of the body—**axial** adj.

**axolemma** n the membrane of an axon, it covers the cytoplasmic extension of the nerve cell body.

**axon** n the long process of a nerve cell conveying impulses away from the cell body—**axonal** adj.

**axon reflex** reflex dilatation of the arterioles occurring when sensory nerves in the skin are stimulated by trauma or massage manipulations. ⇒ triple response.

**axonotmesis** n (*syn* neuronotmesis, neurotmesis) peripheral degeneration as a result of damage to the axons of a nerve, through pinching, crushing or prolonged pressure. The internal architecture is preserved and recovery depends upon regeneration of the axons, and may take many months.

**azoospermia** n sterility of the male through non-production of spermatozoa.

**azotaemia** n ⇒ uraemia.

**azygos** adj occurring singly, not paired. *azygos veins* three unpaired veins of the abdomen and thorax which empty into the inferior vena cava—**azygous** adj.

## B

**Babinski's reflex or sign** (J F Babinski, French neurologist, 1857–1932) movement of the great toe upwards (dorsiflexion) instead of downwards (plantarflexion) on stroking the sole of the foot. It is indicative of disease or injury to upper motor neurons. Babies exhibit dorsiflexion, but after learning to walk they show the normal plantarflexion response.

**baby blues** a colloquial term for the transient low mood and tearfulness experienced by some women a few days after childbirth.

**baby-bottle tooth decay** dental decay in children aged between 12 months and 3 years. It results from a child being given a bottle just before being put to bed and the consequent prolonged exposure to sugars in the milk or fruit juice.

**bacillaemia** *n* the presence of bacilli in the blood—**bacillaemic** *adj.*

**bacille Calmette–Guérin** ⇒ BCG.

**bacilluria** *n* the presence of bacilli in the urine—**bacilluric** *adj.*

*Bacillus* *n* (also a colloquial term for any rod-shaped micro-organism). A genus of bacteria consisting of aerobic, Gram-positive, rod-shaped cells that produce endospores. The majority have flagella and are motile. The spores are common in soil and dust. *Bacillus anthracis* causes anthrax in humans and domestic animals. *B. cereus* produces exotoxins and causes food poisoning. It can occur after eating cooked food, e.g. rice, that has been stored prior to reheating.

**back-slab splint** a splint specifically produced for the posterior part of a limb, used to immobilize a joint. For example, a lower-limb back-slab splint that extends from ankle to hip is designed to prevent movement at the knee. Uses include minimizing the risk of contracture formation.

**bacteraemia** *n* the presence of bacteria in the blood—**bacteraemic** *adj.*

**bacteria** *npl* microscopic unicellular organisms widely distributed in the environment. They may be free-living, sacrophytic or parasitic. Bacteria can be pathogenic to humans, other animals and plants, or non-pathogenic. Pathogens may be virulent and always cause infection, whereas others, known as opportunists, usually only cause infection when the host defences are impaired, such as during cancer chemotherapy. Non-pathogenic bacteria may become pathogenic if they move from their normal site, e.g. intestinal bacteria causing a wound infection. Reproduction is generally by simple binary fission when environmental conditions are suitable. Many bacteria have developed adaptations that allow them to exploit environments and survive unfriendly conditions, e.g. flagella, pili, waxy outer capsules, spore formation and enzymes that destroy antibiotics. Bacteria are classified and identified by features that include shape and staining characteristics with Gram stain (positive or negative). Bacteria shapes may be (Figure B.1): (a) round (cocci), paired (diplococci), in bunches (staphylococci) or in chains (streptococci); (b) rod-shaped (bacilli); or (c) curved or spiral (vibrios, spirilla and spirochaetes)—**bacterium** *sing.*

**bacterial** *adj* pertaining to bacteria. *bacterial vaginosis* ⇒ vaginosis.

**bactericidal** *adj* describes agents that kill bacteria, e.g. some antibiotics—**bactericide** *n*, **bactericidally** *adv.*

**bactericidin** *n* antibody that kills bacteria.

**bacteriologist** *n* an expert in bacteriology.

**bacteriology** *n* the scientific study of bacteria—**bacteriological** *adj*, **bacteriologically** *adv.*

**bacteriolysin** *n* a specific antibody formed in the blood that causes bacteria to break up.

**bacteriolysis** *n* the disintegration and dissolution of bacteria—**bacteriolytic** *adj.*

**bacteriophage** *n* a virus parasitic on bacteria. Some of these are used in phage-typing staphylococci, etc. ⇒ transduction.

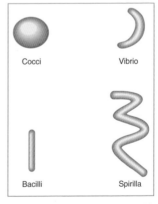

**Figure B.1** Bacterial shapes *(reproduced from Brooker 2006A with permission).*

Cocci

Vibrio

Bacilli

Spirilla

**bacteriostatic** *adj* describes an agent that inhibits bacterial growth, e.g. some antibiotics—**bacteriostasis** *n*.

**bacteriuria** *n* the presence of bacteria in the urine (100 000 or more pathogenic micro-organisms per millilitre). Acute cystitis may be preceded by, and active pyelonephritis may be associated with, asymptomatic bacteriuria.

*Bacteroides* *n* a genus of Gram-negative, anaerobic rod-shaped bacteria, e.g. *Bacteroides fragilis*. They do not form endospores and may be motile or non-motile. They are important commensals in the gastrointestinal flora where they convert complex molecules into simpler substances. The bacteria are also present in the mouth and genital tract. They can cause appendicitis, peritonitis, pelvic inflammatory disease and infections following gastrointestinal and gynaecological surgery. Some species are opportunistic. They are resistant to many antibiotic drugs.

**Bainbridge reflex** *n* (F Bainbridge, British physiologist, 1874–1921) stretch receptors in the heart (right atrium) can increase heart rate through sympathetic stimulation when venous return increases.

**Baker's cyst** (W Baker, British surgeon, 1839–1896) a synovial cyst behind the knee. It may occur with rheumatoid arthritis.

**baker's itch 1.** contact dermatitis resulting from flour or sugar. **2.** itchy papules from the bite of the flour mite *Pyemotes*.

**BAL** *abbr* **1.** British antilewisite. ⇒ dimercaprol. **2.** bronchoalveolar lavage.

**balance** *n* the ability to maintain body equilibrium by controlling the body's centre of gravity over its base of support.

**balance of probabilities** the standard of proof required in civil legal proceedings.

**balanced diet** a diet that contains the correct amount of all nutrients from a wide range of foods. Should also contain the correct proportions of food types, for example, reduced fat, sugar and salt and at least five portions of fruit and vegetables per day.

**balanitis** *n* inflammation of the glans penis. *balanitis xerotica obliterans (BXO)* inflammatory condition involving the glans and prepuce.

**balanoposthitis** *n* inflammation of the glans penis and prepuce.

**balantidiasis** *n* infestation due to ingesting the cysts of the protozoan *Balantidium coli.* Its presence in the large intestine can cause diarrhoea and possibly ulceration of the intestinal wall with abscesses and ulcers.

*Balantidium coli* a parasitic protozoan that causes balantidiasis in humans. It is a commensal micro-organism of the gastrointestinal tract of pigs.

**balanus** *n* the glans of the penis or clitoris.

**baldness** *n* ⇒ alopecia.

**ballism** *n* ⇒ ballismus.

**ballismus** *n* also known as ballism. A neurological condition characterized by uncontrolled ballistic movements. There is jerky, uncoordinated limb movement. It is associated with extrapyramidal conditions. When it affects one side of the body it is termed hemiballismus.

**ballistic movement** high-intensity movement, such as a punch or a tennis serve, which needs the reciprocal activity of agonist and antagonist muscles.

**ballistic stretching** the use of a rapid stretch or repetitive bouncing motions at the end of the available range of movement to increase soft-tissue flexibility.

**ball-and-socket joint** enarthrosis. A synovial joint, e.g. the hip or shoulder, where the ball-shaped head of one bone fits into the cup-like depression in another bone. This type of joint allows the greatest range of motion.

**ballottement** *n* testing for a floating object, especially used to diagnose pregnancy—**ballottable** *adj*.

**balneotherapy** *n* the use of therapeutic bathing in a variety of conditions. It can be used, for instance, to improve mobility or reduce pain. ⇒ hydrotherapy.

**bandage** *n* material applied to a wound or used to bind an injured part of the body. May be used to: (a) retain a dressing or splint; (b) support, compress, immobilize; (c) prevent or correct deformity. Available in strips or circular form in a range of different materials and applying varying levels of pressure. Compression bandages are widely used in the management of venous leg ulceration.

**Bandl's ring** (L Bandl, German obstetrician, 1842–1892) an abnormally enlarged retraction ring that forms between the upper and lower uterine segments, as the lower segment continues to thin if labour is obstructed. It presents as an oblique ridge seen above the symphysis pubis. ⇒ retraction ring.

**Bankart lesion** (A Bankart, British orthopaedic surgeon, 1879–1951) a traumatic detachment of the glenoid labrum, glenohumeral ligaments and damage to the capsular attachment.

**Bankart's operation** (A Bankart) for recurrent dislocation of the shoulder joint: the defect of the glenoid cavity is repaired.

**Banti's syndrome** (G Banti, Italian pathologist, 1852–1925) a syndrome characterized by hepatic portal hypertension, splenomegaly, gastrointestinal bleeding, leucopenia and anaemia. It is associated with liver cirrhosis.

**Barbados leg** (*syn* elephant leg) ⇒ elephantiasis.

**barbiturates** *npl* a group of sedative/hypnotic drugs. They are associated with serious problems of dependence and tolerance, and sudden withdrawal may cause a serious withdrawal syndrome that includes anxiety, convulsions and even death. They have been replaced by safer drugs and their use is limited to anaesthesia and sometimes for epilepsy.

**barbotage** *n* a method of extending the spread of spinal anaesthesia whereby local anaesthetic is directly mixed with aspirated cerebrospinal fluid and reinjected into the subarachnoid space.

**bariatrics** *n* a branch of medicine and surgery that deals with obesity, its effects and control.

**baritosis** *n* a form of pneumoconiosis caused by the inhalation of barium dust.

**barium enema** a radiographic examination of the large bowel using barium sulphate as the contrast medium. Barium sulphate liquid, plus a quantity of air, is introduced into the large bowel by means of a rectal tube, during fluoroscopy. It is used for diagnostic purposes, e.g. for colon cancers, in conjunction with endoscopy. ⇒ barium sulphate, colonoscopy.

**barium meal, swallow** a radiographic examination of the upper gastrointestinal tract (oesophagus and stomach) and the small intestine with follow-through X-rays, using barium sulphate as the contrast medium. The barium sulphate suspension is swallowed and X-rays are taken of the gastrointestinal tract. Pre-examination fasting is required and medicines, e.g. some antacids, that may interfere with the examination should be stopped. Further fasting may be required until follow-through X-rays are completed.

**barium sulphate** a heavy insoluble powder used, in an aqueous suspension, as a contrast medium in X-ray visualization of the alimentary tract.

**Barlow's sign/test** a manoeuvre designed to test for congenitally dislocatable hips in the neonate. Often used in association with the Ortolani sign/test. ⇒ developmental dysplasia of the hip.

**barodontalgia** *n* also called aerodontalgia. Pain in a tooth due to a decrease in atmospheric pressure, such as occurs at high altitude.

**baroreceptors** *npl* sensory nerve endings which respond to pressure changes. They are present in the cardiac atria, aortic arch, venae cavae, carotid sinus and the inner ear.

**barotitis** *n* also called aerotitis. Inflammation affecting the ear caused by changes in atmospheric pressure.

**barotrauma** *n* injury due to unequalized changes in atmospheric or water pressure, e.g. ruptured eardrum.

**Barr body** ⇒ sex chromatin.

**Barrett's oesophagus** (N R Barrett, British surgeon, 1903–1979) columnar-lined oesophagus replacing normal squamous mucosa. Related to chronic gastro-oesophageal reflux disease (GORD). Predisposes to oesophageal cancer. ⊙DVD

**barrier nursing** a method of preventing the spread of infection from an infectious individual to other people. It is achieved by isolation techniques. ⇒ containment isolation, isolation, protective isolation, source isolation.

**Barron's banding apparatus** a device used to treat haemorrhoids by elastic band ligation.

**Barthel index** (D Barthel, American psychiatrist, 20th century) a disability profiles score. It is based on an assessment of a person's ability to self-care in 10 functional areas, which include dressing, hygiene, bladder and bowel control, feeding and walking.

**Bartholin's glands (greater vestibular glands)** (C Bartholin, Danish anatomist, 1655–1738) two small glands situated at each side of the external orifice of the vagina. Their ducts open into the vestibule. They produce lubricating mucus that facilitates coitus.

**bartholinitis** *n* inflammation of Bartholin's (greater vestibular) glands.

***Bartonella*** *n* (A Barton, Peruvian bacteriologist, 1871–1950) a genus of Gram-negative micro-organisms. Various species infect red blood cells, liver, spleen and lymph nodes. *Bartonella bacilliformis* causes bartonellosis; *B. henselae* causes cat-scratch fever. Other species cause trench fever, endocarditis and myocarditis.

**bartonellosis** *n* an infection caused by *B. bacilliformis*. It is transmitted by the bite of a sandfly and causes anaemia, fever and skin lesions. The infection is endemic in valleys of the Andes across Colombia, Peru and Ecuador. Known as Oroya fever, Carrión's disease or verruga peruana.

**Bartter syndrome** (F Bartter, American physician, 1914–1983) a rare genetic syndrome which affects the kidneys resulting in secondary hyperaldosteronism. The blood pressure is usually normal or low even though the levels of renin and angiotensin are raised. There are problems with electrolyte and acid–base balance; hypokalaemia, hypercalciuria and metabolic alkalosis. The infant/child may have excessive thirst (polydipsia) and pass large volumes of urine (polyuria) and life-threatening dehydration can occur if fluids are not replaced. Muscle weakness is a feature and physical growth and mental development may be slowed. Hypercalciuria can lead to kidney stones and possibly end-stage renal failure. Management includes potassium supplements; potassium-sparing drugs, e.g. spironolactone; angiotensin-converting enzyme (ACE) inhibitor drugs; and, for some types of Bartter syndrome, non-steroidal anti-inflammatory drugs (NSAIDs).

**basal cell carcinoma (BCC)** rodent ulcer. A common type of skin cancer, often seen on the face. Although locally invasive, it does not give rise to metastases. ⊙DVD

**basal ganglia** ⇒ basal nuclei.

**basal metabolic rate (BMR)** some authorities use the term resting metabolic rate. The rate at which energy is consumed at complete rest for essential physiological functions. It is the expression of basal metabolism in terms of kilojoules per square metre of body surface per hour. BMR is influenced by nutritional status, age, gender, physiological status, disease, certain drugs and ambient temperature. It is determined by measuring the oxygen consumption when the energy output has been reduced to a basal minimum, that is, the person is fasting and is physically and mentally at rest. In clinical practice it is usually estimated by prediction equations and used to estimate energy requirements. ⇒ metabolic equivalents.

**basal narcosis** the preanaesthetic administration of narcotic drugs which reduce fear and anxiety and induce sleep.

**basal nuclei** a collection of interconnected nuclei (masses of grey matter) deep within the cerebral hemispheres concerned with cognition, and modifying and co-ordinating voluntary muscle movement. Their proper functioning requires the release of the neurotransmitter dopamine. Sometimes erroneously referred to as ganglia, which more properly describes structures in the peripheral nervous system. Site of degeneration in Parkinson's disease. ⇒ dopamine.

**base** *n* **1.** the lowest part, such as the lung. ⇒ Appendix 1, Figure 7. **2.** the major part of a compound. **3.** an alkali—**basal, basic** *adj*.

**base of support** the area between the body part and the surface with which it makes contact. The larger the base of support, the less muscle activity is required. For instance, less muscular activity is needed when sitting in a chair than when standing up, or trying to balance on one foot.

**baseline measurements 1.** the routine recording of vital signs when a person is either admitted to a health care facility, or consults a health professional as an outpatient. These might include temperature, pulse, respiration and blood pressure and they provide an initial baseline from which to compare subsequent recordings. **2.** in sports medicine the initial physical findings which are usually performed while the athlete is in a healthy state.

**basement membrane** *n* the thin layer of tissue that separates epithelium from the underlying structures.

**basic life support (BLS)** a term that describes the application of artificial respiration, usually by rescue breaths (mouth-to-mouth/nose breathing) and chest compressions (external cardiac massage) to save life without the use of artificial aids or equipment in the case of cardiac or respiratory arrest. Techniques differ between adult BLS, paediatric BLS and newborn life support. ⊙DVD

**basilar artery** *n* forms part of the circulus arteriosus (circle of Willis); it supplies blood to the brainstem.

**basilar membrane** *n* the membrane between the scala media and the scala tympani in the cochlea of the inner ear. It has the specialized cochlear hair cells that contain the auditory receptors. ⇒ Reissner's membrane.

**basilic** *adj* prominent.

**basilic vein** *n* a superficial vein that begins on the ulnar aspect of the back of the hand and carries blood up the medial side of the forearm to empty into the deep veins of the arm. ⇒ Appendix 1, Figure 10.

**basophil** *n* **1.** a cell which has an affinity for basic dyes. **2.** a polymorphonuclear granulocyte (white blood cell) which takes up a particular dye: it is phagocytic and has granules containing heparin and histamine.

**basophilia** *n* **1.** increase in the number of basophils in the blood. **2.** basophilic staining of red blood cells.

**Batchelor plaster** a type of double abduction plaster, with the legs encased from groins to ankles, in full abduction and medial rotation. The feet are then attached to a wooden pole or 'broomstick'. Alternative to frog plaster, but the hips are free. ⇒ developmental dysplasia of the hip.

**bat ears** the outer/external ear protrudes away from the head. They can be corrected by surgery if the child/parent or person is unhappy about appearance.

**bath** *n* **1.** the apparatus used for bathing. **2.** the immersion of the body or any part of it in water or any fluid; or the application of spray, jet or vapour of such a fluid to the body. The term is modified according to: (a) temperature, e.g. cold, contrast, hot, tepid; (b) medium used, e.g. mud, water, wax; (c) medicament added, e.g. potassium permanganate; (d) function of medicament, e.g. astringent, antiseptic. ⇒ balneotherapy, hydrotherapy.

**Batten's disease** (F Batten, British neurologist, 1865–1918) one of a group of genetic diseases characterized by disordered metabolism of fatty acids leading to visual impairment, encephalopathy and progressive mental deterioration.

**battery** *n* legal term. An unlawful touching or contact. Constitutes a trespass against the person. ⇒ assault.

**Battle's sign** (W Battle, British surgeon, 1855–1936) ecchymosis or bogginess felt over the mastoid process indicative of a skull fracture.

**Bazin's disease** (*syn* erythema induratum) (P Bazin, French dermatologist, 1807–1878) a chronic recurrent disorder, involving the skin of the legs of women. There are deep-seated nodules which later ulcerate.

**BBA** *abbr* born before arrival (at hospital).

**BBB** *abbr* **1.** blood–brain barrier. **2.** bundle branch block.

**BBV** *abbr* blood-borne virus.

**BCC** *abbr* basal cell carcinoma.

**B cells** ⇒ lymphocytes.

**BCG** *abbr* bacille Calmette–Guérin. An attenuated form of tubercle bacilli: it has lost its power to cause tuberculosis, but retains its antigenic function; it is the base of a vaccine used for immunization against tuberculosis. In the UK it is offered to groups at increased risk, e.g. all newborns and infants who live in a high-risk area where tuberculosis cases are greater than 40 per 100 000, people in contact with cases of active tuberculosis, etc.

Also used in urology for the treatment of high-risk superficial bladder cancer.

**BDD** *abbr* body dysmorphic disorder.

**bdelygmia** *n* an extreme dislike or loathing for food.

**beam** *n* metal pole attached to a hospital bed to facilitate the use of traction. For example, a Thomas' splint can be slung up, with pulleys and weights attached, to allow movement and provide counterbalance to the weight of the splint and leg.

**bearing-down** *n* **1.** a lay term for the expulsive contractions in the second stage of labour. **2.** a feeling of weight and descent in the pelvis associated with uterine prolapse or pelvic tumours.

**beat** *n* pulsation of the blood in the heart and blood vessels. *apex beat* ⇒ apex. *dropped beat* refers to the loss of an occasional ventricular beat as occurs in extrasystoles. *premature beat* an extrasystole.

**Beau's lines** (J Beau, French physician, 1806–1865) transverse ridges or grooves which reflect a temporary retardation of the normal nail growth following a debilitating illness (Figure B.2). They first appear towards the proximal nail fold and move towards the free edge as the nail grows. The distance the groove has moved indicates quite accurately the length of time since the illness or trauma (nail growth being about 1 mm per week).

**Becker muscular dystrophy** (P Becker, German geneticist, 1908–2000) a type of muscular dystrophy inherited as an X-chromosome recessive condition. It is less severe than Duchenne muscular dystrophy and has a better prognosis. Also known as benign pseudohypertrophic muscular dystrophy.

**Beck's triad** (C Beck, American surgeon, 1894–1971) hypotension, muffled heart sounds and neck vein distension; the three principal physical signs of cardiac tamponade.

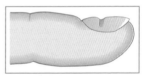

**Figure B.2** Beau's lines *(reproduced from Boon et al. 2006 with permission).*

**becquerel (Bq)** *n* (A H Becquerel, French physicist, 1852–1908) the derived SI unit (International System of Units) for radioactivity. Equals the amount of a radioactive substance undergoing one nuclear disintegration per second. Has replaced the curie. ⇒ Appendix 2.

**bedbug** *n* a blood-sucking insect belonging to the genus *Cimex*. The commonest species are *Cimex lectularius* in temperate zones and *C. hemipterus* in tropical zones. They live and lay eggs in cracks and crevices of furniture and walls. They are active at night and their bites provide a route for secondary infection.

**bedsore** *n* obsolete term. ⇒ pressure ulcer.

**bed-wetting** *n* ⇒ enuresis.

**Beevor's sign** movement of the umbilicus as an athlete performs a half sit-up. It indicates an interruption to the nerve supply (innervation) of the abdominal muscles.

**behaviour** *n* the observable behavioural response of a person to an internal or external stimulus.

**behaviour change** psychological concept generally applied to lifestyle in relation to health. An approach used in health education, whereby individuals are encouraged to make lifestyle changes by providing information, looking at existing health beliefs and values and increasing self-confidence. The change may be the adoption of health-protective behaviour (e.g. healthy eating, regular exercise) or changing health-threatening behaviour (e.g. excessive alcohol intake, smoking).

**behaviourism** *n* in psychology describes an approach which studies and interprets behaviour by objective observation of that behaviour without regard to any subjective mental processes such as ideas, emotions and will. Behaviour is considered to be a series of conditioned reflexes.

**behaviour modification** in a general sense, an inevitable part of living, resulting from the consistent rewarding or punishing of response to a stimulus, whether that response is negative or positive. Some education systems deliberately employ a modification approach to maximize learning.

**behaviour therapy** a type of psychotherapy to modify observable, maladjusted patterns of behaviour by the substitution of a learned response or set of responses to a stimulus. The treatment is designed for a particular patient and not for the particular diagnostic label which has been attached to that patient. Such treatment includes assertiveness training, aversion therapy, conditioning and desensitization.

**Behçet syndrome** (H Behçet, Turkish dermatologist, 1889–1948) a form of systemic vasculitis. There is stomatitis, genital ulceration, retinitis and uveitis. There may also be skin nodules, thrombophlebitis and arthritis affecting one or more of the large joints. Gastrointestinal and neurological complications may occur. The syndrome is associated with the presence of a certain human leucocyte antigen (HLA). Treatment is with non-steroidal anti-inflammatory drugs, corticosteroids and immunosuppressant drugs.

**BEI** *abbr* bioelectrical impedance.

**bejel** *n* a non-venereal form of syphilis mainly affecting children in the Middle East and sub-Saharan Africa. The causative organism is *Treponema pallidum* (ssp. *endemicum*). It usually starts in the mouth and affects mucosae, skin and bones. ⇒ pinta, yaws.

**beliefs** *npl* a set of ideas and thoughts that a person uses to construct attitudes, views and behaviour. They are formed by culture, family, experiences and many other factors.

**belladonna** *n* deadly nightshade. The poisonous alkaloid (*Atropa belladonna*) contains atropine and other muscarinic antagonists.

**bell and pad** a psychological approach to the management of bed-wetting in children. A special pad/sheet is placed on the mattress and when the child starts to void urine, a buzzer or bell sounds. This wakens the child who completes the voiding of urine in a potty or on the lavatory.

**belle indifférence** the incongruous lack of appropriate affect in the presence of incapacitating symptoms commonly shown by patients with dissociative disorders.

**Bell's palsy** (C Bell, British surgeon and anatomist, 1774–1842) usually non-permanent facial hemiparesis due to idiopathic (cause unknown) lesion of the seventh (facial) cranial nerve.

**Bell's phenomenon** a sign present in peripheral facial paralysis. There is upward and outward movement of the eyeball, on the affected side, when the person attempts to close the eye.

**Bence Jones protein** (H Bence Jones, British physician, 1814–1873) an abnormal protein that is excreted in the urine of some patients with multiple myeloma, composed of fragments of immunoglobulin molecules.

**benchmarking** *n* part of quality assurance. Involves the identification of examples of best practice from others engaged in similar practice. From this, best-practice benchmark scores in agreed areas of care are identified, against which individual units can compare their own performance.

**bends** *npl* (*syn* caisson disease) ⇒ decompression sickness/illness.

**beneficence** *n* the principle of doing good that also includes avoiding, removing and preventing harm and promoting good. Ethical dilemmas and problems may arise when the common good is at odds with that for individuals. ⇒ non-maleficence.

**benign** *adj* **1.** non-malignant (of a growth), non-invasive (no capacity to metastasize), non-cancerous (of a growth). **2.** describes a condition or illness which is not serious and does not usually have harmful consequences.

**benign hypotonia** describes infants who are initially floppy but otherwise healthy. Improvement occurs and the infant regains normal tone and motor development.

**benign intracranial hypertension (BIH)** a condition in which there is raised intracranial pressure with papilloedema and which can lead to the loss of vision, typically in young, obese women. Often associated with thrombosis in the sagittal sinus.

**benign paroxysmal positional vertigo (BPPV)** short-lived rotatory vertigo associated with sudden movements of the head. It is a common condition and often occurs after a head injury. It is thought to be caused by chalk-like debris dislodged into the semicircular canals. The vertigo may last for a few seconds to minutes. Typically it happens when the person lies down or gets up from the bed. Specific manoeuvres, such as the Epley manoeuvre, can improve the condition but may need to be repeated.

**benign prostatic enlargement (BPE)** also called benign prostatic hyperplasia/hypertrophy. The increase in the size of the prostate gland due either to an increase in cell size or the growth of new cells; it generally occurs in older men. It leads to urinary problems that include hesitancy, poor stream, dribbling, frequency and retention. Management may be with drugs, e.g. finasteride, to shrink the gland; minimally invasive techniques that include stent insertion, ultrasound, various laser techniques, vaporization and microwave; or by transurethral resection of the prostate gland (TUR, TURP).

**Bennett's fracture** (E Bennett, Irish surgeon, 1837–1907) fracture of proximal end of first metacarpal involving the articular surface.

**benzene** *n* a colourless inflammable liquid obtained from coal tar. Extensively used as a solvent. Continued occupational exposure to it results in aplastic anaemia and, rarely, leukaemia.

**benzodiazepines** *npl* a group of anxiolytic/hypnotic drugs, e.g. diazepam, midazolam. Dependence and withdrawal problems may occur. They may be misused. ⇒ Appendix 5.

**benzoic acid** an antiseptic and antifungal agent used sometimes in an ointment for ringworm.

**benzoin** *n* (*syn* Friar's balsam) a resin of balsam used traditionally in inhalations but of doubtful value.

**bereavement** *n* a response to a life event involving loss. Includes that which happens to a person after the death of another person who has been important in his or her life. It also occurs in other situations of loss, such as redundancy, loss of home, divorce or loss of a body part, e.g. mastectomy, amputation. ⇒ grieving process.

**Berger's disease/nephropathy** (J Berger, French nephrologist, 20th century) also called mesangial IgA nephropathy. A common type of glomerulonephritis characterized by the deposition of immunoglobulin A (IgA) in the glomeruli. There is macroscopic and/or microscopic haematuria and proteinuria, which may progress to renal failure.

**beri-beri** *n* a deficiency disease caused by lack of vitamin $B_1$ (thiamin[e]). It occurs mainly in those countries where the staple diet is polished rice. Beri-beri is usually described as either 'wet' (cardiac) or 'dry' (neurological) depending on the symptoms. The symptoms are pain from neuritis, paralysis, muscular wasting, progressive oedema, mental deterioration and, finally, heart failure.

**berylliosis** *n* an industrial disease: there is impaired lung function because of interstitial fibrosis from inhalation of beryllium. Corticosteroids are used in treatment.

**Best's disease** (F Best, German ophthalmologist, 20th century) ⇒ vitelliform macular degeneration.

**beta (β)-adrenoceptor agonists** (*syn* beta-stimulants, sympathomimetics) a group of drugs that stimulate β-adrenoceptors, e.g. dobutamine, salbutamol. ⇒ Appendix 5.

**beta (β)-adrenoceptor antagonists** (*syn* beta-blockers) a group of drugs that block the stimulation of β-adrenoceptors in the myocardium and other locations, e.g. atenolol, propranolol. ⇒ Appendix 5.

**beta-blockers** *npl* ⇒ beta (β)-adrenoceptor antagonists.

**beta (β)-lactam antibiotics** antibiotics containing a β-lactam ring in their structure (Figure B.3). They include the cephalosporins and penicillins. Many bacteria produce enzymes (β-lactamases) that destroy the β-lactam ring, which renders the antibiotic ineffective.

**beta (β)-lactamases** previously known as penicillinases. The enzymes, produced by certain bacteria, e.g. most staphylococci and *Escherichia coli*, that destroy β-lactam antibiotics.

**beta (β) oxidation** metabolic process whereby fatty acids are converted to acetyl coenzyme A prior to the production of energy (adenosine triphosphate [ATP]).

**beta (β) phase** the period after the alpha redistribution phase of drug administration. There is a slow decrease in drug blood levels during its metabolism and excretion.

**betatron** *n* an accelerator device used to produce a stream of high-energy electrons for use during some types of radiotherapy.

**bezoar** *n* a compacted mass of hair and/or vegetable material found within the stomach. The ingestion of such material can be a feature of some forms of mental distress. The bezoar can eventually obstruct gastric emptying. Strictly speaking, a mass comprising only hair (the person's own hair or that from animals) is called a trichobezoar.

**biacromial measure** the width of the shoulder.

**bibliographical databases** details of papers, etc., but sometimes abstracts and full articles, are available electronically via CD-ROM or the internet, e.g. MEDLINE.

**bicarbonate (hydrogen carbonate) (HCO₃⁻)** *n* an anion. Important in pH regulation and the acid–base balance in the body.

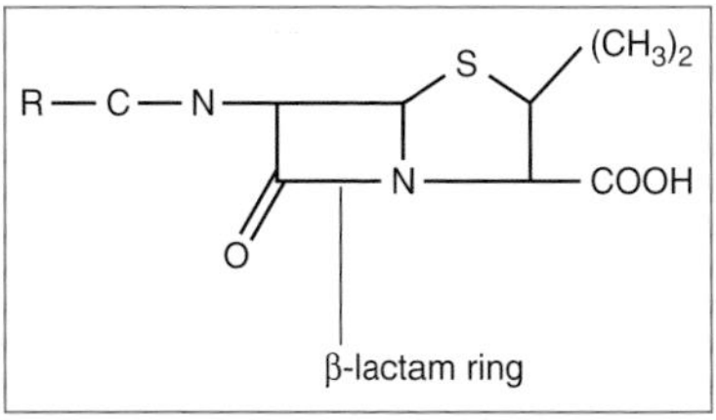

**Figure B.3** Beta-lactam ring *(reproduced from Wilson 1995 with permission).*

Also called hydrogen carbonate. *serum (plasma) bicarbonate* that in the blood. Represents the alkali reserve.

**bicellular** *adj* composed of two cells.

**biceps** *n* two-headed muscle. *biceps brachii* the two-headed muscle on the anterior surface of the upper arm. Its origins are on the coracoid process and the glenoid cavity and it inserts on to the radius. It flexes the elbow joint and supinates the forearm and the hand. ⇒ Appendix 1, Figure 4. *biceps femoris* two-headed muscle, the most lateral on the posterior surface of the thigh. Its origins are on the ischial tuberosity and the femur and it inserts into the fibula and the lateral condyle of the tibia. It extends the thigh and flexes the knee joint. Also rotates the leg laterally when the knee is flexed. It is one of the three hamstring muscles. ⇒ semimembranosus, semitedinosus, Appendix 1, Figure 5.

**biconcave** *adj* concave or hollow on both surfaces, as in the shape of a normal red blood cell, or the shape of a divergent lens used to correct myopia.

**biconvex** *adj* convex on both surfaces, as in the shape of a convergent lens used to correct hypermetropia.

**bicornuate** *adj* having two horns; generally applied to a double uterus or a single uterus possessing two horns.

**bicristal measure** the width of the hip.

**bicuspid** *adj* having two cusps or points. *bicuspid teeth* the premolars. *bicuspid valve* the mitral valve between the left atrium and ventricle of the heart.

**BID** *abbr* brought in (to hospital) dead.

**Bielschowsky's head tilt test** (A Bielschowsky, German ophthalmologist, 1871–1940) a test used to determine a weakness affecting the superior oblique muscle (extraocular/extrinsic muscle of the eye) caused by damage to the fourth (trochlear) cranial nerve.

**bifid** *adj* divided into two parts. Cleft or forked.

**bifidus factor** a carbohydrate constituent of human milk. It stimulates the growth of the bacterium *Lactobacillus bifidus* in the bowel. The presence of this micro-organism reduces the pH within the bowel contents and inhibits the establishment and growth of pathogenic bacteria.

**bifocal lens** a lens with two separate parts that have different focal lengths. This facilitates corrected vision for near and distant objects by using a single pair of spectacles or contact lenses.

**B**

**bifurcation** *n* division into two branches, such as the bifurcation of the trachea to form the two main bronchi—**bifurcate** *adj*, *vt*, *vi*.

**bigeminy** *n* a cardiac arrhythmia in which two rapid beats are followed by a longer pause. Every other beat is premature.

**biguanides** *npl* a group of oral hypoglycaemic drugs, e.g. metformin hydrochloride. ⇒ Appendix 5.

**BIH** *abbr* benign intracranial hypertension.

**bilateral** *adj* pertaining to both sides—**bilaterally** *adv*.

**bile** *n* a bitter, alkaline, viscid, greenish-yellow fluid secreted by the liver and stored in the gallbladder. 500–1000 mL is produced each day. Bile leaves the gallbladder in response to the secretion of cholecystokinin by intestinal cells when fatty foods enter the duodenum. Bile contains water, mineral salts, mucin, lecithin, cholesterol, bile salts (derived from bile acids), the pigments bilirubin and biliverdin and substances (e.g. drug residues) for excretion. Bile emulsifies the fats in food to form smaller particles to allow digestion and absorption, facilitates the absorption of fat-soluble vitamins, stimulates peristalsis and deodorizes faeces.

**bile acids** *npl* organic acids produced by the liver during the metabolism of cholesterol. They include cholic acid, chenodeoxycholic acid, taurocholic acid and glycocholic acid. The bile acids entering the duodenum in the bile are in the form of bile salts, and most of these are reabsorbed to be reused. ⇒ enterohepatic circulation.

**bile ducts** *npl* the ducts forming the biliary tract; the right and left hepatic ducts, common hepatic duct and cystic duct, which join to form the common bile duct that empties bile into the duodenum. ⇒ biliary tract.

**bile pigments** *npl* ⇒ bilirubin, biliverdin.

**bile salts** *npl* sodium glycocholate and sodium taurocholate present in bile are formed from bile acids. They act as surfactants and reduce surface tension to emulsify fats in the small intestine—**bilious**, **biliary** *adj*.

**Bilharzia** *n* ⇒ Schistosoma.

**bilharziasis** *n* ⇒ schistosomiasis.

**biliary** *adj* pertaining to bile.

**biliary atresia** congenital condition characterized by the absence or abnormal development of the bile ducts, resulting in a failure to drain bile with jaundice and, in the absence of effective treatment, irreversible damage to the liver and eventually hepatic portal hypertension. Surgical correction is only possible in a few cases but increasingly a liver transplant is a treatment option.

**biliary colic** pain in the right upper quadrant of abdomen, due to obstruction of the gallbladder or common bile duct, usually by a gallstone (calculus); it may last several hours and is usually steady, which differentiates it from other forms of colic. Vomiting may occur.

**biliary fistula** an abnormal track conveying bile to the surface or to some other organ.

**biliary tract** the bile ducts and gallbladder. The pathway from the canaliculi in the liver, by way of the gallbladder, to the opening of the common bile duct into the duodenum at the hepatopancreatic ampulla (Figure B.4).

**bilious** *adj* **1.** a word usually used to signify vomit containing bile. **2.** a non-medical term, usually meaning 'suffering from indigestion'.

**bilirubin** *n* a red bile pigment mostly derived from haemoglobin during red blood cell breakdown. Unconjugated fat-soluble bilirubin, which gives an indirect reaction with van den Bergh's test, is potentially toxic to metabolically active tissues, particularly the basal nuclei of the immature brain. Unconjugated bilirubin is transported to the liver in the blood attached to albumen to make it less likely to enter and damage brain cells. In the liver the enzyme glucuronyl transferase conjugates fat-soluble bilirubin with glucuronic acid to make it water-soluble, in which state it is relatively non-toxic (reacts directly with van den Bergh's test) and can be excreted in the bile. ⇒ haemolytic disease of the newborn, jaundice, phototherapy.

**bilirubinaemia** *n* the presence of bilirubin in the blood. Sometimes used (incorrectly) for an excess of bilirubin in the blood. ⇒ hyperbilirubinaemia.

**bilirubinuria** *n* the presence of the bile pigment bilirubin in the urine.

**biliverdin** *n* the green pigment formed by oxidation of bilirubin.

**Billings' method** (J & E Billings, Australian physicians, 20th century) a method of natural family planning that uses the changes in cervical mucus during the menstrual cycle to estimate the timing of ovulation. The mucus increases in amount and becomes clear, thinner, slippery and more elastic during the time around ovulation. ⇒ ferning, spinnbarkeit.

**Billroth's operation** (C Billroth, Austrian surgeon, 1829–1894) ⇒ gastrectomy.

**bilobate** *adj* having two lobes.

**bilobular** *adj* having two little lobes or lobules.

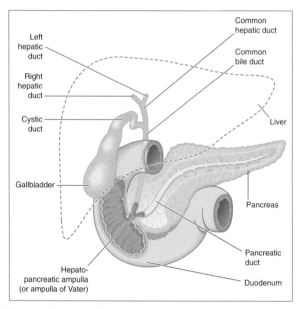

**Figure B.4** Biliary tract *(reproduced from Brooker & Nicol 2003 with permission).*

**bimanual** *adj* performed with both hands. A method of examination sometimes used in gynaecology whereby the internal genital organs are examined between one hand on the abdomen and one or two fingers of the other hand within the vagina.

**binary fission** a method of reproduction common among the bacteria and protozoa. The cell divides into two equal 'daughter' cells.

**binaural** *adj* pertaining to, or having two ears. Applied to a type of stethoscope.

**Binet's test** (A Binet, French psychologist, 1857–1911) a test of mental capacity in children and young people. The answers given to a series of questions (standardized for mental capacity of normal children at different ages) are used to calculate the mental age of the child being tested.

**binge–purge syndrome** ⇒ bulimia.

**binocular vision** the focusing of both eyes on one object at the same time, in such a way that only one image of the object is seen.

**binovular** *adj* derived from two separate ova. Binovular twins may be of different sexes. ⇒ uniovular *opp*.

**bioassay** *n* the measurement of biologically active compounds (e.g. hormones, vitamins and essential amino acids) by their ability to support growth of animals or microorganisms.

**bioavailability** *n* the amount of a drug (or nutrient) that enters the circulation in the active form. It is dependent on the route of administration and the degree to which the drug is metabolized before it reaches the blood stream. Drugs administered intravenously will have 100% bioavailability, whereas those given orally may not be fully absorbed and are subject to first-pass metabolism/effect in the liver. Some drugs are totally metabolized in the liver, e.g. glyceryl trinitrate, so other routes of administration must be used such as sublingually or transdermally.

**biochemistry** *n* the chemistry of life and organic molecules—**biochemical** *adj*.

**biocytin** *n* the main form of the biotin (part of the B-vitamin group) in most foods, bound to lysine, an amino acid.

**bioelectrical impedance (BEI)** a way of measuring the proportion of fat in the body.

59

An electric current is passed through the body and the amount of fat can be calculated by the difference in the resistance to the electric current between fat and lean muscle tissue. Various factors, including hydration status, can affect the result.

**bioethics** *n* the application of ethical principles to biological problems.

**biofeedback** *n* presentation of immediate visual or auditory information about usually unconscious body functions such as blood pressure, heart rate and muscle tension. Either by trial and error or by operant conditioning a person can learn to repeat behaviour which results in a satisfactory level of body functions.

**biofilm** *n* collection of micro-organisms and their products that adhere to a surface, e.g. a urinary catheter.

**bioflavonoids** *npl* ⇒ flavonoids.

**biofortification** *n* improving the nutrient content of plants through genetic modification or selective plant breeding. For example, increasing the essential amino acid content of certain staple cereal crops.

**biohazard** *n* anything that presents a hazard to life. For instance, some specimens for the pathological laboratory are so labelled.

**bioinformatics** *n* the application of computer technology and techniques to extract meaning from complex, multifaceted biological data.

**biological body 'clock'** an inherent timing mechanism that controls physiological processes and is not dependent on external factors.

**biological engineering** designing microelectronic or mechanical equipment for external use by patients: for attachment to patients, or placement inside patients.

**biological response modifier (BRM)** cancer treatment that manipulates the patient's immune response in order to destroy cancer cells. They include colony-stimulating factors, interleukins and interferons.

**biological value (BV)** the quantity of absorbed nitrogen from food that is retained for body maintenance, repair and/or growth.

**biology** *n* the science of life, concerned with the structure, function and organization of all living organisms—**biological** *adj*, **biologically** *adv*.

**biomechanics** *n* the study of the structure and function of biological systems relative to the methods of mechanics.

**biometry** *n* the application of statistical methods to analyse data/measurements obtained in biological research.

**biopsy** *n* excision of tissue to provide a sample for microscopic examination to establish a precise diagnosis, such as the type and degree of differentiation in a malignant tumour.

**biopsychosocial** *adj* relating to biological, psychological and social perspectives.

**biorhythm** *n* the cyclical patterns of biological functions unique to each person, e.g. sleep–wake cycles, body temperature, etc.—**biorhythmic** *adj*.

**biosensors** *npl* non-invasive devices that measure the result of biological processes, e.g. skin temperature or blood oxygen saturation.

**biotechnology** *n* the use of biology in the scientific study of technology and vice versa—**biotechnical** *adj*, **biotechnically** *adv*.

**biotin** *n* a member of vitamin B complex. Dietary sources are liver, soya flour, egg yolk, cereals and yeast. It is also synthesized by commensal bacteria in the colon. Deficiency is rare in humans; symptoms include fatigue, anorexia, muscle pains and dermatitis. ⇒ biocytin.

**BIPAP** *abbr* biphasic positive airways pressure.

**biparous** *adj* producing two offspring at one birth.

**biphasic positive airways pressure (BIPAP)** mode of ventilatory (respiratory) support in which the airway pressure alternates between two levels. The higher pressure ventilates the patient or provides pressure support, whilst the lower pressure acts as positive end-expiratory pressure/continuous positive airway pressure. Can be delivered non-invasively (without intubation) by mask to patients with chronic lung disease or as an aid to weaning from ventilatory support.

**bipolar** *adj* having two poles.

**bipolar affective disorder** (*syn* bipolar depression, manic-depressive illness) a disorder of mood that is characterized by repeated episodes of mania/hypomania and depression.

**bird-fancier's lung** a respiratory disease. It is a type of extrinsic alveolitis that is caused by inhaling avian protein allergens found in bird excreta and feathers. Can occur in individuals who keep birds such as pigeons. ⇒ extrinsic allergic alveolitis.

**birefringence** *n* double refraction, a characteristic of some natural substances, such as crystals of calcite (calcium carbonate) and some biological materials. As a ray of light passes through the material it is split into two light rays.

**birth** *n* the act of expelling the young from the mother's body; delivery; being born. *premature* *birth* one occurring between 24 and 37 weeks of pregnancy.

**birth canal** the cavity or canal of the pelvis through which the fetus passes during labour.

**birth centres** a self-contained unit where the emphasis is on supporting normal births in a more homely (less medical) environment. They may be sited within a hospital, adjacent to a hospital or completely separate from the hospital site.

**birth certificate** in the UK a legal document given on registration, within 42 days of a birth.

**birth control** prevention or regulation of conception by any means; contraception.

**birth injury** any injury occurring during parturition, e.g. fracture of a bone, subluxation of a joint, injury to peripheral nerve, intracranial haemorrhage, etc.

**birth mark** naevus.

**birth rate** the *crude birth rate* is the number of births as a proportion of a population. It is expressed as the number of live births per 1000 population in 1 year. *refined birth rate* ratio of the total number of births to the female population over a 1 year. *true birth rate* the ratio of total births to the female population of child-bearing age (between 15 and 44 years).

**bisexual** *adj* **1.** having some of the physical genital characteristics of both sexes; a hermaphrodite. When there is gonadal tissue of both sexes in the same person, that person is a true hermaphrodite. **2.** describes a person who is sexually attracted to both men and women.

**Bishop's score** (E H Bishop, obstetrician, 1913–1995) an assessment of the cervix used in induction of labour. The score is made up of the sum of individual scores of 0, 1 or 2 assigned for cervical effacement, consistency, dilatation and position along with a score for the station of the presenting part. A score of 4 or less suggests that induction may be difficult. ⇒ cervical effacement.

**bisphosphonates** *npl* drugs that reduce bone turnover, e.g. disodium etidronate. Used in the management of bone diseases and the hypercalcaemia associated with cancer. ⇒ Appendix 5.

**bite** *n* the occlusal record or relationship between the upper (maxillary) and lower (mandibular) teeth. *closed bite* a bite where there is a reduction in the occlusal vertical dimension. *open bite* a bite in which the anterior teeth do not occlude in any mandibular position.

**biteguard** *n* an appliance designed to cover the incisal and occlusal surfaces of the teeth. It provides stability for the teeth and/or provides a flat platform for excursive movements of the mandible and prevents damage to the teeth during nocturnal grinding.

**bite wing radiograph** *n* a type of dental radiograph which demonstrates the coronal parts of the upper teeth (maxillary) and the lower teeth (mandibular) and parts of the interdental septa on a single film.

**Bitot's spots** (*syn* xerosis conjunctivae) (P Bitot, French surgeon, 1822–1888) localized area of thickened, keratinized epithelium, with micro-organisms, at the limbus of the cornea. A manifestation of vitamin A deficiency.

**biuret test** a chemical test for the amount of protein in food. Sodium hydroxide (alkali) and copper sulphate are added to the sample solution. A positive result is indicated by a violet colour as copper sulphate reacts with the peptide bonds in the alkaline solution.

**bivalent** *n* **1.** in chemistry a substance with a valence of two. Also called divalent. **2.** in genetics a pair of synapsed homologous chromosomes.

**bivalve** *adj* having two blades such as in a vaginal speculum. In orthopaedics, the division of a plaster of Paris split into two portions—an anterior and posterior half.

**bivariate statistics** descriptive statistics that compare the relationship between two variables, such as correlations. Can be used to decide whether multivariate statistics are needed.

**blackhead** *n* ⇒ comedone.

**black heel** a discoloured area over the Achilles tendon due to the rupture of small blood vessels in the skin. It is associated with certain sports, including squash.

**blackwater fever** a serious complication of some forms of malaria where there is red blood cell haemolysis. The resultant haemoglobinuria causes dark-coloured urine, jaundice and renal failure.

**bladder** *n* a membranous sac containing fluid or gas. A hollow organ for receiving fluid. ⇒ gallbladder, urinary bladder.

**bladder augmentation** an operation to increase the capacity of the urinary bladder.

**bladder outflow obstruction** pathophysiological obstruction to the lower urinary tract commonly due to benign prostatic enlargement in older males.

**Blalock–Taussig procedure** (A Blalock, American surgeon, 1899–1964; H Taussig,

American physician, 1898–1986) a temporary measure to improve pulmonary blood flow in congenital heart abnormalities, such as tetralogy of Fallot. A shunt is constructed by anastomosing (joining) the subclavian artery to the pulmonary artery to divert blood from the systemic circulation to the lungs.

**bland diet** a diet that does not irritate or overstimulate the digestive tract. Generally, avoiding pickles, spicy food, alcohol and strong tea or coffee.

**blastocyst** *n* stage in early embryonic development in mammals that follows the morula, which becomes cystic and enfolds. Comprises a fluid-filled cavity and inner cell mass surrounded by an outer cell mass, or trophoblast. The inner cell mass is the source of embryonic stem cells from which all body structures are formed. The trophoblastic cells of the outer cell mass are involved in implantation of the blastocyst, and will eventually differentiate into two layers that form the chorion and placenta. ⇒ gastrula.

**blastoderm** *n* a cell layer of the blastocyst. Eventually becomes the three primary germ layers, ectoderm, endoderm and mesoderm, from which the embryo will form.

*Blastomyces* *n* a genus of pathogenic fungi. Species include *Paracoccidioides brasiliensis* in South America and *Blastomyces dermatidis* in North America—**blastomycetic** *adj*.

**blastomycosis** *n* granulomatous condition caused by *Blastomyces dermatidis*; infection usually affects the skin but it can involve the lungs, kidneys, nervous system, bones and joints. It is most common in the south-eastern states of the United States and in Latin America—**blastomycotic** *adj*.

**blastula (blastosphere)** *n* an early stage in embryonic development in lower animals. It follows the morula and comprises a fluid-filled cavity (blastocele) surrounded by a single layer of cells ⇒ blastocyst.

**bleb** *n* a large blister. ⇒ bulla, vesicle.

**bleeding time** the time required for the spontaneous arrest of bleeding from a skin puncture: under controlled conditions this is assessed using the Ivy method.

**blennorrhagia** *n* excessive discharge of mucus, such as from the urethra in urethritis. Also known as blennorrhoea.

**blennorrhoea** *n* ⇒ blennorrhagia.

**blepharitis** *n* inflammation of the eyelids, particularly the lid margins, eyelash follicles and meibomian glands. There is redness, swelling and discharge that forms crusts—**blepharitic** *adj*.

**blepharochalasis** *n* a looseness of the eyelid skin that occurs as supporting tissues atrophy.

**blepharoconjunctivitis** *n* inflammation of the eyelids and the conjunctiva.

**blepharon** *n* the eyelid; palpebra—**blephara** *pl*.

**blepharophimosis** *n* an abnormally narrow palpebral fissure, the gap or aperture between the eyelids.

**blepharoplasty** *n* tarsoplasty. Plastic surgery of the eyelid. An operation in which excess skin is removed from the eyelid.

**blepharoptosis** *n* ⇒ ptosis.

**blepharospasm** *n* spasm of the muscles in the eyelid. Excessive winking. A condition in which there is involuntary shutting of the eye, which can occur in isolation or may be due either to local irritative lesions in the eye or to a movement disorder.

**blighted ovum** a failure of development. There are fetal membranes enclosing a fluid-filled cyst but no embryonic tissue.

**blindness** *n* ⇒ visual impairment.

**blind-loop syndrome** a condition resulting from stasis in the small intestine leading to excessive bacterial growth, thus producing diarrhoea and malabsorption (e.g. due to surgical anastomosis or dysmotility).

**blind spot** the spot at which the optic nerve leaves the retina. Without any cones or rods it is insensitive to light. May also describe an abnormal gap in the visual field caused by pathology affecting the optic nerve or retina. ⇒ optic disc.

**blister** *n* an elevated lesion of the skin containing fluid, usually serum. ⇒ bulla, vesicle.

**blood** *n* a fluid connective tissue. It is the red fluid filling the heart and blood vessels. It consists of a colourless fluid, plasma, in which are suspended the red blood cells (erythrocytes), the white cells (leucocytes), and the platelets (thrombocytes). The plasma contains a great many substances in solution, including factors which enable the blood to clot. In adults the blood volume is normally around 7–8% of body weight.

**blood bank** the area or department of a hospital responsible for the selection, testing and storage of blood for later transfusion to patients.

**blood-borne viruses (BBV)** viruses transmitted via blood to cause infection. Include human immunodeficiency virus (HIV) and several hepatitis viruses.

**blood–brain barrier (BBB)** the protective arrangement that prevents many substances crossing from the blood to the brain. It comprises the capillary endothelial cells and astrocytes (neuroglial cells) that ensure that the capillary wall is relatively impermeable. The barrier allows the passage of nutrients and metabolic waste. However, some drugs, alcohol and other toxic substances, e.g. lead in young children, can pass from the blood through this barrier to the cerebrospinal fluid.

**blood coagulation** ⇒ coagulation.

**blood count** calculation of the number of red blood cells (erythrocytes), white blood cells (leucocytes) and platelets (thrombocytes) in a given volume of blood, using automated cell counting or a haemocytometer. *differential blood count* the estimation of the relative proportions of the different white blood cells in the blood. A normal differential count is: neutrophils (polymorphonuclear cells) 65–70%, lymphocytes 20–25%, monocytes 5%, eosinophils 0–3%, basophils 0–0.5%. In childhood the proportion of lymphocytes is higher.

**blood culture** a sample of venous blood is incubated in a suitable medium at an optimum temperature, so that any micro-organisms can multiply and so be isolated and identified microscopically. ⇒ septicaemia.

**blood donor** in the UK a healthy volunteer who donates blood or blood components for transfusion.

**blood doping** a prohibited ergogenic aid, which is used illicitly by some athletes to increase aerobic performance. It involves the removal and subsequent reinfusion of blood, which in the short term increases the number of red blood cells and hence the oxygen-carrying capacity of the blood.

**blood film** the result of spreading a droplet of blood very thinly on a microscope slide. The blood can then be stained with dyes and examined for abnormalities under a microscope.

**blood formation** haemopoiesis.

**blood gases** ⇒ arterial blood gases.

**blood glucose** the amount of glucose in the blood; varies within the normal range. It is regulated by hormones, e.g. insulin. ⇒ continuous glucose monitoring (CGM), hyperglycaemia, hypoglycaemia, self-monitoring blood glucose (SMBG).

**blood groups** a way of classifying blood by the presence or absence of certain genetically determined factors called antigens (agglutinogens) on the red blood cell membrane. There are many blood-grouping systems including ABO, Rhesus, Duffy, Kell, Lewis, etc. The ABO and Rhesus are clinically significant in transfusion, maternal–fetal compatibility and transplantation. There are four groups in the ABO system: A, B, AB and O. The red cells of these groups contain the corresponding antigens (agglutinogens): group A has A; group B has B; group AB has both antigens; and group O has neither. In the plasma there are antibodies (agglutinins) which will cause agglutination (clumping) of any cell carrying the corresponding antigen. Group A plasma contains anti-B; group B plasma contains anti-A; group O plasma contains both anti-A and anti-B; and group AB plasma contains no agglutinins. This grouping is determined by: (a) testing a suspension of red cells with anti-A and anti-B serum or (b) testing serum with known cells. Transfusion with an incompatible ABO group will cause a severe haemolytic reaction and death may occur unless the transfusion is promptly stopped. For most transfusion purposes, group A can receive groups A and O; group B can receive groups B and O; group AB can have blood of any group; and group O can only have group O (Table B.1). The terms 'universal donor' and 'recipient' are outdated and confusing because of the many other blood groups that exist. *Rhesus blood group* a further three pairs of antigens coded for by genes designated by the letters Cc, Dd and Ee are present on the red cells. The letters denote allelomorphic genes which are present in all cells except the gametes where, for instance, a chromosome can carry C or c, but not both. In this way the Rhesus genes and blood groups are derived equally from each parent. When the cells contain only the cde groups, then the blood is Rhesus-negative (Rh); when the cells contain C, D or

**Table B.1** ABO blood group compatibility

| Recipient | Donor | | | |
|---|---|---|---|---|
| | A | B | AB | O |
| A | Yes | No | No | Yes |
| B | No | Yes | No | Yes |
| AB | Yes | Yes | Yes | Yes |
| O | No | No | No | Yes |

Reproduced from Brooker & Nicol (2003) with permission.

E singly or in combination with cde, then the blood is Rhesus-positive (Rh+). For general purposes, only the Dd antigens are of clinical significance. About 85% of the Caucasian population have the D antigen. In contrast to the ABO system, there are no preformed antibodies to the D antigen but these groups are antigenic and can, under suitable conditions, produce the corresponding antibody in the serum. Antibodies are formed if there is: (a) transfusion of Rhesus-positive blood to a Rhesus-negative person; or (b) immunization during pregnancy by Rhesus-positive fetal red cells, with the D antigen, entering the maternal circulation where the woman is Rhesus-negative. This can cause haemolytic disease of the newborn (erythroblastosis fetalis). ⇒ ABO blood group system, anti-D, Rhesus incompatibility.

**blood letting** venesection.

**blood plasma** ⇒ plasma.

**blood pressure (BP)** the pressure exerted by the blood on the blood vessel walls. Usually refers to the pressure within the arteries. Arterial blood pressure is usually measured in millimetres of mercury (mmHg). The arterial blood pressure fluctuates with each heart beat, having a maximum value (the systolic pressure) which is related to the ejection of blood from the heart into the aorta and the systemic arteries and a minimum value (diastolic pressure) when the aortic and pulmonary valves are closed and the heart is relaxed. Usually values for both systolic and diastolic pressures are recorded (e.g. 120/70 mmHg). The factors that contribute to blood pressure include: cardiac output, blood volume, blood viscosity, elasticity of the arterial walls, the venous return (the amount of blood returning to heart) and the peripheral resistance in the arterioles. The normal BP range varies with age; in healthy adults the normal BP is below 130 mmHg systolic and below 85 mmHg diastolic, and an optimum BP is below 120 mmHg systolic and below 80 mmHg diastolic. BP also varies during the 24-hour period and is influenced by factors such as body position, physical activity, stress levels, etc. Arterial blood is measured indirectly using a stethoscope with an anaeroid or mercury sphygmomanometer, or by using an automatic electronic device with a digital display. It may also be recorded directly in critical care situations by using an intra-arterial cannula with a pressure transducer. ⇒ hypertension, hypotension, Korotkoff sounds.

**blood sugar** ⇒ blood glucose.

**blood transfusion** ⇒ transfusion.

**blood urea** the amount of urea (the end-product of protein metabolism) in the blood; varies within the normal range. This is virtually unaffected by the amount of protein in the diet when the kidneys, which are the main organs of urea excretion, are functioning normally. When they are diseased the blood urea quickly rises. ⇒ uraemia.

**Bloom's syndrome** (D Bloom, American dermatologist, 20th century) a rare inherited disorder. It is transmitted as an autosomal recessive trait and mainly affects Ashkenazi Jews. Affected individuals have short stature, abnormalities of the capillaries in the arms and face, increased sensitivity to sunlight, recurrent infections and a higher than normal risk of leukaemia.

**blow-out fracture** fracture of the orbital wall due to blunt trauma.

**BLS** abbr basic life support.

**'blue baby'** cyanotic appearance at birth, often attributed to congenital cyanotic heart defects.

**blue pus** bluish/green discharge from a wound infected with *Pseudomonas aeruginosa*.

**B lymphocyte (B cell)** ⇒ lymphocyte.

**BMD** abbr bone mineral density.

**BMI** abbr body mass index.

**BMR** abbr basal metabolic rate.

**BMT** abbr bone marrow transplantation/transplant.

**BNF** abbr British National Formulary. ⇒ formulary.

**Boari flap** method of extending one side of the bladder to compensate for a shortened/pathological distal ureter.

**Boas' sign** (I Boas, German gastroenterologist, 1858–1938) hyperaesthesia (increased sensitivity) of the skin overlying the wing of the right scapula, a feature of cholecystitis.

**Bobath concept** the concept of treatment of abnormal muscle tone and movement disorder, seen in children with cerebral palsy and adults after a stroke, and now widely applied to similar dysfunction caused by multiple sclerosis and other neurological conditions.

**body density** the density of lean body mass is 1.10, whereas that of body fat is 0.90. A calculation of the proportions of lean body tissue and fat can be made once density has been determined. This is either by weighing in air and in water, or by measuring body weight and volume.

**body dysmorphic disorder (BDD)** a disorder where individuals experience a pervasive feeling that they have a physical defect when, in fact, they look normal and others confirm this.

**body image** the image present in an individual's mind of his or her own body. Distortions of this occur in anorexia nervosa. ⇒ mutilation.

**body language** non-verbal symbols that express a person's current physical, emotional and mental state. They include body movements, postures, gestures, facial expressions, spatial positions, clothes and other bodily adornments.

**body mass index (BMI)** also known as Quetelet's index. Used as an index of adiposity and obesity. It is calculated by dividing an individual's weight (kg) by his or her height (m) squared. Separate charts are available for adults and children; adult charts should not be used for children. A BMI of less than 18.5 is underweight, BMI 18.5–24.9 is normal weight (some authorities use 20–24.9), BMI 25–29.9 is overweight, BMI over 30 is obese, BMI greater than 35 is morbidly obese, and BMI over 40 is extreme obesity. BMI has some limitations; for example, BMI is inaccurate in athletes with particularly well-developed muscle tissue. ⇒ waist:hip ratio.

**body temperature** the balance between heat produced and heat lost in the body. It is maintained around 37°C throughout the 24 hours, but varies between 0.5 and 1.0°C during that period. Most heat is produced by metabolism, voluntary and involuntary muscular activities, and heat loss occurs through convection, conduction and evaporation of sweat; small amounts are lost during expiration, urination and defecation. *core body temperature* that in the organs of the central cavities of the body (cranium, thorax and abdomen). *shell body temperature* that outside the body core. Varies between sites, e.g. 36°C at the shoulder and 28°C at the forearm (Figure B.5).

**body type, somatotype** the physical appearance of the body. There are three basic types. ⇒ ectomorph, endomorph, mesomorph.

**Boeck's disease** (C Boeck, Norwegian dermatologist, 1845–1917) a form of sarcoidosis.

**Bohn's nodules** tiny white nodules on the palate of the newly born.

**Bohr effect** (C Bohr, Danish physiologist, 1855–1911) the effect of hydrogen ion concentration (pH) on the oxygen dissociation

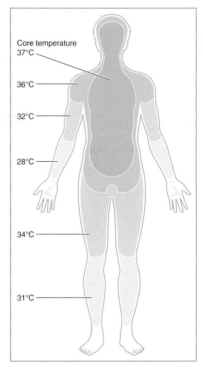

**Figure B.5** Core/shell body temperature *(reproduced from Brooker & Nicol 2003 with permission).*

curve. An increase in carbon dioxide in the blood or hydrogen ion concentration (i.e. a fall in pH) and also increased temperature causes the curve to 'shift to the right' and decreases the affinity of haemoglobin for oxygen. This means that more oxygen is unloaded to metabolically active tissues. The Bohr effect is particularly important in supplying oxygen to contracting muscle and in the placenta where oxygen passes from maternal to fetal vessels. ⇒ oxygen dissociation curve.

**boil** *n* (*syn* furuncle) an acute inflammatory condition, surrounding a hair follicle; often caused by *Staphylococcus aureus*. Usually attended by suppuration; it has one opening for drainage, in contrast to a carbuncle.

**Bolam test** the test laid down in the case of Bolam *v.* Friern HMC on the standard of care

**B**

expected of a professional in cases of alleged negligence.

**bolus** *n* **1.** a soft, pulpy mass of masticated food. **2.** a large dose of a drug given at the beginning of a treatment regimen to raise the blood concentration rapidly to a therapeutic level.

**bonding** *n* the emotional tie one person forms with another, making an enduring and special emotional relationship. There is a fundamental biological need for this to occur between an infant and its parents, particularly the mother. When newborn babies are cared for in an intensive care setting, special arrangements have to be made to encourage bonding between the parents and their new baby.

**bone** *n* connective tissue in which salts, such as calcium carbonate and calcium phosphate, are deposited in an organic matrix to make it hard and dense. Bone tissue is of two types: hard dense compact bone (Figure B.6) and spongy cancellous bone. The separate bones make up the skeleton.

**bone mineral density (BMD)** a measure of bone density. It decreases as part of normal ageing and is changed with osteoporosis (Figure B.7). ⇒ peak bone density.

**bone graft** the transplantation of a piece of bone from one part of the body to another, or from one person to another. Used to repair bone defects or to supply osteogenic tissue.

**bone marrow** the substance contained within bone cavities. At birth the cavities are filled with blood-forming *red marrow* but later in life, deposition of fat in the long bones converts the red marrow into *yellow bone marrow.*

**bone marrow biopsy (sampling)** an investigation of blood cell production whereby a sample of marrow is obtained by aspiration or trephine. Usually the site used is the iliac crest or sometimes the sternum.

**bone marrow transplantation (BMT)** ⇒ haemopoietic stem cell transplantation (HSCT).

**Bonnevie–Ullrich syndrome** (K Bonnevie, Norwegian zoologist, geneticist, 1872–1948; O Ullrich, German paediatrician, 1894–1957) ⇒ Noonan's syndrome, Turner's syndrome.

**borborygmi** *npl* rumbling noises caused by the movement of gas in the intestines.

**borderline substances** *npl* foods and toiletries that possess the characteristics of medication for specified disorders. These may be supplied to patients as an NHS prescription in the UK. Examples of foods include gluten-free products for gluten-sensitive enteropathies, liquid feeds for short-bowel syndrome, dysphagia, inflammatory bowel disease, etc. Toiletries include emollient bath oil for dermatitis, sunblocks/sunscreens for photodermatoses, etc.

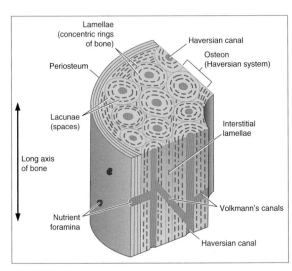

**Figure B.6** Bone tissue *(reproduced from Brooker 2006A with permission).*

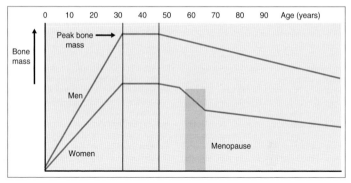

**Figure B.7** Bone mineral density *(reproduced from Porter 2005 with permission).*

**B**

*Bordetella* n (J Bordet, Belgian bacteriologist, 1870–1961) a genus of Gram-negative coccobacilli bacteria. Species that are pathogenic to humans include *B. pertussis* that causes whooping cough (pertussis).

**Borg dyspnoea scale** a validated scale (0–10) used by patients to quantify their perception of the severity of dyspnoea. The scale records no breathlessness at 0 up to maximal breathlessness at 10.

**Bornholm disease** *(syn* epidemic myalgia, epidemic pleurodynia) an epidemic pleurodynia usually associated with the B group of coxsackieviruses. It was first identified on Bornholm, a Danish island. Incubation is 2–14 days. There is sudden onset of severe pain in lower chest and/or abdominal and/or lumbar muscles. Breathing may be difficult, because of the pain, and fever is common. May last up to 1 week. There is no specific treatment.

*Borrelia* n (A Borrel, French bacteriologist, 1867–1936) a genus of coiled spirochaetes. Various species are responsible for louse-borne and tick-borne relapsing fevers. Lyme disease is caused by the bacterium *Borrelia burgdorferi.*

**BOS** *abbr* bronchiolitis obliterans syndrome.

**botulism** n an intoxication with the preformed exotoxin of *Clostridium botulinum.* Vomiting, respiratory, ocular and pharyngeal paralysis occurs within 24–72 h of eating food contaminated with the spores, which require anaerobic conditions to produce the toxin. Associated with home preserving of vegetables and meat and improperly treated tinned food.

**Bouchard's node** (C Bouchard, French physician, 1837–1915) bony enlargement of the proximal interphalangeal finger joints. Characteristic of osteoarthritis. ⇒ Heberden's nodes.

**bougie** n a cylindrical instrument made of gum elastic, metal or other material. Used in varying sizes for dilating strictures, e.g. oesophageal or urethral.

**Bourneville's disease** (D Bourneville, French neurologist, 1840–1909) ⇒ tuberous sclerosis.

**boutonneuse fever** also known as Mediterranean spotted fever. A rickettsial infection caused by *Rickettsia conorii*, it is transmitted by tick bites. The infection is endemic in areas around the Mediterranean. The clinical features include the bite site turning black (tache noire), high fever, chills, headache, photophobia, joint and muscle pain and a rash, which may become petechial.

**boutonnière deformity** a deformity of the finger occurring in rheumatoid arthritis. There is flexion of the proximal interphalangeal joint with hyperextension affecting the distal interphalangeal joint.

**bovine** *adj* relating to the cow or ox. *bovine tuberculosis* ⇒ tuberculosis.

**bovine somatotropin (BST)** a natural growth hormone of cattle. The administration of biosynthetic BST to dairy herds to increase milk production is prohibited in the European Union.

**bovine spongiform encephalopathy (BSE)** a fatal, infective (prion) neurological disease of cattle. ⇒ Creutzfeldt–Jakob disease.

**bowel** *n* the large intestine. ⇒ intestine.

**bowleg** *n* genu varum.

**bowler's finger** in sports medicine a colloquial term used to describe compression of the digital nerve on the medial aspect of the thumb leading to paraesthesia of the thumb.

**Bowman's capsule** (W Bowman, British anatomist, 1816–1892) glomerular capsule. The cup-like end of the renal tubule that encloses the glomerulus.

**boxer's fracture** in sports medicine a colloquial term used to describe a fracture of the fifth metacarpal bone secondary to a compressive force when the head of the metacarpal rotates over the neck leading to a flexion deformity.

**Boyle's anaesthetic machine** apparatus for delivering anaesthetic agents mixed with oxygen and nitrous oxide or air. ⇒ pin index.

**Boyle's law** (R Boyle, English scientist, 1627–1691) a gas law that states that the volume of a quantity of a dry gas is inversely proportional to the pressure, if the temperature is constant.

**BP** *abbr* **1.** blood pressure. **2.** British Pharmacopoeia.

**BPD** *abbr* bronchopulmonary dysplasia.

**BPE** *abbr* benign prostatic enlargement.

**BPH** *abbr* benign prostatic hyperplasia.

**BPPV** *abbr* benign paroxysmal positional vertigo.

**brachial** *adj* pertaining to the arm. Applied to vessels in this region and a nerve plexus at the root of the neck. *brachial artery* the main artery of the upper arm. It forms the radial and ulnar arteries. Used for indirect blood pressure recording. ⇒ Appendix 1, Figure 9. *brachial vein* the vein accompanying the brachial artery; it drains blood into the axillary vein. ⇒ Appendix 1, Figure 10.

**brachial plexus** formed from the four lower cervical nerves (C5–C8) and the first thoracic nerve (T1). Branches supply the muscles and skin of the arm and some chest muscles.

**brachialis** *n* a muscle of the upper arm. Its origin is on the humerus and it inserts on the coronoid process of the ulna. It is deep to the biceps brachii and flexes the forearm. ⇒ Appendix 1, Figure 4.

**brachiocephalic** *adj* pertaining to the arm and head. *brachiocephalic (innominate) artery* large artery branching from the aortic arch which forms the right common carotid and right subclavian arteries. ⇒ Appendix 1, Figure 9. *brachiocephalic (innominate) veins* two large veins derived from the internal jugular and subclavian veins. Convey blood to the heart via the superior vena cava. ⇒ Appendix 1, Figure 10.

**brachioradialis** *n* a superficial muscle of the forearm involved in forearm flexion. Its origin is on the lateral aspect of the distal humerus and it inserts on the styloid process of the radius. ⇒ Appendix 1, Figure 4.

**brachium** *n* the arm (especially from shoulder to elbow), or any arm-like appendage—**brachia** *pl*, **brachial** *adj*.

**brachycephaly** *n* a congenital malformation that results in a short, broad skull.

**brachygnathia** *n* also called micrognathia. There is underdevelopment of the mandible.

**brachytherapy** *n* radiotherapy delivered from a small radioactive source or sources which are implanted in or close to the tumour. The technique may be used to treat cancers of the anus, breast, cervix, lung, oesophagus, prostate gland and the tongue.

**bracket** *n* orthodontic attachment. The metal attachment bonded to the teeth on which the arch wire is secured.

**Bradford frame** (E Bradford, American surgeon, 1848–1926) a stretcher type of bed used for: (a) immobilizing the spine; (b) resting trunk and back muscles; (c) preventing deformity. It is a tubular steel frame fitted with two canvas slings allowing a 100–150 mm gap to facilitate personal care and elimination.

**bradycardia** *n* slow rate of heart contraction. Defined in adults at rest as a pulse rate less than 60 beats/min.

**bradykinesia** abnormally slow or retarded movement associated with difficulty initiating and then stopping a movement; typically seen in Parkinson's disease.

**bradykinin** *n* a kinin. A polypeptide mediator of the inflammatory process. It causes vasodilation, increases blood vessel permeability and smooth-muscle contraction and induces pain. ⇒ kinins.

**bradyphagia** *n* very slow eating.

**Braille** *n* (L Braille, French teacher, 1809–1852) a printing system that produces a series of raised dots representing the alphabet. People with visual impairment are able to read by touch.

**brain** *n* the encephalon; the largest part of the central nervous system: it is contained in the cranial cavity and is surrounded by three membranes called meninges. It comprises the cerebral hemispheres, brainstem (midbrain, pons and medulla oblongata) and the cerebellum. The brainstem connects the cerebral hemispheres to the cerebellum and the spinal cord. The cerebrospinal fluid inside the brain is contained in the ventricles, and outside in the subarachnoid space acts as a shock absorber to the delicate nerve tissue. ⇒ Appendix 1, Figure 1.

**brain death** a situation where the brainstem is fatally and irreversibly damaged. The brainstem is responsible for maintaining vital functions, including breathing. Strict criteria must be met before the patient is declared dead. These include testing certain reflexes, e.g. gag and pupillary, and the absence of factors that could depress brainstem activity. Suitable patients may become organ donors if this coincides with the wishes of the family and those of the patient if known. ⇒ death.

**bran** *n* the husk of grain. The coarse outer part of cereals, especially wheat, high in non-starch polysaccharide (NSP) and the vitamin B complex.

**branchial** *adj* relating to the gills. Embryonic clefts or fissures either side of the neck from which the nose, ears and mouth will eventually develop. *branchial cyst* a cyst in the neck resulting from a developmental abnormality of the branchial clefts.

**Brandt–Andrews method** (T Brandt, Swedish obstetrician, 1819–1895; H Andrews, British obstetrician, 1871–1942) a method of delivering the placenta during the third stage of labour. The contracted uterus is pushed upwards away from the placenta with the other hand on the abdomen while controlled cord traction is applied.

**Braun's frame** a metal frame, bandaged for use, and equally useful for drying a lower-leg plaster and for applying skeletal traction (Steinmann's pin or Kirschner wire inserted through the calcaneus) to a fractured tibia, after reduction.

**Braxton Hicks contractions** (J Braxton Hicks, British physician, 1823–1897) painless uterine contractions occurring during pregnancy. They facilitate uterine blood flow through the placenta, thereby promoting oxygen delivery to the fetus.

**BRCA1, BRCA2** genes that normally protect against abnormal cell growth. A defective version of the gene does not prevent cell proliferation and the individual is at risk of developing breast cancer.

**break-bone fever** ⇒ dengue.

**break test** an isometric contraction against manual resistance (provided by the examiner) with the joint in its mid-range position; used to determine the athlete's ability to generate a static force within a muscle or muscle group.

**breast** *n* **1.** the anterior upper part of the thorax. **2.** the milk-secreting mammary gland. *breast bone* the sternum.

**breast awareness** the activities undertaken by the woman in order to detect abnormal breast changes. These include change in breast size or shape, lumps in the breast or axilla, thickening, skin changes such as dimpling, nipple inversion, nipple discharge or itching, or pain.

**breath holding** involuntary breath holding in otherwise healthy toddlers. This typically occurs when the child is upset or startled, and starts to cry.

**breath sounds** the sounds generated in the larger airways, mainly during inspiration and for a short time during expiration. They can be heard using a stethoscope. Abnormal breath sounds include diminished, rhonchi (wheeze), a pleural rub and crepitations (crackles).

**breath tests** non-invasive investigations for gastrointestinal conditions such as the presence of *Helicobacter pylori* or malabsorption.

**breathing** *n* ventilation. The alternate cycle of inspiration and expiration as air is moved in and out of the lungs.

**breech** *n* the buttocks. ⇒ buttock.

**breech presentation** refers to the position of a baby in the uterus such that the buttocks, knee or foot would be born first: the normal position is head first (Figure B.8).

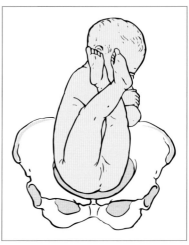

**Figure B.8** Frank breech presentation
*(reproduced from Fraser & Cooper 2003 with permission).*

**B**

**bregma** *n* the anterior fontanelle. ⇒ fontanelle.

**Breslow's depth** (A Breslow, American pathologist, 1928–1980) the depth to which a malignant melanoma has infiltrated. ⇒ Clark's level.

**bridge** *n* in dentistry, restoration to replace one or more teeth using artificial crowns connected to natural teeth.

**British sign language (BSL)** a type of sign language (signing) used in the UK.

**brittle diabetes** poor glycaemic control of diabetes mellitus. Blood glucose levels are unstable.

**BRM** *abbr* biological response modifier.

**broad ligaments** lateral ligaments; not a ligament but a double fold of parietal peritoneum which hangs over the uterus and outstretched uterine (fallopian) tubes, forming a lateral partition across the pelvic cavity. Also called the mesometrium. ⇒ Appendix 1, Figure 17.

**broad-thumb syndrome** Rubinstein–Taybi syndrome.

**Broca's area** (P Broca, French neurologist, 1824–1880) the motor speech area, situated in the dominant cerebral hemisphere (usually the left). Injury to this centre can result in an inability to speak.

**Brodie's abscess** (B Brodie, British surgeon, 1783–1862) chronic abscess in bone.

**Brodmann areas** (K Brodmann, German neurologist, 1868–1918) areas of the cerebral cortex that are associated with specific neurological functions such as movement (motor cortex) or vision (visual cortex), etc. Each area is distinguished histologically by the different staining characteristics of the neurons.

**bromatology** *n* the science concerned with foods.

**bromidrosis** *n* a profuse, fetid perspiration, especially associated with the feet—**bromidrotic** *adj*.

**bromism** *n* chronic poisoning due to continued or excessive use of bromides.

**bromopnoea** *n* bad breath. ⇒ halitosis.

**bronchi** *npl* the two tubes into which the trachea divides at its lower end. ⇒ Appendix 1, Figures 6 and 7—**bronchus** *sing*.

**bronchial** *adj* pertaining to the bronchi. *bronchial cancer* ⇒ non-small cell carcinoma, oat cell carcinoma. *bronchial tree* network of bronchi and bronchioles as they subdivide within the lungs.

**bronchial asthma** ⇒ asthma.

**bronchiectasis** *n* abnormal dilatation of the bronchi which, when localized, is usually the result of pneumonia or lobar collapse in childhood, but when generalized is due to some inherent disorder of the bronchial mucous membrane as in cystic fibrosis. Characterized by recurrent respiratory infections with profuse purulent sputum and digital clubbing. Eventually leads to respiratory failure. Mainstay of treatment is prompt treatment with appropriate antibiotics and regular physiotherapy to optimize sputum clearance—**bronchiectatic** *adj*.

**bronchiole** *n* one of the minute subdivisions of the bronchi which terminate in the alveoli (air sacs) of the lungs—**bronchiolar** *adj*.

**bronchiolitis** *n* inflammation of the bronchioles, usually due to viral infection in infants in the first year of life—**bronchiolitic** *adj*.

**bronchiolitis obliterans syndrome (BOS)** progressive scarring and loss of function seen in the lungs, in part as a result of chronic rejection of a transplanted lung over time.

**bronchitis** *n* inflammation of the bronchi. *acute bronchitis* as an isolated incident is usually a primary viral infection occurring in children as a complication of the common cold, influenza, whooping cough, measles or rubella. Secondary infection occurs with bacteria, commonly *Streptococcus pneumoniae* or *Haemophilus influenzae*. Acute bronchitis in adults is usually an acute exacerbation of chronic bronchitis precipitated by a viral infection but sometimes by a sudden increase in atmospheric pollution. *chronic bronchitis* is defined as a cough productive of sputum for at least three consecutive months in two consecutive years. The bronchial mucus-secreting glands are hypertrophied with an increase in goblet cells and loss of ciliated cells due to irritation from tobacco smoke, or atmospheric pollutants. ⇒ chronic obstructive pulmonary disease (COPD), pulmonary emphysema—**bronchitic** *adj*.

**bronchoalveolar lavage (BAL)** endoscopic diagnostic irrigation of the lungs with small volumes of saline which are then aspirated and examined for cancer, infection and other abnormalities; occasionally large-volume lavage may be therapeutic.

**bronchoconstrictor** *n* any agent which constricts the bronchi.

**bronchodilator** *n* any agent which dilates the bronchi, e.g. the drug salbutamol. ⇒ beta (β)-adrenoceptor agonists, muscarinic antagonists. ⇒ Appendix 5.

**bronchogenic** *adj* arising from one of the bronchi.

**bronchography** *n* obsolete radiological demonstration of the bronchial tree.

**bronchomycosis** *n* general term describing a variety of fungal infections of the bronchi and lungs, e.g. pulmonary candidiasis—**bronchomycotic** *adj*.

**bronchophony** *n* abnormal transmission of voice sounds heard over consolidated lung or over a thin layer of pleural fluid.

**bronchopleural fistula** pathological communication between the pleural cavity and one of the bronchi.

**bronchopneumonia** *n* describes a type of pneumonia in which areas of consolidation are distributed widely around bronchi and not in a lobar pattern. Generally affects patients at the extremes of age, those who are debilitated or secondary to existing condition—**bronchopneumonic** *adj*.

**bronchopulmonary** *adj* pertaining to the bronchi and the lungs—**bronchopulmonic** *adj*.

**bronchopulmonary dysplasia (BPD)** a chronic condition that occurs in infants who required long-term respiratory support with mechanical ventilation or oxygen. It is characterized by thickening of pulmonary blood vessels and scarring of lung tissue, resulting in a ventilation/perfusion mismatch.

**bronchorrhoea** *n* an excessive discharge of mucus from the bronchial mucosa—**bronchorrhoeal** *adj*.

**bronchoscope** *n* an endoscope used for examining, photographing and taking biopsies from the interior of the bronchi. Also used for removal of inhaled foreign bodies. Bronchoscopes are either flexible fibreoptic instruments or rigid tubes—**bronchoscopic** *adj*, **bronchoscopically** *adv*.

**bronchoscopy** *n* endoscopic examination of the tracheobronchial tree.

**bronchospasm** *n* sudden constriction of the bronchial tubes due to contraction of involuntary smooth muscle in their walls—**bronchospastic** *adj*.

**bronchostenosis** *n* narrowing of one of the bronchi—**bronchostenotic** *adj*.

**bronchotracheal** *adj* pertaining to the bronchi and trachea.

**bronchus** *n* ⇒ bronchi.

**bronze diabetes** ⇒ haemochromatosis.

**brought in dead (BID)** describes a situation where the person has died prior to arriving at the hospital.

**brow** *n* the forehead; the region above the supraorbital ridge. *brow presentation* a situation where the fetal brow/forehead is the presenting part at the pelvic brim The presenting diameter (mentovertical) of 13.5 cm exceeds the size of the average pelvis. It may convert to a face presentation but delivery by caesarean section is the likely outcome.

**brown adipose tissue (brown fat)** present in newborns and rarely in adults. It is metabolically highly active adipose tissue with a greater thermogenic activity than ordinary white fat. Provides the heat energy needed by infants to maintain body temperature.

**Brown-Séquard syndrome** (C Brown-Séquard, French physiologist, 1817–1894) a condition resulting from compression of one side of the spinal cord above the 10th thoracic vertebra. There is spastic paralysis on the same side of the body, loss of proprioception and loss of pain and temperature sensation on the other side.

***Brucella*** *n* a genus of bacteria causing brucellosis (undulant fever in humans; contagious abortion in cattle). *Brucella abortus* is the bovine strain, *B. melitensis* the sheep/goat strain, both transmissible via infected milk.

**brucellosis** *n* (*syn* melitensis) a generalized infection in humans resulting from one of the species of *Brucella*: *B. abortus* in cattle, *B. suis* in pigs and *B. melitensis* in sheep and goats. It is transmitted by contaminated milk or contact with the carcass of an infected animal. High-risk groups include farmers, abattoir workers and veterinary surgeons. There are recurrent attacks of continuous or undulating fever and low mood. It may last for months with relapses. The condition is also known as Malta fever, abortus fever, Mediterranean fever and undulant fever.

**Bruch's membrane** (K Bruch, German anatomist, 1819–1884) the innermost layer of the choroid. It has contact with the retinal pigment epithelium. ⇒ age-related macular degeneration.

**Brudzinski's sign** (J Brudzinski, Polish physician, 1874–1917) immediate flexion of knees and hips on raising head from pillow. Seen in meningitis.

**bruise** *n* (*syn* contusion, ecchymosis) a discoloration of the skin due to an extravasation of blood into the underlying tissues; there is no break of the skin.

**bruit** *n* ⇒ murmur.

**Brunner's glands** (J Brunner, Swiss anatomist, 1856–1927) mucus-secreting glands of the small intestine.

**brush border** microvilli present on the surface of absorptive cells in the small intestine and those in the proximal convoluted tubule of the nephron.

**Brushfield's spots** (T Brushfield, British physician, 1858–1937) white, grey or yellow spots on the iris of the eye. Typically associated with Down's syndrome but occasionally seen in other infants.

**Bruton's agammaglobulinaemia** (O Bruton, American physician, 1908–2003) a congenital condition in boys, in which B lymphocytes are absent but cellular immunity remains intact. ⇒ dysgammaglobulinaemia.

**bruxism** *n* abnormal grinding of teeth, often producing attrition.

**Bryant's 'gallows' traction** (T Bryant, British physician, 1828–1914) skin traction applied to the lower limbs; the legs are then suspended vertically (from an overhead beam), so that the buttocks are lifted just clear of the bed. Formerly used for fractures of the femur in children up to 4 years. Now largely replaced by hoop traction.

**BSE** *abbr* **1.** bovine spongiform encephalopathy. **2.** breast self-examination.

**BST** *abbr* bovine somatotropin.

**bubo** *n* enlargement of lymph nodes, especially in the groin. A feature of chancroid, lymphogranuloma venereum and bubonic plague— **bubonic** *adj*.

**bubonic plague** ⇒ plague.

**buccal** *adj* relating to the cheek or mouth. *buccal drug administration* a method where a drug, usually in tablet form, is dissolved between the cheek and gum or the top lip and gum. The buccal mucosa has a plentiful blood supply which allows the drug to be absorbed into the circulation, thereby overcoming first-pass metabolism/first-pass effect in the liver. Sometimes a spray containing the drug is used. ⇒ sublingual.

**buccinator** *n* a cheek muscle, important in the mastication of food. Its origin is on the maxilla and mandible and it inserts on to the orbicularis oris muscle.

**bucket-handle tear** a description given to a type of tear of the meniscus of the knee joint that extends along the length of the meniscus.

**Budd–Chiari syndrome** (G Budd, British physician, 1808–1882; H Chiari, German pathologist, 1851–1916) a liver condition. Obstruction of the hepatic vein leads to hepatic portal hypertension.

**Buerger's disease** (*syn* thromboangiitis obliterans) (L Buerger, American physician, 1879–1943) a chronic obliterative vascular disease of peripheral vessels that results in ischaemia, intermittent claudication, skin changes and gangrene. The incidence is associated with the presence of human leucocyte antigen HLA-A9 and HLA-B5. It affects young and middle-aged men. *Buerger's exercises* were designed to treat this condition. The legs are placed alternately in elevation and dependence to assist perfusion of the extremities with blood.

**buffer** *n* **1.** substances that limit pH change by their ability to accept or donate hydrogen ions as appropriate. In biological systems they limit pH changes that would inhibit cell functioning. The important buffer systems in the body include: bicarbonate (hydrogen carbonate) system, hydrogen phosphates and proteins, e.g. haemoglobin. **2.** any agent that reduces shock or jarring due to contact.

**bulbar** *adj* pertaining to the medulla oblongata. *bulbar palsy or paralysis* paralysis which involves the labioglossopharyngeal (lips, tongue and pharynx) region and results from degeneration of the motor nuclei in the medulla oblongata. There are problems with swallowing and speech. Individuals are at risk of inhaling fluids and food, with the development of pneumonia.

**bulbourethral (Cowper's) glands** two mucus-secreting glands which open into the bulb of the male urethra. Their secretion is part of seminal fluid.

**bulimia** *n* an eating disorder involving repeated uncontrolled consumption of large quantities of food. Many people with anorexia have a history of such episodes. *bulimia nervosa* (*syn* binge–purge syndrome) self-induced vomiting after binge eating. ⇒ anorexia, eating disorders.

**bulk-forming laxatives** ⇒ laxatives. ⇒ Appendix 5.

**bulla** *n* (*syn* blister) a fluid-filled skin blister with a diameter greater than 5 mm. In dermatology, multiple bullae may suggest pemphigoid or pemphigus, but they sometimes occur in other diseases of the skin, e.g. in impetigo, in dermatitis herpetiformis, etc.—**bullae** *pl*, **bullate**, **bullous** *adj*.

**bullous keratopathy** ⇒ Fuchs endothelial dystrophy.

**bundle branch block (BBB)** a disorder affecting the conducting fibres of the heart. The cardiac impulses are not transmitted, leading to changes to the QRS complex. Commonly seen following an anterior myocardial infarction.

**bundle of His** (W His, Swiss anatomist, 1863–1934) atrioventricular bundle. Part of the cardiac conduction system. ⇒ atrioventricular.

**bunion** *n* ⇒ hallux valgus.

**buphthalmos** *n* (ox eye) enlarged eye, usually secondary to congenital glaucoma.

**Burch colposuspension operation** the vagina is suspended from the iliopectineal ligament. Carried out for severe stress incontinence of urine.

**Burkitt's lymphoma** (D Burkitt, British surgeon, 1911–1993) a highly malignant lymphoma frequently of the jaw but other sites as well. Most commonly diagnosed in areas of Africa and New Guinea where malaria is endemic.

**burn** *n* tissue damage (necrosis) due to chemicals, moist heat, dry heat, electricity, flame, friction or radiation; classified as partial or full-thickness according to the depth of skin destroyed: full-thickness burns usually require skin graft(s). Analgesia, fluid replacement and the prevention of shock, infection and malnutrition are important aspects of treatment.

**burnout syndrome** a condition resulting from exposure to stressors. The stressors are often chronic and work-related, but burnout may occur after exposure to an acute stressor and may also result from stressful family roles such as caring for a relative, or a combination. Health professionals are at particular risk of burnout because of their prolonged contact with ill people. It has been described as emotional exhaustion, isolation, becoming indifferent to others, and a lack of ability to deal with problems. The adverse effects may be physical, emotional, intellectual, social and spiritual, and may include anxiety, poor coping strategies, insomnia, inability to make decisions, appetite and weight changes, excessive tiredness, apathy, lack of motivation, relationship difficulties and possible misuse of alcohol and drugs. ⇒ general adaptation syndrome, stress, stressor.

**Burns Marshall manoeuvre** a manoeuvre used to deliver the after-coming head in a breech presentation.

**burr** *n* an attachment for a surgical drill which is used for cutting into tooth or bone.

**burrow** *n* a tunnel in the skin that may house an ectoparasite, e.g. acarus of scabies.

**bursa** *n* a fibrous sac lined with synovial membrane and containing a small quantity of synovial fluid. Bursae are found between: (a) tendon and bone; (b) skin and bone; (c) muscle and muscle. Their function is to facilitate movement by reducing friction between these surfaces—**bursae** *pl*.

**bursitis** *n* inflammation of a bursa. *olecranon bursitis* inflammation of the bursa over the point of the elbow. *prepatellar bursitis* (*syn* housemaid's knee) a fluid-filled swelling of the bursa in front of the kneecap (patella). It is frequently associated with excessive kneeling. A blow can result in bleeding into the bursa and there can be infection with pyogenic pathogens. *retrocalcaneal bursitis* inflammation of an anatomical bursa located between the posterior angle of the calcaneus and the Achilles tendon near to its insertion. There is a fluctuant soft-tissue swelling on both sides of the tendon.

**butterfly rash** an erythematous butterfly-shaped rash occurring over the cheeks, connected by a narrow area of rash over the nose. A feature of systemic lupus erythematosus.

**buttock** *n* nates. The two projections posterior to the hip joints. Formed mainly of the gluteal muscles, gluteus maximus, gluteus medius and gluteus minimus.

**butyric acid** a saturated fatty acid.

**BV** *abbr* biological value.

**BXO** *abbr* balanitis xerotica obliterans.

**bypass** *n* describes a surgical procedure that usually diverts or provides a shunt for blood, other fluids or gastrointestinal contents. ⇒ cardiac bypass operation, cardiopulmonary bypass, coronary artery bypass graft, extracorporeal membrane oxygenation.

**byssinosis** *n* an occupational disease caused by inhalation of flax, hemp or cotton fibres. Symptoms that include wheeziness, cough, dyspnoea and chest tightness are often more pronounced on return to work following a break. There is bronchitis, fibrosis, chronic airways obstruction and pulmonary hypertension. Eventually this may lead to respiratory and cardiac failure.

# C

**CA-125** *abbr* cancer cell surface antigen 125. Levels in the blood may be used as a tumour marker for ovarian and other cancers.

**CABG** *abbr* coronary artery bypass graft.

**cachexia** *n* a constitutional disorder: malnutrition and general ill health caused partly by inadequate food intake but mainly the effects of disease that lead to hypermetabolism and the breakdown of lean (protein) tissue. There is debility, muscle weakness and anaemia. The chief signs of this condition are emaciation, wasting, sallow unhealthy skin and heavy lustreless eyes. A feature of advanced disease such as cancer and AIDS—**cachectic** *adj*.

**cacosmia** *n* an abnormality of smell. There is a perception of a foul stench or odour which others do not notice. It may occur with disorders affecting the brain or olfactory nerve, or as an olfactory hallucination.

**cadaver** *n* a corpse. In a medical context it implies a dead body which is dissected in a medical school, or in a mortuary at a postmortem examination.

**cadaverine** *n* a molecule produced when protein breaks down during the putrefaction of animal tissue. It results from the decarboxylation of lysine, an amino acid, and has an extremely foul odour. ⇒ putrescine.

**cadence** *n* the rhythm of a movement or the voice. In physiotherapy practice it also refers to the number of steps taken in a specific time period, frequently used as an outcome measure.

**cadmium (Cd)** *n* a poisonous metallic element. *cadmium poisoning* may occur as an occupational hazard. The inhalation of fumes during industrial processes such as welding or smelting can lead to lung damage and kidney disease. Ingestion of cadmium causes gastrointestinal effects that include vomiting.

**caecostomy** *n* a surgically established fistula between the caecum and anterior abdominal wall, usually to achieve drainage and/or decompression of the caecum. It is usually created by inserting a wide-bore tube into the caecum at operation.

**caecum** *n* the blind, pouch-like commencement of the colon in the right iliac fossa. To it is attached the vermiform appendix; it is separated from the ileum by the ileocaecal valve—**caecal** *adj*.

**caesarean section, c-section (CS)** delivery of the fetus through an abdominal incision. It is said to be named after Caesar, who is supposed to have been born in this way.

**caesium-137 ($^{137}$Cs)** *n* a radioactive substance which, when sealed in needles or tubes, can be used for interstitial and surface applications during radiotherapy. It can also be employed as a source for treatment by Selectron. Historically has been used for external beam therapy.

**café au lait spots** pale brown (like milky coffee) patches or spots on the skin. Some isolated spots may be normal but the appearance of several spots may be indicative of neurofibromatosis.

**caffeine** *n* the central nervous system stimulant that is present in tea, coffee, chocolate and cola drinks. It causes diuresis, increases heart rate and may cause restlessness and difficulty sleeping. It has been given as a diuretic, but its main use is in analgesic preparations such as with codeine. Excess intake may result in caffeine poisoning with anxiety, tremor, nausea, tachycardia, cardiac arrhythmias and insomnia.

**Caffey's disease** (J Caffey, American paediatrician, 1895–1978) ⇒ infantile cortical hyperostosis.

**CAH** *abbr* congenital adrenal hyperplasia.

**caisson disease** ⇒ decompression sickness/ illness.

**calamine** *n* zinc carbonate with ferric oxide. Used in lotions and creams for the relief of itching; however, it is not generally effective.

**calcaneus** *n* (*syn* calcaneum, os calcis) the largest of the tarsal bones, it forms the heel bone. It articulates distally with the cuboid and proximally with the talus. ⇒ Appendix 1, Figure 3.

**calcareous** *adj* chalky. Relating to lime or calcium.

**calcidiol** *n* 25-hydroxycholecalciferol, a derivative of vitamin D. It is the main circulating and storage form of vitamin D in the body.

**calciferol** *n* ⇒ ergocalciferol. Sometimes used as a general term for vitamins $D_2$ and $D_3$.

**calcification** *n* the hardening of an organic substance by a deposit of calcium salts within it. May be physiological, as in the formation of bone, or pathological, as in arteries.

**calcinosis** *n* the abnormal deposition of calcium salts in tissues and organs. Some cases are caused by an excessive intake of vitamin D.

**calciol** *n* cholecalciferol (vitamin $D_3$), the naturally occurring form of vitamin D.

**calcitonin** *n* (*syn* thyrocalcitonin) hormone secreted by the thyroid gland. It has a fine-tuning role in calcium homeostasis. It opposes the action of parathyroid hormone and reduces levels of calcium and phosphate in the serum by its action on the kidneys and bone. It inhibits calcium reabsorption from bone and stimulates the excretion of calcium and phosphate in the urine. Calcitonin is released when the concentration of calcium in serum rises. Synthetic calcitonin is used in the management of metastatic bone cancer, Paget's disease and osteoporosis.

**calcitriol** *n* 1,25-dihydroxycholecalciferol. Formed in the kidneys from 25-hydroxycholecalciferol (calcidiol). It is the active form of vitamin D (vitamin D₃) concerned with calcium homeostasis. It controls calcium levels by increasing calcium absorption from the small intestine.

**calcium (Ca)** *n* a metallic element. Needed by the body for neuromuscular conduction. It is factor IV of blood coagulation where it is essential for the conversion of prothrombin to thrombin, and the activation of factor XII, which stabilizes the fibrin clot. Also as an important component of the bone and teeth. An essential nutrient. *calcium carbonate* a calcium salt used in many antacid medicines. *calcium chloride* a calcium salt administered intravenously in the treatment of hypocalcaemic tetany. Also used during cardiopulmonary resuscitation. *calcium gluconate* a calcium salt used orally to treat calcium deficiencies and disorders such as rickets. Used intravenously to treat hypocalcaemic tetany. *calcium sulphate* gypsum, plaster of Paris.

**calcium channel blockers (antagonists)** a group of drugs that block the flow of calcium ions in smooth muscle, e.g. nifedipine. They are negatively inotropic and may reduce myocardial contractility. ⇒ inotropes. ⇒ Appendix 5.

**calculus** *n* a stone. An abnormal concretion composed chiefly of mineral substances and formed in the passages which transmit secretions, or in the cavities which act as reservoirs for them. Examples include gallstones and renal calculi—**calculi** *pl*, **calculous** *adj*. ⇒ dental calculus, gallstones, renal calculus.

**Caldicott guardian** every NHS establishment, e.g. NHS trust or health authority, must appoint a board member to take responsibility for the security and confidentiality of all patient-identifiable information. The guardian will be involved with approving and reviewing local protocols, and controlling the use and protection of patient-identifiable information.

The guardian also fulfils a strategic role, for example, in the development of confidentiality and security policies and representing confidentiality issues at board level.

**Caldwell–Luc operation** (*syn* radical antrostomy) a radical operation previously used for sinusitis.

**caliper** *n* 1. a two-pronged instrument for measuring the diameter of a round body. Used chiefly in pelvimetry. 2. a two-pronged instrument with sharp points which are inserted into the lower end of a fractured long bone. A weight is attached to the other end of the caliper, which maintains a steady pull on the distal end of the bone. 3. *Thomas' walking caliper* is similar to the Thomas' splint, but the W-shaped junction at the lower end is replaced by two small iron rods which slot into holes made in the heel of the boot. The ring should fit the groin perfectly, and all weight is then borne by the ischial tuberosity.

**callosity** *n* a local hardening of the skin. ⇒ callus.

**callus** *n* 1. the partly calcified tissue which forms about the ends of a broken bone during fracture healing and ultimately accomplishes repair of the fracture. When this is complete the bony thickening is known as *permanent callus*. 2. (*syn* callosity, corn, keratoma, mechanically induced hyperkeratosis) a yellowish plaque of hard skin caused by pressure or friction. The stratum corneum becomes hypertrophied. Most commonly seen on the feet and palms of the hands. A painful, cone-shaped overgrowth and hardening of the epidermis, with the point of the cone in the deeper layers. Corns on the sole of the foot and over joints are often described as hard corns, and those occurring between the toes are described as soft corns.

**calmodulins** *npl* a group of intracellular calcium-binding proteins, important in mediating many biochemical processes including signalling functions within cells.

**calor** *n* heat: one of the five classic local signs and symptoms of inflammation—the others are dolor, loss of function, rubor and tumor.

**caloric test** irrigation of the outer/external ear canal with water at 30°C and then at 44°C to assess vestibular function by stimulating the lateral semicircular canals. Each ear is tested separately. When the ear is normal the test produces nystagmus, whereas nystagmus may not be produced if the ear is diseased.

**calorie** *n* a unit of heat. In practice the calorie is too small a unit to be useful and 1000 calories, the kilocalorie (kcal), is the preferred unit in studies in metabolism. A kilocalorie is the amount of heat required to raise the temperature of 1 kg of water by 1°C. In medicine, science and technology generally, the calorie has been replaced by the joule (derived SI unit) as a unit of energy, work and heat. For approximate conversion 4.2 kJ = 1 kcal.

**calorific** *adj* describes any phenomena that relate to heat production.

**calorimeter** *n* an instrument used to measure the heat gain or loss occurring during physical and chemical changes. A calorimeter is used to determine the amount of oxidizable energy in a specific food, by burning it in oxygen and measuring heat production.

**calorimetry** *n* in nutrition the measurement of energy expenditure by the body. *direct calorimetry* is the measurement of heat produced from the body, as an index of energy expenditure, and hence the individual's energy requirements. *indirect calorimetry* measures the heat produced during oxidation of nutrients by determining the consumption of oxygen, or by measuring the carbon dioxide or nitrogen released and converting the values into a heat equivalent.

**calvaria** *n* the superior part of the skull, the vault.

**CAM** *abbr* **1.** cell adhesion molecule. **2.** complementary and alternative medicine.

**cAMP** *abbr* cyclic adenosine monophosphate.

**Campylobacter** *n* a genus of Gram-negative, non-spore-forming motile bacteria. They are spirally curved rods with a flagellum at either or both ends. *Campylobacter jejuni* is a common cause of bacterial food poisoning. It causes abdominal pain and blood-stained diarrhoea that may last for 10–14 days. The microorganism is associated with raw meat and poultry, the fur of infected pet animals and unpasteurized milk. No reported person-to-person spread. *C. fetus* causes abortion in cattle. It is an opportunistic organism and causes bacteraemia in humans, this can lead to local infections, e.g. involving the meninges. Immunocompromised individuals and neonates may develop septicaemia, which, in rare cases, results in death.

**canaliculus** *n* a minute capillary passage. Any small canal, such as the passage leading from the edge of the eyelid to the lacrimal sac or one of the numerous small canals leading from the Haversian canals and terminating in the lacunae of bone—**canaliculi** *pl*, **canalicular** *adj*, **canaliculization** *n*.

**canal of Schlemm** (F Schlemm, German anatomist, 1795–1858). ⇒ scleral venous sinus. ⇒ Appendix 1, Figure 15. ⇒ glaucoma.

**canbra oil (canola oil)** ⇒ canola oil.

**cancellous** *adj* resembling latticework; light and spongy; like a honeycomb. Describes a type of bone tissue (cancellous, spongy or trabecular). ⇒ bone.

**cancer** *n* a general term which covers any malignant growth in any part of the body. The growth is purposeless, parasitic, and flourishes at the expense of the human host. Characteristics are the tendency to cause local destruction, to invade adjacent tissues and to spread by metastasis. Frequently recurs after removal. Carcinoma refers to malignant tumours of epithelial tissue, sarcoma to malignant tumours of connective tissue—**cancerous** *adj*. ⇒ grading, staging.

**cancer cell surface antigen 125 (CA-125)** ⇒ CA-125.

**cancerophobia** *n* obsessive fear of cancer—**cancerophobic** *adj*.

**cancrum oris** gangrenous stomatitis of cheek in debilitated children. Often called noma. Associated with measles in malnourished African children. ⇒ noma.

**candela (cd)** *n* one of the seven base units of the International System of Units (SI). Measures luminous intensity. ⇒ Appendix 2.

**Candida** *n* (*syn* Monilia) a genus of fungi. They are widespread in nature. *Candida albicans* is a commensal of the mouth, gastrointestinal tract, vagina and skin in humans.

**candidiasis** *n* (*syn* candidosis, moniliasis, thrush) infections caused by a species of *Candida*, usually *Candida albicans*. Infection may involve the mouth, gastrointestinal tract, skin, nails, respiratory tract or genitourinary tract (vulvovaginitis, balanitis), especially in individuals who are debilitated, e.g. by cancer or diabetes mellitus, or immunosuppressed, and after long-term or extensive treatment with antibiotics, which upsets the microbial flora, and other drugs, e.g. corticosteroids. Candidiasis is also a feature of immunodeficiency conditions such as human immunodeficiency virus (HIV). Oral infection can be caused by poor oral hygiene, including carious teeth and ill-fitting dentures.

**canicola fever** leptospirosis.

**canine** *adj* of or resembling a dog. *canine tooth* pointed tooth with a single cusp (cuspid), placed third from the midline in both primary and secondary dentitions (see Figure T.4B, p. 482). A lay term for the upper permanent canine is 'eye tooth'. There are four in all.

**canities** *n* a loss of pigment, as in the greying of hair, or the formation of white streaks in the nails.

**cannabinoids** *npl* a group of antiemetic drugs derived from cannabis, e.g. nabilone. ⇒ Appendix 5.

**cannabis** *n* (*syn* marijuana, pot, hashish, etc.) a psychoactive drug that produces euphoria and hallucinations. It is usually smoked. In the UK the cultivation, possession and supply of cannabis are criminal offences (⇒ Appendix 5). There is, however, considerable interest in possible medicinal uses and trials are ongoing.

**cannula** *n* a hollow tube, usually plastic, for the introduction of fluid, such as intravenous fluids, or withdrawal of fluid from the body (Figure C.1). In some types the lumen is fitted with a sharp-pointed trocar to facilitate insertion, which is withdrawn when the cannula is in situ—**cannulae** *pl.*

**cannulation** *n* insertion of a cannula, such as into a vein to facilitate the administration of intravenous fluids or drugs.

**canola oil (canbra oil)** oil obtained from a variety of rapeseed, which is low in glucosinolates. Developed to contain no more than 2% erucic acid.

**canthoplasty** *n* plastic surgery either to refashion canthus or correct a defect.

**canthus** *n* palpebral commissure. The angle formed by the junction of the eyelids. The inner one is known as the *nasal* or *medial canthus* and the outer as the *temporal* or *lateral*

canthus—**canthi** *pl.* **canthal** *adj.* ⇒ epicanthus.

**CAPD** *abbr* continuous ambulatory peritoneal dialysis.

**CAPE** *acron* **C**lifton **A**ssessment **P**rocedures for the **E**lderly.

**capelline bandage (divergent spica)** a bandage applied in a circular fashion to the head or an amputated limb.

**Capgras syndrome** (J Capgras, French psychiatrist, 1873–1950) characterized by a delusion, whereby the person believes that the people around have been replaced by doubles or impostors.

**capillarization** *n* a long-term adaptation to endurance exercise where the number and usage of blood capillaries in muscle tissue increase to meet the need for oxygenated blood. ⇒ aerobic adaptations.

**capillary** *n* (literally, hair-like) any tiny thin-walled vessel forming part of a network which facilitates rapid exchange of substances between the contained fluid and the surrounding tissues. For example, the exchange of oxygen and waste carbon dioxide between the blood and the cells. *bile capillary* begins in a space in the liver and joins others, eventually forming a bile duct. *blood capillaries* unite an arteriole and a venule. *capillary bed* the network of capillaries between the arteriole and the venule (Figure C.2). *capillary fragility* an expression of the ease with which blood

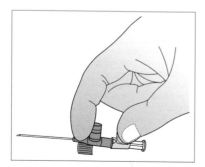

**Figure C.1** Intravenous cannula *(reproduced from Nicol et al. 2004 with permission).*

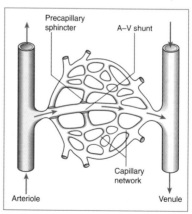

**Figure C.2** Capillary bed *(reproduced from Brooker 2006B with permission).*

capillaries may rupture. *capillary refill time* used for the assessment of skin perfusion and cardiac output. Pressure is applied to a nail bed (peripheral area) or a central area such as the skin over the sternum if the patient has poor peripheral circulation or a low cardiac output. Normal skin colour should return within 2 seconds of the removal of pressure. A prolonged capillary refill time can indicate that the cardiac output is low. *lymph capillary* begins in the tissue spaces throughout the body and joins others, eventually forming a lymphatic vessel.

**capital budget** financial allocation for the purchase of items, such as equipment, that will last longer than 12 months, or items that cost more than an agreed level. ⇒ revenue budget.

**capitate** *adj* shaped like a head.

**capitate bone** *n* one of the carpal bones of the wrist. It articulates with other carpal bones, scaphoid, lunate, hamate and trapezoid, and the second, third and fourth metacarpal bones.

**capitation funding** method of allocating money and other resources based on the number of people living in a geographical area. *weighted capitation* the allocation of resources based on the number of people in an area but adjusted for the age profile or the relative economic and social conditions, e.g. areas with a high level of social deprivation would be allocated extra resources.

**capitulum** *n* a rounded prominence on the end of a bone where it articulates with another bone. For example the *capitulum humeri*, the prominence at its distal end that articulates with the radius at the elbow.

**capsaicin** *n* a irritant chemical present in sweet peppers. It prevents the transmission of pain impulses. Used topically to relieve the pain of postherpetic neuralgia, which follows an attack of herpes zoster (shingles).

**capsid** *n* the protein layer that encloses viral nucleic acid.

**capsule** *n* **1.** the ligaments which surround a joint. **2.** a gelatinous or rice paper container for a drug. **3.** the outer membranous covering of certain organs, such as the kidney, liver. **4.** the outer covering of certain bacteria— **capsular** *adj*.

**capsulectomy** *n* the surgical excision of a capsule. Refers to a joint or lens, less often to the kidney.

**capsulitis** *n* inflammation of a capsule. Sometimes used as a synonym for frozen shoulder.

**capsulotomy** *n* incision of a capsule, usually referring to that surrounding the crystalline lens of the eye, which remains after modern cataract surgery. Usually created by a laser.

**caput** *n* the head.

**caput medusae** dilated knot of veins around the umbilicus, associated with hepatic portal hypertension.

**caput succedaneum** an oedematous swelling covering the fetal scalp at birth. Results from the pressure of the cervix on the fetal head during labour. The swelling is diffuse, not delineated by skull suture lines and resolves spontaneously after delivery. ⇒ cephalhaematoma, moulding.

**carbaminohaemoglobin** *n* a compound formed between carbon dioxide and haemoglobin. Some carbon dioxide in the blood is normally carried in this form.

**carbapenems** *npl* a group of β-lactam antibiotics, e.g. imipenem. ⇒ Appendix 5.

**carbohydrate** *n* an organic compound containing carbon, hydrogen and oxygen. Formed in nature by photosynthesis in plants. Carbohydrates are the major source of energy in most diets; on average 1 g of carbohydrate is metabolized to produce 16 kJ heat. They include saccharides, starches, glycogen and cellulose, and are often classified in groups— monosaccharides (e.g. glucose, fructose, galactose), disaccharides (maltose, sucrose, lactose), polysaccharides (e.g. starch, glycogen) and non-starch polysaccharides (NSP) (e.g. cellulose).

**carbohydrate loading (carboloading, glycogen loading)** a term used in sports medicine to describe the dietary regimens intended to increase glycogen stores in the liver and muscles before a major endurance activity such as running a marathon. Athletes may increase their carbohydrate intake for a few days before the event while decreasing the intensity of training.

**carbol fuchsin** a stain used in microbiology and to stain cell nuclei prior to microscopic examination.

**carbolic acid** ⇒ phenol.

**carboloading** *n* ⇒ carbohydrate loading.

**carbon** *n* a non-metallic element found in all organic molecules and living matter. Carbon can bond with four other atoms and is able to form a huge number of complex molecules. Carbon is a constituent of important biochemical molecules, including amino acids (proteins), carbohydrates, lipids, hormones, enzymes and nucleic acids.

**carbon dioxide** a gas; a waste product of many forms of combustion and metabolism, excreted via the lungs. Carbon dioxide retention occurs in respiratory insufficiency or failure, due for instance to alveolar hypoventilation. The carbon dioxide tension in arterial blood ($PaCO_2$) rises above normal levels and acid–base balance is adversely affected. ⇒ hypercapnia.

**carbonic anhydrase** a zinc-containing enzyme involved in maintaining acid–base balance in the body. It increases the rate of transfer of carbon dioxide from tissues to blood and then to alveolar air in the lungs. This is achieved by reversibly catalysing the interconversion of carbon dioxide and water from the tissues to carbonic acid, which dissociates into bicarbonate and hydrogen ions. Once in the lungs the reactions are reversed, thereby facilitating the excretion of acid carbon dioxide by the lungs. The enzyme is involved in acid–base balance and the regulation of pH by the kidneys. For example, the conservation and reabsorption of bicarbonate (hydrogen carbonate) ions by the renal tubule in order to replenish the alkaline reserve, and the secretion of hydrogen ions.

**carbonic anhydrase inhibitors** drugs that reduce the production of aqueous humour, thereby reducing intraocular pressure, e.g. acetazolamide. They also have some diuretic effects. ⇒ Appendix 5.

**carbon monoxide (CO)** a poisonous gas that is odourless and colourless. Carbon monoxide is produced by the incomplete combustion (oxidation) of organic fuels in situations where there is limited oxygen. The gas is produced by the internal combustion engine and is present in exhaust fumes; by wood-burning stoves; in faulty central heating boilers (furnace) and other heaters. It combines with haemoglobin to form a stable compound. This blocks the normal reversible oxygen-carrying function and leads to hypoxia. The onset of hypoxia may be insidious but it is associated with confusion, headache, increasing respiratory rate, cherry-pink flushed appearance, changes in conscious level, seizures, cardiac arrhythmias and, without treatment, death. Exposure to carbon monoxide may occur intentionally during suicide attempts or accidentally through inhalation of vehicle exhaust fumes or from a faulty central heating boiler.

**carbon tetrachloride** colourless volatile liquid used in dry cleaning and some types of antifreeze. Exposure may result in toxicity and liver damage.

**carboxyhaemoglobin** n a stable compound formed by the union of carbon monoxide and haemoglobin; the red blood cells thus lose their respiratory function. Large amounts are present in carbon monoxide but smaller amounts are also present in smokers' blood.

**carboxyhaemoglobinaemia** n carboxyhaemoglobin in the blood—**carboxyhaemoglobinaemic** adj.

**carboxyhaemoglobinuria** n carboxyhaemoglobin in the urine—**carboxyhaemoglobinuric** adj.

**carboxylase** n an enzyme that catalyses the reaction that adds carbon dioxide to a substance to create a carboxyl group (COOH).

**carboxylation** n the process by which a carboxyl group (COOH) replaces a hydrogen atom.

**carboxypeptidase** n a pancreatic enzyme, secreted as inactive procarboxypeptidase, which hydrolyses amino acids from the carboxyl end of proteins and polypeptides during digestion in the small intestine.

**carbuncle** n an acute inflammation (usually caused by *Staphylococcus*). There is a collection of boils causing necrosis in the skin and subcutaneous tissue. ⊙DVD

**carcinoembryonic antigen (CEA)** an oncofetal antigen. Its presence in the serum of adults can be a tumour marker for colorectal cancers and those of the stomach, pancreas, breast and lung, and for non-malignant conditions, such as liver cirrhosis caused by alcohol misuse and pancreatitis. ⇒ oncofetal antigens.

**carcinogen** n agent, substance or environment causing cancer—**carcinogenic** adj, **carcinogenicity** n.

**carcinogenesis** n the production of cancer—**carcinogenetic** adj.

**carcinoid syndrome** cluster of symptoms including flushing, palpitation, diarrhoea and bronchospasm from histological (usually low-grade) malignancy; often originates in the appendix or in the bronchial tree. ⇒ APUD cells, apudoma, argentaffinoma, 5-hydroxyindoleacetic acid.

**carcinoma** n a cancerous growth of epithelial tissue (e.g. mucous membrane) and derivatives such as glands.

**carcinoma in situ (CIS)** condition with cells closely resembling cancer cells. A very early cancer (premalignant) where the abnormal cell growth has not invaded the basement membrane. Well described in uterine cervix and endometrium, lip, oral mucosa, oesophagus, anus, prostate and bronchi. Previously called preinvasive carcinoma—**carcinomata** *pl*, **carcinomatous** *adj*.

**carcinomatosis** *n* widespread malignancy affecting many organs.

**cardia** *n* the oesophageal opening into the stomach.

**cardiac** *adj* **1.** pertaining to the heart. **2.** pertaining to the cardia of the stomach.

**cardiac arrest** complete cessation of effective output (of blood) from heart activity. Failure of the heart action to maintain an adequate circulation. The clinical picture of cessation of circulation in a patient who was not expected to die at the time. There are several forms: asystole, pulseless electrical activity/electromechanical dissociation, pulseless ventricular tachycardia or ventricular fibrillation. ⇒ arrhythmia. ⊙DVD

**cardiac bed** one which can be manipulated so that the patient is supported in a sitting position.

**cardiac bypass operation** the bypassing of atheromatous vessels (coronary arteries) supplying heart muscle (myocardium). ⇒ coronary artery bypass graft.

**cardiac catheterization** ⇒ catheterization.

**cardiac cycle** the rhythmic contraction (systole) and relaxation (diastole) of the heart as it fills with blood and pumps it around the body and to the lungs. The cycle provides an adequate output of blood from the heart. There are a series of stages that occur during a single heart beat, which is normally completed in less than 1 second. Cycles follow on without pause to maintain a continuous flow of blood. ⇒ diastole, systole.

**cardiac enzymes** released from damaged myocardial cells. Abnormal levels found in the blood are suggestive of a diagnosis of myocardial infarction. Used to confirm or refute the diagnosis of myocardial infarction. The enzymes usually measured are cardiac troponins (I and T) and creatine kinase (CK). Elevated levels of troponins indicate myocardial damage from any cause and they are used to differentiate between chest pain caused by unstable angina and myocardial infarction. Aspartate aminotransferase (AST) and lactate dehydrogenase (LDH) may also be measured.

**cardiac index (CI)** the measure of cardiac output in relation to body surface area, i.e. L/min per $m^2$.

**cardiac massage** ⇒ cardiopulmonary resuscitation (CPR), chest compressions.

**cardiac muscle** a distinct muscle type that forms the myocardium. It has common features with both skeletal and smooth muscle. Its short branching fibres may have a single nucleus or two, are striated, but contraction is involuntary. The presence of an inherent 'pacemaker' produces rhythmic contractions that are modified to meet changing physiological needs by the autonomic nervous system and hormones. The boundaries between individual fibres, which are not well defined, are formed by intercalated discs—a feature that ensures that the wave of contraction passes easily across the myocardium, which behaves like a syncytium. ⇒ muscle.

**cardiac oedema** gravitational oedema. Such patients secrete excessive aldosterone which increases excretion of potassium and conserves sodium and chloride. Antialdosterone (aldosterone antagonists) drugs may be useful, e.g. spironolactone. ⇒ oedema.

**cardiac output (CO)** the volume of blood ejected by the heart per minute, typically 4–5 L/min at rest. It can be expressed as the cardiac index (CI), cardiac output divided by body surface area.

**cardiac pacemaker** an electrical device for maintaining myocardial contraction by stimulating the heart muscle. A pacemaker may be permanent or temporary. They are programmed in a variety of modes. Nowadays pacemakers can be programmed to alter their rate in response to physical activity.

**cardiac reflex** an automatic neural process that alters heart rate. It functions through stretch receptors in the right side of the heart which respond to the volume of venous blood returning to the heart.

**cardiac rehabilitation** provided primarily for patients after a myocardial infarction or revascularization but also for those with angina or heart failure. Programmes involve a multidisciplinary team (specialist nurse, exercise expert, dietitian, physiotherapist, occupational therapist and physician) and are likely to involve education about risk factor modification, exercise, counselling and psychological and social support. The aim is to enable the person to manage the activities of daily living independently.

**cardiac tamponade** excessive fluid surrounding the heart, usually blood when the cause is traumatic. Can occur in surgery and penetrating wounds or cardiac rupture. Causes compression of the heart leading to heart failure from haemopericardium. ⇒ Beck's triad.

**cardiac veins** several small veins that carry most venous blood from the myocardium. They unite to form the coronary sinus.

**cardialgia** *n* literally, pain in the heart. Often used to mean heartburn (pyrosis).

**cardinal ligaments** ⇒ transverse cervical ligaments.

**cardiogenic** *adj* of cardiac origin, such as the shock that may be due to low cardiac output following an extensive acute myocardial infarction.

**cardiograph** *n* an instrument for recording graphically the force and form of the heart beat—**cardiographic** *adj*, **cardiogram** *n*, **cardiographically** *adv*. ⇒ electrocardiograph.

**cardiologist** *n* a medically qualified person who specializes in diagnosing and treating diseases of the heart.

**cardiology** *n* study of the structure, function and diseases of the heart.

**cardiomegaly** *n* enlargement of the heart.

**cardiomyopathy** *n* a disease of the myocardium associated with cardiac dysfunction. It is classified as dilated cardiomyopathy, hypertrophic cardiomyopathy, arrhythmogenic right ventricular cardiomyopathy or restrictive cardiomyopathy. Management includes treatment of the cause (if possible), treatment of heart failure and sometimes heart transplantation—**cardiomyopathic** *adj*.

**cardiomyoplasty** *n* a surgical procedure whereby ventricular contraction is augmented by the use of stimulated skeletal muscle.

**cardiomyotomy** *n* cutting or dissection of the muscular tissue at the gastro-oesophageal junction for achalasia.

**cardiophone** *n* a microphone strapped to a patient which allows audible and visual signal of heart sounds. By channelling pulses through an electrocardiograph, a graphic record can be made. Can be used for the fetus.

**cardioplegia** *n* **1.** paralysis of the heart. **2.** the use of an electrolyte solution to induce cardiac arrest. *cold cardioplegia* cardioplegia combined with hypothermia to reduce the oxygen consumption of the myocardium during open-heart surgery.

**cardiopulmonary** *adj* pertaining to the heart and lungs. *cardiopulmonary bypass* used in open-heart surgery. The heart and lungs are excluded from the circulation and replaced by a pump oxygenator (heart–lung machine)—**cardiopulmonic** *adj*.

**cardiopulmonary resuscitation (CPR)** the techniques used to maintain circulation and respiration following cardiopulmonary arrest. It involves: (a) the maintenance of a clear airway; (b) rescue breaths (artificial respiration) using mouth-to-mouth or mouth-to-nose respiration, or with a bag and face mask, or by an endotracheal tube; and (c) maintenance of the circulation of blood by chest compressions (external cardiac massage). ⇒ resuscitation. ⊙DVD

**cardiorenal** *adj* pertaining to the heart and kidney.

**cardiorespiratory** *adj* pertaining to the heart and the respiratory system.

**cardiorrhaphy** *n* stitching of the heart wall; usually reserved for traumatic surgery.

**cardiospasm** *n* the failure of the gastro-oesophageal (cardiac) sphincter between the oesophagus and stomach to relax and allow food or fluids through. A type of achalasia.

**cardiothoracic** *adj* pertaining to the heart and thoracic cavity. A specialized branch of surgery.

**cardiotocograph** *n* the instrument used in cardiotocography.

**cardiotocography (CTG)** *n* fetal monitoring. A procedure whereby the fetal heart rate is measured either by an external microphone or by the application of an electrode to the fetal scalp, recording the fetal electrocardiograph and from it the fetal heart rate. Fetal movements are also recorded. An external transducer placed on the woman's abdomen or an intrauterine catheter measures the frequency and strength of the uterine contractions. Used for the early detection of fetal distress caused by hypoxia and other departures from normal. ⇒ fetal blood sampling, tocography.

**cardiotomy** *n* **1.** incision into the heart. **2.** surgical procedure in which the cardiac orifice of the stomach is incised.

**cardiotomy syndrome** pyrexia, pericarditis and pleural effusion following heart surgery. It may develop weeks or months after the operation and is thought to be an autoimmune reaction.

**cardiotoxic** *adj* describes any agent that has an injurious effect on the heart.

**cardiovascular** *adj* pertaining to the heart and blood vessels. *cardiovascular endurance* the ability to sustain exercise without undue fatigue, cardiac distress or respiratory distress. *cardiovascular disease (CVD)* includes disease affecting the heart or blood vessels, for example coronary heart disease, strokes, peripheral vascular disease, etc.

C

**cardioversion** *n* use of an electrical direct current (DC) countershock for restoring the heart rhythm to normal, such as slowing a rapid heart rate or converting atrial fibrillation to sinus rhythm. It may be accomplished with either an external or an internal defibrillator implanted in the chest.

**carditis** *n* inflammation of the heart. A word seldom used without the appropriate prefix, e.g. endo-, myo-, peri-. Often more than one layer is involved. ⇒ endocarditis, myocarditis, pericarditis.

**care pathway** an integrated plan or pathway agreed locally by the multidisciplinary team for specific patient/client groups or disorder. The agreed pathway is based on available evidence and guidelines. ⇒ integrated care pathway.

**caries** *n* inflammatory decay of bone, usually associated with pus formation—**carious** *adj*. ⇒ dental caries.

**carina** *n* a keel-like structure exemplified by the keel-shaped cartilage at the bifurcation of the trachea into two bronchi—**carinal** *adj*.

**cariogenic** *adj* causing caries, by convention referring to dental caries. Examples include soft drinks with high levels of sugar and confectionary.

**cariostatic** *adj* agents such as the oils and fats in food that coat the teeth and prevent acids and sugars from forming plaque.

**carminative** *adj, n* having the power to relieve flatulence and associated colic. They include cinnamon, nutmeg, peppermint.

**carneous mole** a fleshy mass in the uterus comprising blood clot and a dead fetus or parts thereof that have not been expelled with miscarriage.

**carnitine** *n* a substance formed from the amino acid lysine, needed for the transport of fatty acids within cells prior to their oxidation.

**Caroli's disease II** (J Caroli, French gastroenterologist, 1902–1979) congenital dilatation of the small intrahepatic bile ducts. It is associated with an increased risk of cholangitis (inflammation of the bile ducts), liver abscess and septicaemia.

**carotenaemia, carotinaemia** *n* also called xanthaemia. Abnormally high amounts of carotene in the blood, which leads to yellow coloration of the skin. May be due to an excessive intake of foods high in carotene such as carrots, or certain diseases.

**carotenes** *npl* a group of naturally occurring pigments within the larger group of carotenoids. They are fat-soluble and have antioxidant properties. Carotene occurs in three forms—alpha (α), beta (β) and gamma (γ). The β form is converted in the body to vitamin A; it is therefore a provitamin.

**carotenoids** *npl* a group of about 100 naturally occurring yellow to red pigments found mostly in plants, some of which are carotenes. Heating of foods before eating usually improves carotenoid availability.

**carotid artery** the principal artery on each side of the neck supplying the head and neck. The right and left common carotid arteries each divide into an internal carotid that supplies blood to the cerebrum, nose, forehead and eyes, and the external carotid that supplies the scalp and the structures of the face and neck. ⇒ Appendix 1, Figure 9.

**carotid bodies** a collection of chemoreceptors associated with each common carotid artery at its bifurcation. They are sensitive to changes in the level of oxygen and carbon dioxide in the blood and stimulate the respiratory centre in the medulla oblongata to make the necessary respiratory adjustments.

**carotid sinuses** a collection of baroreceptors sited at the bifurcation of each common carotid artery; they are sensitive to pressure changes and when blood pressure changes they signal the vasomotor centre in the medulla oblongata to make the necessary adjustments to blood pressure through, for example, peripheral vasodilation and reducing heart rate when blood pressure rises.

**carotid sinus massage** firm rubbing over the area of carotid sinus is used to stimulate reflex vagal slowing of the heart. The technique can be used by a competent practitioner to slow the heart rate in certain supraventricular tachyarrhythmias.

**carpal 1.** *adj* pertaining to the wrist. **2.** *n* one of the eight bones of the wrist.

**carpal tunnel syndrome** nocturnal pain, numbness, weakness of the thumb and tingling in the area of distribution of the median nerve in the hand. Due to compression as the nerve passes through the carpal tunnel. Most common in middle-aged women.

**carphology** *n* involuntary picking at the bedclothes, as seen in exhaustive or febrile delirium.

**carpometacarpal** *adj* pertaining to the carpal and metacarpal bones.

**carpopedal** *adj* pertaining to the hands and feet. *carpopedal spasm* painful spasm of hands and feet in tetany. ⇒ Chvostek's sign, hypocalcaemia, Trousseau's sign.

**carpus** *n* the wrist. Comprises eight bones: trapezium, trapezoid, capitate, hamate, scaphoid, lunate, triquetral and pisiform, in two rows. ⇒ Appendix 1, Figure 2.

**carrier** *n* **1.** a person who, without manifesting an infection, harbours the micro-organism which can cause the overt infection, and who can transmit infection to others. **2.** a person who carries a recessive gene at a specific chromosome location (locus).

**carrier molecule** a cell membrane protein that assists the transfer of drugs, ions and nutrients into the cell.

**cartilage** *n* a dense connective tissue capable of withstanding pressure. There is relatively more cartilage in a child's skeleton but much of it has been converted into bone by adulthood. There are three basic types of cartilage, each with a different function to fulfil. *fibrocartilage (white)* forms the pads between the vertebrae, ligaments, the semilunar cartilages in the knee and the rim or labrum that deepens the sockets of the shoulder and hip joints; *elastic fibrocartilage (yellow)* is found in the pinna of the ear, the middle coat of blood vessels and in the epiglottis; and *hyaline cartilage* forms part of the larynx, trachea and bronchi, the costal cartilages that join the ribs to the sternum, and covers the articular surfaces of long bones—**cartilaginous** *adj.*

**cartilaginous joint** amphiarthrosis. One of the three main classes of joint. A slightly movable joint where the two bones are connected by cartilage. There are two types: symphysis and synchondrosis. ⇒ symphysis, synchondrosis.

**caruncle** *n* a red fleshy projection. Hymenal caruncles surround the entrance to the vagina after rupture of the hymen. The lacrimal caruncle is the fleshy prominence at the inner canthus (angle) of the eye.

**case control study** an epidemiological approach comprising a retrospective research study that compares outcomes for a group with a particular condition with those of a control group matched for age, gender, etc. who do not have the condition.

**case study** research that studies data from one case, or a small group of cases.

**caseation** *n* the formation of a soft, cheese-like mass, as occurs in tuberculosis—**caseous** *adj.*

**casein** *n* a protein produced when milk enters the stomach. Coagulation occurs and is due to the action of rennin upon the caseinogen in the milk, splitting it into two proteins, one being casein. The casein combines with calcium and a clot is formed. Casein is known as paracasein in the USA.

**casein hydrolysate** predigested protein food derived from casein; can be added to other foods to increase the protein content.

**caseinogen** *n* the principal protein in milk. It is not soluble in water but is kept in solution in milk by inorganic salts. The proportion to lactalbumin is much higher in cows' milk than in human milk. In the presence of rennin it is converted into insoluble casein. Caseinogen is known as casein in the USA.

**caseous degeneration** cottage cheese-like tissue resulting from atrophy in a tuberculoma or gumma.

**Casoni test** intradermal injection of fresh, sterile hydatid fluid. A white papule indicates a hydatid cyst.

**cast** *n* **1.** material or exudate that has been moulded to the form of the cavity or tube in which it has collected. **2.** a rigid casing, often made with plaster of Paris and applied to immobilize a part of the body.

**castor oil** a vegetable oil previously used as a stimulant laxative. ⇒ laxatives. Used with zinc ointment as a barrier cream for napkin and urinary rash.

**castration** *n* surgical removal of the testes in the male, or of the ovaries in the female. Castration can be part of the treatment for a hormone-dependent cancer—**castrated** *adj*, **castrate** *n*, *vt.*

**CAT** *acron* **c**omputed **a**xial **t**omography.

**catabolic hormones** natural or synthetic hormones that stimulate the breakdown of complex chemical substances in order to release energy. They include cortisol, adrenaline (epinephrine), glucagon and cytokines. Others, including the excitatory neuropeptides hypocretins (orexins), appear to be involved in balancing sleep–wake–activity cycles and hence the expenditure of energy by the body and appetite. Compare with anabolic hormones.

**catabolism (or katabolism)** *n* the series of chemical reactions in the living body whereby complex substances are broken down into simpler ones accompanied by the release of energy. This energy is needed for anabolism, heat production, work and the other activities of the body. ⇒ adenosine diphosphate, adenosine triphosphate, anabolism, hypercatabolism, metabolism—**catabolic** *adj.*

**catagen** *n* a short interval in the hair growth cycle between active growth and the resting stage. ⇒ anagen, telogen.

**catalase** *n* a cellular enzyme that catalyses the breakdown of hydrogen peroxide into oxygen and water.

**catalysis** *n* an increase in the rate at which a chemical reaction proceeds to equilibrium through the medium of a catalyst or catalyser. Reaction retardation is termed negative catalysis—**catalytic** *adj*.

**catalyst** *n* any substance that regulates or accelerates the rate of a chemical reaction without itself undergoing a permanent change.

**cataplexy** *n* a condition of muscular rigidity induced by severe mental shock or fear. The patient remains conscious—**cataplectic** *adj*.

**cataract** *n* an opacity of the crystalline lens. Usually age-related, but there are many causes, including congenital, traumatic or metabolic, such as diabetes mellitus—**cataractous** *adj*.

**cataract extraction** removal of the affected lens and usually the insertion of an intraocular lens. ⇒ phacoemulsification.

**catarrh** *n* chronic inflammation of a mucous membrane with constant flow of a thick sticky mucus. Usually applied to the inflammation of the nasal air passages and the trachea—**catarrhal** *adj*.

**catatonic schizophrenia** a form of schizophrenia characterized by psychomotor disturbances (e.g. stupor, posturing, negativism, hyperkinesis). ⇒ schizophrenia.

**catchment area** the geographic area and its population served by a particular health provider or other organization, e.g. a health centre, school, NHS trust.

**cat cry syndrome** ⇒ 'cri du chat' syndrome.

**catecholamines** *npl* a group of important physiological amines, such as adrenaline (epinephrine), noradrenaline (norepinephrine) and dopamine. They act as hormones and neurotransmitters and affect blood pressure, heart rate, respiratory rate and blood glucose (sugar). Abnormally high levels are secreted by adrenal and other tumours and can be detected in the urine. ⇒ phaeochromocytoma.

**categorical data** data that can be categorized, e.g. hair colour. ⇒ nominal data, ordinal data.

**catgut** *n* a form of ligature and suture of varying thickness, strength and absorbability, prepared from animal tissue. The plain variety is usually absorbed in 5–10 days, whereas chromic catgut takes 10–21 days to be absorbed.

**catharsis** *n* in psychology, it describes the purging or outpouring of emotion through experiencing it deeply—**cathartic** *adj*.

**cathepsins (kathepsins)** *npl* group of intracellular enzymes that break down proteins. They function in the normal cellular turnover of tissue protein, and result in the changes that occur when meat and game are hung.

**catheter** *n* a hollow tube of variable length and bore, usually having one fluted end and a tip of varying size and shape according to function. Catheters are made of many substances, including soft plastics and silicone, with various coatings, soft and hard rubber, gum elastic, glass, silver and other metals, some of which are radiopaque. They have many uses, including insufflation of hollow tubes, cardiac catheterization, introduction of contrast medium for angiography, withdrawal of fluid from body cavities, e.g. urinary catheter, and the administration of drugs, fluids and nutrients.

**catheterization** *n* insertion of a catheter, most usually into the urinary bladder. *cardiac catheterization* a long plastic catheter or tubing is inserted into an artery or vein and moved under X-ray guidance until it reaches the heart. A catheter inserted into the brachial or femoral artery gives access to the left side of the heart and those inserted into the brachial or femoral vein can be guided into the right atrium, ventricle and the pulmonary artery. Cardiac catheterization can be used for: (a) recording pressures and cardiac output, ⇒ pulmonary artery occlusion pressure; (b) the introduction of radiopaque contrast medium for angiography; (c) treatments such as angioplasty and stent insertion, ⇒ angioplasty—**catheterize** *vt*.

**cathetron** *n* a high-rate dose, remotely controlled, afterloading device for radiotherapy. Hollow steel catheters are placed in the desired position. They are then connected to a protective safe by hollow cables. The radioactive cobalt moves from the safe into the catheters. After delivery of the required dose, the cobalt returns to the safe, thus avoiding radiation hazard to staff. Currently superseded by units such as the Selectron.

**cation** *n* an ion with a positive electrical charge, e.g. calcium ($Ca^{2+}$). They move towards the negative electrode (cathode) during electrolysis. ⇒ anion.

**cation exchange resin** one of several high-molecular-weight, insoluble organic substances which exchange cations with other ions. ⇒ ion exchange resin.

**cat-scratch fever** a virus infection resulting from a cat scratch or bite. There is fever and lymph node swelling about a week after the incident. Recovery is usually complete, although an abscess may develop.

**cauda** *n* a tail or tail-like appendage. *cauda equina* lower part of the spinal cord where the nerves for the legs and bladder originate—**caudal, caudate** *adj*.

**caudal anaesthesia** injection of local anaesthetic into the epidural space at the level of the sacrum causing loss of sensation in the lower abdomen and pelvis.

**caul** *n* the amnion, instead of rupturing as is usual to allow the baby through, persists and covers the baby's head at birth.

**cauliflower ear** in sports medicine a colloquial term used to describe deformity of the pinna that may follow auricular haematoma (collection of blood between the perichondrium and cartilage of the outer/external ear) caused by repeated trauma sustained during contact sports.

**causalgia** *n* ⇒ complex regional pain syndrome.

**caustic** *adj, n* corrosive or destructive to organic tissue; the agents which produce such results. Usually a strong alkali or acid, they are used to destroy overabundant granulation tissue, warts or polyps. Carbolic acid, carbon dioxide snow and silver nitrate are most commonly employed.

**cauterize** *vt* to cause tissue destruction by applying a heated instrument, a cautery—**cauterization** *n*.

**cautery** *n* an agent or device, e.g. electricity, chemicals or extremes of temperature, which destroys cells and tissues. Uses include the prevention of blood loss during surgery, or to remove abnormal tissue.

**cavernous** *adj* having hollow spaces.

**cavernous sinus** a channel for venous blood, on either side of the sphenoid bone. Contains many veins, several nerves, e.g. oculomotor (cranial nerve III) and the internal carotid artery. Its veins drain blood from the cerebral hemispheres, orbits and the bones of the skull. Sepsis around the eyes or nose can cause cavernous sinus thrombosis, a very serious condition.

**cavitation** *n* the formation of a cavity, as in pulmonary tuberculosis.

**cavity** *n* a hollow; an enclosed area. *abdominal cavity* that below the diaphragm; the abdomen. *buccal cavity* the mouth. *cerebral cavity* the ventricles of the brain. *cranial cavity* the brain box formed by the bones of the cranium. *dental cavity* a space or hole in a tooth caused by caries (decay). *medullary cavity* the hollow centre of a long bone, containing yellow bone marrow or medulla. *nasal cavity* that in the nose, separated into right and left halves by the nasal septum. *oral cavity* buccal cavity. *pelvic cavity* that bounded by the pelvic bones, more particularly the part below the iliopectineal line. *peritoneal cavity* a potential space between the parietal and visceral layers of the peritoneum. Similarly, the *pleural cavity* is the potential space between the visceral and parietal pleurae which in health are in contact in all phases of respiration. *synovial cavity* the potential space in a synovial joint. *uterine cavity* that of the uterus, the base extending between the orifices of the uterine tubes.

**CBA** *abbr* cost–benefit analysis.

**C cells** parafollicular cells in the thyroid gland. They produce a hormone calcitonin (thyrocalcitonin) which has a regulatory role in calcium and phosphate homeostasis.

**CCK** *abbr* cholecystokinin.

**CCPNS** *abbr* cell cycle phase non-specific.

**CCPS** *abbr* cell cycle phase specific.

**CCU** *abbr* coronary care unit. ⇒ high-dependency unit, intensive care/therapy unit.

**CD** *abbr* controlled drug.

**CDC** *abbr* Centers for Disease Control and Prevention.

**CD4 cells** denotes the immune helper T cells (lymphocytes) which have the specific CD4 glycoprotein surface antigen. ⇒ delayed-sensitivity T cells, helper T cells.

**CD4/CD8 count** the ratio of the CD4+ helper T cells to the CD8+ cytotoxic or suppressor T cells. It is used to monitor the immune system in people with viral infections such as human immunodeficiency virus (HIV) or following transplant. HIV and acquired immunodeficiency syndrome (AIDS) are associated with declining numbers of CD4+ helper T cells.

**CD8 cells** denotes the immune cytotoxic/suppressor T cells (lymphocytes) which have the specific CD8 glycoprotein surface antigen. ⇒ cytotoxic T cells, suppressor T cells.

**CDH** *abbr* congenital dislocation of the hip. ⇒ developmental dysplasia of the hip.

**CEA** *abbr* **1.** carcinoembryonic antigen. **2.** cost-effectiveness analysis.

**cell** *n* basic structural unit of living organisms. A mass of protoplasm (cytoplasm) and usually a nucleus within a plasma or cell membrane. Some cells, e.g. erythrocytes, are non-nucleated whereas others, such as voluntary muscle, may be multinucleated. The cytoplasm contains various subcellular organelles—mitochondria,

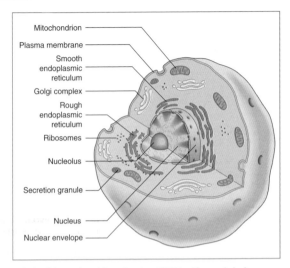

**Figure C.3** A typical cell *(reproduced from Brooker 2006A with permission).*

ribosomes, etc. (Figure C.3)—that undertake the metabolic processes of the cell—**cellular** *adj.*

**cell adhesion molecules (CAM)** *npl* protein molecules located on the cell membrane, which either bind cells together or bind cells with the extracellular matrix. There are several types of molecules that facilitate cell adhesion, for example immunoglobulins.

**cell cycle** the events occurring within a cell from one mitotic division to the next. Comprises the dynamic course of division of normal and cancer cells incorporating phases of DNA synthesis (S-phase), growth phases ($G_1$ and $G_2$), mitosis (M) and 'rest phase' ($G_0$) (Figure C.4).

**cell cycle phase non-specific (CCPNS)** describes a cytotoxic drug that acts at any time in the cell cycle.

**cell cycle phase specific (CCPS)** describes a cytotoxic drug that acts during a specific phase of the cell cycle.

**cell-mediated immunity** ⇒ immunity.

**cell-surface molecules** a diverse group of molecules present on the surface of cells. They facilitate and regulate cell functions and allow cells to communicate with each other and with the environment. They include cell recognition proteins; immune proteins; ion channels and other transport proteins for moving

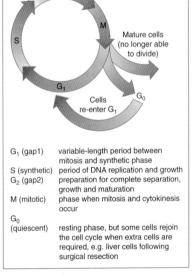

| | |
|---|---|
| $G_1$ (gap1) | variable-length period between mitosis and synthetic phase |
| S (synthetic) | period of DNA replication and growth |
| $G_2$ (gap2) | preparation for complete separation, growth and maturation |
| M (mitotic) | phase when mitosis and cytokinesis occur |
| $G_0$ (quiescent) | resting phase, but some cells rejoin the cell cycle when extra cells are required, e.g. liver cells following surgical resection |

**Figure C.4** Cell cycle *(reproduced from Brooker 2006A with permission).*

material in or out of the cell; receptors that respond to a specific ligand (e.g. hormone, growth factor, neurotransmitter or enzyme); and complexes of cell adhesion molecules forming desmosomes.

**cellulitis** *n* a diffuse acute inflammation of the skin and connective tissue, especially the loose subcutaneous tissue. ⊙DVD Often caused by group A beta-haemolytic streptococci. When it occurs in the floor of the mouth it is called Ludwig's angina.

**cellulose** *n* a carbohydrate forming the outer walls of plant and vegetable cells. A polysaccharide which cannot be digested by humans but supplies non-starch polysaccharides (NSP) for stimulation of peristalsis.

**Celsius** (A Celsius, Swedish scientist, 1701–1744) the derived SI unit (International System of Units) for temperature. ⇒ centigrade, Appendix 2.

**cementoblast** *n* the cell that forms the organic component of cementum.

**cementocyte** *n* the cell located within the lacunae of the cementum. They form from cementoblasts that are trapped during the formation of cementum.

**cementoma** *n* any benign endontogenic cementum-producing tumour that affects the apical part of the root of a tooth.

**cementopathia** *n* poor condition of the teeth due to diseased or deficient cementum. It is implicated in periodontal disease.

**cementum** *n* calcified organic hard tissue forming on the surface of a root of a tooth, and providing attachment for the periodontal ligament. ⇒ tooth.

**censor** *n* term used by Freud to describe the resistance that prevents repressed material from easily re-entering the conscious mind from the subconscious (unconscious) mind.

**Centers for Disease Control and Prevention (CDC)** a federal agency in the USA (Atlanta). Its functions include the investigation, identification, prevention and control of disease.

**centigrade** *n* a scale with 100 divisions or degrees. Most often refers to the thermometric scale, in which the freezing point of water is fixed at 0° and the boiling point at 100°. It is usually called Celsius for medical and scientific purposes. ⇒ Celsius.

**centile** *n* the numbered points that divide a set of scores into 100 points. *centile chart* used to compare, for instance, a child's growth compared with children of the same sex and age. The chart shows the line for the average weight, height, etc. The individual child's measurements are charted on the appropriate centile and health professionals are able to predict the percentage of children of the same age and sex who would be bigger or smaller. For example, the 90th percentile would mean that 90% of children would be smaller and 10% of children would be bigger. Serial measurements will detect if a child's growth moves into another centile, or falls outside the 97th or 3rd centile which needs further investigation.

**central auditory processing disorder** ⇒ auditory processing disorder.

**central cyanosis** ⇒ cyanosis.

**central limit theorem** in research. Sampling distribution becomes more normal the more samples are taken.

**central nervous system** comprises the brain and spinal cord. ⇒ peripheral nervous system.

**central sterile supplies department (CSSD)** designated area where packets are prepared containing the equipment and/or swabs and dressings necessary to perform activities requiring aseptic technique. ⇒ hospital sterilization and disinfection unit (HSDU).

**central tendency statistic** averages. The tendency for observations to centre around a specific value rather than across the entire range (Figure C.5). ⇒ mean, median, mode.

**central venous catheter/line** specialized intravenous cannula which is placed in a large vein (internal jugular, subclavian), or inserted into a peripheral vein in the arm. The cannula is advanced until the tip is in the superior vena cava or the right atrium of the heart. ⇒ Appendix 1, Figure 10. Used for the measurement of central venous pressure and central venous oxygen saturation ($CVSO_2$), and also for the administration of drugs and fluids. Also used for long-term

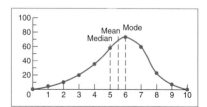

**Figure C.5** Central tendency statistic *(reproduced from Gunn 2001 with permission).*

vascular access for the administration of drugs, blood products or nutritional support.

**central venous pressure (CVP)** the pressure of the blood within the right atrium. It is measured using a central venous catheter attached to a pressure transducer or occasionally a manometer is used. Serial readings are used in the assessment of circulatory function, circulating blood volume and fluid replacement needs.

**centrifugal** *adj* efferent. Having a tendency to move outwards from the centre, as the nerve impulses from the brain to the peripheral structures.

**centrifuge** *n* an apparatus which subjects solutions to centrifugal forces by high-speed rotation, thereby separating substances of different densities into discrete bands within the liquid phase. It is usually used to separate ('spin down') particulate material (e.g. subcellular particles) from a suspending liquid.

**centriole** *n* a subcellular organelle that aids spindle formation during nuclear division. ⇒ meiosis, mitosis.

**centripetal** *adj* afferent. Having a tendency to move towards the centre, such as the rash occurring in chickenpox.

**centromere** *n* the structure that joins the double chromosome (two chromatids) and eventually attaches to the spindle during nuclear division. ⇒ meiosis, mitosis.

**centrosome** *n* a region adjacent to the cell nucleus that contains the centrioles.

**cephalalgia** *n* pain in the head; headache.

**cephalhaematoma** *n* a collection of blood in the subperiosteal tissues of the scalp of an infant. It is usually caused by pressure on the scalp during a long labour. ⇒ caput succedaneum, moulding.

**cephalic** *adj* pertaining to the head; near the head. *cephalic version* ⇒ version.

**cephalic vein** *n* a superficial vein that drains blood from the arm. ⇒ Appendix 1, Figure 10.

**cephalin** *n* a phospholipid present in nervous tissue—the white matter of the brain, spinal cord and nerves.

**cephalocele** *n* hernia of the brain; protrusion of part of the brain through the skull.

**cephalohaematoma** *n* cephalhaematoma.

**cephalometry** *n* measurement of the living human head.

**cephalopelvic disproportion** a disparity between the size of the fetal head and the size of the woman's pelvis. Either the fetal head is too large or the woman's pelvis is too small

to allow a vaginal delivery, necessitating a caesarean section.

**cephalosporins** *npl* a large group of beta-lactam antibiotics, closely related to the penicillins, e.g. cefaclor. ⇒ Appendix 5.

**cerclage** *n* **1.** a technique used to correct a detached retina in which a taut band is applied around the sclera to restore the contact between the retina and choroid. **2.** a technique whereby a wire or metal band is used to secure the bone ends or fragments of certain fractures such as a fractured patella. ⇒ cervical cerclage.

**cereal** *n* the grains or edible seeds obtained from the grass family, e.g. rice, wheat, barley, oats, rye, maize and millet.

**cerebellar gait** a staggering, unsteady, wide-based walk seen in patients with damage to the cerebellum or its connections. ⇒ gait.

**cerebellum** *n* that part of the brain which lies behind and below the cerebrum (⇒ Appendix 1, Figures 1 and 11). Its chief functions are the co-ordination of fine voluntary movements and the control of posture—**cerebellar** *adj*.

**cerebral** *adj* pertaining to the cerebrum.

**cerebral compression** arises from any space-occupying intracranial lesion, for example tumour, swelling, haemorrhage, etc.

**cerebral cortex** the outer layer of cells (grey matter) of the cerebral hemispheres.

**cerebral embolism** the presence of an embolus impeding blood flow in a cerebral blood vessel resulting in cerebral ischaemia. The embolus can originate in the heart such as in atrial fibrillation. ⇒ cerebrovascular accident.

**cerebral function monitor (CFM)** equipment for continuous monitoring of brain wave activity, e.g. to detect seizures in sedated and paralysed patients.

**cerebral haemorrhage** bleeding from a cerebral blood vessel into the substance of the brain. It may arise from degenerative disease affecting the vessel or from hypertension, as in a stroke (cerebrovascular accident); from the rupture of a congenital aneurysm or other vessel abnormality; or as a result of trauma. Traditional management of cerebral bleeding caused by an aneurysm was to clip the aneurysm to prevent further bleeding but newer and less invasive treatments are now available. A neuroradiologist inserts tiny platinum coils into the aneurysm through a microcatheter passed via the blood vessels in the groin through the body and into the aneurysm.

The coils cause the blood in the aneurysm to clot, preventing it from rupturing. ⇒ cerebrovascular accident, embolization, extradural haematoma, subarachnoid haemorrhage, subdural haematoma.

**cerebral hemisphere** one side of the cerebrum, right or left.

**cerebral palsy** non-progressive brain damage that typically occurs at, or shortly after, birth resulting in a range of mainly motor conditions ranging from clumsiness to severe spasticity. ⇒ Little's disease.

**cerebral perfusion pressure (CPP)** the pressure which drives blood through the brain. It is the difference between the mean arterial blood pressure and the intracranial pressure. If CPP is too low, the blood flow to the brain may be inadequate and the brain deprived of oxygen.

**cerebral thrombosis** the presence of a blood clot impeding blood flow in a cerebral vessel resulting in cerebral ischaemia. The clot forms within the cerebral blood vessel.

**cerebration** *n* mental activity.

**cerebroside** *n* one of a group of glycolipids found in the brain and the myelin sheath covering nerves. ⇒ ganglioside, glycosphingolipids.

**cerebrospinal** *adj* pertaining to the brain and spinal cord.

**cerebrospinal fluid** the clear fluid found within the ventricles (cavities) of the brain, central canal of the spinal cord and beneath the cranial and spinal meninges in the subarachnoid space. Protects and nourishes the brain and spinal cord. It is formed by the choroid plexuses in the ventricles and circulates around the brain and spinal cord before being returned to the blood through the arachnoid villi/granulations, which project into the venous sinuses of the brain.

**cerebrovascular** *adj* pertaining to the blood vessels of the brain.

**cerebrovascular accident (stroke) (CVA)** interference with the cerebral blood flow due to embolism, haemorrhage or thrombosis. Signs and symptoms vary according to the duration, extent and site of tissue damage; there may be only a passing, even momentary inability to move a hand or foot; weakness or tingling in a limb; stertorous breathing; incontinence of urine and faeces; coma; paralysis of a limb or limbs; and speech deficiency (aphasia). ⇒ transient ischaemic attack.

**cerebrum** *n* the largest and uppermost part of the brain (⇒ Appendix 1, Figures 1 and 11).

The longitudinal fissure divides it into two hemispheres, each containing a lateral ventricle. A mass of nerve fibres (white matter) is covered by a thin layer of nerve cells (grey matter). It controls the higher functions and contains major motor and sensory areas. The outer surface is convoluted—**cerebral** *adj*.

**certified** *adj* a redundant psychiatric term. In the UK patients detained under current mental health legislation are said to be formally detained or 'sectioned'.

**ceruloplasmin** *n* plasma protein involved in copper transport.

**cerumen** *n* ear wax, sticky brown secretion from glands in the external auditory meatus/canal. Traps dust and other particles entering the ear—**ceruminous** *adj*.

**cervical** *adj* **1.** pertaining to the neck. **2.** pertaining to the cervix (neck) of an organ, such as the uterine cervix.

**cervical amnioscopy** ⇒ amnioscopy.

**cervical canal** the lumen of the cervix uteri that reaches from the internal os to the external os.

**cervical cerclage** the insertion of a non-absorbable pursestring suture (stitch) in the cervix to keep it from opening. It is indicated for women who have a cervix which does not fully close (incompetent cervix), which may lead to miscarriage or preterm birth. The suture is inserted at 14 weeks' gestation and removed at 38 weeks' gestation or sooner if labour commences.

**cervical effacement** thinning, softening and shortening of the cervix, as the internal os is taken up to become part of the lower uterine segment, and have contact with the forewaters and the presenting part. The cervical canal becomes a circular orifice with extremely thin edges (Figure C.6). Usually it occurs in the last

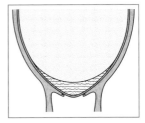

**Figure C.6** Cervical effacement *(reproduced from Fraser & Cooper 2003 with permission).*

C

2 weeks before labour in a primigravida, and during labour in a multigravida.

**cervical eversion (ectropion)** erroneously called an erosion. It is caused by high levels of oestrogen during pregnancy that cause a proliferation of columnar epithelium in the cervical canal which encroaches over the squamous epithelium which is normally present over the vaginal portion of the cervix. The junction where the two epithelial tissue types meet everts into the vagina. The eversion usually resolves after the birth.

**cervical nerves** the eight pairs of spinal nerves that arise from the cervical part of the spinal cord. The first nerve exits above the atlas (first cervical vertebra) and the others exit from below each of the seven cervical vertebrae. The cervical nerves C1–C4 innervate the head and neck, and cervical nerves C5–C8 innervate the arms, back and scalp. *cervical plexus* the complex network of deep and superficial branches formed by the anterior rami of cervical nerves C1–C4. They supply the skin over the front of the neck, the back and side of the head, the neck muscles and one branch—the phrenic nerve—supplies the diaphragm. ⇒ Appendix 1, Figure 11.

**cervical rib** ⇒ thoracic inlet syndrome.

**cervical smear** microscopic examination of cells obtained from the surface of the cervix. ⇒ cervical intraepithelial neoplasia, Papanicolaou test.

**cervical vertebrae** the first seven vertebrae. The first vertebra or atlas supports the skull and rotates around the odontoid process (dens) of the second vertebra or axis. ⇒ Appendix 1, Figure 3.

**cervical intraepithelial neoplasia (CIN)** staging of cellular changes in the uterine cervix that occur prior to the development of carcinoma in situ and invasive cancer. Abnormal cells are detected by a smear test and the diagnosis is confirmed by colposcopy and biopsy. CIN1, mild dysplasia; CIN2, moderate dysplasia; CIN3, severe dysplasia, carcinoma in situ. ⇒ conization.

**cervicectomy** *n* amputation of the uterine cervix.

**cervicitis** *n* inflammation of the uterine cervix.

**cervix** *n* a neck. *cervix uteri, uterine cervix* the neck of the uterus (⇒ Appendix 1, Figure 17)—**cervical** *adj*.

**cestode** *n* tapeworm. ⇒ *Taenia*.

**cetrimide** *n* a disinfectant with detergent properties. Used for wound cleansing and skin preparation.

**CF** *abbr* cystic fibrosis.

**CFM** *abbr* cerebral function monitor.

**CFS/ME** *abbr* chronic fatigue syndrome/myalgic encephalomyelitis.

**CFT** *abbr* complement fixation test.

**CFTR** *abbr* cystic fibrosis transmembrane regulator.

**CGM** *abbr* continuous glucose monitoring.

**Chagas' disease** ⇒ trypanosomiasis.

**chaining** *n* a skills training technique used for people with a learning disability. Each small step in a skilled task, such as dressing or making a sandwich, is taught in sequence. It may be *forward*, where the skill is learnt from the beginning in the sequence it normally occurs, with each step linking to the next, or *backward*, where the skill is learnt by working backwards from the final step of the finished task.

**chalazion** *n* a cyst in the eyelid caused by chronic inflammation of retained secretion of a meibomian gland.

**chalcosis** *n* a condition that results from an intraocular copper foreign body. The serious chemical reaction that occurs causes endophthalmitis and rapid visual impairment.

**chalone** *n* a substance that inhibits rather than stimulates, e.g. enterogastrone inhibits gastric secretions and motility.

**chancre** *n* the primary syphilitic ulcer developing at the site of infection with *Treponema pallidum*. It is associated with swelling of local lymph nodes. The chancre is painless, indurated, solitary and highly infectious. It heals spontaneously without treatment.

**chancroid** *n* (*syn* soft sore) a type of sexually transmitted infection prevalent in warmer climates. Caused by the bacillus *Haemophilus ducreyi*. Causes multiple, painful, ragged ulcers on the genitalia, often with bubo formation.

**character** *n* the sum total of the known and predictable mental characteristics of an individual, particularly his or her conduct. *character change* denotes change in the form of conduct, to one foreign to the patient's natural disposition, e.g. violent or indecent behaviour.

**charcoal** *n* used therapeutically for its adsorptive and deodorant properties. Oral administration of activated charcoal is used for certain types of poisoning. It binds to some poisons in the gastrointestinal tract and prevents their absorption, and may also be used for active elimination techniques once the poison has been absorbed into the body. Activated charcoal when incorporated into dressings is used to reduce odour in malodorous discharging wounds.

**Charcot's joint** (J M Charcot, French neurologist, 1825–1893) complete disorganization of a joint associated with syringomyelia, diabetes mellitus, or advanced cases of tabes dorsalis (locomotor ataxia). The condition is painless.

**Charcot's triad I** (J M Charcot) sometimes seen as a manifestation of multiple sclerosis—nystagmus, intention tremor and scanning or staccato speech.

**CHD** *abbr* coronary heart disease.

**Chédiak–Higashi syndrome** (A M Chédiak, Cuban physician, 20th century; O Higashi, Japanese physician, 20th century) an inherited autosomal recessive disorder of the immune system. The leucocytes are abnormal and result in chronic infection. There is decreased pigmentation in skin and eyes, neurological disease, photophobia and early death.

**cheek biting** damage to the buccal mucosa that results from malocclusion, poor chewing co-ordination or habit.

**cheilitis** *n* inflammation of the lip.

**cheiloplasty** *n* any plastic operation on the lip.

**cheilosis** *n* maceration at the angles of the mouth; fissures occur later. May be due to riboflavin deficiency.

**cheiropompholyx** *n* symmetrical eruption of skin of hands (especially fingers) characterized by the formation of tiny vesicles and associated with itching or burning. On the feet the condition is called podopompholyx.

**chelating agents** soluble organic compounds that combine with certain metallic ions, such as iron, to form complexes that are safely excreted in the urine. For example, desferrioxamine used for iron overload or poisoning. ⇒ DTPA, haemochromatosis, thalassaemia. ⇒ Appendix 5.

**chemokines** *npl* small cytokines that induce chemotaxis and the recruitment and activation of leucocytes during the inflammatory response. They are released from many different cells in response to infection with bacteria or viruses and physical damage. Chemokines act upon cells of both innate and adaptive immunity. They attract leucocytes (neutrophils, monocytes and lymphocytes) to areas of damage or infection and some may stimulate the formation of new blood vessels (angiogenesis).

**chemonucleolysis** *n* injection of an enzyme, usually into an intervertebral disc, for dissolution of same—**chemonucleolytic** *adj*.

**chemopallidectomy** *n* the chemical destruction of a predetermined section of globus pallidus.

**chemoprophylaxis** *n* the prevention of disease (or recurrent attack) by administration of drugs such as antibiotics following some surgical procedures and for people exposed to infection, and antimalarial drugs. For example the administration of rifampicin to the contacts of patients with meningococcal meningitis—**chemoprophylactic** *adj*.

**chemoreceptor** *n* a sensory nerve ending or a cell having an affinity for, and capable of reacting to, a chemical stimulus, e.g. taste, oxygen levels in the blood. ⇒ carotid bodies.

**chemoreceptor trigger zone (CTZ)** a vomiting centre in the medulla of the brain that is stimulated by chemical stimuli present in the blood, such as toxins; and impulses from the higher centres of the cerebral cortex, gastrointestinal tract and the vestibular apparatus and centres. ⇒ vomiting centre.

**chemoresistant** *adj* describes a tumour that does not usually shrink with chemotherapy.

**chemosensitive** *adj* describes a tumour that shrinks following chemotherapy administration.

**chemosis** *n* oedema or swelling of the bulbar conjunctiva—**chemotic** *adj*.

**chemotaxis** *n* movements of a cell (e.g. leucocyte) or a micro-organism in response to chemical stimuli; attraction is termed *positive chemotaxis*, repulsion is *negative chemotaxis*—**chemotactic** *adj*. ⇒ chemokines.

**chemotherapy** *n* chemical agents of various types; prescribed to delay or arrest growth of cancer cells through interruption/inhibition of cell cycle; usually given in combination rather than as single agents. They are non-selective and non-specific and therefore affect all cycling cells, whether benign or malignant. Administration is by oral, intramuscular, intravenous, intracavitary or intra-arterial routes. ⇒ alkylating agents, antimetabolites, antitumour antibiotics, vinca alkaloids. ⇒ Appendix 5.

**chenodeoxycholic acid** a bile acid. It can be taken orally to dissolve certain types of gallstones.

**chest compressions** external cardiac massage. Performed during cardiac arrest. With the person lying on his or her back on a firm surface, the lower part of the sternum (breastbone) is depressed to compress the heart and force blood into the circulation (Figure C.7). ⇒ basic life support. ⊙DVD

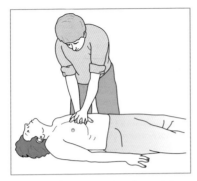

**Figure C.7** Chest compressions in an adult (*reproduced from Brooker & Waugh 2007 with permission*).

**Cheyne–Stokes respiration** cyclical waxing and waning of breathing, characterized at one extreme by deep fast breaths and at the other by apnoea: it generally has an ominous prognosis.

**CHF** *abbr* congestive heart failure.

**CHI** ⇒ Qi energy.

**chiasma** *n* an X-shaped crossing or decussation, such as the optic chiasma—**chiasmata** *pl*. ⇒ optic chiasma.

**chickenpox** *n* (*syn* varicella) a generally mild, specific infection with varicella-zoster virus (VZV), a herpes virus, mainly affecting children. Immunization against varicella is part of the routine childhood programme in the USA. The incubation is 12–21 days. Successive crops of vesicles appear first on the trunk; they scab and usually heal without scars. The disease can be much more severe in adults, especially those who are immunocompromised, such as those with human immunodeficiency virus (HIV) disease, or those having immunosuppression treatment, e.g. after transplant, when it may be fatal. Treatment with antiviral drugs is indicated. ⊙ DVD

**chief cells** cells in the gastric mucosa that secrete pepsinogen, the inactive precursor of the digestive enzyme pepsin.

**chikungunya** *n* a mosquito-transmitted haemorrhagic fever occurring in Africa.

**chilblain** *n* (*syn* erythema pernio) seasonal vasospasm (spasm of blood vessels) caused by cold. It mainly affects children and older people, and leads to congestion and swelling of the feet or hands. In the short, acute stage there is redness with severe itching and burning sensation. The chronic stage is characterized by dull redness and congestion in the affected area. The affected skin is easily damaged and healing is prolonged. ⇒ perniosis.

**child abuse** physical, sexual or emotional abuse or neglect of children by relatives, other carers or health and social care staff. ⇒ non-accidental injuries.

**Chinese-restaurant syndrome (Kwok's syndrome)** postprandial disturbance once thought to be caused by eating the flavour enhancer monosodium glutamate, which is used as a food additive and to enhance flavours in Chinese cooking. It is characterized by flushing, headache, palpitations, numbness and abdominal symptoms. The cause is not known.

**chiropodist** *n* ⇒ podiatrist.

**chiropody** *n* ⇒ podiatry.

**chiropractic** *n* a technique of spinal manipulation, based on the principle that defects in vertebral alignment may result in various problems caused by functional changes in the nervous system. In the UK chiropractic is subject to statutory regulation, which means that practitioners must be registered with the General Chiropractic Council in order to practise.

**chiropractor** *n* a person who uses chiropractic techniques.

**chi-square statistic ($\chi^2$)** a technique used to analyse the relationship between expected frequency and the actual frequency of data obtained. A test of statistical significance used to determine the probability of results occurring by chance. ⇒ non-parametric tests.

**chlamydiae** *npl* micro-organisms of the genus *Chlamydia*. They are intracellular parasites and have features common to both bacteria and viruses. *Chlamydia psittaci* infects birds and causes psittacosis in humans. ⇒ ornithosis. Subgroups of *C. trachomatis* cause genital tract infection in adults, and are sexually transmitted. In men, may be associated with urethritis, but infection is often symptomless; epididymitis may be a complication. In women, most infections are symptomless; about 20% of untreated women develop pelvic inflammatory disease with subsequent scarring of the uterine (fallopian) tubes with risk of infertility or of ectopic pregnancy. Reactive arthritis is an uncommon complication. Autoinoculation from the genital tract can cause conjunctivitis in adults. Chlamydial conjunctivitis and pneumonia in infants can result from infection during birth. Lymphogranuloma venereum is caused by a different subgroup of *C. trachomatis*. The micro-organism also causes trachoma. ⇒ trachoma.

**chloasma** *n* patchy brown discoloration of the skin, especially the face. Can appear during pregnancy and during use of the oral contraceptive. ⇒ melasma.

**chlorhexidine** *n* a disinfectant solution which is effective against a wide range of bacteria. Used for general skin cleansing and disinfection, and hand decontamination, etc.

**chloride** *n* a salt of hydrochloric acid. A major anion in extracellular fluid. *chloride shift* the movement of chloride ions into the red blood cells to restore electrical balance, as bicarbonate (hydrogen carbonate) ions move out into the blood during the transport of carbon dioxide.

**chlorine** *n* a greenish-yellow, irritating gaseous element. Powerful disinfectant, bleaching and deodorizing agent in the presence of moisture when nascent oxygen is liberated. Mainly used as hypochlorites, or other compounds which slowly liberate active chlorine.

**chloroform** *n* a heavy liquid, once used extensively as a general anaesthetic. Used as chloroform water as a flavouring and preservative in aqueous mixtures.

**chlorolabe** *n* a pigment contained in one group of cones; responds to green light.

**chloropsia** *n* an abnormality of vision where all objects are seen as green.

**CHM** *abbr* Commission on Human Medicines.

**choanae** *npl* funnel-shaped openings. ⇒ nares—**choana** *sing*, **choanal** *adj*.

**chocolate cyst** an endometrial cyst containing altered blood. The ovaries are the most usual site. ⇒ endometriosis.

**cholagogue** *n* a drug which increases the flow of bile into the intestine.

**cholangiography** *n* rarely performed radiographic examination of hepatic, cystic and bile ducts (biliary tract). Can be performed: (a) after oral or intravenous administration of contrast medium; (b) by direct injection at operation to detect any further stones in the ducts; (c) during or after operation by way of a T-tube in the common bile duct; or (d) percutaneously by means of an injection via the skin on the anterior abdominal wall and the liver. ⇒ endoscopic retrograde cholangiopancreatography, percutaneous transhepatic cholangiography (PTC).

**cholangitis** *n* inflammation of the bile ducts.

**cholecalciferol** *n* vitamin $D_3$. An essential precursor of the active forms of vitamin D.

**cholecystectomy** *n* surgical removal of the gallbladder. *laparoscopic cholecystectomy* removal of the gallbladder using minimally invasive surgical techniques.

**cholecystenterostomy** *n* literally, the establishment of an artificial opening (anastomosis) between the gallbladder and the small intestine. Specific terminology more frequently used.

**cholecystitis** *n* acute or chronic inflammation of the gallbladder, most often associated with the presence of gallstones.

**cholecystoduodenal** *adj* pertaining to the gallbladder and duodenum as an anastomosis between them.

**cholecystoduodenostomy** *n* the establishment of an anastomosis between the gallbladder and the duodenum.

**cholecystography** *n* rarely performed radiographic examination of the gallbladder after administration of opaque contrast medium. Superseded by computed tomography and magnetic resonance imaging scanning.

**cholecystojejunostomy** *n* an anastomosis between the gallbladder and the jejunum.

**cholecystokinin (CCK)** *n* a hormone that contracts the gallbladder and relaxes the sphincter of Oddi, thus allowing bile into the duodenum, and stimulates the secretion of pancreatic enzymes. Secreted by the duodenal mucosa.

**cholecystolithiasis** *n* the presence of a gallstone or stones in the gallbladder.

**cholecystostomy** *n* a surgically established fistula between the gallbladder and the abdominal surface; used to provide drainage, in empyema of the gallbladder.

**cholecystotomy** *n* incision into the gallbladder.

**choledochoduodenal** *adj* pertaining to the bile ducts and duodenum, e.g. *choledochoduodenal fistula*.

**choledochography** *n* cholangiography.

**choledochojejunostomy** *n* an anastomosis between the bile duct and the jejunum.

**choledocholithiasis** *n* the presence of a gallstone or gallstones in the extrahepatic bile ducts.

**choledocholithotomy** *n* surgical removal of a stone from the common bile duct.

**choledochoscope** *n* endoscopic instrument used to examine the lumen of the biliary tree (bile ducts).

**choledochoscopy** *n* endoscopic examination of the biliary tree.

**choledochostomy** *n* drainage of the common bile duct using a T-tube, usually after exploration for a gallstone.

**choledochotomy** *n* incision into the common bile duct.

**cholelithiasis** *n* the presence or formation of gallstones in the gallbladder or bile ducts.

**cholera** *n* acute enteritis occurring in Africa and Asia, where it is endemic and epidemic. It is caused by the bacterium *Vibrio cholerae* and is associated with faecal contamination of water, overcrowding and insanitary conditions. There is diarrhoea (rice-water stools) accompanied by agonizing cramp and vomiting, resulting in dehydration, electrolyte imbalance and severe collapse. There are high mortality rates without adequate fluid and electrolyte replacement.

**choleric temperament** one of the four classic types of temperament, hasty and with a propensity to emotional outbursts.

**cholestasis** *n* an obstruction to the flow of bile. It produces jaundice, dark urine, pale stools, metallic taste and pruritus. *extrahepatic cholestasis* caused by a blockage to a large duct, e.g. the common bile duct, by a gallstone or cancer involving the head of the pancreas. *intrahepatic cholestasis* caused by blockage of the small bile ducts within the liver, such as in hepatitis or due to cirrhosis—**cholestatic** *adj*.

**cholesteatoma** *n* a benign encysted tumour containing squamous epithelial debris. Mainly occurs in the middle ear—**cholesteatomatous** *adj*.

**cholesterol** *n* a sterol found in many tissues. It is an important component of cell membranes and is the precursor of many biological molecules such as steroid hormones and is concerned with the absorption and transportation of fatty acids. High levels of low-density lipoprotein cholesterol in the blood are linked with the development of arterial disease and some types of gallstones. It is present in some foods and is processed by the liver. ⇒ hypercholesterolaemia.

**cholesterosis** *n* abnormal deposition of cholesterol.

**cholic acid** a bile acid produced from cholesterol in the liver.

**choline** *n* a chemical found in animal tissues as a component of phospholipids, e.g. lecithin (phosphatidylcholine); has an important influence on the production of the neurotransmitter acetylcholine. Choline is involved in the transportation of fats and the entry of fats into cells.

**cholinergic** *adj* applied to nerves that release acetylcholine as the neurotransmitter at their synapses. They include the somatic motor nerves innervating voluntary skeletal muscle, all parasympathetic nerves (preganglionic and postganglionic), preganglionic sympathetic nerves and a few postganglionic sympathetic nerves (the innervation to some sweat glands and the blood vessels supplying the skin and skeletal muscle). ⇒ adrenergic.

**cholinergic crisis** severe muscle weakness, flaccid paralysis and respiratory failure caused by an excess of acetylcholine at the neuromuscular junction. It can result from overtreatment with the anticholinesterase drugs used to treat myasthenia gravis, or from organophosphate poisoning.

**cholinergic receptors** receptor sites on the effector structures innervated by parasympathetic and voluntary motor nerves. The receptors may be muscarinic or nicotinic depending on their response to acetylcholine. They may be excitatory or inhibitory depending on their location. Both muscarinic and nicotinic receptors are further subdivided. ⇒ edrophonium test.

**cholinesterase** *n* an enzyme that inactivates acetylcholine at nerve endings. It catalyses the reaction whereby acetylcholine is broken down into choline and water.

**choluria** *n* bile in the urine.

**chondritis** *n* inflammation of cartilage.

**chondroblast** *n* a mesenchymal cell that produces cartilage. Particularly important in endochondral ossification.

**chondroblastoma** *n* a benign tumour of the precursor cells of cartilage.

**chondrocalcinosis** *n* an arthritic condition characterized by calcium deposits in joints, especially the knee. It usually affects people over 50 years of age.

**chondrocostal** *adj* pertaining to the costal cartilages and ribs.

**chondroclast** *n* a cell involved in the reabsorption of cartilage.

**chondrocyte** *n* a cartilage cell.

**chondrodynia** *n* pain in a cartilage.

**chondrodystrophy** *n* a group of conditions in which cartilage is converted to bone. Commonly occurs in the epiphyses of long bones. Affected individuals have short stature with shortened limbs and normal trunk size.

**chondroectodermal dysplasia** also known as Ellis–van Creveld syndrome. A rare genetic disorder transmitted by an autosomal recessive gene. It is characterized by polydactyly; acromelic dwarfism with abnormally short limb bones; heart defects; and defects affecting the nails, hair, the upper and lower jaw and the teeth, which may erupt prenatally.

**chondrolysis** *n* dissolution of cartilage—**chondrolytic** *adj*.

**chondroma** *n* a benign tumour of cartilage. It may be on the surface of the cartilage (ecchondroma) or within the cartilage (enchondroma).

**chondromalacia** *n* softening of cartilage.

**chondrosarcoma** *n* malignant tumour of cartilage or its precursor cells—**chondrosarcomata** *pl*, **chondrosarcomatous** *adj*.

**chondrosternal** *adj* pertaining to the costal cartilages and sternum.

**chordae tendineae** structures that stabilize the atrioventricular valves (bicuspid and tricuspid) of the heart by attaching them to the papillary muscles.

**chordee** *n* angulation of the penis associated with hypospadias.

**chordotomy** *n* ⇒ cordotomy.

**chorea** *n* describes irregular and jerky dance-like movements, beyond the patient's control. Chorea may follow childhood rheumatic fever *Sydenham's chorea*, but usually results from a disorder or drug affecting the basal nuclei. In adults, chorea is a feature of the inherited condition Huntington's disease and the administration of drugs including the phenothiazines and L-dopa used in parkinsonism—**choreal, choreic** *adj*.

**choreiform** *adj* resembling chorea.

**choriocarcinoma** *n* (*syn* chorionepithelioma) a malignant tumour of chorionic cells; develops following normal pregnancy (rarely), miscarriage or evacuation of a hydatidiform mole. A sensitive (though not specific) tumour marker is human chorionic gonadotrophin (hCG). Choriocarcinoma is usually chemosensitive and curable.

**chorion** *n* the outer extraembryonic membrane comprising trophoblast and mesoderm. It forms the placenta and the sac that contains the amniotic fluid and the fetus—**chorial, chorionic** *adj*. *chorion biopsy* ⇒ amnion, chorionic villus sampling.

**chorionepithelioma** *n* ⇒ choriocarcinoma.

**chorionic** *adj* pertaining to the chorion. *chorionic gonadotrophin* ⇒ human chorionic gonadotrophin. *chorionic villi* vascular projections from the chorion that invade the decidua, eventually forming the fetal part of the placenta. Through it substances such as nutrients and waste diffuse between maternal and fetal blood and vice versa.

**chorionic villus sampling (CVS)** also known as chorion or chorionic villus biopsy. A prenatal screening test for chromosomal (e.g. Down's syndrome) and other inherited disorders (e.g. haemoglobinopathies, Tay–Sachs disease). Samples of fetal tissue are obtained under ultrasound control either via a catheter passed through the cervix into the uterus (Figure C.8) or through a transabdominal puncture. It is used for the detection of genetic abnormalities during early pregnancy (around 11 weeks).

**chorioretinal** *adj* pertaining to the choroid and the retina.

**chorioretinitis** *n* (*syn* retinochoroiditis) inflammation involving both the choroid and retina. It may be an autoimmune disorder, or bacterial, viral, fungal or parasitic in origin.

**choroid** *n* the middle pigmented, vascular coat of the posterior five-sixths of the eyeball, continuous with the iris in front (⇒ Appendix 1, Figure 15). It lies between the sclera externally and the retina internally. It prevents the passage of light rays, thus preventing blurred vision. The choroid is part of the uveal tract—**choroidal** *adj*. ⇒ Bruch's membrane, ciliary body, iris.

**choroiditis** *n* inflammation of the choroid layer of the eye. It causes blurring of vision.

**choroid plexus** an area of specialized capillaries surrounded by modified ependymal cells that line the cerebral ventricles. They produce

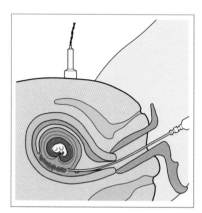

**Figure C.8** Transcervical chorionic villus sampling *(reproduced from Rodeck & Whittle 1999 with permission)*.

cerebrospinal fluid (CSF) from blood. ⇒ cerebrospinal fluid.

**CHRE** *abbr* Council for Healthcare Regulatory Excellence.

**Christmas disease** haemophilia B. ⇒ haemophilias.

**Christmas factor** factor IX (or antihaemophiliac factor B) in the coagulation cascade. It is involved in the intrinsic coagulation system. Deficiency causes Christmas disease (haemophilia B).

**chromaffin** *n* an affinity for staining with chromium salts, such as the cells of the adrenal medulla. *chromaffin cells* neuroendocrine cells that form from the neural crest in the embryo. They are present in the adrenal medulla and sympathetic nervous system ganglia. The cells in the adrenal medulla release the catecholamines adrenaline (epinephrine) and noradrenaline (norepinephrine) when stimulated by the splanchnic nerve.

**chromatid** *n* one of the strands that result from the duplication of chromosomes during nuclear division.

**chromatin** *n* the threads of DNA and protein that form the substance of chromosomes.

**chromatography** *n* analytical methods used to separate and identify substances in a complex mixture based on their differential movement through a two-phase system. Include: gel filtration chromatography, gas chromatography and ion exchange chromatography.

**chromatopsia** *n* a disorder of colour vision. It may be a type of colour blindness where people have abnormal perception of various colours or a condition in which colourless objects may appear to be tinged with a particular colour.

**chromium (Cr)** *n* an essential trace element required in very small amounts in the diet. It potentiates the action of insulin in carbohydrate, lipid and protein metabolism. Symptoms of chromium deficiency include impaired glucose tolerance.

**chromosome** *n* the genetic material present in the nucleus of the cell. During the preparation for cell division chromosomes appear as microscopic threads. They contain strands of DNA molecules or genes. Each species has a constant number; humans have 23 pairs (46) in each somatic cell: 22 pairs of autosomes and 1 pair of sex chromosomes—males have XY (Figure C.9) and females have XX. Mature gametes, however, have half the usual number (haploid), which results from the reduction division during meiosis. The 23 unpaired chromosomes inherited from each parent unite to produce an embryo with 46 chromosomes (diploid). Genetic sex is determined by the male gamete and depends on

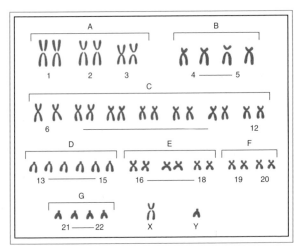

**Figure C.9** Chromosomes—normal male *(reproduced from Brooker 2006A with permission).*

whether the oocyte is fertilized by a sperm that contributes a Y chromosome (genetic male) or an X chromosome (genetic female). Some genetic material is also present in organelles, such as the mitochondria—**chromosomal** *adj.* ⇒ meiosis, mitochondrial genes, mitosis.

**chronic** *adj* lingering, lasting, opposed to acute. The word does not imply anything about the severity of the condition. *chronic heart failure* ⇒ congestive heart failure. *chronic leukaemia* ⇒ leukaemia. ⇒ chronic obstructive pulmonary disease—**chronicity** n, **chronically** adv.

**chronic energy deficiency** a term used to describe malnutrition occurring in adults. Generally defined by a body mass index below the normal range or wasting. ⇒ protein–energy malnutrition.

**chronic fatigue syndrome/myalgic encephalomyelitis (CFS/ME)** sometimes referred to as postviral fatigue. A flu-like illness characterized by disabling fatigue, with varied signs and symptoms including dizziness, adenopathy, muscle fatigue and spasm, myalgia, joint pain, sore throat, headaches and other neurological pain, poor concentration and impaired memory. The cause is unclear but may be associated with a viral infection, or a poorly functioning immune system. Management is directed towards symptom relief, including the use of complementary therapies. Cognitive-behavioural therapy or physiotherapy can be helpful for some people.

**chronic injury** an injury with long onset and duration.

**chronic obstructive pulmonary disease (COPD)** also known as chronic airflow limitation or chronic obstructive airways disease. A group of obstructive lung diseases where airway resistance is increased with impaired airflow, e.g. pulmonary emphysema, chronic bronchitis. Some authorities include asthma in the COPD group. Defined on spirometric grounds as a forced expiratory volume in 1 second ($FEV_1$) <80% and an $FEV_1$:forced vital capacity ratio <70%. Usually seen as a long-term sequela of smoking. Genetic factors include $\alpha_1$-antitrypsin deficiency, and, more recently, family clustering studies suggest other genetic susceptibility factors.

**chronic pain** pain that does not resolve, usually lasting longer than 3 months. Chronic pain can be subdivided into non-malignant pain (not life-threatening) such as that associated with arthritis or phantom-limb pain, and malignant pain, which is associated with terminal diseases, especially cancer. Chronic pain affects every aspect of a person's life and can lead to relationship problems, financial problems, social isolation, depression and, in extreme cases, suicidal ideation. ⇒ acute pain, neuropathic pain, nociceptive pain.

**chronic suppurative otitis media (CSOM)** chronic inflammation of the middle ear. It is classified as either tubotympanic, a 'safe' condition that leads to fewer intracranial problems, or atticoantral, which is classified as an 'unsafe' condition as it is associated with an increased risk of intracranial problems.

**chronic wound** a wound that is slow to heal and displays delayed healing, such as a venous leg ulcer. ⇒ acute wound, wound healing.

**chronological age** a person's age in years.

**chronotherapy** *n* the administration of treatment modalities, such as chemotherapy or radiotherapy, at the most effective time.

**chunking** *n* the organization and coding of 'chunks' of data/information that facilitates an increase in the effective capacity of short-term memory, which can only store around seven items of information.

**Churg–Strauss syndrome** (J Churg, American pathologist, 20th century; L Strauss, American pathologist, 1913–1985) an allergic condition characterized by vasculitis associated with asthma.

**Chvostek's sign** (F Chvostek, Austrian surgeon, 1835–1884) spasm or twitching of the face on tapping the facial nerve, seen with hypocalcaemia: a sign of tetany.

**chyle** *n* fatty, milky fluid formed from chylomicrons within the lymphatic lacteals of the intestinal villi—**chylous** adj.

**chylomicron** *n* tiny particles formed from triglycerides, lipoproteins and cholesterol within the intestinal mucosa following the absorption of digested fat. They form chyle within the lacteals.

**chylothorax** *n* leakage of chyle from the thoracic duct into the pleural cavity.

**chyluria** *n* chyle in the urine, which can occur in some nematode infestations, either when a fistulous communication is established between a lymphatic vessel and the urinary tract or when the distension of the urinary lymphatics causes them to rupture—**chyluric** adj.

**chyme** *n* partially digested food which passes from the stomach to the duodenum. Its acidity controls the pylorus to regulate the amount entering the duodenum.

**chymotrypsin** *n* the active proteolytic enzyme secreted as inactive chymotrypsinogen by the pancreas: it is activated by trypsin.

**CI** *abbr* cardiac index.

**cicatrix** *n* ⇒ scar.

**cilia** *npl* **1.** the eyelashes. **2.** microscopic hair-like projections from certain epithelial cells. Membranes containing such cells, e.g. those lining the trachea and uterine (fallopian) tubes, are known as ciliated membranes—**cilium** *sing*, **ciliary, ciliated, cilial** *adj*.

**ciliary** *adj* hair-like. *ciliary body* part of the uveal tract. A specialized structure in the eye connecting the anterior choroid to the iris (⇒ Appendix 1, Figure 15); it is composed of the ciliary muscles and processes. ⇒ choroid, iris. *ciliary muscles* fine muscle fibres arranged in a circular manner. They control accommodation. *ciliary processes* about 70 in number, they secrete aqueous humour.

***Cimex*** *n* a genus of insects of the family Cimicidae. *Cimex lectularius* is the common bedbug.

**CIN** *abbr* cervical intraepithelial neoplasia.

**cinchona** *n* the bark from which quinine is obtained.

**cinchonism** *n* quininism.

**C1 inhibitor (C1 INH)** an essential regulator of the classical complement pathway.

**circadian rhythm** any rhythm with a periodicity of about 24 h, such as the sleep–wake cycle, body temperature, the secretion of some hormones, etc. ⇒ ultradian.

**circinata** *n* ⇒ tinea.

**circinate** *adj* in the form of a circle or segment of a circle, e.g. the skin eruptions of late syphilis, ringworm, etc.

**circle of Willis** (T Willis, English physician, 1621–1675) ⇒ circulus arteriosus.

**circuit training** training that includes a number of specific exercises/activities targeted at working specific muscle groups and often the associated skills involved in the target activity.

**circulation** *n* passage in a circle. Usually means circulation of the blood—**circulatory** *adj*, **circulate** *vi, vt. circulation of bile* ⇒ enterohepatic circulation; *circulation of blood* the passage of blood from heart to arteries to capillaries to veins and back to heart; *circulation of cerebrospinal fluid* takes place from the ventricles of the brain to the cisterna magna, whence the fluid bathes the surface of the brain and the spinal cord, including its central canal. It is absorbed into the blood in the cerebral venous sinuses. *circulation of lymph* lymph is collected from the tissue spaces and passed in the lymphatic capillaries, vessels, nodes and ducts to be returned to the blood stream. *pulmonary circulation* circulation of deoxygenated blood from right ventricle to pulmonary artery, to lungs and back to left atrium of heart (Figure C.10). *systemic circulation*

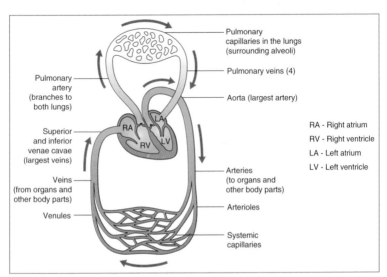

**Figure C.10** Systemic and pulmonary circulation (*reproduced from Brooker and Waugh 2007 with permission*).

circulation of oxygenated blood from left ventricle to aorta, to tissues and back to right atrium of heart (Figure C.10).

**circumcision** *n* excision of the prepuce or foreskin of the penis, usually for religious or cultural reasons. The operation is sometimes required for phimosis or paraphimosis. *female circumcision* excision of the clitoris, labia minora and labia majora. The extent of cutting varies from country to country. The simplest form is clitoridectomy; the next form entails excision of the prepuce, clitoris and all or part of the labia minora. The most extensive form, infibulation, involves excision of clitoris, labia minora and labia majora. The vulval lips are sutured together but total obliteration of the vaginal introitus is prevented by inserting a piece of wood or reed to preserve a small passage for urine and menstrual fluid.

**circumcorneal** *adj* (*syn* limbal) around the cornea.

**circumduction** *n* the circular movement comprising abduction, flexion, extension and adduction, such as when the arm traces a cone in space.

**circumoral** *adj* surrounding the mouth. *circumoral pallor* a pale appearance of the skin around the mouth, in contrast to the flushed cheeks. A characteristic of scarlet fever—**circumorally** *adv*.

**circumvallate** *adj* surrounded by a raised ring or ridge, as the large circumvallate papillae at the base of the tongue. *circumvallate placenta* one with a well-defined ring or edge on the fetal surface. It is formed from the chorion and amnion.

**cirrhosis** *n* hardening of an organ. There are degenerative changes in the tissues with resulting fibrosis. *cirrhosis of liver* increasing in prosperous countries. Damage to liver cells can be from viruses, other micro-organisms or toxic substances and dietary deficiencies interfering with the nutrition of liver cells—often the result of alcohol misuse. Associated developments include ascites, obstruction of the circulation through the hepatic portal vein with haematemesis from oesophageal varices, jaundice and enlargement of the spleen—**cirrhotic** *adj*.

**CIS** *abbr* carcinoma in situ.

*cis* **configuration** means on the same side. In chemistry, describes an isomerism in which the two substituent groups are on the same side of a carbon–carbon double bond. ⇒ *trans* configuration.

**cissa** *n* desire for extraordinary or abnormal foods. Also known as allotriophagy, cittosis and pica.

**cisterna** *n* any closed space serving as a reservoir for a body fluid. *cisterna chyli* the pear-shaped commencement of the thoracic duct. It receives lymph. *cisterna magna* is a subarachnoid space in the cleft between the cerebellum and medulla oblongata—**cisternal** *adj*.

**cisternal puncture** insertion of a special hollow needle with stylet between the occiput and atlas, into the cisterna magna. One method of obtaining cerebrospinal fluid but rarely used. ⇒ lumbar puncture.

**cistron** *n* the smallest fragment of DNA that codes for the amino acids needed for a particular polypeptide chain during the synthesis of proteins. A cistron is in effect a gene.

**citric acid** an organic acid present in citrus fruit such as lemons and oranges and in soft fruit. *citric acid cycle* ⇒ Krebs cycle.

**citrullinaemia** *n* an inborn error of metabolism in which the enzyme argininosuccinic acid synthetase is deficient. Untreated, the presence of citrulline and other metabolites in the blood results in seizures, poor development and learning disability. Management includes a low-protein diet, which still provides the essential nutrients.

**citrulline** *n* an amino acid formed as a metabolic intermediate in the urea cycle. It is normally converted to arginine.

**cittosis** *n* desire for extraordinary or abnormal foods. Also known as allotriophagy, cissa and pica.

**civil law** law relating to non-criminal matters. *civil action* proceedings brought in the civil courts. *civil wrong* act or omission which can be pursued in the civil courts by the person who has suffered the wrong.

**CJD** *abbr* Creutzfeldt–Jakob disease.

**clamps** *npl* a variety of instruments with locking handles used in surgical procedures. They can be used to grip, hold or compress vessels, ducts or organs. Used mainly to compress blood vessels to prevent bleeding (haemostasis).

**clap** *n* a slang term for gonorrhoea.

**Clark level** (W Clark, American dermatologist, b. 1924) vertical levels (anatomical landmarks) that determine the stage of a melanoma. ⇒ Breslow's depth.

**clasp-knife phenomenon** a pathological manifestation of the stretch reflex in which great resistance at the beginning of passive movement suddenly collapses; characteristic of spasticity.

**class** *n* the socioeconomic diversity between groups that explains the differences in their level of wealth and influence. ⇒ social class.

**classical conditioning** ⇒ conditioning.

**claudication** *n* literally limping. Cramp-like pain caused by interference with the blood supply to the muscles of the legs. The cause may be spasm or disease of the vessels themselves. In *intermittent claudication* the patient experiences severe pain in the legs (calves or thighs) when walking; after a short rest the patient is able to continue. ⇒ peripheral vascular disease.

**claustrophobia** *n* a fear of enclosed spaces—**claustrophobic** *adj*.

**clavicle** *n* the collar bone (⇒ Appendix 1, Figure 2)—**clavicular** *adj*.

**clavus** *n* a corn. ⇒ callus.

**claw-foot** *adj, n* ⇒ pes cavus.

**claw-hand** *n* the hand is flexed and contracted giving a claw-like appearance; the condition may be due to injury or disease.

**clean intermittent self-catheterization** ⇒ intermittent self-catheterization.

**cleanser** *n, adj* (describes) agents that have cleansing properties. Substances such as cetrimide are both disinfectant and cleansing. Used to remove dirt, grease, etc., from the skin or wounds, and for removing crusts and other debris from skin lesions.

**clearance** *n* the ability of the kidney to remove a specific substance from the blood. *renal clearance* used to measure glomerular filtration rate (GFR) and kidney function by calculating the volume of blood cleared of a substance such as creatinine or inulin, in a given time, usually 1 minute. ⇒ creatinine, inulin.

**cleavage** *n* the mitotic divisions that occur immediately following fertilization of the oocyte (ovum). This converts the single-celled zygote into a ball of cells that will eventually develop into an embryo with the capability to differentiate into many different cell types.

**cleft lip** a congenital defect in the lip; a fissure extending from the margin of the lip to the nostril; may be single or double, and is often associated with cleft palate. It may be surgically repaired soon after birth, or when the infant is a few weeks old.

**cleft palate** congenital failure of fusion between the right and left palatal processes. Often associated with cleft lip. It is usually surgically repaired when the infant is around 6 months old. The child may need regular reviews and referral to a speech and language therapist and/or an orthodontist as necessary.

**cleidocranial dysostosis** a congenital condition in which there is faulty ossification of the cranial bones and the partial or complete absence of the clavicles (collar bones).

**client-centred practice** practice that requires a partnership between the practitioner and the client. The aim is to empower the client in order to reach fulfilment in everyday life.

**Clifton Assessment Procedures for the Elderly (CAPE)** a series of tests which measure cognitive function in older people as well as behavioural aspects.

**climacteric** *n* the perimenopause and postmenopause. A period of time during which ovarian activity declines and eventually ceases. In most women it occurs between the mid-40s to mid-50s. Cessation of menstruation is a single event during the climacteric. ⇒ menopause.

**clinical** *adj* pertaining to a clinic. Describes the practical observation and treatment of sick persons as opposed to theoretical study.

**clinical audit** critical and systematic analysis of the quality of clinical care and treatment. It includes diagnostic procedures, treatment, resource use and outputs, including quality of life.

**clinical governance** the framework within which all NHS organizations are accountable for their services, and are required to operate an active programme of continuous quality improvement within an overall coherent framework of cost-effective service delivery.

**clinical guidelines** systematically developed statements that help the practitioner and patient in making decisions about care. ⇒ evidence-based practice.

**clinical reasoning** the thought processes used by the practitioner in order to evaluate data, make decisions, identify problems, set goals and plan appropriate action concerning a patient/client. Clinical reasoning may lead to the selection of a conceptual model or frame of reference or be directed by a previously used approach.

**clinical thermometer** previously, glass and mercury thermometers of various types were used. These have mostly been replaced by safer alternatives, such as electronic probes, e.g. tympanic membrane thermometers, and single-use thermometers.

**clitoridectomy** *n* the surgical removal of the clitoris. ⇒ circumcision.

**clitoriditis** *n* inflammation of the clitoris.

**clitoris** *n* a small erectile organ situated at the anterior junction of the labia minora. Involved in the female sexual response. Homologous to the corpora cavernosa of the penis.

**clitoromegaly** *n* an abnormal enlargement of the clitoris. It may lead to confusion regarding a newborn's gender. ⇒ congenital adrenal hyperplasia.

**CLL** *abbr* chronic lymphocytic leukaemia.

**CLO** *abbr* columnar-lined oesophagus. ⇒ Barrett's oesophagus.

**cloaca** *n* in osteomyelitis, the opening through the involucrum which discharges pus—**cloacal** *adj*.

**clone** *n* a group of genetically identical cells or organisms derived from a single cell or common ancestor. ⇒ monoclonal.

**clonic** *adj* ⇒ clonus.

**clonorchiasis** *n* infestation with the hepatobiliary (liver and biliary tract) fluke, *Clonorchis sinensis*. The adult fluke lives in the bile ducts and, although it may produce cholangitis, hepatitis and jaundice, it may be asymptomatic or be blamed for vague digestive symptoms. ⇒ fluke.

*Clonorchis sinensis* (*syn Opisthorchis sinensis*) the Chinese or oriental fluke. A trematode fluke that infests the liver and biliary tract. It is caused by eating raw or partially cooked fish, or smoked, salted or pickled fish. Can cause serious liver and biliary disease. ⇒ fluke.

**clonus** *n* a series of intermittent muscular contractions and relaxations. ⇒ tonic *opp*, ankle clonus—**clonic** *adj*, **clonicity** *n*. ⇒ myoclonus.

**closed-chain exercise** ⇒ closed kinetic chain.

**closed fracture** ⇒ fracture.

**closed kinetic chain** in sports medicine or physiotherapy describes a motion during which the distal segment of the extremity is weight-bearing or otherwise fixed, e.g. a squat (lower limb) or a press-up (upper limb) (Figure C.11). ⇒ kinematic chain exercises, open kinetic chain.

*Clostridium* *n* a genus of bacteria. They are large Gram-positive, spore-forming anaerobic bacilli of the Bacillaceae family. They are present as commensals in the gut of animals and humans and as saprophytes in the soil. Many species are pathogenic due to the production of exotoxins, e.g. *Clostridium botulinum* (botulism); *C. difficile* (pseudomembranous

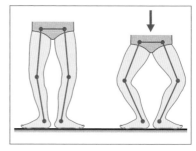

**Figure C.11** Closed kinetic chain *(reproduced from Porter 2005 with permission).*

colitis); *C. perfringens*, previously known as *C. welchii* (gas gangrene); *C. tetani* (tetanus).

**clotting time** the time taken for blood to form a clot. Also called coagulation time. Mostly replaced by the activated partial thromboplastin time.

**clotting/coagulation factors** ⇒ coagulation, factor.

**clubbing** *n* enlargement of the distal phalanges particularly of the fingers. There is thickening and broadening of the bulbous fleshy portion of the fingers under the nails (Figure C.12). The cause is not known but it occurs in people who have reduced oxygen tension in the blood such as with chronic heart and/or lung disease. Also occurs in other conditions, e.g. biliary cirrhosis, colitis, etc., and as a benign congenital abnormality.

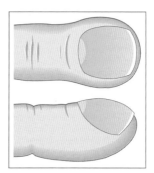

**Figure C.12** Finger clubbing *(reproduced from Boon et al. 2006 with permission).*

**club foot** *n* a congenital malformation, either unilateral or bilateral. ⇒ talipes.

**clue cell** epithelial cell to whose surface Gram-variable, Gram-negative and Gram-positive bacteria adhere. A microscopical feature of bacterial vaginosis.

**clumping** *n* agglutination.

**clunk test** a test used to diagnose a glenoid tear affecting the shoulder.

**cluster headache** an uncommon migraine variant, which occurs more often in men. There is intense unilateral pain, commonly around one eye. It may be accompanied by Horner's syndrome with nasal congestion and a watering eye. The attacks of excruciating pain occur in clusters and typically last for a short time (30–90 minutes).

**Clutton's joints** (H Clutton, British surgeon, 1850–1909) joints which show symmetrical swelling usually painless, the knees often being involved. Associated with congenital syphilis.

**CML** *abbr* chronic myeloid leukaemia.

**CMV** *abbr* **1.** controlled mandatory ventilation. **2.** cytomegalovirus.

**CNS** *abbr* central nervous system.

**CO** *abbr* cardiac output.

**coach's finger** in sports medicine a colloquial term used to describe the dislocation of the proximal interphalangeal joint leading to a fixed flexion deformity of the finger.

**coagulant** *n* a drug or other agent that causes blood to coagulate (clot).

**coagulase** *n* an enzyme produced by some staphylococci: it coagulates plasma and is used to classify staphylococci as coagulase-negative or coagulase-positive.

**coagulation** *n* the third of four overlapping processes involved in haemostasis. Coagulation (clotting) occurs through a series of complex reactions that use enzyme cascade amplification to start the formation of a fibrin clot to stop bleeding. There are two pathways/systems, intrinsic and extrinsic, which converge to follow a common final pathway. Coagulation starts when platelets break down, tissue is damaged and thromboplastins are released. Various factors are involved in coagulation: I, fibrinogen; II, prothrombin; III, thromboplastin (tissue factor); IV, calcium ions; V, labile factor (proaccelerin); VII, stable factor (proconvertin); VIII, antihaemophilic factor (AHF); IX, Christmas factor; X, Stuart–Prower factor; XI, plasma thromboplastin antecedent; XII, Hageman factor; and XIII, fibrin-stabilizing factor. During the final common pathway, inactive prothrombin is converted to thrombin, the active enzyme. Thrombin converts soluble fibrinogen to insoluble fibrin, which forms a network of fibres in which blood cells are caught to form the clot. ⇒ fibrinolysis, haemostasis, platelet plug, vasoconstriction.

**coagulation time** ⇒ clotting time.

**coalesce** *vi* to grow together; to unite into a mass. Often used to describe the development of a skin eruption, when discrete areas of affected skin coalesce to form sheets of a similar appearance—**coalescence** *n*, **coalescent** *adj*.

**coal-miners/worker's pneumoconiosis** ⇒ anthracosis.

**coal tar** obtained by the distillation of coal. Used in topical preparations for the treatment of psoriasis and eczema.

**coarctation** *n* contraction, stricture, narrowing; applied to a vessel or canal. *coarctation of the aorta* congenital narrowing of the aorta, commonly affecting the area just after the origin of the left subclavian artery. ⇒ Appendix 1, Figure 9.

**coarse tremor** violent trembling.

**Coats' disease** (G Coats, British ophthalmologist, 1876–1915) exudative retinopathy/retinitis. Retinopathy characterized by the presence of massive exudates on the retina caused by an abnormality of the retinal blood vessels.

**cobalamins** *npl* a group of molecules containing a cobalt atom and four pyrrole units. A constituent of substances having vitamin $B_{12}$ activity. ⇒ cyanocobalamin.

**cobalt (Co)** *n* an essential trace element, utilized as a constituent of vitamin $B_{12}$ (cobalamins). Required for healthy red blood cell production and proper neurological function. *cobalt-60* ($^{60}$Co) a radioactive isotope of cobalt which is used as a source of radiation in teletherapy.

**COC** *abbr* combined oral contraceptive. ⇒ oral contraceptive.

**cocaine** *n* a powerful local anaesthetic obtained from the leaves of the coca plant. It is a controlled drug which is highly addictive and subject to considerable criminal misuse. ⇒ Appendix 5. Toxic, especially to the brain; may cause agitation, disorientation and convulsions. *crack cocaine* a highly potent and addictive form.

**cocarcinogen** *n* a substance that potentiates the action of a carcinogen.

***Coccidioides*** *n* a genus of pathogenic fungi, such as *C. immitis*, that causes coccidioidomycosis and pneumonia.

**coccidioidomycosis** *n* infection caused by the fungus *Coccidioides immitis*. The infection is endemic in Central and South America, and the southern USA, and causes opportunistic infection in people with human immunodeficiency virus (HIV) disease. Inhalation of fungal spores leads initially to a flu-like illness but the secondary infection is characterized by dyspnoea, haemoptysis, fever, weight loss, skin lesions, and bone and joint pain.

**coccobacilli** *npl* rod-shaped bacteria which are slightly elongated. They include the genus *Brucella* and the bacterium *Haemophilus influenzae*.

**coccus** *n* a spherical bacterium, such as staphylococcus—**cocci** *pl*, **coccal, coccoid** *adj*.

**coccydynia** *n* pain in the region of the coccyx.

**coccygeal nerves** the last of the spinal nerves. ⇒ Appendix 1, Figure 11.

**coccygeal plexus** a small plexus formed by a branch of the fourth sacral nerve, the fifth sacral nerve (S4–S5) and the coccygeal spinal nerves (Co). It innervates the skin over the coccyx, the anal area and the pelvic floor.

**coccygectomy** *n* surgical removal of the coccyx.

**coccyx** *n* the last bone of the vertebral column (⇒ Appendix 1, Figure 3). It is composed of four or five rudimentary vertebrae, cartilaginous at birth, ossification being completed at about the 30th year—**coccygeal** *adj*.

**cochlea** *n* a spiral canal resembling the interior of a snail shell, in the anterior part of the bony labyrinth of the inner ear. It contains the organ of Corti (the organ of hearing). (⇒ Appendix 1, Figure 13)—**cochlear** *adj*.

**cochlear implant** the insertion of an electronic device into the cochlea of people who have profound deafness or severe hearing loss. It comprises an external microphone; a transmitter outside the skin; a receiver/stimulator inserted under the skin behind the ear; and electrodes that feed through to the cochlea from where impulses are conveyed to the brain.

**Cochrane collaboration** (A Cochrane, British epidemiologist, 1909–1988) a not-for-profit organization that provides accurate, authorative systematic literature reviews of health care interventions. Important in the provision of evidence-based practice.

**Cockayne's syndrome** (E Cockayne, British physician, 1880–1956) a condition with autosomal recessive inheritance. It is characterized by dwarfism, learning disability, retinal atrophy, hearing impairment and a type of epidermolysis bullosa simplex. ⇒ epidermolysis bullosa.

**cockup splint** a splint that immobilizes the wrist joint while leaving the fingers free.

**code of conduct/practice** the guidelines setting out how health care professionals should fulfil their roles, duties, obligations and responsibilities, such as those produced by the statutory bodies whose functions are to regulate the standards, registration and practice of health care professionals, e.g. Health Professions Council, General Medical Council.

**Codex Alimentarius** part of the United Nations Food and Agriculture Organization/World Health Organization Commission on Food Standards used since the early 1960s to simplify and integrate food standards for international adoption.

**Codman's exercises** (E Codman, American surgeon, 1869–1940) gentle exercises that aim to restore normal range of motion in the shoulders and arms.

**codominance** *n* in genetics, a situation where both alleles of a pair are expressed in the phenotype of the heterozygous individual. For example, if the A and B blood group alleles are inherited, the person will have type AB blood.

**codon** *n* in genetics, the three complementary bases carried by messenger RNA (mRNA) involved in protein synthesis (transcription stage). ⇒ anticodon.

**coeliac** *adj* relating to the abdominal cavity; applied to arteries and a nerve plexus.

**coeliac disease** (*syn* gluten-induced enteropathy) due to intolerance to the protein gluten in wheat and rye, the gliadin fraction being harmful. This results in subtotal villous atrophy of the mucosa of the small intestine and the malabsorption syndrome. Symptoms may become apparent at any age or patients may be asymptomatic. Treatment is with a gluten-free diet.

**coelom** *n* the body cavity in the embryo.

**coenzyme** *n* a non-protein enzyme activator, e.g. substances formed from the B vitamins. *coenzyme A* a cofactor important in metabolism, it is a carrier molecule for acyl groups. ⇒ acetyl coenzyme A. *coenzyme Q* ⇒ ubiquinone.

**cofactor** *n* substances, such as metal ions and coenzymes, required for certain enzyme activation.

**coffee-ground vomit** vomit containing blood, which in its partially digested state resembles coffee grounds. Indicative of slow upper gastrointestinal bleeding ⇒ haematemesis.

**Cogan's syndrome** (D Cogan, American ophthalmologist, 1908–1993) keratitis and iridocyclitis occurring with vertigo, tinnitus and sensorineural deafness. Also describes a form of oculomotor apraxia that occurs during childhood.

**cognition** *n* awareness; one of the three aspects of mind. A general term that describes all the psychological processes by which individuals gain awareness and knowledge about their environment. Includes perception, reasoning, understanding, making judgements, problem-solving—**cognitive** *adj.* ⇒ affection, conation.

**cognitive psychology** the study of the development of intelligence, language, thought processes and the acquisition, storage and use of knowledge.

**cognitive therapy** an approach to the psychological treatment of some mental health problems such as anxiety-related disorders. It concentrates on, and is effective through, correcting the individual's cognitive dysfunctions, such as errors in thinking and poor problem-solving.

**cogwheel rigidity** a pathological pattern of resistance to passive movement of a limb which yields in a series of jerks, observed in people with Parkinson's disease, thought to be due to tremor superimposed on lead-pipe rigidity.

**cohort** *n* a group of people who have some common feature or characteristic, e.g. year group at university. *cohort study* research that studies a population that shares a common feature, such as occupation.

**coitus** *n* insertion of the erect penis into the vagina; the act of sexual intercourse or copulation.

**coitus interruptus** removal from the vagina of the penis before ejaculation of semen as a means of contraception. The method is considered unsatisfactory as it is not only unreliable but can lead to sexual disharmony—**coital** *adj.*

**cold abscess** ⇒ abscess.

**cold flow** *n* ⇒ creep.

**cold sore** *n* oral herpes simplex.

**colectomy** *n* excision of part or the whole of the colon.

**colic** *n* severe pain resulting from periodic spasm in an abdominal organ. *biliary colic* ⇒ biliary. *intestinal colic* abnormal peristaltic movement of an irritated gut. *uterine colic* dysmenorrhoea—**colicky** *adj.* ⇒ renal colic.

**coliform** *adj* describes any of the enterobacteria (intestinal bacteria) such as *Escherichia coli.*

**colitis** *n* inflammation of the colon. May be acute or chronic, and may be accompanied by ulcerative lesions. ⇒ inflammatory bowel disease, ulcerative colitis.

**collagen** *n* the main protein constituent of white fibrous tissue of skin, tendon, bone, cartilage and all connective tissue.

**collagen diseases** a term used for some connective tissue diseases.

**collapse** *n* **1.** the 'falling in' of a hollow organ or vessel, e.g. collapse of lung from change of air pressure inside or outside the organ (pneumothorax). **2.** a vague term describing physical or nervous prostration.

**collapsing pulse** also known as Corrigan's pulse. The water-hammer pulse of aortic regurgitation with high initial upthrust which quickly falls away.

**collar-bone** *n* the clavicle.

**collateral circulation** an alternative route provided for the blood by secondary blood vessels when a primary vessel is blocked.

**Colles' fracture** (A Colles, Irish surgeon/anatomist, 1773–1843) a break at the lower end of the radius following a fall on the outstretched hand. The backward displacement of the hand produces the 'dinner fork' deformity (Figure C.13). A common fracture in older women and associated with osteoporosis.

**collimator** *n* a device used in radiography and radiotherapy to reduce the size and shape of a beam of radiation, thereby reducing the scatter radiation. This enhances the quality of the radiographic image and decreases the radiation dose needed to investigate or treat a patient. ⇒ multileaf collimation.

**collision sport** individual or team sports during which the participants use their bodies to deter or block opponents, thereby relying on

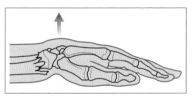

**Figure C.13** Colles' fracture *(reproduced from Porter 2005 with permission).*

the physical dominance of one athlete over another.

**collodion** *n* a solution forming a flexible film on the skin. Previously used as a protective dressing.

**colloid** *n* glue-like. A non-crystalline chemical; diffusible but not soluble in water; unable to pass through a semipermeable membrane. Some drugs can be prepared in their colloidal form. *colloid degeneration* that which results in the formation of gelatinous material, as in tumours. *colloid goitre* enlargement of the thyroid gland caused by the presence of viscid, iodine-containing colloid within the gland.

**colloid solutions** ones containing large particles (solutes). When administered intravenously they stay in the blood because they are too large to pass through capillary membranes. Colloid solutions, such as human albumin solution or those containing gelatin or starch, are used to increase blood volume. ⇒ crystalloid solutions.

**coloboma** *n* a developmental discontinuity in a layer of the eyeball caused by failure of closure of the optic fissure. Can also occur in the eyelids—**colobomata** *pl.*

**colon** *n* the large bowel extending from the caecum to the rectum (⇒ Appendix 1, Figure 18B). Comprises the ascending, transverse, descending and sigmoid colon. ⇒ flexure; *spasmodic colon* ⇒ megacolon—**colonic** *adj.*

**colonization** *n* the installation of micro-organisms in a specific environment, such as a body site with only minimal or no response. There is no disease or symptoms, but colonization leads to the formation of a reservoir of micro-organisms that may be a source of infection—**colonize** *vt.*

**colonoscopy** *n* use of an endoscope to view, biopsy or photograph the colonic mucosa—**colonoscopic** *adj*, **colonoscopically** *adv.*

**colony** *n* a mass of bacteria resulting from the multiplication of one or more micro-organisms. Containing many millions of individual micro-organisms, it may be visible to the unaided eye; its physical features are often characteristic of the species.

**colony-stimulating factor (CSF)** growth factors, such as granulocyte colony-stimulating factor (G-CSF), which cause blood stem cells to produce a specific white cell line.

**colorectal** *adj* pertaining to the colon and the rectum.

**colorimeter** *n* an instrument that uses colour intensity to measure the amount of a substance

present. Can be used to determine the level of haemoglobin in the blood.

**colostomy** *n* a surgically established fistula between the colon and the surface of the abdomen; a type of stoma that discharges faeces. May be temporary, such as when an anastomosis (join) in the bowel is healing, or permanent, when the colon and rectum have been removed.

**colostrum** *n* fluid secreted by the breasts during late pregnancy and in the 3 days following parturition. It is a rich source of maternal immunoglobulins, and has a different composition to true milk, i.e. more protein, but less fat and lactose.

**colotomy** *n* incision into the colon.

**colour blindness** dysfunction in or absence of a photoreceptor subtype (cones) stimulated by red, green or blue light, leading to difficulty distinguishing between certain colours. ⇒ achromatopsia, chloropsia, chromatopsia, cyanopsia, deuteranopia, dichromatic vision, erythropsia, hemichromatopsia, xanthopsia.

**colpitis** *n* inflammation of the vagina.

**colpocele** *n* protrusion or prolapse of either the bladder or rectum so that it presses on either the anterior or the posterior vaginal wall.

**colpocentesis** *n* withdrawal of fluid from the vagina, as in haematocolpos.

**colpohysterectomy** *n* removal of the uterus through the vagina. ⇒ hysterectomy.

**colpoperineorrhaphy** *n* the surgical repair of vaginal injury and deficient perineum.

**colpophotography** *n* filming the cervix using a camera and colposcope.

**colporrhaphy** *n* surgical repair of the vagina. An anterior colporrhaphy repairs a cystocele and a posterior colporrhaphy repairs a rectocele.

**colposcope** *n* a binocular instrument used to obtain a high-power view of the cervix in cases of abnormal cervical smears. Used for diagnostic procedures and local treatments to the cervix—**colposcopy** *n*, **colposcopically** *adv.*

**colposuspension** *n* surgical procedure involving placement of sutures between the vaginal fornices and the pectineal ligaments for genuine stress incontinence.

**colpotomy** *n* incision of the vaginal wall. A posterior colpotomy drains an abscess in the rectovaginal pouch (pouch of Douglas) through the vagina.

**coma** *n* a state of unrousable unconsciousness, the severity of which can be assessed by corneal and pupillary reflexes and withdrawal responses to painful stimuli. ⇒ Glasgow Coma Scale—**comatose** *adj.*

**comedone, comedo** *n* a worm-like cast formed of sebum which occupies the outlet of a hair follicle in the skin, a feature of acne vulgaris. Open comedones have a black colour because of pigmentation (blackheads). Closed comedones are closed cysts (whiteheads)—**comedones** *pl.*

**commensals** *npl* parasitic micro-organisms adapted to grow on the skin and mucous surfaces of the host, forming part of the normal flora. Some commensals are potentially pathogenic, e.g. bowel commensals that include *Escherichia coli* cause urinary tract infection.

**comminuted fracture** ⇒ fracture.

**Commission for Health Improvement** ⇒ Healthcare Commission.

**Commission on Human Medicines (CHM)** established in 2005, it combines the functions and roles of the Committee on Safety of Medicines and the Medicines Commission. The Commission advises ministers and the licensing authority about the safety, quality and efficacy of human medicines; promotes the collection and investigation of information about adverse drug reactions; and considers representation from applicants or licence holders. ⇒ adverse drug reactions, European Medicines Agency, yellow card reporting.

**commissioning** *n* a complex process that aims to ensure that a specific population has an appropriate level of service provision. The stages include a needs assessment that is used to determine priorities, taking into account the overall national policy guidance from government. On completion of this process, an appropriate range of services are purchased from relevant providers. The final stage is evaluation.

**commissure** *n* **1.** the site at which two anatomical structures unite, such as the labia. **2.** a connecting structure such as the band of nervous tissue connecting the two sides of the brain, the corpus callosum or the spinal cord.

**Committee on Safety of Medicines (CSM)** in the UK the body that previously monitored drug safety and advised the licensing authority regarding the safety, efficacy and quality of medicines. ⇒ Commission on Human Medicines.

**common bile duct** the bile duct formed by the merging of the right and left hepatic ducts and the cystic duct. It is joined by the pancreatic duct at the opening into the duodenum (hepatopancreatic ampulla). ⇒ Appendix 1, Figure 18B.

**common law** case law. Law made by judges rather than by statute.

**common variable immunodeficiency (CVID)** one of the primary antibody deficiency syndromes, presenting in childhood or adulthood and associated with recurrent infections, autoimmunity and an increased risk of malignancy.

**communicable** *adj* transmissible directly or indirectly from one person to another.

**communicating** *n* the exchange of information between at least two individuals. Most often accomplished by the use of language: (a) verbal, which can be spoken, handwritten, word-processed/typed, printed or displayed on a screen; or (b) non-verbal, which allows the transmission of attitudes, values and beliefs that are appropriate and relevant to the information exchanged.

**community** *n* a social group defined by geographical boundaries and/or common values and interests. Also implies shared relationships, lifestyles and a greater frequency and intimacy of contact among those who live in a community.

**community care** the care and support of individuals in community settings. Such care is delivered by health and social care professionals and unpaid carers such as family and neighbours. The community or primary care setting is increasingly important in the development and delivery of health services. ⇒ primary care trust.

**community development** whole-community initiatives that enable individual communities to assess their particular needs, such as for health care, and decide on what action should be taken by the community. In the broadest sense, community care services could be provided by the 'community' on a voluntary basis, or by statutory organizations in residential settings or by professionals working in the community. For example, the development of adequate provision of (community) care services such as the treatment of long-term sick and frail people in their own homes. This can be interpreted to cover personal, domiciliary and social care as well as medical or nursing care. The community includes family, friends and community self-help.

**community therapists** therapists including occupational therapists, physiotherapists and speech and language therapists who work in community settings, for example based in a health centre or attached to a primary care team. They visit clients in their own homes, schools, care homes, etc., to undertake assessments or to provide professional services such as the provision of adaptive equipment and adaptations to the environment.

**comorbidity** *n* coexistence of two or more diseases.

**comparative study** research study that compares two separate populations.

**compartment syndrome 1.** swelling of the muscles in one of the limb compartments leading to ischaemia and necrosis of muscle tissue. It may follow traumatic injury, or compression caused by bandages or plaster casts. Treatment is fasciotomy. ⇒ Volkmann's ischaemic contracture. **2.** in sports medicine a term used to describe a condition where increased intramuscular pressure brought on by activity impedes blood flow and function of the tissues within that intermuscular compartment.

**compatibility** *n* suitability; congruity. The ability of a substance to mix with another without unfavourable results, e.g. two medicines, blood plasma and cells—**compatible** *adj.*

**compensation** *n* **1.** a mental mechanism, employed by a person to cover up a weakness, by exaggerating a more socially acceptable behaviour trait. **2.** the state of counterbalancing a functional or structural defect, e.g. cardiac compensation, where the heart muscle enlarges by hypertrophy to maintain cardiac output in chronic heart failure.

**compensatory techniques** adaptive techniques using relatively intact skills to compensate for physical or cognitive deficits in performance. This might include the provision of adaptive equipment, adaptations to the environment or new methods of performing tasks.

**complement** *n* a system of over 20 serum proteins involved in cytolysis, opsonization, phagocytosis and anaphylaxis. Several cascading systems, including the classical pathway (antibody-mediated), alternate pathway and a third pathway, converge, resulting in the formation of a multimeric (composed of multiple parts) membrane attack complex capable of lysing cells. The system is regulated by numerous proteins and cell surface receptors.

**complement fixation test (CFT)** a test in which complement fixation is found. It indicates the presence of a particular specific antigen.

**complemental air** the extra air that can be drawn into the lungs during deep inspiration.

**complementary and alternative medicine (CAM)** health-related therapies that are not considered to be part of conventional (allopathic) medicine. Some therapies offered in conjunction with conventional medical interventions are described as complementary, e.g. aromatherapy, whereas others, such as osteopathy, provide diagnostic information and are offered as an alternative to conventional medicine. ⇒ integrated medicine.

**complementary feed** a bottle feed of infant formula milk given to an infant to complement breast-feeding.

**complementation** *n* describes a situation when a relative deficiency of an amino acid in one protein is compensated by a relative surplus from another protein consumed in the same meal.

**complete abortion** ⇒ miscarriage.

**complex** *n* a psychodynamic term meaning a series of emotionally charged ideas repressed because they conflict with ideas acceptable to the individual. ⇒ Electra complex, Oedipus complex.

**complex regional pain syndrome (CRPS)** a chronic pain syndrome of which there are two types. *CRPS 1* is caused by a chronic nerve problem that follows an injury. It most often affects the arms or legs. Previously known as reflex sympathetic dystrophy. *CRPS 2* causes excruciating pain, resulting from an identified injury to a cutaneous nerve. Previously known as causalgia.

**compliance** *n* the acceptance (understanding and remembering) of and following health (medical) advice or specific regimens of treatment. Two main models are proposed for health professionals to increase compliance when giving health (medical) advice: (a) the adherence model, suggesting that there are patient-centred factors that affect the process of following advice, such as locus of control, social support and disruption of lifestyle; (b) the cognitive model, where compliance is influenced by the level of understanding, satisfaction with, and recall of, the advice given. ⇒ concordance.

**complicated fracture** ⇒ fracture.

**complication** *n* in medicine, an accident or second disease arising in the course of a primary disease; may worsen the prognosis or can be fatal.

**composite resin** a type of tooth-coloured resin used in restorative dentistry to fill defects in teeth. They are formed from inorganic filler particles within an organic resin, and are generally hard-wearing, resistant to fractures and easy to polish.

**compos mentis** of sound mind. Mentally competent is now the preferred term.

**compound** *n* a substance composed of two or more elements, chemically combined in a definitive proportion to form a new substance which displays new properties.

**compound (open) fracture** ⇒ fracture.

**comprehension** *n* mental grasp of ideas, their meaning and relationships.

**compress** *n* usually refers to a folded pad of lint, gauze or other material used to arrest haemorrhage or apply pressure, cold, heat, moisture or medication. Used to reduce swelling or pain, such as a cold compress to ease a headache.

**compression** *n* the state of being compressed. Pressing or squeezing together. ⇒ intermittent pneumatic compression.

**compression fracture** ⇒ fracture.

**compression therapy** various types of bandaging technique or compression hosiery used in the management of venous leg ulceration. The application of graduated linear compression to the lower limb reduces venous hypertension and increases venous return from the legs. Compression hosiery can be used to prevent venous leg ulcers occurring where there is venous insufficiency, or to reduce the risk of ulcer recurrence. ⇒ antiembolism hosiery/stockings, venous ulcer.

**compressive force** a force applied along the length of a structure, causing the tissues to approximate one another. This force can be caused by muscular activity, weight bearing, gravity or external loading down the length of the bone. It is necessary for the development and growth of bone. If a large compressive force, which surpasses the stress limits of the structure, is applied, a fracture will occur.

**compromise** *n* in psychoanalysis, a mental mechanism whereby a conflict is evaded by disguising the repressed wish to make it acceptable in consciousness.

**compulsion** *n* an urge to carry out an act, recognized to be irrational. Resisting the urge leads to increasing tension which is only relieved by carrying out the act.

**computed axial tomography (CAT)** ⇒ computed tomography.

**computed tomography (CT)** computer-constructed imaging technique of a thin slice through the body, derived from X-ray absorption data collected during a circular scanning motion.

**conation** *n* the will, desire or volition. The conscious tendency to action. One of the three aspects of mind. ⇒ affection, cognition.

**concentric** *adj* having a common centre or point.

**concentric muscle work** the shortening of a muscle to pull its attachments closer together and produce movement at a joint. For example, the quadriceps femoris muscle group of the anterior and lateral thigh work concentrically to straighten the knee. ⇒ eccentric muscle work.

**concept** *n* the abstract idea or image of the properties of a class of objects. Results from the mental process of abstracting and recombining certain qualities or characteristics of a number of ideas.

**conception** *n* **1.** the creation of a state of pregnancy: impregnation of the oocyte by the spermatozoon. **2.** an abstract mental idea of anything—**conceptive** *adj*.

**conceptual model of practice** in occupational therapy practice the theoretical understanding of the significance of occupation in human life. Conceptual models develop through research and often have associated assessment frameworks and instruments that have been developed along with the conceptual model and assist in the implementation of theory into practice.

**conceptus** *n* the product of conception. It comprises the developing embryo/fetus and the enclosing fetal membranes throughout the developmental stages from implantation to the birth of the infant.

**concha** *n* any shell-like structure—**conchae** *pl. concha auris* the external part of the ear surrounding the external auditory meatus/canal. *nasal concha* one of three bones (turbinates) that protrude into the nasal cavity. ⇒ Appendix 1, Figure 14.

**concordance** *n* **1.** the expression of one or more specific physical traits in both twins. **2.** an approach to prescribing medicines and other treatments which respects the beliefs and wishes of the patient/client in determining whether a treatment should be used and how it should be used. An agreement is reached through negotiation between the patient/client and the health professional.

**concrescence** *n* a growing together of structures that are normally separate. In dentistry, the growing together of two teeth after eruption, or the fusion of the roots of adjacent teeth.

**concretion** *n* a deposit of hard material; a calculus, such as in the kidney.

**concussion** *n* a condition resulting from a blow to the head characterized by headache, nausea, confusion, amnesia and visual symptoms. ⇒ Glasgow Coma Scale.

**condensation** *n* the process of becoming more compact, e.g. the changing of a gas to a liquid.

**conditioned reflex** a reaction acquired by practice or repetition. A reflex in which the response occurs, not to the sensory stimulus which caused it originally, but to another stimulus which the subject has learned to associate with the original stimulus: it can be acquired by training and repetition. In Pavlov's classic experiments, dogs learned to associate the sound of a bell with the sight and smell of food: even when food was not presented, salivation occurred at the sound of a bell (I Pavlov, Russian physiologist, 1849–1936).

**conditioning** *n* the encouragement of new (desirable) behaviour by modification of the stimulus/response associations. *classical conditioning* where the conditioned reflex occurs in response to a neutral stimulus, i.e. a conditioned reflex. *operant conditioning* the term used when there is a programme to reward (or withhold the reward) a response each time it occurs, so that, given time, it occurs more (or less) frequently. ⇒ deconditioning.

**condom** *n* a latex sheath used as a male contraceptive. It also protects both partners against sexually transmitted infections (STIs). *female condom* a polyurethane tube that fits inside the vagina to provide contraception and protection against STIs.

**conduct disorder** characterized by repetitive behaviour that is usually evident during childhood. The behaviour neither meets the prevailing social norms nor shows consideration for the feelings and rights of other people. The child may be physically aggressive or cruel to other people or animals; damage or destroy property; tell lies or steal; and seriously disregard rules or laws. The condition can progress to an antisocial personality disorder in adulthood.

**conduction** *n* the transmission of heat, light or sound waves through suitable media; also the passage of electrical currents and nerve impulses through body tissues—**conductivity** *n*.

**conductor** *n* a substance or medium which transmits heat, light, sound, electric current, etc. The degree of conductivity varies, some substances being good conductors, whereas others are non-conductors.

**condyle** *n* a rounded projection situated at the end of some bones, e.g. tibia.

**condyloid** *adj* resembling a knuckle.

**condyloma** *n* papilloma. *condylomata acuminata* fleshy, viral warts, caused by the human papillomavirus (HPV), affecting the genital or anal areas. *condylomata lata* wart-like lesions found in moist areas of the body during the secondary stage of syphilis—**condylomata** *pl*, **condylomatous** *adj*.

**cone biopsy** cone-shaped excision of the cervix, performed using a colposcope, for certain stages of cervical intraepithelial neoplasia.

**cones** *npl* three types of photoreceptors in the retina, each containing a different pigment, responsible for high-definition colour vision in good light. ⇒ rods.

**confabulation** *n* a symptom common in delirium when there is impairment of memory for recent events. The gaps in the patient's memory are filled in with fabrications. ⇒ amnesic syndrome, dysmnesic syndrome, Korsakoff's (Korsakov's) syndrome.

**confidence interval** in statistics, a level, e.g. 95%, that indicates the level of confidence that the test result, such as a mean, will occur within a specified range.

**confidentiality** *n* a legal and professional requirement to protect all confidential information concerning patients/clients obtained in the course of professional practice, and make disclosures only with consent, where required by specific legislation, or a court order, or where disclosure in the wider public interest is justified.

**conflict** *n* in psychoanalysis, the presence of two incompatible and contrasting wishes or emotions. When the conflict becomes intolerable, repression of the wishes may occur. Mental conflict and repression form the basic causes of many mental health problems and distress.

**confluence** *n* becoming merged; flowing together; a uniting, as of adjacent lesions of a rash.

**conformal therapy** a system that allows the radiotherapy treatment volume to be shaped to conform to the shape of the tumour, permitting a high dose to be given to the tumour and a lesser dose to surrounding tissue than with conventional radiotherapy. Employs the use of a multileaf collimator.

**conformity** *n* a propensity to alter views and/or behaviour to match better the prevailing social norms in response to social pressure.

**confounding factors** extraneous factors, apart from the variables already allowed for, that distort research findings.

**C**

**confusion** *n* being out of touch with reality—associated with a clouding of consciousness. Occurs in a wide variety of mental health problems, particularly organic disorders. Acute confusional states may have an acute medical cause, such as infection, electrolyte imbalance, anaemia, inappropriate medication, etc. Chronic confusion may have an insidious onset and be caused by an unnoticed chronic condition, e.g. hypothyroidism. ⇒ acute confusional state.

**congenital** *adj* of abnormal conditions, present at birth, often genetically determined. ⇒ genetic. Existing before or at birth, usually associated with a defect or disease, e.g. developmental dysplasia of the hip (DDH) (previously known as congenital dislocation of the hip [CDH]).

**congenital adrenal hyperplasia (CAH)** an inherited group of conditions characterized by excessive secretion of adrenal androgen (male) hormones. It is caused by a deficiency of one of the enzymes needed to synthesize the hormones cortisol and aldosterone. Adrenal crisis can result from the lack of hormones. Excessive secretion of adrenocorticotrophic hormone (ACTH) causes adrenal enlargement (through hyperplasia) and the secretion of androgen (male) hormones. This leads to virilization, which may not be evident in male infants, but in severe cases a female infant will develop external male sexual characteristics. Late onset causes virilization in females and precocious puberty in males.

**congenital heart disease** developmental abnormalities in the anatomy of the heart, resulting postnatally in imperfect circulation of blood and often manifested by murmurs, cyanosis, breathlessness, poor feeding and sweating. For example, Fallot's tetralogy, septal defects, patent ductus arteriosus, etc. ⇒ 'blue baby'.

**congenital syphilis** ⇒ syphilis.

**congestion** *n* hyperaemia. Passive congestion results from obstruction or slowing down of venous return, as in the lower limbs or the lungs—**congestive** *adj*, **congest** *vi, vt. congestive dysmenorrhoea* ⇒ dysmenorrhoea.

**congestive heart failure** a chronic inability of the heart to maintain an adequate output of blood from one or both ventricles, resulting in pulmonary congestion and overdistension of certain veins and organs with blood, and in an inadequate blood supply to the body tissues.

**congruent** *adj* when describing a visual field defect implies the defect affects the same area of the field in both eyes.

**conization** *n* removal of a cone-shaped part of the cervix by knife or cautery.

**conjoined twins** identical twins where the normal separation during early development has not occurred. They may be joined, for instance, at the head, chest or abdomen. There may be sharing of vital organs such as the heart or liver. Surgical separation is undertaken successfully in some cases.

**conjugate** *n* a measurement of the bony pelvis. *diagonal conjugate* the clinical measurement taken in pelvic assessment, from the lower border of the symphysis pubis to the sacral promontory = 111–126 mm. It is 18.5 mm greater than *obstetrical conjugate*, the available space for the fetal head, i.e. the distance from the sacral promontory to the posterior surface of the top of the symphysis pubis = 108–114 mm. *true conjugate* the distance from the sacral promontory to the summit of the symphysis pubis = 110.5 mm.

**conjugation** *n* **1.** a process whereby unicellular organisms, such as bacteria, are able to transfer or exchange genetic material by means of sex pili. It allows the genes that confer antibiotic resistance to be passed between bacteria. **2.** the joining together of molecules. It is an important physiological process, usually occurring in the liver, where toxic substances such as drug residues are conjugated with molecules that include glucuronic acid, glutathione, etc., to allow their safe excretion from the body.

**conjunctiva** *n* the delicate transparent mucous membrane which lines the inner surface of the eyelids (palpebral conjunctiva) and reflects over the anterior part of the eyeball (bulbar or ocular conjunctiva)—**conjunctival** *adj*.

**conjunctivitis** *n* inflammation of the conjunctiva. Usually infective or allergic. Follicular and papillary types may indicate cause.

**connective tissue** the diverse group of tissue that includes adipose, areolar, bone, cartilage, blood and blood-producing tissue, elastic, fibrous and lymphoid (reticular tissue).

**connective tissue diseases** a group of diseases often characterized by inflammation affecting collagen and elastin, the structural protein molecules found in connective tissue. Many involve autoimmune responses and include dermatomyositis, myositis, polyarteritis nodosa, rheumatoid arthritis, scleroderma,

Sjögren syndrome, systemic lupus erythematosus (SLE) and a category of mixed connective tissue diseases. Some are also known as collagen diseases.

**connective tissue massage** manipulations that stretch the superficial and deep connective tissue in order to stimulate the circulation.

**Conn's syndrome** (J Conn, American physician, 1907–1994) primary hyperaldosteronism. ⇒ hyperaldosteronism.

**Conradi–Hünermann syndrome** (E Conradi, German physician, 20th century; C Hünermann, German physician, 20th century) a skeletal dysplasia which is inherited as an autosomal dominant trait. Skeletal abnormalities are variable; they are present at birth. After the first few weeks, life expectancy is normal.

**consanguinity** *n* blood relationship. May be close (as between parent and child) or less so (as between cousins)—**consanguineous** *adj*.

**conscientious objection** a legal recognition that an individual is not bound to take part in some specific activities such as termination of pregnancy. It may also apply to other strongly held beliefs that are not acknowledged by law.

**consciousness** *n* a complex concept which implies that a person is consciously perceiving the environment through the five sensory organs, and responding to the perceptions. ⇒ anaesthesia, sleep.

**consent** *n* patients are legally required to consent to treatment, surgery and any intervention that requires physical contact. Consent may be verbal, written, or implied i.e. by non-verbal communication. However, where there are likely to be risks or disputes, written consent is advisable. It is the responsibility of the health care professional undertaking the procedure to provide a full explanation to the patient prior to treatment or surgery about what is involved and any additional measures that may be required and to obtain written consent. Previously the health care professional was the doctor concerned, but increasingly other health care professionals are undertaking treatments, e.g. endoscopy by nurses. If the patient is a minor, or incapable of giving informed consent, the next of kin must sign the consent form.

**consequentialist ethics** an ethical theory that considers the consequences of actions or inactions.

**conservative treatment** aims at preventing a condition from becoming worse without using radical measures. For example, the use of drug therapy rather than surgery.

**consolidation** *n* becoming solid, such as, for instance, the state of the lung due to exudation and organization in lobar pneumonia.

**constipation** *n* an implied chronic condition of infrequent and often difficult evacuation of faeces due to insufficient high-fibre food or fluid intake, immobility, or to sluggish or disordered action of the bowel musculature or nerve supply, or to habitual failure to empty the rectum. Other causes include pain on defecation, inability to respond to the urge to defecate, hypokalaemia, drugs such as iron preparations, pregnancy (hormonal), depression, colorectal cancer (alternating with diarrhoea) and some systemic diseases. *Acute constipation* signifies obstruction or paralysis of the gut of sudden onset.

**consumption** *n* **1.** act of consuming or using up. **2.** a once popular term for pulmonary tuberculosis, which 'consumed' the body—**consumptive** *adj*.

**contact** *n* **1.** direct or indirect exposure to infection. **2.** a person who has been so exposed.

**contact lens** of glass or plastic, worn under the eyelids in direct contact with conjunctiva (in place of spectacles) for therapeutic or cosmetic purposes. Some are designed to be disposable and are worn for a single day, but the standard type must be soaked in special cleaning solutions when not in use to prevent infection.

**contact tracer** ⇒ health adviser.

**contact sports** individual or team sports in which contact between two players, although not an integral part of the game, is unavoidable.

**contagious** *adj* capable of transmitting infection or of being transmitted.

**containment isolation** separation of a patient with any type of infection to prevent spread of the condition to others. ⇒ protective isolation, source isolation.

**contaminants** *npl* describes any undesirable chemicals present in foodstuffs. These include residues of agricultural chemicals, e.g. fertilizers, herbicides, pesticides, fungicides, etc., occurring during processing or caused by pollution, or the result of a malicious act.

**continent diversion** surgical technique of bladder reconstruction by the creation of a pouch that can be emptied using a catheter.

**contingency fund** an amount of money included in the costings of a project that would be used for some unplanned or unpredictable expense.

**continuous ambulatory peritoneal dialysis (CAPD)** peritoneal dialysis carried out every day, by patients needing renal replacement therapy, at home.

**continuous glucose monitoring (CGM)** use of a subcutaneous probe to monitor tissue glucose concentrations giving a continuous profile over 48 to 72 hours; useful for adjustment of insulin doses.

**continuous passive motion (CPM)** type of passive mobilization, used to help the recovery of cartilage after knee surgery.

**continuous positive airways pressure (CPAP)** the application of gas at a constant positive pressure, to the airway of a spontaneously breathing patient, via an endotracheal tube, a tightly fitting face mask that covers both the mouth and nose, or a nasal mask. It reduces alveolar collapse at the end of expiration and reduces the work of breathing; used at night in patients with sleep apnoea syndromes. CPAP is increasingly used to correct hypoxaemia.

**continuous subcutaneous insulin infusion (CSII)** the use of a pump to deliver insulin continuously, either with a fixed or variable basal rate, and with a facility for bolus dosing, to achieve almost physiological control of diabetes mellitus.

**contraceptive** *n, adj* (describes) an agent used to prevent conception, e.g. condom, spermicidal vaginal pessary or cream, rubber cervical cap, intrauterine device. ⇒ combined oral contraceptive, emergency contraception, intrauterine device—**contraception** *n*.

**contract** *v* **1.** draw together; shorten; decrease in size. **2.** acquire by contagion or infection.

**contractile** *adj* having the ability to shorten— usually following stimulation; a property of muscle tissue—**contractility** *n*.

**contraction** *n* shortening, e.g. in muscle fibres.

**contracture** *n* shortening of scar or muscle tissue, causing deformity ⇒ Dupuytren's contracture, Volkmann's ischaemic contracture.

**contraindication** *n* any factor or condition indicating that a certain type of treatment (usually used for that condition) should be discontinued or not used.

**contralateral** *adj* on the opposite side—**contralaterally** *adv*. ⇒ homolateral.

**contrast medium** substance used to improve the visibility of body structures during imaging. Examples include barium sulphate, gases including air and iodine-containing substances, etc.

**contrecoup** *n* injury or damage at a point opposite the impact, resulting from transmit-

ted force. It can occur in an organ or part containing fluid. For example, the brain inside the skull.

**control group** in research, the group that is not exposed to the independent variable, such as a therapeutic intervention or experimental drug. ⇒ experimental group, variable.

**controlled-dose transdermal absorption of drugs** application of a drug patch to the skin: gradual absorption gives a constant level in the blood. Examples include analgesics such as fentanyl, various types of hormone replacement and nicotine for smoking cessation.

**controlled drugs (CD)** drugs that are subject to statutory control, e.g. barbiturates, cocaine, morphine. ⇒ Appendix 5.

**Control of Substances Hazardous to Health (COSHH)** regulations relating to obligatory risk assessment and action to be taken, such as during the use of certain anaesthetic agents.

**contusion** *n* ⇒ bruise—**contuse** *vt*.

**convection** *n* transfer of heat from the hotter to the colder part; the heated substance (air or fluid), being less dense, tends to rise. The colder portion, flowing in to be heated, rises in its turn; thus *convection currents* are set in motion.

**convergence** *n* the inward movement of the eyes to focus on near objects.

**conversion** *n* a mental defence mechanism. A psychological conflict being expressed as a physical symptom. *conversion disorder* an old term for dissociative disorders.

**convolutions** *npl* folds, twists or coils as found in the intestine, renal tubules and the surface of the brain—**convoluted** *adj*.

**convulsions** *npl* involuntary contractions of muscles resulting from abnormal electrical activity in the brain: there are many causes. They occur with or without loss of consciousness. ⇒ epilepsy, febrile seizures, seizures. *clonic convulsions* show alternating contraction and relaxation of muscle groups. *tonic convulsions* reveal sustained muscle rigidity—**convulsive** *adj*.

**Cooley's anaemia** (T Cooley, American paediatrician, 1871–1945) ⇒ thalassaemia.

**Coombs' test** (R Coombs, British immunologist, b. 1921) a highly sensitive test designed to detect antibodies to red blood cells, such as those found in Rhesus incompatibility or haemolytic anaemia. The indirect method detects unbound antibodies in the serum, whereas the direct method detects those bound to the red cells.

**co-ordination** *n* moving in harmony. The body's ability to execute smooth, fluid, accurate and controlled movements.

**COPD** *abbr* chronic obstructive pulmonary disease.

**coping** *n* the way in which a person deals with a circumstance which can be either negative or positive. The coping response can be negative, e.g. reducing social activities because of failing sight or the odour of a chronic wound; or it can be positive, e.g. increasing participation in sport although the person uses a wheelchair.

**copper (Cu)** *n* essential trace element widely distributed in the body tissues; an important component of metalloenzymes involved in protein synthesis. Copper deficiency can develop in preterm infants and full-term infants who have been fed cows' milk instead of infant formula milk.

**coprolalia** *n* the excessive use of obscene speech. Occurs as a sign most commonly in cerebral deterioration or trauma affecting frontal lobes of the brain. ⇒ Tourette's syndrome.

**coprolith** *n* faecolith.

**coproporphyrin** *n* nitrogenous substance derived from the breakdown of bilirubin produced when haemoglobin is decomposed, normally excreted in the faeces.

**copulation** *n* coitus, sexual intercourse.

**cor** *n* the heart or pertaining to the heart.

**coracobrachialis muscle** a muscle of the upper arm which causes adduction and flexion of the humerus. Its origin is on the scapula and the insertion on the medial aspect of the humerus. ⇒ Appendix 1, Figure 4.

**coracoid process** beak-like process of the scapula; provides attachment for the pectoralis minor muscle and other muscles.

**cord** *n* a thread-like structure. *spermatic cord* that which suspends the testes in the scrotum. *spinal cord* a structure which lies in the spinal column, reaching from the foramen magnum to the first or second lumbar vertebra. It is a direct continuation of the medulla oblongata. *umbilical cord* attaching the fetus to the placenta. It contains two arteries and a vein. *vocal cord* the membranous bands in the larynx, vibrations of which produce the voice.

**cord presentation** a situation where the umbilical cord is below the presenting part of the fetus.

**cord prolapse** an obstetric emergency occurring as a complication of a cord presentation. Once the fetal membranes rupture the umbilical cord may prolapse and the umbilical blood vessels become compressed between the presenting part and the cervix, thus depriving the fetus of oxygen and causing hypoxia.

**cordectomy** *n* surgical excision of a cord, usually reserved for a vocal cord.

**cordotomy** *n* (*syn* chordotomy) division of the anterolateral nerves in the spinal cord to relieve intractable pain in the pelvis or lower limbs.

**core** *n* central portion, usually applied to the slough in the centre of a boil.

**core skills** competencies. The basics of professional practice which remain relatively constant. In occupational therapy practice they include therapeutic use of self-assessment, environmental analysis and adaptation, and occupational analysis and adaptation.

**corectopia** *n* the displacement of the pupil of the eye from the normal position in the centre of the iris.

**Cori cycle** (C Cori, American biochemist, 1896–1984; G Cori, American biochemist, 1896–1957) a biochemical process whereby lactic acid, formed in contracting muscle, is converted to glucose for cell use in the liver.

**corium** *n* the dermis of the skin.

**corn** *n* ⇒ callus.

**cornea** *n* the outwardly convex transparent three-layer structure forming part of the anterior outer coat of the eye. It has no blood vessels and comprises the outer epithelium, the stroma and the inner endothelium. It is situated in front of the iris and pupil and merges backwards into the sclera (⇒ Appendix 1, Figure 15)—**corneal** *adj*. ⇒ Descemet's membrane.

**corneal graft** (*syn* keratoplasty) replacement of the cornea with a healthy cornea from a human donor.

**corneal reflex** a reaction of blinking when the cornea is touched.

**corneal topography** a technique used to determine the exact shape of the cornea and its refractive power. Important in the surgical correction of refractive errors, such as with the use of lasers.

**corneoscleral** *adj* pertaining to the cornea and sclera, as the circular junction of these structures.

**cornu** *n* a horn-shaped structure, such as the upper angles of the uterus, where the uterine tubes join, or part of the thyroid cartilage—**cornua** *pl*.

**corona** *n* **1.** a crown. **2.** crown-like encircling structure or projection.

**coronal** *adj* in dentistry relating to a crown. Also pertains to the crown of the head.

**coronal plane** ⇒ frontal plane.

**corona radiata 1.** the follicular cells surrounding the zona pellucida in the ovum. **2.** a network of fibres associated with the internal capsule in the cerebral hemispheres and the fibres of the corpus callosum.

**coronary** *adj* crown-like; encircling, as of a vessel or nerve.

**coronary angiography** demonstration of the coronary arteries that supply the myocardium following the injection of a contrast medium.

**coronary arteries** those supplying the myocardium, the first pair of arteries to branch from the aorta as it leaves the left ventricle (Figure C.14). Spasm, narrowing or blockage of these vessels causes angina pectoris or myocardial infarction (heart attack). Diseased vessels may be cleared by balloon angioplasty or lasers or replaced with veins taken from the legs. ⇒ angioplasty.

**coronary artery bypass graft (CABG)** a technique used to revascularize the myocardium, thereby relieving anginal pain and decreasing the risk of myocardial infarction. A healthy portion of saphenous vein from the leg or the mammary artery is grafted between the aorta and a point beyond the blockage in a coronary artery. Often more than one artery is bypassed. Increasingly the procedure is undertaken using minimally invasive techniques.

**coronary care unit (CCU)** high-dependency area in a hospital specialized in the care of patients with acute heart problems, particularly those with cardiac arrhythmias, unstable angina pectoris and after a myocardial infarction.

**coronary heart disease (CHD)** also known as coronary artery disease and, more rarely, ischaemic heart disease. It includes angina pectoris and myocardial infarction. A deficient supply of oxygenated blood to the myocardium, causing central chest pain of varying intensity that may radiate to arms and jaws.

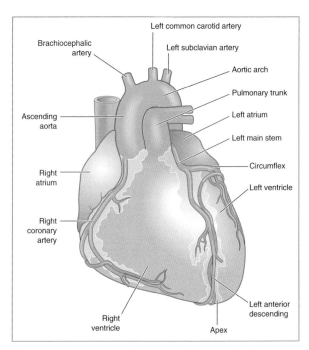

**Figure C.14** Coronary arteries *(reproduced from Brooker & Nicol 2003 with permission).*

The lumen of the blood vessels is usually narrowed by atheromatous plaques. If treatment with drug therapy is unsuccessful, percutaneous transluminal angioplasty, or bypass surgery, may be considered. ⇒ angina pectoris, angioplasty, coronary artery bypass graft, myocardial infarction.

**coronary sinus** channel receiving most venous blood from the myocardium and opening into the right atrium.

**coronary thrombosis** occlusion of a coronary artery by a thrombus. The area deprived of blood becomes necrotic and is called an infarct. ⇒ coronary heart disease, myocardial infarction.

**coronaviruses** *npl* a group of RNA viruses responsible for acute respiratory infections such as the common cold.

**coroner** *n* in England and Wales, an officer of the Crown, usually a solicitor, barrister or doctor, who presides over the Coroner's Court responsible for establishing the cause of death in cases where violence may be a possibility or suspected. Where doubts exist about the cause of death the doctor should consult the coroner and act on his or her advice. The coroner must be notified if a patient dies within 24 hours of admission to hospital. In addition all theatre/anaesthetic deaths must be reported. Any death where the deceased has not been seen by a doctor recently requires that a coroner's postmortem is undertaken. In Scotland, reports about such deaths are submitted to the Procurator Fiscal but a postmortem is normally only ordered if foul play is suspected. The Scottish equivalent of the Coroner's inquest is the fatal accident inquiry, presided over by the Sheriff.

**coronoid fossa** a fossa on the distal dorsal aspect of the humerus, it receives the coronoid process of the ulna when the elbow is bent to flex the forearm.

**coronoid process 1.** a process on the ramus of the mandible which provides attachment for the temporalis muscle. **2.** a process at the proximal end of the ulna; it forms part of the trochlear notch that articulates with the humerus at the elbow.

**cor pulmonale** enlargement of the right ventricle and right-sided heart disease resulting from primary disease of the lung (emphysema, fibrosis, silicosis, etc.) or pulmonary blood vessels, which strains the right ventricle.

**corpus** *n* a body, any mass of tissue which is easily distinguishable from its surroundings—**corpora** *pl*.

**corpus albicans** the white scar remaining on the ovary once the corpus luteum has degenerated.

**corpus cavernosum** one of two lateral columns of spongy erectile tissue in the penis and also the clitoris. ⇒ Appendix 1, Figure 16.

**corpus luteum** a yellow mass which forms in the ovary after ovulation. It secretes progesterone and persists to maintain pregnancy should it occur.

**corpus spongiosum** the single ventral column of erectile tissue in the penis. ⇒ Appendix 1, Figure 16.

**corpus striatum** part of the basal nuclei (basal ganglia).

**corpuscle** *n* outdated term for blood cells—**corpuscular** *adj*. ⇒ erythrocytes, leucocytes.

**corrective** *adj, n* something which changes, counteracts or modifies something harmful.

**correlation** *n* in statistics. The relationship between variables, i.e. how one characteristic influences another, or in other words, a measure of cause and effect. The two types of correlation are positive and negative (inverse). The *correlation coefficient* ($r$) illustrates the degree of association between a pair of variables. Correlation coefficient values range between $+1$ (perfect positive) to $-1$ (perfect negative), with a value of 0 indicating that there is no linear relationship.

**Corrigan's pulse** (D Corrigan, Irish physician, 1802–1880) ⇒ collapsing pulse.

**cortex** *n* the outer layer of an organ or structure beneath its capsule or membrane such as the cerebral cortex, adrenal cortex or renal cortex—**cortices** *pl*, **cortical** *adj*.

**corticosteroids** *npl* hormones produced by the adrenal cortex. ⇒ glucocorticoids, mineralocorticoids, sex hormones. The word is also used for synthetic steroids such as prednisolone and dexamethasone. ⇒ Appendix 5.

**corticotrophin** *n* ⇒ adrenocorticotrophic hormone.

**corticotrophin-releasing hormone (CRH)** a polypeptide hormone produced by the hypothalamus. It stimulates the release of adrenocorticotrophic hormone (corticotrophin) from the anterior lobe of the pituitary gland.

**cortisol** *n* hydrocortisone, one of the principal adrenal cortical steroids. It is essential to life. There is decreased secretion in Addison's disease and increased amounts in Cushing's disease and syndrome.

**cortisone** *n* one of the hormones of the adrenal gland. It is converted into cortisol before use by the body. Used therapeutically as

C

replacement in conditions that include Addison's disease.

**Corynebacterium** *n* a bacterial genus of Gram-positive, curved rod-shaped bacteria. Many strains colonize the upper respiratory tract, and some are pathogenic and produce exotoxins such as *Corynebacterium diphtheriae* that causes diphtheria.

**coryza** *n* the 'common cold'. Rhinoviruses, coronaviruses and adenoviruses cause an acute upper respiratory infection of short duration; highly contagious.

**COSHH** *abbr* Control of Substances Hazardous to Health.

**cosmetic** *adj, n* or aesthetic. (That which is) performed to improve the appearance or prevent disfigurement. ⇒ plastic surgery.

**cosmetic orthodontics** limited orthodontic treatment which aims to improve appearance, such as the closing of a diastema (gap) between central incisors.

**costal** *adj* pertaining to the ribs. *costal cartilages* those which attach the ribs to the sternum and each other.

**cost–benefit analysis (CBA)** method of analysis used in the economic evaluation of health care interventions (programmes or procedures). Health outcomes are measured in monetary terms to enable comparisons between interventions from a variety of disciplines. There are problems with valuing life and health in monetary terms, so this method is not widely used.

**cost centre** a department, for example, physiotherapy or catering, for which a budget covering staff and other resources has been set.

**cost-effectiveness analysis (CEA)** analytical technique used in the economic evaluation of health care interventions (programmes and procedures). A cost-effectiveness analysis is used when the outcomes of the procedures are not necessarily the same, but can be measured in the same natural units. For example, the outcomes may be measured in death rates, healthy years of life gained, symptom-free days or even blood pressures. The output of this type of analysis is 'cost per unit increase', for example, cost of intervention against cost per life year gained. Health benefits are measured in natural units (e.g. mortality rates, survival rates) or final clinical outcomes (e.g. cost per life-years gained, reduced cost per days off sick). Intermediate clinical outcomes are sometimes used (e.g. number of cancers detected in a screening programme) but this is not valid if a clear

association between cancer detected and survival or quality of life cannot be demonstrated.

**costive** *adj* lay term for constipated. ⇒ constipation—**costiveness** *n*.

**cost minimization** analytic technique used in economic evaluation of health care interventions (programmes or procedures). A cost minimization analysis is used when the outcomes or consequences of the procedures are the same. A prerequisite for such a study is that there is evidence (preferably from a randomized clinical trial) that the different procedures are equally effective. A cost minimization analysis therefore solely consists of the analyses of costs. Common examples include comparisons of home and hospital care for chronic and terminal conditions.

**costochondral** *adj* pertaining to a rib and its cartilage.

**costochondritis** *n* inflammation of the costochondral cartilage. ⇒ Tietze syndrome.

**costoclavicular** *adj* pertaining to the ribs and the clavicle. *costoclavicular syndrome* is a synonym for cervical rib/thoracic inlet syndrome.

**cost utility analysis (CUA)** analytic technique used in economic evaluation of health care interventions (programmes or procedures). A cost utility analysis is used when the outcomes cannot be measured in natural units, so a utility or value scale has to be employed. This may be because the important outcomes of the procedures are not directly comparable or they are multifaceted, e.g. a comparison of amputation against waiting for the treatment of a gangrenous foot—outcomes could be pain, mobility and/or survival. The commonly used utility scale is quality-adjusted life years (QALYs), which use survey tools such as the Nottingham Health Profile to allocate 'relative qualities' to different health states. However, different people value their health differently, therefore utility ratings are not unique. Research has provided 'average' utility. Cost utility analyses report results as 'costs per QALY (gained)'.

**cot death** ⇒ sudden unexpected death in infancy (sudden infant death syndrome).

**cotton-wool spot** white swelling in the nerve fibre layer of the retina caused by microinfarction.

**cotyledon** *n* one of the subdivisions of the uterine surface of the placenta.

**cough** *n* explosive expulsion of air from the lungs. It may be voluntary, or as a protective reflex that expels a foreign body such as food or sputum. Cough is a feature of numerous respiratory and cardiac conditions. It can be defined as dry, where no sputum is expectorated, or wet if sputum is present. ⇒ postural drainage.

**coumarins** *npl* a group of anticoagulant drugs, e.g. warfarin. ⇒ Appendix 5.

**Council for Healthcare Regulatory Excellence (CHRE)** a UK-wide statutory body that oversees the regulation of health care professionals by several individual statutory regulatory bodies, including the General Medical Council, Health Professions Council, Nursing and Midwifery Council, etc.

**counselling** *n* a professional helping relationship with a client who is experiencing psychological problems. The counsellor listens actively and helps the client to identify and clarify the problems and supports the client in making a positive attempt to overcome the problems.

**counterextension** *n* extension by means of holding back the upper part of a limb while pulling down on the other end.

**counterirritant** *n* an agent which, when applied to the skin, initiates a mild inflammatory response (hyperaemia) and relief of pain and congestion associated with deep-seated inflammation—**counterirritation** *n*.

**countertraction** *n* traction upon the proximal extremity of a fractured limb opposing the pull of the traction apparatus on the distal extremity.

**counter-transference** *n* the emotional response (unconscious or conscious) of a therapist to a client/patient, for example interacting with the client as if a close relative. Such responses are inappropriate in the therapeutic relationship.

**couvade** *n* exhibiting the symptoms of pregnancy and childbirth by the father. Common in some cultures.

**Couvelaire uterus** (A Couvelaire, French obstetrician, 1873–1948) 'uterine apoplexy'. Bruising and swelling due to bleeding into the uterine muscle associated with serious placental abruption (abruptio placentae).

**cover test** test used to diagnose a squint (strabismus).

**Cowper's glands** (W Cowper, English surgeon, 1666–1709) ⇒ bulbourethral glands.

**COX-2 inhibitors** cyclo-oxygenase-2 inhibitors, e.g. celecoxib, are selective non-steroidal anti-inflammatory drugs (NSAIDs). They have a lower incidence of gastrointestinal disturbances, but there are worries regarding cardiovascular safety. ⇒ Appendix 5.

**coxa** *n* the hip joint—**coxae** *pl*. *coxa valga* an increase in the normal angle between neck and shaft of femur. *coxa vara* a decrease in the normal angle plus torsion of the neck, e.g. slipped femoral epiphysis.

**coxalgia** *n* pain in the hip joint.

*Coxiella* *n* a microbial genus closely related to *Rickettsia*, including *Coxiella burnetii*, which causes Q fever.

**coxitis** *n* inflammation of the hip joint.

**coxsackievirus** *n* one of the three groups of viruses included in the family of enteroviruses. Divided into groups A and B. Cause conditions that include: aseptic meningitis, herpangina, Bornholm disease, gastroenteritis and myocarditis.

**CPAP** *abbr* continuous positive airways pressure.

**C-peptide** an inactive peptide formed when proinsulin is converted to insulin in the beta cells of the pancreas. The amount of C-peptide in the blood can be measured to give an indication of pancreatic beta-cell function.

**CPK/CP** *abbr* creatine phosphokinase ⇒ creatine kinase.

**CPM** *abbr* continuous passive motion.

**CPP** *abbr* cerebral perfusion pressure.

**CPR** *abbr* cardiopulmonary resuscitation.

**crab louse** phthirus pubis.

**cracked-tooth syndrome** transient pain during eating can indicate a crack in a tooth. Often occurs in people who crush ice or crack nuts with their teeth.

**cradle cap** *n* scaling of the scalp of infants, often due to atopic dermatitis or seborrhoeic dermatitis.

**cramp** *n* spasmodic contraction of a muscle or group of muscles; involuntary and painful; may result from fatigue.

**cranial** *adj* pertaining to the cranium.

**cranial nerves** twelve pairs of nerves that arise from the brain and exit through openings in the skull (Figure C.15). They have names and are designated by Roman numerals—olfactory (I); optic (II); oculomotor (III); trochlear (IV); trigeminal (V); abducens (abducent) (VI); facial (VII); vestibulocochlear (auditory/acoustic) (VIII); glossopharyngeal (IX); vagus (X); accessory (XI); hypoglossal (XII).

**craniofacial** *adj* pertaining to the cranium and the face.

**craniometry** *n* the science which deals with the measurement of skulls.

**craniopharyngioma** *n* a tumour which develops between the brain and the pituitary gland.

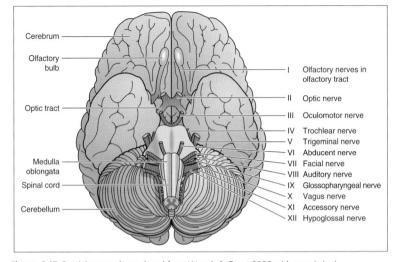

**Figure C.15** Cranial nerves *(reproduced from Waugh & Grant 2006 with permission).*

**cranioplasty** *n* operative repair of a skull defect—**cranioplastic** *adj*.

**craniosacral** *adj* pertaining to the skull and sacrum. Applied to the outflow of the parasympathetic nervous system.

**craniostenosis** *n* a condition in which the skull sutures fuse too early and the fontanelles close. It may cause increased intracranial pressure requiring surgery.

**craniosynostosis** *n* craniostosis. Premature fusion of cranial sutures resulting in abnormal skull shape and craniostenosis. Deformities depend on which sutures are affected. Often associated with other skeletal abnormalities.

**craniotabes** *n* a thinning or wasting of the cranial bones occurring in infancy. May persist in infants/children who later have rickets—**craniotabetic** *adj*.

**craniotomy** *n* a surgical opening of the skull in order to remove a growth, relieve pressure, evacuate blood clot or arrest haemorrhage.

**cranium** *n* the part of the skull enclosing the brain. It comprises eight bones: the occipital, two parietals, frontal, two temporals, sphenoid and ethmoid—**cranial** *adj*.

**crank test** a test used to assess shoulder stability.

**craquelé** *adj* describes cracked skin resembling crazy paving. A term used in association with a certain type of eczema seen in older people.

**C-reactive protein (CRP)** an acute-phase protein. Elevated amounts are present in the plasma in response to inflammation and tissue damage. It is a very sensitive progress indicator of many inflammatory conditions, such as infective endocarditis.

**creatine** *n* a nitrogenous compound produced in the body. *phosphorylated creatine* the important storage form of high-energy phosphate.

**creatine kinase (CK)** (*syn* ATP:creatine phosphokinase [CPK, CP]) an enzyme occurring as three isoenzymes. It is found in brain tissue, skeletal muscle, blood and in myocardial tissue. *creatine kinase test* increased levels of the myocardial isoenzyme in serum are indicative of acute myocardial infarction.

**creatinine** *n* a byproduct of the metabolism of creatine phosphate in muscle tissue. The amount produced daily is fairly constant and depends on the muscle mass, which is influenced by age, gender and body weight. Creatinine is normally cleared by the kidneys and excreted in the urine. Serum creatinine is raised in renal failure, hyperthyroidism and muscle-wasting disorders, but the interpretation of the results must take account of age, gender and body weight. *creatinine clearance test* measures the rate at which the kidneys clear creatinine from the blood. The relationship between age, gender, body weight and serum creatinine may be used to calculate the creatinine clearance rate, which can be used to provide an estimate of the glomerular filtration rate.

**creatinuria** n excess amount of creatine present in the urine, as in situations where muscle protein is rapidly broken down.

**creep** n (*syn* cold flow) the continued change in the size of the lumen of plastic tubing in intravenous giving sets after release of the clamp. It can change the rate of the fluid passing along the tube.

**crenation** n the shrinkage of red blood cells when they are placed in a hypertonic solution.

**crepitation** n ⇒ crepitus.

**crepitus** n **1.** (crepitation) grinding noise or sensation within a joint, as in osteoarthritis. A feature of fracture and overuse injury. **2.** crackling sound heard via stethoscope. **3.** crackling sound elicited by pressure on tissue containing air (surgical emphysema).

**cresol** n chemically related to phenol. Used in many general environmental disinfectants.

**CREST syndrome** *acron* **c**alcinosis, **R**aynaud's phenomenon, (o)**e**sophageal dysfunction, **s**clerodactyly and **t**elangiectasis. A form of systemic sclerosis.

**crest** n in anatomy a ridge or elevation, e.g. iliac crest.

**cretinism** n obsolete term. ⇒ hypothyroidism.

**Creutzfeldt–Jakob disease (CJD)** (H Creutzfeldt, German neurologist, 1885–1964; A Jakob, German neurologist, 1884–1931) a progressive dementia transmissible through prion protein. New-variant vCJD, mainly affecting young adults, is possibly linked with the prion causing bovine spongiform encephalopathy (BSE). CJD follows a rapid degenerative course, often with myoclonus, and is usually fatal.

**CRF** *abbr* chronic renal failure. ⇒ renal failure.

**CRH** *abbr* corticotrophin-releasing hormone.

**cribriform** *adj* perforated, like a sieve. *cribriform plate* that portion of the ethmoid bone allowing passage of fibres of olfactory nerve.

**cricoid** *adj* ring-shaped. Applied to the cartilage forming the inferior anterior/posterior part of larynx. ⇒ Appendix 1, Figure 6.

**cricoid pressure (Sellick's manoeuvre)** a manoeuvre in which manual pressure is applied over the cricoid cartilage to occlude the oesophagus to prevent regurgitation and aspiration of gastric contents during induction of anaesthesia.

**cricothyroid membrane** fibroelastic membrane that joins the cricoid and thyroid cartilages.

**cricothyroidotomy** n (*syn* cricothyrotomy) incision through the skin and cricothyroid membrane into the larynx to secure a patent airway for emergency relief of upper-airway obstruction. ⇒ minitracheostomy, tracheostomy.

**'cri du chat' syndrome** caused by the partial deletion of one arm of chromosome number 5 leading to learning disability and shortened lifespan. There are certain physical abnormalities and a curious flat, toneless cat-like cry in infancy.

**Crigler–Najjar syndrome** (J Crigler, American paediatrician, b. 1919; V Najjar, American microbiologist, b. 1914) an inherited condition, in which the enzyme glucuronyl transferase is absent or deficient. There is jaundice and unconjugated hyperbilirubinaemia, resulting in damage to the central nervous system.

**criminal abortion** ⇒ abortion.

**criminal law** the law that creates offences heard in the criminal courts such as theft. *criminal wrong* an act or omission that can be pursued in the criminal courts.

**crisis** n **1.** the turning point of a disease—as the point of defervescence in fever. ⇒ lysis *opp*. **2.** muscular spasm in tabes dorsalis referred to as visceral crisis (gastric, vesical, rectal, etc.)—**crises** *pl*.

**crista** n **1.** an anatomical crest. **2.** the crista ampullaris, sensory structure in the ampulla of the semicircular canals within the inner ear. **3.** the infolding of the inner membrane of a mitochondrion.

**critical appraisal** the process of making an objective judgement regarding a research study. Includes research design, methodology, analysis, interpretation of results and the applicability of the study findings to a particular area of health care.

**critical care (outreach) team** in hospital the provision of an outreach team of specialist critical care practitioners with three objectives: to prevent admissions to critical care facilities; to share critical care skills with ward-based staff; and to facilitate timely discharges from critical care.

**critical pH** the pH below which tooth enamel is demineralized.

**Crohn's disease** (B Crohn, American physician, 1884–1983) a chronic recurrent granulomatous inflammation affecting any part of the bowel from mouth to anus. Inflammation may be discontinuous ('skip lesions') with normal bowel in between. May be complicated by fistulae and strictures. ⇒ inflammatory bowel disease.

**Crosby capsule** a special tube which is passed through the mouth to the small intestine. Allows biopsy of jejunal mucosa. Endoscopic biopsy is often used in preference to this time-consuming investigation.

**crossbite** *n* occlusion with the line of occlusion of the mandibular (lower) teeth anterior and/or buccal to the maxillary (upper) teeth.

**cross-infection** *n* ⇒ infection.

**cross-over studies** a research study where the participants are exposed to both the experimental intervention and the placebo, one after another.

**croup** *n* viral infection leading to laryngeal narrowing. The child has 'croupy', stridulous (noisy or harsh-sounding) breathing. Narrowing of the airway which gives rise to the typical attack with crowing inspiration may be the result of oedema or spasm, or both.

**crown** *n* the top part of a structure. *artificial crown* in dentistry, restoration used to cover the part of the tooth that projects above the gum line, usually made of metal, porcelain, or a combination of both. *crown of a tooth* that part of the tooth covered with enamel. ⇒ tooth.

**crowning** *n* the time during the second stage of labour when the fetal head is visible at the vaginal introitus.

**CRP** *abbr* C-reactive protein.

**CRPS** *abbr* complex regional pain syndrome.

**cruciate** *adj* shaped like a cross, such as the ligaments stabilizing the knee joint.

**crural** *adj* relating to the thigh.

**crus** *n* a structure which is leg-like or root-like. Applied to various parts of the body, e.g. crus of the diaphragm—**crura** *pl*, **crural** *adj*.

**'crush' syndrome** traumatic uraemia. Following extensive trauma to muscle, there is a period of delay before the effects of renal damage manifest themselves. There is an increase of non-protein nitrogen in the blood, with oliguria, proteinuria and urinary excretion of myohaemoglobin. Loss of blood plasma to damaged area is marked. Where hypotension has occurred the renal failure will be exacerbated by tubular necrosis.

**crutch palsy** paralysis of extensor muscles of wrist, fingers and thumb from repeated pressure of a crutch upon the radial nerve in the axilla.

**cryaesthesia** *n* **1.** the sensation of coldness. **2.** exceptional sensitivity to a low temperature.

**cryoanalgesia** *n* the relief of pain symptoms by blocking peripheral nerve conduction with extreme cold.

**cryogenic** *adj*, *n* produced by low temperature. Also used to describe any means or apparatus involved in the production of low temperature.

**cryoglobulin** *n* an immunoglobulin that precipitates on cooling, and redissolves on warming; associated with numerous pathological conditions, including occlusion of peripheral blood vessels, ulceration and gangrene. Type 1 cryoglobulins are monoclonal and are associated with lymphoproliferative disorders. Type 2 cryoglobulins are monoclonal with reactivity against polyclonal immunoglobulins, i.e. they are rheumatoid factors. Type 3 are polyclonal with rheumatoid factor activity.

**cryokinetics** *n* use of cold treatments prior to activity.

**cryopexy** *n* surgical fixation by freezing, of a detached retina.

**cryoprecipitate** *n* a preparation of factor VIII obtained by rapid freezing and thawing of plasma. Used in the treatment of haemophilia.

**cryoprobe** *n* freezing probe which can be used to destroy tumours.

**cryosurgery** *n* the use of intense, controlled cold to remove or destroy diseased tissue.

**cryothalamectomy** *n* freezing applied to destroy groups of neurons within the thalamus in the treatment of Parkinson's disease and other hyperkinetic conditions.

**cryotherapy** *n* the use of cold for the treatment of disease.

**cryococcosis** *n* the disease resulting from infection with the yeast *Cryptococcus neoformans*, which is present in soil and pigeon excreta. It most commonly causes meningitis but may also affect the lungs, skin and bones. Immunocompromised individuals, such as those with acquired immunodeficiency syndrome (AIDS), are at increased risk.

**Cryptococcus** *n* a genus of fungi. *Cryptococcus neoformans* occasionally causes disease in humans.

**cryptogenic** *adj* of unknown or obscure cause.

**cryptogenic fibrosing alveolitis** interstitial lung disease characterized by cellular infiltration and thickening of the alveolar walls. Pulmonary macrophages are implicated in fibrosis, and in recruiting other cell types such as neutrophils to the lung.

**cryptomenorrhoea** *n* retention of the menses due to a congenital obstruction, such as an imperforate hymen or atresia of the vagina. ⇒ haematocolpos.

**cryptophthalmos** *n* ⇒ Fraser syndrome.

**cryptorchism** *n* a developmental defect whereby the testes do not descend into the scrotum; they are retained within the abdomen or inguinal canal—**cryptorchid, cryptorchis** *n*.

**cryptosporidiosis** *n* infection caused by *Cryptosporidium* species (protozoa). The organisms are present in the faeces of both domestic and farm animals, and transmission to humans occurs through contaminated water and food. Infection may be symptomless or result in profuse watery diarrhoea. Immunocompromised individuals may be seriously affected.

**crystalline** *adj* like a crystal. *crystalline lens* a biconvex body, oval in shape, which is suspended just behind the iris of the eye, and separates the aqueous humour from the vitreous body (humour). It is slightly less convex on its anterior surface and it contributes to refraction of light rays so that they focus directly on to the retina.

**crystallins** *npl* proteins forming the lens of the eye.

**crystalloids** *npl* substances in solution that will diffuse through a semipermeable membrane.

**crystalloid solutions** clear solutions containing small molecules that are able to pass through the capillary membrane, thereby moving between the blood stream and the tissue fluid. They are used intravenously to maintain hydration and electrolyte balance, for example 0.9% sodium chloride. ⇒ colloid solutions.

**crystalluria** *n* excretion of crystals in the urine—**crystalluric** *adj*.

**crystal violet** (*syn* gentian violet) a brilliant, violet-coloured, antiseptic aniline dye, used as 0.5% solution as a stain. It is only licensed for application to intact skin, the exception being marking the skin before surgery.

**CS** *abbr* caesarean section.

**CSF** *abbr* **1.** cerebrospinal fluid. **2.** colony-stimulating factor.

**CSII** *abbr* continuous subcutaneous insulin infusion.

**CSM** *abbr* Committee on Safety of Medicines.

**CSOM** *abbr* chronic suppurative otitis media.

**CSSD** *abbr* central sterile supplies department.

**CSSU** *abbr* central sterile supply unit.

**CT** *abbr* computed tomography.

**CTG** *abbr* cardiotocography.

**CTZ** *abbr* chemoreceptor trigger zone.

**CUA** *abbr* cost–utility analysis.

**cubital** *adj* pertaining to the elbow, such as the *cubital fossa* in the front of the elbow.

**cubital tunnel external compression syndrome** ulnar paralysis resulting from compression of the ulnar nerve within the cubital tunnel situated on the inner and posterior aspect of the elbow—sometimes referred to as the 'funny bone'.

**cubital vein (median cubital vein)** a superficial vein at the front of the elbow. ⇒ Appendix 1, Figure 10.

**cubitus** *n* the forearm; elbow—**cubital** *adj*.

**cuboid** *adj* shaped like a cube. Lateral tarsal bone, it articulates with the lateral cuneiform bone, sometimes with the navicular, and with the fourth and fifth metatarsals to form the lateral longitudinal arch of the foot.

**cue** *n* during communication, a verbal or non-verbal signal from another individual that is perceived by the observer to require sensitive exploration (by prompting or reflection) as to its meaning for the individual exhibiting it.

**culdocentesis** *n* aspiration of the rectovaginal pouch (pouch of Douglas) via the posterior vaginal wall.

**culdoscope** *n* an endoscope used via the vaginal route.

**culdoscopy** *n* a form of peritoneoscopy or laparoscopy. Passage of a culdoscope through the posterior vaginal fornix, behind the uterus to enter the peritoneal cavity, for viewing same—**culdoscopic** *adj*, **culdoscopically** *adv*.

**Cullen's sign** (T Cullen, American gynaecologist, 1868–1953) blue-black discoloration of the skin around the umbilicus, a sign seen in acute pancreatitis. ⇒ Grey Turner's sign.

**culture** *n* the growth of micro-organisms on artificial media under ideal conditions. ⇒ medium.

**cumulative action** when a dose of a slowly excreted drug is repeated too frequently, an increasing action occurs. This may lead to an accumulation of the drug in the system and toxic symptoms, such as with digoxin.

**Cumulative Index to Nursing and Allied Health Literature (CINAHL)** computerized database of literature relevant to nursing and allied health.

**cuneiform bones** three tarsal bones. All three articulate with the navicular bone and each one articulates with the corresponding metatarsal bone (first, second or third) to complete the medial longitudinal arch of the foot.

**cupola** *n* **1.** gelatinous material surrounding the 'hair' cells projecting from the ampulla of a semicircular canal. ⇒ crista. **2.** gelatinous material surrounding the 'hair' cells and oto-liths in the maculae of the utricle and saccule in the inner ear.

**cupping** *n* space within the optic nerve head due to absence of nerve fibres, often due to glaucoma.

**cupula** *n* ⇒ cupola.

**curettage** *n* the scraping of unhealthy or exu-berant tissue from a cavity. This may be treat-ment or may be done to establish a diagnosis after laboratory analysis of the scrapings.

**curette** *n* a spoon-shaped instrument or a metal loop which may have sharp and/or blunt edges for scraping out (curetting) cavities.

**curettings** *npl* the material obtained by scrap-ing or curetting and usually sent for histologi-cal examination.

**Curling's ulcer** (T Curling, British surgeon, 1811–1888) acute peptic ulceration which occurs either in the stomach or duodenum as a response to physiological stress. First identi-fied after extensive burns but also occurs fol-lowing other physiological stressors, such as severe haemorrhage and hypovolaemia.

**Cusco's speculum** a bivalve speculum used for inspection of the cervix and vagina and for holding the vaginal walls apart while tak-ing high vaginal swabs and cervical smears.

**cushingoid** *adj* a description of the moon face, central obesity and facial plethora common in people with elevated levels of plasma glucocor-ticoids from whatever cause.

**Cushing's disease** (H Cushing, American neurosurgeon, 1869–1939) a rare disorder, mainly of females, characterized principally by a cushingoid appearance, proximal myo-pathy, hyperglycaemia, hypertension and osteoporosis; due to excessive cortisol produc-tion by hyperplastic adrenal glands as a result of increased adrenocorticotrophic hormone (ACTH) secretion by a tumour or hyperplasia of the anterior pituitary gland.

**Cushing's reflex** a rise in blood pressure and a fall in pulse rate; occurs in cerebral space-occupying lesions.

**Cushing's syndrome** clinically similar to Cushing's disease but including all causes: (a) adrenocortical hyperplasia, adenoma or carcinoma, which can be associated with hir-sutism and hypokalaemia due to excess of other adrenal steroids; (b) ectopic adreno-corticotrophic hormone (ACTH) secretion by tumours, e.g. small cell lung cancer, often associated with hyperpigmentation; (c) iatro-genic, due to treatment with glucocorticoids.

**cusp** *n* a projecting point, such as the edge of a tooth or the segment of a heart valve. The cardiac tricuspid valve has three, the mitral (bicuspid) valve two cusps.

**cutaneous** *adj* relating to the skin. *cutaneous nerve* any mixed nerve supplying a region of the skin. ⇒ Appendix 1, Figure 12. *cutaneous ureterostomy* the ureters are transplanted so that they open on to the skin of the abdominal wall.

**cuticle** *n* **1.** the epidermis. **2.** the eponychium. The epidermis or dead epidermis, which covers the proximal part of a nail—**cuticular** *adj.* ⇒ nail.

**CVA** *abbr* cerebrovascular accident.

**CVD** *abbr* cardiovascular disease.

**CVID** *abbr* common variable immunodeficiency.

**CVP** *abbr* central venous pressure.

**CVS** *abbr* **1.** cardiovascular system. **2.** chorionic villus sampling.

**CVVH** *abbr* continuous veno-venous haemofil-tration. ⇒ haemofiltration.

**CVVHD** *abbr* continuous veno-venous haemo-diafiltration (haemodialysis). ⇒ haemodiafil-tration.

**cyanocobalamin** *n* the most stable form of vitamin $B_{12}$, which is produced commercially by bacterial fermentation. This synthetic form must be converted in the body to a naturally occurring form before it can be utilized by the body. ⇒ cobalamins.

**cyanolabe** *n* a pigment contained in one group of cones; responds to blue light.

**cyanopsia** *n* an abnormality of vision where all objects are seen as blue.

**cyanosis** *n* a bluish tinge manifested by hypoxic tissue, observed most frequently under the nails, lips and skin. It is always due to lack of oxygen, and the causes of this are legion—**cyanosed, cyanotic** *adj. central cyanosis* blueness seen on the warm surfaces such as the oral mucosa and tongue. It increases with exertion. *peripheral cyanosis* blueness of the limb extremities, the nose and the earlobes.

**cycle** *n* a regular series of movements or events; a sequence which recurs. ⇒ cardiac, men-strual—**cyclical** *adj.*

**cyclic adenosine monophosphate (cAMP)** a metabolic molecule that acts as a 'second messenger' for many hormones and in pro-cesses where many reactions are occurring simultaneously (enzyme cascade).

**cyclical syndrome** an alternative term preferred by some people to that of premenstrual syndrome.

**cyclical vomiting** periodic attacks of vomiting in children, usually associated with ketosis and usually with no demonstrable pathological cause. Occurs mainly in highly strung children.

**cyclist's nipples** a colloquial expression used in sports medicine to describe the irritation of the nipple due to the combined effects of perspiration and windchill.

**cyclist's palsy** a colloquial expression used in sports medicine to describe the paraesthesia of the ulnar nerve distribution of the forearm and hand due to prolonged leaning on the handlebars when cycling.

**cyclitis** *n* inflammation of the ciliary body of the eye. ⇒ iridocyclitis.

**cyclodestruction** *n* destruction of the ciliary body by heat (usually laser-induced) or freezing.

**cyclodialysis** *n* the formation of a communication between anterior chamber and suprachoroidal space. May be used for the relief of glaucoma.

**cyclo-oxygenase-2 inhibitors** ⇒ COX-2 inhibitors.

**cycloplegia** *n* paralysis of the ciliary muscle of the eye—**cycloplegic** *adj*.

**cycloplegics** *npl* drugs which paralyse the ciliary muscle of the eye, e.g. atropine, cyclopentolate. ⇒ mydriatics.

**cyclothymia** *n* a tendency to alternating but relatively mild mood swings between elation and depression—**cyclothymic** *adj*.

**cyclotron** *n* a device that produces high-energy positive ion beams used to bombard a suitable target resulting in the production of radioisotopes (radionuclides). These can then be used as a source of neutrons or protons for therapeutic purposes.

**cyesis** *n* pregnancy. When there are signs and symptoms of pregnancy in a woman who believes she is pregnant, and this is not so, it is called pseudocyesis. ⇒ phantom pregnancy.

**cylindroma** *n* a tumour of the endothelial element of apocrine tissue such as a sweat gland or a salivary gland. The supporting stroma is hyalinized.

**cyst** *n* a closed cavity or sac, usually with an epithelial lining, enclosing fluid or semisolid matter—**cystic** *adj*.

**cystadenoma** *n* an innocent cystic new growth of glandular tissue. Liable to occur in the female breast.

**cystalgia** *n* pain in the urinary bladder.

**cystathioninuria** *n* inherited disorder of cystathionine metabolism marked by excessive excretion of cystathionine in the urine, an intermediate product in conversion of methionine to cysteine. Sometimes associated with learning disability.

**cystectomy** *n* usually refers to the removal of part or the whole of the urinary bladder. This may necessitate urinary diversion.

**cysteine** *n* a sulphur-containing conditionally essential (indispensable) amino acid. It is synthesized from the amino acids methionine and serine. Cysteine is needed for the synthesis of coenzyme A, glutathione and taurine.

**cystic duct** the bile duct that transports bile between the gallbladder and the common bile duct.

**cysticercosis** *n* infection of humans with cysticercus, the larval stage of the pork tapeworm (*Taenia solium*). After ingestion, the ova do not develop further, but form cysts in subcutaneous tissues, voluntary muscle and the brain, where they cause seizures.

**cysticercus** *n* the larval form of *Taenia solium*.

**cystic fibrosis (CF)** (*syn* fibrocystic disease of the pancreas, mucoviscidosis) an autosomal recessive disorder affecting the exocrine glands; diagnosis may be confirmed by high levels of sodium in sweat. It is the commonest genetically determined disease in Caucasian populations. Meconium ileus in newborns may be an early physical effect. The affected glands produce viscous mucus which leads to blocked dilated ducts, stasis of mucus, infection and fibrosis. The lungs and pancreas are primarily affected, giving rise to digestive problems, including steatorrhoea and malabsorption, repeated chest infections and respiratory and cardiac deterioration, leading ultimately to respiratory and cardiac failure. Current treatment involves physiotherapy, antimicrobial drugs and replacement of pancreatic enzymes, but advances in management include: heart/lung transplants, identification of the defective gene, antenatal testing, gene therapy and genetic counselling for affected couples. ⇒ sweat test.

**cystic fibrosis transmembrane regulator (CFTR)** also known as cystic fibrosis membrane conductance regulator. A protein required for the transport of chloride ions across epithelial cell membranes in the respiratory tract, gastrointestinal tract, pancreas, the skin and the reproductive tract. The gene that encodes for the CFTR protein is located on chromosome number 7. Mutations occurring in the CFTR protein cause abnormal chloride channels that result in cystic fibrosis. Other mutations cause congenital absence of the deferent duct (vas deferens).

**cystine** *n* a sulphur-containing amino acid, produced by the breakdown of proteins during the digestive process. It is readily reduced to two molecules of cysteine.

**cystinosis** *n* a recessively inherited metabolic disorder in which crystalline cystine is deposited in the body. Cystine and other amino acids are excreted in the urine.

**cystinuria** *n* metabolic disorder in which cystine and other amino acids appear in the urine. A cause of renal stones—**cystinuric** *adj*.

**cystitis** *n* inflammation of the urinary bladder; the cause is usually bacterial. The condition may be acute or chronic, primary or secondary to stones, etc. More frequent in females, as the urethra is short.

**cystocele** *n* prolapse of the posterior wall of the urinary bladder into the anterior vaginal wall (Figure C.16). ⇒ colporrhaphy, procidentia, rectocele.

**cystodiathermy** *n* the application of a cauterizing electrical current to the walls of the urinary bladder through a cystoscope, or by open operation.

**cystography** *n* radiographic examination of the urinary bladder, after it has been filled with a contrast medium—**cystographic** *adj*, **cystograph** *n*, **cystogram** *n*, **cystographically** *adv*.

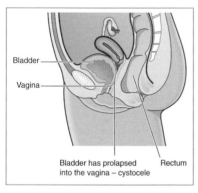

Bladder

Vagina

Bladder has prolapsed into the vagina – cystocele

Rectum

**Figure C.16** Cystocele *(reproduced from Brooker & Nicol 2003 with permission).*

**cystoid macular oedema** oedema of the macula of the retina with cyst formation. Caused by a collection of fluid and protein under the macula. Leads to visual disturbances.

**cystolithiasis** *n* the presence of a stone or stones in the urinary bladder.

**cystometer** *n* an apparatus for measuring the pressure under various conditions in the urinary bladder.

**cystometrogram** *n* a record of the changes in pressure within the urinary bladder under various conditions; used in the study and diagnosis of voiding disorders.

**cystometry** *n* the study of pressure changes within the urinary bladder—**cystometric** *adj*.

**cystopexy** *n* surgical procedure to secure the urinary bladder in a specific position.

**cystoplasty** *n* surgical repair or augmentation of the urinary bladder.

**cystosarcoma phylloides** a malignant connective tissue tumour of the breast. It is characterized by rapid growth and recurrence if surgical removal is incomplete.

**cystoscope** *n* an endoscope used to visualize the inside of the urinary bladder—**cystoscopic** *adj*, **cystoscopically** *adv*.

**cystoscopy** *n* use of a cystoscope to view the internal surface of the urinary bladder. Also used in biopsies, photographing areas of interest and for some treatments.

**cystostomy** *n* (*syn* vesicostomy) an operation whereby a fistulous opening is made into the urinary bladder via the abdominal wall. Usually the fistula can be allowed to heal when it is no longer needed.

**cystotomy** *n* incision into the urinary bladder via the abdominal wall.

**cystourethritis** *n* inflammation of the urinary bladder and urethra.

**cystourethrogram** *n* radiographic examination of the urinary bladder and urethra. *micturating cystourethrogram* a dynamic X-ray performed during micturition, often to assess the degree of ureteric reflux—**cystourethrographic** *adj*, **cystourethrograph** *n*, **cystourethrographically** *adv*. ⇒ vesicoureteric reflux.

**cystourethropexy** *n* operation used for some types of urinary incontinence. The bladder and upper urethra are fixed in a forward position. ⇒ Marshall–Marchetti–Krantz operation.

**cytochemistry** *n* the study of the biochemical compounds within living cells and their action and function in cellular processes.

**cytochromes** *npl* a series of haem proteins containing iron or copper. They have a similar structure to haemoglobin and are involved in mitochondrial oxidation-reduction reactions (electron transport chain) that produce adenosine triphosphate. *cytochrome* $P_{450}$ a family of liver enzymes important in the oxidation and clearance of a variety of compounds, including cholesterol and lipid-soluble drugs. The drugs are made more water-soluble, thereby allowing them to be safely excreted by the kidney. $\Rightarrow P_{450}$ enzymes.

**cytodiagnosis** *n* diagnosis by the microscopic study of cells—**cytodiagnostic** *adj*.

**cytogenetics** *n* the scientific study of cells; particularly of chromosomes, genes and their behaviour. Chromosomes can be studied by culture techniques, using either tissue such as skin or lymphocytes, or fetal cells obtained by chorionic villus sampling or amniocentesis—**cytogenesis** *n*.

**cytokines** *npl* large group of proteins which act either on the cytokine-producing cell, or on other cells, via cell surface receptors. The term is usually applied to proteins which act on immune cells (T cells, B cells, monocytes, etc.). Cytokines have many diverse effects on many different cell types. Examples include interleukins (e.g. IL-1, IL-2), tumour necrosis factor, interferon-alpha and interferon-gamma.

**cytokinesis** *n* the division of the cell cytoplasm into two daughter cells following nuclear division. $\Rightarrow$ meiosis, mitosis.

**cytology** *n* the microscopic study of cells. The term *exfoliative cytology* is used when the cells studied have been shed, or sampled, from the surface of an organ or lesion—**cytological** *adj*.

**cytolysis** *n* the degeneration, destruction, disintegration or dissolution of cells—**cytolytic** *adj*.

**cytomegalovirus (CMV)** *n* a herpesvirus. Can cause latent and asymptomatic infection. The virus is excreted in urine and saliva. It can be passed to the fetus in utero and may cause miscarriage, stillbirth or serious neonatal disease, characterized by hepatosplenomegaly, purpura, encephalitis and microcephaly with learning disability, or death. In adults it causes an illness similar to infectious mononucleosis (glandular fever) and pneumonia. The virus is a serious threat to immunocompromised individuals.

**cytometer** *n* a device for counting and measuring cells, such as blood cells.

**cytoplasm** *n* (*syn* protoplasm) the complex chemical compound constituting the main part of the living substance of the cell, other than the contents of the nucleus—**cytoplasmic** *adj*.

**cytoplasmic inheritance** inheritance of diseases or traits through the genetic material present in mitochondria rather than that on the chromosomes.

**cytoscreening** *n* the process of carefully evaluating cells on a cytological preparation for the detection of malignancy.

**cytosine** *n* a nitrogenous base derived from pyrimidines. With other bases, one or more phosphate groups and a sugar, it is part of the nucleic acids DNA and RNA. $\Rightarrow$ deoxyribonucleic acid, ribonucleic acid.

**cytospin** *n* process of centrifuging fluid in order to separate the cells for cytological evaluation.

**cytostasis** *n* arrest or hindrance of cell development—**cytostatic** *adj*.

**cytotoxic** *n, adj* any substance which kills cells.

**cytotoxic drugs** drugs used mainly for the treatment of malignant diseases, but sometimes for other conditions, e.g. methotrexate may be used for severe psoriasis. They work in different ways, but they all eventually cause cancer cell death by either disrupting DNA or causing apoptosis. Some are cell cycle phase specific (CCPS) whereas others work at any point in the cell cycle and are termed cell cycle phase non-specific (CCPNS). They also harm some normal cells and some have longer-term side-effects. $\Rightarrow$ chemotherapy. There are five groups: (a) alkylating agents that disrupt DNA, e.g. busulfan, cyclophosphamide; (b) antimetabolites that disrupt DNA by blocking enzymes required for its synthesis, e.g. 5-fluorouracil, methotrexate; (c) antitumour antibiotics that disrupt DNA and the cell membrane, e.g. bleomycin; (d) vinca alkaloids and etoposide disrupt microtubules during cell division, e.g. vincristine; and (e) miscellaneous group of antineoplastic drugs that work in a variety of ways, including crisantaspase; platinum-containing drugs such as carboplatin; taxanes, e.g. paclitaxel; topoisomerase I inhibitors, e.g. irinotecan hydrochloride and trastuzumab, etc. $\Rightarrow$ Appendix 5.

**cytotoxic T cell** T lymphocytes that destroy certain cells, such as virus-infected cells. $\Rightarrow$ CD8 cells, suppressor T cells.

**cytotoxins** *npl* antibodies which are toxic to cells.

125

**D**

**dacr(y)oadenitis** *n* inflammation of a lacrimal gland. May occur in mumps.

**dacryocystectomy** *n* excision of any part of the lacrimal sac.

**dacryocystitis** *n* infective inflammation of the lacrimal sac.

**dacryocystography** *n* rarely used radiographic examination of the tear drainage apparatus after it has been rendered radiopaque. Superseded by computed tomography and magnetic resonance imaging.

**dacryocystorhinostomy (DCR)** *n* an operation to establish drainage from the lacrimal sac into the nose when there is obstruction of the nasolacrimal duct.

**dacryolith** *n* a concretion in the lacrimal passages.

**dactyl** *n* a digit, finger or toe—**dactylar, dactylate** *adj*.

**dactylitis** *n* inflammation of finger or toe. The digit becomes swollen due to periostitis. Associated with congenital syphilis, tuberculosis, sarcoid.

**dactylology** *n* finger spelling. Used in conjunction with British sign language to communicate with hearing impaired people. ⇒ British sign language, Makaton.

**DADL** *abbr* domestic activities of daily living.

**D and C** *abbr* dilatation and curettage.

**D and E** *abbr* dilatation and evacuation.

**dalton** *n* (J Dalton, British chemist/mathematician, 1766–1844) unit (kilodaltons) used to express the molecular weight of important biological molecules, such as nucleic acids and proteins. Also used as a unit for atomic mass. ⇒ atomic mass unit.

**daltonism** *n* a form of inherited red–green colour blindness. ⇒ deuteranopia, protanopia.

**Dalton's law of partial pressures** a gas law that states that the pressure of a mixture of gases is the sum of the partial pressures that each gas would exert if it alone completely filled the space.

**dandruff** *n* (*syn* scurf) the common scaly condition of the scalp. May be the forerunner of skin diseases of the seborrhoeic type, such as seborrhoeic dermatitis, or psoriasis.

**dandy fever** dengue.

**Dandy–Walker syndrome** (W Dandy, American neurosurgeon, 1886–1946; A Walker, Canadian/American surgeon, 1907–1995) a congenital brain malformation of the cerebellum and the fourth ventricle leading to hydrocephalus.

**Dane particle** the complete hepatitis B virus particle.

**Darier's disease** (*syn* keratosis follicularis) (F-J Darier, French dermatologist, 1852–1938) an autosomal dominant condition characterized by greasy scaled papules on the flexures, trunk and face.

**dark adaptation** adjustments made by the eye in reduced light or darkness. The pupils dilate, cone function ceases, rhodopsin is formed and the rod activity increases. ⇒ light adaptation.

**DAS** *abbr* disease activity score.

**data** *npl* items of information, usually collected for a specific purpose—**datum** *sing*. *data analysis* describes statistical analyses on data. *data processing* storage, sorting and analysis of data, usually electronically with specific computer software. *data set* the data relating to a specific group such as a particular age group.

**data protection** rules relating to information held about individuals, such as in Data Protection Act 1998. ⇒ Caldicott guardian.

**dawn phenomenon** experienced by some people with type 1 diabetes. There is an increase in blood glucose during the early hours of the morning caused by increased secretion of growth hormone and cortisol during the night.

**day-case surgery** ⇒ ambulatory surgery.

**day hospital** a centre which people attend on a daily basis or for some days in the week. Recreational and occupational therapy and physiotherapy are often provided. Greatest use is in the services for older people and those with learning disability or mental health problems. The day hospital provides vital respite for family, neighbours and other carers.

**DC** *abbr* direct current.

**DCIS** *abbr* ductal carcinoma in situ.

**DCR** *abbr* dacryocystorhinostomy.

**DDH** *abbr* developmental dysplasia of the hip.

**deafness** *n* a partial or complete loss of hearing. *conductive deafness* is due to interruption of the conduction of sound waves from the atmosphere to the inner ear. *congenital deafness* present at birth, e.g. caused by maternal rubella in early pregnancy. *sensorineural (perceptive)* or *nerve deafness* is due to a lesion in the inner ear, the auditory nerve or the auditory centres in the brain. ⇒ hearing impairment.

**deamination** *n* removal of an amino group (NH$_2$) from organic compounds such as excess amino acids.

**death** *n* irreversible cessation of vital functions usually assessed by the absence of heart beat and breathing. Mechanical ventilation may maintain vital functions despite the fact that the brainstem is fatally and irreversibly damaged. Consequently stringent tests are necessary to diagnose death in such cases. Death may be expected and occurs when the failure of one or more organs and/or systems fails to maintain homeostasis. This may be due, for example, to cancer, chronic heart failure or chronic respiratory diseases. Sudden death occurs when the flow of blood to the brain ceases. This might be due to serious haemorrhage such as following a road traffic accident or other trauma, severe acute illness, cerebrovascular accident, myocardial infarction, cardiac arrest, or suicide. ⇒ brainstem death, coroner.

**death certificate** official document, issued by the registrar of deaths to relatives or other authorized person, that allows for the disposal of the body. It is issued after a notification of probable cause of death is completed by the doctor in attendance upon the deceased or the appropriate documentation from the coroner.

**debility** *n* a condition of weakness with lack of muscle tone.

**debonding** *n* the removal of bonding resin and brackets previously bonded to the teeth during orthodontic treatment. The surface of the teeth is restored to its pretreatment condition.

**débridement** *n* the removal of foreign matter and contaminated or devitalized tissue from or adjacent to a wound. Required before wound healing can progress. *biological débridement* using larval (maggot) therapy for wound débridement. ⇒ larval therapy. *chemical/medical débridement* is accomplished by the external application of enzymes, e.g. streptokinase. *moist wound environment débridement* through using certain dressings, e.g. hydrocolloids, which augment natural débridement processes. *sharp débridement* using scalpel and scissors. *surgical débridement* is accomplished in theatre.

**debulking** *n* removal of a significant proportion of a pathological mass, as in the reduction of tumour bulk prior to chemotherapy or radiotherapy.

**decalcification** *n* the removal of mineral salts, as from teeth in dental caries, bone in disorders of calcium metabolism.

**decannulation** *n* the removal of a cannula such as an intravenous cannula.

**decapsulation** *n* the surgical removal of a capsule.

**decay** *n* a psychological term that describes the loss of information from the memory that occurs spontaneously over time.

**decerebrate** *adj* without cerebral function; a state of deep unconsciousness. *decerebrate posture/rigidity* a condition of the usually unconscious patient in which all four limbs are spastic and extended and which indicates severe damage to the cerebrum. The jaw is clenched and the neck retracted. There is hypertonus of the extensor muscles in both upper and lower limbs following severe decerebrating brain injury. ⇒ Glasgow Coma Scale, opisthotonos.

**decibel (dB)** *n* a unit of sound intensity (loudness).

**decidua** *n* the endometrial lining of the uterus thickened and altered for the potential reception of the fertilized ovum. It is shed at the end of pregnancy. *decidua basalis* that part which lies under the embedded ovum and forms the maternal part of the placenta. *decidua capsularis* that part that lies over the developing ovum. *decidua vera* the decidua lining the rest of the uterus—**decidual** *adj*.

**deciduous** *adj* by convention refers to the 20 teeth of the primary dentition.

**decompensation** *n* a failure of compensation, usually referring to heart failure.

**decompression** *n* removal of pressure or a compressing force. *decompression of brain* achieved by trephining the skull in order to evacuate clot. *decompression of bladder* in cases of chronic urinary retention, by continuous or intermittent drainage via catheter inserted per urethra.

**decompression sickness/illness** results from sudden reduction in atmospheric pressure, as experienced by divers on return to surface and aircrew ascending to great heights. Caused by bubbles of nitrogen which are released from solution in the blood; symptoms vary according to the site of these. The condition is largely preventable by proper and gradual decompression technique. Variously described as 'bends, chokes and creeps' depending on the symptomatology. Originally called caisson disease when identified as a hazard for divers. Later recognized as a complication of high altitude.

**deconditioning** *n* eliminating an unwanted particular response to a particular stimulus ⇒ aversion therapy, conditioning.

**decongestants** *npl* agents which decrease congestion, usually referring to nasal congestion, e.g. ephedrine hydrochloride locally. Administered orally, or locally as drops or sprays. ⇒ Appendix 5.

**decongestion** *n* relief of congestion—**decongestive** *adj*.

**decorticate posture/rigidity** a condition of the unconscious patient in which there is marked extension of the lower limbs and body, and flexion of the upper limbs (wrists and elbows). It results from a severe brain injury. ⇒ Glasgow Coma Scale.

**decortication** *n* surgical removal of cortex or outer covering of an organ such as the lung or kidney.

**decubitus** *n* the recumbent position; lying down. *decubitus ulcer* ⇒ pressure ulcer—**decubiti** *pl*, **decubital** *adj*.

**decussation** *n* intersection; a crossing of nerve fibres at a point beyond their origin, as in the optic and pyramidal tracts.

**deep-vein thrombosis (DVT)** thrombus forming in a deep vein such as those in the legs or pelvis. It is associated with the slowing of blood flow, abnormal or inappropriate coagulation processes, or damage to veins (known collectively as Virchow's triad). A thrombus may break off to form an embolus that travels in the venous circulation, through the heart to the lungs. Factors increasing the risk of DVT include obesity, >40 years of age, smoking, previous DVT, and pregnancy and during the puerperium. ⇒ pulmonary embolus, thromboembolic deterrents.

**DEF index** *abbr* decayed, extracted, filled index applied to the primary dentition (deciduous) in order to classify the overall condition. Missing teeth are not included in this index because they may have come out naturally. ⇒ DMF index.

**defecation** *n* voiding of faeces from the colon, through the rectum and anal canal—**defecate** *vi*.

**defence mechanisms 1.** the general protective measures by which the body is defended against a huge range of potentially harmful agents, e.g. viruses, bacteria, cancer cells, foreign cells. The measures are divided into two broad groups: (a) non-specific (innate), e.g. intact skin and mucous membranes, natural antimicrobial substances, inflammatory response and phagocytosis; (b) specific (adaptive) measures which are known as immunity, i.e. humoral immunity (antibody-mediated) or cell-mediated immunity. **2.** the unconscious processes by which the ego can prevent disturbing or unpleasant emotions from troubling the conscious mind. They all involve some degree of self-deception, distort the real situation and can only provide a temporary relief from the problem. They include compensation, conversion, denial, displacement, identification, intellectualization, projection, rationalization, reaction formation, regression, repression, sublimation, suppression, withdrawal.

**deferent duct** (*syn* vas deferens) the excretory duct of the testis. Continuous with the epididymis, it carries spermatozoa to the ejaculatory ducts. ⇒ Appendix 1, Figure 16.

**defervescence** *n* the time during which a fever is declining. If the body temperature falls rapidly it is spoken of as crisis; if it falls slowly the term 'lysis' is used.

**defibrillation** *n* the application of a direct current (DC) electric shock to correct ventricular fibrillation of the heart and restore normal cardiac rhythm (Figure D.1)—**defibrillate** *vt*.

**defibrillator** *n* equipment for the application of direct current (DC) electric shock to the heart. ⇒ automatic implantable cardioverter defibrillator, automated external defibrillator, implantable defibrillator.

**defibrinated** *adj* rendered free from fibrin. A necessary process in the preparation of serum from whole blood. ⇒ blood—**defibrinate** *v*.

**deficiency disease** disease resulting from deficiency of any essential nutrient. Can be caused by a diet that is deficient in a particular nutrient, e.g. iron, or because the nutrient present in the diet cannot be absorbed and metabolized by that individual.

**degeneration** *n* deterioration in quality or function. Regression from more specialized to less specialized type of tissue—**degenerative** *adj*, **degenerate** *vi*.

**deglutition** *n* swallowing, a complex process that is partly voluntary, partly involuntary.

**dehiscence** *n* the process of splitting or bursting open, as of a wound. Usually associated with wound infection.

**dehydration** *n* loss or removal of fluid. In the body this condition arises when the fluid intake fails to replace fluid loss. This is liable to occur when there is bleeding, diarrhoea, excessive exudation from a raw area as in burns, excessive sweating, polyuria, vomiting or inadequate fluid intake for any number of reasons. It is accompanied by disruption to the electrolyte balance. If suitable fluid replacement cannot be achieved orally, then

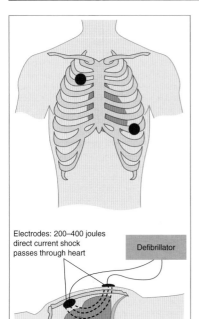

Electrodes: 200–400 joules
direct current shock
passes through heart

Defibrillator

**Figure D.1** Defibrillation *(reproduced from Hinchliff et al. 1996 with permission).*

other routes must be used. These include subcutaneous infusion (hypodermoclysis), rectal infusion (proctoclysis) or by the intravenous route—**dehydrate** *vt, vi.*

**7-dehydrocholesterol** *n* a sterol found in the skin. It is converted to a form of vitamin D by the action of ultraviolet radiation from exposure to sunlight.

**dehydroepiandrosterone (DHEA)** *n* a steroid hormone produced by the adrenal glands, the ovaries/testes, the brain and fatty tissue; the precursor of all the sex hormones, e.g. oestrogens, testosterone. The secretion of dehydroepiandrosterone varies across the lifespan. Secretion is high before birth, low during infancy and early childhood until it increases again from 6 to 8 years of age to peak in the mid-20s. Thereafter it declines until it reaches very low levels in older people. ⇒ adrenarche.

**déjà vu phenomenon** occurs in epilepsy involving temporal lobes of the brain and in certain epileptic dream states. An intense feeling of familiarity, as if everything had happened before.

**delayed-onset muscle soreness (DOMS)** appears 24–48 hours after exercise; may be caused by severe, unaccustomed exercise, particularly that involving eccentric muscle contractions.

**delayed hypersensitivity T cell** a T lymphocyte involved with macrophages and other T cells in cell-mediated delayed hypersensitivity and chronic inflammation. ⇒ CD4 cells.

**delayed union** longer than expected healing of a fracture.

**deletion** *n* in genetics, a mutation involving the loss of part of a chromosome or a sequence of genetic material. An example of a condition caused by chromosome deletion is cri du chat syndrome, which results from a deletion affecting chromosome number 5.

**Delhi boil** ⇒ oriental sore.

**deliberate self-harm (DSH)** wilful non-fatal act(s) carried out in the knowledge that it was potentially harmful. Examples include self-poisoning (overdose), self-cutting and self-mutilation.

**deliquescent** *adj* capable of absorption, thus becoming fluid.

**delirium** *n* abnormal mental condition based on hallucinations or illusion. May occur in high fever, in mental health problems, or be toxic in origin.

**delirium tremens (DTs)** acute psychosis, usually associated with the withdrawal of alcohol after a period of excessive intake over a considerable time. It is characterized by terror, hallucinations, confusion, disorientation and tremor—**delirious** *adj.*

**dellen** *npl* small areas of reduced thickness in the cornea.

**Delphi technique** a research method where a consensus of expert opinion is obtained during a multiple-step process where the contributors are asked to rate a number of items, e.g. research priorities, in order of importance.

**deltoid** *adj* triangular. *deltoid muscle* a thick muscle acting at the shoulder. Its origin is on the clavicle, the acromion and the spine of the scapula, and it inserts on to the humerus. It is the prime mover of arm abduction when the main part of the muscle contracts. The anterior fibres cause flexion and the posterior fibres extend and cause lateral rotation of the shoulder. ⇒ Appendix 1, Figures 4 and 5.

**delusion** *n* a fixed, usually false belief, inconsistent with an individual's culture and intelligence, which cannot be altered by argument or reasoning. A type of psychotic symptom.

**demarcation** *n* an outlining of the junction of diseased and healthy tissue, often used when referring to gangrene.

**dementia** *n* (*syn* organic brain syndrome—OBS) an irreversible organic brain disease causing progressive disturbance of memory and disintegration of personality, deterioration in personal care, impaired cognitive ability and disorientation. *presenile dementia* occurring in people between 50 and 60 years of age. ⇒ Alzheimer's disease, Creutzfeldt–Jakob disease, multi-infarct dementia, Pick's disease.

**demographic indices** such as age distribution, birth and mortality rates, occupation and geographical distribution. They are used to obtain a profile of a given population, compare different areas and plan services to meet specific needs. For example, an area with a large population of retired people will, along with other priorities, need to plan and provide services for degenerative conditions more common in an ageing population, and specific health-promoting activities such as falls prevention.

**demography** *n* the study of population, such as gender and age distribution—**demographic** *adj*.

**demulcent** *n* a slippery, mucilaginous fluid that alleviates irritation and inflammation, especially of mucous membranes.

**demyelination** *n* destruction of the myelin sheaths surrounding nerve fibres. Can occur in the peripheral nerves (e.g. Guillain–Barré syndrome) or in the central nervous system (e.g. multiple sclerosis).

**denaturation** *n* a change in the basic structure or nature of a substance. As in proteins exposed to acids, alcohols, radiation or heat, such as the change in egg albumen (white of the egg) during cooking.

**dendrite** *n* (*syn* dendron) one of the branched filaments which are given off from the body of a nerve cell. That part of a neuron which transmits an impulse to the nerve cell—**dendritic** *adj*.

**dendritic cell** an antigen-presenting cell that presents a processed antigen to B and T lymphocytes bearing antigen-specific receptors. They are thought to be the cells important in determining the type of immune response generated against an antigen. ⇒ antigen-presenting cell.

**dendritic ulcer** a linear corneal ulcer that sends out tree-like branches. Usually caused by herpes simplex virus.

**dendron** *n* ⇒ dendrite.

**denervation** *n* the means by which a nerve supply is cut off. Usually refers to incision, excision or blocking of a nerve.

**dengue** *n* (*syn* 'break-bone fever') a mosquito-transmitted viral haemorrhagic fever occurring in tropical regions. The severity varies but may cause fever, headache, limb pains, vomiting and a rash. Mortality is high in cases where disseminated intravascular coagulation and acute circulatory collapse occur.

**denial** *n* a complex unconscious defence mechanism in which difficult situations, or unacceptable or distressing facts, are not acknowledged, so as to avoid distress, anxiety and emotional conflict. It may occur in response to drastically changed circumstances, e.g. sudden incapacitating illness, or terminal illness.

**Dennis Browne splints** (D Browne, Australian surgeon, 20th century) splints used to correct congenital talipes equinovarus (club foot).

**dens** *n* a tooth or tooth-like structure. Also the odontoid process of the second cervical vertebra (axis).

**dens in dente** an anomaly of teeth characterized by invagination of the enamel. This gives a radiographic appearance suggestive of a 'tooth within a tooth'.

**dental** *adj* relating to teeth.

**dental amalgam** a compound of a basal alloy of silver and tin with mercury, used for restoring teeth. ⇒ amalgam.

**dental arch** describes the curved structure comprising the teeth and the alveolar ridge in each jaw.

**dental attrition** non-carious, mechanical wearing of teeth, either through normal mastication or as a result of parafunctional habits, e.g. bruxism.

**dental calculus** or tartar. A deposit of calcified dental plaque, containing calcium carbonate and phosphate, which forms on the surface of the teeth. Its presence is associated with periodontal disease and gum recession, which may lead to the loss of teeth.

**dental caries** a microbial disease of the calcified tissues of the teeth, characterized by demineralization of the inorganic portion and destruction of their organic substance.

**dental cement** substances used in dentistry to effect temporary restorations prior to longer-term solutions.

**dental dam** device placed in the mouth during dental treatment to prevent the passage of saliva or water. Used to keep a tooth or teeth dry during treatment.

**dental enamel** hard, acellular calcified tissue covering the crown of a tooth. ⇒ tooth.

**dental erosion** non-carious wearing away of the surfaces of the teeth due to chemical causes.

**dental floss/tape** waxed or unwaxed thread or tape used for removing plaque from interproximal surfaces and contact areas of the teeth. Regular use promotes oral hygiene and reduces the risk of dental caries and periodontal disease.

**dental hygienist** dental auxiliary trained to scale and clean teeth, carry out certain preventive procedures and give oral hygiene instruction to the prescription of a dentist.

**dental implant** a device inserted in the jawbone to provide an abutment to support a crown, denture or a bridge.

**dental pantomography** *n* panoramic radiography that gives a view of all the teeth in both jaws on a single radiograph.

**dental plaque** soft deposit of bacteria and cellular debris that rapidly forms on the surface of a tooth in the absence of effective oral hygiene.

**dental pulp** tissue consisting of blood vessels, nerves and connective tissue that occupies the core of the crown and the root canal(s) of a tooth.

**dental restoration** the process of replacing part or all of a tooth by artificial means; also the term given to the type of replacement used, e.g. filling, crown, bridge.

**dental scaling** the removal of calculus, using special instruments, from the surfaces of the teeth.

**dental therapist** dental auxiliary who is trained to carry out certain dental operative procedures to the prescription of a dentist.

**dentate** *adj* having natural teeth present.

**denticle** *n* calcified material found in the pulp chamber of a tooth.

**dentine** *n* calcified organic hard tissue forming the bulk of the crown and roots of teeth. ⇒ tooth.

**dentinogenesis** *n* dentogenesis. The production of dentine by the odontoblasts during tooth development. *dentinogenesis imperfecta* **1.** localized mesodermal dysplasia that disrupts dentine formation. It may be inherited. **2.** an inherited disorder where the dentine is defective but the enamel is normal. **3.** a genetic disorder of dentine, in which there is early calcification of the root canals and pulp chambers, excessive wear and a characteristic hue to the teeth.

**dentist** *n* any person who practises dentistry, and is qualified and licensed to do so.

**dentistry** *n* profession concerned with the diagnosis, prevention and treatment of diseases of the teeth and their supporting tissues, including their restoration and replacement. *conservative dentistry* the diagnosis, treatment and restoration of diseased or injured teeth. *cosmetic dentistry* the restoration or enhancement of dental aesthetics. *forensic dentistry* the examination, interpretation and presentation of dentally related evidence in a legal context. *paediatric dentistry* the diagnosis, prevention and treatment of dental and related diseases in children. *preventive dentistry* the prevention of, and preventive treatment for, dental disease and the promotion of good oral health. *prosthetic dentistry* the restoration of the function and aesthetics of missing teeth using artificial dentures.

**dentition** *n* the natural teeth collectively in an individual.

**dentoalveolar abscess** a 'gumboil'. Localized collection of pus within the alveolar bone, of dental origin.

**dentofacial deformity** any malformation involving the dentofacial complex—the mouth and jaw. Examples include cleft lip and palate, malocclusion and other skeletal anomalies.

**dentogenesis** *n* ⇒ dentinogenesis.

**dentulous** *adj* having natural teeth.

**denture** *n* a removable dental prosthesis. May be partial or full (replacing some, or all, of the teeth in either jaw respectively).

**Denver II** previously known as the Denver Developmental Screening Test (DDST). A tool for assessing infants'/children's developmental progress by comparing their behaviours with those shown by the majority of their age group. Comparative grids are used to assess milestones, which are arranged in four categories: personal and social; fine motor—adaptive; language; and gross motor.

**deodorant** *n, adj* a substance which destroys or masks an (unpleasant) odour. Deodorants are used for personal hygiene and within the environment. Topical antibiotics and charcoal dressings can be used to deodorize malodorous infected wounds—**deodorize** *vt*.

**deontological** *adj* ethical theory based on the science of deontology that supports the view that there is a duty to act within certain

131

universal rules of morality. A theory associated with the work of Immanuel Kant. ⇒ utilitarianism.

**deoxygenation** *n* the removal of oxygen—**deoxygenated** *adj*.

**deoxycholic acid** a bile acid produced by the liver. It emulsifies fats in the small intestine and aids their absorption. Ursodeoxycholic acid is rarely used to dissolve gallstones.

**deoxyribonucleases (DNase)** enzymes that cleave deoxyribonucleic acid linkages at particular points on the strand. *recombinant human deoxyribonuclease* (rhDNase) a genetically engineered form of the natural enzyme called dornase alfa. It is administered, by jet nebulizer, to improve lung function in some people with cystic fibrosis.

**deoxyribonucleic acid (DNA)** a double-strand nucleic acid molecule found in the chromosomes of all organisms (except some viruses). DNA (as genes) carries the coded instructions for passing on hereditary characteristics. DNA is a polymer formed from many nucleotides. These consist of the sugar deoxyribose, phosphate groups and four nitrogenous bases: adenine (A), guanine (G), thymine (T) and cytosine (C). Adenine and guanine are purine bases, and thymine and cytosine are pyrimidine bases. The nucleotide units are bound together to form a double helix with the adenine of one strand opposite the thymine of the other and the same for guanine and cytosine.

**dependency** *n* the state of needing help from others to meet physical and/or emotional needs.

**dependency culture** a sociological term that describes the opinion that unlimited state welfare provision may reduce individuals' ability to be assertive and support themselves.

**depersonalization** *n* a subjective feeling that one no longer feels that one is real or exists. Occurs in a wide range of disorders, including depressive states, anxiety disorder, with psychoactive substance misuse, etc.

**depilate** *vt* to remove hair from—**depilatory** *adj*, *n*, **depilation** *n*.

**depilatories** *npl* substances usually made in pastes (e.g. barium sulphide) which remove excess hair only temporarily; they do not act on the papillae, consequently the hair grows again. ⇒ epilation—**depilatory** *sing*. *Preoperative depilation* lessens the risk of wound infection because it is non-abrasive, unlike shaving the skin.

**depolarization** *n* in excitable cells the inside of the membrane becomes electrically positive with respect to the outside. Occurs during the transmission of a nerve impulse. ⇒ polarized.

**depot** *n* a body area where a drug is deposited or stored, and from where it can be released and distributed, such as hormone therapy. *depot injection* drugs, usually psychotropic, that are given by deep intramuscular injections. Used when clients are unable to take their drugs on a regular basis.

**depressed fracture** ⇒ fracture.

**depression** *n* **1.** a hollow place or indentation. **2.** a downward or inward movement or displacement. **3.** diminution of power or activity. **4.** a mental health disorder characterized by feelings of profound sadness. May be classified by severity (mild/moderate/severe), by the presence of somatic symptoms (anorexia, weight loss, impaired libido, sleep disturbance, etc.) and by the presence or absence of psychotic symptoms. Recognized cognitive symptoms include hopelessness, helplessness, guilt, low self-esteem and suicidal ideation. The previous description of reactive versus endogenous depression is outdated and not thought to be relevant to treatment or prognosis.

**deprivation indices** a set of census variables and weightings used to assess levels of deprivation within a specific community or population. They include: levels of unemployment, lone-parent households, pensioners living alone and households without a car. ⇒ Jarman index, Townsend index.

**De Quervain's thyroiditis** *n* (F De Quervain, Swiss surgeon, 1868–1940) an inflammatory condition of the thyroid gland. Often follows a viral infection of the upper respiratory tract. It is characterized by tenderness and swelling of the thyroid gland, pyrexia, neck pain and dysphagia.

**Derbyshire neck** goitre.

**derealization** *n* feelings that people, events or surroundings have changed and are unreal. These sensations may occur in normal people during dreams, in states of fatigue or after sensory deprivation. May sometimes occur in schizophrenia and depressive states. Also experienced with the use of hallucinogenic drugs.

**dereistic** *adj* of thinking, not adapted to reality. Describes autistic thinking.

**dermabrasion** *n* removal of superficial layers of the skin by abrasive methods.

**dermatitis** *n* inflammation of the skin (by custom limited to an eczematous reaction). ⇒ eczema. *atopic dermatitis* that variety of infantile eczema that may be associated with asthma or hayfever. *dermatitis herpetiformis* (*syn* hydroa) an intensely itchy skin eruption of unknown cause, most commonly characterized by papules and vesicles which remit and relapse. Associated with coeliac disease (gluten-induced enteropathy). *industrial dermatitis* a term used in the National Insurance (Industrial Injuries) Act to cover occupational skin conditions.

**dermatochalasia** *n* loose, superfluous eyelid skin which causes the eyelid to droop. A feature of normal ageing, it occurs in older people.

**dermatoglyphics** *n* study of the ridge patterns of the skin of the fingertips, palms and soles to identify certain chromosomal anomalies.

**dermatographia** *n* ⇒ dermographia.

**dermatologist** *n* medically qualified individual who studies skin diseases and is skilled in their treatment. A skin specialist.

**dermatology** *n* the science which deals with the skin, its structure, functions, diseases and their treatment—**dermatological** *adj*, **dermatologically** *adv*.

**dermatome** *n* **1.** an instrument for cutting slices of skin of varying thickness, usually for grafting. **2.** the area of skin supplied by a single spinal nerve (Figure D.2).

**dermatomycosis** *n* a superficial fungal infection of the skin—**dermatomycotic** *adj*.

**dermatomyositis** *n* an autoimmune connective tissue disease mainly affecting the skin and muscles. Presents with a characteristic skin rash and muscle weakness. Can be associated with an underlying malignancy in older people—a paraneoplastic syndrome. ⇒ collagen, connective tissue diseases.

**dermatophytes** *npl* a group of fungi (*Epidermophyton*, *Microsporum* or *Trichophyton*) that cause superficial infections of skin, hair and nails.

**dermatophytosis** *n* infection of the skin caused by one of the dermatophyte species—*Epidermophyton*, *Microsporum* or *Trichophyton*.

**dermatosis** *n* generic term for skin disease—**dermatoses** *pl*.

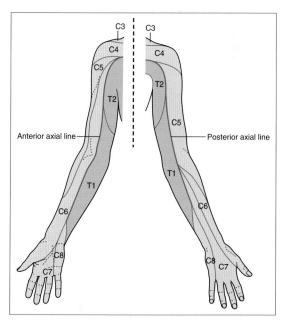

**Figure D.2** Dermatomes of the upper limb (C, cervical, T, thoracic) *(reproduced from Porter 2005 with permission).*

**dermis** *n* the true skin; the cutis vera; the layer below the epidermis ⇒ Appendix 1, Figure 12—**dermal** *adj*.

**dermographia** *n* (*syn* dermatographia, factitial urticaria) a condition in which weals occur on the skin after a blunt instrument or fingernail has been lightly drawn over it. Seen in vasomotor instability and urticaria—**dermographic** *adj*.

**dermoid** *adj* pertaining to or resembling skin. *dermoid cyst* a cyst which is congenital in origin and usually occurs in the ovary. It contains elements of hair, nails, skin, teeth, etc.

**Descemet's membrane** (J Descemet, French physician, 1732–1810) the deepest layer of the corneal stroma, it is in contact with the endothelium.

**descending colon** ⇒ Appendix 1, Figure 18B.

**descriptive statistics** that which describes or summarizes the observations of a sample. ⇒ inferential statistics.

**desensitization** *n* **1.** process of reducing subsequent immediate-type hypersensitivity reactions to venoms and other allergens by repeated injection of minute quantities of allergen in order to modulate the immune response away from the harmful allergic-type reaction to a less pathological response. **2.** a behavioural therapy used for phobias where people are helped to overcome their irrational fear. There is a gradual introduction to the object or situation through imagining the object, looking at pictures or by eventually confronting the real thing—**desensitize** *vt*.

**desiccation** *n* drying out. As in desiccation of the nucleus pulposus, thus diminishing the cushioning effect of a healthy intervertebral disc.

**designer foods** ⇒ functional foods.

**desloughing** *n* the process of removing slough from a wound. ⇒ débridement.

**desmoid tumour** a benign tumour of fibrous connective tissue. Occurs on the neck, arms, legs and within the abdomen.

**desmosines** *npl* compounds forming the cross-linkages between chains of elastin, the structural protein of connective tissue.

**desmosome** *n* also known as macula adherens. A complex junction that aids adhesion between cells. They are composed of proteins that span the gap between squamous epithelial cells such as those in the skin. Desmosomes are able to prevent structural damage from shearing forces.

**desquamation** *n* shedding; flaking off; casting off, as of the skin—**desquamate** *vi, vt*.

**detached retina** separation of the neurosensory retina from the pigment epithelium. May be caused by retinal tears or holes, fibrous traction on the retina, or by exudation of fluid under the neurosensory retina.

**detained patient** a person with a mental disorder who has been detained under the relevant legislation such as the Mental Health Act in England and Wales, or in Scotland the Mental Health (Care and Treatment) (Scotland) Act. ⇒ informal patient.

**detergent** *n, adj* (describes) a cleansing agent. ⇒ cetrimide.

**deterioration** *n* progressive impairment of function: worsening of the patient's condition.

**determinants of health** factors that may influence the health of an individual, or differences in health between individuals, apart from age, sex and constitution (physiological, genetic factors). These could be social and economic, environmental or psychological factors that increase the risk of ill health or disease (e.g. heart disease, cancers, diabetes). These determinants, or indicators, are associated with better or worse health of populations as measured by mortality (standardized mortality ratios), valid measures of morbidity or self-reported health status (e.g. health surveys, census, standardized illness ratios). For example, higher infant mortality may be associated with environmental factors, health care provision, social and community support, maternal deprivation and poverty. There may also be a cultural and behavioural perspective. ⇒ morbidity, mortality.

**detoxication** *n* the removal of the poisonous property of a substance—**detoxicant** *adj, n*, **detoxicate** *vt*.

**detritus** *n* matter produced by detrition; waste matter from disintegration.

**detrusor** *n* an expelling muscle such as that of the urinary bladder. *detrusor instability* failure to inhibit reflex detrusor contraction. ⇒ incontinence.

**detumescence** *n* subsidence of a swelling.

**deuteranopia** *n* a rare form of colour blindness, in which the affected male lacks medium-wavelength cones in the retina and is unable to distinguish between greens, yellows and reds. ⇒ daltonism, protanopia.

**developmental dysplasia of the hip (DDH)** also known as congenital dislocation of the hip. The term DDH is useful in describing the varying causes and severity of the condition. There is poor development of the acetabulum which allows the head of the femur to dislocate. ⇒ Barlow's sign/test, Ortolani's sign/test.

**developmental milestones** the skills or competencies usually attained by the infant or child by a given age, e.g. walking by 18 months. The skills are usually grouped in categories—fine motor, gross motor, personal and social and language. ⇒ Denver II.

**deviance** *n* a variation from normal. A sociological term that describes a change from the accepted social norm.

**deviation** *n* abnormal position of the eyes, for example, both eyes deviated to right or left when the person is facing to the front. May be a feature of some neurological disorders. ⇒ sexual deviation.

**DEXA** *abbr* dual-energy X-ray absorptiometry.

**dexamethasone suppression tests** tests using different doses and duration of dexamethasone treatment to identify patients producing excess glucocorticoid, Cushing's syndrome and the source.

**dextran** *n* a colloid solution obtained by the action of a specific bacterium on sugar solutions. Previously used for replacing fluids in hypovolaemia. It is no longer routinely used as a colloid. Dextran may cause allergic reactions. It also affects clotting and interferes with blood cross-matching. ⇒ colloid solutions.

**dextrin** *n* a soluble polysaccharide resulting from the hydrolysis of starch.

**dextrocardia** *n* transposition of the heart to the right side of the thorax—**dextrocardial** *adj*.

**dextrose** *n* (*syn* glucose) a soluble carbohydrate (monosaccharide) widely used in intravenous infusion solutions. Also given orally as a readily absorbed sugar in rehydration fluids for fluid and electrolyte replacement, and for hypoglycaemia.

**DHA** *abbr* docosahexaenoic acid.

**DHEA** *abbr* dehydroepiandrosterone.

**dhobie itch** tinea cruris.

**diabetes** *n* a disease characterized by polyuria, with consequent polydipsia; used without qualification implies diabetes mellitus—**diabetic** *adj, n*.

**diabetes insipidus** diabetes caused by disordered water homeostasis. It may be *cranial* due to deficiency of antidiuretic hormone (ADH), either idiopathic or due to trauma, tumour or inflammation affecting posterior pituitary lobe function, or *nephrogenic* due to renal tubular resistance to the action of ADH.

**diabetes mellitus** diabetes due to glycosuria and osmotic diuresis resulting from hyperglycaemia; defined as fasting plasma glucose ≥ 7.0 mmol/L, or a glucose level 2 hours following 75 g glucose load (oral glucose tolerance test) ≥ 11.1 mmol/L. Diabetes mellitus is classified as: *type 1*, due to autoimmune destruction of insulin-producing cells in the pancreatic islets: uncontrolled, it leads to ketoacidosis; *type 2*, due to varying degrees of insulin resistance, often due to obesity, and impaired insulin secretion: if uncontrolled, it leads to hyperglycaemic hyperosmolar non-ketotic coma (HHNK)/hyperosmolar non-ketotic coma (HONK); may also be *secondary* to other diseases, e.g. pancreatitis, Cushing's syndrome, haemochromatosis; or *genetic* e.g. maturity-onset diabetes of the young (MODY), mitochondrial diabetes; or *gestational diabetes* ⇒ gestational diabetes.

**diabetic amyotrophy** a complication of poorly controlled diabetes. A mononeuropathy affecting the lower limb caused by pathology affecting the tiny blood vessels that supply the femoral nerve and the lumbar plexus. It typically occurs in one leg and causes tenderness, weakness and wasting of the anterior thigh muscles (quadriceps femoris) and absence of the knee-jerk reflex. Slow recovery and improvement can occur if diabetic control improves.

**diabetic 'honeymoon' period** a phenomenon occurring, in some people, soon after the diagnosis of type 1 diabetes. It occurs because there are often a few beta cells remaining in the pancreas and these can recover sufficiently after insulin therapy is started so that they produce insulin. Some people need less insulin and, more uncommonly, other people need no insulin for a variable time period. However long this period lasts, all those who have a 'honeymoon' period will require larger doses of insulin in the future.

**diabetic nephropathy** a long-term microvascular complication of diabetes characterized by glomerulosclerosis caused by damage to the glomerular capillaries. There is microalbuminuria, hypertension, and eventually loss of glomeruli and end-stage renal failure in some cases.

**diabetic neuropathy** a long-term microvascular complication of diabetes characterized by damage to nerves (motor, sensory and autonomic). It may present as a sensorimotor neuropathy in the lower limbs ('stocking' distribution); neuropathic foot ulcers; mononeuropathies, such as diabetic amyopathy: and nerve compression, e.g. carpal tunnel syndrome. The effects of autonomic nerve damage depend on the structures affected and can cause erectile dysfunction, sweating after eating, gastroparesis, diarrhoea, constipation, incomplete bladder emptying and postural hypotension.

**diabetic retinopathy** a long-term microvascular complication of diabetes characterized by retinal changes, which can lead to sight impairment or blindness. Early changes may cause no symptoms so annual examination is vital. In the early stages the retinal changes include haemorrhages (blots), microaneurysms (dots), hard exudates and small areas of retinal ischaemia (cotton-wool spots). Later there is worsening retinal ischaemia with neovascularization (growth of abnormal new retinal blood vessels) and fibrosis. This leads to vitreous haemorrhages and detachment of the retina. Damage close to the macula can result in the loss of central vision.

**diagnosis** *n* the art or act of distinguishing one disease from another. *differential diagnosis* is the term used when making a correct decision between diseases presenting a similar clinical picture—**diagnoses** *pl*, **diagnose** *vt*.

**diagnostic** *adj* **1.** pertaining to diagnosis. **2.** serving as evidence in diagnosis—**diagnostician** *n*.

***Diagnostic and Statistical Manual of Mental Disorders (DSM-IV)*** a manual that lists the official classification of mental disorders. It is published by the American Psychiatric Association. ⇒ *International Classification of Diseases* (ICD).

**dialysate** *n* exogenous fluid used in dialysis to promote diffusion and removal of waste products.

**dialyser** *n* (*syn* artificial kidney) used in haemodialysis; consists of blood and dialysate compartments separated by a semipermeable membrane.

**dialysis** *n* a renal replacement therapy. The process by which solutes are removed from solution by diffusion across a porous membrane; requires the presence of a favourable solute gradient. ⇒ haemodialysis, peritoneal dialysis—**dialyses** *pl*, **dialyse** *vt*.

**diapedesis** *n* the passage of cells from within blood vessels through the vessel walls into the tissues, such as during the inflammatory response—**diapedetic** *adj*.

**diaphoresis** *n* perspiration.

**diaphoretic** *adj, n* (*syn* sudorific) an agent which induces diaphoresis (sweating).

**diaphragm** *n* **1.** the dome-shaped muscular partition between the thoracic cavity above and the abdominal cavity below. **2.** any partitioning membrane or septum. **3.** a cap which encircles the cervix to act as a barrier contraceptive. Reliable when correctly fitted and used with a spermicidal chemical—**diaphragmatic** *adj*.

**diaphysis** *n* the shaft of a long bone—**diaphyses** *pl*, **diaphyseal** *adj*. ⇒ epiphysis.

**diarrhoea** *n* deviation from established bowel habit characterized by an increase in frequency and fluidity of the stools. May cause dehydration, hypokalaemia, acidosis (metabolic), malabsorption of nutrients and perianal soreness. Causes include infection, food sensitivity, laxative misuse, drugs such as antibiotics, dietary change or indiscretion, anxiety, colorectal cancer (alternating with constipation) and some systemic diseases. ⇒ spurious diarrhoea.

**diarthrosis** *n* a synovial, freely movable joint—**diarthroses** *pl*, **diarthrodial** *adj*.

**diastasis** *n* **1.** the forcible separation of bones without fracture. **2.** the separation of two muscles, for example, the rectus muscles. ⇒ diastasis recti abdominis.

**diastasis recti abdominis** separation of the two rectus muscles. It can occur following pregnancy, especially after multiple births or multiple pregnancies. In neonates it is caused by a developmental abnormality.

**diastasis symphysis pubis** ⇒ symphysis pubis dysfunction.

**diastema** *n* a naturally occurring but abnormally large space between two teeth.

**diastole** *n* the relaxation filling period of the cardiac cycle; usually refers to ventricular filling—**diastolic** *adj*. ⇒ systole.

**diastolic blood pressure** the lowest blood pressure measured between cardiac contractions, i.e. when the aortic and pulmonary valves are closed and the heart is relaxed. ⇒ systolic blood pressure.

**diathermy** *n* the passage of a high-frequency electric current through the tissues whereby heat is produced. When both electrodes are large, the heat is diffused over a wide area according to the electrical resistance of the tissues. In this form it is widely used in the treatment of inflammation, especially when deeply seated (e.g. sinusitis, pelvic cellulitis). When one electrode is very small the heat is concentrated in this area and becomes great enough to destroy tissue. In this form (surgical diathermy) it is used to stop bleeding at operation

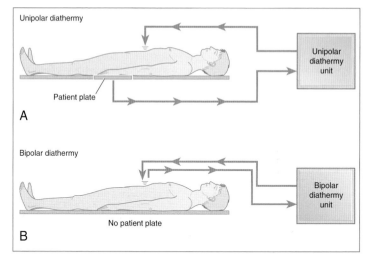

**Figure D.3** (A) Unipolar and (B) bipolar diathermy *(reproduced from Brooker & Nicol 2003 with permission).*

by coagulation of blood, or to cut through tissue (Figure D.3).

**dibenzodiazepines** *npl* a group of atypical antipsychotic drugs (neuroleptics), e.g. clozapine. ⇒ Appendix 5.

**DIC** *abbr* disseminated intravascular coagulation.

**dicephalous** *adj* two-headed.

**dichorionic twins** twins who have separate chorions.

**dichromatic vision** dichromatopsia. A defect of colour vision in which the person can only perceive two of the three primary colours.

**Dick test** (G F Dick, 1881–1967; G R Dick, 1881–1963; American physicians) a skin test used to determine whether an individual is sensitive to the toxin produced by the group A streptococci that cause scarlet fever.

**dicrotic** *adj, n* (pertaining to, or having) a double beat, as indicated by a second expansion of the artery during diastole. *dicrotic notch* the second rise in the arterial tracing caused by the closure of the aortic valve (that between the left ventricle and the aorta). ⇒ anacrotic.

**DIDMOAD syndrome** *abbr* diabetes insipidus, diabetes mellitus, optic atrophy and deafness. ⇒ Wolfram syndrome.

**diencephalon** *n* the part of the brain between the mesencephalon and telencephalon. It contains the third ventricle, thalamus, hypothalamus and epithalamus.

**diet** *n* **1.** the foods and drink normally consumed by a person. **2.** the nutrient intake prescribed or restricted (type and amount) for treatment or management of conditions. For example, a low salt intake for hypertension.

**dietary fibre** ⇒ non-starch polysaccharides.

**diet-induced thermogenesis** increase in heat production in the body after consuming food. It is caused by the metabolic energy used during digestion and the energy used in forming glycogen and fat, etc. It is around 10% of the energy intake but this depends on the type of foods eaten.

**dietary reference intakes (DRI)** used in the United States for dietary reference values.

**dietary reference values (DRVs)** in the UK a set of tables that estimate a range of nutritional requirements for different groups of the population (healthy individuals). Usually three values are given—estimated average requirement (EAR), lower reference nutrient intake (LRNI) and reference nutrient intake (RNI).

**dietary supplementation** a term in sports medicine used to describe the food supplements (above what is required to ensure the intake of nutrients for a balanced diet) taken as an ergogenic aid. For example, carbohydrate loading, creatine supplements and isotonic sports drinks.

**dietetic foods** foods specially prepared or modified to meet specific nutritional needs.

For example, for people who cannot digest or metabolize a food/nutrient, e.g. gluten-free foods, or those who need to have a controlled intake of certain foods/nutrients, e.g. low-fat foods.

**dietetics** *n* the interpretation and application of the scientific principles of nutrition to feeding in health and disease.

**dietitian** *n* one who applies the principles of nutrition to the feeding of an individual or a group of individuals. Dietitians are employed in a range of hospital and community settings, the food industry, by local authorities and by national and international agencies, e.g. World Health Organization.

**Dietl's crisis** (J Dietl, Polish physician, 1804–1878) sudden severe pain in the kidney, due to distension of the renal pelvis, or ureteric obstruction such as kinking of the ureter.

**Dieulafoy's lesion** (P Dieulafoy, French physician, 1839–1911) an abnormality of small blood vessels (arterioles) in the gastric mucosa, which usually occur in the area adjacent to the gastro-oesophageal junction but can occur elsewhere in the digestive tract. An uncommon cause of gastrointestinal bleeding. Treatment is usually by endoscopic coagulation techniques, sclerotherapy or banding.

**differential blood count** ⇒ blood count.

**differential diagnosis** ⇒ diagnosis.

**differentiation** *n* the process whereby cells and tissues expand the ability to perform specialized functions that distinguish them from other cell types. Cancer cells are graded by their degree of differentiation.

**diffusion** *n* **1.** the process whereby gases and liquids of different concentrations mix when brought into contact, until their concentration is equal throughout. ⇒ active transport, filtration, osmosis. **2.** dialysis.

**DiGeorge's syndrome** (A DiGeorge, American paediatrician, b. 1921) also known as thymic-parathyroid aplasia. An inherited condition characterized by immunodeficiency, hypocalcaemia and various physical abnormalities. These include the absence of the thymus and parathyroid glands, cardiovascular abnormalities, oesophageal atresia, abnormal facies with small mouth, low-set ears and hypertelorism. Death, caused by an infection, usually occurs during early childhood.

**digestion** *n* the process by which food is rendered absorbable—**digestible, digestive** *adj*, **digestibility** *n*, **digest** *vt*.

**digestibility** *n* the fraction of a foodstuff that is absorbed from the gastrointestinal tract to

enter the bloodstream. It is the difference between the food intake and faecal output, minus that part of faeces that is not derived from undigested food residues, such as microorganisms, intestinal cells and digestive juices.

**digestive system** comprises the structures of the gastrointestinal tract (alimentary tract) and the accessory organs. The mouth, oesophagus, stomach and small and large intestine and the salivary glands, the pancreas and the liver and biliary tract. The digestive system is concerned with ingestion, propulsion, digestion, absorption and elimination. ⇒ Appendix 1, Figure 18B.

**digit** *n* a finger or toe—**digital** *adj*.

**digital compression** pressure applied by the fingers, usually to an artery to stop bleeding.

**digital radiography (DR)** a method of producing radiographic images that utilize computer technology to store and manipulate data.

**digital subtraction** an advanced technique that uses digital technology to produce radiographic images, especially of blood vessels. It can also be used to locate tumours of the parathyroid glands. *digital subtraction angiography* (DSA) an image (the mask) taken before the administration of contrast medium is digitized. Contrast is then introduced into the blood vessel and further images are obtained and digitized. Computer software subtracts the mask from the postcontrast images, thus leaving an enhanced image of only those vessels that contain contrast medium.

**digitalis** *n* leaf of the common foxglove containing glycosides, such as digoxin. ⇒ glycosides.

**digitalization** *n* physiological saturation with digitalis to obtain optimum therapeutic effect.

**digiti minimi quinti varus** (*syn* congenital overlapping fifth toe) the smallest toe lies on the dorsum of the base of the fourth toe in a medially deviated position. It may be bilateral or unilateral.

**diglyceride** *n* diacylglycerol. A lipid substance that comprises a glycerol molecule and two fatty acids. Produced during the digestion of triglycerides (triacylglycerols).

**dilatation** *n* stretching or enlargement. May occur physiologically or pathologically or be induced artificially.

**dilatation and curettage (D and C)** by custom refers to dilating the uterine cervix to obtain an endometrial sample by curettage. ⇒ hysteroscopy.

**dilatation and evacuation (D and E)** dilatation of the cervix and evacuation of the products of conception under anaesthetic for therapeutic termination of pregnancy or for the removal of a dead fetus in the second trimester of pregnancy.

**dimercaprol (BAL)** *n* an organic compound used as an antidote for poisoning by heavy metals such as arsenic, bismuth, gold and mercury. It forms soluble but stable compounds with the metals, which are then rapidly excreted by the kidneys.

**diode laser** a laser used in the treatment of retinal diseases.

**Diogenes syndrome** gross self-neglect. Most frequently seen in older people who are living in appalling conditions of squalor, sometimes with many companion animals or other livestock. The person concerned usually rejects offers of help, and strenuously resists any measures to change the situation.

**dioptre** *n* a unit of measurement in refraction. A lens of 1 dioptre has a focal length of 1 metre.

**dioxide** *n* oxide containing two atoms of oxygen in each molecule, e.g. $CO_2$.

**dipeptidases** *npl* digestive enzymes that split dipeptides (paired amino acids) into individual amino acids.

**dipeptide** *n* a pair of amino acids linked by a peptide (dehydration) bond.

**2,3-diphosphoglycerate (2,3-DPG)** *n* substance present in red blood cells that decreases the affinity of haemoglobin for oxygen, thus allowing oxygen to be released to the tissues.

**diphtheria** *n* an acute, specific, infectious notifiable disease caused by *Corynebacterium diphtheriae*. Characterized by a grey, adherent, false membrane growing on a mucous surface, usually that of the upper respiratory tract. Locally there is pain and swelling, and there may be airway obstruction. Bacterial exotoxins may cause serious damage to nerves and heart muscle. Immunization is available as part of routine programmes during childhood. Close contacts with infected people are immunized and given antibiotic prophylaxis—**diphtheritic** *adj*.

**diphyllobothriasis** *n* infestation with the fish tapeworm *Diphyllobothrium latum*.

**Diphyllobothrium** *n* a genus of large tapeworm that parasitizes the intestine. Human infestation is often with the *Diphyllobothrium latum* present in fish. Infestation occurs through eating raw fish, and is common in certain countries: the Baltic states, Scandinavia, parts of Russia, and the north-west states of the United States. Infestation may lead to

gastrointestinal symptoms, such as diarrhoea and malabsorption of vitamins.

**diplacusis** *n* a condition in which a single sound is heard as two.

**diplegia** *n* symmetrical paralysis of legs, usually associated with cerebral damage—**diplegic** *adj*.

**diplococcus** *n* a coccal bacterium that occurs in pairs. *Diplococcus* may be used in a binomial to describe a characteristically paired coccus, e.g. *Diplococcus pneumoniae* (*Streptococcus pneumoniae* or pneumococcus).

**diploë** *n* the layer of cancellous bone sandwiched between two layers of compact bone in the skull.

**diploid (2n)** *adj* describes a cell with a full set of paired chromosomes. In humans the diploid number is 46 chromosomes (44 autosomes and 2 sex chromosomes) arranged in 23 pairs in all cells except the gametes. ⇒ haploid.

**diplopia** *n* the seeing of two objects when only one exists (double vision).

**dipsesis** *n* dipsosis. Experiencing extreme thirst, such as wanting abnormal fluids.

**dipsetic** *n* tending to cause thirst.

**dipsogen** *n* any agent such as food or drug that causes thirst.

**dipsomania** *n* an uncontrollable morbid craving for alcohol.

**Dipylidium** *n* a genus of tapeworm. Dogs and cats are the definitive host of *Dipylidium caninum*, which can cause disease in humans.

**direct cost** a cost that can be directly attributed to the budget of a specific department, for example, pharmacy costs in a given department.

**directly observed treatment** may be used in situations where patient compliance with a drug therapy may be poor. For example, the treatment of tuberculosis in rough sleepers.

**disability** *n* the limitations experienced by a person with an impairment (e.g. chronic lung disease) when undertaking normal functions. ⇒ International Classification of Functioning, Disability and Health.

**disaccharidases** *npl* enzymes that catalyse the hydrolysis reactions whereby disaccharides are split into their constituent monosaccharides within the intestinal mucosa. They include lactase, sucrase and maltase.

**disaccharide** *n* a carbohydrate made up of two monosaccharide molecules, e.g. lactose, sucrose, maltose, which yields two molecules of monosaccharide on hydrolysis.

**disarticulation** *n* amputation at a joint.

**discectomy** *n* surgical removal of a disc, usually an intervertebral disc.

**discogenic** *adj* arising in or produced by a disc, usually an intervertebral disc.

**discrete** *adj* distinct, separate, not merging. For example, used to describe some types of skin lesions.

**disease** *n* any deviation from or interruption of the normal structure and function of any part of the body. It is manifested by a characteristic set of signs and symptoms and in most instances the aetiology, pathology and prognosis is known.

**disease activity score (DAS)** a tool used to measure disease activity in rheumatic joint disease on a scale between 1 and 10, depending on the erythrocyte sedimentation rate and the number of tender, swollen joints.

**disease-modifying antirheumatic drugs (DMARDs)** a group of drugs that influence the immune response, which may be used to suppress the disease process in rheumatoid arthritis and other conditions. They include chloroquine, gold, penicillamine and sulfasalazine.

**disease prevention** reducing the risk of a disease process, illness, injury or disability. Includes preventive services, e.g. immunization and screening, preventive health education, e.g. advice about sensible drinking, and preventive health protection, e.g. taxing tobacco and fluoridating water. Preventive activities are classified as primary, secondary or tertiary prevention. *primary prevention* (1°) includes all activities to eradicate the cause of disease or decrease the susceptibility of the individual to the causative agent. Examples include smoking cessation advice, immunization programmes. *secondary prevention* (2°) is the detection and treatment of disease before symptoms or disordered function develop, i.e. before irreversible damage occurs, generally achieved through screening. Examples include cervical cytology screening, hypertension screening. *tertiary prevention* (3°) is the monitoring and management of established disease in order to prevent the complications of the disease process, disability or handicap. For example, monitoring of patients with diabetes in order to detect and treat early complications.

**disengagement theory** a psychosocial theory of ageing. It describes a process whereby older people gradually disengage from social life and physical activity as they become older. ⇒ activity theory.

**disimpaction** *n* separation of the broken ends of a bone that have been driven into each other during the impact which caused the fracture. Traction may then be applied to maintain the bone ends in good alignment and separate.

**disinfectants** *npl* the term usually reserved for liquid, chemical germicides that are too corrosive or toxic to be applied to tissues, but which are suitable for application to inanimate objects. They are used to destroy most or all pathogenic micro-organisms but not bacterial spores.

**disinfection** *n* the removal or destruction of pathogenic micro-organisms but not usually bacterial spores. It is commonly achieved by using heat or chemicals.

**disinfestation** *n* eradication of an infestation, especially of lice (delousing).

**disjunction** *n* in genetics, the separation of paired homologous chromosomes during the first meiotic division, or the separation of the chromatids of a chromosome during mitosis and the second division in meiosis. ⇒ nondisjunction.

**dislocation** *n* displacement of organs, or the articular surfaces of joints, so that all apposition between them is lost. The disruption of the joint is such that the bony components no longer form a working joint. It may be congenital, spontaneous, traumatic or recurrent. Treatment may include reduction under anaesthetic—**dislocated** *adj*, **dislocate** *vt*.

**disobliteration** *n* rebore. Removal of that which blocks a vessel, most often intimal plaques in an artery, when it is called endarterectomy.

**disorientation** *n* loss of orientation.

**dispensing practice** a general practice where prescribed medications are dispensed by the practice, rather than patients taking their prescription to a local pharmacy. May be used in rural areas.

**displacement** *n* **1.** a mental defence mechanism whereby a painful emotion is transferred to a another person or object. **2.** describes the loss of pieces of information from short-term memory as new information is added.

**disposable soma theory** a theory of ageing attributed to Tom Kirkwood that posits that reproductive potential in early years is maximized at the expense of ageing in later years.

**dissection** *n* separation of tissues by cutting. When a group of lymph nodes are totally excised it is referred to as a *block dissection of nodes*; it is usually part of the treatment for cancer.

**disseminated** *adj* widely spread or scattered.

**disseminated intravascular coagulation (DIC)** an abnormal overstimulation of coagulation processes characterized by a rapid consumption of clotting factors which leads to microvascular thrombi and bleeding. It is associated with conditions leading to inadequate organ perfusion, such as hypovolaemia and/or sepsis. ⇒ multiple-organ dysfunction syndrome, systemic inflammatory response syndrome.

**dissociation** *n* **1.** separation of complex substances into their components. **2.** ionization; when ionic compounds dissolve in water they dissociate or ionize into their ions.

**dissociative disorder** formerly known as conversion/hysteria disorders. Loss of conscious integration between control of body movement, sensory perceptions, self-identity and memory. Generally considered to be of psychogenic aetiology. Usually of sudden onset/termination and short duration. Often associated with striking denial.

**distal** *adj* farthest from the head or source. ⇒ proximal *opp*—**distally** *adv*.

**distichiasis** *n* extra eyelashes at the posterior lid margin, which turn inwards against the eye.

**distomolar** *n* a supernumerary fourth molar.

**distractibility** *n* a mental health disorder of the power of attention, when it can only be applied momentarily.

**distraction test** a crude hearing test used to screen infants for hearing impairment. While the infant is distracted by a parent, the health professional makes a sound to the side/behind the infant and observes whether the infant turns toward the sound. Increasingly superseded by tests using more sophisticated computer-based equipment. ⇒ automated auditory brainstem response, otoacoustic emission testing.

**distress** *n* ⇒ stress.

**diuresis** *n* increased production/secretion of urine.

**diuretics** *npl* substances that increase the secretion of urine by the kidney. ⇒ caffeine, carbonic anhydrase inhibitors, loop diuretics, osmotic diuretics, potassium-sparing diuretics, thiazide diuretics. ⇒ Appendix 5.

**diurnal rhythm** a process that follows a daily pattern, such as the sleep–wake cycle. ⇒ circadian rhythm. Also relates to a daily process, or a process occurring during daylight.

**diurnal variation** the changes that occur during a usual average day, such as changes in body temperature and the level of certain hormones.

**divagation** *n* discursive, digressing, rambling speech. The speaker is unable to stick to the main topic. May be present in a variety of serious mental health problems.

**divalent** *adj* bivalent. Having a valency of two.

**divarication** *n* separation of two points on a straight line.

**divers' paralysis** ⇒ decompression sickness/illness.

**diverticular disease** the presence of small pouch-like sacs (diverticula) in the wall of the colon. It is common in developed countries where the diet is highly refined and lacks dietary fibre (non-starch polysaccharides). The incidence increases with age and is associated with chronic constipation. It may be asymptomatic, cause bleeding, or become inflamed to cause diverticulitis, or the colon may perforate causing faecal contamination and peritonitis (Figure D.4).

**diverticulitis** *n* inflammation of a diverticulum. Faecal contamination can cause abscess formation around the bowel (pericolic). Repeated attacks of inflammation can lead to fistula formation, or scarring and narrowing of the lumen of the colon, which eventually leads to intestinal obstruction.

**diverticulosis** *n* a condition in which there are many diverticula, especially in the colon. Colonic diverticula increase in frequency with age. ⇒ diverticular disease.

**diverticulum** *n* a pouch or sac protruding from the wall of a tube or hollow organ. May be congenital or acquired—**diverticula** *pl*.

**dizygotic** *adj* relating to two zygotes. Describes non-identical twins that develop from two separate zygotes. ⇒ monozygotic *opp*.

**dizziness** *n* a feeling of unsteadiness, usually accompanied by anxiety.

**DMARD** *abbr* disease-modifying antirheumatic drug.

**DMD** *abbr* Duchenne muscular dystrophy.

**DMF index** *abbr* decayed, missing, filled index. A way to manage statistically the numbers of decayed, missing or teeth with fillings in the mouth. ⇒ DEF index.

**DNA** *abbr* deoxyribonucleic acid.

**DNA polymerase** an enzyme that catalyses the reactions needed to form double-stranded deoxyribonucleic acid from the single-stranded template.

**DNAR** *abbr* do not attempt resuscitation.

**DNase** *abbr* deoxyribonuclease.

**DNR** *abbr* do not resuscitate.

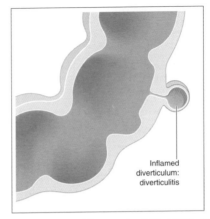

Inflamed
diverticulum:
diverticulitis

**Figure D.4** Diverticular disease *(reproduced from Brooker & Nicol 2003 with permission).*

**DO₂** *abbr* oxygen delivery.

**docosahexaenoic acid (DHA)** a 22-carbon, omega-3 polyunsaturated fatty acid. It is present in oily fish and can also be made in the body from alpha-linolenic acid.

**docosanoids** *npl* a group of polyunsaturated fatty acids with 22 carbon atoms in their structure.

**docosapentaenoic acid** a 22-carbon polyunsaturated fatty acid.

**Döderlein's bacillus** (A Döderlein, German obstetrician/gynaecologist, 1860–1941) a non-pathogenic Gram-positive rod, normally part of the vaginal flora in women of reproductive age. It contributes to the protective acidic environment by the production of lactic acid. ⇒ lactobacillus.

**Doering rule** the first fertile day of a woman's menstrual cycle is calculated from the earliest previous temperature change. Used as a back-up check for recognizing the start of the fertile days.

**dolichocephaly** *n* an abnormally long skull. ⇒ scaphocephaly.

**doll's-eye reflex** oculocephalic reflex. A normal reflex present in newborns. The eyes remain stationary when the infant's head is moved from side to side. It normally disappears when ocular fixation is achieved by the infant. It may be present in children and adults with problems affecting the brain, vestibular apparatus, the cranial nerves III, VI, extraocular/extrinsic eye muscles, etc.

**dolor** *n* pain; usually used in the context of being one of the five classical signs and symptoms of inflammation—the others being calor, loss of function, rubor and tumor.

**domestic activities of daily living (DADL)** include activities such as cooking and cleaning.

**dominant** *adj* describes a gene with the ability to override the expression of other recessive genes. Dominant genes are expressed in both the homozygous state and the heterozygous state. Examples of dominant gene expression include normal skin and hair pigmentation and Huntington's disease. ⇒ Mendel's law, recessive.

**dominant hemisphere** on the opposite side of the brain to that of the preferred hand. The dominant hemisphere for language is the left in most right-handed and around a third of left-handed people.

**DOMS** *abbr* delayed-onset muscle soreness.

**donor** *n* a person who gives blood for transfusion, or semen for artificial insemination by donor (AID), or donates tissue for transplantation.

**Donovan bodies** (C Donovan, Irish physician, 1863–1951) Leishman–Donovan bodies.

**donovanosis** *n* chronic granulomatous ulceration of the genitalia or anal region, caused by *Klebsiella granulomatis.* Prevalent in warmer climates.

**dopa** *n* a compound formed in an intermediate stage during the synthesis of catecholamines, e.g. adrenaline (epinephrine) from tyrosine.

**dopamine** *n* a monoamine neurotransmitter. It functions in the central nervous system, especially the basal nuclei (basal ganglia). Reduced levels are associated with Parkinson's disease. Used intravenously in some types of shock to increase cardiac output and blood flow to the kidneys.

**Doppler technique** (C Doppler, Austrian physicist and mathematician, 1803–1853) can be used to measure the velocity of blood flow through a vessel to determine the degree of occlusion or stenosis. *Doppler scanning* combines ultrasonography with pulse echo. *Doppler ultrasound technique* is widely used to assess the arterial blood flow to the lower limb in patients with leg ulcers. It can be used to calculate cardiac output and stroke volume by measuring blood flow in the aorta via a probe passed into the oesophagus. Used to monitor haemodynamic status and response to treatment. ⇒ ankle–brachial pressure index.

**dorsal** *adj* pertaining to the back, or the posterior part of an organ.

**dorsalis pedis artery** *n* an artery passing over the dorsum of the foot; supplying blood to the muscles of the foot and toes. The dorsalis pedis pulse, which can be palpated on the top of the foot, is used to check blood flow to the foot, such as when arterial obstruction is suspected or following arterial surgery. ⇒ Appendix 1, Figure 9.

**dorsiflexion** *n* bending backwards. In the case of the great toe, upwards. ⇒ Babinski's reflex or sign.

**dorsocentral** *adj* at the back and in the centre.

**dorsolumbar** *adj* pertaining to the lumbar region of the back.

**dorsoventral** *adj* pertaining to the dorsal (back) and the ventral (front) surfaces.

**dorsum** *n* the back of the body or the upper surface of a body part, such as the foot.

**dosimeter, dosemeter** *n* a device worn by personnel or placed within equipment to measure incident X-rays or gamma rays. Thermoluminescent dosimeters, using lithium fluoride powder impregnated into plastic discs, are used in personnel monitoring, as part of health and safety requirements. Previously, photographic film in a special filter holder was used.

**double-blind study** a randomized controlled trial in which neither the subjects (experimental and control) nor the investigators know which group is having the drug/treatment being investigated, or the placebo.

**double contrast** in radiology, the use of two contrast agents to produce the image. For example, the use of barium sulphate and air

during a barium enema to produce a detailed image of the mucosal lining of the colon.

**double vision** ⇒ diplopia.

**doubling time** time over which a tumour will double in size. A mark of tumour virulence and occasionally an indicator of chemoresponsiveness (faster doubling time often associated with high growth fraction and occasionally with higher chemoresponsiveness).

**douche** *n* a stream of fluid directed against the body externally or into a body cavity.

**downregulation** *n* **1.** in assisted conception, a phase in an in vitro fertilization (IVF) cycle, whereby drugs are used to suppress the release of the hormone that stimulates oocyte production in order to establish a baseline prior to the drug-induced stimulation of the ovaries. **2.** in genetics, the processes that regulate gene activity.

**Down's syndrome** (J Down, British physician, 1828–1896) a genetic condition in which there is mild to moderate learning disability and facial characteristics that include oval tilted eyes, squint and a flattened occiput. The chromosome abnormality is of two types: (a) primary trisomy, caused by abnormal division of chromosome 21 (at meiosis). This results in an extra chromosome instead of the normal pair: the infant has 47 chromosomes and is often born of an older mother; (b) structural abnormality, involving chromosome 21, with a total number of 46 chromosomes, one of which has an abnormal structure as the result of a special translocation. Such infants are usually born of younger mothers and there is a higher risk of recurrence in subsequent pregnancies.

**2,3-DPG** *abbr* 2,3-diphosphoglycerate.

**DR** *abbr* digital radiography.

**dracontiasis** *n* infestation with *Dracunculus medinensis* common in Africa, Middle East and Asia. It is transmitted through contaminated drinking water. The female worm moves from the intestine to emerge through the skin surface in order to deposit larvae. There is inflammation, thickening and ulceration.

**Dracunculus medinensis** (*syn* Guinea worm) a nematode parasite (tissue-dwelling) that infests humans.

**drain** *n* ⇒ wound drains.

**dreaming** *vi* altered state of consciousness where fantasies and remembered events are confused with reality.

**D₂-receptor antagonists** a group of antiemetic drugs that act by blocking the dopamine receptors, e.g. metoclopramide. ⇒ Appendix 5.

**dressings** *npl* ⇒ wound dressings.

**Dressler's syndrome** (W Dressler, American physician, 1890–1969) ⇒ postmyocardial infarction syndrome.

**DRI** *abbr* dietary reference intakes.

**drive** *n* a compelling urge to satisfy a need. It may be an innate primary drive which is concerned with homeostasis, such as thirst. Secondary drives involve a wider range of human activities that evolve during growth and development, such as social activities.

**drop attacks** periodic falling because of sudden loss of postural control of the lower limbs, without vertigo or loss of consciousness. Usually followed by sudden return of normal muscle tone, allowing the person to rise, if uninjured. ⇒ vertebrobasilar insufficiency.

**droplet infection** pathogen transmission in droplets of moisture such as during coughing or talking.

**dropsy** *n* ⇒ oedema—**dropsical** *adj*.

**drug** *n* the generic name for any substance used for the prevention, diagnosis and treatment of diagnosed disease and also for the relief of symptoms. The term 'prescribed drug' describes such usage. ⇒ prescription-only medicine (POM). The word 'medicine' is usually preferred for therapeutic drugs to distinguish them from the addictive drugs which are used illegally. For alleviating unpleasant symptoms of self-limiting illnesses, any remedy which does not require a medical prescription is termed an 'over-the-counter' (OTC) medicine. ⇒ general sales list (GSL). *drug reaction* ⇒ adverse drug reactions.

**drug dependence** a state arising from repeated administration of a drug on a periodic or continuous basis. Now a preferable term to drug addiction and drug habituation.

**drug errors** are described as preventable prescribing, dispensing or administration mistakes.

**drug interaction** occurs when the action of one drug is affected by another drug, beverage or food taken previously or simultaneously.

**drug misuse** term increasingly used to describe the illegal use of drugs. Substance misuse includes solvents and alcohol, as well as drugs such as cocaine or heroin.

**drug resistance** the increasing problem caused by the ability of many micro-organisms to develop resistance to certain antibiotics, e.g. vancomycin-resistant enterococci and meticillin (methicillin)-resistant *Staphylococcus aureus*.

**drug tolerance** a situation where the therapeutic effects of a drug lessen over time, which necessitates the administration of a larger dose to achieve the same benefit.

**drug trials** several levels of testing occurring during the development of new drugs: (a) phase I trials, where small numbers of healthy volunteers (usually male) are given small doses and monitored for adverse reactions. Blood samples are tested to determine drug distribution and excretion; (b) phase II trials involve patients, and the new drug's efficacy is compared with existing treatments; (c) phase III trials involve large multiple-centre studies carried out before the drug is approved and licensed for use by the appropriate bodies. ⇒ Commission on Human Medicines, Committee on Safety of Medicines, Medicines and Healthcare products Regulatory Agency; (d) phase IV trials take place after the drug has been approved for clinical use, and aim to monitor and report adverse and idiosyncratic reactions not seen earlier.

**drusen** *npl* yellow or white spots present beneath the neurosensory retina, usually in the macula.

**DRVs** *abbr* dietary reference values.

**dry-eye syndrome** ⇒ Sjögren syndrome.

**DSA** *abbr* digital subtraction angiography.

**DSH** *abbr* deliberate self-harm.

**DSM** *abbr* *Diagnostic and Statistical Manual of Mental Disorders*.

**DTPA** *abbr* diethylenetriamine-penta-acetic acid. A chelating agent used to remove the radioactive substances americium, curium and plutonium. Calcium DTPA or zinc DTPA is administered following internal contamination with the radioactive materials. They bind to the radioactive material prior to its excretion by the kidney.

**DTs** *abbr* delirium tremens.

**dual-energy X-ray absorptiometry (DEXA)** an imaging technique used to measure bone mineral density. Used in the diagnosis of osteoporosis and to assess response to treatment.

**dualism** *n* in psychology, a view that mind and body are separate.

**Duane's syndrome** (A Duane, American ophthalmologist, 1858–1926) an autosomal dominant disorder characterized by limitation of eye movement. There is retraction of the eye into the socket on adduction and a narrowed opening between the eyelids (palpebral fissure) during adduction.

**Dubowitz score** (V Dubowitz, South African paediatrician, b. 1931) assesses gestational age, using physical and neurological characteristics, such as ankle dorsiflexion, posture, etc. ⇒ New Ballard Score.

**Duchenne muscular dystrophy (DMD)** (G Duchenne, French neurologist, 1806–1875) an X-linked recessive disorder affecting only boys. The disorder usually begins to show between 3 and 5 years and is characterized by progressive muscle weakness and loss of locomotor skills. Death usually occurs during the teens or early twenties from respiratory or cardiac failure.

**Ducrey's bacillus** (A Ducrey, Italian dermatologist, 1860–1940) *Haemophilus ducreyi.*

**duct** *n* a tube for carrying away the secretions from a gland. For example, the bile ducts carry bile away from the liver.

**ductal carcinoma in situ (DCIS)** a precancerous condition confined to the lactiferous (milk) ducts in the breast.

**ductless glands** endocrine glands.

**ductus arteriosus** a fetal blood vessel connecting the left pulmonary artery to the aorta, to bypass the lungs in the fetus. At birth the duct closes, but if it remains open it is called *persistent or patent ductus arteriosus*, a congenital heart defect.

**ductus venosus** a vessel of the fetal circulation. It bypasses the fetal liver by shunting blood from the umbilical vein to inferior vena cava. Closes at birth.

**Dukes' staging** (C Dukes, British pathologist, 1890–1977) a system for the staging of colorectal cancer. It has four categories, A–D, and is based on the degree of tissue invasion and metastasis.

**DUB** *abbr* dysfunctional uterine bleeding.

**dumbness** *n* ⇒ mutism.

**'dumping syndrome'** the name given to the symptoms of epigastric fullness and a feeling of faintness and sweating after meals that sometimes follow partial gastrectomy. Rapid movement of hypertonic gastric contents into the duodenum causes fluid to move from the blood to the bowel lumen. Rapid absorption of glucose leads to rebound insulin secretion and hypoglycaemia.

**Duncan disease/syndrome** named for the original family in which the condition was described. ⇒ X-linked lymphoproliferative syndrome.

**duodenal intubation** ⇒ intubation.

**duodenal ulcer** a peptic ulcer occurring in the duodenal mucosa. The majority are associated with the presence of the bacterium *Helicobacter pylori* in the stomach. Other factors include non-steroidal anti-inflammatory drugs (NSAIDs), smoking and genetic factors. Epigastric pain may occur some time after meals or during the night. The pain may be relieved by food, antacids and vomiting. The ulcer can bleed, leading to haematemesis and/or melaena, or it can perforate, causing peritonitis. Severe scarring following chronic ulceration may produce pyloric stenosis and gastric outlet obstruction. Management includes: (a) general measures—smoking cessation, avoiding foods that cause pain, avoiding aspirin and NSAIDs; (b) eradication of *H. pylori*; (c) drugs to reduce gastric acid; $H_2$-receptor antagonists, e.g. ranitidine, proton pump inhibitors, e.g. omeprazole, antacids based on calcium, magnesium or aluminium salts; (d) rarely, surgical treatment, e.g. after perforation.

**duodenitis** *n* inflammation of the duodenum.

**duodenojejunal** *adj* pertaining to the duodenum and jejunum.

**duodenopancreatectomy** *n* ⇒ pancreaticoduodenectomy.

**duodenoscope** *n* a side-viewing flexible fibreoptic endoscope—**duodenoscopic** *adj*, **duodenoscopy** *n*.

**duodenostomy** *n* a surgically made fistula between the duodenum and another cavity, e.g. cholecystoduodenostomy.

**duodenum** *n* the fixed, curved, first portion of the small intestine, connecting the stomach above to the jejunum below. The pyloric sphincter at the lower end of the stomach controls the amount of partially digested food entering the duodenum. The common bile duct and the pancreatic duct unite and enter the duodenum at the hepatopancreatic ampulla (⇒ Appendix 1, Figure 18B)—**duodenal** *adj*.

**Dupuytren's contracture** (G Dupuytren, French surgeon, 1777–1835) painless chronic flexion of the digits of the hand, especially the third and fourth, towards the palm. The aetiology is uncertain but some cases are associated with hepatic cirrhosis.

**dural sinuses** sinuses or channels enclosed by layers of dura mater that drain venous blood from the different parts of the brain. They are the occipital, superior and inferior petrosal, superior and inferior sagittal, sigmoid, straight and transverse sinuses. ⇒ cavernous sinus.

**dura mater** the fibrous outer meningeal membrane covering the brain and spinal cord. ⇒ falx cerebri, falx cerebelli, meninges, tentorium cerebelli—**dural** *adj*.

**duty of care** the legal responsibility in the law of negligence that a person must take reasonable care to avoid causing harm.

**DVT** *abbr* deep-vein thrombosis.

**dwarf** *n* person of stunted growth. May be due to growth hormone deficiency. Also occurs in untreated congenital hypothyroidism and juvenile hypothyroidism, achondroplasia and other conditions.

**dwarfism** *n* arrested growth and development, as occurs in congenital hypothyroidism, and in some chronic diseases such as intestinal malabsorption, renal failure and rickets.

**dynamic flexibility** active range of motion exercises used to increase flexibility.

**dynamic psychology** a psychological approach which stresses the importance of (typically unconscious) energy or motives, as in Freudian or psychoanalytic theory.

**dynamic splinting** the use of modified splints that provide active forces and facilitate some controlled movement that counteracts the unwanted forces of the splint.

**dynamometer** *n* a device used to measure strength of muscle contraction.

**dysaesthesia** *n* impairment of touch sensation.

**dysarthria** *n* a speech disorder that results from a problem in muscular control of the mechanisms of speech. It is caused by damage to either the central or the peripheral nervous system, or both. Loss of muscular control may involve inco-ordination and/or slowness and weakness. The problem may affect articulation, phonation, prosody, resonance and respiration—**dysarthric** *adj.*

**dysbarism** *n* any condition caused by changes in atmospheric pressure. ⇒ decompression sickness/illness.

**dyschezia** *n* painful defecation. Causes include constipation, anal fissure, haemorrhoids, etc.

**dyschondroplasia** *n* Ollier's disease. A disorder of bone growth resulting in normal trunk, short arms and legs.

**dyscoria** *n* abnormality of the shape of the pupil.

**dyscrasia** *n* an abnormality in the cellular composition of the blood, as in leukaemia, agranulocytosis, aplastic anaemia, etc.

**dysdiadochokinesia** *n* impairment of the ability to perform alternating movements, such as pronation and supination, in rapid, smooth and rhythmical succession; a sign of cerebellar disease but also seen in the so-called 'clumsy child' with minimal brain damage.

**dysentery** *n* inflammation of the bowel with evacuation of blood and mucus, accompanied by tenesmus and colic—**dysenteric** *adj. amoebic dysentery* is caused by the protozoon *Entamoeba histolytica* ⇒ amoebiasis. *bacillary dysentery* is caused by bacilli of the genus

*Shigella*: *S. dysenteriae*, *S. flexneri*, *S. boydii* or *S. sonnei* (the commonest cause in the UK). The organism is excreted by cases and carriers in their faeces, and contaminates hands, food and water, from which new hosts are infected.

**dysfunction** *n* **1.** a temporary, or permanent, inability to adapt to the demands of a normal situation in a normal environment. **2.** abnormal functioning of a body part or organ.

**dysfunctional uterine bleeding (DUB)** heavy bleeding from the uterus for which no organic cause is found. ⇒ menorrhagia.

**dysgammaglobulinaemia** *n* impaired immunoglobulin production in terms of quantitative or qualitative humoral immunity. There are numerous primary and secondary causes, including common variable immunodeficiency, X-linked agammaglobulinaemia, X-linked hyper-IgM syndrome, myeloma and transient hypogammaglobulinaemia of infancy.

**dysgenesis** *n* malformation during embryonic development—**dysgenetic** *adj*, **dysgenetically** *adv.*

**dysgerminoma** *n* ovarian tumour, benign or of low-grade malignancy. It originates from primitive/undifferentiated gonadal cells.

**dysgeusia** *n* impaired or abnormal sense of taste. Impaired taste is associated with fluid deficits and poor oral/dental health. Changes during normal ageing diminish the sense of taste. Abnormal taste may be due to drug side-effect, such as with angiotensin-converting enzyme inhibitors, anticancer drugs and metronidazole. Disease processes can alter taste—some people experience strange taste sensations during an aura that precedes an epileptic seizure, and gustatory (taste) hallucinations may occur in some mental health disorders.

**dysgnathia** *n* an abnormality of the maxilla or mandible, or both.

**dysgraphia** *n* an acquired problem of written language caused by brain damage. The affected person's ability to spell familiar and/or unfamiliar words is altered in one or many modes, e.g. word-processing or hand-writing. Several different types of dysgraphia are described—**dysgraphic** *adj.*

**dyshidrosis** *n* a vesicular skin eruption on the palms and soles, formerly thought to be caused by blockage of the sweat ducts at their orifice; histologically an eczematous process.

**dyskaryosis** *n* abnormality of nuclear chromatin, indicating a malignant or premalignant condition.

**dyskeratosis** *n* abnormal keratin production by epithelial cells; may indicate malignancy.

**dyskinesia** *n* **1.** (clumsy-child syndrome) impairment of voluntary movement—**dyskinetic** *adj.* **2.** involuntary purposeless movement. ⇒ tardive dyskinesia.

**dyslalia** *n* a disorder of articulation characterized by poor pronunciation or the replacement of one sound for another, for instance, 'g' is replaced by 'd'.

**dyslexia** *n* a disorder affecting the ability to read. There are a number of different types of dyslexia, for example, *deep dyslexia* and *surface dyslexia*. Many individuals with dyslexia may also exhibit dysgraphia—**dyslexic** *adj.*

**dyslogia** *n* disordered speech, an inability to express thoughts in speech. May be due to dementia, mental health problem, or learning disability, etc.

**dysmaturity** *n* signs and symptoms of growth retardation at birth. ⇒ low birth weight.

**dysmelia** *n* limb malformation, including deficiency.

**dysmenorrhoea** *n* painful menstruation. It may be *spasmodic or primary dysmenorrhoea*, most often affecting young women once ovulation has become established, or *congestive or secondary dysmenorrhoea*, usually affecting women in their late twenties, and may be associated with pelvic pathology, such as fibroids or endometriosis.

**dysmetria** *n* difficulty in assessing and achieving the correct distance and range of movement, causing undershooting or overshooting of a target and the appearance of homing in on it.

**dysmnesic syndrome** a disorder of memory characterized by an inability to learn basic new skills. The person, however, retains the ability to perform high-level skills learned before the illness. The patient may confabulate, creating false memory to fill the gaps in memory. The disorder is caused by damage to those parts of the brain concerned with memory.

**dysmorphogenic** *adj* ⇒ teratogen.

**dysmorphophobia** *n* **1.** a morbid fear of deformity of a body part. **2.** the fixed belief that a part of the body is deformed or appears repulsive to others.

**dysmotility** *n* abnormality of intestinal peristalsis.

**dysostosis** *n* a disorder caused by faulty ossification. ⇒ cleidocranial dysostosis.

**dyspareunia** *n* painful or difficult coitus, experienced by the woman.

**dyspepsia** *n* indigestion. Epigastric discomfort and feeling of fullness after eating with heartburn, often exacerbated by stressful situations. The numerous causes include peptic ulceration, gallstones and chronic cholecystitis—**dyspeptic** *adj.*

**dysphagia** *n* difficulty in swallowing. Dysphagia can occur in a variety of medical conditions, including oesophageal cancer, cerebral palsy, motor neuron disease, cerebrovascular accident, dementia and head and neck cancer. The difficulty in swallowing may be experienced with fluids and/or solid food. The extent of difficulty can range from a mild to a very severe problem. Assessment and management of dysphagia are best conducted by a multidisciplinary team that may include a gastroenterologist, specialist nutrition nurse, dietitian and speech and language therapist. The composition of the team will be determined by the needs of the patient, the medical condition underlying the swallowing problem, whether surgery is indicated, the clinical setting and the aim of treatment (curative or palliative)—**dysphagic** *adj.*

**dysphasia** *n* also sometimes known as aphasia. Dysphasia is a disorder of language and has nothing to do with intelligence level or an intellectual disorder. It is most commonly associated with cerebrovascular accident affecting the left side of the brain, but can occur after a brain injury or brain surgery. Dysphasia can affect the ability to understand language and also the use of language for expression. The presentation of dysphasia varies greatly and those affected have very different skills and difficulties. It is important that detailed, individual consideration is given to their difficulties. The understanding of language includes understanding both what is said and what is written. Likewise, expression includes both verbal expression and written expression. Discrepancies between the level of understanding and expression of language are common. Most often, people with dysphasia have problems both in comprehension and in expression, although the degree of impairment in each may vary. Assessment and treatment of dysphasia need a detailed understanding and breakdown of language. Speech and language therapists can provide therapy to assist individuals and their carers to improve their communication. Dysphasia has a considerable impact on most areas of life, such as relationships, work and leisure activities. Rehabilitation takes time and may last many months. People affected by dysphasia can become very withdrawn and isolated if they do not receive sufficient support. ⇒ aphasia.

**dysphemia** *n* a disorder of speech. ⇒ stammering.

**dysphonia** *n* a voice production disorder, e.g. hoarseness. It may have a neurological, behavioural, organic or psychogenic cause.

**dysphoria** *n* low mood characterized by profound feelings of depression, unrest and anguish.

**dysplasia** *n* developmental abnormality, often referring to a premalignant condition and graded according to severity—**dysplastic** *adj*.

**dyspnoea** *n* difficulty in, or laboured, breathing; can be mainly of an inspiratory or expiratory nature. Causes include respiratory disease, cardiovascular disease, anaemia, etc.—**dyspnoeic** *adj*. ⇒ orthopnoea.

**dyspraxia** *n* lack of voluntary control over muscles, particularly the orofacial ones—**dyspraxic** *adj*.

**dysreflexia autonomic** ⇒ autonomic dysreflexia.

**dysrhythmia** *n* ⇒ arrhythmia.

**dyssynergia** *n* loss of fluency of movement; poor sequencing and timing of movements; loss of co-ordination of muscles that normally act in unison, particularly the abnormal state of muscle activity due to cerebellar disease.

**dystaxia** *n* difficulty in controlling voluntary movements—**dystaxic** *adj*.

**dystocia** *n* difficult labour characterized by slow progress or failure to progress. Causes include ineffective dilatation of the cervix, unco-ordinated uterine contraction and lack of expulsion, unfavourable presentation of the fetus and pelvic abnormalities.

**dystonia** *n* a movement disorder in which there is the abnormal posturing of a part of the body, examples of which are spasmodic torticollis and writer's cramp.

**dystrophy** *n* defective nutrition of an organ or tissue, usually muscle. The word is applied to several unrelated conditions. ⇒ muscular dystrophy, Duchenne muscular dystrophy.

**dysuria** *n* painful micturition. Usually associated with bacterial infection, such as cystitis, urethritis and prostatitis, or bladder tumours or urinary calculi causing obstruction and gynaecological disorders—**dysuric** *adj*.

# E

**Eagle–Barrett syndrome** ⇒ prune-belly syndrome.

**Eales' disease** (H Eales, British ophthalmologist, 1852–1913) a condition affecting the retinal vessels. It is characterized by recurrent haemorrhages into the retina and the vitreous. It affects both eyes and causes sudden visual impairment.

**ear** *n* the sensory organ concerned with hearing and balance. It has three parts: the outer (external), middle (tympanic cavity) and inner (internal) ear. The outer/external ear comprises the auricle (pinna) and the external auditory meatus/canal, along which sound waves pass to vibrate the tympanic membrane, which separates it from the middle ear. The middle-ear cavity is air-filled and contains three tiny bones or ossicles: malleus, incus and stapes. The ossicles transmit the sound waves to the inner ear via the oval window. The middle ear communicates with the nasopharynx via the pharyngotympanic (eustachian or auditory) tube. The fluid-filled inner ear comprises the cochlea (organ of hearing) and the semicircular canals, which are concerned with balance. The cochlea and semicircular canals contain the nerve endings of the cochlear and vestibular branches of the vestibulocochlear or auditory nerve (eighth cranial). ⇒ cerumen, cochlea. ⇒ Appendix 1, Figure 13.

**EAR** *acron* **e**stimated **a**verage **r**equirement.

**eardrum** *n* the tympanic membrane at the end of the external auditory meatus/canal. The first auditory ossicle is attached to the inner surface. ⇒ Appendix 1, Figure 13.

**ear wax** ⇒ cerumen.

**eating disorders** a term used to describe the range of conditions in which an individual's eating behaviour and nutrient intake are inappropriate for their needs. Anorexia nervosa is characterized by distorted body image and a deliberate restriction of food intake, resulting in severe weight loss, malnutrition, endocrine disorders and electrolyte disturbances. Bulimia nervosa—body weight is controlled by periods of restricted eating, purging and binge eating. Weight usually remains stable and within normal range. Binge-eating disorder—periods of binge eating without periods of food restriction or purging which result in the development of obesity. A complex mixture of social and psychological factors and life events predispose to and precipitate the development of eating disorders. Consequently they are best treated by a multidisciplinary team.

**EBM** *abbr* **1.** evidence-based medicine. **2.** expressed breast milk.

**Ebola** *n* a serious viral haemorrhagic fever that occurs sporadically in Africa. The first known outbreak occurred near the Ebola river in Zaire (now the Democratic Republic of the Congo). It is caused by a Filovirus and mortality rates can be as high as 90%. The mechanism for the primary infection is not known but secondary infection occurs through direct contact with infected body fluids, or by droplets. Initially there is high temperature, headache, muscle pain, etc.; later there is diarrhoea and vomiting and internal bleeding that leads to shock and multiple-organ dysfunction syndrome. Treatment is supportive only. ⇒ Marburg disease.

**EBP** *abbr* evidence-based practice.

**Ebstein's anomaly** (W Ebstein, German physician, 1836–1912) a congenital heart defect affecting the right atrioventricular (tricuspid) valve. Surgical correction may be necessary.

**eburnation** *n* the changes that occur in the articular cartilage of a joint affected by osteoarthritis. Caused by the extra stresses.

**EBV** *abbr* Epstein–Barr virus.

**ecbolic** *adj* describes any agent that causes contraction of the gravid uterus and accelerates expulsion of its contents, e.g. oxytocin used to induce and/or augment labour. ⇒ oxytocin.

**eccentric** *adj* positioned off-centre.

**eccentric muscle work** paying out of a muscle, allowing attachments to be moved further apart. For example, when going downstairs, the hamstring muscles of the posterior thigh work eccentrically to control straightening of the knee. ⇒ concentric muscle work.

**ecchondroma** *n* a benign tumour composed of cartilage which protrudes from the surface of the bone in which it arises—**ecchondromata** *pl*.

**ecchymosis** *n* ⇒ bruise—**ecchymoses** *pl*.

**eccrine** *adj* describes the most abundant type of sweat gland. ⇒ apocrine glands.

**ecdemic** *adj* describes an occurrence, such as a disease, which is not normally present in a population, i.e. it is not endemic.

**ecdysis** *n* the shedding or 'moulting' of the outer skin layer. ⇒ desquamation.

**ECF** *abbr* extracellular fluid.

**ECG** *abbr* electrocardiogram ⇒ electrocardiograph.

**echinococciasis** *n* infestation with the larval stage of a tapeworm of the genus *Echinococcus*. ⇒ hydatid cyst.

**Echinococcus** *n* a genus of cestodes, tapeworms, e.g. *Echinococcus granulosa*; the adult worms infest dogs and other canines as the primary host. The larval stage can infect humans through contaminated drinking water or handling affected dogs. The encysted larvae cause hydatid disease in humans and animals such as cattle and sheep who are secondary hosts. ⇒ hydatid cyst.

**echocardiogram** *n* an ultrasound-produced image of the movements that take place in the heart.

**echocardiography** *n* ultrasound cardiography. The use of ultrasound for studying the structure and motion of the heart. Useful for measuring the ventricles, cardiac output, myocardial contraction and ejection fraction, and in the diagnosis of pericardial effusion, endocarditis, septal defects and other congenital defects, valve dysfunction and checking prosthetic valves. It can be performed through the chest wall as a non-invasive procedure (transthoracic echocardiography) by placing the ultrasound probe (transducer) on the chest, or by passing the ultrasound probe into the oesophagus (transoesophageal echocardiography). The transoesophageal route produces clearer images of some structures, e.g. heart valves and the atria.

**echoencephalography** *n* passage of ultrasound waves across the head to investigate intracranial structures. Can detect midline shift caused by space-occupying lesions such as an abscess or blood clot, etc., within the brain. Mostly superseded by magnetic resonance imaging and computed tomographic imaging.

**echolalia** *n* repetition, almost automatically, of words or phrases heard. Occurs most commonly in people who have schizophrenia and dementia and sometimes in delirium—**echolalic** *adj*.

**echopraxia** *n* the copying or repetition of the body movements of another person. Can be a feature of schizophrenia.

**echoviruses** *npl* name originates from **e**nteric **c**ytopathic **h**uman **o**rphan. A group of RNA viruses of the genus *Enterovirus* that cause conditions that include: gastroenteritis, respiratory infection, aseptic meningitis, encephalitis and rashes.

**echoxia** *n* involuntary mimicking of another's movements.

**eclampsia** *n* **1.** new onset of convulsions in a pregnant woman or postpartum, which is not related to other cerebral conditions, occurring in a woman with pre-eclampsia. **2.** a sudden convulsive attack—**eclamptic** *adj*. ⇒ HELLP syndrome, pre-eclampsia.

**ECM** *abbr* extracellular matrix.

**ECMO** *abbr* extracorporeal membrane oxygenator.

**ecmnesia** *n* impaired memory for recent events with normal memory of remote ones. Common in older adults and in early cerebral deterioration.

**ECoG** *abbr* electrocochleography.

**ecological study** a research study where a particular group of individuals rather than an individual, e.g. schools, towns, etc., form the unit being observed.

**economy** *n* describes spending or using as little as possible whilst still maintaining quality services. One of the three 'Es' of value for money. ⇒ effectiveness, efficiency, value for money.

**Ecstasy** *n* colloquial term for an amphetamine derivative methylenedioxymethamphetamine (MDMA) that causes euphoria and hallucinations. Use is widespread at 'raves' and clubs. It is considered by many users to be safe, but serious effects from excessive physical activity and dehydration, which leads to hyperpyrexia and possibly death, have occurred.

**ECT** *abbr* electroconvulsive therapy.

**ectasis, ectasia** *n* dilatation or distension of a hollow organ, duct or tube.

**ecthyma** *n* a crusted eruption of pyogenic infection, usually on the legs, producing necrosis of the skin, which heals with scarring.

**ectoderm** *n* the outer of the three primary germ layers of the early embryo. It gives rise to some epithelial and nervous tissues, e.g. skin structures, inner ear, mammary glands, pituitary gland, the central nervous system, cranial, spinal and autonomic nerves, adrenal medulla and the lens and retina of the eye—**ectodermal** *adj*. ⇒ endoderm, mesoderm.

**ectogenesis** *n* the growth of the embryo outside the uterus (in vitro fertilization).

**ectomorph** *n* a frail body type (physique) in which the person is slender—**ectomorphic** *adj*. ⇒ endomorph, mesomorph.

**ectoparasite** *n* a parasite that lives on the exterior surface of its host, such as head lice—**ectoparasitic** *adj*.

**ectopia** *n* malposition of an organ or structure, usually congenital. *ectopia vesicae* an abnormally placed urinary bladder which protrudes through or opens on to the abdominal wall—**ectopic** *adj*.

**ectopic beat** ⇒ extrasystole.

**ectopic pregnancy** (*syn* tubal pregnancy) extrauterine gestation, the uterine (fallopian) tube being the most common site (Figure E.1). Other, less common sites include the ovary, external os of the cervix and the abdominal cavity.

**ectrodactyly, ectrodactylia** *n* congenital absence of one or more fingers or toes or parts of them.

**ectropion** *n* an eversion or turning outward, especially of the lower eyelid. It may be due to age-related tissue changes, trauma to the eyelids, facial nerve damage or Bell's palsy.

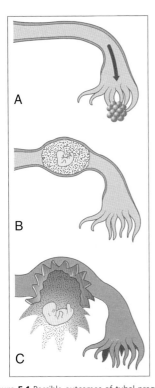

**Figure E.1** Possible outcomes of tubal pregnancy: (A) tubal abortion; (B) tubal mole; (C) tubal rupture *(reproduced from Fraser & Cooper 2003 with permission)*.

The eyelids do not close fully, which exposes the eyeball and disrupts the tear film. The tears cannot drain into the punctum and the eye waters. ⇒ entropion.

**ECV** *abbr* external cephalic version.

**eczema** *n*
an inflammatory skin reaction that may begin with erythema, then vesicles appear. These rupture, forming exudative areas that may crust. Scaling may occur. In chronic forms the skin becomes thickened. Some authorities limit the word 'eczema' to cases with internal (endogenous) causes while those caused by external (exogenous) contact factors are called dermatitis. The skin of patients with eczema may be colonized or infected with *Staphylococcus aureus*. ⇒ dermatitis—**eczematous** *adj*.

**eczema herpeticum** also known as Kaposi's varicelliform eruption. A serious condition that occurs when the herpes simplex virus (HSV-1) infects existing eczema. There are clusters of small vesicles on areas of eczema and normal skin. It is accompanied by systemic effects and patients may feel very unwell. Management includes the administration of antiviral drugs, and in severe cases the person is hospitalized for intravenous administration. Patients are isolated as eczema herpeticum is infectious. ⊙DVD

**ED** *abbr* erectile dysfunction.

**EDD** *abbr* expected date of delivery.

**edentulous** *adj* without natural teeth.

**EDRF** *abbr* endothelium-derived relaxing factor. ⇒ nitric oxide.

**edrophonium test** a test for myasthenia gravis: a small intramuscular dose of edrophonium chloride will immediately relieve symptoms, albeit temporarily, while quinine sulphate will increase the muscular weakness. Resuscitation drugs and equipment must be available, as respiratory depression may occur.

**EDTA** *abbr* ethylene diamine tetra-acetic acid.

**EDV** *abbr* end-diastolic volume.

**Edwards' syndrome** (J Edwards, British medical geneticist, b. 1928) an autosomal trisomy of chromosome number 18 associated with abnormal facial appearance (e.g. low-set ears, small eyes and micrognathia), growth retardation and learning disability. The cells have 47 chromosomes.

**EEG** *abbr* electroencephalogram ⇒ electroencephalograph.

**EFAs** *abbr* essential fatty acids.

**EFSA** *abbr* European Food Safety Authority.

**effacement of cervix** ⇒ cervical effacement.

**effective dose** the amount of a drug that can be expected to initiate a specific intensity of effect in people taking the drug.

**effectiveness** *n* describes using the available resources to achieve the required outcomes. One of the three 'Es' of value for money. ⇒ economy, efficiency, value for money.

**effector** *n* a motor or secretory nerve ending in a muscle, gland or organ. They stimulate muscle contraction or glandular secretion.

**efferent** *adj* carrying, conveying, conducting away from a centre, such as motor nerves that carry nerve impulses away from the brain and spinal cord (central nervous system). ⇒ afferent *opp*.

**efficiency** *n* describes the use of minimum resources to achieve the maximum outcomes. One of the three 'Es' of value for money. ⇒ economy, effectiveness, value for money.

**effleurage** *n* a massage manipulation, using long, whole-hand strokes in the direction of venous and lymphatic drainage, that aims to help venous return to the heart and the reduction of oedema. Deep effleurage causes dilatation of the arterioles by stimulating the axon reflex.

**effort continua** subjective response that occurs to an exercise stimulus that involves the three elements—physiological, perceptual and performance.

**effort syndrome** a form of anxiety disorder, manifesting itself in a variety of cardiac symptoms, including chest pain, palpitations, dizziness, for which no pathological explanation can be discovered.

**effusion** *n* extravasation of fluid into body tissues or cavities, such as a pleural effusion, or into joints where it causes swelling.

**ego** *n* one of the three main aspects of the personality (the others being the id and superego); refers to the conscious self, the 'I', which, according to Freud, deals with reality; is influenced by social forces and controls unconscious instinctual urges. ⇒ id, superego. ⇒ Freud, Sigmund.

**ego strength** the ability of the ego to deal with the demands of the id as well as the real-world constraints. Traits, such as tolerance of disappointment and loss, forgiveness, compassion, being able to defer gratification, flexibility, perseverance, etc., are considered to contribute to good mental health.

**ego support** the defences utilized by the ego to ensure that inner conflicts are resolved without overwhelming.

**EHEC** *abbr* enterohaemorrhagic *Escherichia coli*.

**Ehlers–Danlos syndrome** (E Ehlers, Danish dermatologist, 1863–1937; H Danlos, French physician, 1844–1921) a group of inherited conditions affecting connective tissues. Abnormal collagen production leads to skin that is very elastic, fragile and easily damaged. There is joint hypermobility that leads to joint injuries—sprains, dislocation and joint effusion.

**EIA** *abbr* exercise-induced asthma. ⇒ asthma.

**eicosanoids** *npl* a variety of compounds formed from long-chain polyunsaturated fatty acids, e.g. arachidonic acid. They include prostaglandins, prostacyclins, thromboxanes and leukotrienes. They are all important as intercellular signalling molecules and for platelet aggregation, inflammation and many other physiological processes.

**eicosapentaenoic acid (EPA)** a 20-carbon long-chain omega-3 polyunsaturated fatty acid. Present in fish oils.

**eicosenoic acids** a group of 20-carbon long-chain polyunsaturated fatty acids.

**eidetic image** a vivid image, usually visual but it can be auditory. The image, which is very detailed, is very close to actual perception. The person is still able to scan a visual display even after the display is no longer present. The image may be recalled with photographic accuracy, long after the original experience. It is one form of illusion. ⇒ illusion, pareidolic.

**EIEC** *abbr* enteroinvasive *Escherichia coli*.

**Eisenmenger's complex** (V Eisenmenger, German physician, 1864–1932) congenital heart defect with an abnormal shunt between the left and right sides of the heart, malposition of the aorta and an abnormal pulmonary artery.

**Eisenmenger's syndrome/reaction** a syndrome associated with a ventricular septal defect or Eisenmenger's complex. The increased blood flow through the left-to-right shunt damages the pulmonary blood vessels, changes pulmonary vascular resistance and leads to pulmonary hypertension. This eventually leads to back flow that increases the pressure in the right side of the heart. At a certain point the shunt is reversed to a right-to-left shunt. The affected individual will also develop polycythaemia.

**ejaculation** *n* sudden emission of semen from the penis at the moment of male orgasm. *retrograde ejaculation* a situation where semen is discharged backwards into the bladder. It may follow prostate surgery or be associated with diabetic neuropathy.

**ejaculatory ducts** two ducts formed from the combining of the deferent duct (vas deferens) and the duct from the seminal vesicle. They go through the prostate gland, conveying seminal fluid containing spermatozoa to the urethra. ⇒ Appendix 1, Figure 16.

**ejection fraction** the fraction or percentage of the total ventricular filling volume of blood that is pumped out in each ventricular contraction. A reduced ejection fraction may indicate systolic heart failure.

**elastic fibrocartilage (yellow)** one of the three types of cartilage, comprising yellow fibres in a solid matrix. It is flexible and is present in the pinna of outer/external ear, the middle coat of blood vessels and in the epiglottis, where it supports and maintains shape. ⇒ cartilage.

**elastin** *n* the protein forming the principal constituent of elastic tissue.

**elder abuse** physical (including neglect), sexual, psychological, pharmacological or financial abuse of older people. May be carried out by family and other carers, neighbours, or by health and social care staff.

**elective surgery** planned surgery rather than that undertaken as an emergency.

**Electra complex** excessive emotional attachment of daughter to father. The name is derived from Greek mythology.

**electrocardiogram (ECG)** *n* a recording of the electrical activity of the heart muscle during the cardiac cycle made by an electrocardiograph. The normal heart produces a typical waveform, sinus rhythm, which consists of five deflection waves, known universally as P-QRS-T. ⇒ P-QRS-T complex. *ambulatory ECG (Holter monitoring)* recording heart rhythm and rate over a 24-hour period to detect transient ischaemia or arrhythmias. The person continues with normal activities and keeps a record of times and activities. *exercise (stress) ECG* performed during increasing levels of exertion, such as on a treadmill or static cycle, to detect arrhythmias or ischaemic changes caused by physical stress. Frequently used for the diagnosis or prognosis of heart disease or to guide cardiac rehabilitation, or as part of an athletic fitness assessment.

**electrocardiograph** *n* an instrument that records the electrical activity of the heart from electrodes placed on the limbs, and on several positions on the chest (Figure E.2) —**electrocardiographic** *adj*, **electrocardiography** *n*, **electrocardiographically** *adv*.

**electrocardiophonography** *n* a combined investigation that simultaneously records heart sounds during the cardiac cycle, and the electrical activity with an electrocardiogram.

**electrocoagulation** *n* technique of surgical diathermy. Coagulation, especially of bleeding points, by means of electrodes.

**electrocochleography (ECoG)** *n* direct recording of the action potential generated following stimulation of the cochlear nerve. ⇒ vestibulocochlear nerve.

**electroconvulsive therapy (ECT)** a physical treatment used in psychiatry, mainly in the treatment of severe/life-threatening depression or psychotic states. A device is used that delivers a definite electrical voltage for a precise fraction of a second to electrodes placed on the head, producing a convulsion. The convulsion is modified by use of an intravenous anaesthetic and a muscle relaxant prior to treatment. *unilateral ECT* avoids the sequela of amnesia for recent events. Memory for recent events is probably in the dominant cerebral hemisphere. ECT is therefore applied to the right hemisphere to reduce memory disturbance.

**electrode** *n* in medicine or therapy, a conductor in the form of a pad or plate, whereby electricity enters or leaves the body.

**electrodesiccation** *n* fulguration. A technique of surgical diathermy. There is drying and subsequent removal of tissue. Used to remove superficial skin growths.

**electrodiagnosis** *n* recording the electrical activity of electrically excitable body structures (spontaneous activity or following stimulation) as an aid to diagnosis, e.g. electrocardiogram, electromyogram, etc.

**electroencephalogram (EEG)** *n* a graphic recording of the various types of electrical activity occurring in the brain, made by an electroencephalograph. The device produces a trace of the brain waves—alpha, beta, delta and theta rhythms. It is used to investigate seizures and sleep disorders.

**electroencephalograph** *n* an instrument by which electrical activity derived from the brain can be amplified and recorded, in a fashion similar to that of the electrocardiograph. Electrodes are applied to various parts of the scalp—**electroencephalographic** *adj*, **electroencephalography** *n*, **electroencephalographically** *adv*.

**electrolysis** *n* **1.** chemical decomposition by electricity, with ion movement shown by changes at the electrodes. **2.** term used for

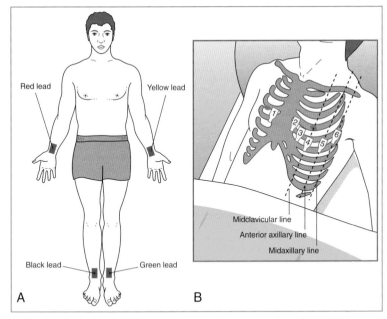

**Figure E.2** Electrocardiograph. Position of (A) limb leads and (B) chest leads for 12-lead ECG *(reproduced from Nicol et al. 2004 with permission)*.

the destruction of individual hairs (epilation), removal of moles, spider naevi, etc., using electricity.

**electrolyte** *n* a solution of a substance, such as sodium chloride, which dissociates into ions with an electrical charge—anions (negative charge) and cations (positive charge). In medicine it describes the individual ion, e.g. potassium and bicarbonate (hydrogen carbonate) ions in the body.

**electrolyte balance** the balance of relative amounts of electrolytes, e.g. potassium, sodium, magnesium, calcium, chloride, bicarbonate and phosphate in blood, other fluids and tissues. The balance between ions with a positive charge (cations), e.g. potassium, and those with a negative charge (anions), e.g. chloride, ensures overall electrical neutrality in the body. Many conditions and diseases cause electrolyte imbalance, which is often associated with loss of fluid and pH homeostasis—**electrolytic** *adj*. ⇒ anion, anion gap, cation.

**electromechanical dissociation (EMD)** older term for pulseless electrical activity. ⇒ cardiac arrest, pulseless electrical activity.

**electromotive force (EMF)** measures the force needed for an electric current to flow between two points. A derived SI unit (International System of Units), the volt (V), is used. ⇒ Appendix 2.

**electromyography (EMG)** *n* the use of an instrument which records electric currents generated in contracting muscle—**electromyographical** *adj*, **electromyogram** *n*, **electromyograph** *n*, **electromyographically** *adv*.

**electron** *n* a negatively charged subatomic particle.

**electron microscopy** the use of a beam of electrons to visualize very small structures, such as virus particles. It may involve a transmission electron microscope or a scanning electron microscope.

**electron transfer chain** a series of mitochondrial oxidation–reduction reactions that transfer electrons in order to generate cellular energy as adenosine triphosphate.

**electronically evoked twitch** an investigation that involves the application of an electrical stimulus to a motor nerve adjacent to the muscle. Used to provide information about the maximal inherent muscle force.

**electro-oculography** *n* the use of an instrument which records eye position and movement, and potential difference between front and back of the eyeball using electrodes placed on the skin near the eye. Can be used as a diagnostic test of retinal function—**electro-oculogram (EOG)** *n*.

**electrophoresis** *n* a technique where charged particles are separated in a liquid medium by their characteristic speed and direction of migration in an electrical field.

**electroretinography** *n* the use of an instrument to measure electrical currents generated in the retina stimulated by light—**electroretinogram (ERG)** *n*.

**electrosurgery** *n* the use of electrical devices that work on high-frequency electrical current during surgical procedures. ⇒ electrocoagulation, electrodesiccation.

**electrotherapy** *n* in physiotherapy, electrophysical agents in treatments, e.g. short-wave diathermy and transcutaneous electrical nerve stimulation, may be used for musculoskeletal problems.

**element** *n* one of the constituents of a compound. The elements, such as carbon, oxygen, hydrogen, sodium are the primary substances which, in pure form, or in combinations as compounds, constitute all matter. They cannot be broken down into another substance.

**elephantiasis** *n* the swelling of a limb, usually a leg, as a result of lymphatic obstruction (lymphoedema), followed by thickening of the skin (pachyderma) and subcutaneous tissues. A complication of filariasis in tropical countries. ⇒ *Filaria*, filariasis, lymphoedema.

**elevation** *n* an upward movement such as the scapulae when the shoulders are lifted. Or the positioning of a body part, such as a limb to reduce swelling.

**elimination** *n* the passage of waste from the body—urine and faeces—**eliminate** *vt*.

**ELISA** *abbr* enzyme-linked immunosorbent assay.

**elixir** *n* a sweetened, aromatic solution of a drug, often containing alcohol.

**elliptocytosis (ovalocytosis)** *n* elliptical red blood cells. Characteristic of hereditary elliptocytosis, a rare congenital haemolytic anaemia. Also a feature of some anaemias, and a few (<15%) may be present in normal blood.

**Ellis–van Creveld syndrome** (R Ellis, British paediatrician, 1902–1966; S van Creveld, Dutch paediatrician, 1894–1971). ⇒ chondroectodermal dysplasia.

**emaciation** *n* excessive leanness, or wasting of body tissue, such as that caused by malnutrition or widespread cancer—**emaciate** *vt*.

**emasculation** *n* castration.

**embolectomy** *n* surgical removal of an embolus from an artery, such as a limb artery, carotid artery, the aorta or pulmonary artery. Usually a fine balloon (Fogarty) catheter is used to extract the embolus, or the artery is opened during arteriotomy to facilitate removal of the obstruction.

**embolic** *adj* pertaining to an embolism or an embolus.

**embolism** *n* obstruction of a blood vessel by a body of undissolved material. Usually caused by a thrombus (clot), but other causes include cancer cells, fat, amniotic fluid, gases, bacteria and parasites. Rarer emboli, such as fat, may follow long bone fractures, air may enter the circulation via a penetrating chest wound or during surgery, and amniotic fluid during labour. The most common type is a thromboembolus that originates in the deep veins of the legs or pelvis, which travels in the veins, through the right side of the heart to lodge in a pulmonary artery—a pulmonary embolus. *arterial (systemic) embolism*, originating from the left side of the heart, such as with atrial fibrillation, or as a result of arterial disease, may travel to various sites including brain, bowel or a limb; the effects are dependent on the size of vessel affected and site, e.g. gangrene of a limb or a portion of bowel. ⇒ cerebrovascular accident, deep-vein thrombosis, pulmonary embolism.

**embolization** *n* therapeutic occlusion of a blood vessel using a foreign substance, such as polyvinyl alcohol or tiny coils. The minimally invasive technique is used to reduce menorrhagia caused by uterine fibroids, treat severe or recurrent epistaxis, aneurysms and arteriovenous malformations.

**embologenic** *adj* capable of producing an embolus.

**embolus** *n* solid body or gas bubble transported in the circulation. ⇒ embolism—**emboli** *pl*.

**embrasure** *n* an opening, such as that between the proximal surfaces of the teeth.

**embrocation** *n* a liquid applied topically by rubbing.

**embryo** *n* developmental stage starting 2 weeks after fertilization until the end of week 8 of gestation. The stage marked by rapid increase in size, cell differentiation and organ formation (organogenesis)—**embryonic** *adj*.

**embryo/fetal reduction** a number of healthy embryos/fetuses in a multiple pregnancy are destroyed (but remain in the uterus until the end of pregnancy) in order to increase the chances of survival for the one, two or three embryos left in place. It may be offered to couples who have conceived triplets or more, either naturally or after assisted conception treatments.

**embryology** *n* study of embryonic development—**embryological** *adj*, **embryologically** *adv*.

**embryoma** *n* ⇒ teratoma.

**embryopathy** *n* abnormality or disease of the embryo—**embryopathic** *adj*.

**embryoscopy** *n* visualization of the embryo around the ninth week of gestation. It uses a small, specialized fibreoptic endoscope to examine the embryo through the intact sac of membranes. The endoscope may be inserted transabdominally or transcervically. Usually used for couples from families who suffer from genetic disorders that can be identified from the appearance of the embryo. ⇒ fetoscopy.

**embryotomy** *n* a procedure that involves the destruction of the fetus to facilitate delivery. Very rarely performed.

**EMD** *abbr* electromechanical dissociation.

**EMEA** *abbr* European Medicines Agency.

**emergency contraception** postcoital contraception. Popularly referred to as the 'morning-after' pill. A single dose of levonorgestrel (available without prescription) administered orally within 72 hours of unprotected intercourse, or the insertion of a copper-containing intrauterine contraceptive device within 5 days.

**emesis** *n* vomiting.

**emetic** *n* any agent used to produce vomiting.

**emetogenic** *adj* term that describes substances that cause vomiting, such as ipecacuanha used after certain types of poisoning, or may do so, e.g. cancer chemotherapy.

**EMF** *abbr* electromotive force.

**EMG** *abbr* electromyogram.

**eminence** *n* a rounded projection on a bone, such as the iliopectineal eminence on the hip bone.

**emissary veins** *npl* veins that connect the venous sinuses in the dura mater to veins on the outside of the skull.

**emission** *n* an ejaculation or sending forth, especially an involuntary ejaculation of semen.

**EMLA** *abbr* eutectic mixture of local anaesthetics.

**emmetropia** *n* normal refractive power of the eye, such that light from a distant object forms a clear image on the retina without accommodative effort—**emmetropic** *adj*.

**emollient** *adj*, *n* (an agent) which moisturizes and soothes skin or mucous membrane. Emollients are oil-based substances that are used when dry skin is a problem, such as in some skin diseases (e.g. eczema) and that resulting from normal age changes. The emollient replaces the natural substances that normally waterproof the skin and minimize water loss from the skin surface.

**emotion** *n* the tone of feeling recognized in ourselves by certain physiological changes, and in others by tendencies to certain characteristic behaviour. Aroused usually by ideas or concepts.

**emotional** *adj* characteristic of or caused by emotion. *emotional bias* tendency of emotional attitude to affect logical judgement. *emotional lability* ⇒ lability. *emotional state* effect of emotions on normal mood, e.g. agitation, depressed mood.

**empathy** *n* identifying oneself with another person or understanding the meaning and significance of the actions of another person. Having some understanding of their situation, feelings and experiences. Described as having awareness of and insight into the biopsychosocial experiences of another person. A vital component of a therapeutic relationship—**empathic** *adj*.

**emphysema** *n* gaseous distension of the tissues. ⇒ crepitation, pulmonary emphysema, surgical emphysema—**emphysematous** *adj*.

**empirical** *adj* describes treatment or management based on observation and experience rather than on scientific reasoning.

**empowerment** *n* the acquisition of knowledge and skills leading to personal development and growth. The enabling processes whereby people increase the control and power that they have over decisions that influence how they live. For example, when individuals with a learning disability acquire the skills needed to live independently, or make individual decisions about, for example, what clothes they select to wear.

**empyema** *n* pus within a pleural cavity.

**EMRSA** *abbr* epidemic meticillin (methicillin)-resistant *Staphylococcus aureus*.

**emulsifying agents** substances soluble in both water and fat. They facilitate the formation of an emulsion as fat is uniformly dispersed in water.

**emulsion** *n* the mixture of two immiscible liquids, e.g. water and fat. The uniform suspension of fat or oil particles in an aqueous continuous phase (*O/W emulsion*) or aqueous droplets in an oily continuous phase (*W/O emulsion*).

**enablement** *n* in health care and/or social care the active involvement of patients or clients in their therapy or care.

**enamel** *n* ⇒ dental enamel.

**enarthrosis** *n* a ball-and-socket joint in which the head of one bone articulates in a depression on another. For example, the head of femur articulates in the cup-like acetabulum of the pelvis. A type of freely movable joint or diarthrosis, which allows the greatest range of motion.

**encapsulation** *n* enclosure within a capsule, such as an organ, a cancer, or a micro-organism.

**encephalins** *npl* ⇒ enkephalins.

**encephalitis** *n* inflammation of the brain; usually viral but can be bacterial. It may follow an infectious illness such as measles or influenza. A serious condition in which severe inflammation can result in neurological sequelae such as seizures or even death. *encephalitis lethargica* also known as epidemic encephalitis or 'sleepy/sleeping sickness'. A worldwide pandemic (1917–1928) killed many millions of people and left others with severe neurological problems, including postencephalitic Parkinson's disease. Sporadic cases still occur.

**encephalocele** *n* protrusion of brain substance through a congenital defect in the skull. Also associated with hydrocephalus when the protrusion occurs at a suture line. ⇒ neural tube defects.

**encephalography** *n* a general term for techniques used to examine the brain. ⇒ echoencephalography, electroencephalography, pneumoencephalography, ventriculography—**encephalogram** *n*.

**encephaloid** *adj* resembling brain tissue.

**encephalomalacia** *n* softening of the brain.

**encephalomyelitis** *n* inflammation of the brain and spinal cord. ⇒ encephalitis.

**encephalomyelopathy** *n* disease affecting both brain and spinal cord—**encephalomyelopathic** *adj*.

**encephalon** *n* the brain and its component parts—cerebrum, cerebellum, pons and medulla oblongata.

**encephalopathy** *n* any disease of the brain causing reduced levels of arousal and cognitive function, such as Wernicke's encephalopathy—**encephalopathic** *adj*.

**enchondroma** *n* a benign tumour of cartilage—**enchondromata** *pl*.

**encopresis** *n* the repeated involuntary or voluntary passage of faeces in inappropriate places, such as faecal soiling of clothing, or on the floor, by a child over 4 years of age who was previously continent. In many cases it is associated with prolonged constipation, with faecal impaction and leakage of liquid faeces. It may also be associated with neurological problems, surgery or psychological disorders that include conduct disorder and oppositional defiant disorder—**encopretic** *adj, n*.

**encounter group** a form of psychotherapy. Small groups of individuals focus on becoming aware of their feelings and developing the ability to express them openly, honestly and with clarity. The objectives are to increase self-awareness, promote personal growth and improve interpersonal skills.

**encysted** *adj* contained within a cyst or capsule.

**endarterectomy** *n* the surgical removal of an atheromatous core from an artery, along with the intimal lining, sometimes called disobliteration or 'rebore'. It may be a *disobliterative endarterectomy*, or carbon dioxide gas can be used to separate the occlusive core in a *gas endarterectomy*.

**endarteritis** *n* inflammation of the intima or inner lining coat of an artery. *endarteritis obliterans* the new intimal connective tissue obliterates the lumen.

**end artery** a terminal artery. An artery that does not join another blood vessel; it terminates in a body structure or organ, e.g. the retinal artery, which is completely dependent on the artery for its blood supply. Occlusion of an end artery leads to tissue damage due to ischaemia.

**end-diastolic volume (EDV)** the volume of blood in the cardiac ventricles at the end of diastole. ⇒ stroke volume.

**endemic** *adj* recurring in an area, particularly a disease that is always present in an area, e.g. a particular communicable disease such as the common cold. ⇒ epidemic *opp.*

**endemic syphilis** also known as non-venereal syphilis. Usually found in children, the infection is spread by skin-to-skin contact or from contaminated drinking vessels. Features similar to those of syphilis. ⇒ bejel, pinta, yaws.

**endemic treponematoses** the non-venereal treponemal diseases—bejel, yaws and pinta. They generally affect people living in rural communities in underdeveloped countries. Transmission occurs by skin contact in childhood.

**endemiology** *n* the special study of endemic diseases.

**end-feel** *n* the quality of the feel or sensation felt by the examiner when pressure is applied to the joint at the end of its range of movement.

**endobronchial tube** plastic double-lumen tube introduced via the mouth into either of the two main bronchi in thoracic anaesthesia.

**endocardial mapping** the recording of electrical potentials from various sites on the endocardium to determine the origin of cardiac arrhythmias.

**endocarditis** *n* inflammation of the inner lining of the heart (endocardium) and heart valves due to infection by micro-organisms (bacteria, fungi or *Rickettsia*), or to rheumatic fever. There may be temporary or permanent damage to the heart valves. ⇒ infective endocarditis.

**endocardium** *n* the smooth layer of endothelial cells that line the chambers of the heart. In health the smoothness of the endocardium prevents turbulence, which could lead to the formation of blood clots. It is continuous with the endothelium lining the blood vessels that carry blood to and from the heart.

**endocervical** *adj* pertaining to the inside of the cervix uteri.

**endocervicitis** *n* inflammation of the mucous membrane lining the cervix uteri.

**endochondral** *adj* relating to the tissue within the cartilage.

**endocrine** *adj* secreting internally. ⇒ autocrine, exocrine *opp*, paracrine—**endocrinal** *adj. endocrine glands* the ductless glands that produce hormones which pass directly into the blood or lymph to influence distant structures. They include the hypothalamus, pineal body (gland), pituitary, thyroid, parathyroids, thymus, adrenal cortex and medulla, ovaries, testes and pancreas. Other structures also produce hormones, e.g. placenta, gastrointestinal tract, kidneys and the heart.

**endocrinology** *n* the study of the endocrine structures and their internal secretions.

**endocrinopathy** *n* abnormality of one or more of the endocrine glands or their secretions. For example, an overactive thyroid gland—hyperthyroidism.

**endocytosis** *n* a term for the bulk transport of large molecules into cells. ⇒ exocytosis *opp*, phagocytosis, pinocytosis.

**endoderm** *n* inner layer of the three primary germ layers of the early embryo. It gives rise to some epithelial tissue, e.g. that of the pharynx, middle ear, respiratory tract, gastrointestinal tract and bladder. ⇒ ectoderm, mesoderm.

**endodontics** *n* branch of dentistry concerned with the diagnosis and treatment of diseases of the dental pulp and periapical tissues.

**end-of-life care** the care given at the very end of life, during the last week, days and hours before death. Appropriate and effective care requires several members of the multidisciplinary team (MDT) to be involved in the care and support of patients with advanced disease, their families and friends. End-of-life care is part of the much broader palliative care provided for people with life-limiting diseases, such as heart failure and cancer.

**endogenous** *adj* originating within the organism. ⇒ ectogenous, exogenous *opp*.

**endolymph** *n* the fluid within the membranous labyrinth of the inner ear. ⇒ perilymph.

**endolymphatic duct** *n* the duct that connects the endolymphatic sac to the saccule and utricle.

**endolymphatic hydrops** excess endolymph in the endolymphatic system. Distension of the endolymphatic system is associated with Ménière's disease.

**endolymphatic sac** *n* the dilated part of the endolymphatic duct.

**endometrial** *adj* pertaining to the endometrium.

**endometrial ablation/destruction** transcervical destruction of the basal layer of the endometrium by resection, laser ablation, microwaves, radiofrequency, or by using heat. Frequently used instead of hysterectomy in the treatment of menorrhagia. ⇒ embolization.

**endometrial hyperplasia** abnormal overgrowth of the endometrium resulting from prolonged contact with unopposed oestrogens. These may be endogenous oestrogens, such as occurs in anovulatory cycles, or exogenous if oestrogen-only hormone replacement therapy (without progesterone) is prescribed for women with an intact uterus. It may progress to endometrial cancer.

**endometrioma** *n* a tumour of misplaced endometrium ⇒ chocolate cyst—**endometriomata** *pl.*

**endometriosis** *n* the presence of endometrium in abnormal sites, i.e. outside the uterus. The tissue outside the uterus is influenced by hormones during the menstrual cycle, resulting in bleeding and the formation of adhesions. The commonest sites are the peritoneum of the rectovaginal pouch (pouch of Douglas), ovary, sigmoid colon, broad ligament and uterosacral ligament, but it can affect other pelvic structures, such as the bladder. The cause is unknown but two theories suggest that either endometrium travels along the uterine tubes during menstruation instead of being lost through the cervix, or that peritoneal mesothelium is transformed into tissue similar to endometrium. Signs and symptoms vary considerably, but commonly there is pelvic pain, which can be associated with menstruation or can occur at any other time due to adhesions. Treatment options include the use of drugs to reduce oestrogen secretion or oppose its action, or laparoscopic destruction of the ectopic endometrium. ⇒ chocolate cyst.

**endometritis** *n* inflammation of the endometrium.

**endometrium** *n* the specialized lining mucosa of the uterus. It contains many blood vessels and glands. During the reproductive years the endometrium undergoes cyclical changes in response to ovarian hormones. This prepares the endometrium to receive an embryo if fertilization occurs. The endometrium comprises two layers—the permanent stratum basalis, and the stratum functionalis, which regenerates after being lost every 28 days or so during menstruation (Figure E.3)—**endometrial** *adj.*

**endomorph** *n* a soft, round body type (physique), with large thighs and trunk, and fat accumulation—**endomorphic** *adj.* ⇒ ectomorph, mesomorph.

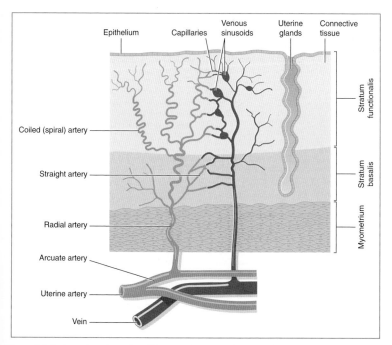

**Figure E.3** Endometrium *(reproduced from Brooker & Nicol 2003 with permission).*

**endomyocardial** *adj* relating to the endocardium and myocardium—**endomyocardium** *n*.

**endomyocarditis** *n* inflammation involving both the endocardium and myocardium.

**endomysium** *n* thin, inner connective tissue surrounding the muscle fibres. ⇒ epimysium, perimysium.

**endoneurium** *n* the delicate, inner connective tissue surrounding the nerve fibres. ⇒ epineurium, perineurium.

**endoparasite** *n* any parasite living within the host, such as threadworms—**endoparasitic** *adj*.

**endopeptidase** *n* an enzyme that catalyses the breakdown of internal peptide bonds between amino acids in a polypeptide or protein.

**endophthalmitis** *n* enophthalmia. A serious inflammation (bacterial or fungal) of the internal eye involving the anterior chamber and vitreous body (humour) and the layers of the wall of the eye. Rarely it may follow eye trauma or eye surgery. Urgent treatment to prevent blindness involves intensive use of topical and intravenous antibiotics. Antibiotics may also be injected into the eye (intracameral route).

**endoplasmic reticulum (ER)** part of the endomembrane system comprising interconnected membranous tubules within the cell cytoplasm. There are two distinct types: rough ER, which have associated ribosomes, and smooth ER, without ribosomes. They are concerned with the synthesis of proteins, lipids and other macromolecules and their transport within the cell.

**end organ** a specialized encapsulated nerve ending in a structure such as the taste buds on the tongue.

**endorphins** *npl* a group of opioid-like neuropeptides. Found in the brain, pituitary gland and the gastrointestinal tract. The three types are alpha, beta and gamma. They are active in both central and peripheral nervous functions where they modulate pain interpretation and induce feelings of euphoria. Also have neurotransmitter properties. ⇒ enkephalins.

**endoscope** *n* instrument for visualization of the interior of hollow tubular structures such as the urinary, respiratory and gastrointestinal tracts, or body cavities, e.g. abdominal cavity and joints. The older ones were rigid metal tubes. Modern ones use fibreoptic technology: light is transmitted by means of very fine glass fibres along a flexible tube (Figure E.4). It permits examination, photography, biopsy and treatment of the cavities or organs of a relaxed (sedated) conscious person—**endoscopic** *adj*, **endoscopy** *n*.

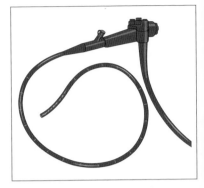

**Figure E.4** Endoscope *(reproduced from Brooker & Nicol 2003 with permission).*

**endoscopic retrograde cholangiopancreatography (ERCP)** introduction of a contrast medium into the pancreatic and bile ducts via a catheter from an endoscope located in the duodenum.

**endoscopy** *n* visualization of hollow organs or structures by use of the appropriate endoscope. ⇒ amnioscopy, antroscopy, arthroscopy, bronchoscopy, choledochoscopy, colonoscopy, culdoscopy, cystoscopy, duodenoscopy, embryoscopy, fetoscopy, hysteroscopy, laparoscopy, laryngoscopy, mediastinoscopy, oesophagogastroduodenoscopy, proctoscopy, sigmoidoscopy, ureteroscopy.

**endospore** *n* a bacterial spore that has a solely vegetative function. It forms during adverse environmental conditions, such as drying. Its metabolism is minimal, thus allowing the micro-organism to resist heat, desiccation and disinfectants. Endospores can remain dormant for long periods and can become active when environmental conditions are suitable for growth and reproduction. The only genera which include spore-forming pathogenic species are *Bacillus* and *Clostridium*.

**endosteum** *n* the membrane that lines the medullary cavity of a long bone. ⇒ periosteum.

**endothelin** *n* a naturally occurring peptide that causes vasoconstriction, found in the smooth muscle of blood vessels. It is important, along with other vasoconstrictor substances and vasodilators (e.g. prostacyclins, nitric oxide), in the balance between vasoconstriction and vasodilation. Abnormal activity of endothelin is associated with conditions that include pulmonary arterial hypertension. Drugs, such as bosentan, which act as endothelin receptor antagonists, can be used for patients with pulmonary arterial hypertension.

**endothelioid** *adj* resembling endothelium.

**endothelioma** *n* a tumour derived from endothelial cells.

**endothelium** *n* a type of specialized epithelial tissue with flat cells. A single layer of endothelium lines the heart, all blood vessels and lymph vessels. Endothelial cells are important in vasoconstriction/vasodilation, haemostasis, the inflammatory response and angiogenesis (growth of new blood vessels). Movement of substances through the capillary walls is facilitated by a wall comprising a single layer of endothelial cells. Highly specialized endothelial cells are part of the blood–brain barrier and the glomerular filtration membrane in glomerulus of the nephron—**endothelial** *adj*.

**endothelium-derived relaxing factor (EDRF)** ⇒ nitric oxide.

**endothermic** *adj* describes a chemical reaction in which there is heat absorption. ⇒ exothermic.

**endotoxin** *n* a toxin found within the cell wall of certain bacteria, e.g. *Neisseria meningitidis*. It is only released if the cell wall is destroyed. ⇒ exotoxin—**endotoxic** *adj*.

**endotracheal** *adj* within the trachea. *endotracheal anaesthesia* the administration of an anaesthetic through an endotracheal tube. *endotracheal tube* a plastic tube introduced via the nose or mouth into the trachea to maintain an airway during general anaesthesia and to facilitate short-term intermittent positive-pressure ventilation.

**endovascular** *adj* intraluminal (within the lumen) surgical approach to correction of vascular abnormalities, e.g. *endovascular stenting* of an abdominal aortic aneurysm.

**end-plate** *n* also known as myoneural junction. The junction between the axon membrane of a motor nerve and the membrane of the muscle fibres. ⇒ motor end-plate.

**end-stage renal disease/failure (ESRD)** the deterioration of chronic renal failure (CRF) to the point of irreversible loss of renal function. Patients with CRF may or may not need renal replacement therapy, but once ESRD is reached they must have replacement therapy, such as haemodialysis, to survive. The causes of ESRD include any condition that disrupts normal kidney structure and function, e.g. diabetes mellitus, reflux nephropathy

(chronic pyelonephritis), glomerulonephritis, adult polycystic kidney disease and hypertension.

**end-systolic volume (ESV)** the volume of blood remaining in the cardiac ventricles at the end of systole. ⇒ stroke volume.

**end-tidal carbon dioxide (ETCO$_2$)** partial pressure of carbon dioxide measured in the breath at the end of expiration. Used to monitor the adequacy of ventilation in mechanically ventilated patients.

**endurance performance** in simple terms, continuous physical activity that lasts between 5 minutes and 4 hours. Although this includes a huge range of physical activities and sports, most of the adenosine triphosphate is produced by aerobic processes.

**enema** *n* the introduction of a liquid into the bowel via the rectum, to be returned or retained. The word is usually preceded by the name of the liquid used. It can be further designated according to the function of the fluid. The evacuant enemas are usually prepared commercially in small bulk as a disposable enema: the chemicals attract water into the bowel, promoting cleansing and peristaltic contractions of the lower bowel. The enemas to be retained are usually drugs, the most common being corticosteroids. ⇒ barium enema, laxatives.

**energy** *n* the capacity to undertake vigorous physical activity or to do work. The SI unit of energy is the joule, but in nutrition the kilojoule (kJ) or megajoule (MJ) is more appropriate.

**energy conservation** techniques, including time management, problem solving and lifestyle planning, that enable an individual to make the best possible use of limited energy reserves. Commonly used in occupational therapy practice.

**energy metabolism** a general term for the chemical reactions involved in the oxidation of metabolic fuels (mainly carbohydrates, fats and proteins under certain circumstances), which provide energy in the form of adenosine triphosphate for body processes.

**enervation** *n* **1.** the surgical removal of an entire nerve, or a part of a nerve. **2.** lack of strength, weakness, lassitude.

**engagement** *n* in obstetrics, when the widest transverse diameter of the presenting part passes through the pelvic brim. In a vertex (head-first) presentation this will be the biparietal diameter, and the bitrochanteric diameter in a breech presentation. In a primigravida, the infant's head normally engages any time after the 36th week of gestation, whereas in multiparous women engagement may not happen until they are in labour.

**enkephalins** *npl* (*syn* encephalins) peptide neurotransmitters present in the central nervous system, and also present in the pituitary gland and gastrointestinal tract. They have opioid-like analgesic effects. ⇒ endorphins.

**enophthalmos** *n* sunken position of an eyeball within its socket.

**enrichment** *n* enriching foods by adding nutrients, e.g. cream or milk powder to soups, in order to increase the amount of nutrients present. Often used interchangeably with the term fortification.

**ensiform** *adj* sword-shaped; xiphoid.

**ENT** *abbr* ear, nose and throat.

**Entamoeba** *n* (*syn* Endamoeba) a genus of protozoon parasites. There are three species infesting humans. Two are non-pathogenic: *Entamoeba coli* in the intestinal tract and *E. gingivalis* in the mouth, whereas *E. histolytica* is pathogenic, causing amoebic dysentery.

**enteral** *adj* within the gastrointestinal tract.

**enteral diets** those which are taken by mouth or through a nasogastric tube; low-residue enteral diets can be whole protein/polymeric, or amino acid/peptide.

**enteral feeding** method of providing nutrition when there is some gastrointestinal tract function. Includes via nasogastric and nasoduodenal tubes or via gastrostomy or jejunostomy tubes. Enteral feeding can be administered by bolus, gravity or pump-controlled methods. ⇒ parenteral feeding, percutaneous endoscopic gastrostomy (PEG).

**enterectomy** *n* excision of part of the intestine.

**enteric** *adj* relating to the small intestine.

**enteric coating** a coating applied to a pill that prevents drug release until it reaches the small intestine. Crushing tablets can alter the way in which the drug is absorbed and metabolized with deleterious effects. A liquid preparation of the drug should always be prescribed in situations where swallowing is difficult.

**enteric fevers** includes typhoid and paratyphoid fever.

**enteritis** *n* inflammation of the intestinal mucosa.

**enteroanastomosis** *n* intestinal anastomosis, a surgical join.

**Enterobacter** *n* a genus of Gram-negative bacilli of the family Enterobacteriaceae, they are facultative anaerobes. Includes two species, *Enterobacter aerogenes* and *E. cloacae*. They

cause infection in hospital, especially of wounds, urinary and respiratory tract. They may cause opportunistic infection in immuno-compromised individuals.

**Enterobacteriaceae** *npl* a family of coliform bacteria that includes *Enterobacter* spp., *Escherichia* spp., *Klebsiella* spp., *Proteus* spp., *Salmonella* spp., *Serratia* spp., *Shigella* spp. and *Yersinia* spp.

**enterobiasis (oxyuriasis)** *n* infestation with *Enterobius vermicularis* (threadworm, pinworm). Because of the autoinfective life cycle, treatment aims at complete elimination. Everyone in the household is given an anthelmintic, mebendazole or, less commonly, piperazine citrate, and hygiene measures, such as hand-washing, not sharing towels or flannels, etc., are also necessary to prevent reinfestation during treatment.

**Enterobius** *n* a genus of parasitic nematode worms. Includes *Enterobius vermicularis* (threadworm, pinworm) which infests the small and large intestine.

**enterocele** *n* prolapse of intestine. Can prolapse into the upper third of vagina.

**enteroclysis** *n* the introduction of fluid into the intestine, such as contrast medium. ⇒ proctoclysis.

**Enterococcus** *n* a genus of Gram-positive cocci commensal in the bowel, e.g. *Enterococcus faecalis*, *E. faecium*. They are facultative anaerobes. They cause urinary tract infection and wound infection and occasionally meningitis in neonates. It is increasingly common as a cause of health care-associated infection, and many strains are developing resistance to antibiotics. ⇒ vancomycin-resistant enterococci (glycopeptide-resistant enterococci).

**enterocolitis** *n* inflammation of the small intestine and colon. ⇒ necrotizing enterocolitis.

**enterocystoplasty** *n* an operation to increase the capacity of the urinary bladder by using part of the small intestine.

**enteroglucagon** *n* one of the glucagon-like peptides, e.g. oxyntomodulin, glicentin, produced by special intestinal cells. They are released in response to the intake of food and are hyperglycaemic.

**enterohepatic circulation** the recycling of bile salts and other substances including drugs that are secreted into bile. They are absorbed from the intestine and returned to the liver via the hepatic portal vein. The returning bile salts stimulate more bile and bile acid production, but recycled drugs, such as morphine, create a pool of active drug that prolongs drug activity and can lead to toxic levels.

**enterokinase** *n* (*syn* enteropeptidase) a proteolytic (protein-splitting) enzyme produced by duodenal mucosa. It converts inactive trypsinogen (pancreatic enzyme) into active trypsin.

**enterolithiasis** *n* the presence of intestinal stones known as enteroliths.

**enteron** *n* the gut.

**enteropathy** *n* any disorder affecting the small intestine, such as gluten-induced enteropathy (coeliac disease).

**enteropeptidase** *n* ⇒ enterokinase.

**enteroscope** *n* an endoscope for visualization of the small intestine—**enteroscopically** *adv*.

**enterostomy** *n* a surgically established fistula between the small intestine and some other surface. ⇒ gastroenterostomy, ileostomy, jejunostomy—**enterostomal** *adj*.

**enterotomy** *n* an incision into the small intestine.

**enterotoxin** *n* a toxin which has its effect on the gastrointestinal tract, causing vomiting, diarrhoea and abdominal pain.

**enterovesical** *adj* pertaining to the intestine and the urinary bladder. *enterovesical fistula* an abnormal communication between the intestine and the urinary bladder. Also called vesicoenteric.

**enteroviruses** *npl* a group of picornaviruses that enter the body by the gastrointestinal tract. Comprise the polioviruses, echoviruses and coxsackieviruses.

**enthesis** *n* the point at which a tendon inserts into a bone.

**Entonox**® *n* proprietary name for a gaseous mixture of oxygen and nitrous oxide in equal measures that is inhaled by the patient to provide analgesia, e.g. in obstetrics, during painful procedures and in intensive care.

**entoptic phenomena** visual phenomena that arise from within the eye itself, such as 'floaters' or flashes.

**entropion** *n* inversion of an eyelid, usually the lower, so that the lashes are in contact with the globe of the eye. It may be caused by spasm of the muscle that normally closes the eyelids (orbicularis oculi), or trauma or disease affecting the conjunctiva or eyelids. Irritation by the eyelashes causes discomfort and tearing (watering). Untreated it can cause corneal ulceration. Treatment is either surgical or the repeated injection of botulinum toxin to relieve the muscle spasm. ⇒ ectropion.

**enucleation** *n* the removal of an organ or tumour in its entirety, as of an eyeball from its socket.

**E numbers** identification numbers used in the European Union for permitted food additives. The categories include antioxidants (e.g. E300 ascorbic acid); colours (e.g. E102 tartrazine); emulsifiers, gelling agents, stabilizers and thickeners (e.g. E460 cellulose); preservatives (e.g. E211 sodium benzoate); sweeteners (e.g. E951 aspartame); and others such as E570 fatty acids. The food additive may be identified by name or E number on food labelling.

**enuresis** *n* incontinence of urine, especially bed-wetting. *nocturnal enuresis* bed-wetting during sleep.

**environment** *n* external surroundings. Living organisms are influenced by the physical and chemical conditions of the environment external to them, and by those within the organism—**environmental** *adj*.

**environmental adaptation** in occupational therapy, the modifications made to the physical or social characteristics of an environment so as to improve performance, encourage or discourage a behaviour or provide therapy.

**enzyme** *n* a protein that functions as a catalyst for specific biochemical reactions involving specific substrates. Many reactions in the body would proceed too slowly without an enzyme, e.g. waste carbon dioxide would not be removed from the tissues without the enzyme carbonic anhydrase. Enzyme names often reflect their function, e.g. dehydrogenases catalyse the removal of hydrogen in oxidation reactions.

**enzyme activation assays** techniques used to assess the level of certain vitamins, for example vitamins $B_1$, $B_2$ and $B_6$.

**enzyme induction** the ability of some chemicals, e.g. alcohol, environmental chemicals and drugs, to increase the secretion of liver enzymes. ⇒ cytochromes. The increase in enzyme production can speed up the rate at which the inducer drug and others are metabolized and excreted. There is loss of drug effectiveness, e.g. the oral contraceptive is inactivated by rifampicin (antituberculosis drug). In some situations the induction of enzyme production may increase drug effects such as the toxic metabolites formed in paracetamol overdose.

**enzyme inhibitors** chemicals, including many drugs that inhibit specific enzymes in the body. The inhibition may be reversible or irreversible. Some inhibitors are false substrates (very similar to the normal substrate of the enzyme) and act as competitive inhibitors, e.g. some cytotoxic drugs inhibit the enzyme needed by cancer cells for folic acid use. Others inhibit liver enzymes and increase the effects of other drugs. For example, aspirin inhibits the enzymes needed to metabolize oral anticoagulants, which causes increased anticoagulation with the risk of bleeding.

**enzyme-linked immunosorbent assay (ELISA)** an assay technique for measuring soluble substances based on recognition of the target antigen by specific antibodies, linked to an enzyme which causes a colour change in a substrate solution. The degree of colour change is proportional to the concentration of the substance being examined. It is used to test for the presence of antibodies to human immunodeficiency virus (HIV). All positive tests for HIV are confirmed by the more precise Western blot test before HIV infection is established.

**EOG** *abbr* electro-oculogram.

**eosin** *n* a red staining agent used in histology and laboratory diagnostic procedures.

**eosinopenia** *n* a reduction in the number of eosinophils (leucocytes) in the blood.

**eosinophil** *n* **1.** cells having an affinity for eosin. **2.** a type of polymorphonuclear leucocyte containing eosin-staining granules. It is associated with immune responses that involve allergies and immunoglobulin E (IgE)—**eosinophilic** *adj*.

**eosinophilia** *n* increased number of eosinophils in the blood. Indicative of an allergic condition, a parasitic infestation and a rarer form of leukaemia.

**EPA** *abbr* eicosapentaenoic acid.

**EPEC** *abbr* enteropathic *Escherichia coli*.

**ependymal cells** part of the macroglia. A type of neuroglial cell that lines the fluid-filled cavities of the central nervous system (cerebral ventricles and the central canal of the spinal cord).

**ependymoma** *n* neoplasm arising in the lining of the cerebral ventricles or central canal of spinal cord. Occurs in all age groups.

**ephelides** *npl* freckles caused by an increase in pigment granules with a normal number of pigment cells. ⇒ lentigo—**ephelis** *sing*.

**ephebiatrics** *n* a branch of medicine that specializes in the care of older children and adolescents.

**epicanthus** *n* epicanthal or epicanthic fold. The congenital occurrence of a variable-size fold of skin that obscures the inner canthus of the eye. A normal feature in some racial groups in Asia, it may also be seen abnormally in infants with Down's syndrome—**epicanthal** *adj*.

**epicardium** *n* the visceral layer of the pericardium—**epicardial** *adj*.

**epicondyle** *n* an eminence on some bones situated above the condyles, e.g. femoral epicondyles.

**epicondylitis** *n* inflammation of the muscles and tendons around the elbow. Can occur if the structures are subjected to excess or repetitive stress. It may affect the structures at the lateral (outer) or medial (inner) aspect of the elbow. *lateral epicondylitis* (*syn* tennis elbow) is associated with tennis, other racquet sports and weight training. *medial epicondylitis* (*syn* golfer's elbow) is primarily an overuse injury associated with golf and poor lifting techniques. ⇒ bursitis.

**epicranium** *n* the structures comprising the scalp—muscles, aponeuroses and the skin.

**epicritic** *adj* describes cutaneous nerve fibres which are sensitive to fine variations of touch and vibration. Concerned with proprioception and two-point discrimination. ⇒ protopathic *opp*.

**epidemic** *n* a disease, such as measles or influenza, simultaneously affecting many people in an area (more than the expected number). ⇒ endemic *opp*.

**epidemic myalgia, epidemic pleurodynia** ⇒ Bornholm disease.

**epidemiology** *n* the scientific study of the distribution of diseases, risk factors and determinants. It is concerned with the incidence, distribution and control of disease—**epidemiological** *adj*, **epidemiologically** *adv*.

**epidermal growth factor (EGF)** a protein growth factor that promotes cell growth and differentiation. Its role is important during embryonic development and in wound healing. ⇒ transforming growth factor. *epidermal growth factor receptors* some cancers produce EGF, e.g. some metastatic colorectal cancers. A monoclonal antibody cetuximab is used, in some cases, to 'block' the EGF receptors, thereby preventing EGF from stimulating further abnormal cell growth. ⇒ human epidermal growth factor receptor-2.

**epidermis** *n* the outer avascular layer of the skin. It comprises several layers and is constantly being renewed as cells in the deeper layers divide, move upwards and are shed as flat, keratinized cells from the skin surface.

(⇒ Appendix 1, Figure 12); the cuticle—**epidermal** *adv.*

**epidermolysis bullosa** a group of inherited diseases where the skin is very fragile and even very minor trauma results in bulla or blister formation. ⇒ Cockayne's disease.

*Epidermophyton* *n* a genus of fungi affecting the skin and nails. ⇒ dermatophytes, tinea.

**epidermophytosis** *n* infection with fungi of the genus *Epidermophyton* such as ringworm.

**epididymectomy** *n* surgical removal of the epididymis.

**epididymis** *n* a small oblong body attached to the posterior surface of the testes (⇒ Appendix 1, Figure 16). It consists of the seminiferous tubules which carry the spermatozoa from the testes to the deferent ducts (vas deferens).

**epididymitis** *n* inflammation of the epididymis. It is a bacterial infection usually caused by *Escherichia coli* or *Chlamydia trachomatis*; there is acute pain and swelling. Rarely due to tuberculosis and possibly secondary to urological surgery. It is vital to differentiate between epididymitis and testicular torsion, as the latter requires urgent surgical correction.

**epididymo-orchitis** *n* inflammation of the epididymis and the testis.

**epididymovasostomy** *n* an operation to join the epididymis to the deferent duct (vas deferens) in order to bypass a mechanical blockage in a man with azoospermia, and occasionally to reverse a vasectomy.

**epidural** *adj* upon or external to the dura mater (outer meningeal membrane). *epidural anaesthesia* local anaesthetic injected into the space external to the dura either by single injection or intermittently via a catheter, causing loss of sensation in an area determined by the site of the injection and volume of local anaesthetic used (Figure E.5). Used extensively in obstetrics, and increasingly during and after surgery. *epidural space* the region through which spinal nerves leave the spinal cord. It can be approached at any level of the spine, but the administering of anaesthetic is commonly done at the lumbar level or through the sacral cornua for caudal epidural block. ⇒ patient-controlled analgesia.

**epigastrium** *n* the upper, central abdominal region lying directly over the stomach (⇒ Appendix 1, Figure 18A)—**epigastric** *adj.*

**epigastrocele** *n* epigastric hernia. The protrusion of internal structures through the linea alba.

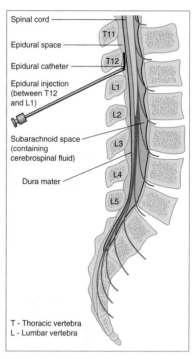

**Figure E.5** Epidural (reproduced from Brooker & Waugh 2007 with permission).

**epiglottis** *n* the thin leaf-shaped flap of cartilage attached to the top of the larynx which, during the act of swallowing, covers the opening leading into the larynx, thus preventing food or fluids entering the larynx and trachea. ⇒ Appendix 1, Figure 6.

**epiglottitis** *n* inflammation of the epiglottis. Acute epiglottis, caused by the bacterium *Haemophilus influenzae* type B, is a serious condition that usually affects young children. There is fever, sore throat, croupy cough and inspiratory stridor. Swelling of the epiglottis may compromise the airway necessitating an emergency tracheostomy. ⇒ Hib vaccine.

**epikeratophakia** *n* surgical introduction of a biological 'lens' into the cornea to correct hypermetropia or keratoconus.

**epilation** *n* extraction or destruction of hair roots, e.g. by coagulation necrosis, electrolysis or forceps. ⇒ depilation—**epilate** *vt.*

**epilatory** *adj, n* (describes) an agent which produces epilation.

**epilepsy** *n* correctly called the epilepsies, a group of conditions resulting from disordered electrical activity in the brain and manifesting as epileptic seizures or 'fits'. The seizure is caused by an abnormal electrical discharge that disturbs cerebration and results in a generalized or partial seizure, depending on the area of the brain involved. (a) *Generalized seizures* may be *tonic–clonic (grand mal)*, the commonest type of epileptic seizure with loss of consciousness and generalized convulsions; or *absences (petit mal)* where there is a brief alteration in consciousness. (b) *Partial seizures* occur when the electrical disturbance is limited to a particular focus of the brain and are manifested in a variety of ways, including motor problems characterized by limb twitching that may spread, known as Jacksonian epilepsy. In *complex partial seizures* (also known as *psychomotor epilepsy* or *temporal lobe epilepsy*) there may be altered consciousness, paraesthesia, visual hallucinations, such as coloured patterns, and psychomotor seizures where there are changes to mood, behaviour, perception and memory with more complex hallucinations and physical manifestations, such as nausea. ⇒ uncinate epilepsy. *Secondary generalized seizures* occur when partial seizure activity spreads to involve other areas of the brain and awareness is lost. ⇒ status epilepticus.

**epileptic 1.** *adj* pertaining to epilepsy. **2.** *n* a person with epilepsy. *epileptic aura* premonitory subjective phenomena (tingling in the hand or visual or auditory sensations) that precede an attack of major epilepsy. ⇒ aura.

**epileptiform** *adj* resembling epilepsy.

**epileptogenic** *adj* capable of causing epilepsy.

**epiloia** *n* ⇒ tuberous sclerosis.

**epimenorrhoea** *n* reduction of the length of the menstrual cycle.

**epimysium** *n* outer fibrous coat surrounding an entire muscle. ⇒ endomysium, perimysium.

**epinephrine** *n* ⇒ adrenaline.

**epineurium** *n* outer fibrous coat enclosing a nerve trunk. ⇒ endoneurium, perineurium.

**epiphora** *n* tearing. The pathological overflow of tears on to the cheek.

**epiphysis** *n* the end of a bone. During growth the epiphysis is separated from the shaft (diaphysis) by the epiphyseal plate (cartilage), from which growth in length occurs. The epiphyseal plate is replaced with bone (ossification) when growth ceases—**epiphyses** *pl*, **epiphyseal** *adj*. ⇒ diaphysis.

**epiphysitis** *n* inflammation of an epiphysis; can cause abnormal bone growth and deformity.

**episclera** *n* loose connective tissue between the sclera and conjunctiva—**episcleral** *adj*.

**episcleritis** *n* inflammation of the episclera.

**episiorrhaphy** *n* surgical repair of a lacerated perineum.

**episiotomy** *n* a perineal incision made during the birth of an infant to enlarge the vulval outlet. It may be performed to avoid maternal trauma with tearing of the perineum, or to hasten the delivery if the infant is distressed. It may also be required for a forceps delivery.

**episodic memory** the part of long-term memory responsible for storing personal experiences. It is organized with respect to when and where the experience occurred, e.g. an episode from the last performance review interview.

**epispadias** *n* a congenital opening of the urethra on the dorsal aspect of the penis, often associated with ectopia vesicae. ⇒ hypospadias.

**epistasis** *n* a particular interaction between genes. One gene modifies the action of a gene at a different locus. It may, for instance, suppress the expression of that gene.

**epistaxis** *n* bleeding from the nose. Local causes include nasal trauma such as from a punch or nose picking, tumours, nasal infections and sudden changes in atmospheric pressure. Bleeding from the nose may be a feature of coagulation disorders, hypertension, arteriosclerosis and anticoagulant drugs—**epistaxes** *pl*. ⇒ Little's area.

**epistemology** *n* theory of the grounds of knowledge. The discussion about knowledge and 'truth' and how it varies between different disciplines.

**epithalamus** *n* part of the diencephalon. It is above and behind the thalamus. Contains the pineal body (gland) and forms part of the third ventricle.

**epithelialization** *n* the growth of epithelium over a raw area; the final stage of wound healing.

**epithelioma** *n* a tumour arising from any epithelium.

**epithelium** *n* one of the four basic tissues. It lines cavities, covers the body and forms glands. It is classified according to the arrangement and shape of the cells it contains (Figure E.6). It may be simple, a single layer of squamous, cuboidal or columnar, or stratified with many layers, e.g. stratified or transitional—**epithelial** *adj*.

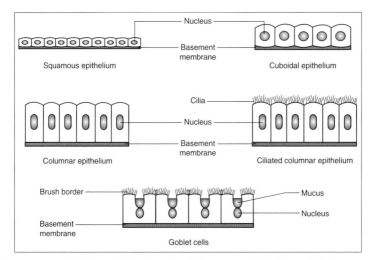

**Figure E.6** Types of simple epithelium *(reproduced from Watson 2000 with permission)*.

**epitope** *n* also known as antigenic determinant. The part (or region) of an antigen recognized by a specific antibody or T-cell receptor. The location at which the paratope of the antibody binds to and acts on the antigen. ⇒ paratope.

**Epley manoeuvre** particle-repositioning manoeuvre. A specific cycle of positions and movements used to relieve benign paroxysmal positional vertigo. The aim is to move debris in the semicircular canals to a more favourable location.

**EPO** *abbr* erythropoietin.

**EPOC** *abbr* excess postexercise oxygen consumption.

**eponychium** *n* the cuticle of the nail. It covers the thickened proximal edge of the nail—the lunula.

**eponym** *n* a place, anatomical structure, biochemical process, micro-organism, sign, a species or a disease/condition, etc., named after a person. For example, Bartholin's glands, Cori cycle, *Borrelia*, Cullen's sign, Addison's disease, etc. Increasingly replaced by a standard descriptive nomenclature, for example, Bartholin's glands are the greater vestibular glands—**eponymous** *adj*.

**epoophoron** *n* vestigial remains of the embryonic mesonephric duct located between the ovary and uterine tube. ⇒ paroophoron.

**Epsom salts** ⇒ magnesium sulphate.

**Epstein–Barr virus (EBV)** (M Epstein, British pathologist and virologist, b. 1921; Y Barr, British pathologist and virologist, b. 1932) a herpesvirus, the causative agent of infectious mononucleosis (glandular fever). Also linked with the formation of some malignant tumours, including Burkitt's lymphoma and nasopharyngeal cancer.

**equality of opportunity** equal access to opportunities for decent housing, education, a job, health care, etc., regardless of age, gender, race, religion, ability or social class.

**equinus** *n* a condition in which the toes point down and the person walks on tiptoe. ⇒ talipes.

**equity** *n* fairness of distribution of resources such as health care. Access to resources is based on need and the ability to receive benefit. The ability of a health care system to provide a comparable level of health care across the entire population. Covers the following dimensions: need for health care in the population (dependent on epidemiology of disease, determinants of health); availability, accessibility of health care resources; distribution of health care resources; use (utilization) of health care resources; geographic variation in need and health care utilization.

**epulis** *n* a tumour growing on or from the gums.

**ER** *abbr* endoplasmic reticulum.

**Erb's palsy** (W Erb, German neurologist, 1840–1921) paralysis involving the shoulder and arm muscles from a lesion of the fifth and sixth cervical nerve roots. The arm hangs loosely at the side with the forearm pronated ('waiter's-tip position'). Most commonly caused by a birth injury.

**ERCP** *abbr* endoscopic retrograde cholangiopancreatography.

**erectile** *adj* upright; capable of being elevated. *erectile dysfunction* (ED) a common condition defined as the inability of a man to gain an erection of sufficient quality for intercourse. The aetiology and associated risk factors are often multiple and include psychological, drug side-effects, vascular, neurological, endocrinological and traumatic. Psychological problems are self-perpetuating, as each failure increases the associated anxiety and can lead to the continual inability to achieve an erection. *erectile tissue* vascular tissue, which, under stimulus, becomes rigid and erect from hyperaemia.

**erection** *n* the state accomplished when erectile tissue is hyperaemic.

**erector** *n* a muscle which achieves erection of a part. *erector spinae* three muscles of the back—iliocostalis, longissimus and spinalis. ⇒ Appendix 1, Figure 5.

**ERG** *abbr* **1.** electroretinogram. **2.** epidermal growth factor.

**ergocalciferol** *n* vitamin $D_2$ obtained from the diet. It is formed from the plant sterol ergosterol.

**ergogenic** *adj* a propensity to increase the output of work.

**ergogenic aids** measures taken to enhance sporting performance. Some aids may be allowed within the rules of the sport but others may be prohibited. The methods include mechanical, dietary supplementation, pharmaceutical, hormonal and psychological. ⇒ blood doping, anabolic steroids.

**ergometry** *n* measurement of work done by muscles—**ergometric** *adj*.

**ergonomics** *n* the study of the work environment and efficient energy use.

**ergosterol** *n* a sterol provitamin found in plants and fungi, particularly yeast. It is converted to ergocalciferol (vitamin $D_2$) by ultraviolet radiation, which is used to fortify foodstuffs with vitamin D.

**ergot** *n* a fungus, *Claviceps purpurea*, which infects rye. There are two important derivatives: (a) ergometrine, used to stimulate uterine contraction, thus preventing or minimizing postpartum haemorrhage; and (b) ergotamine, which may occasionally be used for migraine. It has been mostly replaced by simple analgesics or specific and more effective medications. ⇒ 5-HT$_1$ agonists.

**ergotism** *n* poisoning by ergot, which may cause gangrene, particularly of the fingers and toes.

**erosion** *n* a gradual wearing away of a surface caused by chemical processes or physical events. For example, erosion of the tooth enamel from acidic foods and beverages.

**ERPC** *abbr* evacuation of retained products of conception.

**errorless learning** methods of learning in which trial and error, and hence the making of mistakes, is avoided.

**erucic acid** a toxic fatty acid, found in rapeseed and mustard seed oils. Varieties of rapeseed (canola) with low levels of erucic acid have been developed for food use. ⇒ canola.

**eructation** *n* belching. The bringing-up of air from the stomach, with a characteristic sound. ⇒ aerophagia.

**eruption** *n* **1.** the process by which a tooth emerges through the alveolar bone and gingiva. **2.** the rapid formation of skin lesions, such as a rash occurring following the administration of a drug.

**erysipelas** *n* an acute infectious disease, usually caused by haemolytic streptococci. There is a spreading inflammation of the skin and subcutaneous tissues, accompanied by systemic effects such as fever. ⊙DVD

**erysipeloid** *n* a skin condition resembling erysipelas. It occurs in butchers, fishmongers or cooks. The infecting organism is *Erysipelothrix rhusiopathiae* (*E. insidiosa*), which causes a type of erysipelas that affects pigs, sheep, birds, reptiles and fish, etc.

***Erysipelothrix*** *n* a genus of parasitic bacteria that includes *Erysipelothrix rhusiopathiae* (*E. insidiosa*).

**erythema** *n* reddening of the skin due to vascular congestion—**erythematous** *adj*. *erythema induratum* Bazin's disease. *erythema multiforme* a form of acute toxic or allergic eruption. The lesions are in the form of target-like papules often on the hands. A severe form, called Stevens–Johnson syndrome, may involve mucous membranes. ⊙DVD *erythema nodosum* an eruption of painful red nodules on the front of the legs. It may be a symptom of internal disease, including tuberculosis and sarcoidosis. *erythema pernio* ⇒ chilblain.

**erythrasma** *n* a skin infection caused by the bacterium *Corynebacterium minutissimum*. It tends to occur in the axilla and the groin.

**erythroblast** *n* a nucleated erythrocyte precursor found in the red bone marrow—**erythroblastic** *adj*.

**erythroblastosis** *n* the abnormal presence of nucleated erythrocyte precursors in the blood. This may occur in situations when erythropoiesis (production of erythrocytes) is increased, such as in severe anaemia or when the bone marrow is affected by leukaemia or secondary cancer.

**erythroblastosis fetalis** ⇒ haemolytic disease of the newborn.

**erythrocyanosis** *n* a mottled red or purplish discoloration and swelling of the legs, particularly in cold weather. It commonly affects children, adolescents and older women.

**erythrocyte glutathione reductase** an enzyme present in erythrocytes. It is used for an enzyme activation assay to determine riboflavin (vitamin B$_2$) status.

**erythrocyte sedimentation rate (ESR)** citrated blood is placed in a narrow tube. The erythrocytes (red cells) fall, leaving a column of clear supernatant serum, which is measured at the end of an hour and reported in millimetres. It varies according to age and gender. Inflammation and tissue destruction cause an elevation in the ESR.

**erythrocytes** *npl* red blood cells. Non-nucleated red cells of the circulating blood. They carry oxygen and some carbon dioxide, and buffer pH changes in the blood. They are highly specialized for transporting oxygen from the lungs to the tissues and cells. Without a nucleus they are full of haemoglobin. In addition erythrocytes have no mitochondria (or other organelles) and rely on anaerobic glycolysis for energy production and therefore do not use the oxygen, which they carry. Mature erythrocytes are biconcave discs with a diameter of 7.0 μm and 2.2 μm thick (Figure E.7). Their surface-area-to-volume ratio optimizes the transport of oxygen and carbon dioxide to and from the cells. Various genetically determined antigens are present on the surface of the erythrocytes, including those for the ABO blood groups—**erythrocytic** *adj*.

**erythrocytopenia** *n* deficiency in the number of erythrocytes (red blood cells)—**erythrocytopenic** *adj*.

**erythrocytosis** *n* ⇒ polycythaemia.

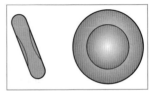

**Figure E.7** Mature erythrocytes *(reproduced from Watson 2000 with permission).*

**erythroderma** *n* excessive redness of the skin, typically involving more than 90% of the skin surface.

**erythroedema polyneuropathy** (*syn* acrodynia, pink disease) a condition of infancy characterized by red, swollen extremities, generalized skin rash, photophobia and irritability. May be caused by mercury poisoning.

**erythrolabe** *n* a pigment contained in one group of cones; responds to light at the red end of the spectrum.

**erythropoiesis** *n* the production of erythrocytes (red blood cells) by the bone marrow. ⇒ erythropoietin, haemopoiesis.

**erythropoietin (EPO)** *n* a glycoprotein hormone/growth factor secreted mainly by kidney cells in response to reduced oxygen content in the blood, and also secreted by fetal liver cells. It acts on the bone marrow, stimulating erythropoiesis. A recombinant human form is used therapeutically to treat anaemia associated with chronic renal failure and platinum-containing chemotherapy.

**erythropsia** *n* an abnormality of vision where all objects are seen as red.

**eschar** *n* a slough, as results from a burn, application of caustics, diathermy, etc.

**escharotomy** *n* surgical incision into eschar to relieve restriction around a limb that could compromise the blood supply, or the chest to allow chest expansion.

***Escherichia*** *n* (T Escherich, German physician, 1857–1911) a genus of bacteria of the family Enterobacteriaceae. Motile, Gram-negative bacilli that are widely distributed in nature. *Escherichia coli* is part of the normal flora in humans. Some strains are pathogens, causing gastroenteritis, peritonitis and wound infections, meningitis and urinary tract infections. The serotypes responsible for gastroenteritis are: (a) enterohaemorrhagic *E. coli* (EHEC), e.g. *E. coli* O157, a virulent micro-organism that produces a toxin (verocytotoxin) and causes a variety of effects from mild diarrhoea to severe haemorrhagic bowel inflammation. It may cause life-threatening haemolytic–uraemic syndrome; (b) enteroinvasive *E. coli* (EIEC), which causes blood-stained diarrhoea; (c) enteropathic *E. coli* (EPEC), which causes serious diarrhoea in babies, especially in developing countries; (d) enterotoxigenic *E. coli* (ETEC), responsible for outbreaks of gastroenteritis in developing countries. Leads to watery diarrhoea with fluid and electrolyte imbalance.

**Esmarch's bandage** (J von Esmarch, German surgeon, 1823–1908) a rubber roller bandage sometimes used to procure a bloodless operative field in the limbs.

**esophoria** *n* latent convergent strabismus.

**esotropia** *n* manifest convergent strabismus.

**ESP** *abbr* **1.** extended-scope physiotherapy practitioner. **2.** extrasensory perception.

**espundia** *n* ⇒ leishmaniasis.

**ESR** *abbr* erythrocyte sedimentation rate.

**ESRD/F** *abbr* end-stage renal disease/failure. ⇒ renal failure.

**essential amino acids** also known as indispensable. The amino acids that cannot be synthesized in the body and therefore have to be provided by the diet. They are isoleucine, leucine, lysine, methionine, phenylalanine, threonine, tryptophan and valine in adults. Infants need these amino acids plus histidine and arginine. Other amino acids are considered to be conditionally essential because they become essential if the diet does not contain enough of the precursor amino acid from which they are synthesized: arginine, cysteine, glycine and tyrosine. ⇒ amino acids.

**essential fatty acids (EFAs)** the linoleic and alpha (α)-linolenic families of fatty acids. Polyunsaturated fatty acids (PUFAs) that cannot be synthesized in the body so must be supplied by the diet. Arachidonic, eicosapentaenoic and docosahexaenoic acids can all be synthesized from linoleic and α-linolenic acids, and become essential if linoleic and α-linolenic acids are in short supply. They have diverse functions, which include being the precursors for many regulatory lipids, e.g. prostaglandins; they fulfil an important role in lipid metabolism and are required for the integrity of cell membranes. They are present in oily fish and natural vegetable and seed oils.

**essential oil** the undiluted oil extracted from plants, usually diluted in a carrier oil prior to use during aromatherapy.

**establishment** *n* describes the planned staffing levels in a particular area. Usually described as the number of whole-time equivalents (WTEs).

**ester** *n* an organic compound (a 'salt') formed from an organic acid and an alcohol. For instance, acetates are formed when the acid is acetic acid.

**esterase** *n* an enzyme that splits esters into an acid and an alcohol.

**estimated average requirement (EAR)** one of the UK dietary reference values. It estimates the average requirement for a group of people, usually for energy requirements. It follows that 50% of people in the group will need more and 50% will need less. ⇒ dietary reference values.

**estradiol** *n Am* ⇒ oestradiol.

**estrogen** *n Am* ⇒ oestrogen.

**ESWL** *abbr* extracorporeal shock-wave lithotripsy.

**ESV** *abbr* end-systolic volume.

**ETCO$_2$** *abbr* end-tidal carbon dioxide.

**ETEC** *abbr* enterotoxigenic *Escherichia coli*.

**ethanol** *n* ethyl alcohol. The alcohol in alcoholic beverages.

**ether** *n* early volatile anaesthetic agent (now rarely used).

**ethics** *n* a code of moral principles derived from a system of values and beliefs. It is concerned with rights and obligations.

**ethics committees** bodies that operate in academic institutions, Health Authorities and NHS Trusts to consider proposals for research projects. The approval of the appropriate ethics committee is usually a prerequisite for obtaining a research grant.

**ethmoid** *n* a spongy bone at the base of the cranium. It contains the ethmoidal air sinuses and forms the lateral walls of the nose and the upper portion of the bony nasal septum, the cribriform plate. ⇒ cribriform.

**ethmoidectomy** *n* surgical removal of a part or all of the ethmoid bone.

**ethnic** *adj* relating to a social group who have common customs and culture. Frequently used incorrectly to describe race.

**ethnocentrism** *n* the belief that one's own culture and lifestyle are superior to those of other groups. Often makes the assumption that the beliefs, values, priorities and views of one's culture are universal.

**ethnography** *n* a study of individuals in their usual surroundings. Used in qualitative research by anthropologists to describe customs, culture and social life through observation, informal interviews, etc.

**ethnology** *n* a branch of anthropology that studies mainly the cultural differences between social groups, particularly the beliefs, attitudes and values pertaining to life events that include birth, marriage, health care, death, etc.—**ethnological** *adj*, **ethnologically** *adv*.

**ethyl chloride** a volatile liquid used to test the onset of regional anaesthesia by reason of the intense cold sensation produced when applied to the skin.

**ethylene diamine tetra-acetic acid (EDTA)** a chelating agent that binds to metals such as calcium, mercury, iron, lead, etc. Used to treat severe hypercalcaemia and occasionally for mercury poisoning. Used in food processing and in many other industrial applications.

**ethylene oxide** a gas used to sterilize delicate equipment that would be damaged by high temperatures.

**EUA** *abbr* examination under anaesthetic.

*Eubacterium* *n* a genus of Gram-positive anaerobic bacteria with rigid cell walls, normally present in water and soil. They are of low pathogenicity but do sometimes cause soft-tissue infections and may be implicated in periodontal disease.

**eugenics** *n* the study of genetics aimed at improving future generations—**eugenic** *adj*.

**eugnathia** *n* a normal jaw, one in which the maxilla and mandible are in correct alignment.

**eunuch** *n* a human male from whom the testes have been removed; a castrated male.

**eupepsia** *n* normal digestion.

**euphoria** *n* in psychiatry, an exaggerated sense of well-being—**euphoric** *adj*.

**euploidy** *n* having a deviation in chromosome number, which is a precise multiple of the haploid (n) number.

**European Food Safety Authority (EFSA)** the agency in the European Union that assesses risks to food safety and issues independent scientific advice about food safety. Its remit covers the entire food chain.

**European Medicines Agency (EMEA)** an agency of the European Union tasked with protecting and promoting the health of people and animals by evaluating and supervising human and veterinary medicines.

**eustachian tube** (B Eustachio, Italian anatomist, 1524–1574). ⇒ pharyngotympanic (auditory) tube.

**eustress** *n* ⇒ stress.

**euthanasia** *n* literally, an 'easy death'. Inferring a painless death. Frequently interpreted as the act of causing a painless and planned death, such as relieving a person's extreme suffering from an incurable disease. Presently illegal in UK and opposed by many professional groups, it is practised legally in some European countries. ⇒ homicide.

**euthyroid state** denoting normal thyroid function.

**eutocia** *n* a natural and normal labour and childbirth without any complications.

**eutrophia** *n* normal nutrition.

**evacuant** *n* an agent which initiates an evacuation, such as of the bowel. ⇒ enema, laxatives.

**evacuation** *n* the act of emptying a cavity; generally refers to the discharge of faecal matter from the rectum. *manual evacuation* digital removal of faeces from the rectum. *evacuation of retained products of conception (ERPC)* emptying the uterus following an incomplete miscarriage.

**evacuator** *n* an instrument for procuring evacuation, e.g. the removal from the bladder of a stone, crushed by a lithotrite.

**evaporate** *vt, vi* to convert from the liquid to the gaseous state by the application of heat.

**evaporating lotion** one which, applied as a compress, absorbs heat in order to evaporate and so cools the skin.

**evening primrose oil** a source of γ-linoleic acid. Sometimes used to relieve the symptoms of premenstrual syndrome.

**eventration** *n* the protrusion of the intestines through a wound in the abdominal wall. ⇒ dehiscence.

**eversion** *n* a turning outwards, as of the upper eyelid to expose the palpebral conjunctiva.

**evidence-based medicine (EBM) practice (EBP)** describes the practice of medicine or delivery of health care interventions that are based on systematic analysis of information available in terms of effectiveness in relation to cost-effective health outcomes. The highest level of evidence (based on the robustness of the research methodology) is that gained from meta-analysis of randomized controlled trials (RCTs). Sometimes this level of evidence is not available and at the lowest level may be based on evidence from expert committee reports or opinions and/or clinical experience of respected practitioners.

**evisceration** *n* removal of internal organs.

**evulsion** *n* forcible tearing away of a structure.

**Ewing's tumour** (J Ewing, American pathologist, 1866–1943) sarcoma involving a long bone, usually diagnosed in a child or young adult.

E

**exacerbation** *n* increased severity, as of symptoms.

**exanthema** *n* a skin eruption—**exanthemata** *pl*, **exanthematous** *adj*.

**excess postexercise oxygen consumption (EPOC)** ⇒ oxygen debt.

**exercise-induced asthma** bronchospasm caused by exercise in a cold, dry climate.

**exercise physiology** involves the description and explanation of functional changes in the body brought about by either a single or repeated exercise sessions. ☞

**excision** *n* removal of a part by cutting—**excise** *vt*.

**excitability** *n* rapid response to stimuli; easily irritated, such as nerve and muscle cells—**excitable** *adj*.

**excitation** *n* the act of stimulating an organ or tissue.

**exchange list** food portions which contain the same amount of energy, carbohydrate, fat and/or protein. Used to simplify meal, snack and diet planning for people with special dietary requirements.

**exchange transfusion** ⇒ transfusion.

**excimer laser** a type of laser that removes very thin layers of tissue. Used to treat certain corneal pathologies, and in the surgical correction of refractive errors.

**exclusion diet** excluding foods that commonly cause food intolerance, then adding specific foods in order to test for intolerance.

**exclusion isolation** ⇒ protective isolation.

**excoriation** *n* ⇒ abrasion.

**excrement** *n* faeces.

**excrescence** *n* an abnormal protuberance or growth of the tissues.

**excreta** *n* the waste material that is normally cleared from the body, particularly urine and faeces.

**excretion** *n* the elimination of waste material from the body, and also the eliminated material—**excretory** *adj*, **excrete** *vt*.

**exenteration** *n* removal of the viscera from its containing cavity, e.g. the eye from its socket, the pelvic organs from the pelvis.

**exercise** *n* physical activity that aims to improve or maintain health, increase mobility during rehabilitation and improve strength, stamina, suppleness and physical performance. ⇒ aerobic exercise, anaerobic exercise, isometric exercise, isotonic exercise.

**exercise economy** the oxygen uptake needed to generate a specific speed or power output.

**exfoliation** *n* **1.** the scaling-off of tissues in layers. **2.** the shedding of the primary teeth—**exfoliative** *adj*.

**exfoliative cytology** ⇒ cytology.

**ex gratia** as a matter of favour, e.g. without admission of liability, of payment offered by an NHS Trust to a claimant.

**exhalation** *n* expiration, breathing out.

**exhibitionism** *n* **1.** any kind of 'showing off'; extravagant behaviour to attract attention. **2.** a psychosexual disorder confined to males and consisting of repeated exposure of the genitalia to a stranger who is usually an adult female or a child. The act of exposure is sufficient and usually no further contact is sought with the victim—**exhibitionist** *n*.

**exocrine** *adj* describes glands from which the secretion passes via a duct; secreting externally, e.g. sweat glands. ⇒ endocrine *opp*—**exocrinal** *adj*.

**exocytosis** *n* a term for the process by which some molecules, e.g. some hormones and mucus, leave cells. ⇒ endocytosis *opp*.

**exodontics** *n* the practice of removing teeth from the mouth.

**exoenzyme** *n* an enzyme that acts outside the cell from which it was secreted, e.g. pepsin.

**exogenous** *adj* of external origin. ⇒ endogenous *opp*.

**exomphalos** *n* (*syn* omphalocele) a condition present at birth and due to failure of the gut to return to the abdominal cavity during fetal development. The intestines and sometimes other structures, including the liver, protrude through a defect in the abdominal wall around the umbilical cord.

**exon** *n* a gene segment that is represented in the messenger RNA product. It is involved in protein production, with each exon coding a specific part of the finished protein. ⇒ intron.

**exopeptidase** *n* an enzyme that catalyses the breaking of the terminal peptide bonds between amino acids in a polypeptide or protein.

**exophoria** *n* latent divergent strabismus.

**exophthalmos** *n* protrusion of the eyeball—**exophthalmic** *adj*.

**exophthalmometer/proptometer** *n* an instrument that measures the degree of exophthalmos.

**exostosis** *n* an overgrowth of bone tissue forming a benign tumour.

**exothermic** *adj* describes a chemical reaction in which there is release of heat. ⇒ endothermic.

**exotoxin** *n* a toxin released through the cell wall of a living bacterium, e.g. *Clostridium tetani*. They have extensive systemic effects, which include muscle spasm. ⇒ endotoxin—**exotoxic** *adj*.

**exotropia** *n* manifest divergent strabismus.

**expected date of delivery (EDD)** usually calculated as 280 days from the first day of the last normal menstrual period.

**expectorant** *n* a drug which may promote expectoration.

**expectoration** *n* **1.** the elimination of secretions from the respiratory tract by coughing. **2.** sputum—**expectorate** *vt*.

**experimental group** a research term that describes the group exposed to the independent variable (the intervention or experimental agent such as a drug). ⇒ control group, variable.

**expiration** *n* the process of breathing out air from the lungs—**expiratory** *adj*, **expire** *vt, vi*.

**expressed emotion** a research concept that sought to establish how certain environments might influence the course of schizophrenia.

**expression** *n* **1.** expulsion by force as of the placenta from the uterus, milk from the breast, etc. **2.** a genetic term for the appearance of a particular trait or characteristic. **3.** facial disclosure of feelings, mood, etc.

**expressive motor aphasia** a type of aphasia where there is difficulty in language production. Those affected have word-finding difficulties and may have problems producing sentence structures. May coexist with receptive aphasia.

**exsanguination** *n* the process of rendering bloodless—**exsanguinate** *vt*.

**exsiccation** *n* ⇒ desiccation.

**exstrophy** *n* a congenital anomaly in which the interior surface of an organ, such as the bladder, communicates with the outside. In this situation the abdominal wall and the anterior wall of the bladder are absent and the inside of the bladder is exposed on the surface of the abdomen.

**extended family** the wider group of family relations, including grandparents, aunts, uncles, cousins, etc. ⇒ nuclear family.

**extended-scope physiotherapy practitioner (ESP)** a specialist physiotherapist whose role has been extended to include assessment, ordering certain investigations, making referrals, etc. Practice in areas that include orthopaedics, rheumatology and with neurosurgical patients.

**extension** *n* **1.** traction upon a fractured or dislocated limb. **2.** the straightening of a flexed limb or part.

**extensor** *n* a muscle which on contraction extends or straightens a part, e.g. extensor carpi ulnaris ⇒ Appendix 1, Figures 4 and 5, flexor *opp*.

**exterioration** *n* a surgical procedure whereby an internal structure is repositioned on the body surface, such as the ileum or colon to form a stoma.

**external auditory meatus/canal** the canal between the pinna and eardrum. ⇒ Appendix 1, Figure 13.

**external cephalic version (ECV)** ⇒ version.

**external fixation** a method of fracture immobilization by inserting pins above and below the fracture. External rods are used to secure the pins. The tension on parts of the device can be adjusted during healing. ⇒ Ilizarov frame.

**external (lateral) rotation** a limb or body movement where there is rotation away from the vertical axis of the body.

**extinction** *n* in psychology. The decline, over time, of a conditioned response unless it is reinforced.

**extirpation** *n* complete removal or destruction of a part.

**extra-articular** *adj* outside a joint.

**extracapsular** *adj* outside a capsule. ⇒ intracapsular *opp*.

**extracardiac** *adj* outside the heart.

**extracellular** *adj* outside the cell membrane.

**extracellular fluid (ECF)** that fluid outside the cells, such as plasma, interstitial fluid, lymph, gastrointestinal secretions and cerebrospinal fluid. In an adult with an ideal weight of 70 kg there will be around 12 L of plasma and interstitial fluid. ⇒ intracellular *opp*.

**extracellular matrix (ECM)** the material outside the cells, which supports cells and influences intercellular communication. It contains many different substances, including elastin, collagen, hyaluronic acid, etc. ⇒ fibronectin.

**extracorporeal** *adj* outside the body.

**extracorporeal circulation** blood is taken from the body, directed through a machine ('heart–lung' or 'artificial kidney') and returned to the general circulation. ⇒ cardiopulmonary bypass, extracorporeal membrane oxygenation (ECMO), haemodialysis.

**extracorporeal membrane oxygenation (ECMO)** a cardiopulmonary bypass device which uses a membrane oxygenator (artificial lung). Venous blood from the patient circulates through the device. A fresh flow of oxygen into the device passes through a semipermeable membrane that allows the diffusion of oxygen whilst simultaneously removing carbon dioxide and water. Once the blood is oxygenated it is returned to the patient through an artery or a vein.

**extracorporeal shock-wave lithotripsy (ESWL)** the use of shock waves produced by a lithotriptor to fragment renal calculi or gallstones. ⇒ lithotriptor.

**extract** *n* a preparation obtained by evaporating a solution of a drug.

**extraction** *n* the removal of a tooth. *extraction of lens* surgical removal of the lens from the eye. It may be *extracapsular extraction*, when the capsule is ruptured prior to delivery of the lens and preserved in part, or *intracapsular extraction*, when the lens and capsule are removed intact.

**extradural** *adj* external to the dura mater.

**extradural haematoma** a collection of blood external to the dura mater (Figure E.8).

**extrahepatic** *adj* outside the liver.

**extramural** *adj* outside the wall of a structure—**extramurally** *adv*.

**extraocular** *adj* outside the eyeball. *extraocular muscles of the eye* also called extrinsic muscles. Six muscles that move the eye. There are four rectus (straight) muscles (medial, lateral, superior and inferior) and two oblique muscles (superior and inferior) attached to the eyeball.

**extraperitoneal** *adj* outside the peritoneum—**extraperitoneally** *adv*.

**extrapleural** *adj* outside the pleura, i.e. between the parietal pleura and the chest wall—**extrapleurally** *adv*.

**extrapyramidal** *adj* outside the pyramidal tracts. *extrapyramidal effects/disturbances* include the tremor and rigidity seen in parkinsonism and the side-effects of drugs, such as phenothiazine antipsychotic drugs (neuroleptics), which may cause a parkinsonian-like syndrome. ⇒ tardive dyskinesia. *extrapyramidal*

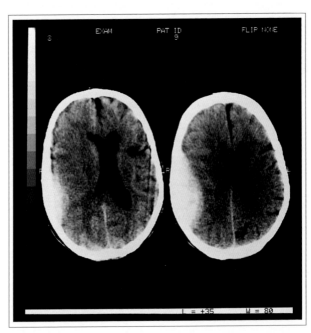

**Figure E.8** Extradural haematoma *(reproduced from Parsons & Johnson 2001 with permission).*

*tracts* motor pathways that pass outside the internal capsule. They modify pyramidal tract motor functions and influence coarse voluntary movement and affect posture, co-ordination and balance.

**extrarenal** *adj* outside the kidney—**extrarenally** *adv*.

**extrasensory** *adj* outside the normally accepted senses. *extrasensory perception (ESP)* response to an external stimulus without normal contact or communication.

**extrasystole** *n* premature beats (ectopic beats) in the pulse rhythm: the cardiac impulse is initiated by an abnormal focus.

**extrathoracic** *adj* outside the thoracic cavity.

**extrauterine** *adj* outside the uterus. *extrauterine pregnancy* ⇒ ectopic pregnancy.

**extravasation** *n* an escape of fluid from its normal enclosure into the surrounding tissues.

**extremophiles** *npl* a general term for microorganisms that can grow and reproduce in extreme environmental conditions, e.g. high temperature, extreme cold, extremes of pH, high pressure and high salt concentrations. ⇒ halophiles, osmophiles, psychrophiles, thermophiles.

**extrinsic** *adj* developing or having its origin from without; not internal.

**extrinsic allergic alveolitis** (*syn* 'farmer's lung' or 'bird-fancier's lung') an inflammatory response in the lungs to the inhalation of organic dusts. The two main causes are microbial spores present in vegetable produce, such as mouldy hay, and animal proteins, most commonly from pigeons and budgerigars. In an acute attack flu-like symptoms and breathlessness develop several hours after exposure; the symptoms generally subside spontaneously. If exposure continues a chronic condition with pulmonary fibrosis will develop.

**extrinsic factor** vitamin $B_{12}$, essential for the maturation of erythrocytes and nerve function, cannot be synthesized in the body and must be supplied in the diet, hence it is called the extrinsic factor. Its absorption in the terminal ileum requires the presence of the intrinsic factor secreted by the stomach.

**extrinsic muscles of the eye** ⇒ extraocular.

**extrinsic sugars** sugars, such as lactose in milk and sucrose as table sugar, that are not contained within cell walls.

**extroversion** *n* turning inside out. *extroversion of the bladder* ectopia vesicae. In psychology, the direction of thoughts to the external world.

**extrovert (extravert)** *adj* Jungian description of an individual whose characteristic interests and behaviour are directed outwards to other people and the physical environment. ⇒ introvert *opp*.

**extrusion** *n* in dentistry, the movement of a tooth/teeth outside the normal occlusal plane.

**extubation** *n* removal of an endotracheal tube.

**exudate** *n* the product of exudation—**exudates** *pl*. Wound exudate is a protein-rich fluid produced during healing. It bathes the wound, keeps it moist and transports substances required for healing. In ophthalmology, the yellow spots within the retina which accumulate secondary to fluid leakage from vessels.

**exudation** *n* the oozing out of fluid through the capillary walls in situations such as inflammation which increase vessel permeability—**exude** *vt, vi*.

**eye** *n* organ of vision. There are three layers, from outside in the sclera, the uvea, which forms the pigmented choroid, ciliary body and iris, and the inner light-sensitive retina containing photoreceptors (cones and rods) and pigment cells. ⇒ Appendix 1, Figure 15.

**eyeball** *n* the globe of the eye.

**eyebrows** *npl* the supraorbital margin of the frontal bone and the hairs projecting from the overlying skin. They help to protect the eye from foreign bodies and sweat.

**eye contact** looking at the face of the person to whom one is talking. In many instances, it is a reciprocal activity and is such an important part of most cultures' non-verbal language that blind people are advised to turn their faces in the direction of the voice being heard. In some cultures, however, it may be perceived as bad manners or offensive to make or maintain eye contact during conversation, or when acknowledging a person.

**eyelashes** *npl* the row of hairs on each eyelid. They protect the eye from foreign bodies and injury.

**eye teeth** *n* the canine teeth in the upper jaw.

**F**

**fabella** *n* a sesamoid bone sometimes present in the lateral head of the gastrocnemius muscle.

**faber test** a test for problems affecting the sacroiliac joint/ligaments. It comprises **f**lexion, **ab**duction and **e**xternal **ro**tation of the hip. A positive result is pain felt in the area of the sacroiliac joint.

**Fabry's disease** (J Fabry, German dermatologist, 1860–1930). ⇒ angiokeratoma corporis diffusum.

**face presentation** the head of the fetus is fully extended with the back of the head in contact with the spine, and the face presents first at the vulva during labour.

**facet** *n* a small, smooth, flat surface of a bone or a calculus.

**facial** *adj* pertaining to the face.

**facial nerve** seventh pair of cranial nerves. They supply the facial muscles, the salivary, lacrimal and nasal glands, and part of the tongue. Damage or disease affecting the facial nerves results in paralysis of facial muscles. ⇒ Bell's palsy.

**facies** *n* the appearance or the expression of the face. *adenoid facies* open-mouthed, vacant expression due to deafness from enlarged pharyngeal tonsils (adenoids). *Parkinson facies* a mask-like appearance; saliva may trickle from the corners of the mouth.

**facilitated diffusion** process whereby larger, non-fat-soluble molecules such as glucose pass into the cell by using a protein carrier molecule. No energy is required but there must be a concentration gradient.

**facilitation** *n* in occupational therapy, the interaction between the therapist and a client, whereby the performance of function becomes possible and easier.

**factitious disorder** a disorder of illness behaviour in which an individual feigns symptoms repeatedly and consistently. As a result there are often repeated investigations and treatment (including surgery) in spite of repeated negative findings. ⇒ Munchausen syndrome.

**factor I** a factor in the blood coagulation cascade. ⇒ fibrinogen.

**factor II** a factor in the blood coagulation cascade. ⇒ prothrombin.

**factor III** thromboplastin (tissue factor). A factor in the blood coagulation cascade. ⇒ thromboplastin.

**factor IV** calcium ions. A factor in the blood coagulation cascade. ⇒ calcium.

**factor V** a factor in the blood coagulation cascade. ⇒ labile factor (proaccelerin).

**factor VII** a factor in the blood coagulation cascade. ⇒ stable factor (proconvertin).

**factor VIII** a factor in the blood coagulation cascade. ⇒ antihaemophilic factor A, haemophilias.

**factor IX** Christmas factor, antihaemophilic factor B. A factor in the blood coagulation cascade. ⇒ Christmas factor, haemophilias.

**factor X** a factor in the blood coagulation cascade. ⇒ Stuart–Prower factor.

**factor XI** a factor in the blood coagulation cascade. ⇒ plasma thromboplastin antecedent.

**factor XII** a factor in the blood coagulation cascade. ⇒ Hageman factor.

**factor XIII** a factor in the blood coagulation cascade. ⇒ fibrin-stabilizing factor.

**factor V Leiden** a genetic abnormality of factor V (a blood coagulation factor), which results in failure of one of the system's inbuilt antithrombotic safety mechanisms. The abnormality is found in 3–5% of populations in northern European countries, but under certain circumstances it may cause a predisposition to venous thrombosis.

**facultative** *adj* conditional; having the power of living under different conditions.

**FAD/FADH₂** *abbr* flavin adenine dinucleotide (oxidized and reduced forms respectively).

**faecal impaction** severe constipation caused by a mass of dried hardened faeces in the colon and rectum.

**faecal incontinence** simply defined as the leakage of liquid faeces. There is a lack of consensus about a precise definition but it is involuntary or inappropriate defecation. There may be faecal soiling of clothing such as when passing flatus, or being unaware of the urge to defecate. Constipation and impaction are common causes of incontinence.

**faecalith** *n* a concretion formed in the bowel from faecal matter: it can cause obstruction and/or inflammation.

**faecal occult blood (FOB)** a test used to detect minute amounts of blood in faeces that occurs as a result of bleeding in the gastrointestinal tract. It is used as a screening test for colorectal cancers in certain older age groups. People who have a positive FOB test are invited to have a diagnostic colonoscopy. ⇒ occult blood test.

**faecal–oral route** describes the ingestion of micro-organisms from faeces which can be transmitted directly or indirectly. Often results in diarrhoeal disease.

**faecal softeners** ⇒ laxatives. ⇒ Appendix 5.

**faeces** *n* the waste material eliminated from the bowel, consisting mainly of indigestible cellulose, unabsorbed food, intestinal secretions, water, electrolytes and micro-organisms, etc.—**faecal** *adj*.

**fahrenheit** *n* (D Fahrenheit, German physicist, 1686–1736) a thermometric scale; the freezing point of water is 32°F and its boiling point 212°F.

**failure to thrive** failure to develop and grow at the expected rate for age and gender, ascertained by consistent measurement of height and weight plotted on a growth chart. It may result from an organic disorder, such as metabolic diseases, acute illness or kidney disease, or have non-organic causes, such as poor feeding, maternal deprivation or psychological problems.

**faint** *n* syncope—**faint** *vi*.

**falciform** *adj* sickle-shaped.

**falciform ligament** also called the broad ligament of the liver. The fold of peritoneum between the right and left lobes of the liver, which helps to support the liver in position.

**fallopian tubes** ⇒ uterine tubes.

**Fallot's tetralogy** (E-L Fallot, French physician, 1850–1911) a cyanotic congenital heart defect comprising a ventricular septal defect, narrowing of the right ventricular outflow tract (subvalvular pulmonary stenosis), right ventricular hypertrophy and malposition of the aorta overriding the ventricular septum. Amenable to corrective surgery.

**false substrate** chemicals, including some drugs, that compete with the normal substrate in a metabolic pathway. The pathway is disrupted. ⇒ enzyme inhibitors.

**falx** *n* a sickle-shaped structure. *falx cerebri* that portion of the dura mater separating the two cerebral hemispheres. *falx cerebelli* the portion of dura mater between the hemispheres of the cerebellum.

**familial** *adj* relating to the family, as of a condition such as Huntington's disease that affects several members of the same family.

**familial adenomatous polyposis** a dominantly inherited condition in which multiple polyps occur throughout the large bowel and which invariably leads to colon cancer. Polyps also occur in the stomach and duodenum. ⇒ Gardner's syndrome, Peutz–Jeghers syndrome. ⊙DVD

**familial Mediterranean fever** a rare genetic disease. It is inherited as an autosomal recessive trait. It usually affects Sephardic Jews and Armenians and is characterized by episodes of inflammatory arthritis, pyrexia, pleurisy and peritonitis. There may be secondary amyloidosis. Should not be confused with boutonneuse fever (Mediterranean spotted fever) caused by a rickettsial infection.

**Family Health Services (FHS)** community-based services provided by family doctors, dentists, opticians and pharmacists as independent contractors. They are not directly employed by the NHS, but have contractual arrangements to practise in the NHS.

**family planning** the methods used to space or limit the number of children born to a couple, or for enhancing conception.

**family therapy** in psychotherapy, a therapy that focuses on the family relationships and communication between individuals in order to understand the problems experienced by a single member. The aims are to clarify issues and help family members to modify their interactions with each other.

**Fanconi anaemia** (G Fanconi, Swiss paediatrician, 1892–1979) a rare autosomal recessive disorder with the insidious onset of aplastic anaemia during childhood. Other abnormalities include short stature, polydactyly, abnormal kidneys, etc. Affected children may develop cancers, including leukaemia. A haemopoietic stem cell transplantation may be a treatment option for some people, but most patients will die.

**Fanconi syndrome** an inherited or acquired dysfunction of the proximal renal tubules. Large amounts of amino acids, phosphates and glucose are excreted in the urine, and there is proximal renal tubular acidosis. Adults may develop osteomalacia, and children have rickets and fail to grow properly.

**fantasy, phantasy** *n* a 'daydream' in which the person's conscious or unconscious desires and impulses are fulfilled. May be accompanied by feelings of unreality. Occurs pathologically in schizophrenia.

**farad (F)** *n* (M Faraday, British scientist, 1791–1867) the SI unit of capacitance.

**farmer's lung** ⇒ extrinsic allergic alveolitis.

**FAS** *abbr* fetal alcohol syndrome.

**fascia** *n* a connective tissue sheath consisting of fibrous tissue and fat which unites the skin to the underlying tissues. It also surrounds and separates many of the muscles, and, in some cases, holds them together—**fascial** *adj*.

**fasciculation** *n* visible flickering of muscle; can occur in the upper and lower eyelids.

**fasciculus** *n* a little bundle, as of muscle or nerve—**fascicular** *adj.* **fasciculi** *pl.*

**fasciitis** *n* inflammation of fascia (connective tissue). It may be caused by micro-organisms, such as streptococci, or be part of an inflammatory condition. ⇒ Fournier's gangrene, necrotizing fasciitis.

**Fasciola** *n* a genus of liver flukes, such as *Fasciola hepatica*. ⇒ flukes.

**fascioliasis** *n* infestation with *Fasciola hepatica*. The ova of the fluke is present in the faeces of sheep and cattle, and snails are an intermediate host. Human infestation occurs through eating contaminated aquatic plants such as watercress. Infestation causes serious hepatobiliary disease: there is fever, malaise, a large tender liver and eosinophilia.

**fasciolopsiasis** *n* infestation with *Fasciolopsis buski*. It is prevalent in Asia and the Indian subcontinent. It affects humans and pigs and is acquired from ingesting contaminated aquatic plants. There is abdominal pain, diarrhoea, constipation, oedema and associated eosinophilia.

**Fasciolopsis** *n* a genus of large intestinal flukes, such as *Fasciolopsis buski*. ⇒ flukes.

**fasciotomy** *n* incision of muscle fascia. ⇒ compartment syndrome.

**fastigium** *n* the summit, such as the highest temperature occurring in a fever.

**fat** *n* **1.** complex organic molecule composed of carbon, hydrogen and oxygen atoms. Fats are formed by the combination of one molecule of glycerol with three fatty acids forming a triacylglycerol (triglyceride). May be of animal or vegetable origin, and may be fats or oils. *fat embolus* ⇒ embolism. ⇒ adipose, brown fat, fatty acid, glycerol, kilojoule, triacylglycerol. **2.** adipose tissue, which acts as a reserve supply of energy and protects some organs—**fatty** *adj.*

**fat-soluble vitamin** vitamins A, D, E and K are fat-soluble. ⇒ water-soluble vitamins.

**Fatal Accident Enquiry** ⇒ coroner.

**fatigue** *n* weariness. Physiological term for diminishing muscle reaction to stimulus applied. In sports medicine the failure of muscle(s) to maintain force (or power output) during sustained or repeated contractions—**fatigability** *n.*

**fatigue index** the decline in power divided by the time (in seconds) interval between maximum (peak) and minimum power, recorded during an anaerobic power exercise test.

**fatigue fracture** ⇒ stress fracture.

**fatty acid** the hydrocarbon component of lipids. May be unsaturated (monounsaturated or polyunsaturated) or saturated depending on the number of double chemical bonds in their structure. ⇒ essential fatty acids.

**fatty degeneration** tissue degeneration that leads to the appearance of fatty droplets in the cytoplasm; found especially in disease of heart, liver and kidney.

**fauces** *n* the opening from the mouth into the pharynx, bounded above by the soft palate, below by the tongue. Pillars of the fauces, anterior and posterior, lie laterally and surround the palatine tonsil—**faucial** *adj.*

**favism** *n* increased breakdown of erythrocytes (red blood cells) precipitated by eating fava beans, in individuals deficient in the enzyme glucose-6-phosphate dehydrogenase (G6PD).

**favus** *n* a type of ringworm not common in the UK, caused by *Trichophyton schoenleini*. Yellow cup-shaped crusts (scutula) develop, especially on the scalp.

**FBS** *abbr* fetal blood sampling.

**fear** *n* an intense emotional state involving a feeling of unpleasant tension, and a strong urge to escape, which is a normal and natural response to a threat of danger but is abnormal when it exists without danger or is a continuous state. ⇒ anxiety, general adaptation syndrome.

**febrile** *adj* feverish; accompanied by fever.

**febrile seizures (convulsions)** occur in children who have an increased body temperature; they do not usually result in permanent brain damage. Most common between the ages of 6 months and 5 years. ⇒ convulsions, seizures.

**fecundation** *n* impregnation. Fertilization. ⇒ superfecundation.

**fecundity** *n* the power of reproduction; fertility.

**feedback** *n* a homeostatic control mechanism. It is usually *negative feedback*, in which a physiological process is slowed or 'turned off' by an increasing amount of product, e.g. hormone secretion, temperature control (Figure F.1). Much more rarely in *positive feedback*, the process is speeded up by high levels of the product, e.g. normal blood clotting, the events of labour. *feedback treatment* ⇒ biofeedback.

**Felty's syndrome** (A Felty, American physician, 1895–1963) enlargement of the spleen and low white blood cell count (leucopenia) associated with rheumatoid arthritis in adults.

**female athlete triad** a syndrome comprising amenorrhoea, eating disorders and osteoporosis. It results from a reduction in energy intake such as decreasing food intake or an increase in energy use by extra training or exercise.

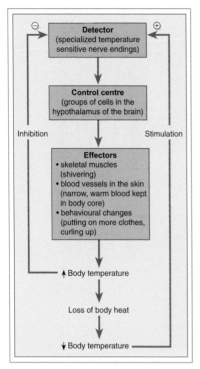

**Figure F.1** Negative feedback—temperature *(reproduced from Waugh & Grant 2006 with permission).*

**feminization** *n* **1.** normal development of female secondary sexual characteristics during puberty. **2.** the presence of female sexual characteristics in a male. May be due to a faulty production of, or an inability to respond to, testosterone. Males with chromosomal anomalies, such as Klinefelter's syndrome, have breast development. Other causes include oestrogen-secreting adrenal tumours; certain testicular tumours; treatment with female hormones for some cancers; drugs, e.g. spironolactone; and, when a diseased liver fails to metabolize natural endogenous oestrogens.

**femoral** *adj* pertaining to the femur or thigh. *femoral artery* the large artery that extends from the external iliac artery to supply arterial blood to the groin and thigh. *femoral nerve* one of the largest branches arising from the lumbar plexus (lumbar nerve roots 2, 3, 4). It innervates the skin and muscles of the anterior thigh. *femoral triangle* also known as Scarpa's triangle. An area at the top, inner part of the thigh. It is bounded by the inguinal ligament, the sartorius and adductor longus muscles, and contains the femoral artery, vein and nerve. *femoral vein* the large vein that extends from the popliteal vein. It carries venous blood from the leg to the external iliac vein having been joined in the groin by the great saphenous vein. ⇒ Appendix 1, Figures 9 and 10.

**femoropopliteal** *adj* usually referring to the femoral and popliteal vessels.

**femur** *n* the thigh bone (⇒ Appendix 1, Figures 2 and 3) the longest and strongest bone in the body. The femoral head articulates in the acetabulum to form the hip joint, and the femoral condyles articulate with the tibia and patella to form the knee joint—**femora** *pl,* **femoral** *adj.*

**fenamates** *npl* a group of non-steroidal anti-inflammatory drugs. ⇒ Appendix 5.

**fenestra** *n* a window-like opening. *fenestra ovalis* an oval opening between the middle and inner ear. Below it lies the *fenestra rotunda,* a round opening.

**fenestration** *n* **1.** a perforation, opening or pore. The glomerular capillaries of the nephron, which form part of the filtration membrane, are adapted for permeability and filtration by the presence of fenestrations. **2.** a surgical opening (or fenestra) in the inner ear to ease the deafness caused by otosclerosis.

**Ferguson's reflex** (J Ferguson, Canadian physiologist, b. 1907) an important reflex involved in labour. A surge of oxytocin is released, which increases uterine contractions, when the cervix and upper vagina are stimulated.

**fermentation** *n* the process whereby microbial (yeasts and bacteria) enzymes break down sugars (glycolysis) and other substrates. For example, in the production of bread, cheese, alcohol and vinegar.

**ferning** *n* arborization. A characteristic of cervical mucus containing high levels of oestrogen, the dried mucus forms a fern-like pattern on a slide. May be used to ascertain when ovulation occurs. ⇒ spinnbarkeit.

**ferric** *adj* relating to trivalent iron and its salts. Ferric iron is converted to the ferrous state by gastric acid.

**ferritin** *n* an iron–protein (apoferritin) complex. It is a storage form of iron found in the liver, spleen and bone marrow. The level of ferritin in serum can indicate the total amount of iron stored in the body. Ferritin levels may be raised in disease processes, such as inflammation, which are linked to the synthesis of acute-phase proteins.

**ferrous** *adj* pertaining to divalent iron, as of its salts and compounds. *Ferrous carbonate, ferrous fumarate, ferrous gluconate, ferrous succinate* and *ferrous sulphate* are prescribed orally in the treatment of iron-deficiency anaemias.

**fertility rate** known as the general fertility rate. A rate obtained by dividing the number of live births by the number of women of child-bearing age (15 to 44 years). Typically expressed as live births per 1000 women. ⇒ total fertility rate.

**fertilization** *n* the penetration of an oocyte by a spermatozoon.

**FESS** *abbr* functional endoscopic sinus surgery.

**fester** *vi* to become inflamed; to suppurate.

**festinating gait** rapid, short shuffling steps continuing until stopped by an object that gets in the way. Caused by lack of control of forward tilt of the pelvis with appearance of feet 'catching up' with centre of gravity that is too far ahead, instead of over them; characteristic of Parkinson's disease.

**fetal alcohol syndrome (FAS)** a range of problems that include stillbirth, fetal abnormality and learning disability due to intrauterine growth restriction/retardation caused by excessive maternal alcohol consumption during pregnancy. Infants with fetal alcohol syndrome have typical facial features, and may have neurological problems and cardiac defects.

**fetal blood sampling (FBS) 1.** blood taken from the fetus during pregnancy to test for abnormalities, mostly superseded by newer diagnostic methods. Or to check fetal haemoglobin levels in Rhesus incompatibility to determine whether an intrauterine transfusion is required. **2.** blood from a fetal scalp vein obtained during labour is tested to detect acidosis if the fetal heart rate pattern is abnormal. The presence of acidosis indicates that the baby should be delivered. ⇒ cardiotocography.

**fetal circulation** circulation adapted for intrauterine life. Extra shunts and vessels (ductus venosus, ductus arteriosus, foramen ovale and umbilical vein) allow blood largely to bypass the liver, gastrointestinal tract and lungs, as their functions are covered by maternal systems and the placenta (Figure F.2).

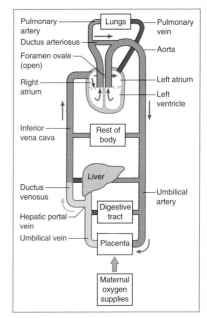

**Figure F.2** Fetal circulation *(reproduced from Rutishauser 1994 with permission)*.

**fetal reduction** ⇒ embryo/fetal reduction.

**feticide** *n* the deliberate destruction of a fetus. Medically it is used during fetal reduction or late termination. It may be achieved by injecting potassium chloride or saline into the fetal thorax.

**fetishism** *n* a condition in which a particular material object is regarded with irrational awe or a strong emotional attachment. Can have a psychosexual dimension in which such an object is repeatedly or exclusively used in achieving sexual excitement.

**fetofetal transfusion syndrome** also called twin-to-twin transfusion syndrome. Blood from one monozygotic twin transfuses into the other twin through the placental blood vessels.

**fetor** *n* offensive odour, stench. *fetor oris* bad breath.

**fetoscopy** *n* direct visual examination of the fetus by using an appropriate fibreoptic endoscope. It is performed transabdominally after the 11th week of gestation. The examination may be used to confirm possible abnormalities detected using ultrasound. It can be combined with amniocentesis, and increasingly for other interventions such as biopsies of abnormal tissue. ⇒ embryoscopy.

**fetus** *n* the developmental stage from the eighth week of gestation until birth—**fetal** *adj*.

**fetus-in-fetu** an abnormality in which the parts of one monozygotic twin are within the other twin.

**fetus papyraceus** a dead fetus, one of a twin which has become flattened and mummified.

**Feulgen stain** (R Feulgen, German biochemist, 1884–1955) a stain used in histology to identify deoxyribonucleic acid or chromosomal material in specimens.

**FEV** *abbr* forced expiratory volume. ⇒ respiratory function tests.

**fever** *n* (*syn* pyrexia) an elevation of body temperature above normal. Designates some infectious conditions, e.g. *paratyphoid fever, scarlet fever, typhoid fever*, etc.

**FHS** *abbr* Family Health Services.

**fibre** *n* a thread-like structure—**fibrous** *adj*. ⇒ non-starch polysaccharide.

**fibreoptics** *n* light is transmitted through flexible glass fibres which enable the user to 'see round corners'. The technology utilized in modern fibreoptics endoscopic equipment.

**fibril** *n* a component filament of a fibre; a small fibre.

**fibrillation** *n* unco-ordinated quivering contraction of muscle; usually referring to myocardial muscle. ⇒ atrial fibrillation, cardiac arrest, ventricular fibrillation.

**fibrin** *n* the insoluble matrix on which a blood clot is formed. Produced from soluble fibrinogen by the action of thrombin—**fibrinous** *adj*.

**fibrinogen** *n* factor I of blood coagulation. A soluble plasma protein that is converted to fibrin by the action of the proteolytic enzyme thrombin.

**fibrinolysin** *n* ⇒ plasmin, plasminogen.

**fibrinolysis** *n* the last of the four overlapping processes of haemostasis. The dissolution of the fibrin clot by the proteolytic enzyme plasmin. There is normally a balance between blood coagulation and fibrinolysis in the body. ⇒ coagulation, platelet plug, thrombolytic, vasoconstriction.

**fibrinolytic drugs** a group of drugs that disperse thrombi by acting as thrombolytics, e.g. alteplase. ⇒ Appendix 5, thrombolytic therapy.

**fibrin-stabilizing factor** an enzyme that causes polymerization leading to the formation of the insoluble stabilizing network within the fibrin clot. It is activated by thrombin in the presence of calcium ions that act as a cofactor. Factor XIII in the blood coagulation cascade.

**fibroadenoma** *n* a benign tumour containing fibrous and glandular tissue, such as in the breast.

**fibroblast** *n* (*syn* fibrocyte) a blast cell that forms connective tissues. Involved during growth and tissue repair—**fibroblastic** *adj*.

**fibrocartilage** (white) *n* one of the three types of cartilage. It comprises white collagen fibres within a matrix. It is a strong and slightly flexible tissue that provides support in a variety of locations. These include the intervertebral pads, ligaments between bones, the semilunar cartilages in the knee and deepening the sockets of the shoulder and hip joints—**fibrocartilaginous** *adj*.

**fibrocaseous** *adj* a soft, cheesy mass infiltrated by fibrous tissue, formed by fibroblasts.

**fibrochondritis** *n* inflammation of fibrocartilage.

**fibrocyst** *n* a fibroma which has undergone cystic degeneration.

**fibrocystic** *adj* pertaining to a fibrocyst. *fibrocystic disease of bone* cysts may be solitary or generalized. If generalized and accompanied by decalcification of bone, it is symptomatic of hyperparathyroidism. *fibrocystic disease of breast* the breast feels lumpy due to the presence of cysts, usually caused by hormone imbalance. *fibrocystic disease of pancreas* ⇒ cystic fibrosis.

**fibrocyte** *n* ⇒ fibroblast—**fibrocytic** *adj*.

**fibroid 1.** *adj* having fibres. **2.** *n* fibromyoma, leiomyoma, uterine fibroid. A fibromuscular benign tumour usually found in the uterus. The location of uterine fibroids can be described as *intramural* (embedded in the wall of the uterus), *subserous* (protruding from the serosal surface into the peritoneal cavity) or *submucous* (protruding into the endometrial surface). Common pathology in women between 35 and 45 years of age. They cause menorrhagia, dysmenorrhoea, subfertility and problems if pregnancy does occur, such as miscarriage and preterm labour. Large fibroids cause abdominal swelling and may cause urinary frequency. The fibroid may become twisted on its stalk, bleed, degenerate or, rarely, become malignant. ⇒ embolization, hysterectomy, myomectomy.

**fibroma** *n* a benign tumour composed of fibrous tissue—**fibromata** *pl*, **fibromatous** *adj*.

**fibromuscular** *adj* pertaining to fibrous and muscle tissue.

**fibromyalgia** *n* a condition characterized by widespread pain and tender points. Many patients also complain of tiredness and of waking feeling unrefreshed.

**fibromyoma** *n* a benign tumour consisting of fibrous and muscle tissue—**fibromyomata** *pl*, **fibromyomatous** *adj*.

**fibromyositis** *n* general term for inflammation of fibrous and muscle tissue.

**fibronectin** *n* a glycoprotein present in the plasma, it occurs in several forms. It is important in the integrity of the extracellular matrix, proliferation of new epithelial cells, cell migration and adhesion. Thus, it is of importance in embryonic development and wound healing. Also involved with platelet aggregation during haemostasis and as part of the body's host defences.

**fibroplasia** *n* the production of fibrous tissue which is a normal part of healing. *retrolental fibroplasia* older term for retinopathy of prematurity.

**fibrosarcoma** *n* a form of sarcoma. A malignant tumour derived from fibroblastic cells—**fibrosarcomata** *pl*, **fibrosarcomatous** *adj*.

**fibrosis** *n* the formation of excessive fibrous tissues in a structure, such as pulmonary fibrosis caused by radiation, certain cytotoxic drugs and pneumoconiosis—**fibrotic** *adj*.

**fibrositis** *n* a lay term (now seldom used) that denotes non-specific soft-tissue pain. ⇒ fibromyalgia.

**fibrous dysplasia** *n* an abnormality of bone, whereby bone tissue is replaced by fibrous tissue. The onset generally occurs during childhood. There are several types and sometimes there are associated endocrine abnormalities. The effects include pain, pathological fractures and bony deformities. ⇒ Albright's syndrome.

**fibrous joint** one of the three main classes of joints. Usually an immovable joint or synarthrosis, e.g. the sutures of the skull. A joint, e.g. a tooth in the jaw, in which a tiny amount of movement occurs is called a gomphosis. Those joints where an interosseous ligament connects two bones are termed syndesmosis, e.g. tibiofibular joint. They allow some 'give'.

**fibrovascular** *adj* relating to fibrous tissue which is well supplied with blood vessels.

**fibula** *n* one of the longest and thinnest bones of the body, situated on the outer side of the leg and articulating at the upper end with the lateral condyle of the tibia and at the lower end with the lateral surface of the talus

(astragalus) and tibia (⇒ Appendix 1, Figures 2 and 3). It provides a surface for muscle attachments, e.g. soleus, peroneus longus and brevis—**fibular** *adj*.

**field of vision** ⇒ visual field.

**FIGLU** *abbr* formiminoglutamic (FIGLU) acid, an intermediate metabolite in histidine metabolism. *FIGLU test* a test for folic acid deficiency, vitamin $B_{12}$ deficiency or the absence of an enzyme, which are all needed for histidine metabolism. Following a dose of histidine, the urine is tested for FIGLU and its presence in the urine indicates that either of the vitamins or the enzyme may be deficient.

**FIGO** *abbr* the International Federation of Gynaecology and Obstetrics provides a classification staging cancer of the cervix from 0 (pre-invasive disease) to IVb (distant metastasis). A similar staging classification, based on locality and extent of disease, is available for ovarian and uterine cancer.

**filament** *n* a fine, threadlike structure, such as the filaments of contractile proteins in muscle fibres.

*Filaria* *n* a genus of parasitic, thread-like nematode worms found mainly in the tropics and subtropics. They include *Brugia malayi*, *Loa loa*, *Onchocerca volvulus* and *Wuchereria bancrofti*. ⇒ filariasis.

**filariasis** *n* infestation with *Filaria*. The adult worms may live in the lymphatics, connective tissues or mesentery, where they may cause obstruction, but the microfilariae migrate to the blood stream and some infiltrate the eye, skin or pulmonary capillaries. The completion of the life cycle of some types is dependent upon passage through a mosquito. ⇒ elephantiasis, loiasis, onchocerciasis.

**filaricide** *n* an agent, such as ivermectin and diethylcarbamazine, which destroys *Filaria*.

**filiform** *adj* thread-like. *filiform papillae* small projections ending in several minute processes; found on the tongue.

**filter** *n* a device designed to remove particles over a certain size or rays of specific wavelength while allowing others to pass through. Examples include intravenous fluid filters and optical filters.

**filtrate** *n* substance that passes through the filter.

**filtration** *n* the process of straining through a filter under gravity, pressure or vacuum. *filtration under pressure* occurs in the nephron due to high-pressure blood in the wide-bore afferent arteriole of the glomerulus. ⇒ active transport, diffusion, osmosis.

**filum** *n* any filamentous or thread-like structure. *filum terminale* a strong, fine cord blending with the spinal cord above, and the periosteum of the sacral canal below.

**FIM** *abbr* Functional Independence Measure.

**fimbria** *n* a fringe, e.g. of the uterine tubes (⇒ Appendix 1, Figure 17)—**fimbriae** *pl*, **fimbrial**, **fimbriated** *adj*.

**fine motor control** the specific control of the muscles allowing for completion of small, delicate tasks, such as picking up a pin.

**fine-needle aspiration** a diagnostic test whereby a thin needle is used to obtain a tissue sample for examination. For example, it may be used to determine whether a breast lump or a thyroid swelling is benign or malignant.

**fine tremor** slight trembling, as seen in the outstretched hands or tongue of a patient suffering from hyperthyroidism.

**finger** *n* a digit. ⇒ clubbed finger.

**finger–nose test** the person is asked to touch the tip of the nose with an extended index finger. It tests voluntary eye–motor coordination and may be used to check cerebellar function.

**finger spelling** communication by spelling words using the fingers to make the letters of the alphabet. It may be either one-handed or two-handed finger spelling.

**FiO₂** *abbr* fractional inspired oxygen concentration.

**first aid** the immediate treatment or assistance given to a person after injury or sudden illness prior to the arrival of a qualified health care professional, e.g. paramedic. First aid aims are to preserve life, stop deterioration and encourage recovery.

**first-degree tear** ⇒ perineal tear.

**first intention** ⇒ primary intention, wound healing.

**first-pass metabolism (first-pass effect)** occurs when orally administered drugs are rapidly metabolized in the liver. This leads to a situation where the amount of the active drug reaching the circulation is insufficient to produce a therapeutic effect, such as with glyceryl trinitrate. Other routes of administration are used to overcome the problem, e.g. transdermal, or tablets or sprays that can be absorbed through the buccal, sublingual or nasal mucosa.

**fission** *n* ⇒ binary fission.

**fissure** *n* a split or cleft. Can be moist or dry cracks in the epidermis or mucosa. They usually develop at 90° to the direction of the tension stress. Common sites include the anal mucosa and interdigitally for moist fissures, and the heel margins for dry fissures. ⇒ anal fissure. *palpebral fissure* the opening between the eyelids.

**fistula** *n* an abnormal communication between two epithelial surfaces (e.g. enterovesical between bowel and bladder). May occur in conditions such as Crohn's disease, diverticulosis and cancer—**fistulae** *pl*, **fistular**, **fistulous** *adj*. ⇒ anal fistula, arteriovenous fistula, biliary fistula, bronchopleural fistula, enterovesical, tracheo-oesophageal fistula, vesicocolic, vesicovaginal.

**fistulotomy** *n* incision of a fistula.

**fitness** *n* general term used to describe a person's ability to undertake a series of different physical exercises.

**fits** *npl* ⇒ convulsions, seizures.

**fixation** *n* **1.** in optics, the direct focusing of one or both eyes on an object so that the image falls on the fovea centralis. **2.** the point on the retina used to look directly at an object of interest, usually the fovea centralis. **3.** as a psychoanalytical term, an emotional attachment, generally sexual, to a parent, causing difficulty in forming new attachments later in life.

**fixed costs** the costs incurred regardless of the level of activity, e.g. related to the buildings and land, equipment maintenance.

**flaccid** *adj* soft, flabby, not firm.

**flaccidity** *n* loss of muscle tone due to disturbance of the lower motor neuron, with varying degrees of paralysis depending on the extent of loss of motor supply to the muscles and associated with weakness due to lack of use.

**flagellate** *n* a protozoon that has flagella for propulsion. Examples include *Giardia*, *Leishmania* and *Trichomonas*.

**flagellation** *n* the act of whipping oneself or others to gain sexual pleasure. Can be a component of masochism and sadism.

**flagellum** *n* a fine, hair-like appendage capable of whip-like movements that moves the cell through fluid. Characteristic of spermatozoa, certain bacteria and protozoa—**flagella** *pl*.

**flail chest** unstable thoracic cage and chest wall due to multiple rib fractures. ⇒ paradoxical respiration.

**flap** *n* a unit of skin and other subcutaneous tissues that maintains its own blood and nerve supply, used to repair defects in other parts of the body. Common in plastic surgery to treat burns and other injuries; skin flaps used to cover amputation stumps.

F

**flare** *n* **1.** skin redness at the periphery of an urticarial hypersensitivity reaction. **2.** a sudden escalation of an existing condition. **3.** expanding reddening of the skin around an area of irritation, or an infective lesion.

**flashback** *n* involuntary phenomenon whereby people relive past traumatic events, or the abnormal perceptions, such as hallucinations, associated with previous use of hallucinogenic drugs. ⇒ derealization, hallucination, posttraumatic stress disorder.

**flat foot** *n* ⇒ pes planus.

**flat pelvis** a pelvis in which the anteroposterior diameter of the brim is reduced.

**flat worm** platyhelminth. Includes the cestodes (tapeworms) and trematodes (flukes).

**flatulence** *n* gastric and intestinal distension with gas—**flatulent** *adj*.

**flatus** *n* gas in the gastrointestinal tract.

**flavin adenine dinucleotide (FAD/FADH₂)** coenzyme synthesized from riboflavin. One of the major electron carrier/transfer molecules in the oxidation of fuel molecules in the mitochondria. ⇒ electron transfer chain.

**flavin mononucleotide (FMN/FMNH₂)** coenzyme synthesized from riboflavin. An electron carrier/transfer molecule involved in the oxidation of fuel molecules in the mitochondria. ⇒ electron transfer chain.

*Flavivirus* *n* a genus of RNA viruses that include those that cause dengue, St Louis encephalitis and West Nile fever.

**flavonoids** *npl* also known as bioflavonoids. A large group of plant pigments that occur naturally in many vegetables and fruit (e.g. tomatoes, broccoli, cherries, plums, etc.). Bioflavonoids are also present in tea and wine. Many are antibacterial, some others have antioxidant properties and may offer protection against heart disease and cancer, and others are phyto-oestrogens.

**flavoproteins** *npl* proteins combined with either flavin adenine dinucleotide or flavin mononucleotide. They function in the mitochondrial processes in which energy is produced from the oxidation of fuel. ⇒ cytochrome, electron transfer chain, oxidative phosphorylation.

**flea** *n* a blood-sucking wingless insect; it operates as a host and can transmit disease. Its bite provides an entry point for infection. *Pulex irritans* is the human flea. The rat flea *Xenopsylla cheopis* is a transmitter of plague.

**Fleischer ring** (B Fleischer, German ophthalmologist, 1874–1965) a green/brown line around the cone of the cornea in keratoconus.

**flexibilitas cerea** literally, waxy flexibility. A condition of generalized hypertonia of muscles found in catatonic schizophrenia. When fully developed, the patient's limbs retain positions in which they are placed, remaining immobile for hours at a time. Occasionally occurs in hysteria as hysterical rigidity.

**flexibility** *n* the range of movement possible around a joint or series of joints. Determined by the size and shape of the bones, normal joint mechanics, mobility of soft tissues and muscle extensibility.

**flexion** *n* the act of bending by which the shafts of long bones forming a joint are brought towards each other, such bending the elbow.

**Flexner's bacillus** (S Flexner, American pathologist and bacteriologist, 1863–1946). ⇒ *Shigella flexneri.*

**flexor** *n* a muscle which on contraction flexes or bends a part. For example, flexor carpi radialis, which flexes the hand and assists in hand abduction. ⇒ Appendix 1, Figures 4 and 5, extensor *opp.*

**flexure** *n* a bend, as in a tube-like structure, or a fold, as on the skin—it can be obliterated by extension or increased by flexion in the locomotor system—**flexural** *adj. left colic (splenic) flexure* is situated at the junction of the transverse and descending parts of the colon. It lies at a higher level than the *right colic* or *hepatic flexure,* the bend between the ascending and transverse colon, beneath the liver. *sigmoid flexure* ⇒ sigmoid colon.

**flight of ideas** succession of thoughts with no rational connection. A feature of manic disorders.

**floaters** *npl* floating bodies in the vitreous body (humour) of the eye, which are visible to the person.

**flocculation** *n* the coalescence of colloidal particles in suspension, resulting in their aggregation into larger discrete masses which are often visible to the naked eye as turbidity (cloudiness).

**flooding** *n* **1.** a popular term to describe excessive bleeding from the uterus. **2.** a behavioural technique that may be used to reduce anxiety in people with phobias. Individuals are exposed to the particular stimulus that causes them anxiety while being supported and encouraged to remain until the anxiety reduces and they feel calmer, thus reducing the fear and consequent anxiety.

**floppy-baby syndrome** may be due to nervous system or muscle disorder as opposed to benign hypotonia.

**flora** *n* used in microbiology to describe the colonization of various areas of the body by micro-organisms, e.g. *Staphylococcus epidermidis* on the skin. In most instances they are non-pathogenic, but can become pathogenic.

**flossing** *n* mechanical cleaning of the interproximal tooth surfaces by waxed or unwaxed thread (floss) or dental tape. Special floss is available for used with fixed orthodontic appliances.

**flow cytometer** a laboratory instrument used to measure the proportions and absolute numbers of cell populations in, for example, blood. Cells of interest are stained with monoclonal antibodies against particular cell surface markers. The monoclonal antibodies are conjugated to fluorescent dyes and are detected once illuminated by a laser inside the flow cytometer. CD4+ T-cell counts in human immunodeficiency virus (HIV) patients are commonly measured using flow cytometry.

**flowmeter** *n* a measuring instrument for flowing gas or liquid.

**fluctuation** *n* a wave-like motion felt on digital examination of a fluid-containing tumour, e.g. abscess—**fluctuant** *adj*.

**fluke** *n* a trematode worm of the order Digenea. Different flukes infest the hepatobiliary system, the lungs, blood and the intestine. The *hepatobiliary flukes Clonorchis sinensis* (Chinese fluke) and *Opisthorchis viverrini* (South-east Asia) are usually ingested with raw fish. ⇒ clonorchiasis, *Clonorchis sinensis*, opisthorchiasis, *Opisthorchis*. The *hepatobiliary fluke* present in Europe is the *European* or *sheep fluke* (*Fasciola hepatica*), which is usually ingested from watercress. ⇒ *Fasciola hepatica*, fascioliasis. The *lung fluke Paragonimus westermani* is usually ingested with raw crab and other shellfish in China and Far East. ⇒ paragonimiasis, *Paragonimus*. The *blood flukes* from the genus *Schistosoma* are present in Africa, Middle East, Philippines, Japan, Eastern Asia, the Caribbean and South America, they are *Schistosoma haematobium, S. japonicum and S. mansoni.* ⇒ *Schistosoma*, schistosomiasis. An example of an *intestinal fluke* is *Fasciolopsis buski*, it is endemic in Asia and tropical regions. ⇒ fasciolopsiasis, *Fasciolopsis buski*.

**fluorescein** *n* orange substance which fluoresces green when exposed to blue light. Used as eye drops to detect corneal lesions. Also used in retinal angiography, by injection into a peripheral vein, to demonstrate the retinal and choroidal circulation, and chorioretinal disease. ⇒ angiography.

**fluorescein string test** *n* used to detect the site of obscure upper gastrointestinal bleeding. The patient swallows a radiopaque knotted string. Fluorescein is injected intravenously and after a few minutes the string is withdrawn. If staining has occurred the site of bleeding can be determined.

**fluorescent antibody test** *n* a technique for visualizing an antibody by coating it with a fluorescent dye which can then be viewed by use of a fluorescent microscope with a source of ultraviolet light. ⇒ immunofluorescence.

**fluorescent treponemal antibody absorbed test (FTA-Abs)** *n* a specific serological test for syphilis.

**fluoridation** *n* ⇒ fluoride.

**fluoride** *n* an ion sometimes present in drinking water, toothpastes, tea, vegetables and sea food. It can be incorporated into the structure of bone and teeth, where it provides protection against dental caries but in gross excess it causes mottling of the teeth. As a public health preventive measure it can be added to a water supply (fluoridation).

**fluorine (F)** *n* halogen element.

**fluoroquinolones** *npl* a group of synthetic antibiotics, e.g. ciprofloxacin. ⇒ Appendix 5.

**fluoroscopy** *n* dynamic X-ray examination of the human body, observed by means of fluorescent screen and TV system.

**fluorosis** *n* a condition caused by excessive intake of fluorine over a long period. It leads to the mottling and pitting of the teeth and bone disorders.

**FM** *abbr* Fugel–Meyer.

**FMN/FMNH₂** *abbr* flavin mononucleotide (oxidized and reduced form respectively).

**FOB** *abbr* faecal occult blood.

**focal injuries** those injuries that occur in a small concentrated area, usually due to a high-velocity, low-mass force, e.g. ice hockey puck making contact with an unguarded area of the player's body.

**focus** *n* **1.** in optics, the point at which light rays converge after passing through a lens. **2.** the main site of an infection.

**focus groups** in research, a method of obtaining data that involves interviewing people in small interacting groups.

**foetor** *n* ⇒ fetor.

**folate** *n* (*syn* pteroylglutamic acid) collective name for the B vitamin compounds derived from folic acid. Folates occur naturally in foods such as liver, yeasts and leafy green vegetables and are absorbed from the small intestine. They are coenzymes involved in many biochemical reactions in the body, e.g. purine and pyrimidine synthesis, and adequate amounts, along with vitamin $B_{12}$, are required for normal red cells and cell division generally. A deficiency results in a megaloblastic anaemia. It is recommended that supplements are taken before and during the first weeks after conception, to reduce the risk of neural tube defects (NTDs) in the fetus.

**folic acid** the molecule that gives rise to a large group of molecules known as folates that form part of the vitamin B complex. ⇒ folate.

**folie à deux** a rare psychiatric syndrome, in which one member of a close pair suffers a psychotic illness and eventually imposes his or her delusions on the other.

**follicle** *n* **1.** a small secreting sac. **2.** a simple tubular gland—**follicular** *adj.*

**follicle-stimulating hormone (FSH)** secreted by the anterior pituitary gland; it is trophic to the ovaries in the female, where it develops the oocyte-containing (Graafian) follicles; and to the testes in the male, where it stimulates spermatogenesis.

**folliculitis** *n* inflammation of follicles, such as the hair follicles. ⇒ alopecia.

**fomentation** *n* a hot, wet application used to produce hyperaemia when applied to the skin.

**fomites** *npl* any article that has been in contact with infection and is capable of transmitting same, e.g. bed linen, surgical instruments.

**fontanelle** *n* a membranous space between the cranial bones. The diamond-shaped anterior fontanelle (bregma) is at the junction of the frontal and two parietal bones. It usually closes in the second year of life. The triangular posterior fontanelle (lambda) is at the junction of the occipital and two parietal bones. It closes within a few weeks of birth.

**food allergy** an abnormal immunological response to food that can be severe and life-threatening. Signs and symptoms include swelling of the mouth and throat, breathing difficulties, skin rashes and gastrointestinal disturbances. The term is often used erroneously to describe any adverse reactions to food, whether or not the underlying mechanism has been identified. ⇒ allergy.

**food intolerance** an abnormal reaction to a food that is not immunological in origin, e.g. the effects of lactose intake in a person with lactase deficiency. Symptoms can be chronic or acute; identification of the food can be difficult and may require an exclusion diet.

**food poisoning** a notifiable disease characterized by vomiting, with or without

diarrhoea. It results from eating food contaminated with preformed bacterial toxin (e.g. from *Escherichia coli* O157, *Staphylococcus aureus* and *Clostridium perfringens*) or multiplication of live micro-organisms in food (e.g. *Campylobacter jejuni*, *Salmonella typhimurium*, *Bacillus cereus* and viruses) or poisonous natural vegetation, e.g. berries, toadstools (fungi) or chemical poisons.

**Food Standards Agency (FSA)** in the UK a body set up by the government to oversee food standards and safety.

**foot** *n* that portion of the lower limb below the ankle.

**foot drop** inability to dorsiflex foot due usually to damage affecting the nerve supply to the foot. Can be a complication of bedrest.

**foramen** *n* a hole or opening. Generally used with reference to bones—**foramina** *pl. foramen magnum* the opening in the occipital bone through which the spinal cord passes. *foramen ovale* a fetal cardiac interatrial communication which normally closes at birth.

**force couple** a single movement that is produced by the integrated activity of two or more muscles, such as rotation of the scapula.

**forced expiratory volume (FEV)** volume of air exhaled during a given time (usually the first second: $FEV_1$).

**forced vital capacity (FVC)** the maximum gas volume that can be expelled from the lungs in a forced expiration. ⇒ respiratory function tests.

**forceps** *n* surgical instruments with two opposing blades which are used to grasp or compress tissues, swabs, needles and many other surgical appliances. The two blades are controlled by direct pressure on them (tong-like), or by handles (scissor-like). *forceps delivery* the use of various specialized obstetric forceps, e.g. Wrigley's forceps, Kielland forceps, applied to the infant to facilitate delivery during the second stage of labour.

**forensic medicine** (*syn* medical jurisprudence, or 'legal medicine') the application of medical science to questions of law.

**forebrain** *n* the part of the brain comprising the cerebral hemispheres, basal nuclei and the structures of the diencephalon.

**foregut** *n* the front part of the embryonic alimentary tract. It is endodermal tissue and will form the pharynx, oesophagus, stomach, some of the small intestine, the liver and pancreas. ⇒ hindgut, midgut.

**foreskin** *n* the prepuce or skin covering the glans penis.

**forewaters** *n* the sac of amniotic fluid situated in front of the fetal head. The pressure from the well-flexed head on the cervix creates a dam so that some amniotic fluid becomes trapped in front of the head. ⇒ hindwaters.

**formaldehyde** *n* toxic gas used as a disinfectant. Dissolved in water (formalin), it is mainly used for disinfection and the preservation of histological specimens.

**forme fruste 1.** an inherited condition in which there is only minimal expression of the faulty gene. **2.** a disease presentation which is atypical or incomplete and resolves earlier than is usual.

**formication** *n* a sensation as of ants running over the skin. Occurs in nerve lesions, particularly in the regenerative phase.

**formiminoglutamic acid** ⇒ FIGLU test.

**formula** *n* a prescription. A series of symbols denoting the chemical composition of a substance, e.g. NaCl is the formula for sodium chloride—**formulae, formulas** *pl*.

**formula diet** a diet that requires only minimal digestion and is easily absorbed. It comprises amino acids or peptides, glucose and mono- and diglycerides.

**formulary** *n* a collection of formulas. The *British National Formulary* describes licensed pharmaceutical products available in the UK.

**fornix** *n* an arch; particularly referred to the vagina, i.e. the space between the vaginal wall and the cervix of the uterus—**fornices** *pl*.

**fortification** *n* the addition of specific nutrients to foods, such as vitamins A and D to margarine. Or, as in the United States, the addition of folic acid to all cereal products, thus increasing intake levels in the population.

**forward parachute reflex** ⇒ parachute reflex.

**fourth-degree tear** ⇒ perineal tear.

**fossa** *n* a depression or furrow—**fossae** *pl*.

**fostering** *n* placing a vulnerable child with a suitable family, either as a short- or long-term measure. The aims are to provide a child with the security of a home environment, and to reunite the child with his or her natural family as soon as practical. Long-term fosterings can be 'with a view to adoption'.

**Fothergill's operation** ⇒ Manchester operation.

**fourchette** *n* a membranous fold connecting the posterior ends of the labia minora.

**'four-day blues'** ⇒ postnatal depression.

**Fournier's gangrene** (J Fournier, French dermatologist, 1832–1914) a fulminating gangrene of the scrotum. ⇒ fasciitis.

**fovea** *n* a small depression or fossa; particularly, the *fovea centralis* in the macula lutea of the retina. The fovea contains many cones and is important for sharp central vision and high-quality colour vision.

**fractional inspired oxygen concentration ($FiO_2$)** the concentration of oxygen in inspired gas, expressed as a fraction of 1 (e.g. $FiO_2$ 0.6 equals 60% inspired oxygen concentration).

**fractional utilization** the percentage of maximum oxygen consumption/uptake ($VO_{2max}$) that can be sustained during exercise at competition/race pace. It is affected by the duration of exercise and the level of training.

**fractionation** *n* in radiotherapy, the division of the total prescribed radiation dose into smaller doses to be given over a period of time to minimize tissue damage.

**fracture** *n* breach in continuity of a bone as a result of injury (Figure F.3). ⇒ Bennett's fracture, Colles' fracture. *closed fracture* there is no communication with external air. *comminuted fracture* a breach in the continuity of a bone which is broken into more than two pieces. *complicated fracture* a breach in the continuity of a bone when there is injury to surrounding organs and structures. *compression fracture* usually of lumbar or dorsal region of the spine; the anterior vertebral bodies are crushed together. *depressed fracture* the broken bone presses on an underlying structure, such as brain or lung. *impacted fracture* one end of the broken bone is driven into the other. *incomplete fracture* the bone is only cracked or fissured—called *greenstick fracture* when it occurs in children. *open (compound) fracture* there is a wound permitting communication of broken bone end with air. *pathological fracture* occurring in abnormal bone as a result of force which would not break a normal bone. *spontaneous fracture* one occurring without appreciable violence; may be synonymous with pathological fracture. *stress* or *fatigue fracture* ⇒ march fracture, stress fracture.

**fraenotomy** *n* frenotomy.

**fraenum** *n* frenum.

**fragile X syndrome** X-linked disorder, mainly affecting males. During childhood there is relatively normal appearance, but some degree of learning disability. Physical features include large ears and a long and narrow face, enlarged testes and, in a smaller percentage, very smooth skin, flat feet and mitral valve prolapse and which usually come to prominence after puberty.

187

F

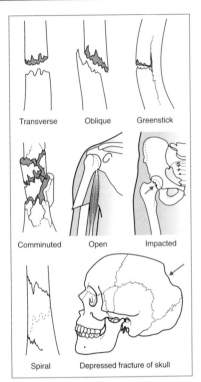

Transverse    Oblique    Greenstick

Comminuted    Open    Impacted

Spiral    Depressed fracture of skull

**Figure F.3** Types of fractures *(reproduced from Brooker 2006A with permission).*

**fragilitas ossium** ⇒ osteogenesis imperfecta.

**framboesia** *n* yaws.

*Francisella* *n* (E Francis, American microbiologist, 20th century) a genus of Gram-negative bacteria. The species *Francisella tularensis* causes tularaemia in humans. ⇒ tularaemia.

**Fraser syndrome** (G Fraser, American geneticist, b. 1932) a congenital absence of the opening between the eyelids. It is an autosomal recessive condition and is associated with other abnormalities that include abnormal eyeball development, cleft palate, heart problems, etc.

**FRC** *abbr* functional residual capacity.

**freckle** *n* small brown macules on the skin, especially after sun exposure. An inherited trait that is particularly common in people with red hair. ⇒ ephelis, lentigo.

**free-floating anxiety** generalized pervasive anxiety with no link to a specific situation or object. The person feels persistent fear and unease.

**free radical** reactive oxygen species, such as the superoxide ion and hydroxyl radical. They are extremely reactive chemicals produced during normal metabolism. Normally they are dealt with by complex antioxidant enzyme systems but they can cause oxidative damage to cells. ⇒ antioxidant nutrients.

**free text term** in literature searching, a list of words that describe each part of the search question more fully. These may include alternative spellings (including American spelling), abbreviations, plurals and synonyms.

**freezing** *n* the sudden inability of a parkinsonian patient to take another step while walking until an external visual, auditory or cutaneous stimulus is appreciated. It is due to co-contraction of antagonistic muscle groups; a manifestation of dystonia.

**Freiberg's infarction** (A Freiberg, American surgeon, 1868–1940) an aseptic necrosis of bone tissue which most commonly occurs in the head of the second metatarsal bone.

**fremitus** *n* a trembling vibration of a body structure, usually the chest wall. It can be palpated during examination or heard by auscultation when the patient speaks, breathes or coughs.

**Frenkel's exercises** (H Frenkel, Swiss neurologist, 1860–1931) special repetitive exercises to improve muscle and joint sense.

**frenotomy** *n* surgical severance of a frenum or frenulum, particularly for tongue tie.

**frenulum or frenum** *n* a small fold of mucous membrane that checks or limits the movement of an organ, e.g. tongue, prepuce of the penis. *frenulum linguae* from the undersurface of the tongue to the floor of the mouth.

**frequency distribution** in statistics, the number of times (frequency) each value in a variable is observed.

**frequency** *n* **1.** electromagnetic frequencies. The number of cycles per second, now measured in hertz (Hz). **2.** the voiding of urine more often than is acceptable to the person, usually more often than previously experienced and in smaller volumes. **3.** the number of repetitions in a set time, e.g. respirations in 1 minute.

**Fresnel zone** (A Fresnel, French physicist, 1788–1827) also called the near field. The area closest to the head of an ultrasound transducer. It is irregular in intensity but is generally the area which produces images with the best resolution, and the most beneficial therapeutic effects.

**Freud, Sigmund** (Austrian neurologist, 1856–1939) the originator of psychoanalysis and the psychoanalytical theory of the causation of neuroses. He first described the existence of the unconscious mind, censor, repression and the theory of infantile sexuality, and worked out in detail many mental mechanisms of the unconscious which modify normal, and account for abnormal, human behaviour.

**friable** *adj* easily crumbled; readily pulverized.

**friction** *n* rubbing. Can cause abrasion of skin, leading to a superficial pressure ulcer; the adhesive property of friction, increased in the presence of moisture, can contribute to a shearing force which can cause a more severe pressure ulcer. *friction murmur/rub* heard through the stethoscope when two rough or dry surfaces rub together, as in pleurisy and pericarditis.

**frictions** *npl* small, accurately localized, penetrating massage manipulations using the pads of the fingers and thumb. Used in a circular direction on connective tissue and muscle, or transversely across tendons, to mobilize tissues, for example to maintain and restore mobility of tissues at risk of developing adhesions following strain or injury.

**Friedreich's ataxia** (N Friedreich, German physician, 1825–1882) a recessively inherited progressive disease of childhood, in which there is sclerosis of the sensory and motor columns in the spinal cord, with consequent muscular weakness and staggering (ataxia). The heart may also be affected.

**frigidity** *n* absence of normal sexual desire.

**frog plaster** conservative treatment of developmental dysplasia of the hip (congenital dislocation of the hip), whereby the dislocation is reduced by gentle manipulation and both hips are immobilized in plaster of Paris, both hips abducted to 80° and externally rotated.

**Fröhlich's syndrome** (A Fröhlich, Austrian neurologist/pharmacologist, 1871–1953). ⇒ adiposogenital dystrophy.

**Froin's syndrome** (G Froin, French physician, 1874–1932) characterized by yellow cerebrospinal fluid which has an increased amount of protein.

**frontal** *adj* pertaining to the front of a structure.

**frontal bone** the cranial bone that forms the forehead.

**frontal lobe** the lobe of each cerebral hemisphere that lies under the frontal bone.

Contains the primary motor area, the motor speech area and functions in higher mental activities.

**frontal plane** vertical plane running from head to foot. It divides the body into front and back parts and is at right angles to the median plane. Also called the coronal plane (Figure F.4).

**frontal sinus** the paranasal air sinus at the inner aspect of each orbital ridge on the frontal bone. ⇒ Appendix 1, Figure 14.

**frostbite** *n* freezing of the skin and superficial tissues resulting from exposure to extreme cold. The lesion is similar to a burn and may become gangrenous with loss of fingers and toes, and other extremities. ⇒ trench foot.

**frozen shoulder** shoulder capsulitis. There is initial pain followed by stiffness, lasting several months. As pain subsides, exercises are intensified until full recovery is gained. Cause unknown.

**fructo-oligosaccharide** *n* a short chain of fewer than 10 fructose units.

**fructosan** *n* general term for polysaccharides comprising fructose units, such as inulin.

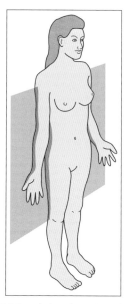

**Figure F.4** Frontal plane *(reproduced from Hinchliff et al. 1996 with permission)*.

**fructose** n (*syn* laevulose) fruit sugar, a monosaccharide found in some fruit and vegetables and in honey. Sucrose in the diet is digested to 1 molecule of fructose and 1 of glucose. Fructose can be converted to glycogen in the body, without the presence of insulin.

**fructosuria** n presence of fructose in the urine. Caused by an enzyme deficiency.

**fruitarian** *adj, n* an extremely restrictive diet whereby the person will only eat fruit, nuts and seeds.

**FSA** *abbr* Food Standards Agency.

**FSH** *abbr* follicle-stimulating hormone.

**Fuchs' corneal endothelial dystrophy** (E Fuchs, German ophthalmologist, 1851–1913) an inherited degenerative condition of the eye characterized by corneal clouding. It occurs more commonly in females.

**Fuchs' heterochromic cyclitis** a disorder of the eye with the lighter-coloured iris. There is uveitis of the lighter-coloured iris, iridocyclitis and keratitic precipitates. Often there is cataract formation.

**Fugel–Meyer (FM)** an assessment used after a cerebrovascular accident to assess sensorimotor recovery. It includes balance, sensation, pain, joint function and motor recovery.

**fugue state** an apparently purposeful journey takes place with associated loss of memory. The behaviour of the person involved may appear normal or unspectacular to the casual observer. Occurs in dissociative disorder or postictally in some forms of epilepsy.

**fulguration** n destruction of tissue by diathermy.

**full-term** *adj* mature—describes a pregnancy that has lasted 40 weeks.

**fulminant** *adj* developing quickly and with an equally rapid termination.

**fumigation** n disinfection using the fumes of a vaporized disinfectant.

**function** n **1.** the ability to adapt consistently and competently to the demands of any normal situation in any normal environment. **2.** describes the specific work done by a structure or organ in its normal state.

**functional** *adj* **1.** relating to function. **2.** of a disorder, of the function but not the structure of an organ. **3.** as a psychiatric term, describes a condition without primary organic disease.

**functional assessment** evaluation of the occupational performance components that are required in order to perform activities of daily living consistently and competently.

**functional endoscopic sinus surgery (FESS)** minimally invasive sinus surgery using a fine nasal endoscope.

**functional exercise** in sports medicine the activity(ies) that mimic the stresses, demands and skills of a particular sport.

**functional foods** foods that have a high level of a nutrient, e.g. omega-3 fatty acids, or non-nutrients, which may confer health benefits if included in the diet.

**Functional Independence Measure (FIM)** a widely used measure for assessing a person's ability to function independently. The 18-item scale is used in rehabilitation settings, for example following a stroke, brain injury, spinal injury or after limb amputation.

**functional limitations** the inability to perform functional tasks.

**functional residual capacity (FRC)** the volume of air remaining in the lungs following a normal expiration.

**functional tests** in sports medicine the assessment of the athlete's ability to move a body part actively, passively and against resistance. Also encompasses the normal activity of the internal and sensory organs. *functional tests (sport-specific)* the use of activities and motions that closely represent the athlete's sport and position to assess a body part's readiness to return to competition.

**fundoplication** n surgical folding of the gastric fundus to prevent reflux of gastric contents into the oesophagus. ⇒ gastro-oesophageal reflux disease.

**fundoscopy** n examination of the fundus of the eye ⇒ ophthalmoscope.

**fundus** n **1.** the basal portion of a hollow structure; the part which is distal to the opening. **2.** in ophthalmology the inner surface of the eye as viewed through the pupil using an ophthalmoscope (Figure F.5)—**fundi** *pl*, **fundal** *adj*.

**fungi** *npl* simple plants. Mycophyta, including mushrooms, yeasts, moulds and rusts, many of which cause superficial and systemic disease in humans, such as actinomycosis, aspergillosis, candidiasis and tinea—**fungus** *sing*, **fungal** *adj*.

**fungicide** n an agent that kills fungi—**fungicidal** *adj*. ⇒ antifungal.

**fungiform** *adj* resembling a mushroom, like the fungiform papillae of the tongue.

**fungistatic** *adj* describes an agent which inhibits the growth of fungi.

**fungoid** *adj* similar to a fungus in appearance, such as some cancers.

**funiculitis** n inflammation of a cord, including the spermatic cord.

**funiculus** n a cord-like structure.

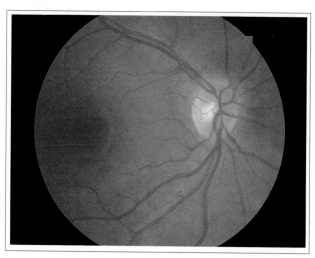

**Figure F.5** Normal fundus of the eye *(reproduced from Kanski 1999 with permission).*

**funnel chest** (*syn* pectus excavatum) a congenital deformity in which the breast bone is depressed towards the spine.

**furuncle** *n* a boil originating in a hair follicle. ⇒ boil.

**furunculosis** *n* an affliction due to boils.

**fusiform** *adj* resembling a spindle with tapering ends. For example, a fusiform aneurysm (Figure A.7, p. 26).

**FVC** *abbr* forced vital capacity.

**F v. West Berkshire Health Authority (1989)** a professional who acts in the best interests of an incompetent person (incapable of giving consent) does not act unlawfully if he/she follows the accepted standard of care according to the Bolam test.

# G

**GABA** *abbr* gamma-aminobutyric acid.

**gag** *n* **1.** the reflex causing contraction of the pharyngeal muscles and elevation of the palate when the soft palate or posterior pharynx is stimulated. **2.** an instrument used to keep the mouth open.

**gait** *n* a manner or style of walking. *ataxic gait* an inco-ordinate or abnormal gait. *cerebellar gait* reeling, staggering, lurching. *scissors gait* one in which the legs cross each other in progressing. *spastic gait* stiff, shuffling, the legs being held together. *tabetic gait* the foot is raised high, then brought down suddenly, the whole foot striking the ground.

**galactagogue** *n* an agent inducing or increasing the flow of milk.

**galactans** *npl* polysaccharides. Polymers comprising many galactose units.

**galactocele** *n* a cyst containing milk, or fluid resembling milk.

**galactorrhoea** *n* excessive flow of milk. Usually reserved for abnormal or inappropriate secretion of milk.

**galactosaemia** *n* excess of galactose in the blood and other tissues. Normally the enzyme lactase in the small intestine converts lactose into glucose and galactose. In the liver another enzyme system converts galactose into glucose. Galactosaemia is an inherited autosomal recessive condition that results from a deficiency of the enzyme galactose-1-phosphate uridyltransferase. The infant has diarrhoea, vomiting and anorexia and fails to gain weight. There is hepatomegaly, cataract formation and learning disability. Management centres on excluding lactose and galatose from the diet. Female carriers of the mutant gene should also exclude these substances from their diet during pregnancy. A milder form of the condition exists where individuals produce some of the enzyme, and may not experience ill effects—**galactosaemic** *adj*.

**galactose** *n* a monosaccharide that is produced by the digestion of the disaccharide lactose found in milk. ⇒ galactosaemia.

**galactosuria** *n* the presence of galactose in the urine.

**Galeazzi's fracture** (R Galeazzi, Italian surgeon, 1866–1952) a fracture of the distal radius and subluxation of the distal radioulnar joint.

**gall** *n* bile.

**gallbladder** *n* a pear-shaped, muscular sac/bag on the undersurface of the liver (⇒ Appendix 1, Figure 18B). It concentrates and stores bile.

**gallipot** *n* a small vessel for lotions.

**gallium (Ga)** *n* a metallic element. Many gallium compounds are toxic. *gallium scan* a radioactive isotope of gallium may be administered intravenously in a total body scan to detect metastatic spread, lymphomas or a focus of infection.

**gallop rhythm** a heart rhythm with a third or fourth heart sound.

**gallows traction** ⇒ Bryant's 'gallows' traction.

**gallstones** *npl* concretions formed within the gallbladder or bile ducts; they are often multiple and faceted. They may contain cholesterol, bile pigments, or both in varying proportions.

**galvanometer** *n* an instrument for measuring an electrical current.

**Gamblers Anonymous** an organization for compulsive gamblers.

**gamekeeper's thumb** (*syn* skier's thumb) a colloquial expression used in sports medicine to describe forced abduction of the metacarpophalangeal joint whilst the thumb is extended, leading to rupture of the ulnar collateral ligament.

**gamete** *n* a female or male reproductive cell with the haploid (n) chromosome number; oocyte or spermatozoon.

**gamete intrafallopian transfer (GIFT)** a technique used in assisted conception for couples where the woman has at least one patent uterine tube (fallopian). The oocyte and sperm are placed in the uterine tube laparoscopically. Fertilization occurs as normal within the uterine tube and the ovum subsequently implants in the lining of the uterus.

**gametogenesis** *n* production of gametes (oocytes and spermatozoa) within the gonads (ovaries or testes). ⇒ oogenesis, spermatogenesis.

**gamma-aminobutyric acid (GABA)** an inhibitory neurotransmitter present in the central nervous system.

**gamma camera** a device used in radioisotope (radionuclide) imaging. It detects concentrations of gamma radiation in body locations following the introduction of a radioactive isotope into the body. The device contains a crystal (the scintillator) in which scintillation events convert gamma rays to light.

**gamma-carboxyglutamate** *n* a substance synthesized in the liver from the amino acid glutamic acid (glutamate) in reactions requiring vitamin K. It is an important component of proteins, e.g. osteocalcin, present in the bone matrix, and in blood coagulation factors, such as prothrombin.

**gamma encephalography** a small dose of a radioactive isotope (radionuclide) is given, which is concentrated in many cerebral tumours. The pattern of radioactivity is then measured.

**gamma globulins** *npl* a group of plasma proteins that have antibody activity, referred to as immunoglobulins (IgA, IgD, IgE, IgG and IgM). They are responsible for the humoral aspects of immunity.

**gamma-glutamyltransferase** (GGT, **gamma-GT, γ-GT**) an enzyme. Increased levels in the plasma reflect liver cell dysfunction, which may be indicative of liver and/or biliary disease, but the level may be affected by the intake of alcohol and by some drugs.

**gamma (γ)-linolenic acid (GLA)** a polyunsaturated fatty acid. ⇒ linolenic acids.

**gamma (γ)-rays** short-wavelength, penetrating rays of the electromagnetic spectrum produced by disintegration of the atomic nuclei of radioactive elements.

**ganglion** *n* **1.** a mass of nerve cell bodies in the peripheral nervous system such as those of the autonomic nervous system and those ganglia containing the cell bodies of sensory nerves. **2.** localized cyst-like swelling near a tendon, sheath or joint. Sometimes occurs on the back of the wrist due to strain such as excessive use of a word processor keyboard—**ganglia** *pl*, **ganglionic** *adj*. *Gasserian ganglion* deeply situated within the skull, on the sensory root of the fifth cranial nerve. It is involved in trigeminal neuralgia.

**ganglionectomy** *n* surgical excision of a ganglion.

**ganglioside** *n* a glycosphingolipid present in the brain and elsewhere in the nervous system. They belong to a group of cerebrosides that contain a sugar and have a basic composition of ceramide-glucose-galactose-N-acetyl-neuraminic acid. Important as a component of the cell membrane.

**gangliosidosis** *n* ⇒ Tay–Sachs disease.

**gangrene** *n* death of part of the tissues of the body. Usually the results of inadequate blood supply, but occasionally due to direct injury (traumatic gangrene) or infection (e.g. gas gangrene caused by species of *Clostridium*). Deficient blood supply may result from pressure on blood vessels (e.g. tourniquets, tight bandages and swelling of a limb); from obstruction within healthy blood vessels (e.g. arterial embolism, frostbite where the capillaries become blocked); from spasm of the vessel wall (e.g. ergot poisoning); or from thrombosis due to disease of the vessel wall (e.g. arteriosclerosis in arteries, phlebitis in veins)—**gangrenous** *adj*. *dry gangrene* occurs when the drainage of blood from the affected part is adequate; the tissues become shrunken and black. *moist gangrene* occurs when venous drainage is inadequate so that the tissues are swollen with fluid.

**gangrenous stomatitis** ⇒ cancrum oris.

**Ganser's syndrome** (S Ganser, German psychiatrist, 1853–1931) a rare dissociative disorder characterized by 'approximate answers' to questions, disorientation/changes in consciousness, amnesia and pseudohallucinations. Sometimes associated with head injury.

**gap junction** a junction between cells that contains pores or channels that allow the passage of ions and molecules, e.g. sugars, vitamins, amino acids, hormones. The passage of ions is particularly important in excitable tissues, such as the myocardium. ⇒ tight junction.

**Garden classification** a four-part classification of fractures of the femoral neck. Type 1, inferior cortex not completely fractured; type 2, cortex fractured but without angulation; type 3, a degree of displacement and rotation of the femoral head; and type 4, complete displacement (Figure G.1).

*Gardnerella vaginalis* (F Gardner, American bacteriologist, b. 1919) a bacterium normally present in the vagina, but is found in increased concentrations in bacterial vaginosis.

**Gardner's syndrome** (E Gardner, American physician, geneticist, 1909–1989) a type of familial adenomatous polyposis that affects the large bowel. Associated abnormalities include epidermal cysts, fibromas and osteomas.

**gargle** *n, vi* a solution used for washing the throat; to wash the throat.

**gargoylism** *n* mucopolysaccharidoses. A congenital disorder of mucopolysaccharide metabolism with either autosomal recessive or sex-linked inheritance. The polysaccharides chondroitin sulphate B and heparitin sulphate are excreted in the urine. Characterized by skeletal abnormalities, coarse features, enlarged liver and spleen and a learning disability. ⇒ Hunter's syndrome, Hurler's syndrome.

**GAS** *abbr* general adaptation syndrome.

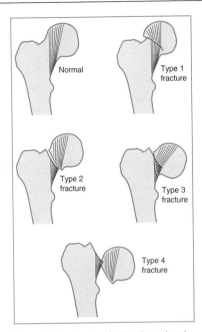

**Figure G.1** Garden classification *(reproduced from Porter 2005 with permission).*

**gas** *n* one of the three states of matter, the others being solid and liquid. A gas retains neither shape nor volume when released— **gaseous** *adj.*

**gas gangrene** a serious wound infection caused by anaerobic organisms of the genus *Clostridium*, especially *Clostridium perfringens (welchii)*, a soil microbe often present in the intestine of humans and animals. It may follow traumatic wounds or surgery. The wound is swollen and discoloured with necrotic tissue and there is foul discharge and gas formation. The systemic effects include fever, tachycardia and hypotension with circulatory collapse. Fatal without effective antibiotic and supportive therapy. ⇒ gangrene.

**gastralgia** *n* pain in the stomach.

**gas transfer factor** measure of the lung's ability to exchange gases. Particularly useful in the diagnosis and surveillance of interstitial lung diseases, sarcoidosis and emphysema.

**gastrectasia** *n* abnormal dilatation of the stomach. The causes include gastric outlet

obstruction due to pyloric stenosis, following gastrointestinal surgery or overeating. ⇒ acute dilatation of the stomach.

**gastrectomy** *n* removal of a part or the whole of the stomach. Usually for cancers but may occasionally be used for gastric ulcers that do not respond to drug therapy. *Billroth I gastrectomy* is a partial gastrectomy where the remaining portion of the stomach is anastomosed to the duodenum. *Polya partial gastrectomy* (known in the USA as *Billroth II gastrectomy*) involves removal of part of the stomach and duodenum and anastomosing the remaining part of the stomach to the jejunum. *total gastrectomy* a radical operation that may be performed for cancer in the upper part of the stomach. ⇒ Roux-en-Y operation.

**gastric** *adj* pertaining to the stomach.

**gastric aspiration or suction** the intermittent or continuous aspiration of gastric contents via a nasogastric tube. It may be used to keep the stomach empty after some gastrointestinal or abdominal operations, when the bowel is obstructed, or to obtain samples.

**gastric glands** glands in the gastric mucosa containing different cells (chief, parietal [oxyntic]) that secrete pepsinogen (precursor of pepsin), rennin, hydrochloric acid (HCl), the intrinsic factor, water and salts; and mucus from goblet cells. ⇒ chief cells, parietal (oxyntic) cells.

**gastric juice** approximately 2 L of acidic (pH 1.5–3) gastric juice is secreted by the gastric glands every day. Apart from hydrochloric acid, gastric juice contains protective mucus, water, salts, two proteolytic enzymes pepsin and rennin, which is important in milk-fed infants, and the intrinsic factor needed for the absorption of vitamin $B_{12}$.

**gastric-inhibitory peptide (GIP)** a regulatory peptide hormone secreted by the small intestine mucosa when fatty acids and glucose are present in the duodenum. It inhibits gastric acid secretion and stimulates insulin secretion.

**gastric ulcer** a peptic ulcer in the gastric mucosa. The majority are associated with the presence of the bacterium *Helicobacter pylori* in the stomach. Other factors include a genetic predisposition, drugs such as non-steroidal anti-inflammatory drugs (NSAIDs) and smoking. The ulcer can bleed, leading to haematemesis and/or melaena, or it can perforate, constituting an abdominal emergency. Severe scarring following chronic ulceration may produce pyloric stenosis and gastric outlet

G

obstruction. For management ⇒ duodenal ulcer.

**gastrin** *n* a local hormone. Polypeptide hormones secreted by special cells in the gastric mucosa of the antrum of the stomach, by fibres of the vagus nerve and to a lesser extent in the duodenum; stimulates the secretion of hydrochloric acid when food enters the stomach.

**gastrinoma** *n* a gastrin-secreting tumour of the pancreas or duodenum. ⇒ islet cell tumours, Zollinger–Ellison syndrome.

**gastritis** *n* inflammation of the stomach, such as that caused by an excessive intake of alcohol.

**gastrocele** *n* a hernia of the stomach.

**gastrocnemius** *n* the large two-headed superficial muscle of the calf. It has two origins, one on each femoral condyle and inserts into the calcaneus by the Achilles (calcaneal) tendon (see Figure A.1, p. 4). It acts at both knee and ankle joints to cause knee flexion and plantar flexion of the foot. ⇒ Appendix 1, Figures 4 and 5.

**gastrocolic** *adj* pertaining to the stomach and the colon.

**gastrocolic reflex** sensory stimulus arising on entry of food into stomach, resulting in strong peristaltic waves (mass movement) in the colon.

**gastroduodenal** *adj* pertaining to the stomach and the duodenum.

**gastroduodenoscopy** *n* endoscopic examination of the stomach and duodenum.

**gastroduodenostomy** *n* a surgical anastomosis between the stomach and the duodenum.

**gastrodynia** *n* pain in the stomach.

**gastroenteritis** *n* food poisoning. Inflammation of mucous membranes of the stomach and the small intestine; usually due to microorganisms, but may be caused by chemicals, poisonous fungi, etc. There is vomiting and diarrhoea due to either the multiplication of micro-organisms (invasive intestinal gastroenteritis) ingested in food or from bacterial toxins (intoxication). Microbial causes include: the bacteria *Bacillus cereus*, *Campylobacter jejuni*, *Clostridium perfringens* and *C. botulinum*, *Escherichia coli*, *Salmonella enteritidis*, *Staphylococcus aureus*, or viruses such as Norovirus (Norwalk-like virus), or rotavirus, a common cause of gastroenteritis in infants. Gastroenteritis is generally transmitted by the faecal–oral route, either directly or indirectly. However, droplet spread is a feature of some viruses.

**gastroenterology** *n* study of the digestive tract, including the liver, biliary tract and pancreas and the associated diseases—**gastroenterological** *adj*, **gastroenterologically** *adv*.

**gastroenteropathy** *n* disease of the stomach and intestine—**gastroenteropathic** *adj*.

**gastroenteroscope** *n* an endoscope for visualization of stomach and intestine—**gastroenteroscopic** *adj*, **gastroenteroscopically** *adv*.

**gastroenterostomy** *n* a surgical anastomosis between the stomach and small intestine.

**gastrointestinal** *adj* pertaining to the stomach and intestine.

**G**

**gastrojejunostomy** *n* a surgical anastomosis between the stomach and the jejunum.

**gastrolith** *n* a solid 'stone' in the stomach, which forms around a mass of hair or vegetable matter. ⇒ bezoar.

**gastro-oesophageal** *adj* pertaining to the stomach and oesophagus.

**gastro-oesophageal reflux disease (GORD)** a condition caused by a malfunctioning lower oesophageal sphincter which allows the acidic gastric contents to move into the oesophagus. This results in pain ('heartburn'), vomiting and potential complications that include oesophagitis, ulceration, scarring with stricture formation and Barrett's oesophagus. There is also the risk of aspiration pneumonia. Reflux is associated with factors that include: gastric distension, increased abdominal pressure, e.g. during coughing, central nervous system disease, hiatus hernia, delayed gastric emptying and the presence of a gastrostomy. A fairly common condition in children, those at increased risk include children with asthma, cystic fibrosis, neurological conditions or previous oesophageal surgery. Conservative treatment includes small frequent thickened feeds for infants and frequent small meals for children and adults, sitting up after eating and elevating the head of the bed/cot at night. $H_2$-receptor antagonist drugs that reduce gastric acid, e.g. ranitidine, may be prescribed. Surgical treatment, such as a fundoplication, may be necessary if conservative measures fail, or if complications occur.

**gastro-oesophagostomy** *n* a surgical operation in which the oesophagus is joined to the stomach to bypass the natural junction.

**gastroparesis** *n* delayed gastric emptying due to poor motility.

**gastropathy** *n* any disease of the stomach.

**gastropexy** *n* surgical fixation of a displaced stomach.

**gastrophrenic** *adj* pertaining to the stomach and diaphragm.

**gastroplasty** *n* previously any reconstructive operation on the stomach to repair damage or deformity. More recently it also includes surgical procedures, e.g. gastric banding, which seek to reduce stomach size as a treatment for morbid obesity.

**gastroschisis** *n* a congenital incomplete closure of the abdominal wall with consequent protrusion of the viscera uncovered by peritoneum.

**gastroscope** *n* a fibreoptic endoscope used to examine the inside of the stomach. ⇒ endoscope—**gastroscopic** *adj*, **gastroscopy** *n*.

**gastrostomy** *n* a surgically established fistula between the stomach and the external abdominal wall. A feeding tube is inserted endoscopically, surgically or radiologically into the stomach. Allows feeding with liquid feeds. ⇒ percutaneous endoscopic gastrostomy.

**gastrotomy** *n* incision into the stomach during an abdominal operation for such purposes as removing a foreign body, securing a bleeding blood vessel, approaching the oesophagus from below to pull down a tube through a constricting growth.

**gastrula** *n* the stage following the blastocyst in embryonic development.

**gastrulation** *n* in early embryonic development the immense changes occurring as the blastocyst becomes the gastrula. The three primary germ layers are formed and cells move to their appointed locations in readiness for the start of structural development.

**gate control theory** a theory that proposes that there is active processing of pain sensation when it first enters the central nervous system at the dorsal horn of the spinal cord. The 'gate' in the spinal cord is opened or closed by a variety of ascending sensory impulses from the peripheral nerves and the descending impulses from the brain. Pain is reduced when the 'gate' is shut but increases when it is open.

**Gaucher's disease** (P Gaucher, French physician, 1854–1918) a rare inherited autosomal recessive disorder. There are three types, of which types 1 and 3 mainly affect Jewish children. It is characterized by a disordered fat metabolism (lipid reticulosis) due to an enzyme deficiency, which leads to very marked enlargement of the spleen and liver, involvement of the bones and lymph nodes. Diagnosis follows biopsy of the bone marrow, liver or spleen. Abnormal histiocytes are found in the marrow. In type 2 disease the central nervous system is involved and the child has seizures and learning disability.

**gauze** *n* a thin, open-meshed absorbent material used in operations to dry the operative field and facilitate the procedure.

**gavage** *n* feeding liquids by a nasogastric tube directly into the stomach.

**GBM** *abbr* glomerular basement membrane.

**GBS** *abbr* Guillain–Barré syndrome.

**GCS** *abbr* Glasgow Coma Scale.

**G-CSF** *abbr* granulocyte colony-stimulating factor.

**GDC** *abbr* General Dental Council.

**GDS** *abbr* geriatric depression scale.

**Geiger–Müller counter** *n* (H Geiger, German physicist, 1882–1945; W Müller, German physicist, 20th century) a device for detecting and registering radioactivity.

**gelatin(e)** *n* the glue-like substance found in animal connective tissue, used in capsules, suppositories and culture medium and in food preparation. Alternative medicines may be needed for vegans, vegetarians and others who will not accept medicines containing gelatin—**gelatinous** *adj*.

**gemellus muscles** a pair of muscles with origins, one on the ischial spine and the other on the ischial tuberosity. The insertion is on the greater trochanter of the femur. They stabilize the hip and rotate the thigh laterally. ⇒ Appendix 1, Figure 5.

**gender** *n* more than just biological sex. The term encompasses the socially constructed views of feminine and masculine behaviour within individual cultural groups.

**gene** *n* a hereditary factor consisting of DNA located at a specific locus of a specific chromosome. Genes are responsible for determining specific characteristics or traits. ⇒ dominant, recessive.

**gene expression** all the processes whereby information encoded by a gene is converted to a physical manifestation of the trait, as observable in the phenotype, usually in the form of a protein.

**gene therapy** the techniques that deliver a normal version of a gene to replace the defective mutant gene, which causes diseases such as cystic fibrosis. The process, which is termed somatic cell gene therapy, aims to treat or cure the condition.

**general adaptation syndrome (GAS)** proposed by Hans Selye (Austrian/Canadian physician/endocrinologist, 1907–1982). It describes a three-phase (triphasic) response of the body to a stressor. Comprising: alarm, resistance/adaptation and exhaustion.

**General Dental Council (GDC)** the statutory body that regulates the practice of dentistry in the UK. It oversees professional quality and continuing professional development standards for professional practice, discipline and conduct. It is responsible for the establishment and maintenance of a professional register for all dentists, dental therapists, dental hygienists, and, from 2008, dental nurses and technicians working in the UK, and has the power to remove individuals from the register.

**General Medical Council (GMC)** the statutory body that regulates the practice of medicine in the UK. It oversees professional quality and continuing professional development standards for professional practice, discipline and conduct. It is responsible for the establishment and maintenance of a professional register for all doctors working in the UK, and currently has the power to remove individuals from the register in cases of professional misconduct, or in some cases to restrict practice or order specific training.

**General Medical Services** the medical services provided by family doctors.

**general paralysis of the insane (GPI)** a manifestation of neurosyphilis in which the brain is principally affected. ⇒ neurosyphilis.

**general practice** in the UK the services provided by generalist doctors in first-contact health care. First defined in 1948 at the inception of the NHS. Provides general medical services as opposed to specialist services.

**general sales list (GSL)** in the UK. Drugs on sale, without prescription, to the public through various retail outlets such as supermarkets. Examples include paracetamol and ibuprofen.

**generalizability** *n* the extent to which research findings from a study of a patient/client group can be valid for another group, or within a different context. For example, can research carried out with a nursing home population be applicable to people living in their own homes or to patients in an acute hospital?

**generalization** *n* in occupational therapy, the ability of clients to transfer knowledge and skills learned during therapy to a number of similar situations.

**generalized anxiety disorder** a state characterized by excessive and persistent generalized anxiety and worry. People may feel apprehensive, tense, indecisive and tired with a low mood. There may be physical manifestations such as rapid heart rate, sweating, breathlessness, changes in appetite and insomnia.

**generative** *adj* pertaining to reproduction.

**generic** *adj* denoting a drug name not protected by brand name or manufacturer. ⇒ recommended International Non-proprietary Name.

**generic descriptor** a term that includes the different chemical forms of a vitamin, all with the same biological activity.

**genetic** *adj* that which relates to heredity. For example, disorders, the basis of which resides in abnormalities of the genetic material, genes and chromosomes. ⇒ congenital.

**genetic code** the arrangement of genetic material stored as nucleotides in the DNA molecule (a double-stranded helix) of the chromosome. It is in this coded form that the information contained in the genes is transmitted to individual cells during transcription and translation. Transcription involves the encoding of the nucleotide sequence on to single-strand messenger RNA (mRNA) using the DNA as a template. The mRNA then conveys the code to the ribosomes. During translation the transfer RNA (tRNA) and ribosomal RNA (rRNA) translate the code for the specific amino acid sequences needed for the ribosomes to synthesize the proteins that control cell activity. ⇒ anticodon, codon, transcription, translation.

**genetic counselling** the specialist multidisciplinary services provided for individuals, couples and families with a history of genetic diseases. They provide information about the genetic disease, its implications and the risk of having affected children. The service also provides information about genetic screening to identify carriers of a recessive mutant gene, prenatal diagnosis, termination of pregnancy and the assisted conception techniques such as the use of donated sperm and eggs.

**genetic drift** the random changes in allele frequency that occur in a finite population over time.

**genetic engineering** ⇒ recombinant DNA technology.

**genetics** *n* the science of heredity and variation, namely the study of the genetic material, its transmission and its changes (mutations).

**genetic screening 1.** testing individuals for the presence of an abnormal gene, such as when a relative has the disease, or for carriers of a recessive gene, or where they belong to a group who have a high incidence of a particular genetic disease, e.g. thalassaemia in people from around the Mediterranean, or Tay–Sachs disease in Ashkenazic Jews. **2.** testing a specific population for the presence of a genetic disease, for example testing neonates for cystic fibrosis, congenital hypothyroidism, galactosaemia (in some countries), phenylketonuria, sickle-cell diseases and thalassaemia, and medium-chain acyl-CoA dehydrogenase deficiency (MCADD).

**genioplasty** *n* also called mentoplasty. A surgical procedure to improve the size or shape of the chin. It may involve bone removal, or the use of bone grafts or implants to increase the size.

**genital** *adj* pertaining to the organs of generation.

**genital herpes** ⇒ herpes.

**genital warts** a very common disease caused by certain types of the human papillomavirus (HPV). Cauliflower-like lesions develop in the genital area or in the perianal region after a pre-patent period that varies from several weeks to even years. Some strains of HPV are associated with the development of cervical cancer.

**genitalia** *n* the external organs of generation.

**genitocrural** *adj* pertaining to the genital area and the legs.

**genitourinary** *adj* pertaining to the reproductive and urinary organs. *genitourinary medicine (GUM)* specialty concerned with the management of sexually transmitted infections and other medical conditions of the genital tract.

**genome** *n* the basic set of chromosomes and the genes, equal to the sum total of gene types possessed by different organisms of a species.

**genotype** *n* the total genetic information encoded in the chromosomes of an individual (as opposed to the phenotype). Also, the genetic make-up of a person at a specific locus, namely the alleles present at that locus. ⇒ phenotype.

**gentian violet** ⇒ crystal violet.

**genu** *n* the knee.

**genupectoral position** the knee–chest position, i.e. the weight is taken by the knees, and by the upper chest, while the shoulder girdle and head are supported on a pillow in front.

**genu valgum (bow legs)** abnormal outward curving of the legs resulting in separation of the knees.

**genu varum (knock knee)** abnormal incurving of the legs so that there is a gap between the feet when the knees are in contact.

**genus** *n* a classification ranking between the family and species.

**geophagia** *n* the habit of eating clay or earth.

**geriatric depression scale (GDS)** a test of depression for use with older people.

**geriatrician** *n* one who specializes in geriatrics; the medical care of older people.

**geriatrics** *n* the branch of medical science dealing with old age and its diseases, together with the medical care and nursing required by older people.

**germ** *n* colloquial term for a micro-organism, especially a pathogen.

**German measles** ⇒ rubella.

**germ cell** refers to a reproductive cell during any stage of gametogenesis (formation of gametes, oocytes or spermatozoa), e.g. gametogonia, gametocytes, or to the gametes themselves. A germline cell rather than a somatic (body) cell. ⇒ gamete, gametogenesis, oogenesis, spermatogenesis.

**germicide** *n* any agent capable of killing micro-organisms (germs)—**germicidal** *adj.*

**germinal** *adj* pertaining to a germ cell, or to the first stages in embryonic development.

**germinal epithelium** the outer epithelial layer of the ovary. So called because it was previously thought to be the site of oogonia formation.

**germ layers** the three primordial cell layers responsible for every cell type in the body. The ectoderm, endoderm and mesoderm develop during gastrulation in very early embryonic development. Each layer differentiates into different cell types.

**germ line** the genetic material passed from parents to their offspring through the oocyte and spermatozoa (gametes).

**gerontology** *n* the scientific study of ageing—**gerontological** *adj.*

**Gerstmann's syndrome** (J Gerstmann, Austrian neurologist, 1887–1969) includes right–left disorientation, an inability to identify the fingers (finger agnosia), constructional apraxia, acalculia and agraphia. It may occur after damage to the parietal lobe of the brain or following a stroke.

**Gestalt theory** a German word meaning 'organized whole'. A theory of behaviour developed early in the 20th century. It contends that perception and learning are active, creative processes that are part of an 'organized whole'.

**gestation** *n* ⇒ pregnancy—**gestational** *adj.*

**gestational diabetes** diabetes mellitus that develops, or is first observed during pregnancy. It is due to an intolerance to carbohydrate that leads to hyperglycaemia. The cause is unknown but the hormones of pregnancy may decrease the response to insulin.

Certain groups are at higher risk, such as in women with a family history of type 2 diabetes and increasing age. It resolves following the birth of the infant, but affected women have a greater risk than normal of developing both type 1 and type 2 diabetes. It may be treated with diet alone or with diet and insulin. The insulin is stopped immediately following the birth of the infant.

**GFR** *abbr* glomerular filtration rate.

**GGT, gamma-GT, γ-GT** *abbr* gamma-glutamyltransferase.

**GH** *abbr* growth hormone.

**Ghon's focus/complex** (A Ghon, Czechoslovakian pathologist, 1866–1936). ⇒ primary complex.

**ghrelin** *n* peptide hormone secreted by cells in the stomach and duodenum. It stimulates the secretion of growth hormone and regulates food intake and energy balance through its effects on the hypothalamus.

**GHRH** *abbr* growth hormone-releasing hormone.

**GHRIH** *abbr* growth hormone release-inhibiting hormone.

**giant cell arteritis** ⇒ arteritis.

***Giardia*** *n* (A Giard, French biologist, 1846–1908) a genus of flagellate protozoans. They are parasites that infect the gastrointestinal tract where they cause inflammation in the duodenum and jejunum. In some individuals they may be commensals. Hosts include cats, dogs, cattle and sheep.

**giardiasis** *n* (*syn* lambliasis) infection with the flagellate *Giardia intestinalis*. May be symptomless, especially in adults. Causes crampy pain, bloating, vomiting, anorexia, foul-smelling diarrhoea with steatorrhoea and flatulence. Occurs worldwide but is more common in tropical regions. It particularly affects children, people travelling to other areas and those who are immunocompromised.

**gibbus** *n* an abnormal convex spinal curvature. It may be associated with vertebral body collapse, such as that occurring in tuberculosis affecting the spine.

**GIFT** *abbr* gamete intrafallopian transfer.

**gigantism** *n* abnormal overgrowth, especially in height, due to excess growth hormone in childhood prior to fusion of the epiphyseal plates in the long bones. Almost always due to a pituitary tumour.

**Gilles de Tourette syndrome** (G Gilles de la Tourette, French neurologist, 1857–1904). ⇒ Tourette's syndrome.

**Gillick competence** concerns the decision-making competence of children and young people and their capacity to give valid consent for medical treatment. It arises from the case of Gillick v. West Norfolk and Wisbech Area Health Authority in which the House of Lords ruled that children under 16 years of age can give legally effective consent to medical treatment providing they can demonstrate sufficient maturity and intelligence to understand fully the treatment planned. The capacity to make a decision, which is judged by the health professional, is subject to certain guidelines, for example, that the treatment is in the best interests of the young person. The case in question centred on the provision of contraceptive advice and treatment in a female under 16 years of age.

**gingiva** *n* the keratinized oral mucosa immediately surrounding a tooth, i.e. the gum—**gingivae** *pl*, **gingival** *adj*.

**gingival sulcus** the invagination made by the gingiva as it joins with the tooth surface.

**gingivectomy** *n* surgical excision of infected or otherwise diseased gingiva. Such as for severe periodontal disease.

**gingivitis** *n* inflammation of the gingivae. Characterized by redness, bleeding and swelling.

**ginglymus** *n* a hinge joint. A type of freely movable joint that has angular movement in one plane, such as the elbow.

**GIP** *abbr* gastric inhibitory peptide.

**girdle** *n* usually a bony structure of oval shape such as the shoulder and pelvic girdles.

**GLA** *abbr* gamma (γ)-linolenic acid.

**glabella** *n* the flat triangular part of the frontal bone between the two superciliary ridges.

**gland** *n* an organ or structure capable of making an internal or external secretion. ⇒ endocrine, exocrine—**glandular** *adj*.

**glanders** *n* a contagious, febrile, ulcerative disease communicable from horses, mules and asses to humans. Caused by the bacterium *Burkholderia mallei* (previously called *Pseudomonas mallei*). The disease is characterized by skin nodules and ulceration of the respiratory mucosa. It is endemic in Central and South America, Asia, Africa and the Middle East.

**glandular fever** ⇒ infectious mononucleosis.

**glans** *n* the bulbous termination of the clitoris and penis. ⇒ Appendix 1, Figure 16.

**Glasgow Coma Scale (GCS)** a rating scale of conscious level for trauma and neurological patients that assesses their best motor, verbal and eye-opening response (Table G.1). Used, for example, following brain/head injury and

**Table G.1** Glasgow Coma Scale

| Eye-opening (E) | |
|---|---|
| Spontaneous | 4 |
| To speech | 3 |
| To pain | 2 |
| Nil | 1 |
| **Best motor response (M)** | |
| Obeys | 6 |
| Localizes | 5 |
| Withdraws | 4 |
| Abnormal flexion | 3 |
| Extensor response | 2 |
| Nil | 1 |
| **Verbal response (V)** | |
| Oriented | 5 |
| Confused conversation | 4 |
| Inappropriate words | 3 |
| Incomprehensible sounds | 2 |
| Nil | 1 |
| **Coma score = E + M + V** | |
| Minimum | 3 |
| Maximum | 15 |

Reproduced from Boon et al. (2006) with permission.

**G**

neurosurgery. A modified scale is available for use with preverbal children.

**glaucoma** *n* a group of conditions in which raised intraocular pressure (IOP) causes characteristic damage to the optic nerve head and visual field loss. *acute glaucoma* primary closed-angle glaucoma (PCAG) a very painful condition which generally has a sudden onset, usually with very high IOP. It affects middle-aged and older people and the incidence in females is four times greater than that in males. It is also more common in people from South-east Asia. It is characterized by severe pain around one eye, which is red with an oval semidilated pupil. Visual acuity is reduced, patients may see halos round lights and they are photophobic. Some people may have nausea and vomiting, and feel unwell. It is an emergency situation and requires immediate treatment to lower the IOP, with drugs that reduce the amount of aqueous humour and others to improve drainage, in order to save the sight in the affected eye. A laser iridotomy will usually be undertaken to provide a pathway for the drainage of aqueous humour. *chronic glaucoma* primary open-angle glaucoma (POAG) is a painless insidious condition causing gradual loss of peripheral vision (tunnel vision), usually over many years. It is more common in middle-aged and older people, where there is a family history of glaucoma and in African–Caribbean individuals. Management involves the use of drugs to reduce IOP by decreasing the flow of aqueous humour or increase its drainage. Surgery to increase drainage may be necessary if drug therapy is ineffective—**glaucomatous** *adj*.

**glaucoma valve** various devices sometimes used in glaucoma to reduce raised intraocular pressure. More recent shunts incorporate a valve. The shunt is used to divert aqueous humour from the trabecular meshwork and redirect it to a subconjunctival bleb.

**Gleason grade** (D Gleason, American pathologist, 20th century) a five-stage system used to assess the degree of differentiation in prostate cancer.

**glenohumeral** *adj* pertaining to the glenoid cavity of scapula and the humerus.

**glenoid** *n* a cavity on the scapula into which the head of the humerus fits to form the shoulder joint.

**glia** *n* ⇒ macroglia, microglia, neuroglia—**glial** *adj*.

**gliadin** *n* a protein found in the gluten present in wheat and rye. Intolerance of gliadin causes coeliac disease.

**glicentin** *n* a form of enteroglucagon.

**gliding joint** a freely movable joint that only allows gliding movement, such as those between the wrist and ankle bones.

**glioblastoma multiforme** a highly malignant brain tumour.

**glioma** *n* a malignant tumour that arises from neuroglial tissue, typically an astrocytoma or oligodendroglioma—**gliomata** *pl.* ⇒ astrocyte, oligodendrocyte.

**gliomyoma** *n* a tumour of nerve and muscle tissue—**gliomyomata** *pl*.

**globin** *n* the four protein molecules that join with haem to form haemoglobin.

**globulins** *npl* a large group of proteins. Those in the plasma are classified as alpha and beta, which are concerned with substance transport, and gamma, which provides protection against infection. The gamma globulins comprise the immunoglobulins A, D, E, G and M.

**globulinuria** *n* the presence of globulin in the urine.

**globus pharyngis** also still called globus hystericus. A subjective feeling of a lump in the throat. Can also include difficulty in swallowing and is due to tension of muscles of deglutition. It may be associated with anxiety states, dissociative disorder and depression.

**globus pallidus** literally pale globe; a mass of motor grey matter situated deep within the cerebral hemispheres, lateral to the thalamus. Part of the basal nuclei.

**glomerular filtration rate (GFR)** the volume of plasma filtered by the kidneys in one minute. It is usually around 120 mL/min.

**glomerulitis** *n* inflammation of the glomeruli.

**glomerulonephritis** *n* inflammation of the glomeruli (of the nephron). The term encompasses many different acute and chronic disorders of varying aetiology and prognosis—**glomerulonephritides** *pl.*

**glomerulosclerosis** *n* fibrosis of the glomeruli (of the nephron), often as a result of glomerulonephritis—**glomerulosclerotic** *adj.*

**glomerulus** *n* a coil of capillaries formed from a wide-bore afferent arteriole. It lies within the invaginated blind end of the renal tubule (Figure G.2). Together with the renal tubule it forms a nephron. Part of the filtration membrane involved in the production of urine—**glomerular** *adj*, **glomeruli** *pl.*

**glomus** *n* arterioles which communicate directly with veins.

**glossa** *n* the tongue—**glossal** *adj.*

**glossectomy** *n* excision of the tongue.

***Glossina*** *n* a genus of biting flies. ⇒ tsetse.

**glossitis** *n* inflammation of the tongue. It may be associated with infection, trauma, B vitamin deficiencies or pernicious anaemia.

**glossodynia** *n* painful tongue without visible change.

**glossopharyngeal** *adj* pertaining to the tongue and pharynx. The ninth pair of cranial nerves; they innervate the tongue and pharynx.

**glossoplegia** *n* paralysis of the tongue.

**glossopyrosis** *n* a burning sensation felt in the tongue.

**glottis** *n* the opening between the abducted vocal folds in the larynx. It allows air to enter the respiratory tract and is involved in voice production—**glottic** *adj.*

**glucagon** *n* a catabolic polypeptide hormone secreted in the pancreatic islets by the alpha cells. It causes the release of glucose from liver glycogen and thereby raises the blood glucose (sugar). Its release is stimulated by hypoglycaemia and growth hormone. Used by injection to reverse hypoglycaemia. ⇒ insulin.

**glucagonoma** *n* a glucagon-secreting tumour of the islet cells of the pancreas. Usually malignant and often part of multiple endocrine neoplasia (MEN). It is characterized by hyperglycaemia, skin rash, cheilitis, glossitis, stomatitis, weight loss, diarrhoea and possible mental health problems or a tendency to develop thromboembolic conditions. ⇒ islet cell tumours.

**glucagon stimulation test** a test of pituitary reserve, assessing the response of growth hormone and adrenocorticotrophic hormone (ACTH) and hence cortisol to subcutaneous or intramuscular administration of glucagon.

**glucans** *npl* complex carbohydrates in cereals such as oats, barley and rye. They are soluble but undigested.

**glucocorticoid** *n* any steroid hormone which promotes gluconeogenesis and which antagonizes the action of insulin. Occurring naturally in the adrenal cortex as cortisone and cortisol, and produced synthetically as, for example, prednisolone.

**glucogenesis** *n* production of glucose.

**glucokinase** *n* an enzyme that catalyses the phosphorylation of glucose to glucose-6-phosphate (G6P); the initial reaction in both glycolysis and glycogenesis. It is a hexokinase and is found in the liver, intestine, pancreas and brain.

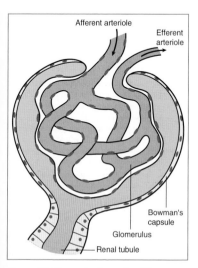

**Figure G.2** Glomerulus *(reproduced from Watson 2000 with permission).*

**gluconeogenesis** *n* the formation of glucose from non-carbohydrate sources, e.g. amino acids, glycerol, lactate, etc.

**glucosamine** *n* an amino sugar that forms the basis of many important glycosylated lipids and proteins, such as those found in cartilage. Individuals with osteoarthritis may choose to take glucosamine supplements.

**glucosan** *n* a term for the group of glucose polysaccharides that include cellulose, glycogen and starch.

**glucose** *n* dextrose. A monosaccharide. The form in which carbohydrates are absorbed through the intestinal tract and circulated in the blood. The amount in the blood is controlled by hormones that include insulin and glucagon. It is stored as glycogen in the liver and skeletal muscle.

**glucose-6-phosphate dehydrogenase (G6PD)** an enzyme. Deficiencies occurring in the red blood cell may be inherited. It affects Africans and their descendants elsewhere, people living around the Mediterranean and in the Middle East. People lacking G6PD develop anaemia when exposed to certain foods or drugs, such as antimalarial agents. ⇒ anaemia, favism.

**glucose tolerance test (oral glucose tolerance test)** after a period of fasting, a measured quantity (75 g) of glucose is taken orally; thereafter blood samples are tested for glucose levels at intervals. A plasma glucose level 11.1 mmol/L 2 h after the oral glucose meets the diagnostic criteria for diabetes mellitus (Figure G.3). ⇒ impaired glucose tolerance.

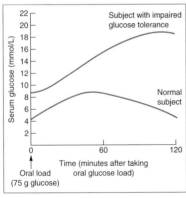

**Figure G.3** Glucose tolerance test *(reproduced from Westwood 1999 with permission)*.

**glucosinolates** *npl* molecules that occur in brassicas, e.g. cabbage, broccoli, Brussels sprouts. They may have anticancer properties by increasing the conjugation and excretion of carcinogenic chemicals.

**glucuronic acid** derived from glucose. It is important in the liver and in other organs for the safe excretion of many compounds, including hormones, bile pigments and drugs. For example, when drug residues are conjugated with glucuronic acid a water-soluble substance (a glucuronide) is produced, which can be safely excreted.

**glue ear** an accumulation of a glue-like substance in the middle ear. A cause of conductive deafness.

**glue sniffing** ⇒ solvent misuse.

**glutamic acid (glutamate)** a non-essential (dispensable) amino acid. At physiological pH glutamic acid is negatively charged and is known as glutamate. Glutamate is an important excitatory neurotransmitter in the central nervous system.

**glutamic oxaloacetic transaminase** ⇒ aminotransferases, AST.

**glutamic pyruvic transaminase** ⇒ aminotransferases, ALT.

**glutamine** *n* a conditionally essential (indispensable) amino acid.

**glutathione** *n* a tripeptide comprising three amino acids (cysteine, glutamic acid [glutamate] and glycine). It functions as a coenzyme, and as an antioxidant to protect cells against free radical damage. Required for conjugation in the liver and for red cell integrity. Paracetamol overdose causes serious depletion of glutathione. In appropriate cases the administration of acetylcysteine or methionine following paracetamol overdose allows the body to replenish glutathione levels.

**gluteal** *adj* pertaining to the buttocks.

**gluten** *n* a protein comprising gliadin and glutenin found in the cereals wheat and rye, and products containing these cereals, e.g. bread. A gluten-free diet, such as gluten-free flour, bread, biscuits and pasta, is used to treat coeliac disease and dermatitis herpetiformis.

**gluten-induced enteropathy** ⇒ coeliac disease.

**gluteus muscles** three muscles of the buttock. *gluteus maximus* the largest of the three: its origin is on the ilium and sacrum and the insertion on the gluteal tuberosity of the femur. It extends the thigh. *gluteus medius* has its origin on the ilium and its insertion on the greater trochanter of the femur. It abducts and medially rotates the thigh. *gluteus minimus* the smallest of the three, its insertion is on the ilium and the insertion on the greater trochanter of the femur. It abducts the thigh. ⇒ Appendix 1, Figure 5.

**glycaemic index** an index used to rank carbohydrate foods based on the effect they have on blood glucose levels. Low-glycaemic-index foods include pulses; high-glycaemic-index foods include confectionery. It is sometimes used in the planning of diets for people with diabetes mellitus.

**glycaemic load** the glycaemic index multiplied by the amount of carbohydrate present in the food.

**glycation** *n* the reaction between glucose and the amino groups in proteins to form a glycoprotein. Linked to the complications associated with poor glycaemic control in people with diabetes. ⇒ glycosylated haemoglobin.

**glycerides** *npl* the esters formed by the addition of one or more fatty acids.

**glycerin(e)** *n* ⇒ glycerol.

**glycerol** *n* also called glycerin(e). Forms esters with three fatty acids to produce simple fats known as triglycerides (triacylglycerols). Glycerol is a clear, syrupy liquid, which has a hydroscopic action. It is used as an emollient and in mouthwashes and suppositories. *glycerol suppositories* act by attracting fluid to soften hardened faeces in the rectum.

**glycine** *n* a conditionally essential (indispensable) amino acid. The amino acid with the simplest chemical structure. Also has neurotransmitter properties.

**glycinuria** *n* excretion of glycine in the urine. Associated with learning disability.

**glycocholic acid** a bile acid.

**glycogen** *n* the main carbohydrate (polysaccharide) storage compound in animals. Many glucose molecules are linked together in a process called glycogenesis occurring in the liver and skeletal muscle. The conversion of liver glycogen back to glucose is called glycogenolysis.

**glycogenesis** *n* glycogen formation from blood glucose.

**glycogenolysis** *n* the breakdown of stored glycogen to glucose.

**glycogenosis** *n* ⇒ glycogen storage disease.

**glycogen storage diseases** also known as glycogenosis. A group of inherited diseases transmitted as an autosomal recessive trait. The metabolic disorder is caused by various enzyme deficiencies. Glycogen accumulates in various organs and tissues. Hypoglycaemia occurs, and the body tends to use fat rather than glucose, leading to ketosis and acidosis.

**glycolipid** *n* a lipid and carbohydrate attached. ⇒ cerebroside, ganglioside, glycosphingolipids.

**glycolysis** *n* metabolic pathway comprising a series of reactions whereby glucose is broken down to form pyruvic acid and some energy (adenosine triphosphate [ATP]) (Figure G.4)—**glycolytic** *adj*. ⇒ Krebs' cycle.

**glyconeogenesis** *n* ⇒ gluconeogenesis.

**glycopeptide antibiotics** a group of antibiotics, e.g. vancomycin. ⇒ Appendix 5.

**glycopeptide-resistant enterococci (GRE)** *n* ⇒ vancomycin-resistant enterococci.

**glycoprotein IIb/IIIa inhibitors** *npl* a group of drugs that reduce blood clotting. They are used in acute coronary syndromes for high-risk patients, and during percutaneous coronary interventions. Examples include abciximab, eptifibatide, tirofiban.

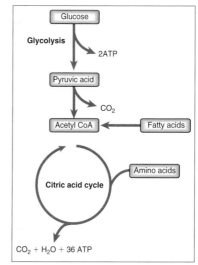

**Figure G.4** Overview of glycolysis and citric acid (Krebs') cycle *(reproduced from Watson 2000 with permission).*

**glycoproteins** *npl* large group of proteins conjugated with one or more carbohydrate residues, e.g. collagen, mucins. The term is often used generically to include proteoglycans and mucoproteins.

**glycosides** *npl* compounds comprising a sugar joined to another molecule. If the sugar is glucose, it is termed a glucoside. Many plant glycosides contain pharmacologically active substances, such as digitalis from foxgloves. *cardiac glycosides* such as digoxin increase myocardial contractility and cardiac output, and are defined as positive inotropes. ⇒ Appendix 5 (inotropes—positive).

**glycosidic bond** a chemical bond between a carbon of one sugar molecule and the carbon of another in a condensation reaction. For example, glycogen is formed by many glucose molecules linked by glycosidic bonds.

**glycosphingolipids** *npl* a group of compounds that contain ceramides (lipids formed from a fatty acid and sphingosine) and a carbohydrate. They are found in the central nervous system and erythrocytes. ⇒ ganglioside.

**glycosuria** *n* the presence of sugar in the urine.

**glycosylated haemoglobin (HbA₁, HbA₁c)** fraction of haemoglobin that non-covalently binds glucose; assay providing a measure of average blood glucose levels and hence control of diabetes over about 8 weeks.

**glycylcycline antibacterials** a new class of antibacterial drugs. Currently tigecycline is the only example available. It is related to the tetracyclines and has demonstrated activity against several antibiotic-resistant strains of bacteria.

**GM-CSF** *abbr* granulocyte–macrophage colony-stimulating factor.

**gnathalgia** *n* jaw pain.

**gnathoplasty** *n* plastic surgery of the jaw or cheek.

**GnRH** *abbr* gonadotrophin-releasing hormone.

**goals** *npl* a clear statement of a defined outcome to be attained at a particular stage in a therapeutic intervention. Goals may be short, medium- or long-term. *goal setting* an essential part of any medical intervention, which occurs after identification of the client's/patient's actual and potential problems. Whenever possible, the client/patient and/or family participate in goal setting. Goals should be SMART, i.e. **s**pecific, **m**easurable, **a**chievable, **r**ealistic and **t**ime-oriented.

**goblet cells** mucus-secreting cells, shaped like a goblet, found in the mucosa lining the gastrointestinal and respiratory tracts.

**Goeckerman regimen** a method of treating psoriasis; exposure to ultraviolet radiation alternating with the application of a tar paste.

**goitre** *n* struma. Thyroid gland enlargement; may be smooth (simple) or nodular, and associated with normal or abnormal thyroid function; hyperthyroid with smooth enlargement in Graves' disease, or nodular enlargement in toxic multinodular goitre; hypothyroid with glandular enlargement in Hashimoto's disease.

**goitrogens** *npl* agents that cause goitre. Some occur in plants, such as brassicas, e.g. cabbage.

**gold (Au)** *n* metallic element used in the management of rheumatoid arthritis. The radioactive isotope gold-198 ($^{198}$Au) is sometimes used in the treatment of some malignant diseases.

**Goldenhar's syndrome** (M Goldenhar, American physician, 1924–2001) a congenital condition characterized by asymmetrical facial abnormalities and associated vertebral abnormalities, low hair line, mandibular hypoplasia, low-set ears, auricular appendages, sensorineural deafness, coloboma affecting the eyelids, dermoid cysts and short neck.

**Goldmann applanation tonometer** a contact method for measuring the intraocular pressure. ⇒ applanation, tonometry.

**golfer's elbow** ⇒ epicondylitis.

**Golgi apparatus/body/complex** (C Golgi, Italian histologist, 1843–1926) a cell organelle comprising a network of membranous sacs within the cytoplasm. Involved in the processing of lipids and proteins synthesized in the cell. Particularly well developed in secretory cells.

**Golgi cells** two types of neurons; Golgi type I neurons which have a long axon and project to other parts of the nervous system, and Golgi type II neurons with short axons.

**Golgi tendon organ** specialized mechanoreceptors in tendons that with skeletal muscle spindles monitor muscle stretching. Involved in proprioception.

**gomphosis** *n* an immovable (fibrous) joint. For example, a tooth with a socket in the jaw.

**gonad** *n* the female or male primary reproductive structure, ovary, testis—**gonadal** *adj*.

**gonadotrophic** *adj* having an affinity for, or influencing, the gonads.

**gonadotrophins** *npl* the gonad-stimulating hormones, e.g. follicle stimulating hormone. ⇒ follicle-stimulating hormone, human chorionic gonadotrophin, luteinizing hormone.

G

**gonadotrophin-releasing hormone** a hypothalamic peptide hormone that stimulates the anterior lobe of the pituitary gland to secrete the gonadotrophins.

**goniometer** *n* protractor used to measure a joint's position and range of movement; uses either a 180° or 360° system—**goniometric** *adj*.

**gonioscope** *n* an instrument used to determine how well aqueous humour is able to drain by assessing the degree to which the drainage angle of the anterior chamber of the eye is open.

**gonioscopy** *n* examination of the anterior-chamber angle of the eye with a special lens. A routine assessment for people suspected of having glaucoma.

**goniotomy** *n* simple operation for congenital glaucoma. Surgical incision or use of a laser to improve the drainage of aqueous fluid. ⇒ trabeculotomy.

**gonococcal** *adj* relating to the gonococcus or an infection caused by *Neisseria gonorrhoeae*.

**Gonococcus** *n* a Gram-negative diplococcus (*Neisseria gonorrhoeae*), the causative organism of gonorrhoea. It is a strict parasite—**gonococci** *pl*, **gonococcal** *adj*.

**gonorrhoea** *n* a sexually transmitted infection in adults. Infants can become infected during delivery, resulting in gonococcal conjunctivitis. Gonococcal vulvovaginitis in girls before puberty may indicate sexual abuse. Chief manifestations of the disease in men are a purulent urethral discharge and dysuria after an average incubation period of about 6 days. The majority of women with uncomplicated infection are symptomless. Acute pelvic inflammatory disease in women, and septic arthritis with or without skin lesions, may complicate untreated gonorrhoea—**gonococcal** *adj*.

**Goodpasture syndrome** ⇒ anti-GBM disease.

**gooseflesh** contraction of the tiny muscles attached to the hair follicles causing the hair to stand on end: it is a reaction to either cold or fear.

**GORD** *abbr* gastro-oesophageal reflux disease.

**gouge** *n* a chisel with a grooved blade for removing bone.

**gout** *n* a form of metabolic disorder in which blood levels of uric acid are raised (hyperuricaemia). It may be due to abnormal purine metabolism or increased purine intake, increased uric acid production or a reduction in the excretion of uric acid by the kidneys. Acute arthritis can result from inflammation in response to urate crystals in the joint. The big toe is characteristically involved and becomes acutely painful and swollen. Drugs that reduce uric acid levels can control the disease. If gout is untreated deposition of urate crystals can cause chronic arthritis, nodules (e.g. in the ear) and kidney damage. ⇒ pseudogout, tophus.

**Graafian follicle** a mature ovarian follicle. A minute vesicle in the ovarian stroma containing a single oocyte which is released when the vesicle ruptures at ovulation. After ovulation, the Graafian follicle forms the corpus luteum which, should fertilization occur, maintains the early pregnancy. In the absence of fertilization the corpus luteum only lasts for 12–14 days, after which it becomes the corpus albicans.

**gracilis muscle** long, thin muscle of the medial thigh. The origin is on the pubis and its insertion is just below the medial condyle of the tibia. It adducts the thigh and rotates (medially) and flexes the leg. ⇒ Appendix 1, Figures 4 and 5.

**grading** *n* **1.** in oncology, a classification of cancers based on histopathological characteristics. The level of malignancy of the tissue is determined by comparing the amount of cellular abnormality and the rate of cell division with normal cells in the same tissue. Low-grade cancer generally has slow tumour growth and spread, whereas high-grade cancer is aggressive with rapid spread. The grade of the disease is more important (for some types of cancer) than the stage as an indicator of prognosis and effective treatment. ⇒ differentiation, staging. **2.** in occupational therapy, the quantifiable change in activity, graded by duration, extent, level of strength or the energy needed. For example, during a therapeutic intervention aimed at increasing a client's activity or a period of time. ⇒ activity diaries.

**graft** *n*, *v* transplanted living tissue, e.g. skin, bone and bone marrow, cornea, kidney, heart, lungs, pancreas and liver; to transplant such tissue. Grafts may involve: tissue moved from one site to another in the same individual (autograft); tissue moved between genetically identical individuals (isograft); tissue obtained from a suitably matched donor (allografts or homografts); and tissue transplanted between different species (xenografts or heterografts).

**graft-versus-host disease (GVHD)** may follow a successful transplant, especially bone

G

marrow, where the graft 'attacks' the tissues of the immunologically compromised host. ⇒ transplant.

**gram (g)** *n* unit of mass. One thousand is equal to 1 kilogram (kg).

**Gram's stain** (H Gram, Danish pharmacologist and pathologist, 1853–1938) a bacteriological stain used in a basic method of identifying micro-organisms. Those staining violet are Gram-positive (+), such as *Staphylococcus aureus*, and those staining pink are Gram-negative (–), e.g. *Escherichia coli*.

**grand mal** ⇒ convulsions, epilepsy.

**granulation** *n* the formation of new capillaries and connective tissue cells in the wound bed of an open wound. *granulation tissue* the new, healthy, soft tissue so formed in the wound bed. Healthy granulation tissue is moist and red—**granulate** *vi*.

**granulocyte** *n* a cell containing granules in its cytoplasm. Describes the polymorphonuclear leucocytes—neutrophil, eosinophil and basophil.

**granulocyte colony-stimulating factor (G-CSF)** a growth factor that stimulates the differentiation of stem cells into granulocyte precursors.

**granulocyte–macrophage colony-stimulating factor (GM-CSF)** a growth factor that stimulates the differentiation of stem cells into myeloid and macrophage precursors.

**granulocytopenia** *n* decrease of granulocytes not sufficient to warrant the term agranulocytosis. ⇒ neutropenia.

**granuloma** *n* a tumour formed of granulation tissue.

**granulomatosis** *n* a disorder characterized by the development of multiple granulomas. ⇒ Wegener's granulomatosis.

**grasp reflex** a primitive reflex normally present in newborns; when the palm or sole is stroked, the digits flex in a grasping action. If the reflex is not symmetrical or persists after 2–3 months of age it may indicate a lesion in the premotor cortex. The grasp reflex, and other primitive reflexes, may reappear in adults following a stroke or traumatic brain injury.

**Graves' disease** (R Graves, Irish physician, 1797–1853) hyperthyroidism due to production of thyroid-stimulating hormone (TSH) receptor antibodies; may also cause ophthalmopathy (eye disease), often evident as prominence of the eyes (exophthalmos) and pretibial myxoedema. ⇒ hyperthyroidism.

**gravid** *adj* pregnant; carrying fertilized eggs or a fetus.

**gravitational** *adj* being attracted by force of gravity. *gravitational ulcer* ⇒ venous ulcer.

**gravity** *n* weight. ⇒ specific gravity.

**Grawitz tumour** (P Grawitz, German pathologist, 1850–1932) ⇒ hypernephroma.

**gray (Gy)** *n* the derived SI unit (International System of Units) for the absorbed dose of radiation. It has replaced the rad. ⇒ Appendix 2.

**GRE** *abbr* glycopeptide-resistant enterococci.

**green-monkey disease** ⇒ Marburg disease.

**greenstick fracture** ⇒ fracture.

**gregarious** *adj* showing a preference for living in a group, liking to mix and fond of company. The herd instinct is an inborn tendency of many species, including humans.

**grey matter** unmyelinated nerve fibres and nerve cell bodies situated in the central nervous system. ⇒ white matter.

**Grey Turner's sign** (G Grey Turner, British surgeon, 1877–1951) bruising around the flanks/loin; a sign of acute haemorrhagic pancreatitis. ⇒ Cullen's sign.

**grief** *n* the emotional reaction to loss, separation or death.

**grieving process** describes the stages—denial, anger, bargaining, depression, acceptance and possibly fear—that an individual may experience in relation to bereavement and dying. Grieving is also associated with other situations of loss, including loss of employment or a companion animal, loss of body function, such as infertility, or of a body part, e.g. limb, breast. ⇒ bereavement.

**Griffith's types** subdivisions of Lancefield group A streptococci based on their antigenic structure.

**gripe** *n* abdominal colic.

**grocer's itch** contact dermatitis, especially from flour or sugar.

**groin** *n* the junction of the thigh with the abdomen.

**grommet** *n* ventilation tube inserted into the tympanic membrane. Frequently used in the treatment of glue ear in children ⇒ myringotomy.

**grounded theory** research study where a hypothesis is elicited from the data gathered.

**group activities** the simultaneous, active participation of a number of people in purposeful, productive, playful and creative tasks with a specific therapeutic goal such as encouraging social skills. Used as part of occupational therapy practice.

**group C meningococcal disease** serious disease caused by group C *Neisseria meningitidis*. It causes meningococcal meningitis and

G

life-threatening septicaemia, usually in children and young adults. Effective immunization is available and is provided as part of routine immunization programmes.

**group psychotherapy** ⇒ psychotherapy.

**growth factor** substances, usually polypeptides and proteins, that stimulate the differentiation and proliferation of new cells. Important, for example, in fetal development and wound healing. They include those that stimulate specific blood cell proliferation such as the colony-stimulating factors, platelet-derived growth factor, interleukins, nerve growth factors, insulin-like growth factor, epidermal growth factor.

**growth hormone (GH)** (*syn* somatotrophin). Hormone secreted by the anterior pituitary gland under the influence of two hypothalamic hormones: growth hormone-releasing hormone (GHRH) and growth hormone release-inhibiting hormone (GHRIH) or somatostatin. Growth hormone has widespread effects on body tissues and influences the metabolism of proteins, fats and carbohydrates. ⇒ acromegaly, dwarfism, gigantism.

**growth hormone test** a test for acromegaly. Growth hormone levels are measured during an oral glucose tolerance test. In acromegaly the level of growth hormone does not show the normal suppression with glucose.

**grunting** *n* an abnormal breath sound heard mainly in newborns. It is a serious sign and indicates respiratory distress.

**GSL** *abbr* general sales list.

**guanine** *n* a nitrogenous base derived from purine. With other bases, one or more phosphate groups and a sugar it is part of the nucleic acids DNA and RNA. ⇒ deoxyribonucleic acid, ribonucleic acid.

**guar** *n* a soluble form of non-starch polysaccharide (NSP) fibre derived from the locust bean. Taken orally, it absorbs water from the intestine and produces a feeling of fullness and slows the rate of carbohydrate absorption. May be used in the management of some types of diabetes mellitus to reduce postprandial blood glucose levels.

**guardian ad litem** an individual from a social work or childcare background who is appointed to ensure that a court is fully informed of the relevant facts that relate to a child, and that the child's wishes and feelings are clearly demonstrated.

**guarding** *n* intense contraction of the abdominal muscles. Occurs involuntarily in the presence of visceral pain, peritonitis or following abdominal surgery if the abdomen is touched, such as during physical examination.

**gubernaculum** *n* one of two strands of fibrous tissue that attach the fetal gonads within the inguinal region—**gubernacula** *pl*.

**Guedel airway** (A Guedel, American anaesthetist, 1883–1956) a plastic oropharyngeal device used to maintain the airway. ⇒ airway.

**Guillain–Barré syndrome (GBS)** (G Guillain, French neurologist, 1876–1951; J Barré, French neurologist, 1880–1967) an acquired acute demyelinating, inflammatory, peripheral neuropathy that can occur after an infection such as *Campylobacter* gastroenteritis. It may lead to pain, weakness, paralysis and, in some patients, respiratory problems. Management involves the prompt administration of intravenous immunoglobulins, possibly plasmapheresis and supportive measures such as respiratory support and physiotherapy.

**guillotine** *n* a surgical instrument for excision of the tonsils.

**Guinea worm** ⇒ *Dracunculus medinensis*.

**Gulf War syndrome/illness** the set of physical and psychological effects observed in individuals who served in the Gulf War in 1991. It includes fatigue, headaches, dizziness, dyspnoea, memory problems, skin rashes, joint pains, dyspepsia.

**gullet** *n* the oesophagus.

**GUM** *abbr* genitourinary medicine. ⇒ sexually transmitted infection.

**gumboil** *n* ⇒ dentoalveolar abscess.

**gumma** *n* a localized area of vascular granulation tissue that develops in the later stages (tertiary) of syphilis. If near the surface of the body, may form chronic ulcers—**gummata** *pl*.

**Gunn's syndrome** (R M Gunn, British ophthalmologist, 1850–1909). ⇒ jaw-winking.

**gustation** *n* the chemical sense of taste. Closely linked to that of olfaction (smell).

**gustatory** *adj* relating to gustation, or to the structures involved in taste sensation. For example the gustatory pathways (via the seventh, ninth and tenth cranial nerves) and the gustatory area of the cortex.

**gut** *n* the intestines, large and small.

**gut decontamination** the use of non-absorbable antibiotics to prevent endogenous infection in patients having intestinal surgery or those who are immunocompromised because of drugs or neutropenia.

**Guthrie test** (R Guthrie, American physician/bacteriologist, 1916–1995) a screening test, originally for phenylketonuria, carried out within the first week of life after the infant has ingested enough phenylalanine (an amino acid) in milk feeds. Drops of blood are collected on special filter paper. Assays are performed to screen for phenylketonuria and, since the development of newer analytical techniques, conditions including congenital hypothyroidism, cystic fibrosis, sickle-cell diseases and, in some countries, galactosaemia. Infants with a positive test must have the diagnosis confirmed.

**guttae** *npl* medication in drop form, usually for use as ear or eye drops—**gutta** *sing.*

**gutta percha** a substance with rubber-like properties used in dentistry for sealing temporary cavity dressings or used in root canals. It is obtained from the sap of rubber trees.

**GVHD** *abbr* graft-versus-host disease.

**gynaecologist** *n* a surgeon who specializes in gynaecology, women's health issues and the diseases of the female reproductive system.

**gynaecology** *n* the science dealing with the diseases of the female reproductive system—**gynaecological** *adj.*

**gynaecomastia** *n* enlargement of the male mammary gland.

**gypsum** *n* plaster of Paris (calcium sulphate).

**gyrus** *n* a convoluted portion of cerebral cortex.

G

# H

**habilitation** *n* the means by which a child gradually progresses towards the maximum degree of independence of which he or she is capable. ⇒ rehabilitation.

**habit** *n* any learnt behaviour that has a relatively high probability of occurrence in response to a situation or stimulus. Acquisition of habits may depend on both reinforcement and associative learning.

**habitual abortion** ⇒ miscarriage.

**habituation** *n* describes a decreasing response to a stimulus when it becomes familiar through repeated presentation, for example, becoming less aware of the feel of clothing on the skin. It is often used in a negative sense in relation to drug use or misuse, when repeated intake of the drug creates psychological dependence. ⇒ drug dependence.

**haem** *n* the non-protein, iron-containing pigment portion of haemoglobin. Each haemoglobin molecule contains four haem groups. A haem group is a porphyrin comprising an atom of ferrous iron ($Fe^{2+}$) surrounded by four pyrrole rings.

**haemagglutination** *n* the agglutination or clumping together of red blood cells, such as that caused by the transfusion of an incompatible blood group. ⇒ agglutination, blood groups.

**haemagglutinin** *n* an antibody that causes red blood cells to agglutinate. They may be autologous, homologous or heterologous, according to the source of the cells affected.

**haemangioma** *n* a malformation of blood vessels which may occur in any part of the body. When in the skin it is one form of birthmark, appearing as a red spot or a 'port wine stain'—**haemangiomata** *pl*.

*Haemaphysalis* *n* a genus of ticks. Many species transmit rickettsial, bacterial and viral infections. These include some types of typhus, tularaemia and encephalitis.

**haemarthrosis** *n* the presence of blood in a joint cavity, such as that caused by minor trauma in people with haemophilia—**haemarthroses** *pl*. ⊙ DVD

**haematemesis** *n* the vomiting of blood, which may be bright red following recent bleeding. Otherwise it is of 'coffee-ground' appearance due to the action of gastric juice. The bleeding is usually from the upper gastrointestinal tract and causes include: peptic ulcer, oesophageal varices, cancers, gastritis, drug erosions and coagulation defects, but blood swallowed from elsewhere, e.g. during epistaxis, or following oral trauma or dental extraction may be vomited.

**haematin** *n* a ferric ($Fe^{3+}$) iron-containing derivative of haemoglobin formed by the oxidation of the ferrous iron molecule.

**haematinuria** *n* dark urine caused by the presence of haematin or haemoglobin in the urine.

**haematinic** *n* a substance required for the production of red blood cells, for example iron, vitamin $B_{12}$ and folic acid.

**haematocele** *n* a swelling filled with blood.

**haematocolpos** *n* retained blood in the vagina such as caused by an imperforate hymen. ⇒ cryptomenorrhoea.

**haematocrit** *n* ⇒ packed cell volume.

**haematogenous** *adj* relating to blood. Originating in the blood or being transported in the blood.

**haematohidrosis** *n* a condition in which the sweat contains blood.

**haematology** *n* the science dealing with the formation, composition, functions and diseases of the blood—**haematological** *adj*, **haematologically** *adv*.

**haematoma** *n* a swelling composed of extravasated blood, usually traumatic in origin—**haematomata** *pl*. ⇒ extradural haematoma, subdural haematoma.

**haematometra** *n* an accumulation of blood (or menstrual fluid) in the uterus.

**haematomyelia** *n* haemorrhage in the spinal cord.

**haematopoiesis** *n* ⇒ haemopoiesis.

**haematosalpinx** *n* (*syn* haemosalpinx) blood in the uterine (fallopian) tube.

**haematospermia** *n* the discharge of blood-stained semen. It may occur in infection of the seminal vesicles.

**haematozoa** *npl* parasites living in the blood—**haematozoon** *sing*.

**haematuria** *n* blood in the urine; may be macroscopic, i.e. visible to the naked eye, when it may be bright red, dark red or smoky in appearance; or microscopic, when it is not and can only be detected by chemical tests or microscopy. Haematuria may be caused by urinary tract problems, such as glomerulonephritis, trauma to the kidney, cancers, stones, infections; or be caused by coagulation defects or anticoagulant drugs—**haematuric** *adj*.

**haemochromatosis** *n* iron storage disease. **1.** primary haemochromatosis (*syn* bronzed diabetes) is an inherited error in iron metabolism, usually increased iron absorption, with iron deposition in tissues, resulting in brown pigmentation of the skin, cirrhosis of the liver and iron damage to other organs such as the heart, pancreatic islet cells (causing diabetes) and endocrine glands. Management includes weekly venesection until the serum iron is normal, and thereafter at intervals that maintain iron stores at normal levels. In addition, treatment is given as necessary for cirrhosis and diabetes mellitus. **2.** secondary haemochromatosis may be associated with any condition requiring multiple blood transfusions, (e.g. thalassaemia and other chronic haemolytic disorders), excess intake of dietary iron and some types of porphyria. Chelating agents such as desferrioxamine are used to remove the excess iron—**haemochromatotic** *adj.*

**haemoconcentration** *n* relative increase of volume of red blood cells to volume of plasma, usually due to loss of the latter but may be caused by excess red blood cell production.

**haemocytometer** *n* an instrument for counting the number of blood cells in a given volume of blood.

**haemodiafiltration (CVVHD)** *n* similar to haemofiltration, but with the addition of dialysate. Diffusion occurs and the removal of unwanted molecules is enhanced. Used as renal replacement therapy.

**haemodialysis** *n* dialysis involving toxin removal directly from the blood stream using a dialyser and dialysate both outside the body. Often requires the use of an arteriovenous fistula. A method of renal replacement therapy used in patients in end-stage renal disease/ failure (irreversible) or in acute renal failure (potentially reversible).

**haemodilution** *n* relative decrease of volume of red blood cells to volume of plasma, usually due to an increase in the volume of blood plasma. *haemodilution of pregnancy* in spite of the normal physiological increase in red blood cell numbers during pregnancy, the concurrent increase in plasma volume leads to haemodilution. There is reduced concentration of haemoglobin, immunoglobulins and other plasma proteins.

**haemofiltration (CVVH)** *n* form of renal replacement therapy (artificial kidney treatment), in which the patient's blood is passed through a filter allowing separation of an ultrafiltrate containing fluid and solutes. This is discarded and replaced with an isotonic solution. Usually continuous, as in continuous veno-venous haemofiltration.

**haemoglobin (Hb)** *n* the red, respiratory pigment in the red blood cells. A molecule comprises four ferrous ($Fe^{2+}$) iron-containing haem groups and four globin chains, two alpha ($\alpha$) chains and two beta ($\beta$) chains (Figure H.1). It combines with oxygen and releases it to the tissues. Some carbon dioxide is carried by haemoglobin, which also acts to buffer pH changes. There is a special form of fetal haemoglobin (HbF) which has a high affinity for oxygen, and two major adult forms (HbA, $HbA_2$). HbF is normally replaced by adult forms during early childhood. However, some individuals have a genetic abnormality whereby fetal haemoglobin production continues into adulthood. There are many different haemoglobins which cause disease, e.g. Hb C, Hb E, Hb H, Hb S, etc. $\Rightarrow$ glycosylated haemoglobin, haemoglobinopathy, oxyhaemoglobin, sickle-cell disease, thalassaemia.

**haemoglobinaemia** *n* free haemoglobin in the blood plasma—**haemoglobinaemic** *adj.*

**haemoglobinometer** *n* an instrument for estimating the percentage of haemoglobin in the blood.

**haemoglobinopathy** *n* usually hereditary abnormality of the haemoglobin molecule. Very common genetic condition worldwide— **haemoglobinopathic** *adj.* $\Rightarrow$ sickle-cell disease, thalassaemia.

**haemoglobinuria** *n* haemoglobin in the urine. It is the result of substantial intravascular haemolysis leading to haemoglobinaemia. Also occurs as an acute transient condition in some infectious diseases. *paroxysmal cold haemoglobinuria* a condition where exposure to cold leads to intravascular haemolysis. *paroxysmal nocturnal haemoglobinuria* an inherited condition caused by a faulty gene on the X chromosome that results in defective blood cells, including red cells. There is haemolysis, haemoglobinuria, anaemia and venous thromboses, and a decrease in the number of neutrophils and platelets in the blood— **haemoglobinuric** *adj.*

**haemolysin** *n* an agent capable of causing disintegration of red blood cells, such as the substances produced by certain bacteria, e.g. streptococci.

**haemolysis** *n* breakdown of red blood cells, with liberation of contained haemoglobin. This happens normally at the end of the cell's lifespan and the constituent parts are dealt with by various physiological processes. Haemolysis occurs pathologically and the causes include red blood cell defects,

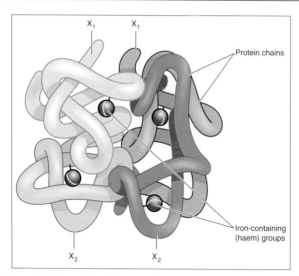

**Figure H.1** Haemoglobin *(reproduced from Waugh & Grant 2006 with permission).*

haemoglobinopathies, transfusion of incompatible blood, infections (e.g. malaria, *Escherichia coli* type O157), disseminated intravascular coagulation, mechanical trauma (e.g. a faulty heart valve), antibodies, hypersplenism (overactive spleen), drugs and exposure to chemicals—**haemolytic** *adj.*

**haemolytic anaemia** ⇒ anaemia.

**haemolytic disease of the newborn** (*syn* erythroblastosis fetalis) a pathological condition in the newborn child due to Rhesus incompatibility between the child's blood and that of the mother. Red blood cell destruction occurs with anaemia, often jaundice and an excess of erythroblasts or primitive red blood cells in the circulating blood. Immunization of women at risk, using anti-D immunoglobulin, can prevent haemolytic disease of the newborn. Treatment of affected infants may include phototherapy, blood transfusion and exchange transfusion in severe cases. ⇒ hydrops fetalis, icterus gravis neonatorum, kernicterus.

**haemolytic–uraemic syndrome (HUS)** intravascular haemolysis and acute renal failure that occur in association with another condition, such as food poisoning due to enterohaemorrhagic *Escherichia coli* type O157. Those affected (mainly children) may need renal replacement therapy. The majority make a full recovery, but others will have residual renal problems.

**haemopericardium** *n* blood in the pericardial sac. ⇒ cardiac tamponade.

**haemoperitoneum** *n* blood in the peritoneal cavity.

**haemophilias** *npl* a group of conditions with inherited blood coagulation defects. In clinical practice the most commonly encountered defects are *haemophilia A*, factor VIII procoagulant deficiency; *haemophilia B* or Christmas disease, factor IX procoagulant deficiency. Both these conditions are X-linked recessive disorders resulting in an increased tendency to bleed, the severity of which depends on the amount of residual factor VIII or IX. Bleeding typically occurs into joints and muscles. ⇒ haemophilic arthropathy, von Willebrand's disease.

**haemophilic arthropathy** joint disease associated with haemophilia. The extent of joint damage has been staged from radiological findings: (a) synovial thickening; (b) epiphyseal overgrowth; (c) minor joint changes and cyst formation; (d) definite joint changes with loss of joint space; and (e) end-stage joint destruction and secondary changes leading to deformity.

**Haemophilus** *n* a genus of bacteria. Small Gram-negative rods which show much variation in shape (pleomorphism). They are strict parasites. *Haemophilus aegyptius* causes acute infectious conjunctivitis. *Haemophilus ducreyi* causes chancroid. *Haemophilus influenzae* causes acute epiglottitis, otitis media and meningitis in young children, and pneumonia in people with chronic lung disease. Effective immunization is available as part of routine programmes. ⇒ Hib vaccine. *Haemophilus pertussis* ⇒ *Bordetella pertussis*.

**haemophthalmia** *n* bleeding into the vitreous of the eye. ⇒ hyphaema.

**haemopneumothorax** *n* the presence of blood and air in the pleural cavity.

**haemopoiesis** *n* (*syn* haematopoiesis) the formation of blood cells. During fetal life haemopoiesis starts in the yolk sac, liver and spleen. As fetal development progresses the active red bone marrow in all bones becomes the main site for haemopoiesis. Most of the active red marrow is replaced by yellow (fatty) marrow during childhood. In adults the red haemopoietic marrow is confined to ends of long bones, the sternum, pelvis and vertebrae. Red marrow contains pluripotent stem cells that are able to self-replicate and differentiate into any type of mature blood cell. Haemopoiesis is controlled by several growth factors, e.g. erythropoietin (EPO), granulocyte colony-stimulating factor (G-CSF), granulocyte–macrophage colony-stimulating factor (GM-CSF), thrombopoietin, interleukins, etc., that cause the stem cells to differentiate into a specific blood cell type. ⇒ erythropoiesis—**haemopoietic** *adj*.

**haemopoietic stem cell transplantation (HSCT)** (*syn* bone marrow transplant) the infusion of stem cells into a patient's vein. The bone marrow may be obtained on an earlier occasion from the patient (autologous transplantation) or from a suitable donor (allogeneic transplantation) or from stem cells obtained from umbilical cord blood. Usually follows myeloablative doses of chemotherapy or radiotherapy as therapy for (most commonly) haematological cancers, other blood disorders, some genetic conditions, although also used therapeutically and experimentally for some solid tumours.

**haemoptysis** *n* the coughing up of blood or blood-stained mucus from the respiratory tract. The amount ranges from blood-streaked mucus up to a life-threatening haemorrhage. The blood may be bright red, frothy or rusty in appearance. Causes include chronic bronchitis, pneumonia, lung abscess, tuberculosis, bronchial cancer, pulmonary infarction, left-sided heart failure, coagulation defects and anticoagulant drugs—**haemoptyses** *pl*.

**haemorrhage** *n* loss of blood from a vessel—**haemorrhagic** *adj*. Usually refers to serious rapid blood loss. This may lead to hypovolaemic shock with tachycardia, hypotension, rapid breathing, pallor, sweating, oliguria, restlessness and changes in conscious level. Haemorrhage can be classified in several ways: (a) according to the vessel involved, arterial, venous, or capillary; (b) timing: *primary haemorrhage* that which occurs at the time of injury or operation. *reactionary haemorrhage* that which occurs within 24 hours of injury or operation. *secondary haemorrhage* that which occurs within some days of injury or operation and usually associated with sepsis; and (c) whether it is internal (concealed) or external (revealed). ⇒ antepartum haemorrhage, intrapartum haemorrhage, placental abruption, postpartum haemorrhage.

**haemorrhagic disease of the newborn** characterized by gastrointestinal, pulmonary or intracranial haemorrhage occurring from the second to the fifth day of life. Caused by a physiological variation in blood clotting resulting from a transient deficiency of vitamin K which is necessary for the formation of some clotting factors. Responds to administration of vitamin K.

**haemorrhagic fever** a group of viral haemorrhagic diseases that include chikungunya, dengue, Ebola, Lassa fever, Marburg disease, Rift Valley fever, yellow fever. ⇒ mosquito-transmitted haemorrhagic fevers, viral haemorrhagic fevers.

**haemorrhoidal** *adj* relating to haemorrhoids or applied to nerves and vessels in the anal region.

**haemorrhoidectomy** *n* surgical removal of haemorrhoids.

**haemorrhoids** *npl* (*syn* piles) varicosity of the veins around the anus. *external haemorrhoids* those outside the anal sphincter, covered with skin. *internal haemorrhoids* those inside the anal sphincter, covered with mucous membrane.

**haemosalpinx** *n* ⇒ haematosalpinx.

**haemosiderin** *n* an iron–protein complex related to the ferritin molecule. Some of the iron in the body is stored in this form.

**haemosiderosis** *n* excess iron deposition in the tissues, especially in the monocyte–

macrophage (reticuloendothelial) system, which eventually affects the liver, heart and endocrine glands. It is associated with excessive haemolysis of red blood cells. Also results from multiple blood transfusions, for example in the management of thalassaemia.

**haemostasis** *n* **1.** the processes that control bleeding from small vessels. Damage to the blood vessels starts a complex series of reactions between substances in the blood and others released from damaged platelets and tissue. There are four overlapping stages: vasoconstriction, platelet plug formation, coagulation and fibrinolysis. **2.** Also includes the measures used to stop bleeding during surgery or following injury.

**haemostatic** *adj* any agent which arrests bleeding. *haemostatic forceps* artery forceps.

**haemothorax** *n* blood in the pleural cavity.

**Hageman factor** also called contact factor. Factor XII of the coagulation cascade. It is produced in the liver and is needed for the production of prothrombin activator (intrinsic system). A rare deficiency is inherited as an autosomal recessive disorder.

**HAI** *abbr* hospital-acquired infection.

**hair** *n* thread-like appendage present on all parts of human skin except palms, soles, lips, glans penis and that surrounding the terminal phalanges. As individual hairs grow within a sheath or hair follicle, each hair grows from a bulb at the bottom of the follicle. The part of the hair within the follicle is the root and the part above the skin is the hair shaft. Types of hair are lanugo, vellus and terminal hair. ⇒ Appendix 1, Figure 12. ⇒ alopecia, anagen, catagen, hirsutism, hypertrichosis, telogen.

**hairball** *n* ⇒ bezoar, trichobezoar.

**hairy-cell leukaemia** an uncommon malignancy of haemopoietic (blood-forming) tissue—the bone and bone marrow. The stem cells are stimulated to produce too many lymphocytes, particularly the B lymphocytes, which are abnormal and have the characteristic hair-like projections seen on microscopy, hence the name 'hairy-cell'. The abnormal cells do not function properly, thus increasing the risk of infections; they also congregate in the spleen which enlarges. There is a reduction in the production of the other blood cells, which leads to anaemia and thrombocytopenia with bruising and infection.

**halal** *n* foods, including meat, permitted by Islamic dietary laws. Meat from herbivorous animals (grazing animals with cloven hooves, thus excluding pigs) slaughtered according to Islamic law. Although there are variations, fish with scales are usually permitted. ⇒ haram.

**half-life ($t_{1/2}$)** *n* amount of time taken for the radioactivity of a radioactive substance to decay by half the initial value. The half-life is a constant for each radioactive isotope, e.g. iodine-131 ($^{131}$I) is 8 days. Or the time taken for the concentration of a drug in the plasma to fall by half the initial level. *biological half-life* time taken by the body to eliminate 50% of the dose of any substance by normal biological processes. *effective half-life* time taken for a combination of radioactive decay and biological processes to reduce radioactivity by 50%.

**halibut liver oil** fish oil. A very rich source of vitamins A and D.

**halitophobia** *n* an intense fear of having halitosis (bad breath), whether it exists or not. May be a feature of some mental health problems.

**halitosis** *n* bromopnoea. Foul-smelling breath. Causes include poor oral hygiene, periodontal disease, a particular food item such as garlic, smoking tobacco, alcohol intake, sinusitis, suppurative respiratory conditions, fetor hepaticus associated with liver failure, uraemia.

**hallucination** *n* a false perception occurring without any true sensory stimulus. A common psychotic symptom that can occur in schizophrenia, affective psychoses, delirium and drug intoxication. The hallucination may be auditory, gustatory, olfactory, tactile or visual.

**hallucinogens** *npl* (*syn* psychotomimetics) chemicals that cause hallucinations. They include cannabis, which is mildly hallucinogenic, lysergic acid diethylamide (LSD) and dimethyltriptamine, which are potent hallucinogens, and certain fungi.

**hallux** *n* the great toe.

**hallux rigidus** ankylosis of the metatarsophalangeal articulation due to osteoarthritis.

**hallux valgus or hallux abductovalgus** (*syn* bunion) a complex deformity of the medial column of the foot involving abduction and external rotation of the great toe and adduction and internal rotation of the first metatarsal (referenced to the midline of the body). Deformity exists when abduction of the hallux on the metatarsal is greater than 10–12°. Friction and pressure of shoes cause a bursa to develop. The prominent bone, with its bursa, is known as a bunion.

**H**

**hallux varus** the great toe deviates toward the midline of the body and is commonly seen with metatarsus adductus.

**halo** *n* **1.** a titanium ring that encircles the head. ⇒ halopelvic traction. **2.** the circle of light seen by people suffering from glaucoma.

**halogen** *n* any one of the non-metallic elements—bromine, chlorine, fluorine, iodine.

**halopelvic traction** a form of external fixation whereby traction can be applied to the spine between two fixed points. The device consists of three main parts: (a) a halo; (b) a pelvic loop; and (c) four extension bars.

**halophiles** *npl* halophilic bacteria and other micro-organisms that are adapted to grow in high concentrations of salt (sodium chloride).

**halophilic** *adj* salt-loving. Needing high levels of salt (sodium chloride) to grow.

**hamartoma** *n* growth of new tissue which looks like tumour but results from disordered tissue development.

**hamate** *n* one of the carpal bones of the wrist. It articulates with other carpal bones—the capitate, lunate and triquetral, and the fourth and fifth metacarpal bones.

**hammer toe** a permanent hyperextension of the first phalanx and flexion of second and third phalanges.

**hamstring muscles** the three flexor muscles of the posterior part of the thigh: the biceps femoris is the most lateral, the semitendinosus and medially the semimembranosus. The origins are on the ischium and they are inserted into the upper end of the fibula and tibia, or the tibia alone. They act to flex the knee. ⇒ biceps (femoris), semimembranosus, semitendinosus.

**hand** *n* that part of the upper limb below the wrist. Comprises the eight carpal bones, five metacarpals and the 14 phalanges forming the thumb and fingers.

**hand–arm vibration syndrome (HAVS)** (*syn* Raynaud's phenomenon) a progressive chronic condition that arises following prolonged use of hand-held vibrating equipment. Early signs are 'white finger', which is caused by constriction of and damage to the digital arteries. Other symptoms include tingling and loss of sensation caused by involvement of the digital nerves leading to loss of manual dexterity.

**handedness** *n* laterality. The use of the preferred hand, either right or left. The vast majority of people are right-handed and this corresponds to cerebral dominance on the left side of the brain, whereas left-handed people

have cerebral dominance on the right side. Very few people are truly ambidextrous (equally skilled with either hand).

**hand, foot and mouth disease** a viral infection that mainly affects children. It is caused by a coxsackievirus. There are painful ulcers on the oral mucosa and vesicles on the hands and feet. Some children will feel unwell. It usually resolves after a week.

**handicapped** *adj* term previously applied to a person with a defect that prevents or limits the normal activities of living and achievement.

**Hand–Schüller–Christian disease** (A Hand, American paediatrician, 1868–1949; A Schüller, Austrian neurologist, 1874–1958; H Christian, American physician, 1876–1951) a rare condition, usually manifesting in early childhood with histiocytic granulomatous lesions affecting many tissues. One of the diseases included in the spectrum of Langerhans' cell histiocytosis. ⇒ Letterer–Siwe disease.

**Hansen's disease** (G Hansen, Norwegian physician, 1841–1912). ⇒ leprosy.

*Hantavirus n* a genus of viruses that cause serious haemorrhagic illnesses associated with kidney damage and failure. It is spread by the faeces of various rodents, including mice and rats. Characterized by a flu-like illness that progresses to high fever, bleeding into the skin, headache, vomiting, shock and kidney failure. Cases have occurred in Korea, Russia, Japan, China and isolated cases in the United States. A *Hantavirus* also infects the respiratory system, causing respiratory distress and respiratory failure.

**hapten** *n* incomplete antigen. Low-molecular-weight substances such as peptides, which combine with body proteins to become antigenic. In combination with the body protein they are able to cause an immunological response, which they could not do alone. Antibiotics such as penicillin can act as haptens in susceptible individuals.

**haptoglobin** *n* a plasma protein produced in several tissues that include the liver, lung and kidney. It binds to free haemoglobin in the plasma and forms a complex that can be safely removed by cells of monocyte–macrophage system (reticuloendothelial system), such as those in the spleen and liver. The level of haptoglobin in the plasma is reduced or absent when red blood cell haemolysis occurs within the circulation, such as haemolytic anaemias, whereas levels may be elevated in some chronic inflammatory diseases.

**haploid** *adj* refers to the chromosome complement of the mature gametes (oocytes or spermatozoa) following the reduction division of meiosis. This set represents the basic complement of 23 (n) unpaired chromosomes in humans (22 autosomes and 1 sex chromosome). The normal multiple is diploid (2n) but abnormally three or more chromosome sets can be found (triploid, tetraploid, etc.). ⇒ diploid.

**haram** *n* foods proscribed according to Islamic dietary laws. They include alcoholic beverages, blood, meat from carnivorous or omnivorous animals, for example pork or any foods containing any product, such as lard, obtained from a pig. ⇒ halal.

**harm reduction** a public health measure that seeks to reduce the harmful effects inherent in some behaviours, rather than concentrating entirely on changing the person's lifestyle. For example, providing clean needle exchange for injecting drug users, or condoms to young people in high schools.

**Harrington rod** used in operations for scoliosis: it provides internal fixation whereby the curve is held by the rod and is usually accompanied by a spinal fusion.

**Harrison's groove/sulcus** (E Harrison, British physician, 1766–1838) a deformity of the lower chest caused by the pull of the diaphragm on the ribs. It may be associated with lung disease during childhood, such as poorly controlled asthma or rickets.

**Hartmann's operation** (H Hartmann, French surgeon, 1860–1952) originally a surgical procedure for colon cancer or diverticulitis in which the diseased colon was resected, the rectal stump closed and a colostomy formed. Usually a second-stage operation is undertaken to restore continuity by anastomosing the distal colon to the rectum and reversing the colostomy.

**Hartmann's solution** (A Hartmann, American paediatrician, 1898–1964) intravenous infusion solution containing sodium lactate and chloride, potassium chloride and calcium chloride. A modified Ringer-lactate solution.

**Hartnup disease** named for the family in whom it was first identified. A rare recessive genetic error of neutral amino acid metabolism. It is associated with dry scaly skin, photosensitivity, hyperaminoaciduria, stomatitis, diarrhoea, ataxia and mental health problems.

**Hashimoto's disease** (H Hashimoto, Japanese surgeon, 1881–1934) firm thyroid gland enlargement, often associated with hypo-thyroidism and rarely with hyperthyroidism, largely in middle-aged females, with high circulating levels of thyroid antibodies and due to autoimmune lymphocytic infiltration.

**hashish** *n* ⇒ cannabis.

**haustration** *n* sacculation, as of the colon— **haustrum** *sing*, **haustra** *pl*.

**HAV** *abbr* hepatitis A virus.

**haversian system/canal** (C Havers, English physician, 1650–1702) the basic unit of compact bone (see Figure B.6, p. 66), an osteon. Tube-shaped structures comprising a central canal surrounded by expanding concentric rings of bone called lamellae. Spaces between the lamellae are called lacunae; these contain osteocytes. The central canal is linked by a network of tunnels to adjacent canals. Each central canal contains blood vessels, lymphatics and nerves.

**HAVS** *abbr* hand–arm vibration syndrome.

**Hawthorne effect** a positive effect occurring from the introduction of change, of which people are less aware as time passes. Researchers doing observation research make allowances for this reaction to their presence by not including data from the first few days in the final data analysis.

**hayfever** *n* a form of allergic rhinitis in which attacks of inflammation of the conjunctiva, nose and throat are precipitated by exposure to pollen.

**hazard analysis critical control process** in the food industry, the identification of critical points in processing that must be controlled for food safety.

**HBIG** *abbr* hepatitis B immunoglobulin.

**HBV** *abbr* hepatitis B virus.

**HCAI** *abbr* health care-associated infection.

**hCG** *abbr* human chorionic gonadotrophin.

**HCV** *abbr* hepatitis C virus.

**HDL** *abbr* high-density lipoprotein.

**HDU** *abbr* high-dependency unit.

**head injury** also know as brain injury. An injury resulting from a blow to the head causing haemorrhage or contusion. ⇒ concussion, extradural haematoma, Glasgow Coma Scale, papilloedema, subdural haematoma.

**head tilt/chin lift** a method of opening the airway in an unconscious casualty by placing a hand on the forehead to tilt the head gently backwards, while using the fingertips to lift the chin (Figure H.2). It is used in the adult to move the tongue forward in order to stop it from blocking the airway. In an adult, head tilt/chin lift needs the neck to be hyperextended and so should not be used when a head

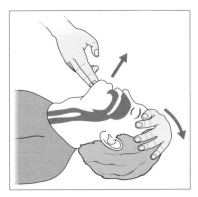

**Figure H.2** Head tilt/chin lift—adult *(reproduced from Mallik et al. 1998 with permission).*

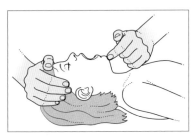

**Figure H.3** Head tilt/chin lift—child *(reproduced from Huband & Trigg 2000 with permission).*

or cervical spine injury is suspected. In infants and children head tilt/chin lift is used but without overextending the neck, as this can cause the airway to close (Figure H.3). ⇒ jaw thrust.

**Heaf test** (F Heaf, British physician, 1894–1973) a tuberculin skinprick test for tuberculosis. Replaced by the Mantoux test in the UK.

**healing** *n* **1.** the natural process of cure or tissue repair. ⇒ wound healing. **2.** in complementary or integrated medicine the term 'healing' refers to a return to health; also the use of a therapy that may assist the healing process; a specific therapeutic form, such as spiritual healing and therapeutic touch—**heal** *vt, vi.*

**health** *n* negatively defined as a state in which no evidence of illness, disease, injury or disability is found. More positively in 1948 the

World Health Organization defined health as 'a state of complete mental, physical and social well-being and not merely the absence of disease or infirmity'. The development of holistic thinking has led to the broadening of definitions of health to include social, environmental and economic influences. Health includes individuals' social and psychological resources as well as their physical capacities. A positive concept of well-being as a subjective feeling, physical fitness, normal functional capacity, resistance, resilience or hardiness. The subjective nature of what constitutes health means that individual definitions will vary from one person to another, from place to place as well as at different times.

**Health and Safety legislation** in the UK the statute and common law that covers health and safety duties. The Health and Safety and Welfare at Work Act 1974 sets out the responsibilities of the employer in relation to their employees, the working environment, equipment and substances, and those of individual employees to themselves and other people. The Health and Safety Commission (HSC) and the Health and Safety Executive (HSE) enforce health and safety law in the UK.

**health care-associated infection (HCAI)** any infection that occurs as a result of the patient's/client's care or treatment by health care staff, or an infection affecting health care staff in the course of their work. ⇒ infection.

**Healthcare Commission** established in England to encourage improvement in care (quality and effectiveness) and its provision (economy and efficiency), inspects and monitors services, investigates serious service failures and acts as an independent review for complaints about the NHS. At the time of writing the government is planning to merge the Healthcare Commission with the Mental Health Act Commission and the Commission for Social Care Inspection in 2008 to create a single regulator.

**health care systems** national or local organizations for providing medical/health care. The structure of the system has to accommodate progress in medical interventions, consumer demand and economic efficiency. Criteria for a successful system have been formulated: (a) adequacy and equity of access to care; (b) income protection (for patients); (c) macroeconomic efficiency (national expenditure measured as a proportion of gross domestic product); (d) microeconomic efficiency (balance of services provided between improving health outcomes and satisfying consumer demand); (e) consumer choice and appropriate autonomy for care providers. There are four basic types of health care systems: (a) socialized (UK NHS); (b) social insurance (Canada, France); (c) mandatory insurance (Germany); and (d) voluntary insurance (USA).

**health centre** premises from which a variety of health care services are provided. Includes general practice, community services such as child health, family planning and some well-woman services. May be owned by local government, Primary Care Trusts or general practitioners or privately owned.

**health determinant** a factor that impacts on the health of individuals and populations. They include genetic inheritance, gender, age, lifestyle choices, level of education, community ties and networks, housing, working conditions, unemployment, social class, accessibility of health care, culture and economic conditions.

**Health Development Agency** ⇒ National Institute for Health and Clinical Excellence.

**health education** providing information to the public or individuals to reduce ill health and enhance positive health by influencing people's beliefs, attitudes and behaviour. The objective is to empower individuals to make appropriate choices for healthy living.

**health gain** an attempt at measuring the benefit of health intervention on the population. For example, health gain from a cervical cytology screening programme may be measured as the reduction in deaths from cervical cancer; coronary heart disease prevention programme measured as a reduction in deaths from coronary heart disease in men under 65 years of age, or the number of deaths avoided over a specified period of time (e.g. 5 years).

**Health Improvement Programme (HImP)** a focused action plan for improving health and health care provision at a local level. Involves a collaborative approach between Primary Care Trust(s), health professionals, local government, voluntary organizations and user groups, etc.

**Health Professions Council (HPC)** a statutory body in the UK which currently regulates 13 professions, including chiropodists/podiatrists, clinical scientists, dietitians, occupational therapists, operating department practitioners, paramedics, physiotherapists, radiographers, speech and language therapists.

**health promotion** efforts to prevent ill health and promote positive health. Five key priority areas for action formulated by the World Health Organization (1986, 1998): (a) building healthy public policy; (b) creating supportive environments for health; (c) strengthening community action for health; (d) developing personal skills for health; and (e) reorienting health services (to focus on whole populations).

**Health Protection Agency (HPA)** in England and Wales an agency established to protect public health and decrease the effects of chemical hazards, infectious diseases, poisons and radiation risks.

**Health Service Commissioner** ⇒ Parliamentary and Health Service Ombudsman.

**hearing impairment** impairment resulting from hearing loss. People can experience hearing loss at any stage of life. Common causes of hearing loss include glue ear, occurring most often during childhood, and presbycusis, which is a permanent sensorineural hearing loss associated with ageing. Communication with hearing-impaired people can be enhanced by some simple steps, including: being in front of, fairly close to, and on the same level as the affected person; reducing background noise; speaking clearly; not shouting and maintaining speech at normal rhythm; using sentences rather than single words; and not covering your face while speaking. Also avoid talking to a hearing person accompanying the patient and always make sure that you have the hearing-impaired person's attention before you start to speak. ⇒ deafness.

**hearing tests** ⇒ acuity.

**heart** *n* the hollow muscular organ which pumps the blood around the pulmonary and general circulations. It is situated behind the sternum, lying obliquely within the mediastinum (⇒ Appendix 1, Figure 6). It weighs around 300 g and is about the size of the person's fist. It is divided into a right and left side by a septum and has four chambers. There are two small upper receiving chambers, the atria, and two large lower pumping chambers, the ventricles. The wall of the heart has three layers: the outer serous pericardium, a middle of cardiac muscle (myocardium) and a lining (endocardium). Valves control blood flow between the atria and ventricles (atrioventricular valves)—tricuspid on the right and bicuspid on the left—and the aortic and pulmonary valves (semilunar) prevent backflow from aorta and pulmonary artery (⇒ Appendix 1,

Figure 8). The normal heart sounds are produced when these valves close during the cardiac cycle.

**heart block** partial or complete block to the passage of impulses through the conducting system of the atria and ventricles of the heart.

**heartburn** *n* pyrosis. Retrosternal burning due to gastro-oesophageal reflux of stomach acid.

**heart failure** an inability of one or both sides of the heart to pump blood effectively into the circulation. ⇒ acute heart failure, congestive heart failure.

**heart–lung machine** *n* a pump oxygenator. A machine that bypasses both the heart and lungs and is used in cardiac surgery in which the heart is stopped, or in critically ill patients to oxygenate the blood. ⇒ cardiopulmonary bypass.

**heart transplant** surgical transplantation of a heart from a suitable donor. May be combined with a lung transplant.

**heat exhaustion** (*syn* heat syncope) collapse, with or without loss of consciousness, occurring in conditions of heat and high humidity: mainly resulting from loss of fluid and electrolytes through sweating. If the surrounding air becomes saturated, the condition progresses to heatstroke.

**heatstroke** *n* (*syn* sunstroke) final stage in heat exhaustion. The body is unable to lose heat, hyperpyrexia occurs and without effective treatment the person may die. ⇒ hyperthermia.

**hebephrenia** *n* a type of schizophrenia characterized by affective disturbance, thought disorder and negative symptoms. Prognosis tends to be poor—**hebephrenic** *adj*.

**Heberden's nodes** (W Heberden, British physician, 1710–1801) small bony swellings at terminal (distal) interphalangeal joints occurring in osteoarthritis. ⇒ Bouchard's node.

**hedonism** *n* excessive devotion to pleasure, so that a person's conduct is determined by an unconscious drive to seek pleasure and avoid unpleasant things.

**heel bruise** (*syn* stone bruise) contusion to the subcutaneous fat pad located over the inferior aspect of the calcaneus.

**heel spurs** occur on the plantar surface of the calcaneus and are considered a variant of the normal point of attachment of the plantar fascia. They are insignificant when small, and may be well defined with smooth, regular cortical contours. However, when enlarged they cause pain on walking.

**Hegar's sign** (E Hegar, German gynaecologist, 1830–1914) extreme softening of the lower segment of the uterus at 8 weeks' gestation detected by bimanual palpation.

**Heimlich's manoeuvre** (H Heimlich, American surgeon, b. 1920) abdominal thrusts. A first-aid measure to dislodge a foreign body (e.g. food) obstructing the glottis, usually performed by holding the patient from behind and jerking the operator's clenched fists up into the victim's epigastrium (Figure H.4). In an unconscious victim it can be performed with the victim lying on the floor.

**Heinz body** (R Heinz, German pathologist, pharmacist, 1865–1924) refractile, irregularly shaped body composed of denatured haemoglobin present in red blood cells in some haemolytic anaemias.

***Helicobacter pylori*** bacterium causing a number of gastrointestinal diseases via gastric infection. These include peptic ulceration, gastric cancer and MALToma. May be diagnosed by urea breath tests, serology or gastric biopsy. Treatment with combination therapy of antibiotics (clarithromycin, with either metronidazole or amoxicillin) and a proton pump inhibitor, e.g. omeprazole, is usually effective, but bacterial resistance does occur.

**helium** *n* an inert gas. Medical uses include pulmonary function tests and to dilute other gases.

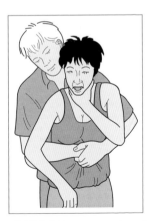

**Figure H.4** Heimlich's manoeuvre *(reproduced from Peattie & Walker 1995 with permission).*

**helix** *n* spiral. **1.** outer ridge on the auricle (pinna) of the outer/external ear. ⇒ Appendix 1, Figure 13. **2.** describes the structure of molecules, such as DNA.

**Heller's operation** ⇒ cardiomyotomy.

**HELLP syndrome** *abbr* **h**aemolysis, **e**levated **l**iver enzymes and **l**ow **p**latelets. A condition associated with pre-eclampsia/eclampsia syndrome. It can be life-threatening through liver failure or rupture of the liver with severe haemorrhage. There is significant perinatal morbidity and mortality.

**helminth** *n* a worm, including cestode, nematodes, taenia, trematoda.

**helminthagogue** *n* an anthelmintic.

**helminthiasis** *n* the condition resulting from infestation with worms.

**helminthology** *n* the study of parasitic worms.

**helper T cells** T lymphocytes which have a key role in the immune response, both cell-mediated and antibody-mediated. Their role includes the production of cytokines and the activation of B cells. ⇒ CD4 cells.

**hemeralopia/day blindness** *n* poor visual acuity with blurring in bright light.

**hemiachromatopsia** *n* a condition in which the person is colour-blind in only half of the visual field.

**hemianopia** *n* loss of vision in the nasal or temporal half of the visual field of one or both eyes.

**hemiatrophy** *n* atrophy of one-half or one side. *facial hemiatrophy* a congenital condition, or a manifestation of scleroderma in which the structures on one side of the face are shrunken.

**hemiballismus** *n* involuntary flailing movements of limbs due in some cases to contralateral damage of the subthalamic (below the thalamus) nucleus in the basal nuclei (ganglia).

**hemicelluloses** *npl* complex carbohydrates such as mucilages and gums. Non-starch polysaccharides, which, with cellulose and lignin, form part of plant cell walls.

**hemichorea** *n* choreiform movements limited to one side of the body. ⇒ chorea.

**hemicolectomy** *n* removal of approximately half the colon. A right hemicolectomy removes the caecum, the ascending colon and part of the transverse colon. A left hemicolectomy removes part of the transverse colon, descending colon, and possibly the sigmoid colon.

**hemicrania** *n* unilateral headache, as in migraine.

**hemidiaphoresis** *n* unilateral sweating of the body.

**hemiglossectomy** *n* removal of approximately half the tongue.

**hemimelia** *n* a congenital developmental abnormality where the lower part of a limb is missing or shortened. It may affect either or both bones of the distal arm (radius and ulna) or leg (tibia and fibula).

**hemiparesis** *n* paralysis or weakness of one side of face or body.

**hemiplegia** *n* paralysis of one side of the body, usually resulting from a stroke (cerebrovascular accident) on the opposite side of the brain—**hemiplegic** *adj*.

**hemizygous** *adj* describes an individual with a genome with only one allele for a given characteristic or trait. Having an allele present on unpaired chromosomes such as those on the X chromosome in males. The characteristic specified by the allele will be expressed whether it is dominant or recessive because there is no corresponding allele on the Y chromosome, e.g. those leading to haemophilia or Duchenne muscular dystrophy.

**Henoch–Schönlein purpura** (E Henoch, German paediatrician, 1820–1910; J Schönlein German physician, 1793–1864) a small-vessel vasculitis, mainly affecting children. Caused by hypersensitivity, which may follow a streptococcal respiratory infection, or a drug allergy, but it may be idiopathic. Immune complexes are formed which damage capillaries in the skin, gut and elsewhere. It is characterized by purpuric bleeding into the skin, particularly shins and buttocks, and from the wall of the gut, resulting in abdominal colic and rectal bleeding; and bruising around joints with arthritis. The kidneys may be affected, leading to haematuria, proteinuria, acute glomerulonephritis, nephrotic syndrome or acute renal failure.

**hepar** *n* the liver—**hepatic** *adj*.

**heparin** *n* a group of naturally occurring anticoagulant substances produced by mast cells and present in liver and lung tissue. Normally it prevents inappropriate blood coagulation in the body. Used therapeutically, it inhibits blood coagulation in several ways, primarily by the prevention of fibrin formation through the inhibition of thrombin activity. Heparin is used subcutaneously or intravenously for existing thromboembolic conditions, such as

219

deep-vein thrombosis, and in prophylaxis, e.g. perioperatively. Bleeding may occur as a side-effect. Its effects can be reversed with the anti-dote protamine sulphate. *low-molecular-weight heparin* given subcutaneously has a longer action and fewer side-effects. ⇒ anticoagu-lant, coagulation. ⇒ Appendix 5.

**hepatalgia** *n* pain in or associated with the liver.

**hepatectomy** *n* excision of the liver, or more usually part of the liver.

**hepatic** *adj* pertaining to the liver. *hepatic artery* the unpaired artery that branches from the coeliac artery to supply the liver with oxy-genated arterial blood. It also supplies blood to the gallbladder, parts of the stomach, duo-denum and pancreas. *hepatic vein* carries deox-ygenated blood from the liver to the inferior vena cava. ⇒ hepatic portal circulation.

**hepatic ducts** two bile ducts, right and left, that carry bile from the liver. They unite to form the common hepatic duct.

**hepatic encephalopathy** altered brain func-tion associated with the wide-ranging meta-bolic disturbances of cirrhosis and liver failure. The liver is unable to detoxify many chemicals, particularly nitrogenous substances.

**hepatic flexure** the right colic flexure. The 90° angle in the colon under the liver.

**hepatic portal circulation** venous blood rich in nutrients is carried to the liver from the small and large intestine, pancreas, spleen, distal oesophagus and stomach by the hepatic portal vein. Once in the liver the blood passes through a second capillary bed (sinusoids) so that nutrients can be modified by liver cells. The blood leaves the liver and returns to the heart via the inferior vena cava.

**hepatic portal hypertension** increased pressure in the hepatic portal vein. Usually caused by cirrhosis of the liver; results in splenomegaly, with hypersplenism and gastro-intestinal bleeding. ⇒ oesophageal varices.

**hepatic portal vein** a vein conveying blood into the liver; it is about 75 mm long and is formed by the union of several veins—the superior mesenteric, inferior mesenteric, splenic and gastric veins.

**hepaticoduodenostomy** *n* anastomosis of the hepatic duct to the duodenum.

**hepaticoenterostomy** *n* anastomosis of the hepatic duct to the small intestine.

**hepaticojejunostomy** *n* anastomosis of the hepatic duct to the jejunum.

**hepatitis** *n* inflammation of the liver, com-monly associated with viral infection but can be due to toxic agents, such as alcohol, drugs and chemicals, or metabolic disorders, e.g. Wilson's disease. Viral hepatitis is currently a serious public health problem. It is associated with a number of different hepatitis viruses that include: hepatitis A virus (HAV), hepatitis B virus (HBV), hepatitis C virus (HCV) and hepatitis D virus (delta virus). Other types of hepatitis identified include: hepatitis E virus, hepatitis F virus and hepatitis G virus. *hepatitis A* is caused by an RNA enterovirus. It is rela-tively common and may be epidemic, espe-cially in institutions, e.g. schools. The virus is transmitted by the faecal–oral route, caused by poor hygiene or contaminated food. *hepati-tis B* is caused by a DNA virus. It is usually transmitted sexually (vaginal or anal inter-course), injection of infected blood or blood products, or via contaminated equipment, such as needles. The virus is shed in vaginal discharge, semen and saliva. Individuals at high risk include: intravenous drug users, homosexual or bisexual men, prostitutes, and health care professionals through needlestick injuries. Hepatitis B virus may persist, causing chronic hepatitis, or a carrier state can develop. Effective vaccine exists. *hepatitis C* is caused by an RNA virus and is most common in intravenous drug users and in those who have had a transfusion of blood or blood pro-ducts. The virus can remain in the blood for many years and 30–50% of infected people develop chronic hepatitis, cirrhosis, liver fail-ure and possibly liver cancer. Some people become carriers of the virus. *hepatitis D (delta virus)* can only replicate in the presence of hepatitis B and is therefore found infecting simultaneously with hepatitis B, or as a super-infection in chronic carriers of hepatitis B. Delta virus may increase the severity of a hep-atitis B infection, increasing the risk of chronic liver disease. *hepatitis E* is transmitted via the faecal–oral route and has been reported in tra-vellers returning from the USA, Mexico, Asia and Africa.

**hepatization** *n* the changes that occur in the lung tissue following lobar pneumonia. The affected tissue becomes a solid mass and takes on the appearance of liver.

**hepatoblastoma** *n* a rare liver cancer of infants and young children. It comprises cells that resemble primitive fetal liver cells. There is an upper abdominal mass and the alphafe-toprotein level in the blood is increased.

**hepatocellular** *adj* pertaining to or affecting liver cells.

**hepatocyte** *n* a parenchymal (functional) liver cell.

**hepatoma** *n* primary cancer of the liver—**hepatomata** *pl.*

**hepatomegaly** *n* enlargement of the liver. It is palpable below the costal margin.

**hepatopancreatic ampulla** *n* the enlargement formed by the union of the common bile duct with the pancreatic duct where they enter the duodenum. Previously known as the ampulla of Vater.

**hepatosplenic** *adj* pertaining to the liver and spleen.

**hepatosplenomegaly** *n* enlargement of the liver and the spleen, so that each is palpable below the costal margin.

**hepatotoxic** *adj* having an injurious effect on liver cells, such as excess alcohol—**hepatotoxicity** *n.*

**HER2** *abbr* human epidermal growth factor receptor-2.

**herbalism** *n* herbal medicine, phytotherapy. The therapeutic use of herbs or mineral remedies. The use of plant material by trained practitioners to promote health and recovery from illness.

**Herbal Medicines Advisory Committee** a UK committee that advises the Medicines and Healthcare Products Regulatory Agency and government ministers regarding the registration of traditional herbal medicines and on the unlicensed herbal remedies.

**hereditary** *adj* inherited; capable of being inherited.

**hereditary angioedema** a genetic disorder characterized by episodes of severe life-threatening angioedema and sometimes abdominal pain. It is caused by a mutation in the gene encoding C1 inhibitor, which may be absent or dysfunctional. It is treated with C1 inhibitor pooled from plasma donations.

**heredity** *n* transmission from parents to children of genetic characteristics by means of the genetic material; the process by which this occurs, and the study of such processes.

**hermaphrodite** *n* individual possessing both ovarian and testicular tissue. Although they may approximate to either male or female type, they are usually sterile from imperfect development of their gonads.

**hernia** *n* the abnormal protrusion of an organ, or part of an organ, through an aperture in the surrounding structures: commonly the protrusion of an abdominal organ through a gap in the abdominal wall (Figure H.5). *diaphragmatic hernia* ⇒ hiatus hernia. *femoral*

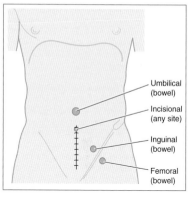

**Figure H.5** Common sites for hernias *(reproduced from Waugh & Grant 2006 with permission).*

*hernia* protrusion through the femoral canal, alongside the femoral blood vessels as they pass into the thigh. *incisional hernia* protrusion through the site of a previous abdominal incision. *inguinal hernia* protrusion through the inguinal canal in the male. *irreducible hernia* when the contents of the sac cannot be returned to the appropriate cavity without surgical intervention. *strangulated hernia* hernia in which the blood supply to the organ involved is impaired, usually due to constriction by surrounding structures. *umbilical hernia* protrusion of a portion of intestine through the area of weakness at the umbilical scar.

**hernioplasty** *n* an operation for hernia in which an attempt is made to prevent recurrence by refashioning the structures to give greater strength—**hernioplastic** *adj.*

**herniorrhaphy** *n* an operation for hernia in which the weak area is reinforced by some of the patient's own tissues or by some other material.

**herniotomy** *n* an operation to cure hernia by the return of its contents to their normal position and removal of the hernial sac.

**heroin** *n* diamorphine. A class A substance which is subject to considerable criminal misuse. Used medicinally as diamorphine to relieve severe pain.

**herpangina** *n* minute vesicles and ulcers at the back of the palate. Short, febrile illness in children caused by coxsackievirus group A.

**herpes** *n* a vesicular eruption caused by infection with the herpes simplex virus. *genital herpes* a sexually transmissible infection, caused by either herpes simplex virus type 1 or type 2 (HSV-1 or HSV-2), that is associated with painful, tender superficial ulcers of the genitalia or anal region. Without treatment first-episode lesions heal within about 1 month; antiviral therapy shortens the duration of the lesions. Recurrences are common, particularly with HSV-2, but the duration of lesions is shorter than during the initial episode. An individual can transmit the virus to a sexual partner even when there are no apparent genital or orolabial lesions.

**herpes gestationis** a rare skin disease peculiar to pregnancy. It clears in about 30 days after delivery.

**herpes simplex virus (HSV)** there are two types of HSV—types 1 and 2 (HSV-1 and HSV-2). HSV-1 is associated with orolabial herpes (cold sores), but either type can cause genital herpes. Following infection, whether or not the individual develops symptoms, the virus becomes latent or hidden for the individual's lifetime in the trigeminal ganglion (in the case of orolabial herpes) or in the sacral ganglia (in the case of genital herpes). Reactivation of the virus can cause recurrent lesions, or the virus can be shed from the mucous membranes or skin without visible signs. ⇒ herpes.

**herpesviruses** *npl* group of DNA viruses that include: cytomegalovirus (CMV), Epstein–Barr virus (EBV), herpes simplex virus (HSV), human herpesvirus 6 (HHV-6) and varicella-zoster virus (VZV).

**herpes zoster** (*syn* shingles) the causative organism is the varicella-zoster virus (VZV), the same virus that causes chickenpox. Herpes zoster occurs when there is reactivation of the VZV that has remained dormant in a sensory nerve ganglion since a much earlier attack of chickenpox, usually during childhood. The reactivation is associated with an event which compromises the immune system, such as stress or serious illness. It occurs in middle-aged and older people, or in individuals who are immunocompromised, especially people with human immunodeficiency virus (HIV) disease. The person with herpes zoster may infect another person with chickenpox. It is characterized by severe pain and usually, some days later, the appearance of vesicles along the distribution of a sensory nerve (usually unilateral). ⊙ DVD Infection of the trigeminal nerve ganglion results in corneal vesicles which can lead to ulceration and corneal scarring. Early treatment, at least 72 hours prior to the development of the rash, with an antiviral drug, such as aciclovir, famciclovir or valaciclovir, can lessen the intensity of the infection. Postherpetic neuralgia may be particularly resistant to treatment. A live virus vaccine that reduces the risk of herpes zoster is available to people over 60 years of age in the USA. ⇒ capsaicin, postherpetic (neuralgia), Ramsay Hunt syndrome.

**herpetiform** *adj* resembling herpes.

**hertz (Hz)** *n* (H Hertz, German physicist, 1857–1894) derived SI unit (International System of Units) for wave frequency. ⇒ Appendix 2.

**Herxheimer's reaction** ⇒ Jarisch–Herxheimer's reaction.

**hesitancy** *n* delay in starting to void urine, even when responding to a strong desire to void. A symptom of outflow obstruction, bladder instability or hypersensitivity.

**Hess test** a sphygmomanometer cuff is applied to the arm and is inflated. Petechial eruption in the surrounding area after 5 min denotes weakness of the capillary walls.

**heterochromia** *n* difference in colour within areas in the same iris, or one iris is different in colour from the other.

**heterogametic** *adj* relating to the sex which produces gametes with different sex chromosomes. Male gametes, spermatozoa, have either the X or Y chromosome. They determine the sex of the offspring. ⇒ homogametic.

**heterogeneity** *n* having variable qualities and characteristics.

**heterogenous** *adj* of unlike origin; not originating within the organism; derived from a different species. ⇒ homogenous *opp*.

**heterograft** *n* ⇒ xenograft.

**heterologous** *adj* of different origin; from a different species. ⇒ homologous *opp*.

**heterometropia** *n* a visual defect in which the refraction in one eye is slightly different from that in the other. Each eye perceives a slightly different image.

**heterophile** *n* a product of one species which acts against that of another, for example human antigen against sheep's red blood cells.

**heterophoria** *n* a latent squint which may become obvious. For example, in bright light or when the person is tired.

**heterosexual** *adj, n* literally, of different sexes; often used to describe an individual who is sexually attracted to members of the opposite sex. ⇒ homosexual *opp*.

**heterotopic transplant** ⇒ transplant.

**heterozygous** *adj* having different genes or alleles at the same locus on corresponding homologous chromosomes (one of paternal origin and one maternal). ⇒ homozygous *opp*.

**hexachlorophene** *n* a phenolic disinfectant used in preoperative skin preparation, and as a dusting powder. It should not be used on children under 2 years of age, during pregnancy, or on excoriated or badly burnt skin.

**hexokinase** *n* enzyme that catalyses the phosphorylation of glucose to glucose-6-phosphate. Important stage in glycolysis and glycogenesis.

**hexosamine** *n* a hexose sugar with an amino group. For example, glucosamine formed from glucose.

**hexoses** *npl* monosaccharides containing six carbon atoms such as glucose, mannose, galactose, fructose.

**HFEA** *abbr* Human Fertilization and Embryology Authority.

**HHNK** *abbr* hyperglycaemic hyperosmolar non-ketotic coma.

**5-HIAA** *abbr* 5-hydroxyindoleacetic acid.

**hiatus** *n* a space or opening. *hiatus hernia* migration of part of the stomach through the diaphragmatic hiatus into the chest. May be asymptomatic, cause gastro-oesophageal reflux disease or strangulate. ⇒ hernia—**hiatal** *adj*.

**Hib vaccine** *abbr Haemophilus influenzae* type B vaccine. An injectable vaccine that protects against the serious infections caused by *H. influenzae* is offered as part of the routine immunization programme at 2, 3 and 4 months of age, with a booster at 12 months.

**hiccough** *n* (*syn* hiccup) an involuntary inspiratory spasm of the diaphragm, ending in a sudden closure of the glottis with the production of a characteristic sound.

**hidradenitis suppurativa** a chronic suppurative condition affecting the axillae, groin and anogenital area. It is characterized by abscess formation with discharge of pus, sinuses, fibrosis and scarring.

**hidrosis** *n* sweat secretion.

**hierarchy of evidence** in evidence-based practice a ranking of types of evidence based on their ability to predict effectiveness, remove bias and control confounders. The highest level is considered to be a systematic review of several high-quality randomized controlled trials, through various levels to the lowest level of expert opinion.

**Higginson's syringe** a rubber bulb with tubes leading to and from it. Compression of the rubber bulb forces fluid forward through the nozzle for irrigation of a body cavity.

Rarely used and now mostly replaced by single-use items of equipment.

**high-density lipoprotein (HDL)** ⇒ lipoprotein.

**high-dependency unit (HDU)** an area within a hospital with augmented levels of staff and equipment in which patients can receive levels of observation, monitoring, nursing and medical care between that available on a general ward and intensive care unit. Generally excludes those needing mechanical ventilation.

**hilum** *n* a depression on the surface of an organ where vessels, ducts, etc. enter and leave—**hili** *pl*, **hilar** *adj*. *hilar adenitis* ⇒ adenitis.

**hindbrain** *n* the part of the brain comprising the fourth ventricle, pons, medulla oblongata and cerebellum.

**hindgut** *n* the caudal or posterior part of the embryonic alimentary tract. It gives rise to the distal transverse colon, descending and sigmoid colon, rectum, part of anal canal and part of the urogenital structures. ⇒ foregut, midgut.

**hindwaters** *n* the sac of amniotic fluid situated beyond the fetal head and surrounding the fetus. ⇒ forewaters.

**hinge joint** ginglymus. A synovial joint, e.g. the elbow or knee, where the bones are moulded in such a way to allow movement in one plane.

**hip bone (innominate bone)** formed by the fusion of three separate bones—the ilium, ischium and pubis.

**hip joint** the ball-and-socket joint formed by the articulation of the head of femur in the acetabulum of the pelvis (Figure H.6).

**hippocampus** *n* a structure located on the medial wall of each temporal lobe and which curves beneath the lateral ventricle. It is the part of the limbic system which is formed from evolutionarily older cortex. It is concerned with the initial processing of new memories and spatial orientation—**hippocampi** *pl*. ⇒ limbic system.

**Hippocrates** *n* Greek physician and philosopher (460–367 BC) who established a school of medicine at Cos, his birthplace. He is often termed the 'father of medicine'.

**hip replacement** ⇒ arthroplasty.

**Hirschsprung's disease** (H Hirschsprung, Danish physician, 1830–1916) congenital intestinal aganglionosis, leading to intractable constipation or even intestinal obstruction. There is marked hypertrophy and dilatation of the colon (megacolon) above the aganglionic

H

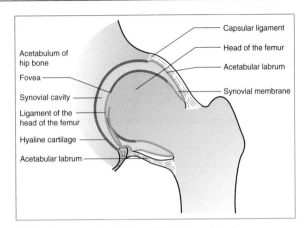

**Figure H.6** Hip joint *(reproduced from Watson 2000 with permission).*

segment. Commoner in boys and children with Down's syndrome.

**hirsute** *adj* hairy or shaggy.

**hirsutism, hirsuties** *n* any abnormal degree of coarse hairiness (usually refers to male pattern of hair growth in a woman). ⇒ hypertrichosis.

**hirudin** *n* a chemical produced by the medicinal leech, which prevents the clotting of blood by acting as an anticoagulant.

**hirudo** *n* ⇒ leech.

**histamine** *n* an amine released in many tissues. It causes smooth muscle contraction, gastric secretion and vasodilation. During the inflammatory response its release from mast cells leads to capillary dilatation and increased vessel permeability. ⇒ allergy, anaphylaxis, inflammation.

**histamine receptors** there are three types in the body—$H_1$ in the bronchial muscle, $H_2$ in the secreting cells in the stomach and $H_3$ in nerve tissue.

**histamine test** test previously used to determine the maximal gastric secretion of hydrochloric acid.

**histidinaemia** *n* an autosomal recessive metabolic condition. The lack of an enzyme needed for the metabolism of histidine leads to an increase in the amount of histidine in blood.

**histidine** *n* an essential (indispensable) amino acid in infants and children which is widely distributed in the proteins present in the diet.

**histiocytes** *npl* macrophages or phagocytic tissue cells.

**histiocytoma** *n* benign tumour of histiocytes.

**histiocytosis** *n* a group of conditions in which histiocytes are abnormal in some way. Known collectively as Langerhans' cell histiocytosis. ⇒ Hand–Schüller–Christian disease, Letterer–Siwe disease.

**histocompatibility** *n* the degree of similarity (compatibility) between the donor and recipient antigens in tissue or organ(s) for transplant. The closer the match, the better chance of a successful transplant. ⇒ human leucocyte antigens, major histocompatibility complex.

**histogram** *n* a bar graph with values for one or more variables plotted against the frequency or time (Figure H.7).

**histology** *n* microscopic study of tissues—**histological** *adj*, **histologically** *adv*.

**histolysis** *n* disintegration of organic tissue—**histolytic** *adj*.

**histones** *npl* proteins closely associated with the chromosomal DNA of higher organisms, which coils around histone molecules.

***Histoplasma*** *n* a genus of fungi. *H. capsulatum* causes the condition histoplasmosis in humans.

**histoplasmosis** *n* an infection caused by inhaling spores of the fungus *Histoplasma capsulatum*. The spores are found in the faeces of some birds, including poultry and in the faeces of bats. It is endemic in parts of the USA, such as the Mississippi valley. The primary lung

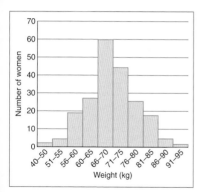

**Figure H.7** Histogram *(reproduced from Gunn 2001 with permission).*

lesion may be asymptomatic or accompanied by raised temperature, malaise, cough and adenopathy. Progressive histoplasmosis can be fatal. Lung involvement increases and the infection can disseminate in the blood to affect organs that include the liver and spleen.

**HIV** *abbr* human immunodeficiency virus. ⇒ AIDS.

**hives** *n* nettlerash; urticaria.

**HLA** *abbr* human leucocyte antigen.

**HMG-CoA reductase inhibitors (3-hydroxy-3-methylglutaryl-coenzyme)** known colloquially as 'statins'. A group of drugs (e.g. pravastatin) that prevent the synthesis of cholesterol in the liver, thereby reducing its level in the blood. ⇒ Appendix 5.

**Hodgkin's disease** (T Hodgkin, British physician, 1798–1866) tumour of lymphoid tissue often originating in the mediastinum. Often occurs in young adults. A diagnostic feature is the presence of the large multinucleated Reed–Sternberg cells in the lymphatic system. The prognosis is related to the histological subtype and stage; cure rate is around 80%. Treatment may consist of radiotherapy and/or chemotherapy. ⇒ lymphoma.

**holandric inheritance** those traits or conditions inherited through the paternal line from father to son. They are transmitted by genes on the non-homologous part of the Y chromosome.

**holistic** *adj* relating to the theory of holism. Describes health care that takes account of physical, psychological, emotional, social and spiritual needs and aspects of care.

**holocrine gland** a type of exocrine gland that disintegrates in order to discharge its secretion. For example, a sebaceous gland of the skin. ⇒ apocrine gland, merocrine (eccrine) gland.

**holoenzyme** *n* enzyme protein combined with a prosthetic group or its coenzyme.

**Homans' sign** (J Homans, American surgeon, 1877–1954) passive dorsiflexion of foot causing pain in calf muscles. Indicative of deep-vein thrombosis affecting the leg.

**home assessment** an evaluation of the suitability of an individual's accommodation in order to identify any adaptations, resources or services needed to enable him or her to perform adequately activities of daily living in the home environment.

**homeopathy** *n* a method of treating disease by prescribing minute doses of drugs which, in maximum dose, would produce symptoms of the disease. The 'law of similars' or 'like cures like' was first adopted by Hahnemann (C Hahnemann, German physician, 1755–1843)—**homeopathic** *adj.* ⇒ allopathy.

**homeostasis** *n* autoregulatory processes whereby functions such as body temperature, blood pressure, blood glucose and electrolyte levels are maintained within set parameters.

**home visit** a visit (such as by an occupational therapist) made to an individual's home in order to assess the ability of an individual to function independently following discharge from hospital or other care setting.

**homicide** *n* killing of another person: intentional killing is murder, whereas accidental (without intent) killing is manslaughter (in Scotland: culpable homicide).

**homocysteine** *n* an intermediate which with serine forms cysteine. It is also a precursor for methionine regeneration in reactions requiring folates and cobalamins. A deficiency in folates and other B vitamins is associated with increased amounts of homocysteine in the blood and a higher risk of coronary heart disease.

**homocystinuria** *n* excretion of homocystine (a sulphur-containing amino acid, homologue of cystine) in the urine. Caused by a recessively inherited metabolic error. Gives rise to slow development or learning disability of varying degree; the lens of the eye may dislocate and there is overgrowth of long bones with thrombotic episodes which are often fatal in childhood—**homocystinuric** *adj.*

**homoeothermic** *adj* describes an animal able to maintain a constant core body temperature despite variations in environmental temperatures.

**homogametic** *adj* relating to the sex which produces gametes with the same-sex chromosomes. Female gametes, oocytes, always have the X chromosome. ⇒ heterogametic.

**homogeneous** *adj* of the same type; of the same quality or consistency throughout.

**homogenize** *vt* to make into the same consistency throughout.

**homogenous** *adj* having a like nature, e.g. a bone graft from another human being. ⇒ heterogenous *opp*.

**homogentisic acid** an intermediate compound formed in the metabolism of the amino acids tyrosine and phenylalanine. It is responsible for the darkly staining urine of individuals with alkaptonuria. ⇒ alkaptonuria.

**homograft** *n* a tissue or organ which is transplanted from one individual to another of the same species. ⇒ allograft.

**homolateral** *adj* on the same side—**homolaterally** *adv*. ⇒ contralateral.

**homologous** *adj* corresponding in origin and structure. ⇒ heterologous *opp*.

**homologous chromosomes 1.** those that synapse (pair) during meiosis. Of the two homologues, one is paternal and the other maternal in origin. **2.** In a diploid (2n) somatic cell a pair of chromosomes which are the same in size and shape and gene loci.

**homonymous** *adj* consisting of corresponding halves. Pertaining to symmetrical halves of the visual fields, i.e. the nasal (inner) half of one field and the temporal (outer) half of the other. When describing a visual field defect implies loss of vision in the same side of the field in the two eyes.

**homosexual** *adj, n* literally, of the same sex; describes an individual who is sexually attracted to members of the same sex. Individuals may prefer to be described as being gay or lesbian.

**homozygous** *adj* having identical genes or alleles in the same locus on both homologous chromosomes of a pair (one is paternal in origin and the other maternal). If a person has inherited a recessive allele from both parents he or she is homozygous for that trait or disease, e.g. cystic fibrosis; it will be expressed and the individual's offspring will be carriers of the recessive allele. ⇒ heterozygous *opp*.

**HONK** *acron* **h**yper**o**smolar **n**on-**k**etotic (coma).

**hookworm** *n* ⇒ Ancylostoma, Necator.

**hoop traction** fixed skin traction used for the treatment of fractures of the femoral shaft in children, and for the gradual abduction of the hip in children with developmental dysplasia of the hip.

**hordeolum** *n* ⇒ stye.

**horizontal plane** ⇒ transverse plane.

**hormone** *n* a specific chemical messenger produced by endocrine glands and other structures. It is transported in the blood or lymph to tissues and organs elsewhere in the body where they regulate metabolic functions and cell growth. Hormones are either lipid-based, e.g. thyroid hormones, or peptides, e.g. insulin, adrenaline (epinephrine). Hormone release is regulated by negative-feedback mechanisms, neurotransmitters, other hormones and releasing and inhibiting factors. Rarely regulation is through positive feedback, such as the release of oxytocin during labour. Other hormones act more locally, such as those secreted in the gastrointestinal tract, e.g. gastrin produced by gastric cells stimulates increased acid secretion by other gastric cells.

**hormone replacement therapy (HRT)** a term usually applied to oestrogen therapy (with progestogens in women who have an intact uterus) given to women to relieve menopausal symptoms and prevent osteoporosis. It is administered orally, by implant or transdermally with patch or gel. The term also applies to a treatment that replaces other missing hormones.

**Horner's syndrome** (J Horner, Swiss ophthalmologist, 1831–1886) loss of sympathetic innervation to the eye and upper face causing myosis (miosis) (small pupil), ptosis (drooping of the eyelid), retraction of the eyeball (enophthalmos) and anhidrosis (loss of sweating) over the forehead on that side. It may be caused by pathology in the hypothalamus or brainstem, and occur with cluster headaches, when it is accompanied by unilateral lacrimation, conjunctival reddening and nasal congestion, carotid artery disease or apical bronchial cancers. ⇒ Pancoast's syndrome.

**horseshoe kidney** an anatomical variation in which the inner lower border of each kidney is joined to give a horseshoe shape. Usually symptomless, but may interfere with drainage of urine into ureters leading to hydronephrosis.

**Horton's syndrome** (B Horton, American physician, 1895–1980) severe headache due to the release of histamine in the body. To be differentiated from migraine.

**hospice care** care provided for those with chronic or terminal illnesses and their families.

The care may be at home, in a day unit and in hospice premises. Individualized symptom (especially pain) control programmes are implemented which aim to minimize the physical, emotional and spiritual distress.

**hospital-acquired infection (HAI)** ⇒ health care-associated infection (HCAI), infection.

**hospital sterilization and disinfection unit (HSDU)** central sterile supply units (CSSUs) that also provide disinfection of equipment.

**host** *n* the organic structure upon which parasites or bacteria flourish. *intermediate host* one in which the parasite passes its larval or cystic stage.

**hourglass contraction** a circular constriction in the middle of a hollow organ (usually the stomach or uterus), dividing it into two portions following scar formation.

**house dust mite** a member of the order Acarina and the genus *Dermatophagoides.* They thrive in controlled environments such as those provided in houses where they are found in carpets, bedding, mattresses, pillows and furniture. They eat exfoliated skin cells, a major part of house dust. Their faecal matter, which contains partially digested food and enzymes, is a major cause of allergic conditions, including asthma.

**housemaid's knee** ⇒ bursitis.

**HPA** *abbr* Health Protection Agency.

**HPC** *abbr* Health Professions Council.

**HPL** *abbr* human placental lactogen.

**HPV** *abbr* human papillomavirus.

**H$_1$-receptor antagonists** *npl* a group of antiemetic drugs, e.g. cinnarizine, that block histamine receptors. ⇒ Appendix 5.

**H$_2$-receptor antagonist** a drug, e.g. ranitidine, which has a selective action against the H$_2$ histamine receptors and thereby decreases, for example, the secretion of gastric juice. ⇒ Appendix 5.

**HR$_{max}$** *abbr* maximum heart rate.

**HRT** *abbr* hormone replacement therapy.

**HSC** *abbr* Health and Safety Commission.

**HSCT** *abbr* haemopoietic stem cell transplantation.

**HSDU** *abbr* hospital sterilization and disinfection unit.

**HSE** *abbr* Health and Safety Executive.

**HSSU** *abbr* hospital sterile supply unit. ⇒ hospital sterilization and disinfection unit.

**HSV** *abbr* herpes simplex virus.

**5-HT$_1$ agonists** *npl* a group of specific antimigraine drugs such as sumatriptan, which is also used for cluster headaches. ⇒ Appendix 5.

**HTLV** *abbr* human T-cell lymphotropic viruses.

**5-HT$_3$-receptor antagonists** a group of antiemetic drugs, e.g. ondansetron, that block 5-hydroxytryptamine$_3$ receptors. ⇒ Appendix 5.

**human chorionic gonadotrophin (hCG)** a hormone produced by the trophoblast cells and later the chorion. Also a tumour marker for testicular and choriocarcinoma.

**human epidermal growth factor receptor-2 (HER2)** some breast cancers overexpress the protein HER2. Around 20% of breast cancers are HER2-positive. Breast cancers that have overexpression of HER2-receptor protein are more likely to return after treatment and have a less favourable outcome because the cancer cells are stimulated to grow by epidermal growth factors. The monoclonal antibody trastuzumab is available for the treatment of early breast cancer with HER2 overexpression with other treatment modalities. It is also used for metastatic breast cancers, which overexpress HER2.

**Human Fertilization and Embryology Authority (HFEA)** a UK statutory body set up in 1991. The primary purpose of the HFEA is to license and monitor clinics that provide in vitro fertilization (IVF) and donor insemination. The HFEA also regulates the storage of sperm, eggs and embryos. It produces a Code of Practice, and information about infertility and treatments for the public. In addition, all UK-based research using human embryos must be licensed and monitored by the HFEA.

**human genome project** the worldwide collaboration between laboratories to decipher and document the DNA sequence of the entire human genome.

**human immunodeficiency virus (HIV)** currently designates the acquired immunodeficiency syndrome (AIDS) virus. There are two types: HIV-1 (many strains), mainly responsible for HIV disease in western Europe, North America and Central Africa, and HIV-2, causing similar disease, mainly in West Africa.

**human leucocyte antigen (HLA)** the major histocompatibility complexes, so called because they were first found on leucocytes. ⇒ major histocompatibility complex.

**human papillomavirus (HPV)** there are many types of HPV, including several that are associated with anogenital warts (particularly types 6 and 11), and a few types (particularly 16 and 18) that are associated with genital tract malignancy such as cervical

**H**

cancer. In the UK, a new vaccine against HPV types 6, 11, 16 and 18 has been added to the routine immunization programme for girls aged 12–13 years starting in 2008 with a catch-up programme for girls aged up to 18 years. As it does not protect against all viral types associated with cancer, normal routine cervical screening continues as before.

**human placental lactogen (human chorionic somatomammotrophin) (HPL)** a peptide hormone produced by the placenta. It is involved in the metabolism of glucose and fatty acids during pregnancy, and may influence the production of human chorionic gonadotrophin and prolactin.

**human T-cell lymphotropic viruses (HTLV)** two retroviruses; HTLV-1 and HTLV-2, both of which are linked with some forms of leukaemia.

**humectant** *n* a substance that aids the retention of water. In the skin a humectant acts as a natural moisturizer. This is protected by lipids that control the transepidermal water loss.

**humerus** *n* the bone of the upper arm, between the elbow and shoulder joint (⇒ Appendix 1, Figure 2)—**humeri** *pl*, **humeral** *adj*.

**humidity** *n* the amount of moisture in the atmosphere, as measured by a hygrometer.

**humoral immunity** ⇒ immunity.

**humour** *n* any fluid of the body. ⇒ aqueous, vitreous body.

**Hunter's syndrome** (C Hunter, Canadian physician, 1873–1955) one of the mucopolysaccharidoses. An X-linked recessive condition.

**Huntington's disease** (G Huntington, American physician, 1851–1916) rare inherited incurable neurodegenerative condition of the brain, for which the gene is known. It is transmitted as an autosomal dominant gene on chromosome 4 and affects both sexes. There is slow progressive degeneration of the nerve cells of the basal nuclei (ganglia) and cerebral cortex. Develops in adult life (30s and 40s) or later, causing a movement disorder (usually chorea), mood changes and dementia. ⇒ chorea.

**Hurler's syndrome** (G Hurler, German physician, 1889–1965) one of the mucopolysaccharidoses. Inherited as an autosomal recessive trait.

**Hürthle cell tumour** (K Hürthle, German histologist, 1860–1945) a new growth of the thyroid gland. It is characterized by large granular cells (Hürthle cells) and may be benign (adenoma) or malignant (carcinoma).

**HUS** *abbr* haemolytic–uraemic syndrome.

**Hutchinson's teeth** (J Hutchinson, British surgeon/pathologist, 1828–1913) defect of the upper central incisors (second dentition) which forms part of the facies of congenital syphilis. The teeth are broader at the gum than at the cutting edge, with the latter showing an elliptical notch.

**hyaline** *adj* like glass; transparent. *hyaline cartilage* a smooth flexible tissue comprising groups of chondrocytes in a solid matrix. It provides support in the larynx, trachea and bronchi, forms the costal cartilages that join the ribs to the sternum and provides a smooth surface over the articular surfaces of long bones to allow movement at joints. ⇒ cartilage. *hyaline degeneration* degeneration of connective tissue, especially that of blood vessels in which tissue becomes formless in appearance. *hyaline membrane disease* ⇒ neonatal respiratory distress syndrome.

**hyalitis** *n* inflammation of the vitreous body of the eye.

**hyaloid** *adj* resembling hyaline tissue. *hyaloid membrane* ⇒ membrane.

**hyaluronic acid** mucopolysaccharide important in the extracellular matrix which holds cells together. Also present in the vitreous body, and the synovial fluid, where it contributes to viscosity. It has some therapeutic uses that include intra-articular injection for osteoarthritis affecting the knee. Increasingly used in cosmetic procedures as a filler/bulking agent in the skin.

**hyaluronidase** *n* enzyme that breaks down hyaluronic acid. It is present in spermatozoa and its release by many spermatozoa allows one to penetrate and fertilize the oocyte. Hyaluronidase may be used therapeutically to improve the absorption of some drugs or fluids administered parenterally.

**hydatid cyst** the cyst formed by larvae of the tapeworm, *Echinococcus granulosa*, found in dogs and other canines. The encysted stage normally occurs in sheep but can occur in humans after eating with hands soiled from contact with dogs or infected sheep. The cysts are commonest in the liver, but can affect the brain, lungs and bone.

**hydatidiform** *adj* pertaining to or resembling a hydatid cyst. *hydatidiform mole* a pregnancy in which the placenta shows degenerative stoma combined with neoplastic chorionic endothelium. A *complete hydatidiform mole* shows abnormal proliferation of the trophoblast and the presence of hydropic placental villi with no fetal parts. An *incomplete hydatidiform mole* or *partial mole* has a chromosomally abnormal fetus (triploid chromosome complement). Malignant transformation to choriocarcinoma may occur, especially in pregnancies affected by a complete hydatidiform mole.

**hydraemia** *n* a greater plasma volume than usual compared with cellular volume of the blood; normally present in late pregnancy—**hydraemic** *adj*.

**hydramnios** *n* ⇒ polyhydramnios.

**hydrarthrosis** *n* a collection of synovial fluid in a joint cavity.

**hydrate** *vi* combine with water—**hydration** *n*.

**hydroa** *n* *hydroa aestivale* a vesicular eruption that affects exposed parts and results from photosensitivity. *hydroa vacciniforme* is a more severe form of this in which scarring ensues.

**hydrocele** *n* a swelling due to accumulation of serous fluid between the tunica vaginalis and tunica albuginea of the testis or in the spermatic cord.

**hydrocephalus** *n* (*syn* 'water on the brain') an excess of cerebrospinal fluid inside the skull due to a disruption in normal cerebrospinal fluid (CSF) circulation, or loss of brain tissue. It may be congenital, when it is often associated with spina bifida, or acquired after trauma, infections or with tumours. *external hydrocephalus* the excess of fluid is mainly in the subarachnoid space. *internal hydrocephalus* the excess of fluid is mainly in the ventricles of the brain. A variety of shunting procedures are available to drain excess CSF and return it to the blood stream—**hydrocephalic** *adj*.

**hydrochloric acid** acid formed from hydrogen and chlorine; secreted by the gastric oxyntic cells and present in gastric juice.

**hydrocolloid** *n* a type of rehydrating wound dressing. A colloid containing substances that include gelatin, cellulose, pectins and adhesives.

**hydrocortisone** *n* ⇒ cortisol.

**hydrogel** *n* a type of rehydrating wound dressing, comprising a soft, water-containing gel.

**hydrogen (H)** *n* a colourless, odourless, combustible gas.

**hydrogenase** *n* an enzyme that catalyses the addition of molecular hydrogen in a reduction reaction.

**hydrogenated oils/fats** oils hardened by the addition of hydrogen, such as in food processing.

**hydrogenation** *n* the addition of hydrogen to a substance. ⇒ reduction.

**hydrogen bond** a weak bond formed between polar water molecules. Or the bonds in large biological molecules such as nucleic acids and proteins. The hydrogen atoms in the bond are already bonded to other atoms such as nitrogen or oxygen. Important in maintaining the three-dimensional structure of biological molecules such as enzymes.

**hydrogen breath test** a non-invasive test to detect disaccharide intolerance or bacterial overgrowth. ⇒ lactase.

**hydrogen ion concentration (pH)** a measure of the acidity or alkalinity of a solution, ranging from pH 0 to 14, 7 being approximately neutral. The lower numbers denote acidity, whereas the higher ones denote alkalinity (Figure H.8).

**hydrogen peroxide ($H_2O_2$)** a powerful oxidizing and deodorizing agent, used in suitable dilution in mouthwashes.

**hydrolase** *n* an enzyme that catalyses hydrolysis, the addition of water.

**hydrolysis** *n* the splitting into more simple substances by adding water—**hydrolytic** *adj*, **hydrolyse** *vt*.

**hydrometer** *n* an instrument for determining the specific gravity of fluids—**hydrometry** *n*.

**hydronephrosis** *n* distension of the renal pelvis with urine, due to an obstructed outflow. If unrelieved, pressure eventually causes atrophy of kidney tissue.

**hydropericarditis** *n* pericarditis with effusion.

**hydropericardium** *n* fluid in the pericardial sac in the absence of inflammation. Can occur in heart and kidney failure.

**hydroperitoneum** *n* ⇒ ascites.

**hydrophilic** *adj* describes an affinity for water.

**hydrophobia** *n* fear of water. ⇒ rabies.

**hydrophobic** *adj* describes an aversion to water.

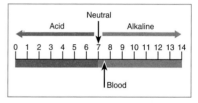

**Figure H.8** Hydrogen ion concentration (pH) *(reproduced from Waugh & Grant 2006 with permission)*.

**hydropneumopericardium** *n* the presence of air and fluid in the pericardial sac surrounding the heart. It may accompany pericardiocentesis.

**hydropneumoperitoneum** *n* the presence of air and fluid and gas in the peritoneal cavity: it may accompany paracentesis of that cavity; it may accompany perforation of the gut; or it may be due to infection with gasforming micro-organisms.

**hydropneumothorax** *n* pneumothorax further complicated by effusion of fluid into the pleural cavity.

**hydrops** *n* oedema—**hydropic** *adj*.

**hydrops fetalis** severe haemolytic disease of the newborn.

**hydrosalpinx** *n* distension of a uterine tube with watery fluid.

**hydrostatic pressure** that exerted by a liquid on the walls of its container, such as blood on an artery.

**hydrotherapy** *n* the science of therapeutic bathing, or exercise for diagnosed conditions.

**hydrothorax** *n* the presence of fluid in the pleural cavity. Also known as a pleural effusion.

**hydroureter** *n* abnormal distension of the ureter with urine.

**hydroxocobalamin** *n* a commercially produced substance with vitamin $B_{12}$ activity. Given by injection for those unable to absorb vitamin $B_{12}$. ⇒ cobalamin, cyanocobalamin, intrinsic factor.

**hydroxyapatite** *n* the calcium salts, carbonate, hydroxide and phosphate, that make bone extremely hard.

**5-hydroxyindoleacetic acid (5-HIAA)** a breakdown product of 5-hydroxytryptamine (serotonin) metabolism. High levels in the blood or urine may confirm the presence of carcinoid syndrome.

**hydroxyl (OH⁻)** *n* a monovalent ion, consisting of a hydrogen atom linked to an oxygen atom. ⇒ free radical.

**hydroxylysine** *n* an amino acid found only in collagen and elastin (proteins of connective tissue). Its formation requires vitamin C.

**hydroxyproline** *n* an amino acid found mainly in collagen and elastin (proteins of connective tissue). Its formation requires vitamin C. Increased excretion of hydroxyproline peptides in the urine occurs during high collagen turnover.

**5-hydroxytryptamine (5-HT)** *n* also known as serotonin. A neurotransmitter. Also present in the gastrointestinal tract and platelets.

**hygiene** *n* the science dealing with the maintenance of health—**hygienic** *adj. communal hygiene* embraces all measures taken to supply the community with pure food and water, good sanitation, housing, etc. *industrial hygiene* (*syn* occupational health) includes all measures taken to preserve the individual's health whilst he or she is at work. *mental hygiene* deals with the establishment of healthy mental attitudes and emotional reactions. *personal hygiene* includes all those measures taken by the individual to preserve his or her own health.

**hygroma** *n* a cystic swelling containing watery fluid, usually situated in the neck and present at birth, sometimes interfering with birth—**hygromata** *pl*, **hygromatous** *adj*.

**hygrometer** *n* an instrument for measuring the amount of moisture in the air. ⇒ humidity.

**hygroscopic** *adj* describes substances that readily absorb water, e.g. glycerol (glycerin [e]).

**hymen** *n* a perforated membrane across the vaginal entrance. *imperforate hymen* a congenital condition leading to haematocolpos. ⇒ cryptomenorrhoea.

**hymenectomy** *n* surgical excision of the hymen.

**hymenolepiasis** *n* heavy infestation with *Hymenolepis nana* or *H. diminuta*. It may cause abdominal pain, anorexia and diarrhoea. Occurs in warm climates such as in the southern United States.

**Hymenolepis** *n* a genus of small tapeworms that are parasitic in birds and mammals such as rats and mice. The worm eggs are eaten by insects where they mature. Humans may be infested by eating food contaminated by insects.

**hymenotomy** *n* surgical incision of the hymen.

**hyoid** *n* a U-shaped bone at the root of the tongue. ⇒ Appendix 1, Figure 6.

**hyperacidity** *n* excessive acidity.

**hyperactivity** *n* excessive activity and distractibility.

**hyperacusis** *n* abnormally acute hearing or excessive sensitivity to sound.

**hyperadrenalism** *n* ⇒ Cushing's disease.

**hyperaemia** *n* excess of blood in an area. *active hyperaemia* caused by an increased flow of blood to a part. *passive hyperaemia* occurs when there is restricted flow of blood from a part—**hyperaemic** *adj*.

**hyperaesthesia** *n* excessive sensitiveness of a part—**hyperaesthetic** *adj*.

**hyperaldosteronism** *n* excessive production of aldosterone causing hypertension, hypokalaemic alkalosis, muscle weakness and rarely tetany. *primary hyperaldosteronism, Conn's disease*: hyperplasia or adenoma of the adrenal cortex; *secondary hyperaldosteronism*, e.g. caused by heart failure, or due to increased renin secretion in renal artery stenosis.

**hyperalgesia** *n* excessive sensibility to pain—**hyperalgesic** *adj.*

**hyperalimentation** *n* literally large amounts of food, in excess of needs. Usually refers to the provision of parenteral nutrition (intravenous).

**hyperandrogenism** *n* excess androgen hormone secretion in women. ⇒ polycystic ovary syndrome.

**hyperbaric** *adj* term applied to gas at greater pressure than normal.

**hyperbaric oxygen therapy** a form of treatment in which a patient is entirely enclosed in a pressure chamber breathing 100% oxygen at greater than one atmosphere pressure. Used for patients with air embolism, gas gangrene, carbon monoxide poisoning, decompression sickness, etc.

**hyperbilirubinaemia** *n* excessive bilirubin in the blood—**hyperbilirubinaemic** *adj.*

**hypercalcaemia** *n* excessive calcium in the blood, usually resulting from bone resorption, as occurs in hyperparathyroidism, metastatic tumours of bone, paraneoplastic syndrome associated with parathyroid hormone production in breast cancer, or Paget's disease. It results in vague symptoms of anorexia, abdominal pain, muscle pain and weakness, which can be easily missed. It is accompanied by hypercalciuria and can lead to nephrolithiasis—**hypercalcaemic** *adj.*

**hypercalciuria** *n* greatly increased excretion of calcium in the urine. Occurs in diseases which result in bone resorption. *idiopathic hypercalciuria* is the term used when there is no known metabolic cause. Hypercalciuria is of importance in the pathogenesis of kidney stones—**hypercalciuric** *adj.*

**hypercapnia** *n* (*syn* hypercarbia) raised $CO_2$ tension in arterial blood, usually due to hypoventilation—**hypercapnic** *adj.*

**hypercarbia** *n* ⇒ hypercapnia.

**hypercatabolism** *n* excessive breakdown of body protein. Amino acids are used as a source of energy. It occurs when energy requirements are not met by dietary sources, such as in situations where nutritional requirements are increased, e.g. major trauma, sepsis,

surgery and burns. ⇒ catabolism, nitrogen balance.

**hyperchloraemia** *n* excessive chloride in the blood. Occurs with hyperkalaemia and leads to metabolic acidosis as acid–base balance is disturbed—**hyperchloraemic** *adj.*

**hyperchlorhydria** *n* excessive hydrochloric acid in the gastric juice—**hyperchlorhydric** *adj.*

**hypercholesterolaemia** *n* excessive cholesterol in the blood. Predisposes to atheroma and gallstones. Also found in hypothyroidism (myxoedema)—**hypercholesterolaemic** *adj.*

**hyperemesis** *n* excessive vomiting.

**hyperemesis gravidarum** severe vomiting during pregnancy that requires medical intervention.

**hyperextension** *n* overextension. Active or passive force which takes the joint into extension beyond its normal physiological range.

**hyperflexion** *n* excessive flexion.

**hyperglycaemia** *n* increased blood glucose, usually indicative of diabetes mellitus or impaired glucose tolerance, but sometimes due to pathological stress, e.g. myocardial infarction—**hyperglycaemic** *adj.*

**hyperglycinaemia** *n* excess glycine in the serum. Can cause acidosis and learning disability—**hyperglycinaemic** *adj.*

**hyperhidrosis** *n* excessive sweating—**hyperhidrotic** *adj.*

**hyperinsulinism** *n* elevated circulating levels of insulin due to pancreatic tumour, insulinoma or factitious administration of hypoglycaemic agents; resulting in hypoglycaemia, which may lead to episodic coma, confusion or even mental health disturbance.

**hyperinvolution** *n* reduction to below normal size, as of the uterus after parturition.

**hyperkalaemia** *n* excessive potassium in the blood as occurs in renal failure. An early sign may be muscle weakness. Severe hyperkalaemia causes arrhythmias and cardiac arrest—**hyperkalaemic** *adj.*

**hyperkeratosis** *n* hypertrophy of the stratum corneum or the horny layer of the skin—**hyperkeratotic** *adj.*

**hyperkinesis** *n* excessive movement—**hyperkinetic** *adj.*

**hyperkinetic disorder/syndrome** usually appears between the ages of 2 and 4 years. The child is slow to develop intellectually and has a marked degree of distractibility. There is an attention deficit and restlessness with uncontrolled activity. There is aggressive behaviour (especially towards siblings) even if unprovoked, and possibly antisocial behaviour. The child is impulsive and may appear to be fearless and undeterred by threats of punishment. The parents complain of the child's cold unaffectionate character and destructive behaviour. ⇒ attention deficit hyperactivity disorder.

**hyperlipaemia** *n* excessive total fat in the blood—**hyperlipaemic** *adj*.

**hyperlipidaemia** *n* abnormally elevated plasma lipid levels. Identified as a risk factor for coronary heart disease.

**hypermagnesaemia** *n* excessive magnesium in the blood; found in renal failure and in people who take excessive amounts of magnesium-containing antacids—**hypermagnesaemic** *adj*.

**hypermetabolism** *n* production of excessive body heat. Characteristic of hyperthyroidism—**hypermetabolic** *adj*.

**hypermetropia** *n* long-sightedness caused by low refractive power or reduced axial length of the eye, with the result that the light rays are focused beyond, instead of on, the retina—**hypermetropic** *adj*.

**hypermobility** *n* excessive mobility. As in a joint that has an increase in the normal range of joint movement, potentially leading to instability.

**hypermotility** *n* increased movement, such as peristalsis in the gastrointestinal tract.

**hypernatraemia** *n* increased sodium concentration in the blood, most often caused by a relative loss or deficit of water. This can be due to polyuria, diarrhoea, excessive sweating or inadequate water intake. Hypernatraemia may also be caused by excessive intake of sodium—**hypernatraemic** *adj*.

**hypernephroma** *n* (*syn* Grawitz tumour) a malignant tumour of the kidney—**hypernephromata** *pl*, **hypernephromatous** *adj*.

**hyperonychia** *n* excessive growth of the nails.

**hyperosmia** *n* abnormally increased sense of smell.

**hyperosmolar non-ketotic coma (HONK)** profound dehydration due to uncontrolled type 2 diabetes leading to hyperosmolar state and ultimately coma. ⇒ diabetes mellitus.

**hyperosmolarity** *n* (*syn* hypertonicity) a solution exerting a higher osmotic pressure than another is said to have a hyperosmolarity, with reference to it. In medicine, the comparison is usually made with normal plasma.

**hyperostosis** *n* exostosis.

**hyperoxaluria** *n* excessive calcium oxalate in the urine—**hyperoxaluric** *adj*.

**hyperparathyroidism** *n* overactivity of one or more parathyroid glands, usually due to parathyroid adenoma, and resulting in elevated serum calcium levels; rarely results in parathyroid bone disease, osteitis fibrosa cystica; may be primary, or secondary/tertiary usually in response to chronic renal failure. ⇒ hypercalcaemia, hypercalciuria, von Recklinghausen's disease.

**hyperperistalsis** *n* excessive peristalsis—**hyperperistaltic** *adj*.

**hyperphagia** *n* overeating. Can be caused by psychological disturbances and lesions of the hypothalamus. It is a symptom of Prader–Willi syndrome. ⇒ obesity.

**hyperphenylalaninaemia** *n* excess of phenylalanine in the blood which results in phenylketonuria. ⇒

**hyperphoria** *n* ⇒ phoria.

**hyperphosphataemia** *n* excessive phosphates in the blood—**hyperphosphataemic** *adj*.

**hyperpigmentation** *n* increased or excessive pigmentation.

**hyperpituitarism** *n* ⇒ acromegaly, Cushing's disease, gigantism, hyperprolactinaemia.

**hyperplasia** *n* excessive formation of new cells—**hyperplastic** *adj*.

**hyperpnoea** *n* rapid, deep breathing; panting; gasping—**hyperpnoeic** *adj*.

**hyperpraxia** *n* restlessness, excessive activity.

**hyperprolactinaemia** *n* elevation in circulating prolactin levels, sometimes due to stress; if pathological, results in galactorrhoea, menstrual irregularity and infertility; may be due to dopamine antagonists, such as metoclopramide or antipsychotic (neuroleptics) drugs, large, often non-functioning pituitary tumours, or prolactinomas.

**hyperpyrexia** *n* body temperature above 40–42°C—**hyperpyrexial** *adj*. ⇒ malignant hyperthermia, neuroleptic malignant syndrome.

**hyperreflexia** *n* exaggerated reflexes.

**hypersecretion** *n* excessive secretion.

**hypersensitivity** *n* an abnormal or exaggerated immune response to an antigen, generally classified as type I, II, III or IV. Type I, or immediate-type, is caused by specific immunoglobulin E (IgE) against an allergen cross-linking Fc receptors on mast cells, causing the mast cell to degranulate and release inflammatory mediators including histamine. Type II hypersensitivity results from antibodies binding to antigens on cell surfaces. Type III reactions are due to the deposition of immune complexes in tissues. Type IV or delayed-type hypersensitivity reactions occur 24–72 hours later and are due to antigen-specific T cells and macrophages—**hypersensitive** *adj*.

**hypersplenism** *n* term used to describe depression of erythrocyte, granulocyte and platelet counts by an enlarged spleen.

**hypertelorism** *n* congenital defect resulting in increased interpupillary distance. May be associated with various genetic disorders.

**hypertension** *n* abnormally high tension, by custom abnormally high blood pressure involving systolic and/or diastolic levels. The consensus view is that hypertension is a systolic blood pressure above 140 mmHg and a diastolic blood pressure above 90 mmHg. Mild hypertension is considered to be systolic pressure between 140 and 159 mmHg and diastolic pressure between 90 and 99 mmHg. Hypertension is considered to be a risk factor for the development of cardiovascular disease. No cause is found in the majority of patients and this condition is termed essential hypertension. Secondary hypertension may result from coarctation of the aorta, renal artery stenosis, renal disease, phaeochromocytoma, Cushing's disease/syndrome, Conn's syndrome, various drugs, such as oral contraceptives, non-steroidal anti-inflammatory drugs (NSAIDs) and the pre-eclampsia of pregnancy. ⇒ hepatic portal hypertension, pulmonary hypertension—**hypertensive** *adj*.

**hyperthermia** *n* very high body core temperature caused by loss of thermoregulatory control. The hypothalamus in the brain malfunctions—**hyperthermic** *adj*. ⇒ hyperpyrexia, malignant hyperthermia.

**hyperthyroid crisis** ⇒ thyroid crisis.

**hyperthyroidism** *n* thyrotoxicosis. A condition due to excessive production of thyroid hormones (thyroxine, triiodothyronine), usually due to Graves' disease, but also multiple or solitary toxic nodules, and resulting classically in anxiety, tachycardia, sweating, increased appetite with weight loss, and a fine tremor of the outstretched hands; much commoner in women than men.

**hypertonia** *n* muscle tone that is too high to permit movement; increased contractility of muscle due to excessive and inappropriate excitation of the motor neuron pools of the anterior horn of the spinal cord setting the bias on the stretch reflex too low (easily triggered), causing the muscles to be more sensitive to stretch. There are two types:

spasticity and rigidity—**hypertonic** *adj*, **hypertonicity** *n*.

**hypertonic** *adj* **1.** pertaining to hypertonia. **2.** a fluid with a higher osmotic pressure relative to another fluid. *hypertonic saline* has a greater osmotic pressure than physiological fluid. ⇒ hyperosmolarity, hypotonic, isotonic.

**hypertrichosis** *n* excessive hairiness in a non-androgenic distribution.

**hypertrophic scar** an unsightly raised red scar showing continued activity and no maturation.

**hypertrophy** *n* increase in the size of tissues or structures, independent of natural growth. It may be congenital, compensatory, complementary or functional—**hypertrophic** *adj*.

**hyperuricaemia** *n* excessive uric acid in the blood. Characteristic of gout. ⇒ Lesch–Nyhan disease—**hyperuricaemic** *adj*.

**hyperuricuria** *n* also known as hyperuricosuria, uricosuria. Excessive amounts of uric acid and urates in the urine. Causes include problems with purine metabolism (e.g. in gout), high intake of purine and renal failure.

**hyperventilation** *n* overbreathing. Increased respiratory rate; may occur during anxiety attacks, in salicylate poisoning or head injury, or passively as part of a technique of general anaesthesia in intensive care. Also associated with alkalosis and tetany.

**hypervitaminosis** *n* any condition arising from an excessive intake of a vitamin. Can develop when large quantities of vitamin supplements are taken.

**hypervolaemia** *n* an increase in the volume of circulating blood.

**hyphaema** *n* blood in the anterior chamber of the eye. ⇒ haemophthalmia.

**hypnogogic stage** the stage between being awake and asleep. Images and hallucinations may occur.

**hypnopompic stage** the stage between being asleep and fully awake. Vivid images and hallucinations may occur.

**hypnosis** *n* a state resembling sleep, brought about by the hypnotist or the individual utilizing the mental mechanism of suggestion to produce a relaxed state and an improvement in well-being. Also used in symptom control or reduction, smoking cessation and forms of anaesthesia, as in skin suturing and pain relief such as in labour—**hypnotic** *adj*.

**hypnotherapy** *n* treatment that uses sleep-like state or hypnosis.

**hypnotic 1.** *n* a drug which produces a sleep similar to natural sleep. ⇒ narcotic. ⇒ Appendix 5. **2.** *adj* pertaining to hypnotism.

**hypoaesthesia** *n* diminished sensitiveness of a part—**hypoaesthetic** *adj.*

**hypobaric** *adj* lower pressure than normal atmospheric pressure.

**hypocalcaemia** *n* decreased calcium level in the blood. Causes include: disturbed kidney function, excess calcium excretion, deficiency of vitamin D, alkalosis and hypoparathyroidism. Leads to tingling in the hands and feet, and stridor and convulsions in children—**hypocalcaemic** *adj.* ⇒ carpopedal spasm, hyperventilation, tetany.

**hypocapnia** *n* reduced $CO_2$ tension in arterial blood; usually produced by hyperventilation—**hypocapnial** *adj.*

**hypochloraemia** *n* reduced chloride level in the blood. Leads to metabolic alkalosis as the acid–base balance is disrupted—**hypochloraemic** *adj.*

**hypochlorhydria** *n* decreased hydrochloric acid in the gastric juice—**hypochlorhydric** *adj.*

**hypochlorite** *n* salts of hypochlorous acid. They are easily decomposed to yield active chlorine, and are extensively used as disinfectants. ⇒ chlorine, sodium hypochlorite.

**hypochondria** *n* unnecessary anxiety about one's health—**hypochondriac, hypochondriacal** *adj*, **hypochondriasis** *n.*

**hypochondriacal disorder** an excessive preoccupation with the possibility of having serious health problems associated with refusal to accept professional reassurance that there is no physical illness underlying the symptoms. Symptoms are often of a bodily nature or concerned with physical appearance.

**hypochondrium** *n* the upper lateral region (left and right) of the abdomen (⇒ Appendix 1, Figure 18A)—**hypochondriac** *adj.*

**hypochromic** *adj* deficient in colouring or pigmentation. Of a red blood cell, having decreased haemoglobin.

**hypocretins** *npl* also known as orexins. Two excitatory neuropeptides which, with other substances, help to regulate sleep–wake cycles and appetite. It is normally produced in the hypothalamus. Low levels have been found in the cerebrospinal fluid of people with narcolepsy. ⇒ orexins.

**hypodermic** *adj* below the skin; subcutaneous—**hypodermically** *adv.*

**hypodermoclysis** *n* the infusion of fluids subcutaneously. Increasingly used to replace fluids and maintain adequate hydration in palliative care and older adults (Figure H.9).

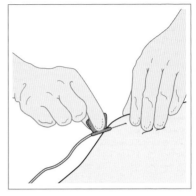

**Figure H.9** Hypodermoclysis—inserting the cannula *(reproduced from Nicol et al. 2004 with permission).*

**hypodontia** *n* congenital absence of some teeth.

**hypofibrinogenaemia** *n* reduced amount of fibrinogen in the blood. May be hereditary or acquired and may result in an increased tendency to bleed—**hypofibrinogenaemic** *adj.*

**hypofunction** *n* diminished performance.

**hypogammaglobulinaemia** *n* decreased gammaglobulin in the blood, occurring either congenitally or, more commonly, as a sporadic disease in adults. Lessens resistance to infection. ⇒ dysgammaglobulinaemia—**hypogammaglobulinaemic** *adj.*

**hypogastrium** *n* that area of the anterior abdomen which lies immediately below the umbilical region (⇒ Appendix 1, Figure 18A)—**hypogastric** *adj.*

**hypogeusia** *n* reduced sensation of taste.

**hypoglossal** *adj* under the tongue.

**hypoglossal nerve** the 12th pair of cranial nerves. They innervate tongue movements and are essential for swallowing and speech.

**hypoglycaemia** *n* decreased blood glucose, attended by anxiety, excitement, sweating, headache, change in personality, delirium or coma. Signs and symptoms vary markedly between individuals and can be mistakenly assumed to be due to another condition. Hypoglycaemia occurs most commonly in diabetes mellitus, when it is due to insulin overdosage, inadequate intake of carbohydrate or excess exercise—**hypoglycaemic** *adj.*

**hypoglycaemic drugs** oral drugs that reduce blood glucose in diabetes mellitus. ⇒ alpha (α)-glucosidases inhibitor, biguanides, glitazones, prandial glucose regulators, sulphonylureas. ⇒ Appendix 5.

**hypogonadism** *n* a condition associated with a deficiency of ovarian or testicular secretions. Often used to mean failure of testicular function.

**hypohidrosis** *n* diminished sweating. ⇒ anhidrosis.

**hypoinsulinism** *n* reduced production of insulin by the pancreatic cells.

**hypokalaemia** *n* abnormally low potassium level of the blood. Causes include: vomiting, gastrointestinal drainage, diarrhoea, starvation, excess renal loss in Cushing's syndrome or aldosteronism and with prolonged use of diuretics and other drugs. Leads to nausea, muscle weakness, arrhythmias and cardiac arrest—**hypokalaemic** *adj*.

**hypokinesia** *n* poverty of movement, including: inability to maintain repetitive movements or perform rapidly alternating movements (dysdiadochokinesis), lack of trunk rotation (e.g. no arm swinging), and loss of amplitude and range of movement (e.g. writing gets smaller).

**hypomagnesaemia** *n* decreased magnesium level in the blood—**hypomagnesaemic** *adj*.

**hypomania** *n* a less intense form of mania with persistent mild elevation of mood, overactivity, increased sociability, overfamiliarity, overtalkativeness, overspending, elevated libido and decreased need for sleep. Hallucinations and delusions are usually absent—**hypomanic** *adj*.

**hypomenorrhoea** *n* small amount of menstrual loss.

**hypometabolism** *n* decreased production of body heat. Characteristic of hypothyroidism.

**hypomobility** *n* decrease in the normal range of joint movement.

**hypomotility** *n* decreased movement, as of the gastrointestinal tract.

**hyponatraemia** *n* decreased sodium concentration in the blood due to a change in the proportion of sodium and water in the blood. It is caused by excess water in the body or a failure to excrete water. In severe cases it leads to cerebral oedema with convulsions and changes in conscious level—**hyponatraemic** *adj*.

**hypo-osmolarity** *n* (*syn* hypotonicity) a solution exerting a lower osmotic pressure than another is said to have a hypo-osmolarity with reference to it. In medicine the comparison is usually made with normal plasma.

**hypoparathyroidism** *n* underactivity of the parathyroid glands resulting in decreased serum calcium levels, producing tetany.

**hypopharynx** *n* that portion of the pharynx lying below and behind the larynx, correctly called the laryngopharynx.

**hypophonia** *n* a weak voice with decreased phonation, which results in whispering. Also known as leptophonia.

**hypophoria** *n* ⇒ phoria.

**hypophosphataemia** *n* decreased phosphate level in the blood—**hypophosphataemic** *adj*.

**hypophysectomy** *n* surgical removal of the pituitary gland.

**hypophysis cerebri** ⇒ pituitary gland—**hypophyseal** *adj*.

**hypopigmentation** *n* decreased pigmentation. ⇒ albinism.

**hypopituitarism** *n* pituitary gland insufficiency, especially of the anterior lobe hormones. When the secretion of all the anterior lobe hormones is decreased it is described as panhypopituitarism or Simmonds' disease. Absence of gonadotrophins leads to failure of ovulation, uterine atrophy and amenorrhoea in women and loss of libido, pubic and axillary hair in both sexes. Lack of growth hormone in children results in short stature and a type of dwarfism. Lack of adrenocorticotrophic hormone (ACTH) and thyrotrophin (thyroid-stimulating hormone [TSH]) may result in lack of energy, pallor, fine dry skin, cold intolerance and sometimes hypoglycaemia. Usually due to tumour of or involving the pituitary gland or hypothalamus but in other cases cause is unknown. Occasionally due to postpartum infarction of the pituitary gland, when it is known as Sheehan's syndrome. ⇒ Sheehan's.

**hypoplasia** *n* defective development of any tissue—**hypoplastic** *adj*.

**hypopnoea** *n* abnormal slow and shallow breathing. ⇒ obstructive sleep apnoea (hypopnoea) syndrome.

**hypopraxia** *n* diminished activity.

**hypoproteinaemia** *n* deficient protein in blood plasma, from dietary deficiency, reduced production or excessive excretion (albuminuria)—**hypoproteinaemic** *adj*.

**hypopyon** *n* a collection of pus in the anterior chamber of the eye.

**hyposecretion** *n* deficient secretion.

**hyposensitivity** *n* lacking sensitivity to a stimulus.

**hyposmia** *n* decrease in the normal sensitivity to smell.

**H**

**hypospadias** *n* a congenital malformation of the male urethra. Subdivided into two types: (a) penile, when the terminal urethral orifice opens at any point along the ventral surface of the penis; and (b) perineal, when the orifice opens on the perineum and may give rise to problems of sexual differentiation. ⇒ epispadias.

**hypostasis** *n* **1.** congestion of blood in a part due to impaired circulation. **2.** a sediment— **hypostatic** *adj.*

**hypotension** *n* low blood pressure that is insufficient for adequate tissue perfusion and oxygenation; may be primary or secondary (e.g. reduced cardiac output, hypovolaemic shock, Addison's disease) or postural—**hypotensive** *adj.*

**hypothalamus** *n* literally, below the thalamus. It consists of an area of grey matter in the brain just above the pituitary gland. It has both endocrine and neural functions. The hypothalamus produces the hormones oxytocin and antidiuretic hormone (vasopressin or arginine vasopressin [AVP]); these are stored in the posterior pituitary prior to release. It is the major centre for the autonomic nervous system and controls physiological functions that include thirst and hunger, circadian rhythms and emotions such as anger—**hypothalamic** *adj.* ⇒ limbic system.

**hypothenar eminence** the eminence on the ulnar side of the palm below the little finger.

**hypothermia** *n* core body temperature below 35°C. It is ascertained by a low-reading thermometer. Occurs particularly at the extremes of age, in hypothyroidism and people exposed to cold environmental conditions such as rough sleepers. An artificially induced hypothermia can be used in the treatment of head injuries and during cardiac surgery. It reduces the oxygen consumption of the tissues and thereby allows greater and more prolonged interference of normal blood circulation. *hypothermia of the newborn* failure of the newborn child to adjust to external cold; may be associated with infection.

**hypothesis** *n* a declaration that can be tested by statistical (inferential) tests. It is a prediction based on the relationship between the dependent and independent variables.

**hypothetico-deductive method** theories are examined and hypotheses for testing are derived in a deductive manner. The particular research study tests the hypotheses by data analysis that either supports or repudiates the original theory.

**hypothyroidism** *n* conditions caused by low circulating levels of one or both thyroid hormones (thyroxine, triiodothyronine). Much more common in women than men and may be: (a) associated with goitre, such as autoimmune thyroiditis, lack of iodine or as a drug side-effect, e.g. with lithium; (b) due to spontaneous atrophy; or (c) after surgical treatment for hyperthyroidism. Some individuals have a subclinical form and in others it may be transient. It results in decreased metabolic rate and may be characterized by some of the following: fatigue, bradycardia, angina, hypertension, aches and pains, carpal tunnel syndrome, low temperature and cold intolerance, weight gain, constipation, hair and skin changes (dry coarse skin), puffy face, anaemia, hoarseness, slow speech, menorrhagia and depression. Treatment is with replacement thyroxine. *congenital hypothyroidism* can be detected (by routine blood testing) soon after birth and treated successfully with thyroxine. Untreated, it leads to impaired mental and physical development. It is recognized by the presence of coarse facies and protruding tongue. The term cretinism was previously used.

**hypotonia** *n* muscle tone that is too low to maintain posture or permit movement against gravity; loss of contractility of muscle due to disturbance of the cerebellum or links between it and other centres in the brain, causing the bias on the stretch reflex to be too high and the muscles to be less sensitive to stretch. ⇒ pendular response—**hypotonicity** *n.*

**hypotonic** *adj* **1.** pertaining to hypotonia. **2.** a fluid with a lower osmotic pressure relative to another fluid. *hypotonic saline* has a lower osmotic pressure than normal physiological fluid. ⇒ hypertonic, hypo-osmolarity, isotonic.

**hypotony** *n* decreased intraocular pressure.

**hypoventilation** *n* diminished breathing or underventilation.

**hypovitaminosis** *n* any condition due to lack of vitamins. For example, lack of vitamin C leading to scurvy.

**hypovolaemia** *n* reduced volume of blood in the circulation—**hypovolaemic** *adj.*

**hypoxaemia** *n* reduced oxygen in arterial blood, shown by decreased $PaO_2$ and reduced oxygen saturation—**hypoxaemic** *adj.*

**hypoxia** *n* reduced oxygen level in the tissues. *anaemic hypoxia* due to inadequate amounts of haemoglobin available to carry oxygen. *histotoxic hypoxia* due to inability of cells to use oxygen, e.g. due to poisoning. *hypoxic hypoxia* due to low oxygen tension in arterial blood.

*stagnant hypoxia* due to insufficient blood flow to deliver oxygen.

**hysterectomy** *n* surgical removal of the uterus. *abdominal hysterectomy* effected via a lower abdominal incision. *laparoscopic-assisted vaginal hysterectomy (LAVH)* a combined approach to vaginal removal of the uterus in which some of the surgical procedure is performed laparoscopically. *subtotal hysterectomy* removal of the uterine body, leaving the cervix in the vaginal vault. *total hysterectomy* complete removal of the uterine body and cervix. *vaginal hysterectomy* carried out through the vagina. *Wertheim's hysterectomy* ⇒ Wertheim's hysterectomy.

**hysteria** *n* **1.** a state of excitement with temporary loss of emotional control. **2.** the term previously used for conversion disorder—**hysterical** *adj*.

**hysterosalpingectomy** *n* excision of the uterus and uterine (fallopian) tube(s).

**hysterosalpingography** *n* ⇒ uterosalpingography.

**hysterosalpingo-oophorectomy** *n* surgical removal of the uterus and one or both uterine tubes and ovaries.

**hysterosalpingosonography** *n* an examination of the uterus and uterine (fallopian) tubes using ultrasound.

**hysterosalpingostomy** *n* anastomosis between a uterine (fallopian) tube and the uterus.

**hysteroscope** *n* an endoscope used to view the cervical canal and uterine cavity.

**hysteroscopy** *n* the passage of a small-diameter endoscope through the cervix to visualize the uterine cavity. Used to obtain tissue for examination, remove polyps, or for treatments such as removal or transcervical resection of endometrium.

**hysterotomy** *n* incision of the uterus to remove a pregnancy. The word is usually reserved for a method of abortion.

**hysterotrachelorraphy** *n* repair of a lacerated cervix uteri.

H

# I

**IABP** *abbr* intra-aortic balloon pump.

**IADL** *abbr* instrumental activities of daily living.

**iatrogenic** *adj* describes a secondary condition arising from treatment of a primary condition.

**I band** the light area visible on electron microscopy in muscle myofibrils when the actin and myosin filaments overlap.

**IBD** *abbr* inflammatory bowel disease.

**IBS** *abbr* irritable bowel syndrome.

**IC** *abbr* inspiratory capacity.

**ICD** *abbr* International Classification of Diseases.

**ICE** *acron* (**i**ce, **c**ompression, **e**levation) a first-aid measure used for swelling and bruising of the limbs. An ice compress is applied to the injury and the limb is elevated to assist venous return. ⇒ RICE.

**ICF** *abbr* **1.** *International Classification of Functioning, Disability and Health*. **2.** intracellular fluid.

**ichthyoses** *npl* a group of usually congenital conditions in which the skin is scaly and feels dry. Fish skin. Xeroderma.

**ICP** *abbr* **1.** integrated care pathway. **2.** intracranial pressure.

**ICSH** *abbr* interstitial cell-stimulating hormone.

**ICSI** *abbr* intracytoplasmic sperm injection (transfer).

**icterus** *n* ⇒ jaundice. *icterus gravis* acute diffuse necrosis of the liver. *icterus gravis neonatorum* one of the clinical forms of haemolytic disease of the newborn. *icterus neonatorum* excess of the normal, or physiological, jaundice occurring in the first week of life as a result of excessive destruction of haemoglobin. ⇒ phototherapy. *icterus index* measurement of concentration of bilirubin in the plasma. Used in diagnosis of jaundice.

**ICU** *abbr* intensive care unit. ⇒ intensive therapy unit.

**id** *n* one of the three main aspects of the personality (the others being the ego and superego): that part of the unconscious mind that comprises a system of biologically determined urges (instincts). It aspires to the immediate fulfilment of all desires and needs. According to Freud, it persists unrecognized into adult life. ⇒ ego, superego.

**IDDM** *abbr* insulin-dependent diabetes mellitus. ⇒ diabetes mellitus type 1.

**idea** *n* a concept or plan of something to be aimed at, created or discovered. *idea of reference* incorrect interpretation of casual incidents and external events as having direct reference to oneself. If of a sufficient intensity may lead to the formation of delusions.

**ideation** *n* the highest function of awareness, process by which ideas are imagined, conceived and formed. It includes intellect, thought and memory.

**identical twins** two offspring of the same sex, derived from a single fertilized ovum. ⇒ monozygotic, uniovular.

**identification** *n* recognition. **1.** in psychology, the way in which personality is formed by modelling it on a chosen person, e.g. identification with the same-sex parent—helping to form one's sex role; identification with a person of own sex such as a footballer or singer in the hero worship of adolescence. **2.** a mental defence mechanism where individuals take on the characteristics of the admired role model figure.

**ideomotor** *adj* pertaining to the motor activity that results from an idea. *ideomotor apraxia* the inability to convert an idea into the action required.

**idiopathic** *adj* of a condition, of unknown or spontaneous origin, e.g. some forms of epilepsy.

**idiopathic thrombocytopenic purpura (ITP)** a syndrome characterized by a low platelet count caused by the presence of autoantibodies. This results in purpura and intermittent bleeding from mucosal surfaces. In children it may appear following a virus infection. The onset in adults tends to be more insidious. Treatment in adults usually involves corticosteroids, with splenectomy in patients who fail to respond.

**idiosyncrasy** *n* a peculiar variation of constitution or temperament. It may relate to an unusual response to a particular protein, drug or food.

**IE** *abbr* infective endocarditis.

**IFG** *abbr* impaired fasting glucose/glycaemia.

**IFN** *abbr* interferon.

**Ig** *abbr* ⇒ immunoglobulin.

**IGF** *abbr* insulin-like growth factors.

**IGT** *abbr* impaired glucose tolerance.

**IHD** *abbr* ischaemic heart disease.

**IL** *abbr* interleukin.

**ileal bladder** ⇒ ileoureterostomy.

**ileal conduit** ⇒ ileoureterostomy.

**ileal pouch** ⇒ ileostomy.

**ileectomy** *n* surgical procedure to remove the ileum.

**ileitis** *n* inflammation of the ileum, such as that caused by Crohn's disease.

**ileoanal reservoir** a two-stage surgical procedure that avoids a permanent ileostomy when it is necessary to remove the colon and rectum (proctocolectomy), for instance in a person with familial polyposis coli. The colon and rectum are removed at the first operation, a temporary ileostomy is formed and a pouch or reservoir is fashioned from the distal small intestine, and this is anastomosed to the anus. Once the ileoanal anastomosis has had time to heal a second operation is performed, during which the ileostomy is reversed to re-establish bowel continuity. This allows the person to pass faeces from the anus.

**ileocaecal** *adj* pertaining to the ileum and the caecum. *ileocaecal valve* the sphincter muscle that controls the rate at which the chyme (contents of the small intestine) enters the caecum (first part of large bowel), and prevents flow in the opposite direction. The valve opens in response to peristalsis in the small intestine and the presence of chyme. It also opens during colonic peristalsis that occurs as part of the gastrocolic reflex.

**ileocolic** *adj* pertaining to the ileum and the colon.

**ileocolitis** *n* inflammation of the ileum and the colon.

**ileocolostomy** *n* a surgically made fistula between the ileum and the colon, usually the transverse colon. Most often used to bypass an obstruction or inflammation in the caecum or ascending colon.

**ileocystoplasty** *n* operation to increase the size of the urinary bladder—**ileocystoplastic** *adj*.

**ileorectal** *adj* pertaining to the ileum and the rectum.

**ileosigmoidostomy** *n* an anastomosis between the ileum and sigmoid colon.

**ileostomy** *n* a surgically made fistula between the ileum and the anterior abdominal wall; a type of stoma discharging liquid faecal matter. Usually permanent when the whole of the large bowel has to be removed, e.g. in severe ulcerative colitis. ⇒ ileoanal reservoir. Special stoma bags are used to collect the liquid discharge from an ileostomy. *continent ileostomy* for some patients it may be possible to fashion an internal pouch/reservoir from the small intestine. A valve is constructed and a stoma brought out through the abdominal wall. Patients are able to use a tube to empty the pouch/reservoir at intervals instead of wearing an external stoma bag.

**ileoureterostomy** *n* (*syn* ureteroileostomy) transplantation of the lower ends of the ureters from the urinary bladder to an isolated loop of small bowel (ileal bladder) which, in turn, is made to open on the abdominal wall (ileal conduit).

**ileum** *n* the lower three-fifths of the small intestine, lying between the jejunum and the ileocaecal valve leading into the caecum. Concerned with the absorption of various nutrients such as vitamin $B_{12}$—**ileal** *adj*.

**ileus** *n* intestinal obstruction. Usually restricted to paralytic as opposed to mechanical obstruction and characterized by abdominal distension, vomiting and the absence of pain. ⇒ meconium.

**iliac** *adj* pertaining to the ilium.

**iliac arteries** *npl* two large arteries, the right and left common iliac, formed when the abdominal aorta divides. They in turn divide into external and internal iliac arteries, which carry arterial blood to the legs and pelvic organs respectively. ⇒ Appendix 1, Figure 9.

**iliac region/fossa** the abdominal region situated either side of the hypogastrium. ⇒ Appendix 1, Figure 18A.

**iliacus** *n* ⇒ iliopsoas muscle.

**iliac veins** the internal iliac veins drain venous blood from the pelvic organs and the external iliac veins carry venous blood from the legs. The internal and external iliac veins unite to form the right and left common iliac veins, which unite to form the inferior vena cava. ⇒ Appendix 1, Figure 10.

**iliococcygeal** *adj* pertaining to the ilium and coccyx.

**iliofemoral** *adj* pertaining to the ilium and the femur, such as the iliofemoral ligament between the ilium and the top of the femur.

**iliopectineal** *adj* pertaining to the ilium and the pubis. *iliopectineal line* bony ridge on the internal surface of the ilium and pubic bones. It is the dividing line between the true and false pelvis.

**iliopsoas** *adj* pertaining to the ilium and the loin. *iliopsoas muscle* comprises two other muscles, the iliacus and psoas major. They insert via a common tendon on to the lesser trochanter of the femur. Act to flex the hip and the lumbar spine.

**ilium** *n* the upper part of the innominate (hip) bone; it is a separate bone in the fetus—**iliac** *adj*.

**Ilizarov frame** (G Ilizarov, Soviet orthopaedic surgeon, 1921–1992) external fixation device

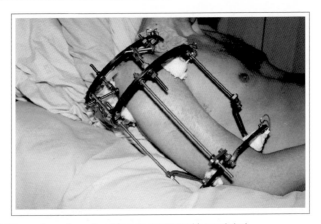

**Figure I.1** Ilizarov frame *(reproduced from Porter 2005 with permission).*

used commonly in the management of fractures and for the correction of skeletal deformities (Figure I.1).

**illusion** *n* a misidentification of existing stimuli, e.g. of sight, a bush or tree being mistaken for a person, the bush being misrepresented in consciousness as a figure. It is a relatively 'normal' phenomenon.

**image** *n* **1.** a revived experience of a percept recalled from memory. **2.** the optical reproduction of an object formed on the retina as light is focused through the eye.

**imagery** *n* imagination. The recall of mental images of various types depending upon the specific sensory organs involved when the images were formed, e.g. smell (olfactory), sound (auditory), sight (visual), touch (tactile). *guided imagery* a technique used as part of a range of coping strategies for pain and other symptom control or anxiety in which patients are asked to imagine a particular situation, feeling or state.

**imaging techniques** diagnostic techniques used to investigate the condition and functioning of organs and structures. They include radiographic examination, radioisotope (radionuclide) scans, ultrasonography, computed tomography, magnetic resonance, positron emission tomography, single-photon emission computed tomography.

**imago** *n* in psychoanalysis, the unconscious, often idealized image of an important/significant person, such as a parent, in the formative time during the patient's childhood.

**imbalance** *n* want of balance. Term refers commonly to the upset of acid–base relationship and the electrolytes in body fluids, or lack of balance in opposing muscle groups.

**immersion foot** ⇒ trench foot.

**immobilization** *n* **1.** a lengthy period of inactivity of a person. **2.** fixation to make a normally mobile part immobile. This includes the use of braces, splints, plaster casts, external and internal fixation of fractures or other conditions. Or surgical techniques to fix a structure permanently.

**immune** *adj* protected against infection by specific or non-specific mechanisms of the immune system. Altered reactivity against an antigen, caused by previous exposure to that antigen. ⇒ defence mechanisms.

**immune response** the specific adaptive responses of the immune system to a perceived threat, either from non-self antigens, or from self antigens during a pathological immune response. This may be against micro-organisms, malignant cells, and damaged or healthy tissues. The response may be humoral, in which the B lymphocytes produce antibodies against specific antigens, or it may be cell-mediated, where T lymphocytes act in a variety of ways to counter the threat. ⇒ immunity.

**immune system** the diverse cells, tissues and organs that protect the body from micro-organisms, foreign cells and abnormal body cells. They include the lymphatic system of vessels, fluid and lymph nodes, lymphoid tissue, the spleen, the mucosal-associated lymphoid tissue, the bone marrow, thymus and the B and T lymphocytes.

**immunity** *n* an intrinsic or acquired state of immune responsiveness to an antigen. *active immunity* is acquired, naturally during an infection or artificially by immunization. It involves the production of antibodies and specific T cells in response to exposure to an antigenic stimulus. The primary response to exposure is followed by a 2–3-week lag phase before enough antibodies are produced, but the secondary response following a subsequent exposure is more intense and has a much reduced lag phase because the memory cells are able to produce antibodies very quickly. This type of immunity tends to be of long duration. *cell-mediated immunity* T-lymphocyte-dependent responses which cause graft rejection, immunity to some infectious agents and tumour rejection. *humoral immunity* from immunoglobulins (antibodies) produced by plasma cells derived from B lymphocytes. Immunity can be innate (from inherited qualities), or it can be acquired, actively or passively, naturally or artificially. *passive immunity* is acquired, naturally when maternal antibodies pass to the fetus via the placenta or after birth in colostrum and breast milk, or artificially by administering immunoglobulins (usually human in origin). This type of immunity tends to be short-lived because the immune response is not stimulated to produce specific antibodies.

**immunization** *n* artificial means by which immunity is initiated or augmented. Achieved by using vaccines containing attenuated micro-organisms or inactive micro-organisms or bacterial products such as toxins. Antibody production (active immunity) occurs and is generally long-lasting. In certain situations, such as during an epidemic, the injection of immunoglobulins obtained from immune humans, or very rarely sera from animals, can give temporary protection (passive immunization). *immunization programme* a routine programme of immunization offered during childhood and to special groups such as health care workers and those travelling abroad.

**immunocompromised patients** (*syn* immunosuppressed patients) patients with defective immune responses, which can be inherited or acquired. Often produced by treatment with cytotoxic drugs or irradiation. Also occurs in some patients with cancer and other diseases affecting the lymphoid system. Depending on

the immune defect, different patterns of infection result. Patients with cellular defects are likely to develop infections with opportunistic organisms such as *Candida*, *Pneumocystis jirovecii* (former name *P. carinii*) and *Cryptococcus neoformans*. Patients with antibody defects are more liable to infections with encapsulated bacteria, such as pneumococcus.

**immunocytochemistry** *n* staining cells with specific antibodies for diagnostic purposes.

**immunodeficiency** *n* the state of having defective immune responses, leading to increased susceptibility to infectious diseases. The problem may be with humoral immune responses, where antibody production is abnormal or cell-mediated responses involving T lymphocytes are deficient.

**immunodeficiency diseases** inherited or acquired disorders of the immune system. They may involve B cells or T cells or both. ⇒ severe combined immunodeficiency.

**immunofluorescence** *n* a procedure used for the identification of an antigen. The antigen is mixed with known antibodies which have been coated with fluorescein (a fluorescent dye) and then checked for precipitation (an antigen–antibody reaction). This is confirmed by the presence of precipitate that is luminous when observed in ultraviolet light from a fluorescent microscope.

**immunogenicity** *n* the ability to produce immunity.

**immunoglobulins (Igs)** *npl* (*syn* antibodies) high-molecular-weight glycoproteins produced by plasma cells (derived from B lymphocytes) in response to specific antigens. The basic structure of immunoglobulins is Y-shaped, consisting of two identical heavy chains, each linked to two identical light chains. Immunoglobulins are found in the blood and other body fluids where they form part of body defences. Immunoglobulins function in a variety of ways, but all involve combining with the antigen to form an immune complex. There are five classes of immunoglobulins, IgG, IgA, IgD, IgM and IgE, each with different characteristics, functions and locations.

**immunohistochemistry** *n* staining tissue with specific antibodies for diagnostic purposes.

**immunological response** ⇒ immune response, immunity.

**immunology** *n* the study of the immune system of lymphocytes, inflammatory cells and associated cells and proteins, which affect an individual's response to antigens—**immuno-logical** *adj*, **immunologically** *adv*.

**immunomodulators** *npl* substances which change the immune response either by augmenting or decreasing part of the response. They include both naturally occurring substances, such as cytokines, and substances used therapeutically, e.g. cytotoxic drugs, corticosteroids and drugs such as infliximab used in rheumatoid arthritis.

**immunopathology** *n* the study of disease involving the immune system.

**immunosuppressant drugs** drugs given to suppress the immune responses, e.g. azathioprine, ciclosporin, tacrolimus. ⇒ Appendix 5.

**immunosuppressed patients** ⇒ immunocompromised patients.

**immunosuppression** *n* treatment which reduces immunological responsiveness.

**immunosuppressive** **1.** *n* that which reduces immunological responsiveness. **2.** *adj* describes an agent such as a drug that suppresses immune system function.

**immunotherapy** *n* can be used to mean desensitization therapy against specific allergens, e.g. insect venom, or can refer to therapeutics which use agonists or antagonists based on immune system components, e.g. treatment based on biological modifiers such as interleukin-2 and lymphokine-activated killer cells. ⇒ immunomodulators.

**impacted** *adj* firmly wedged, abnormal immobility, as of hard constipated faeces in the colon and rectum; fracture such as some types affecting the femoral neck; a fetus in the pelvis; a tooth in its socket or a calculus in a duct. ⇒ fracture.

**impaired fasting glucose/glycaemia (IFG)** fasting plasma glucose levels between 6.1 and 7 mmol/L indicative of a prediabetic state. However, if measured, the 2-hour postglucose load result is less than 7.8 mmol/L .

**impaired glucose tolerance (IGT)** fasting plasma glucose level less than 7 mmol/L. However, plasma levels between 7.8 and 11.0 mmol/L 2 hours after a glucose load are indicative of a prediabetic state and confer a significantly increased risk of cardiovascular disease.

**impalpable** *adj* not palpable; incapable of being felt by touch (palpation).

**imperforate** *adj* lacking a normal opening. *imperforate anus* a congenital absence of an opening into the rectum.

**imperforate hymen** a fold of mucous membrane at the vaginal entrance which has no natural outlet for the menstrual fluid. Rectified by a simple surgical operation. ⇒ cryptomenorrhoea, haematocolpos.

**impetigo** *n* an inflammatory, pustular skin disease usually caused by *Staphylococcus*, occasionally by *Streptococcus*. *impetigo contagiosa* a highly contagious form of impetigo, commonest on the face and scalp, characterized by vesicles which become pustules and then honey-coloured crusts. ⇒ ecthyma—**impetiginous** *adj*.

**implant** *n* any drug, structure or substance inserted surgically into the human body, e.g. implants of progestogens for contraception, or implants used in plastic surgery. Those used to augment tissue contour may be of two types: *alloplastic* synthetic foreign-body implants such as those used in breast reconstruction, or *autologous implants* tissue obtained from the same patient. *dental implant* artificial structure implanted surgically into the alveolar bone, usually made from titanium. It is used as a postorthodontic abutment.

**implantable defibrillator** an implanted device to sense the heart rhythm. Delivers a small electric shock when ventricular tachycardia or ventricular fibrillation is detected. ⇒ automatic implantable cardioverter defibrillator, sudden adult/arrhythmic death syndrome.

**implantation** *n* **1.** the insertion of living cells or solid materials into the tissues, e.g. accidental implantation of cancer cells in a wound. **2.** insertion of a prosthesis into the body such as a pacemaker, breast implant or artificial joint components. **3.** insertion of radioactive material such as iridium-192 ($^{192}$Ir) to treat cancers, or solid drugs that are released over a period of time. **4.** implantation or embedding of the fertilized ovum into the hormone-prepared endometrium or decidua. It occurs around 6–8 days following fertilization when the blastocyst becomes embedded within the decidua. The process, which is also known as nidation, is normally complete around 11 days following ovulation.

**impotence** *n* an outdated term, but still used by the public to describe an inability to participate in sexual intercourse, by custom referring to the male. ⇒ erectile dysfunction, premature ejaculation.

**impregnate** *v* fill; saturate; render pregnant.

**impression** *n* in dentistry or prosthetics, a negative likeness or imprint of teeth, dental arch or other body structures to use when producing a replacement part or prosthesis, such as a denture.

**imprinting** *n* very early learning occurring at a critical developmental stage that results in a newborn becoming attached to a model, usually a parent, but may be a carer.

**impulse** *n* **1.** a sudden inclination, sometimes irresistible urge to act without deliberation. **2.** the electrochemical process involved in neurotransmission of information and stimuli throughout the body. ⇒ nerve impulse.

**IMRT** *abbr* intensity-modulated radiotherapy.

**inanition** *n* a state of starvation characterized by complete exhaustion with wasting. It is caused by total lack of, or inability to assimilate, food.

**inappetence** *n* usually described as having no appetite.

**incarcerated** *adj* describes the abnormal imprisonment of a part, as in a hernia which is irreducible or a pregnant uterus held beneath the sacral promontory.

**incentive spirometry** a method of increasing lung expansion by use of a volumetric or simple flow device. The device provides visual feedback about the level of attainment and whether the agreed target has been met. Incentive spirometry encourages a prolonged and maximal inspiration and increases inflation of the alveoli.

**incest** *n* sexual intercourse between close blood relatives, usually meaning those who are prohibited by law to marry. The most common type of sexual abuse occurs between father and daughter; other types of incest, such as between siblings, also occur. ⇒ abuse.

**incidence** *n* the number of times that an event happens. In epidemiology, the rate of new cases of a disease that occur in a population over a defined time period (usually a year). For example, the number of new cases of a specific cancer or an infectious disease. ⇒ prevalence.

**incipient** *adj* initial, beginning, in its early stages.

**incised wound** one which results from cutting with a sharp knife or scalpel: heals by primary intention in the absence of complications such as infection.

**incision** *n* the result of cutting into body tissue, using a sharp instrument—**incisional** *adj*, **incise** *vt*.

**incisor tooth** tooth with a cutting edge (see Figure T.4B, p. 482), placed first and second from the midline in both dental arches and in both the primary and secondary dentition.

**inclusion bodies** microscopic particles found in the nucleus or cytoplasm of some cells of pathological and normal tissues.

**inclusion conjunctivitis** conjunctivitis caused by the micro-organism *Chlamydia trachomatis*. Also called trachoma inclusion conjunctivitis (TRIC). ⇒ trachoma.

**incompatibility** *n* **1.** refers to the bloods of donor and recipient in transfusion, when antigenic differences in the red cells result in reactions such as haemolysis or agglutination. Or the differences between the donor and recipient tissue types that causes transplanted tissues/organs to be rejected by the recipient's immune system. **2.** When two or more medicaments are given concurrently or consecutively they can attenuate or counteract the desired effect of each.

**incompetence** *n* inadequacy to perform a natural function, e.g. mitral valve regurgitation—**incompetent** *adj*.

**incomplete abortion** ⇒ miscarriage.

**incomplete fracture** ⇒ fracture.

**incontinence** *n* inability to control the evacuation of urine or faeces. **1.** There are various types of urinary incontinence. *functional incontinence* with an erratic pattern of involuntary urinary incontinence. Caused by an impairment of physical or mental ability. It may be associated with cognitive problems, impaired mobility, sensory deficits and with an altered environment. *neurogenic, neurological incontinence* reflex incontinence occurs when the nerve supply to the bladder has been damaged by disease or injury, for example by multiple sclerosis, diabetes mellitus, surgery or spinal injuries. The presentation varies with the cause but may include an atonic or hypotonic bladder with overflow, reflex emptying of the full bladder or urge incontinence. ⇒ neurogenic bladder. *urge incontinence* (overactive bladder, detrusor instability) is caused by detrusor (bladder muscle) instability with unpredictable bladder contraction leading to urgency, frequency and involuntary leakage of urine on the way to the lavatory. It is the commonest cause of incontinence in older people. More common in females, because of the changes following childbirth, but also caused by having a weaker pelvic floor and a shorter urethra. May also occur in neurological conditions. *overflow incontinence* leaking or dribbling of urine from an overfull bladder. It occurs when there is an outflow obstruction such as with benign enlargement of the prostate gland in older men. *stress incontinence* occurs when the intra-abdominal pressure is raised, as in coughing, giggling, laughing, sneezing and during physical exertion; there is usually some weakness of the urethral sphincter muscle coupled with anatomical stretching and displacement of the bladder neck. Stress incontinence generally affects women and is caused by bladder neck displacement due to a weakening of the pelvic floor, which follows childbirth, uterine prolapse and the climacteric. Men may have stress incontinence following prostate surgery. *mixed incontinence* a combination of urge and stress incontinence which is common in postmenopausal women. **2.** faecal incontinence may involve involuntary defecation, lack of awareness of an urge to defecate or faecal soiling. It is commonly due to constipation with faecal impaction and leakage of liquid faeces, but may be caused by rectal prolapse, damage to the anal sphincter, neurological problems such as stroke or multiple sclerosis, episodes of infective diarrhoea, drugs causing diarrhoea and inflammatory bowel diseases. ⇒ encopresis, enuresis.

**inco-ordination** *n* inability to produce smooth, harmonious muscular movements.

**incubation** *n* **1.** the period from entry of infection to the appearance of the first symptom. ⇒ latent period. **2.** the process of development, of an egg, of a bacterial culture.

**incubator** *n* **1.** an apparatus with controlled temperature and oxygen concentration used for preterm or sick babies. **2.** a low-temperature oven in which bacteria are cultured.

**incus** *n* anvil-shaped bone of the middle ear. One of the ossicles, it transmits sound vibrations between the malleus and stapes. (⇒ Appendix 1, Figure 13). ⇒ malleus, stapes.

**indexing term** also called Medical Subject Headings (MESH or MeSH), thesaurus terms, subject headings or descriptors. The word assigned by a database producer to describe the content of a journal article. They are split into subject area and arranged in a hierarchy that moves from a broad subject area to increasing detail and specialism. ⇒ Allied and Complementary Medicine Database (AMED), biographical databases, Cumulative Index to Nursing and Allied Health Literature (CINAHL), MEDLINE.

**Indian hemp** ⇒ cannabis.

**indican** *n* the chemical formed in the intestine from the breakdown of the amino acid tryptophan.

**indicanuria** *n* excess indican in the urine, associated with increased bacterial breakdown of tryptophan (an amino acid) in the bowel or with a high protein intake. ⇒ indole.

**indication** *n* a substantial reason for prescribing a certain course of treatment, for instance surgery, medications or another therapy.

**indicator** *n* a substance used to make visible the completion of a chemical reaction or the achievement of a certain pH.

**indigenous** *adj* of a disease, etc., native to a certain locality or country.

**indigestion** *n* (*syn* dyspepsia) a feeling of gastric discomfort, including fullness and gaseous distension, which is not necessarily a manifestation of disease.

**indirect cost** a cost that cannot be attributed to any one department and its budget. It is shared between various budgets, e.g. the cost of heating a building.

**indole** *n* a product of the decomposition of the amino acid tryptophan in the intestines: it is excreted in urine as indican. ⇒ indicanuria.

**indolent** *adj* a term applied to a sluggish ulcer which is generally painless and slow to heal.

**induced abortion** ⇒ abortion.

**induction** *n* the act of bringing on or causing to occur, as applied to anaesthesia and labour.

**induration** *n* the hardening of tissue, as in hyperaemia, infiltration by tumour, etc.— **indurated** *adj*.

**industrial dermatitis** ⇒ dermatitis.

**industrial disease** (*syn* occupational disease) a disease contracted by reason of occupational exposure to an industrial agent known to be hazardous, e.g. dust, fumes, chemicals, irradiation, etc., the notification of, safety precautions against and compensation for which are controlled by law.

**industrial therapy** simulation of outside industrial working conditions within a psychiatric hospital. The main purpose is preparation for patient return to the community by occupational rehabilitation.

**inequalities in health** differences in the distribution of health associated with social class or poverty (as opposed to physiological processes: age, sex, constitution). A considerable body of evidence shows a clear relationship between poor health and deprivation (measured by income, level of education and type of employment or unemployment). Measures of inequality include differences in standardized mortality ratios, life expectancy, infant and maternal mortality rates. Low-income individuals are more likely to die prematurely, suffer acute and chronic illnesses and experience long-term disability.

**inertia** *n* inactivity. ⇒ uterine inertia.

**inevitable abortion** ⇒ miscarriage.

**in extremis** at the point of death.

**infant** *n* a child of less than 1 year old.

**infanticide** *n* the killing of an infant, by its mother, in the first 12 months after the birth.

**infantile cortical hyperostosis (Caffey's disease)** a condition characterized by tender swellings of bone. Diagnosed radiographically.

**infantile spasms** a form of epilepsy that usually commences in the first year of life. It may be idiopathic or follow a variety of conditions that include hypoxia at birth, meningitis and hypoglycaemia. There is generally a poor prognosis with learning disability, physical problems or death.

**infantilism** *n* child-like behaviour or physical characteristics that persist into adulthood.

**infant mortality/death** the death of an infant under the age of 12 months. The *infant mortality/death rate* is the number of deaths of infants aged under 1 year per 1000 live births in a specific area in a given time. Infant mortality is divided into neonatal deaths occurring in the first 28 days of life and postneonatal deaths. In developed countries most deaths occur in the first 28 days. Infant mortality rates are used as a measure of poverty and deprivation.

**infarct** *n* the localized area of tissue affected by anoxia caused when the end artery supplying it is occluded by atheroma, thrombosis or embolism, e.g. in myocardium or lung.

**infarction** *n* irreversible premature tissue death. Necrosis (death) of a section of tissue because the blood supply has been cut off. ⇒ myocardial infarction, pulmonary infarction.

**infection** *n* the successful invasion, establishment and growth of micro-organisms on the body surfaces or in the tissues of the host, which result in a tissue reaction. It may be acute or chronic—**infectious** *adj*. *autoinfection* infection resulting from commensals becoming pathogenic, or when commensals or pathogens are transferred from one part of the body to another, for example by the hands. *cross-infection* occurs when pathogens are transferred from one person to another. *hospital-acquired (nosocomial) infection (HAI)* one which occurs in a patient who has been in hospital for at least 72 h and did not have signs and symptoms of such infection on admission: around 8% of patients in acute hospitals develop a health care-associated infection. Common sites include the urinary tract, gastrointestinal tract, surgical wounds, respiratory tract and the blood stream. *opportunistic infection* a serious infection with a micro-organism which normally has little or no pathogenic activity but causes disease where host resistance is reduced by a serious disease, invasive treatments or drugs. ⇒ health care-associated infection.

**infectious disease** a disease caused by a specific pathogenic micro-organism and capable of transmission to another individual by direct or indirect contact.

**infectious mononucleosis** (*syn* glandular fever) a contagious self-limiting disease caused by the Epstein–Barr virus (EBV). It mainly affects teenagers and young adults and is characterized by tiredness, headache, fever, sore throat, lymphadenopathy, splenomegaly and appearance of atypical lymphocytes resembling monocytes. Specific antibodies to EBV are present in the blood, as well as an abnormal antibody that forms the basis of the Paul–Bunnell test, which confirms a diagnosis of infectious mononucleosis.

**infective** *adj* infectious. Disease transmissible from one host to another. *infective hepatitis* ⇒ hepatitis.

**infective endocarditis (IE)** previously known as acute, subacute or chronic bacterial endocarditis. Microbial infection affecting the heart lining or the heart valves. It is usually bacterial in origin, e.g. caused by *Staphylococcus aureus*, *S. epidermidis*, *Streptococcus faecalis* and *S. viridans*. Rarely the causative organism is *Rickettsia*, *Chlamydia* or a fungus. IE may occur in people who have a diseased heart valve, after valve replacement, with congenital heart problems, patients with a central line or an intravenous cannula in place and people who inject illegal drugs. Infection from other parts of the body may also travel in the blood stream to affect the endocardium. Vegetations, comprising platelets, fibrin and micro-organisms form on the heart valve or on the endocardium. These may break off and travel in the circulation as emboli to the brain and other sites.

**inferential statistics** also known as inductive statistics. That which uses the observations of a sample to make a prediction about other samples, i.e. makes generalizations from the sample. ⇒ descriptive statistics.

**inferior** *adj* lower; beneath.

**inferiority complex** feelings of being inadequate or inferior to other people. It may be unconscious but still influences behaviour. Individuals may act defensively or can compensate by displaying aggressive extrovert behaviour.

**infertility** *n* lack of ability to reproduce. Psychological and physical causes play their part. The problem can be with either or both partners. Specialist services exist for diagnosis, treatment and counselling. ⇒ assisted conception.

**infestation** *n* the presence of animal parasites such as lice, threadworms or blood flukes such as *Schistosoma haematobium*—**infest** *vt*.

**infibulation** *n* ⇒ circumcision.

**infiltration** *n* the entry into cells, tissues or organs of abnormal substances or cells, e.g. cancer cells, fat. Penetration of the surrounding tissues; the oozing or leaking of fluid into the tissues. *infiltration anaesthesia* analgesia produced by infiltrating the tissues with a local anaesthetic.

**inflammation** *n* a non-specific local defence mechanism initiated by tissue injury. The injury may be caused by trauma, micro-organisms, extremes of temperature and pH, ultraviolet (UV) radiation or ionizing radiation. It is characterized by the cardinal signs of heat (calor), redness (rubor), swelling (tumor), pain (dolor) and often with loss of function. Inflammation is one of the stages of wound healing. ⇒ calor, dolor, inflammatory response, rubor, tumor.

**inflammatory bowel disease (IBD)** idiopathic intestinal inflammation. Commonly due to ulcerative colitis and Crohn's disease, but may also be lymphocytic and collagenous colitis. ⇒ Crohn's disease, ulcerative colitis.

**inflammatory response** in acute inflammation it is the non-specific reaction of the immune system to protect the body against harmful substances or physical agents. It is one of the stages of wound healing. The inflammatory response leads to the tissue changes of inflammation, caused by inflammatory chemical mediators—vasodilation, vascular changes whereby blood flow increases, vessel wall permeability increases with the exudation of fluid from the vessel into the tissue spaces, production of exudate, white blood cell migration into the injured area for phagocytosis of micro-organisms and debris. ⇒ inflammation. *inflammatory chemical mediators* chemicals released from blood cells and tissues that trigger many of the events of the inflammatory response. They include prostaglandins, histamine and kinins.

**influenza** *n* a highly contagious acute viral infection of the nasopharynx and respiratory tract that occurs in epidemics or pandemics. The virus is spread by airborne droplets. There are three main strains of the virus—A, B and C—which all belong to the Orthomyxoviridae, a family of RNA viruses. Influenza is characterized by the sudden onset of cough, headache, anorexia, myalgia and extreme lethargy and fatigue. Antiviral drugs, e.g. oseltamivir and zanamivir, are used for prophylaxis and treatment of influenza, and shorten the duration of symptoms. Complications such as pneumonia may lead to death, especially in the very young, older adults and individuals with chronic diseases, including diabetes, heart and respiratory disease. An annual vaccination programme offers protection to older people (65 years and over); those with chronic conditions of the respiratory system, the heart, kidneys, diabetes and other debilitating conditions; people living in care/nursing homes; and health care workers and carers. Because the influenza virus changes (antigenic drift) over time a new vaccine is required each year—**influenzal** *adj*.

**informal patient** a patient admitted to hospital without any statutory requirements. ⇒ detained patient.

**informatics** *n* information management and technology (IM&T). Information is needed to ensure the effective running of any organization. Data are pieces of material which, when compiled effectively, form information. Information is managed in a number of different ways but increasingly it is managed using technological means (information technology [IT]). Non-technological means may be more appropriate for the target group/recipient. For example, telephone calls and notice boards are all ways in which information might be managed.

**informed choice** in order to make decisions about their own care and management, clients/patients need information from health care professionals. This means the provision of accurate, appropriate information about the person's condition, and about the treatment options available. Health care professionals may disagree with the patient/client's decisions, but the latter takes precedence where an adult patient is deemed to be mentally competent.

**informed consent** in the UK consent forms must include a signed declaration by the doctor or other health care professional that he or she has explained the nature and purpose of the operation or treatment to the patient or parent in non-technical terms. Any questions that the patient may have after signing the form should be referred to the doctor or other health professional who is to carry out the treatment. ⇒ consent.

**infrared rays** invisible, long-wavelength rays of the electromagnetic spectrum.

**infundibulum** *n* any funnel-shaped passage, e.g. the ends of the uterine (fallopian) tubes (⇒ Appendix 1, Figure 17)—**infundibula** *pl*, **infundibular** *adj*.

**infusion** *n* **1.** fluid flowing into the body intravenously, subcutaneously or rectally. **2.** an aqueous solution containing the active principle of a drug.

**ingestion** *n* **1.** taking food or drugs into the stomach. **2.** the means by which a phagocytic cell takes in material such as microorganisms.

**Ingram regimen** a treatment for psoriasis using dithranol paste, tar baths and ultraviolet B radiation.

**ingrowing toenail** ⇒ onychocryptosis.

**inguinal** *adj* pertaining to the groin. *inguinal hernia* ⇒ hernia.

**inguinal canal** a tubular opening through the lower part of the anterior abdominal wall, parallel to and a little above the inguinal (Poupart's) ligament. In the male it contains the spermatic cord; in the female it contains the uterine round ligaments.

**inguinal ligament** Poupart's ligament (F Poupart, French physician, 1616–1708)—a fibrous band running from the pubic bone to the anterior superior iliac spine. It is formed from the aponeurosis of the external oblique abdominal muscle.

**inhalation** *n* **1.** the breathing in of air, or other vapour, etc. **2.** a medicinal substance which is inhaled, such as an inhalation anaesthetic or in the aerosols used for asthma treatment.

**inherent** *adj* innate; inborn.

**inhibin** *n* a protein hormone that inhibits the release of follicle-stimulating hormone.

**inhibition** *n* **1.** in physiology, the reduction of a physiological activity such as hormone secretion, or restraining the action of a cell, tissue or organ. **2.** in chemistry, the slowing or cessation of a chemical reaction. **3.** in psychology, the unconscious restraint of impulses or behaviour as a result of social and cultural influences. **4.** in psychology, the action of the superego to prevent the person expressing the unconscious system of biologically determined instinctive drives and urges of the id.

**injected** *adj* congested, with full vessels.

**injection** *n* **1.** the act of introducing a fluid (under pressure) into the tissues (e.g. intradermal, intramuscularly, subcutaneously), a vessel (e.g. intra-arterial, intravenous), cavity or hollow organ (epidural, intra-articular, intra-osseous, intraperitoneal, intrapleural, intrathecal). **2.** the substance injected.

**injury scoring/severity scale (ISS)** a system used to grade the severity of injuries sustained. Used during triage and to predict the outcome following particular traumas.

**inlay** *n* in dentistry, a restoration made from cast gold or porcelain to fit a prepared cavity, into which it is then cemented.

**innate** *adj* inborn, dependent on genetic make-up.

**inner ear** also called internal ear. That part of the ear which comprises the vestibule, semicircular canals and the cochlea.

**innervation** *n* the nerve supply to a part.

**innocent** *adj* benign; not malignant.

**innominate** *adj* unnamed. Applied to the hip bone formed from the ilium, ischium and pubis. Also the innominate artery and vein. ⇒ hip bone, brachiocephalic (artery and vein).

**inoculation** *n* **1.** the injection of substances, especially vaccine, into the body. **2.** introduction of micro-organisms into culture medium for propagation.

**inorganic** *adj* neither vegetable nor animal in origin. A compound generally containing no carbon or hydrogen.

**inosine monophosphate** a purine nucleotide.

**inositol** *n* a carbohydrate constituent of phospholipids (phosphatidyl inositols). Important in cell membrane structure and in the signalling mechanism for some hormones.

**inositol triphosphate (IP$_3$)** acts with other substances as a 'second messenger' molecule in cells.

**inotropes** *npl* substances, such as drugs, that have an effect on myocardial contractility. Those that decrease contractility are termed negative inotropes. ⇒ beta (β)-adrenoceptor antagonists, calcium channel blockers (antagonists), whereas those that increase contractility are positive inotropes. ⇒ beta (β)-adrenoceptor agonists, glycosides. ⇒ Appendix 5.

**inotropic** *adj* affecting the force of muscle contraction, applied particularly to cardiac muscle.

**inquest** *n* in England and Wales, a legal inquiry by a coroner into the cause of sudden or unexpected death.

**insecticide** *n* an agent which kills insects—**insecticidal** *adj*.

**insemination** *n* introduction of semen into the vagina, normally by sexual intercourse. *artificial insemination* instrumental injection of semen into the vagina. Using donor semen (AID), or semen from the woman's husband or partner (AIH).

**insensible** *adj* without sensation or consciousness. Too tiny or gradual to be noticed. Such as *insensible water loss (perspiration)*, the fluid lost from the body through the skin and during respiration. ⇒ sensible perspiration.

**insertion** *n* **1.** the act of setting or placing in. **2.** the attachment of a muscle to the bone it moves.

**insidious** *adj* having an imperceptible commencement, as of a disease with a late manifestation of definite symptoms.

**insight** *n* ability to accept one's limitations while continuing to develop personally. In psychiatry means: (a) knowing that one is ill; (b) a developing knowledge of one's present attitudes and past experiences and the connection between them.

**in situ** in the normal position, undisturbed.

**insomnia** *n* sleeplessness. A chronic inability to get to sleep, or to stay asleep, or early waking.

**inspiration** *n* inhalation; breathing in—**inspiratory** *adj*, **inspire** *vt*.

**inspiratory capacity (IC)** the maximum volume of air inspired following a normal expiration.

**inspissated** *adj* thickened, as by evaporation or withdrawal of water, applied to sputum and culture media used in the laboratory.

**instep** *n* the arch of the foot on the dorsal surface.

**instillation** *n* insertion of drops into a cavity, e.g. conjunctival sac.

**instinct** *n* an inborn tendency to act in a certain way in a given situation, e.g. *maternal, paternal instinct* to protect children—**instinctive** *adj*, **instinctively** *adv*.

**institutionalization** *n* a condition of apathy resulting from lack of motivation characterizing patients and staff in institutions who have been subjected to a rigid regimen with deprivation of choice and decision-making.

**instrumental activities of daily living (IADL)** include activities such as child care and shopping.

**insufflation** *n* the blowing of air along a tube (pharyngotympanic, uterine) to establish patency. The blowing of powder into a body cavity.

**insula** *n* part of each cerebral hemisphere situated deep within the lateral sulcus.

**insulin** *n* a polypeptide hormone produced by the beta cells of the pancreas. Insulin secretion is regulated by the blood glucose level and it opposes the action of glucagon. It has an effect on the metabolism of carbohydrate, protein and fat by stimulating the transport of glucose into cells. An absolute or relative lack of insulin results in hyperglycaemia, a high blood glucose with decreased utilization of carbohydrate and increased breakdown of fat and protein—a condition known as diabetes mellitus. Three types of insulin are available commercially: bovine insulin, porcine insulin and human insulin, produced using recombinant DNA techniques. Insulin is produced in a single strength, i.e. 100 units per mL, a standardization replacing the previous 20, 40 and 80 unit strengths. ⇒ Appendix 5.

**insulinase** *n* an enzyme that inactivates insulin.

**insulin-dependent diabetes mellitus (IDDM)** ⇒ diabetes mellitus type 1.

**insulin delivery devices** preloaded insulin pens, reusable insulin pens and insulin dosers used by people to inject insulin as an alternative to syringe and needle (Figure I.2).

**insulin-like growth factor (IGF)** also called somatomedin. Two polypeptides, IGF-1 (somatomedin C) and IGF-2 (somatomedin A), similar in structure to insulin. They are involved in early fetal growth and later cell growth and development.

**insulinoma** *n* an insulin-secreting tumour of the pancreatic islet beta cells, usually benign. It causes hypoglycaemia. ⇒ islet cell tumours.

**insulin resistance** an alteration in the functioning of insulin-sensitive peripheral tissues. The body tissues do not respond to available insulin effectively and the pancreas produces more insulin. This results in hyperinsulinaemia (high level of insulin in the blood) and increased blood glucose, which often leads to type 2 diabetes.

**insulin tolerance/stress test** used to assess the hypothalamic–pituitary–adrenal axis and growth hormone deficiency. Intravenous soluble insulin is administered to produce hypoglycaemia (blood glucose <2.2 mmol/L) and serial blood samples are taken to measure glucose, growth hormone and cortisol levels.

**integrated care pathway (ICP)** the multidisciplinary outline of anticipated care, placed in an appropriate timeframe, designed so that patients with a specific condition or pattern

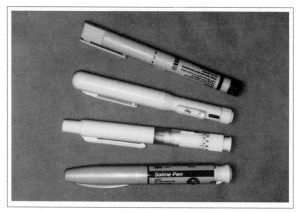

**Figure I.2** Insulin delivery devices—preloaded pens *(reproduced from Brooker & Nicol 2003 with permission).*

of symptoms can move progressively through a clinical experience to a positive outcome.

**integrated medicine** a term used to describe a harmonious integration of particular complementary therapies within conventional medical or other health care practice, where team work and effective therapies (both allopathic and complementary) function together to promote health and well-being.

**integument** *n* a covering, especially the skin.

**intellect** *n* the ability and power of the mind for reasoning, thinking, understanding and knowing, as contrasted with the willing and feeling faculty.

**intellectualization** *n* a mental defence mechanism whereby people attempt to detach themselves from painful emotions or difficult situations by dealing with the issues in an abstract, intellectual manner.

**intelligence** *n* inborn mental ability.

**intelligence quotient (IQ)** the ratio of mental age to chronological (actual) age.

**intelligence tests** various standardized tests designed to determine the level of intelligence. ⇒ Binet test, Stanford Binet Intelligence Scale, Wechsler Intelligence Scales.

**intensity-modulated radiotherapy (IMRT)** the use of a computer system to optimize the radiation delivery technique by evaluating millions of possible beam arrangements to create a clinically optimized treatment plan.

**intensive therapy unit (ITU)** a unit with augmented levels of specialist staff and equipment in which highly specialized monitoring, resuscitation and therapeutic techniques are used to support critically ill patients with actual or impending organ failure, particularly those needing mechanical ventilation. Also called intensive care unit. ⇒ high-dependency unit.

**intention** *n* ⇒ wound healing

**intention-to-treat analysis** ⇒ analysis by intention to treat.

**intention tremor** ⇒ tremor.

**interaction** *n* when two or more things or people have a reciprocal influence on each other. ⇒ drug interaction.

**interarticular** *adj* between joints.

**interatrial** *adj* between the two atria of the heart.

**intercalated** *adj* describes structures inserted between other structures. For example, the intercalated discs between the cardiac muscle cells, which link adjacent cells to form a sheet of muscle with no clear boundaries between cells, thereby allowing the wave of contraction to pass easily across the myocardium, as it behaves like a single unit or syncytium.

**intercellular** *adj* between cells.

**intercostal** *adj* between the ribs. *intercostal muscles* (internal and external) the secondary muscles of respiration situated between the ribs.

**intercourse** *n* **1.** human communication. **2.** coitus.

**intercurrent** *adj* describes a second disease arising in a person already suffering from one disease.

**interdental** *adj* between the teeth.

**interference** *n* a psychological term that describes the contest between pieces of information that may prevent learning and retrieval from long-term memory. It occurs when different pieces of information are linked to the same clue needed for retrieval.

**interferons (IFNs)** *npl* protein mediators that enhance cellular resistance to viruses. They are involved in the modulation of the immune response. Therapeutic use of interferon has caused regression of some cancers and is used in the management of some types of multiple sclerosis.

**interleukins (ILs)** *npl* large group of signalling molecules (cytokines). They are non-specific immune chemicals produced by various cells, such as macrophages. Interleukins are also involved as growth factors in the regulation of haemopoiesis. For example, interleukin-3 (IL-3) is a growth factor for myeloid and platelet precursors in the bone marrow.

**interlobar** *adj* between the lobes.

**interlobular** *adj* between the lobules.

**intermediate care** care provided after primary care and self-care, but before, instead of care or after that level of care available inside acute hospitals. Intermediate care includes preadmission assessment units, fast response specialist teams at home, multidisciplinary community assessment, rehabilitation and treatment teams, early and supported discharge schemes and community hospitals.

**intermenstrual** *adj* between the menstrual periods.

**intermittency** *n* during voiding the flow of urine 'stops and starts'—it is not continuous. May be associated with lower urinary tract pathology.

**intermittent** *adj* occurring at intervals.

**intermittent claudication** ⇒ claudication.

**intermittent peritoneal dialysis** ⇒ dialysis.

**intermittent pneumatic compression** a stocking worn to prevent deep-vein thrombosis of upper and lower limb. ⇒ phlebothrombosis.

**intermittent positive-pressure ventilation (IPPV)** ventilation of the lungs by the intermittent application of gas under positive pressure to the airway. Used for the artificial maintenance of breathing during general anaesthesia and for critically ill patients. Synonymous with artificial, assisted, controlled and mechanical ventilation.

**intermittent self-catheterization (ISC)** the intermittent insertion of a catheter, by the person or carer, to drain urine from the bladder. The procedure is clean rather than one that uses aseptic technique and the catheter is removed once the bladder is empty. It is used by people who are unable to empty their bladder completely, including those with spina bifida or multiple sclerosis, or following damage to the spinal cord. ⇒ self-catheterization.

**internal** *adj* inside. *internal ear* ⇒ inner ear. *internal respiration* ⇒ respiration. *internal secretions* those produced by the endocrine glands; hormones. *internal version* ⇒ version.

**internal (medial) rotation** a limb or body movement where there is rotation towards the vertical axis of the body.

***International Classification of Diseases (ICD)*** list of disease categories produced by the World Health Organization.

***International Classification of Functioning, Disability and Health (ICF)*** used worldwide to classify disability and health. It is the basis for defining, measuring and planning services for health and disability.

**International System of Units (SI)** ⇒ Système International d'Unités, Appendix 2.

**interneuron** *n* connecting neurons in the central nervous system. For example, those in the spinal cord that connect sensory and motor neurons in a reflex arc.

**interosseous** *adj* between bones.

**interpersonal skills** the skills and capabilities required to engage with people in meaningful and appropriate communication.

**interphalangeal** *adj* between the phalanges.

**interphase** *n* in cytology, the phase between two mitotic divisions during which the cell prepares for mitosis whilst performing its normal metabolic activities.

**interpretive approach** a research approach that incorporates the meaning and significance individuals attach to situations and behaviour. May be used in social science research.

**interprofessional** *adj* intense teamwork among practitioners from different health care professions focused on a common problem-solving purpose and requiring recognition of the core expertise and core knowledge of each profession and blending of common core skills to enable the team to act as an integrated whole. ⇒ multiprofessional.

**interprofessional education (IPE)** shared (or common) learning of common (or generic) core skills among students and qualified practitioners of different health care professions that fosters respect for each other's core knowledge and expertise, capitalizes on professional differences and cultivates integrated teamwork to solve patients' problems.

**interserosal** *adj* between serous membrane, as in the pleural, peritoneal and pericardial cavities—**interserosally** *adv*.

**intersexuality** *n* the possession of both male and female characteristics.

**interspinous** *adj* between spinous processes, especially those of the vertebrae.

**interstices** *npl* small spaces.

**interstitial** *adj* situated in the interstices of a part; distributed through the connective structures.

**interstitial cells** also called Leydig cells. Testicular cells that secrete androgen hormones, e.g. testosterone, when stimulated by interstitial cell-stimulating hormone.

**interstitial cell-stimulating hormone (ICSH)** (*syn* luteinizing hormone) a hormone released from the anterior lobe of the pituitary gland; causes production of testosterone in the male.

**interstitial fluid (tissue fluid)** the extracellular fluid situated in the spaces around cells.

**interstitial radiotherapy** therapy achieved by radioactive sources inserted into the tumour.

**intertrigo** *n* superficial inflammation occurring in moist skin folds, such as under the breasts—**intertriginous** *adj*.

**intertrochanteric** *adj* between trochanters such as those on the proximal femur.

**interval cancer** one that is discovered in the time interval between screening episodes, such as breast cancer detected between mammography examinations.

**interval data** measurement data with a numerical value, e.g. temperature, that has an arbitrary zero. The intervals between successive values are the same, e.g. a $1°$ increase from 38 to 39 is exactly the same as one from 39 to 40. $\Rightarrow$ ratio data.

**interval training** a type of training which increases aerobic endurance capacity by the use of repeating bouts of exercise with specific rest periods for recovery.

**interventional radiology** in radiology, the use of imaging techniques to facilitate therapeutic interventions, such as stent insertion to reopen a blood vessel or hollow structure, radiofrequency ablation or embolization by inserting coils into an aneurysm.

**interventricular** *adj* between ventricles, as those of the brain or heart.

**intervertebral** *adj* between the vertebrae, as discs and foramina. $\Rightarrow$ nucleus pulposus, prolapse.

**intestinal failure** failure of the intestine to absorb adequate fluid and nutrients to sustain metabolic needs due to disease or resection. $\Rightarrow$ parenteral nutrition.

**intestinal obstruction** usually refers to a mechanical obstruction that prevents progress of the intestinal contents along the lumen of the intestine. The obstruction can be in the small or large intestine (colon). Causes include strangulated hernia, adhesions, intussusception, volvulus, stenosis caused by inflammatory bowel disease, foreign body, severe impaction of faeces, bowel cancers or cancers outside the bowel. Paralytic ileus also prevents contents moving through the bowel, but in this case there is no mechanical blockage. Obstruction of the small intestine is characterized by vomiting and severe abdominal pain, whereas obstruction in the colon tends to present with less pain, failure to pass faeces and flatus with abdominal distension. However, symptoms depend on the location of the blockage.

**intestine** *n* the part of the alimentary canal extending from the first part of the small intestine, the duodenum, to the anus ($\Rightarrow$ Appendix 1, Figure 18B). Consists of the small and large intestine (bowel)—**intestinal** *adj*.

**intima** *n* the internal coat of a blood vessel—**intimal** *adj*.

**intolerance** *n* the manifestation of various unusual reactions to particular substances such as nutrients or medications.

**intoxication** *n* the condition of being poisoned by a toxic substance, including the inebriation associated with an excess intake of alcohol.

**intra-abdominal** *adj* inside the abdomen.

**intra-amniotic** *adj* within or into the amniotic fluid.

**intra-aortic** *adj* within the aorta.

**intra-aortic balloon pump (IABP)** a counterpulsation device inserted into the aorta. It is used to increase cardiac output in ventricular failure that may follow myocardial infarction or shock.

**intra-arterial** *adj* within an artery—**intra-arterially** *adv*.

**intra-articular** *adj* within a joint.

**intrabronchial** *adj* within a bronchus.

**intracameral** *adj* within a cavity, such as local anaesthetic drugs or antibiotics injected in the cavities of the eye.

**intracanalicular** *adj* within a canaliculus.

**intracapillary** *adj* within a capillary.

**intracapsular** *adj* within a capsule, e.g. that of the lens or a joint. ⇒ extracapsular *opp.*

**intracardiac** *adj* within the heart.

**intracaval** *adj* within the vena cava—**intracavally** *adv.*

**intracellular** *adj* within cells.

**intracellular fluid (ICF)** that fluid inside the cells. In an adult with an ideal weight of 70 kg there will be around 28 L of ICF. ⇒ extracellular *opp.*

**intracerebral** *adj* within the cerebrum, such as a haemorrhage.

**intracranial** *adj* within the skull.

**intracranial pressure (ICP)** the pressure inside the cranial cavity. It is maintained at a normal level by brain tissue, intracellular and extracellular fluid, cerebrospinal fluid and blood. A change in any of these compartments can increase the pressure, e.g. after brain injury. ⇒ raised intracranial pressure.

**intracutaneous** *adj* within the skin tissues—**intracutaneously** *adv.*

**intracytoplasmic sperm injection (ICSI)** a technique used in assisted conception where a single sperm is injected into an oocyte to achieve conception. ⇒ microsurgical epididymal sperm aspiration (MESA).

**intradermal** *adj* within the skin—**intradermally** *adv.*

**intradural** *adj* inside the dura mater.

**intragastric** *adj* within the stomach.

**intragluteal** *adj* within the gluteal muscle of the buttock—**intragluteally** *adv.*

**intrahepatic** *adj* within the liver.

**intralobular** *adj* within the lobule, e.g. vessels draining a hepatic lobule.

**intraluminal** *adj* within the lumen of a hollow tube-like structure—**intraluminally** *adv.*

**intralymphatic** *adj* within a lymphatic node or vessel.

**intramedullary** *adj* within the bone marrow.

**intramural** *adj* within the wall of a hollow tube or organ—**intramurally** *adv.*

**intramuscular** *adj* within a muscle—**intramuscularly** *adv.*

**intranasal** *adj* within the nasal cavity—**intranasally** *adv.*

**intranatal** *adj* ⇒ intrapartum—**intranatally** *adv.*

**intraocular** *adj* within the globe of the eye. *intraocular pressure* (IOP) the pressure inside the eye, normally between 10 and 21 mmHg. It is regulated by the constant production of aqueous humour and its drainage through the trabecular meshwork and into the scleral venous sinus (canal of Schlemm), to be returned to the venous circulation. ⇒ glaucoma.

**intraocular lens implant** an artificial lens is inserted into the eye following cataract surgery.

**intraoral** *adj* within the mouth, such as an intraoral appliance—**intraorally** *adv.*

**intraorbital** *adj* within the orbit.

**intraosseous** *adj* inside a bone.

**intraosseous route** a route for giving fluids and drugs when rapid establishment of vascular access is vital and it is not possible to gain venous access. It provides an alternative route for the administration of drugs and fluids until venous access can be achieved. The intraosseous route can safely be used to administer any intravenous drug or fluid required during a paediatric resuscitation. The onset of action and drug levels are comparable to those achieved when drugs are given intravenously. During paediatric advanced life support it is recommended that intraosseous access should be established if reliable venous access cannot be achieved within 3 attempts or 90 seconds, whichever comes first. A wide-bore needle is inserted into the medullary cavity of a long bone, such as the flat anteromedial surface of the tibia in children under 6 years of age. In children under 6 years of age the marrow cavity is very large and there is less risk of injury to adjacent tissues. The main contraindication to this route is a fracture of the pelvis, or the extremity proximal to or of the chosen site.

**intrapartum** *adj* (*syn* intranatal) at the time of birth; during labour, as asphyxia, or infection.

**intrapartum haemorrhage** that occurring during labour.

**intraperitoneal** *adj* within the peritoneal cavity—**intraperitoneally** *adv.*

**intrapharyngeal** *adj* within the pharynx—**intrapharyngeally** *adv.*

**intraplacental** *adj* within the placenta—**intraplacentally** *adv.*

**intrapleural** *adj* within the pleural cavity—**intrapleurally** *adv.*

**intrapulmonary** *adj* within the lungs, as in intrapulmonary pressure.

**intrapunitive** *adj* self-blaming.

**intraretinal** *adj* within the retina.

**intraspinal** *adj* within the spinal canal—**intraspinally** *adv.*

**intrasplenic** *adj* within the spleen.

**intrasynovial** *adj* within a synovial membrane or cavity—**intrasynovially** *adv*.

**intrathecal** *adj* within the meninges; into the subarachnoid space. A route used for the administration of certain drugs, such as some chemotherapy —**intrathecally** *adv*.

**intrathoracic** *adj* within the cavity of the thorax, such as pressures.

**intratracheal** *adj* within the trachea—**intratracheally** *adv*.

**intrauterine** *adj* within the uterus.

**intrauterine contraceptive device (IUCD, IUD)** a device which is inserted in the cavity of the uterus to prevent conception. Its exact mode of action is not known. Some IUCDs contain a copper component, which increases their effectiveness. These can also be used for emergency contraception up to 5 days after unprotected intercourse. Other IUCDs contain the hormone progesterone and these are also used, in some cases, to manage menorrhagia or provide the progesterone component of hormone replacement therapy.

**intrauterine growth restriction/retardation (IUGR)** the impairment of fetal growth rate commonly arising due to placental insufficiency.

**intrauterine insemination (IUI)** an assisted conception technique in which prepared spermatozoa are introduced into the uterine cavity around the time of ovulation. It may be used if the man has a low sperm count, or in cases where there is an incompatibility with the woman's cervical mucus or the presence of antibodies against sperm.

**intravaginal** *adj* within the vagina—**intravaginally** *adv*.

**intravascular** *adj* within the blood vessels—**intravascularly** *adv*.

**intravenous (IV)** *adj* within or into a vein—**intravenously** *adv*. *intravenous infusion (IVI)* commonly referred to as a 'drip': the closed administration of fluids from a containing vessel into a vein for such purposes as hydrating the body, correcting electrolyte imbalance or introducing nutrients. *intravenous injection* the introduction of drugs, including anaesthetics, into a vein.

**intravenous immunoglobulin (IVIG)** immunoglobulin, mainly IgG, produced from the pooled donations of thousands of individuals, used as replacement therapy for patients with antibody deficiencies, or in higher doses as immunomodulatory therapy for a range of inflammatory and immune-mediated disorders.

**intravenous urogram (IVU)** a radiographic investigation of the urinary tract, formerly known as intravenous pyelogram. ⇒ urography.

**intraventricular** *adj* within a ventricle, especially a cerebral ventricle.

**intrinsic** *adj* inherent or inside; from within; real; natural.

**intrinsic factor** a protein released by gastric parietal cells, essential for the satisfactory absorption of vitamin $B_{12}$ (the extrinsic factor) in the ileum.

**intrinsic sugars** sugars found in the cell walls of foods originating from plants.

**introitus** *n* any opening in the body; an entrance to a cavity, particularly the vagina.

**introjection** *n* the unconscious incorporation of external ideas into one's mind.

**intron** *n* a sequence of non-coding DNA situated between the exons. ⇒ exon.

**inulin** *n* a soluble but undigested non-starch polysaccharide present in root vegetables. It is a fructose polymer. Because it is filtered by the kidney but neither reabsorbed nor secreted by the nephron, it can be used in a clearance test to assess the glomerular filtration rate. ⇒ clearance, creatinine.

**introspection** *n* study of one's own mental processes. May be associated in an exaggerated form in schizophrenia and other serious mental health disorders.

**introversion** *n* **1.** thoughts and interests are directed inwards to the world of ideas, instead of outwards to the external world. **2.** a situation where a hollow structure turns in on itself (invaginates).

**introvert** *n* a person whose interests and behaviour patterns are directed inwards to the self. ⇒ extrovert *opp*.

**intubation** *n* placing of a tube into a hollow organ. Tracheal intubation is used during anaesthesia. ⇒ endotracheal tube. *duodenal intubation* a double-lumen tube is passed as far as the pyloric antrum under fluoroscopy. The inner tube is then passed along to the duodenojejunal flexure.

**intussusception** *n* a condition in which one part of the bowel invaginates (telescopes) into the adjoining distal segment of bowel (Figure I.3). It causes severe colic, vomiting and the passage of blood and mucus rectally ('redcurrant jelly' stools) and intestinal obstruction. It occurs most commonly in

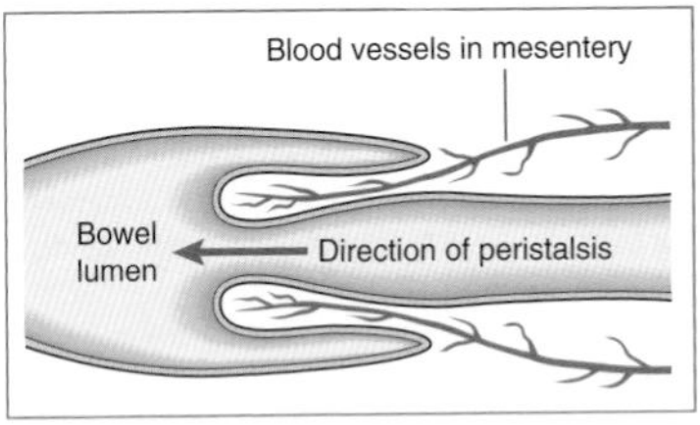

**Figure I.3** Intussusception *(reproduced from Brooker 2006A with permission).*

infants around the time of weaning. It presents as an acute condition and requires emergency treatment. The intussusception is usually reduced hydrostatically using a barium enema, but surgical intervention is sometimes required.

**intussusceptum** *n* the invaginated portion of an intussusception.

**intussuscipiens** *n* the receiving portion of an intussusception.

**inunction** *n* **1.** a drug in an oily base which is rubbed into the skin to be absorbed. **2.** the act of rubbing such an agent into the skin.

**invagination** *n* the act or condition of being ensheathed; a pushing inward, forming a pouch—**invaginate** *vt.*

**invasion** *n* the entry of bacteria into the body or the spread of cancer cells.

**inversion** *n* **1.** turning inside out, as inversion of the uterus. This can occur if the third stage of labour is mismanaged. **2.** a mutation caused by a segment of chromosome breaking off and reattaching to the chromosome in an inverted position. ⇒ procidentia.

**invert sugar** glucose and fructose mixture produced by hydrolysis of sucrose. It is sweeter than sucrose. So called because the process inverts the optical rotation.

**invertase** *n* sucrase, the enzyme that converts sucrose to glucose and fructose.

**in vitro** in glass, as in a test tube.

**in vitro fertilization (IVF)** an assisted conception technique offered by clinics licensed to undertake the technique. Human oocytes are collected following hormone stimulation and are fertilized by spermatozoa in the laboratory. Not all oocytes will fertilize but after a period of incubation a specified number of early embryos are introduced into the uterine cavity where hopefully they will implant into the hormone-primed endometrium. The oocytes and spermatozoa may be those of the couple concerned, or either or both may come from donors. ⇒ Human Fertilization and Embryology Authority (HFEA).

**in vivo** in living tissue.

**involucrum** *n* a sheath of new bone, which forms around necrosed bone, in conditions such as osteomyelitis. ⇒ cloaca.

**involuntary** *adj* independent of the will, such as muscle of the thoracic and abdominal organs.

**involution** *n* the normal shrinkage of an organ after completing its function, e.g. uterus after labour. Or the progressive decline occurring after midlife when tissues and organs reduce in size and functional ability declines. ⇒ subinvolution—**involutional** *adj.*

**iodine (I)** *n* an element required for the formation of thyroid hormones (triiodothyronine [$T_3$], thyroxine [$T_4$]). Oral iodine may be prescribed preoperatively for patients with hyperthyroidism to control the release of thyroid hormones and reduce vascularity of the gland. Radioactive isotopes of iodine, e.g. iodine-131 ($^{131}$I), are used in the diagnosis and treatment of thyroid conditions, such as cancer. Iodine is bactericidal and is used as povidone-iodine for skin disinfection prior to invasive procedures. It is used within several proprietary wound dressings.

**iodism** *n* poisoning by iodine or iodides; presentation is similar to a common cold and the appearance of a rash.

**ion** *n* an atom or radical with an electrical charge—**ionic** *adj.* ⇒ anion, cation.

**ion channel** water-filled channels in the cell membrane that allow certain ions to pass through, as in the transmission of nerve impulses. Some drugs act at the level of the ion channels.

**ion exchange resins** substances administered orally to reduce the level of specific ions (e.g. calcium, sodium and potassium) in the body such as may occur in renal failure. For example, polystyrene sulphonate resins used to reduce mild or moderate hyperkalaemia. Anion exchange resins, such as colestyramine, are used to reduce low-density lipoprotein cholesterol in people with hypercholesterolaemia.

**ionization** *n* the dissociation of a substance in solution into ions.

**ionizing radiation** form of radiation that destabilizes an atom, forming an ion. Examples include gamma rays, X-rays and alpha or beta particle radiation. It has the ability to cause tissue damage and genetic mutations. ⇒ radiation.

**ionophore** *n* a molecule that facilitates the movement of ions across the lipid bilayer of the cell membrane. Some act as carrier molecules, whereas others form ion channels or pores.

**iontophoresis** *n* the introduction of ions of various soluble salts into the tissues by using an electrical current. Pilocarpine is introduced into the skin by this method in order to do a sweat test for the diagnosis of cystic fibrosis.

**IOP** *abbr* intraocular pressure.

**IP₃** *abbr* inositol triphosphate.

**IPE** *abbr* interprofessional education.

**ipecacuanha** *n* dried root from South America. Used in some expectorants. It is sometimes used as an emetic after poisoning but may have limited value.

**IPPV** *abbr* intermittent positive-pressure ventilation.

**ipsilateral** *adj* on the same side—**ipsilaterally** *adv*.

**IQ** *abbr* intelligence quotient.

**iridectomy** *n* excision of a part of the iris. May be performed to improve drainage of aqueous humour in glaucoma.

**iridencleisis** *n* surgical technique previously used to reduce intraocular pressure in glaucoma.

**iridium-192** (**¹⁹²Ir**) *n* a radioactive element used in brachytherapy to treat cancers in the anus, tongue, breast as implanted wires or hair pins. Can also be used as a Selectron source.

**iridocyclitis** *n* inflammation of the iris and ciliary body.

**iridodialysis** *n* a separation of the iris from its ciliary body attachment.

**iridoplegia** *n* paralysis of the muscle of the iris. It may be due to the instillation of drugs used to dilate the pupil, or inflammation or injury of the eye. ⇒ cycloplegia.

**iridotomy** *n* an incision into the iris; usually performed using a laser. It is used in the treatment of primary closed-angle glaucoma (PCAG). The laser is used to make a hole in the iris, thereby allowing aqueous humour to drain through into the anterior chamber and onward into the scleral venous sinus (canal of Schlemm).

**iris** *n* part of the uveal tract. The circular pigmented structure forming the anterior one-sixth of the middle coat of the eyeball (⇒ Appendix 1, Figure 15). It is perforated in the centre by an opening, the pupil. Contraction of its muscle fibres regulates the

amount of light entering the eye through the pupil. ⇒ choroid, iris.

**iris bombe** bulging forward of the iris due to pressure of the aqueous behind, when posterior synechiae are present around the pupil.

**iritis** *n* (*syn* anterior uveitis) inflammation of the iris.

**iron (Fe)** *n* a metallic element needed in the body as a constituent of haemoglobin and several enzymes.

**iron storage disease** the deposition of iron in the tissues and organs. It may be primary or secondary to another disease such as thalassaemia. ⇒ haemochromatosis, haemosiderosis.

**irradiation** *n* exposure to a form of radiant energy such as light, heat or X-rays. Radioactive sources of radiant heat are used in various imaging techniques and medical treatments. Gamma radiation is used to sterilize intravenous fluids, food and various items of medical equipment. Infrared is used for pain relief, muscle relaxation and to improve local blood flow. Ultraviolet light is used in the treatment of skin diseases and in the identification of some micro-organisms.

**irreducible** *adj* unable to be brought to desired condition. *irreducible hernia* ⇒ hernia.

**irrigation** *n* washing out of a body cavity such as the bladder following prostate surgery, or a wound.

**irritable** *adj* capable of being excited to activity; easily stimulated—**irritability** *n*.

**irritable bowel syndrome (IBS)** functional intestinal symptoms not explained by organic bowel disease. Symptoms include abdominal pain, bloating and change in bowel habit (alternating constipation and diarrhoea).

**irritant** *adj, n* describes any agent which causes irritation.

**ISC** *abbr* intermittent self-catheterization.

**ischaemia** *n* deficient blood supply to any part of the body. ⇒ angina, Volkmann's ischaemic contracture—**ischaemic** *adj*.

**ischaemic heart disease (IHD)** ⇒ coronary heart disease.

**ischiorectal** *adj* pertaining to the ischium and the rectum, such as an ischiorectal abscess which occurs between these two structures.

**ischium** *n* the lower part of the innominate bone of the pelvis; the bone on which the body rests when sitting—**ischial** *adj*.

**islet cell tumours** uncommon hormone-secreting tumours of the islet cells of the pancreas. They include gastrinoma, glucagonoma, insulinoma and somatostatinoma.

**islets of Langerhans** (P Langerhans, German pathologist, 1847–1888) collections of special cells scattered throughout the pancreas, mainly concerned with endocrine function. The pancreatic islets contain four types of hormone-secreting cells: alpha cells, which secrete glucagon; beta cells, which secrete insulin and amylin; delta cells, which secrete several substances, including somatostatin or growth hormone release-inhibiting hormone (GHRIH); and other cells that produce regulatory pancreatic polypeptide.

**isoantibody** *n* an antibody to isoantigens present in other individuals of the same species.

**isoantigen** *n* an antigen that reacts with isoantibodies present in other individuals of the same species.

**isodactylism** *n* a condition characterized by having digits of equal length.

**isoenzyme** *n* one that catalyses the same reaction, but exists in several forms and at different body sites, such as lactate dehydrogenase.

**isograft** *n* a graft between individuals with identical genotypes, i.e. identical twins. It can also be used to describe grafts between syngeneic individuals, i.e. inbred strains of laboratory animals.

**isoimmunization** *n* development of anti-Rh agglutinins in the blood of a Rh-negative person who has been given a Rh-positive transfusion, or who is carrying a Rh-positive fetus.

**isokinetic activity** a dynamic activity in which the velocity of the movement remains the same and the resistance varies.

**isokinetic dynamometer** a device that quantitatively measures muscular strength through a preset speed of movement.

**isolation** *n* separation of a patient from others for a number of reasons, e.g. to prevent the spread of an infectious disease. ⇒ containment isolation, protective isolation, source isolation.

**isolator** *n* apparatus ranging from what is virtually a large plastic bag in which a patient can be nursed to that in which surgery can be performed. It aims to prevent pathogenic micro-organisms either gaining entry or leaving the enclosed space.

**isoleucine** *n* an essential (indispensable) branched-chain amino acid.

**isomers** *npl* molecules that have the same mass and formula but have different structures or functional groups. This causes them to have different properties.

**isometric** *adj* of equal proportions.

**isometric contraction** a muscle contraction where its attachments do not move and, therefore, the muscle does not shorten and joints do not move.

**isometric exercises** carried out without movement. Used to maintain muscle tone.

**isometropia** *n* both eyes having the same refractive power.

**isosthenuria** *n* the kidneys are unable to produce concentrated urine; a feature of end-stage renal failure.

**isotonic** *adj* equal tension; applied to any solution which has the same osmotic pressure as the fluid with which it is being compared. ⇒ hypertonic, hypotonic.

**isotonic exercises** carried out with movement. Increases muscle strength and endurance.

**isotonic muscle contraction** muscle contraction that results in a change in muscle length (shortens or lengthens) and movement of its attachments.

**isotonic saline** (*syn* normal saline, physiological saline), 0.9% solution of sodium chloride in water.

**isotopes** *npl* two or more forms of the same element having identical chemical properties and the same atomic number but different mass numbers. Those isotopes with radioactive properties are used in medicine for research, diagnosis and treatment of disease.

**ispaghula husk** a natural dietary fibre supplement. Used as a bulk-forming laxative. ⇒ Appendix 5.

**isthmus** *n* a narrowed part of an organ or tissue such as that connecting the two lobes of the thyroid gland, or the *uterine isthmus*, which with the cervix forms the lower segment of the uterus during pregnancy. *isthmus of the uterine tube*. ⇒ Appendix 1, Figure 17.

**itch** *n* a sensation on the skin which makes one want to scratch. Often accompanies skin disease. *itch mite Sarcoptes scabiei.* ⇒ scabies.

**ITP** *abbr* idiopathic thrombocytopenic purpura.

**ITU** *abbr* intensive therapy unit.

**IUCD** *abbr* intrauterine contraceptive device.

**IUD** *abbr* **1.** intrauterine (contraceptive) device. **2.** intrauterine death (of a fetus).

**IUGR** *abbr* intrauterine growth restriction/retardation.

**IUI** *abbr* intrauterine insemination.

**IVC** *abbr* inferior vena cava.

**IVF** *abbr* in vitro fertilization.

**IVI** *abbr* intravenous infusion.

**IVIG** *abbr* intravenous immunoglobulin.

**IVU, IVP** *abbr* intravenous urogram/pyelogram ⇒ urography.

***Ixodes*** *n* a genus of parasitic hard-bodied ticks. Various species are associated with the spread of diseases that include Lyme disease, tularaemia and Rocky Mountain spotted fever.

## J

**Jacksonian epilepsy** (J Jackson, British neurologist, 1835–1911) ⇒ epilepsy.

**Jacquemier's sign** (J Jacquemier, French obstetrician, 1806–1879) darkening (blue/purple discoloration) of the vaginal mucosa; seen sometimes in early pregnancy from the fourth week. It is a possible indicator of pregnancy rather than definite evidence.

**jactitation** *n* restlessness with muscle spasm and twitching. May accompany an increase in core body temperature.

**Jakob–Creutzfeldt disease** ⇒ Creutzfeldt–Jakob disease.

**jamais vu** a sudden feeling of being a stranger in familiar places or when with people who are known to the individual. It may be associated with temporal lobe epilepsy, but also occurs infrequently as a normal phenomenon.

**Janeway lesions** (E Janeway, American physician, 1841–1911) haemorrhagic spots on the palm or sole. Associated with infective endocarditis.

**jargon** *n* technical or specialized language that is only understood by a particular group, for example health professionals, thereby excluding non-experts such as some patients and carers. Often used to describe the use of obscure and pretentious language, together with a roundabout way of expression.

**Jarisch–Herxheimer's reaction** (A Jarisch, Austrian dermatologist, 1850–1902; K Herxheimer, German dermatologist, 1861–1942) a reaction whereby the symptoms of a disease such as syphilis are initially worsened when antibiotic therapy commences. Typically it is characterized by fever, chills, muscle pain, nausea and headache within a few hours of receiving the antibiotics. The reaction is not harmful and is usually short-lived.

**Jarman index** system for weighting general practice populations according to social conditions. A composite index of social factors that general practitioners considered important in increasing workload and pressure on services. These factors were identified through a survey of one in 10 general practitioners in the UK in 1981. An underprivileged area (UPA) score was then constructed based on the level of each variable in each area, weighted by the weighting assigned from the national general practitioner survey. Eight variables were used: (a) older people living alone; (b) children aged under 5 years; (c) unskilled; (d) unemployed (as % economically active); (e) lone-parent families; (f) overcrowded accommodation (>1 person/room); (g) mobility (moved house within 1 year); (h) ethnic origin (new Commonwealth and Pakistan). Information on the variables were derived from the census. ⇒ Townsend index.

**jaundice** *n* (*syn* icterus) a condition characterized by a raised bilirubin level in the blood (hyperbilirubinaemia). Minor degrees are only detectable chemically. Major degrees are visible in the yellow discoloration of skin, sclerae and mucosae. Pruritus occurs, although the mechanism is not known. Jaundice without the excretion of bilirubin in the urine is termed acholuric. Jaundice may be classified as follows: (a) *haemolytic or prehepatic jaundice* where excessive breakdown of red blood cells (erythrocytes) releases bilirubin into the blood, such as in haemolytic anaemia. ⇒ haemolysis, haemolytic disease of the newborn. (b) *hepatocellular jaundice* arises when liver cell function is impaired, such as with hepatitis or cirrhosis; (c) *obstructive or cholestatic jaundice*, where the flow of bile is obstructed either within the liver (intrahepatic) or in the larger ducts of the biliary tract (extrahepatic). Causes include cirrhosis, cancers, parasites and gallstones. ⇒ cholestasis.

**jawbone** *n* describes either the upper jaw (maxilla) or lower jaw (mandible).

**jaw thrust** a manoeuvre used to open the airway if a head or neck injury is suspected. In adults the index and middle fingers are placed under the angle of the lower jaw and steady gentle pressure used to move the jaw upwards and forwards (Figure J.1); the mouth should then open slightly. The jaw thrust manoeuvre can be used for children and

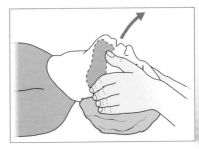

**Figure J.1** Jaw thrust—adult *(reproduced from Mallik et al. 1998 with permission).*

infants, but only the index finger on the lower jaw is used. ⇒ head tilt/chin lift.

**jaw-winking syndrome** also known as Gunn's syndrome and Marcus Gunn's syndrome. Characterized by an involuntary facial movement in which the eyelid droops when the jaw closes but is raised when the jaw opens or moves from side to side. It is usually unilateral.

**JCA** *abbr* juvenile chronic arthritis.

**jejunal biopsy** ⇒ Crosby capsule.

**jejunectomy** *n* surgical removal of all or a portion of the jejunum.

**jejunileostomy** *n* a surgical anastomosis between the jejunum and the ileum.

**jejunostomy** *n* a surgically made fistula between the jejunum and the anterior abdominal wall; used for feeding in cases where passage of food through the stomach is impossible or undesirable.

**jejunum** *n* that part of the small intestine between the duodenum and the ileum— **jejunal** *adj*.

**Jersey finger** a colloquial term used in sports medicine to describe the rupture of the flexor digitorum longus tendon from the distal phalanx of the finger due to rapid extension of the finger while being actively flexed.

**jet lag** disturbance to biological processes that normally have diurnal rhythms; occurs following travel through different time zones. It is characterized by changes in sleep patterns, appetite, concentration and memory, and fatigue for some days until body rhythms return to normal. People working variable shift patterns report similar effects.

**JGA** *abbr* juxtaglomerular apparatus.

**jigger** *n* a sand flea, *Tunga penetrans*, found in the tropics.

**Jod–Basedow phenomenon** (K von Basedow, German physician, 1799–1854) the development of hyperthyroidism following the administration of dietary iodine to a person with endemic goitre living in an iodine-deficient region. May also occur when iodine in large doses is administered to a person with a non-toxic multinodular goitre and who is living in a region which has sufficient levels of iodine.

**Johnstone approach** a treatment approach involving a developmental progression of movement and on sensory stimulation with specific splinting techniques. It is used for patients who have had a stroke.

**joint** *n* the articulation of two or more bones (arthrosis). There are three main classes: (a) fibrous (synarthroses), e.g. the sutures of the skull; (b) cartilaginous (amphiarthroses), e.g. between the manubrium and the body of the sternum; and (c) synovial or freely movable (diarthroses), e.g. shoulder or hip. Freely movable joints are classified by the range of movement possible. They are ball-and-socket, hinge, gliding, pivot, condyloid and saddle joints. ⇒ Charcot's joint.

**joint reaction forces** the forces that are transmitted through a joint's articular surfaces.

**joule (J)** *n* the SI unit for measuring energy, work and quantity of heat. The unit (J) is the energy expended when 1 kg (kilogram) is moved 1 m (metre) by a force of 1 N (newton). The kilojoule (kJ = $10^3$ J) and the megajoule (MJ = $10^6$ J) are used by nutritionists for measuring large amounts of energy.

**JVP** *abbr* jugular venous pressure.

**jugular** *adj* pertaining to the throat.

**jugular veins** internal and external jugular veins pass down either side of the neck. They carry most venous blood from the head and unite with the subclavian veins to form the brachiocephalic veins, which become the superior vena cava. ⇒ Appendix 1, Figure 10.

**jugular venous pressure (JVP)** the pressure of blood in the jugular veins; a guide to the pressure in the right side of the heart.

**jumper's knee** patellar tendinitis. Inflammation of the patellar tendon where it attaches to the patella. An overuse injury associated with repetitive contraction of the quadriceps femoris muscle associated with the movements of athletes and dancers.

**junctional escape rhythm** a cardiac rhythm that usually arises from a focus at the junction between the atrioventricular node and the atrioventricular bundle. If the heart rate is below 50 beats/min the cardiac output is reduced and the blood pressure falls, leading to the person feeling dizzy and faint.

**Jung, Carl** Swiss psychiatrist/psychoanalyst (1875–1961).

**justice** *n* involves the concepts of fairness and justness. May be described as acting within a set of moral laws, respecting the views and rights of others, or equity in the distribution of resources such as health care.

**juvenile chronic arthritis (JCA)** now more commonly termed juvenile idiopathic arthritis.

**juvenile idiopathic arthritis** (*syn* juvenile chronic arthritis) chronic inflammatory arthritis in children. In its systemic form (previously termed Still's disease) systemic features such as fever, rash and anaemia are prominent and may precede the arthritis.

**juxtaglomerular** *adj* close to the glomerulus.

**juxtaglomerular apparatus (JGA)** cells in the distal convoluted tubule and the afferent arteriole of the nephron. They monitor changes in pressure and sodium levels in the blood, and initiate the release of renin. ⇒ macula densa.

**juxtapose** *vt* to place side by side.

Keller's operation ◄

# K

**Kahn reaction** an obsolete serological test for syphilis; used in the 20th century.

**kala-azar** *n* generalized leishmaniasis occurring in the tropics. Characterized by anaemia, fever, splenomegaly and wasting. It is caused by the parasite *Leishmania donovani* and is spread by sandflies.

**kallidin** *n* a kinin. A biologically active polypeptide that is produced in response to tissue injury. It causes vasodilation and the contraction of involuntary smooth muscle. It is similar in structure to bradykinin.

**kallikreins** *npl* a group of enzymes involved in the release of bradykinin and kallidin.

**Kallmann's syndrome** (F Kallmann, German/American psychiatrist and geneticist, 1897–1965) congenital condition in which the olfactory bulbs fail to develop resulting in anosmia. There is also a deficiency of pituitary gonadotrophic hormones and hypogonadism.

**Kanner's syndrome** (L Kanner, Austrian/American psychiatrist, 1894–1981) autism. ⇒ Asperger's syndrome.

**kaolin** *n* natural aluminium silicate. Given orally it absorbs toxic substances, hence it is useful in diarrhoea, food poisoning and colitis. Sometimes used as a poultice.

**Kaposi's disease** (M Kaposi, Austrian dermatologist, 1837–1902) ⇒ xeroderma pigmentosum.

**Kaposi's sarcoma** (M Kaposi) a cancer characterized by new blood vessel growth producing red, purple or brown lesions, often on the skin but with metastatic potential. Originally common in Africa but now often seen in immunocompromised individuals, such as those with acquired immunodeficiency syndrome (AIDS).

**Kaposi's varicelliform eruption** widespread herpes simplex infection complicating atopic dermatitis (eczema). ⇒ eczema herpeticum.

**Kartagener's syndrome** (M Kartagener, Swiss physician, 1897–1975) a rare inherited autosomal recessive condition of primary ciliary dyskinesia and transposition of the viscera, such as the heart being situated on the right side of the body. The abnormal movement of the respiratory cilia leads to chronic sinusitis and repeated respiratory tract infection, which eventually cause bronchiectasis.

**karyolysis** *n* the dissolution of the cell nucleus that occurs prior to cell division during meiosis and mitosis. It also occurs due to pathological changes to cells such as trauma or necrosis.

**karyorrhexis** *n* fragmentation of the cell nucleus and dissemination of nuclear chromatin within the cell cytoplasm.

**karyotype** *n* **1.** the number, size, structure and arrangement of chromosomes in a somatic cell of an individual. **2.** a diagrammatic representation of a set of chromosomes showing an orderly array of chromosomes, the autosomes (groups A–G) and the sex chromosomes (see Figure C.9, p. 96). It is usually derived from the study of cultured cells and may be done for diagnostic purposes, or in individuals at risk of having children with chromosomal abnormalities, or for the prenatal detection of fetal abnormality.

**Kawasaki disease** (T Kawasaki, Japanese physician, 20th century) an inflammatory disease affecting small blood vessels (vasculitis). ⇒ mucocutaneous lymph node syndrome.

**Kayser–Fleischer ring** (B Kayser, German ophthalmologist, 1869–1954; B Fleischer, German ophthalmologist, 1874–1904) a brown/green ring in the outer cornea, a sign of Wilson's disease (hepatolenticular degeneration), that results from disordered copper metabolism. ⇒ Wilson's disease. ⊙DVD

**Kegel exercises** (A Kegel, American gynaecologist, 20th century) a set of pelvic floor exercises used in both women and men to minimize continence problems. Used to retrain the pelvic floor muscles after childbirth, or following prostate surgery. The person learns to identify the muscles of the pelvic floor and undertakes daily contraction of the pelvic floor to strengthen it, thereby strengthening the muscles that surround the internal and external urinary sphincter muscles.

**Kehr's sign** (H Kehr, German surgeon, 1862–1913) acute referred pain felt at the top of the left shoulder caused by blood within the peritoneal cavity irritating the diaphragm. The pain impulses are transmitted by the phrenic nerve. The presence of Kehr's sign is indicative of a ruptured spleen.

**Kell factor/antigen** named for the person in whom the antigen was first identified. A blood group factor/antigen present in about 10% of the Caucasian population. Anti-Kell antibodies can cross the placenta. ⇒ blood groups.

**Keller's operation** (W Keller, American surgeon, 1874–1959) arthroplasty or excision arthroplasty for hallux valgus or rigidus. Excision of the proximal half of the proximal phalanx, plus any osteophytes and exostoses on the metatarsal head. The toe is fixed in the corrected position; after healing a pseudarthrosis results.

**Kelly–Paterson syndrome** ⇒ Plummer–Vinson syndrome.

**keloid scar** excessive scar production extending beyond the site of original injury. An elevated and progressive scar, which may produce contraction deformity. Keloid scarring occurs in some people who have darker skins.

**Kelvin scale (K)** *n* (W Thompson [Lord Kelvin], British physicist, 1824–1907) an absolute temperature scale that uses the cessation of particle vibration for determining zero degrees or absolute zero. It is calculated in degrees Celsius as −273.15°C. The unit, the kelvin, is the SI unit for temperature.

**keratalgia** *n* pain in the cornea.

**keratectomy** *n* surgical excision of a portion of the cornea.

**keratic precipitates (KP)** clusters of inflammatory cells adherent to the posterior surface of the cornea; present following trauma or in inflammation of uvea.

**keratin** *n* a fibrous protein found in nails and the outer part of the skin and horns, etc.

**keratinization** *n* horn-like thickening of the skin. ⇒ keratosis.

**keratinocytes** *npl* the most numerous cells that form the epidermis. The keratinocytes produce keratin from the precursor keratohyalin. They are bound together by desmosomes, and this helps to prevent structural damage to the skin and maintain epidermal cohesion during renewal. Keratinocytes migrate upwards through the layers of the epidermis during epidermal renewal, eventually to be shed from the stratum corneum (surface layer).

**keratitis** *n* inflammation of the cornea. The risk of *microbial keratitis* is increased in immunocompromised individuals, or those with existing eye disease and in eye injuries involving plant substances. It can, however, occur in people who wear soft contact lenses, especially in warmer regions. Keratitis caused by *Fusarium* spp. is treated with antifungal drugs but people who do not respond and suffer corneal damage may need a corneal transplant.

**keratocele** *n* herniation of Descemet's membrane through a structural defect in the cornea such as that caused by an ulcer.

**keratoconjunctivitis** *n* inflammation of the cornea and conjunctiva. *epidemic keratoconjunctivitis* due to an adenovirus. Present as an acute follicular conjunctivitis with preauricular and submandibular adenitis. *keratoconjunctivitis sicca* dry eye, including in Sjögren syndrome.

**keratoconus** *n* a cone-like protrusion of the cornea, usually due to a non-inflammatory thinning.

**keratoectasia** *n* also called kerectasis. A forward bulge or protrusion affecting the cornea.

**keratolytic** *adj* having the property of breaking down keratinized epidermis.

**keratoma** *n* ⇒ callosity—**keratomata** *pl*.

**keratomalacia** *n* frequently caused by lack of vitamin A, there is keratinization of corneal and conjunctival epithelia with loss of mucin-producing cells. May lead to corneal ulceration, secondary infection and corneal perforation.

**keratome** *n* a special knife for incising the cornea.

**keratometer/ophthalmometer** *n* an instrument used to measure the curvature of the cornea.

**keratopathy** *n* any disease of the cornea.

**keratoplasty** *n* ⇒ corneal graft.

**keratoprosthesis** *n* artificial cornea.

**keratosis** *n* thickening of the horny layer of the skin. Also referred to as hyperkeratosis. Has the appearance of warty excrescences. *keratosis palmaris et plantaris* (*syn* tylosis) a congenital thickening of the horny layer of the palms and soles.

**keratotomy** *n* an incision into the cornea.

**keratouveitis** *n* inflammation of the cornea and uvea (uveal tract—iris, ciliary body and choroid), often due to infection.

**kerion** *n* a boggy suppurative mass of the scalp associated with ringworm.

**kernicterus** *n* staining of brain cells, especially the basal nuclei with bilirubin. It is a complication of jaundice affecting preterm babies and haemolytic disease of the newborn. It can lead to a severe encephalopathy with resultant learning disabilities.

**Kernig's sign** (V Kernig, Russian physician, 1840–1917) a sign of meningeal irritation such as occurs in meningitis. The patient is unable to straighten the leg at the knee when the thigh is flexed at right angles to the trunk. There is pain in the lower back and resistance to leg straightening.

**Keshan disease** a condition that occurs in some areas of China where a deficiency of selenium exists. There is cardiomyopathy.

**ketoacidosis** *n* (*syn* ketosis) acidosis due to accumulation of ketone bodies (β-hydroxybutyric acid, acetoacetic acid and acetone), products of the metabolism of fat. Primarily a serious complication of type 1 diabetes, but also occurs in starvation and rarely in alcohol misuse. Symptoms include drowsiness, headache and deep sighing respiration (Kussmaul's). *diabetic ketoacidosis* ketone bodies are formed as fatty acids are incompletely oxidized when glucose is unavailable as an energy source. Acidosis and dehydration accompany hyperglycaemia. ⇒ Kussmaul's respiration.

**ketogenesis** *n* the formation of ketone bodies.

**ketogenic diet** a high-fat, low-carbohydrate diet that produces ketosis (acidosis).

**ketonaemia** *n* ketone bodies in the blood—**ketonaemic** *adj*.

**ketone bodies** include acetone, acetoacetate (acetoacetic acid) and β-hydroxybutyric acid produced normally during fat oxidation. Can be used as fuel but excess production leads to ketoacidosis. This may occur when blood glucose level is high, but unavailable for metabolism, as in poorly controlled diabetes mellitus.

**ketones** *npl* organic compounds (e.g. ketosteroids) containing a keto group.

**ketonuria** *n* ketone bodies in the urine—**ketonuric** *adj*.

**ketose** *n* a monosaccharide that contains a ketone group, for example the hexose fructose.

**ketosis** *n* ⇒ ketoacidosis.

**ketosteroids** *npl* adrenal corticosteroid hormones that contain a ketone group. The 17-ketosteroids are normally present in the blood and excreted in urine and are present in excess in overactivity of the adrenal glands and the gonads.

**key points of control** parts of the body from which movement can be easily controlled. A central key point is described in the upper thorax, proximal key points are the shoulder girdle and the pelvic girdle and the distal key points are the hands and feet.

**keyhole surgery** ⇒ minimally invasive surgery.

**khat** *n* also called chat, miraa, qat, etc. It is obtained from the leaves of the tree *Catha edulis* that grows in the Arabian peninsula and Africa. Khat contains psychostimulants structurally similar to amfetamine. Chewing the leaves is a widespread habit in East Africa and the Middle East. Its effects include excitement, talkativeness and feelings of euphoria. However, users may become hyperactive and serious mental health disturbances can occur. It is becoming increasingly available in the UK.

**kidney** *n* paired retroperitoneal organs situated on the upper posterior abdominal wall in the lumbar region (⇒ Appendix 1, Figures 19 and 20). Vital in the maintenance of homeostasis by the production of urine in the nephrons, the microscopic functional units (comprising the glomerulus and renal tubule). This involves three processes: filtration of the blood contents, reabsorption of substances (e.g. glucose) needed by the body and secretion of unwanted substances. Urine production is vital in the excretion of nitrogenous waste products such as urea and other waste substances, including drug residues, the control and maintenance of fluid balance and electrolyte balance and the maintenance of acid–base balance. The kidneys also secrete renin, which is important in the control of blood pressure. In addition the kidneys produce erythropoietin, which stimulates the production of red blood cells (erythrocytes) in the bone marrow. Also involved in the metabolism of vitamin D. ⇒ horseshoe kidney. *kidney failure* ⇒ renal failure. *kidney machine* ⇒ dialyser.

**kidney function tests** a series of tests that include: routine urine testing, urine concentration/dilution tests, serum urea and electrolytes, serum creatinine and renal clearance to estimate glomerular filtration rate (GFR).

**kidney transplant** surgical transplantation of a kidney from a previously tested suitable live donor or a cadaveric organ. Kidneys may also be transplanted from the renal bed to other sites in the same individual in cases of ureteric disease or trauma.

**Kiesselbach's plexus** (W Kiesselbach, German laryngologist, 1839–1902) a plexus of small blood vessels located on the anterior nasal septum. A common site of bleeding from the nose. ⇒ epistaxis, Little's area.

**kilocalorie (kcal)** *n* one thousand calories. ⇒ calorie, kilojoule.

**kilogram (kg)** *n* one of the seven base units of the International System of Units (SI). A measurement of mass. ⇒ Appendix 2.

**kilojoule (kJ)** *n* a unit equal to 1000 joules. It is used to measure large amounts of energy. It replaces the kilocalorie (kcal), which is still commonly used. ⇒ calorie.

**kinaesthesis** *n* muscle sense; perception of movement—**kinaesthetic** *adj*.

**kinaesthetic sense** the ability to sense body position, weight and movement. Being able to differentiate between static positions and joint action. It involves receptors in structures

**K**

that include muscles, tendons and joints. ⇒ proprioception.

**kinanaesthesia** *n* **1.** loss of the ability to sense movement. **2.** decreased awareness of the position or movement of part of the body.

**kinanthropometry** *n* the utilization of a combination of anthropometry and kinesiology.

**kinase** *n* **1.** an enzyme activator that converts a zymogen (proenzyme) to the active form of the enzyme. **2.** enzymes that catalyse the transfer of a high-energy group of a donor, usually adenosine triphosphate (ATP), to some acceptor, usually named after the acceptor, such as fructokinase.

**kinematic chain exercises** a system of links coupled by joints. ⇒ closed kinetic chain, open kinetic chain.

**kineplastic surgery** operative measures, whereby certain muscle groups are isolated and used to work a modified prosthesis.

**kinesiology** *n* the study of muscle activity that brings together the anatomy, physiology and biomechanics of parts of the body.

**kinetic** *adj* relating to or producing motion.

**kinins** *npl* biologically active proteins and polypeptides such as bradykinin that cause vasodilation, increased vessel permeability, smooth muscle contraction, pain, etc.

**Kirschner wire** (M Kirschner, German surgeon, 1879–1942) a wire drilled into a bone to apply skeletal traction. A hand or electric drill is used, a stirrup is attached and the wire is rendered taut by means of a special wire-tightener.

***Klebsiella*** *n* (T Klebs, German bacteriologist, 1834–1913) a genus of anaerobic Gram-negative non-motile bacteria belonging to the family Enterobacteriaceae. They form part of the normal flora of the mouth and in the gut. They are opportunists and may affect immunocompromised individuals. They are commonly the cause of health care-associated infections of the urinary tract, respiratory tract and wounds. Some strains are resistant to many antibiotics. *Klebsiella pneumoniae* causes serious pneumonia in critically ill patients needing respiratory support.

**Kleine–Levin syndrome** (W Kleine, German psychiatrist, 20th century; M Levin, American neurologist, 20th century) a rare episodic condition characterized by periods of extreme sleepiness and excessive eating.

**kleptomania** *n* a strong impulse to steal.

**Klinefelter's syndrome** (H Klinefelter, American physician, b. 1912) a chromosomal abnormality affecting boys. A type of genetic mosaicism in which there is an extra X chromosome in at least one cell population. The commonest form is XXY, in which the boy/man has 47 chromosomes, but some have more X chromosomes. Puberty is frequently delayed, with small firm testes, often with gynaecomastia. Associated with sterility, which may be the only symptom. The multiple X chromosome forms tend have other abnormalities and learning disability. ⇒ mosaicism.

**Klumpke's paralysis** (A Déjérine-Klumpke, French neurologist, 1859–1927) paralysis and atrophy of forearm and hand muscles, caused by a birth injury. May be accompanied by Horner's syndrome with sensory and pupillary disturbances due to injury to lower roots of brachial plexus and cervical sympathetic nerves. Claw-hand results.

**knee** *n* the hinge joint formed by the lower end of the femur and the head of the tibia. It is a large complex joint formed by the femoral condyles, the tibial condyles and the patella or kneecap (a sesamoid bone in the patellar tendon of the quadriceps femoris muscle), along with associated ligaments, including the cruciate ligaments, semilunar cartilages or menisci, numerous bursae and fat pads. *knee jerk* a reflex contraction of the relaxed quadriceps femoris muscle elicited by a tap on the patellar tendon: usually performed with the lower femur supported behind, the knee bent and the leg limp. Persistent variation from normal usually signifies organic nervous disorder.

**knuckles** *npl* the dorsal aspect of any of the joints between the phalanges and the metacarpal bones, or between the phalanges.

**Kocher's incision** (E Kocher, Swiss surgeon, 1841–1917) an oblique incision in the right upper abdomen previously used for removal of the gallbladder during an open cholecystectomy. ⇒ minimally invasive surgery.

**Kocher's manoeuvre** (E Kocher) a manoeuvre used to reduce a dislocation of the shoulder joint.

**Koebner phenomenon** (H Koebner, Polish dermatologist, 1838–1904) induction of a lesion of certain skin diseases, e.g. psoriasis, following non-specific trauma to the skin.

**Köhler's disease** (A Köhler, German physician, 1874–1947) osteochondritis of the navicular bone. Confined to children of 3–5 years.

**koilonychia** *n* spoon-shaped nails. The normal convex curvature of the nail is lost and it becomes slightly concave. It is more common in fingernails than toenails and is associated with iron-deficiency anaemia.

**Koplik's spots** (H Koplik, American paediatrician, 1858–1927) small white spots inside the mouth, during the first few days of the invasion (prodromal) stage of measles.

**Korotkoff (Korotkov) sounds** (N Korotkoff [Korotkov], Russian physician/surgeon, 1874–1920) the sounds audible when recording non-invasive arterial blood pressure with a sphygmomanometer and stethoscope. The phases are: (I) a sharp thud—systolic pressure; (II) a swishing/blowing sound; (III) sharper noise but softer than in phase I; (IV) a soft blowing that becomes muffled; (V) silence. In the UK the diastolic pressure is normally recorded at the end of phase IV (Figure K.1).

**Korsakoff's (Korsakov's) syndrome** (S Korsakoff [Korsakov], Russian psychiatrist, 1854–1900) chronic amnesia (defect of retrieval of recently acquired information) with denial, lack of insight and confabulation. ⇒ amnesic syndrome, Wernicke's encephalopathy.

**kosher** *n* the choice and preparation of foods which comply with the dietary laws of Judaism. Certain cuts of meat from cud-chewing animals with cloven hoofs, e.g. sheep, goats, cattle and deer, are permitted. The only fish allowed are those with scales and fins. In addition animals must be slaughtered according to the rituals of Judaism. A food that is not kosher is termed traife. ⇒ pareve.

**KP** *abbr* keratic precipitates.

**Krabbe disease** (K Krabbe, Danish neurologist, 1885–1965) genetically determined disorder of lipid metabolism that leads to degenerative changes in the central nervous system. It is associated with learning disability.

**kraurosis vulvae** a degenerative condition of the vaginal introitus associated with postmenopausal lack of oestrogen.

**Krebs' cycle** (*syn* citric acid cycle, tricarboxylic acid cycle) (H Krebs, British biochemist, 1900–1981) the final common pathway for the oxidation of fuel molecules: glucose, fatty acids, glycerol and amino acids. These enter the cycle as acetyl coenzyme A and are oxidized to produce energy (adenosine triphosphate [ATP]), carbon dioxide and water.

**Krukenberg tumour** (F Krukenberg, German pathologist, 1871–1946) a secondary (metastatic) malignant tumour of the ovary, usually spread from primary stomach (gastric) cancer.

**krypton (Kr)** *n* an inert gas. Its radioactive isotope krypton-81m ($^{81m}$Kr) is used in lung ventilation scans.

**KUB** *abbr* kidney, ureter and bladder.

**Küntscher nail** (G Küntscher, German surgeon, 1902–1972) used for intramedullary fixation of fractured long bones, especially the femur. The nail has a 'clover-leaf' cross-section.

**Kupffer cells** (K von Kupffer, German anatomist, 1829–1902) large phagocytic macrophages lining the sinusoids of the liver. Part of the monocyte–macrophage (reticuloendothelial) system, they remove micro-organisms and 'old' red blood cells from the blood and destroy them by phagocytosis.

**kuru** *n* a fatal prion disease with a very long incubation period of many years. It affects the central nervous system and causes dementia, slurred speech, ataxia and paralysis. Probably transmitted by cannibalism. Rare and declining in incidence since the cessation of rituals involving cannibalism of brain tissue. Occurred exclusively among New Guinea highlanders. ⇒ Creutzfeldt–Jakob disease.

**Kussmaul's respiration** (A Kussmaul, German physician, 1822–1902) deep sighing respiration typical of diabetic ketoacidosis.

**Kveim test** (M Kveim, Norwegian physician, 1892–1966) an intracutaneous test for sarcoidosis using tissue prepared from a person known to be suffering from the condition.

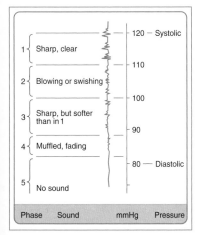

**Figure K.1** Korotkoff (Korotkov) sounds *(adapted from Hinchliff et al. 1996 with permission).*

**kwashiorkor** *n* a nutritional disorder of infants and young children associated with poverty, deprivation and infection. Develops when the diet is deficient in protein; may develop at weaning when a low-protein starchy porridge is fed instead of breast milk. Characteristic features are anaemia, muscle wasting, loss of appetite, pale thin hair, oedema and a fatty liver.

**Kwok's syndrome** ⇒ Chinese-restaurant syndrome.

**Kyasanur forest disease** a viral disease transmitted by ticks in parts of India. It causes headache, myalgia, fever, cough, photophobia and conjunctivitis.

**kymograph** *n* an apparatus for recording movements, e.g. of muscles, columns of blood. Used in physiological experiments—**kymographic** *adj*, **kymographically** *adv*.

**kypholordosis** *n* coexistence of kyphosis and lordosis.

**kyphoscoliosis** *n* coexistence of kyphosis and scoliosis. May prevent proper lung expansion and lead to respiratory problems.

**kyphosis** *n* as in Pott's disease, an excessive backward curvature of the dorsal spine. Commonly associated with osteoporosis—**kyphotic** *adj*.

# L

**labelling theory** process by which socially defined labels or identities are assigned or accepted. Often linked with deviant behaviour and can make it hard for people to escape that identity.

**labia** *npl* lips. *labia majora* two large lip-like folds of skin extending from the mons veneris to form the vulva. *labia minora* two smaller folds lying within the labia majora—**labium** *sing*, **labial** *adj*.

**labile** *adj* unstable; readily changed, such as many drugs when in solution; mood in some mental health problems and blood pressure.

**labile factor (proaccelerin)** *n* factor V in the blood coagulation cascade. It is produced in the liver and is required for the formation of prothrombin activator. A very rare inherited (autosomal recessive) deficiency leads to a bleeding disorder.

**lability** *n* instability. *emotional lability* rapid change in mood.

**labioglossolaryngeal** *adj* relating to the lips, tongue and larynx. *labioglossolaryngeal paralysis* ⇒ bulbar palsy or paralysis.

**labour** *n* (*syn* parturition) the act of giving birth to a child. The first stage lasts from onset until there is full dilatation of the cervical os; the second stage lasts until the baby is delivered; the third stage until the placenta is expelled.

**labyrinth** *n* the convoluted cavities of the inner ear, including the cochlea and semicircular canals, which form the organs concerned with hearing and balance/position sense (vestibular system which responds to changes in head position). The vestibular system conveys information about changes in head position to the muscles that move the eyes, which allows continuous visual focus when the head moves. *bony labyrinth* that part which is directly hollowed out of the temporal bone. *membranous labyrinth* the membrane lining the bony labyrinth—**labyrinthine** *adj*.

**labyrinthectomy** *n* surgical removal of part or the whole of the membranous labyrinth of the inner ear. Sometimes carried out for Ménière's disease.

**labyrinthitis** *n* inflammation of the inner ear which may be caused by viral or bacterial infection, side-effects of some drugs or following head injury. It causes vertigo with dizziness and nausea. Nystagmus may be observed and hearing loss and tinnitus may also occur.

**laceration** *n* a wound in which the tissues are torn, usually by a blunt instrument or pressure: more likely to become infected and to heal by second intention. ⇒ wound healing.

**lacrimal, lachrymal, lacrymal** *adj* pertaining to tears.

**lacrimal apparatus** the lacrimal glands, ducts, sacs and canaliculi involved in the production and drainage of tears (Figure L.1).

**lacrimal bone** a tiny bone at the inner side of the orbital cavity.

**lacrimal duct** tiny ducts that connect the lacrimal gland to the upper conjunctival sac.

**lacrimal gland** situated above the upper, outer canthus of the eye. It produces tears as a continuous process to provide a protective multilayer fluid film across the front of the eyeball. Excess production of tears occurs in response to the presence of foreign bodies, eye injury, inflammation and intense emotions. ⇒ dacryocyst.

**lacrimation** *n* a flow of tears; weeping.

**lacrimonasal** *adj* pertaining to the lacrimal and nasal bones and ducts.

**lactacid (lactic) anaerobic system** a series of chemical reactions occurring within the cells whereby a very small amount of adenosine triphosphate (ATP) for energy use is produced from glucose, without oxygen. The end-product is lactic acid.

**lactacid oxygen debt component** the amount of oxygen required to remove lactic acid from muscle tissue and blood during the process of recovery from intense exercise.

**lactalbumin** *n* one of the whey proteins found in milk. The proportion of protein as lactalbumin is higher in human milk than in cows' milk.

**lactase** *n* (*syn* β-galactosidase) digestive enzyme present in the small intestine mucosa. It catalyses the hydrolysis of lactose to glucose and galactose.

**lactase deficiency** an inherited or acquired deficiency of lactase. Common in African–Caribbean and Asian individuals. Consumption of lactose (milk sugar) results in colic, diarrhoea, bloating and increased flatus. May be acquired in small intestinal conditions such as coeliac disease and Crohn's disease. It may occur temporarily after a gastrointestinal tract infection. The management depends on severity and may involve the exclusion or restriction of lactose-containing foods. Various lactose-free products, such as infant formula milks, are available on prescription in the UK.

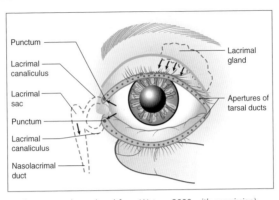

**Figure L.1** Lacrimal apparatus *(reproduced from Watson 2000 with permission)*.

**lactate dehydrogenase (LDH)** an enzyme, of which there are five isoenzymes, that catalyses the interconversion of lactate and pyruvate in the myocardium, skeletal muscle and the liver. The level of lactate dehydrogenase in the serum increases rapidly following necrosis of metabolically active tissue, such as after myocardial infarction.

**lactate threshold ($T_{LAC}$)** the point reached when blood lactate accumulation increases in a non-linear manner in response to progressive physical exertion. ⇒ anaerobic threshold.

**lactation** *n* **1.** production and secretion of milk from the breasts. **2.** the period during which an infant receives nourishment from breast milk.

**lacteals** *npl* the commencing lymphatic ducts in the intestinal villi; they absorb the milky-white fluid chyle that contains digested fats and convey them to the cisterna chyli.

**lactic** *adj* relating to milk.

**lactic acid** a three-carbon organic acid formed from the fermentation of lactose (milk sugar). It is produced when glucose is metabolized anaerobically in vigorously contracting skeletal muscle. Lactic acid is responsible for muscle fatigue occurring during very-high-intensity exercise. The cramp and muscle aches felt the day after exercise may result from a build-up of lactic acid in the muscles.

**lactic acidosis** results from a build-up of lactic acid in the blood and consequent reduction in pH. It is associated with conditions that cause tissue hypoxia, such as shock caused by sepsis, respiratory failure, severe anaemia and poisoning with carbon monoxide. This type of acidosis

is also seen in patients with type 2 diabetes mellitus who are treated with a biguanide hypoglycaemic drug such as metformin. Other causes include liver failure, toxins (e.g. alcohol) and some drugs (e.g. salicylates).

**lactiferous** *adj* conveying or secreting milk. The *lactiferous glands*, the glandular tissue of the alveoli of the breast lobules, produce milk when stimulated by the hormone prolactin. The *lactiferous ducts/tubules* convey milk from the breast lobes to the centre of the breast where they dilate to form temporary reservoirs for milk; these are often described as the *lactiferous sinuses (ampullae)* from which milk flows to the surface of the nipple.

**lactifuge** *n* an agent that decreases the production and secretion of milk.

***Lactobacillus*** *n* a genus of non-pathogenic bacteria. A large Gram-positive rod which ferments carbohydrates, producing lactic acid. They form part of the normal flora of the body, such as in the intestinal tract or the vagina during the reproductive years. ⇒ Döderlein's bacillus.

**lactoferrin** *n* an iron-binding protein with antimicrobial properties. It is a component of non-specific (innate) body defences and is found in colostrum and mature breast milk, saliva, tears and in some white blood cells.

**lactogenic** *adj* stimulating milk production. ⇒ prolactin.

**lacto-ovovegetarian** *adj* describes a diet consisting of milk, milk products, eggs, grain, pulses, fruit and vegetables, but no meat, poultry or fish.

**lactose** *n* milk sugar. A disaccharide of glucose and galactose found in all types of mammalian milk. Less soluble and less sweet than ordinary sugar. *lactose intolerance* ⇒ lactase deficiency.

**lactosuria** *n* the presence of lactose in the urine.

**lactovegetarian** *adj* describes a diet consisting of milk, milk products, grain, pulses, fruit and vegetables, but no meat, poultry, fish or eggs.

**lactulose** *n* a disaccharide that is not absorbed and reaches the colon unchanged. Used as an osmotic laxative. ⇒ Appendix 5.

**lacuna** *n* a space between cells; usually used in the description of bone—**lacunae** *pl*, **lacunar** *adj*.

**laetrile** *n* a substance obtained from apricot stones. It is mostly amygdalin (cyanide-containing glycoside) and was thought by some to have anticancer properties. Research to date has failed to demonstrate any benefits. Also known as 'vitamin B$_{17}$', although it is not a vitamin.

**lagophthalmos** *n* a condition whereby the eyes do not fully close. There is increased risk of corneal damage.

**LAK cells** *abbr* lymphokine-activated killer cells.

**lallation** *n* **1.** speech disorder characterized by problems with pronunciation in which the person uses a child-like substitution of sounds, such as using 'l' in place of 'r' sounds. **2.** unintelligible, repetitive babbling such as in an infant. It may be a feature in some people with a learning disability or in those with serious mental health problems.

**lambda** *n* **1.** The 11th letter of the Greek alphabet (Λ, λ). **2.** The apex of the occipital bone of the skull where the sagittal and lambdoidal sutures unite.

**lambdoidal** *adj* the suture between the occipital and parietal bones of the skull. ⇒ fontanelle.

**lambliasis** *n* ⇒ giardiasis.

**lamella** *n* **1.** a thin plate-like scale or partition. **2.** a gelatin-coated disc containing a drug; it is inserted under the eyelid—**lamellae** *pl*, **lamellar** *adj*.

**lamina** *n* a thin plate or layer, usually of bone. *lamina propria* thin layer of connective tissue situated beneath the epithelium of a mucous membrane—**laminae** *pl*.

**laminate veneer reconstruction** conservative technique undertaken to improve the appearance of the anterior teeth. Materials that include composite resin veneers and acrylic resins are bonded on to the teeth to disguise staining/discoloration, restore malformed teeth, correct minor misalignment and deal with diastemas.

**laminectomy** *n* removal of vertebral laminae—to expose the spinal cord nerve roots and meninges. Most often performed in the lumbar region, for removal of degenerated intervertebral disc.

**Lancefield's groups** (R Lancefield, American bacteriologist, 1895–1981) a serological classification of the bacteria of the genus *Streptococcus* on the basis of antigenic structure. Individual species are allocated to 13 groups on the basis of their characteristic capsular polysaccharide. The streptococci that cause most infections in humans belong to Lancefield group A.

**lancet** *n* a device with a short pointed blade used to obtain capillary blood samples. For example, to obtain blood for checking glucose levels, or for checking haemoglobin prior to the donation of blood.

**lancinating** *adj* describes a cutting, stabbing pain.

**Langerhans' cells** (P Langerhans, German pathologist, 1847–1888) dendritic cells in the epidermis that are part of the biological barrier formed by the skin. They act as antigen-presenting cells, thereby protecting the body from micro-organisms that breach the chemical and physical barriers.

**Langerhans' cell histiocytosis** formally known as histiocytosis X. A group of disorders characterized by the proliferation of histiocytes and the presence of granulomatous changes that mainly affect the lungs and bones. ⇒ Hand–Schüller–Christian disease, histiocytosis, Letterer–Siwe disease.

**Langer's lines** (C von Langer, Austrian anatomist, 1819–1887) a pattern of cleavage lines in the skin. Surgical incisions made parallel to the cleavage lines heal with less scarring than do incisions and other wounds that cross the lines.

**language** *n* a system of communication based on symbols or letters and gestures. The usual interpretation involves verbal language (spoken and written) that uses an 'alphabet' of letters or symbols from which many thousands of words can be formed. Particular groups of people, such as health professionals, may construct a verbal language including jargon to explain their work and inadvertently confuse and exclude clients and patients.

**lanolin** *n* the fat from sheep's wool. Added to ointment bases, as such bases can form water-in-oil emulsions with aqueous constituents,

L

and are readily absorbed by the skin. Contact sensitivity to preparations containing lanolin may develop.

**lanugo** *n* the soft, downy hair sometimes present on newborn infants, especially when they are premature. Usually replaced before birth by vellus hair. ⇒ terminal hair, vellus hair.

**laparoscope** *n* an endoscope used to examine the peritoneal cavity.

**laparoscopy** *n* (*syn* peritoneoscopy) endoscopic examination of the internal organs by the transperitoneal route. A laparoscope is introduced through the abdominal wall after induction of a pneumoperitoneum. A variety of surgical procedures are performed in this way, including biopsy, cyst aspiration, division of adhesions, tubal ligation, assisted conception techniques, appendicectomy and cholecystectomy—**laparoscopic** *adj*, **laparoscopically** *adv*.

**laparotomy** *n* incision of the abdominal wall. Usually the term is reserved for an exploratory operation.

**Larsen's syndrome** (L Larsen, American orthopaedic surgeon, b. 1914) congenital condition characterized by multiple joint dislocations, cleft palate and other skeletal abnormalities.

**larva** *n* an embryo that is independent before developing the characteristic features of its parents.

**larva migrans** itching tracks in the skin with formation of blisters; caused by the burrowing of larvae of some species of fly, and the normally animal-infesting *Ancylostoma*—**larvae** *pl*, **larval** *adj*.

**larval therapy** maggot therapy or biological débridement. The use of sterile blowfly (*Lucilia serricata*) larvae in the débridement of some chronic wounds. Enzymes produced by the larvae break down slough and necrotic tissue, thus providing the conditions for the wound to heal.

**larvicide** *n* any agent which destroys larvae—**larvicidal** *adj*.

**laryngeal** *adj* pertaining to the larynx.

**laryngeal mask airway (LMA)** airway with inflatable cuff placed via the mouth into the oropharynx to maintain the airway during general anaesthesia (Figure L.2). It is used for spontaneously breathing patients or where help with ventilation is appropriate and can be maintained. An LMA is not suitable in all situations, for instance, when patients are repositioned during surgery, which could

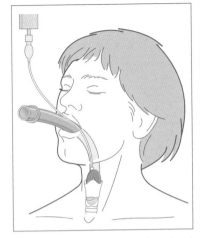

**Figure L.2** Laryngeal mask airway *(reproduced from Brooker & Nicol 2003 with permission).*

dislodge the mask. Furthermore, an LMA is not appropriate when there is a high risk of regurgitation and aspiration of gastric contents, such as in emergency surgery, or in obstetric emergencies.

**laryngectomy** *n* surgical removal of the larynx. Usually for cancer.

**laryngismus** *n* spasm of the larynx. *laryngismus stridulus* sudden laryngeal spasm with closure of the glottis. It is characterized by crowing sounds, respiratory distress and a period of apnoea. It is associated with the administration of an anaesthetic, inflammation, foreign bodies and hypocalcaemia of childhood rickets. ⇒ croup.

**laryngitis** *n* inflammation of the mucosal lining of the larynx. It may be acute, which often follows an acute upper respiratory tract infection. It can be serious in small children who may develop respiratory distress. ⇒ croup, laryngotracheobronchitis. Chronic laryngitis often follows a cold or influenza but precipitating factors include sudden changes in environmental temperature, chronic sinusitis, smoking, exposure to irritant fumes, drinking alcohol and overuse of the voice. It is characterized by hoarseness, dysphonia or aphonia (complete voice loss), sore throat and cough.

**laryngocele** *n* the presence of an air-filled sac/cavity that communicates with the larynx.

**laryngologist** *n* a specialist in disorders of the larynx.

**laryngology** *n* the study of disorders affecting the larynx.

**laryngoparalysis** *n* paralysis of the larynx.

**laryngopharyngectomy** *n* excision of the larynx and part of the pharynx. Usually performed for cancers involving the pharynx, larynx and adjacent structures in the throat.

**laryngopharynx** *n* the hypopharynx. The lower portion of the pharynx below the oropharynx, it gives passage to food and fluids into the oesophagus—**laryngopharyngeal** *adj*.

**laryngoscope** *n* instrument for visualization of the larynx, for diagnostic or therapeutic purposes or to facilitate the insertion of an endotracheal tube into the larynx under direct vision—**laryngoscopic** *adj*.

**laryngoscopy** *n* direct or indirect visual examination of the interior of the larynx.

**laryngospasm** *n* convulsive involuntary muscular contraction of the larynx, usually accompanied by spasmodic closure of the glottis, which prevents air entering the respiratory tract.

**laryngostenosis** *n* narrowing of the glottic aperture.

**laryngotomy** *n* surgical opening in the larynx.

**laryngotracheal** *adj* pertaining to the larynx and trachea.

**laryngotracheitis** *n* inflammation of the mucosal lining of the larynx and trachea.

**laryngotracheobronchitis** *n* inflammation (usually viral) of the mucosal lining of the larynx, trachea and bronchi. May be very serious when it occurs in small children. ⇒ croup.

**laryngotracheoplasty** *n* surgical opening of a stenosed larynx—**laryngotracheoplastic** *adj*.

**larynx** *n* the organ of voice situated below and in front of the pharynx and at the upper end of the trachea. A cartilaginous box formed from nine cartilages (e.g. epiglottis, thyroid, cricoid, arytenoid [2], corniculate [2] and cuneiform [2]), ligaments (e.g. thyrohyoid) and membranes. Inspired air passes through an opening between the vocal folds (vocal cords) and the glottis before entering the trachea. During swallowing several mechanisms prevent food or fluids from entering the trachea and bronchi, for example the upward movement of the larynx which causes the epiglottis to occlude the opening into the larynx. The two vocal folds (vocal cords), which are attached at the front and the back of the larynx, produce sound. (⇒ Appendix 1, Figure 6)—**laryngeal** *adj*.

**laser** *acron* **l**ight **a**mplification by **s**timulated **e**mission of **r**adiation. Energy is transmitted as heat which can coagulate tissue. Has many therapeutic uses that include: endometrial ablation, repair of detached retina, skin lesions and cancer treatments. Health and safety precautions must be taken by those using lasers as eye damage can occur.

**laser-assisted uvulopalatoplasty (LAUP)** the use of lasers to modify the palate in order to relieve obstructive sleep apnoea. ⇒ sleep apnoea (hypopnoea) syndrome.

**laser Doppler flowmeter** a device that utilizes laser technology to measure blood flow.

**LASIK** *abbr* laser in situ keratomileusis. A technique for correcting refractive errors—hypermetropia, myopia or astigmatism. A thin flap of cornea is raised using a microkeratome, prior to reshaping the surface beneath the flap with an excimer laser. Complications may include infections, problems with the flap, night glare, dry eyes and a failure to correct the refractive error (under- or overcorrection).

**Lassa fever** one of the serious viral haemorrhagic fevers. Occurs as isolated cases and small outbreaks, usually in West Africa. The incubation period is 3–16 days; early symptoms resemble typhoid and septicaemia. Mortality is as high as 80%. Strict isolation is required for infected people.

**Lassar's paste** contains zinc oxide, starch and salicylic acid in soft paraffin. Used in hyperkeratotic skin conditions.

**latent period** also known as incubation period. The period of time between exposure to a micro-organism or other agent and the development of symptoms.

**lateral** *adj* at or belonging to the side; away from the median line—**laterally** *adv*.

**latex allergy** an allergic reaction to natural latex or one of the components used in production of latex equipment such as medical gloves and catheters. Latex allergy is increasingly common in patients having repeated invasive interventions, and in health care workers, due to the increased use of gloves as a control of infection measure, particularly following the rise in the incidence of bloodborne viruses.

**latissimus dorsi** large triangular muscle of the lower back. It attaches indirectly via the lumbodorsal fascia into the spines of the lower thoracic and lumbar vertebrae, lower ribs and iliac crest and inserts on to the humerus. It is the prime mover of arm extension. Also causes medial rotation of the arm at the shoulder and is important in arm adduction. ⇒ Appendix 1, Figures 4 and 5.

**laughing gas** ⇒ nitrous oxide.

**LAUP** *abbr* laser-assisted uvulopalatoplasty

**lavage** *n* irrigation of or washing out a body cavity, for example, the stomach, colon, bladder, paranasal sinus, etc.

**LAVH** *abbr* laparoscopic-assisted vaginal hysterectomy. ⇒ hysterectomy.

**laxatives** *npl* (*syn* aperients) drugs used to prevent or treat constipation. Administered orally, or rectally as suppositories or by enema. They may be: bulking agents that retain water and form a large, soft stool; faecal softeners that lubricate or soften the faeces; osmotic laxatives that increase fluid in the bowel lumen; stimulants that increase peristalsis, and combined softeners and stimulants. ⇒ Appendix 5.

**LBC** *abbr* liquid-based cytology.

**LBW** *abbr* low birth weight.

**LD$_{50}$** *abbr* lethal dose in 50% of a population.

**LDH** *abbr* lactate dehydrogenase.

**LDL** *abbr* low-density lipoprotein.

**LE** *abbr* lupus erythematosus. ⇒ systemic lupus erythematosus.

**lead (Pb)** *n* a soft metal with toxic salts. *lead poisoning* (*syn* plumbism) acute poisoning is unusual, but chronic poisoning due to absorption of small amounts over time does occur. For example, young children who suck objects painted with lead paint or made from lead alloys. Lead can be ingested from drinking water contaminated from lead pipes, or from cooking utensils. Abnormally high levels of lead in the environment have been linked to the use of lead in petrol. Presentation varies and may include: abdominal pain, diarrhoea and vomiting, anorexia, anaemia, and the formation of a characteristic blue line round the gums. Neurological manifestations, including convulsions, may occur in severe poisoning.

**Leadbetter–Politano operation** an antireflux procedure by tunnelled reimplantation of the ureter into the urinary bladder.

**lead-pipe rigidity** increased resistance to passive stretch in any direction that is uniform throughout the whole movement, characteristic of Parkinson's disease. ⇒ cogwheel rigidity.

**learned non-use** a situation that can occur when individuals have some recovery in a limb affected, for example, by a stroke. They do not use the limb functionally because they have learnt not to and are not using the motor ability present in activities of daily living.

**learning** *n* **1.** in psychology, the change in behaviour that occurs through training, practice or experience. **2.** specific knowledge, attitudes and/or skills gained through instruction or a course of study. **3.** the activity or process of gaining knowledge.

**learning disability** a general term used to describe the inability to develop intellectually. Individuals may often have problems integrating into society. Learning disability encompasses many conditions, ranging from specific learning disorders such as dyslexia, through to problems of global intellectual impairment.

**learning outcomes** the specific quantifiable results that can be expected to follow involvement in a learning opportunity. Outcomes may focus on cognitive (knowledge), affective (attitudes) or behavioural (skills) aspects that furnish evidence that learning has been achieved.

**learning strategy** the manner in which people approach a learning exercise.

**learning style** the ways in which a person usually thinks, solves problems and remembers new knowledge.

**leather-bottle stomach** ⇒ linitis plastica.

**Leber hereditary optic neuropathy** a condition inherited via mitochondrial DNA that generally affects adult males. It presents with subacute central vision loss caused by degeneration of the optic nerve and the retinal ganglion cells.

**Leber's congenital amaurosis** (T Leber, German ophthalmologist, 1840–1917) a rare condition causing blindness or seriously impaired vision; inherited as an autosomal recessive disorder. The eyes may appear normal at birth but results from electroretinography are abnormal.

**lecithinase** *n* enzyme that catalyses the decomposition of lecithin.

**lecithins** *npl* phosphatidylcholines. A group of phospholipids found in animal tissues. They form a vital component of cell membranes and are involved in the metabolism of fats. They are present in the liver, semen and nervous tissue. Its presence in pulmonary surfactant reduces surface tension and facilitates the exchange of gases in the alveoli.

**lecithin–sphingomyelin ratio (LS)** the ratio of the two substances in the amniotic fluid is used to assess the degree of fetal lung maturity. An unfavourable ratio is indicative of a higher risk of neonatal respiratory distress syndrome.

**lectins** *npl* proteins from legumes such as red kidney beans, and other plants. They bind to the glycolipids and glycoproteins present on animal cell surfaces and can agglutinate red blood cells (erythrocytes) of certain blood groups. Previously known as phytoagglutinins or haemagglutinins.

**leech** *n* *Hirudo medicinalis*. An aquatic worm which can be applied to the human body to suck blood and thereby reduce congestion. Its saliva contains hirudin, an anticoagulant. Used after reconstructive surgery to reduce the congestion and swelling that may compromise the blood supply.

**Le Fort classification** (R Le Fort, French surgeon, 1869–1951) a classification of fractures that involve the upper jaw (maxilla) and the orbit.

**left ventricular assist device (LVAD)** mechanical pump used to increase the output of blood from the left ventricle of the heart. May be used in the short term to support critically ill patients, those waiting for a heart transplant, or to give the heart muscle time to recover from disease.

**leg** *n* lower limb. *leg length discrepancy* a difference of up to 1 cm in true length is considered to be within a normal variation. The effects of discrepancy may either cause a compensatory pelvic tilt and secondary spinal scoliosis, or will force the person to walk on the toes in order to lengthen the leg. The latter will, in time, result in shortening of the Achilles tendon.

**leg ulcer** a wound on the leg, which can be associated with a variety of aetiologies. The vast majority of leg ulcers have a venous aetiology; fewer than 10% have an arterial cause; some ulcers have a mixed venous and arterial aetiology; and a few are associated with other diseases. ⇒ arterial ulcer, venous ulcer.

**Legg–Calvé–Perthes disease** (A Legg, American surgeon, 1874–1939; J Calvé, French orthopaedic surgeon, 1875–1954; G Perthes, German surgeon, 1869–1927) avascular necrosis affecting the upper femoral epiphysis and the head of the femur during childhood. It is usually unilateral and most common in boys from the age of 5 years up to 10 years of age. The child has pain and a limp. Revascularization occurs, but residual deformity of the femoral head may subsequently lead

to arthritic changes. Also known as Perthes' disease.

***Legionella pneumophila*** a small Gram-negative bacillus which causes legionnaires' disease and Pontiac fever.

**legionnaires' disease** a severe and often fatal pneumonia caused by *Legionella pneumophila*; there is pneumonia, dry cough, and often non-pulmonary involvement such as gastrointestinal symptoms, renal impairment and confusion. A cause of both community- and hospital-acquired pneumonia, it is associated with an infected water supply in public buildings such as hospitals and hotels. There is no person-to-person spread.

**legumen** *n* the protein present in peas, beans and lentils.

**legumes** *npl* pulse vegetables—e.g. peas, beans, lentils. Provides valuable protein, B vitamins and iron and soluble dietary fibre. An essential component of a vegetarian and vegan diet but also very useful for people whose diet does contain meat and fish and other animal products.

**Leiden abnormality** ⇒ factor V Leiden, thrombophilia.

**Leigh's disease** (A Leigh, British neuropathologist, b. 1915) a rare inherited disorder that leads to the degeneration of the central nervous system. The disease may be the result of a deficiency of the enzyme pyruvate dehydrogenase, or because of mutations in the DNA found within the mitochondria. Signs of the disease, which progresses rapidly, are usually noticed between the ages of 3 months and 2 years. It is characterized by poor feeding, anorexia, vomiting, deteriorating motor skills, poor head control, irritability and seizures. Later there may be poor muscle tone, weakness and metabolic problems (lactic acidosis) that affect the respiratory system, kidneys and the heart. The prognosis is very poor and most children die within a few years.

**leiomyoma** *n* a benign tumour affecting smooth (involuntary) muscle. Very common benign tumour of the female reproductive tract, where they are generally known informally as fibroids or fibromyoma, as they contain both fibrous connective tissue and muscle tissue. ⇒ fibroid. Leiomyomas also occur in the gastrointestinal tract—**leiomyomas, leiomyomata** *pl*.

**leiomyosarcoma** *n* a rare malignant tumour of smooth muscle tissue. They occur in the myometrium of the uterus, in the stomach and intestine.

**Leishman–Donovan bodies** (W Leishman, British pathologist, 1865–1926; C Donovan, Irish physician, 1863–1951) the rounded resting stage of the protozoan parasite *Leishmania* found in certain cells, e.g. macrophages, of individuals with leishmaniasis.

*Leishmania* *n* genus of flagellated parasitic protozoa. *Leishmania donovani* causes leishmaniasis.

**leishmaniasis** *n* infestation by *Leishmania*, spread by sandflies. Generalized (visceral) manifestation is kala-azar. Old World cutaneous forms are called an oriental sore. New World cutaneous forms may involve the nasal and oral mucosa and the lesion is called an espundia.

**leisure** *n* those activities in which a person chooses to participate during time allocated specially for the activity. The activities are very varied and chosen because they have meaning for the person and are pleasurable, relaxing, allow opportunities for personal fulfilment and achieving ambitions, and have other attributes of worth to the person, such as an activity that includes the whole family.

**lemniscus** *n* a band-like tract of nerve fibres in the central nervous system.

**lens** *n* **1.** the small biconvex crystalline body which is supported by the suspensory ligament immediately behind the iris of the eye (⇒ Appendix 1, Figure 15). On account of its elasticity, the lens can alter in shape, enabling light rays to focus exactly on the retina. **2.** glass or plastic used to correct refractive errors (spectacles or contact lens) or in optical instruments. ⇒ bifocal lens, contact lens.

**lenticonus** *n* an abnormal protrusion on the lens of the eye. Present in Alport's syndrome.

**lenticular** *adj* pertaining to or resembling a lens.

**lenticular nucleus** a biconvex part of the basal nuclei (basal ganglia).

**lentigo** *n* a freckle with an increased number of pigment cells. ⇒ ephelides—**lentigines** *pl*.

**leontiasis** *n* enlargement of the face and head giving a lion-like appearance; associated with some types of leprosy.

**leprologist** *n* one who specializes in the study and treatment of leprosy.

**leprology** *n* the study of leprosy and its treatment.

**lepromata** *npl* the granulomatous cutaneous eruption of leprosy—**leproma** *sing*, **lepromatous** *adj*.

**leprosy (Hansen's disease)** *n* a chronic and contagious disease, endemic in warmer climates and characterized by granulomatous formation in the peripheral nerves or on the skin, mucous membranes and bones with tissue destruction. Caused by *Mycobacterium leprae* (Hansen's bacillus). Bacille Calmette–Guérin (BCG) vaccination conferred variable protection in different trials. Management includes specific care, such as that required for impaired sensation, and long-term treatment with various antimicrobial drugs, including dapsone and rifampicin—**leprous** *adj*.

**leptin** *n* a peptide hormone secreted by adipocytes, which controls appetite and energy use by signalling information about the amount of body fat reserves.

**leptocyte** *n* ⇒ target cell.

**leptomeninges** *npl* the pia and arachnoid mater combined.

**leptophonia** *n* ⇒ hypophonia.

*Leptospira* *n* a genus of bacteria. Very thin, finely coiled bacteria. Common in water as saprophytes; pathogenic species are numerous in many animals. *Leptospira interrogans* serotype *icterohaemorrhagiae* causes Weil's disease in humans; *Leptospira interrogans* serotype *canicola* infects dogs and pigs, and is transmissible to humans. ⇒ leptospirosis.

**leptospiral agglutination tests** serological tests used to diagnose specific leptospiral infections, e.g. Weil's disease.

**leptospirosis** *n* infection of humans by bacteria of the *Leptospira* group found in rats and other rodents, cattle, dogs, pigs and foxes. Those at risk include abattoir and agricultural workers and water sports enthusiasts. Presentation varies according to which leptospira is responsible, but may include: high fever, headache, conjunctival congestion, rash, anorexia, jaundice, severe muscular pains, rigors and vomiting. Severe infections may cause hepatitis, myocarditis, renal tubular necrosis and, less frequently, meningitis with an associated mortality rate of up to 20%. ⇒ Weil's disease.

**Leriche's syndrome** (R Leriche, French surgeon, 1879–1955) a syndrome caused by gradual blockage of the distal aorta. It is characterized by intermittent claudication felt in the buttocks, thighs and lower legs; erectile dysfunction; absent femoral pulses; muscle wastage; cold pale legs and gangrenous toes. Management includes restoring blood flow through the aorta and iliac arteries, e.g. endarterectomy, bypass graft.

**lesbianism** *n* sexual attraction between women.

**Lesch–Nyhan disease** (M Lesch, American paediatrician, b. 1939; W Nyhan, American paediatrician, b. 1926) X-linked recessive genetic disorder. Overproduction of uric acid, associated with brain damage, resulting in cerebral palsy and learning disability. Victims are compelled, by a self-destructive urge, to bite away the sides of their mouth, lips and fingers.

**lesion** *n* pathological change in a bodily tissue.

**lethal dose 50% (LD$_{50}$)** the amount of a substance, such as a drug, that produces death in 50% of the members of a species population when administered as a single dose, within a set time.

**Letterer–Siwe disease** (E Letterer, German pathologist, 1895–1982; S Siwe, Swedish physician, 1897–1966) a disseminated form of Langerhans' cell histiocytosis that affects young children. There is infiltration of the lungs and bones, skin lesions, hepatosplenomegaly and lymphadenopathy.

**leucine** *n* an essential (indispensable) branched-chain amino acid.

**leucocytes** *npl* generic name for white blood cells. They are nucleated, mobile and are all involved with body defences, e.g. some are phagocytic and others produce antibodies. There are two main groups: (a) polymorphonuclear cells or granulocytes (neutrophils, basophils and eosinophils)—these have a many-lobed nucleus and granules in their cytoplasm; (b) monocytes and lymphocytes—these generally have no granules, but some lymphocytes are granular.

**leucocytolysis** *n* destruction and disintegration of white blood cells—**leucocytolytic** *adj*.

**leucocytosis** *n* increased number of leucocytes in the blood. Often a response to infection—**leucocytotic** *adj*.

**leucodepletion** *n* the removal of white blood cells from donated blood for transfusion in order to reduce the risk of transmitting variant Creutzfeldt–Jakob disease.

**leucoderma** *n* absent skin pigmentation, especially when it occurs in patches or bands.

**leucoma** *n* white opaque spot on the cornea—**leucomata** *pl*.

**leuconychia** *n* white areas on the nails. These may be dots, lines, or extend over the entire nail plate (totalis). They are usually indicative of minor trauma, e.g. resulting from short shoes or sporting activities.

**leucopenia** *n* decreased number of white blood cells in the blood—**leucopenic** *adj*.

**leucopheresis** *n* donated blood is separated into its components and the white cells are retained before the remaining blood is returned to the donor. The white cells so obtained are used in the treatment of severe neutropenia.

**leucopoiesis** *n* formation of white blood cells from stem cells. Regulated by colony-stimulating factors and cytokines—**leucopoietic** *adj*.

**leucorrhoea** *n* a sticky, whitish vaginal discharge—**leucorrhoeal** *adj*.

**leukaemia** *n* a group of neoplastic diseases of the haematopoietic tissue with most commonly abnormal proliferation of immature white blood cells (leucocytes). Uncontrolled proliferation of the leukaemic cells causes secondary suppression of other blood components, and anaemia and thrombocytopenia result. The lack of mature neutrophils (polymorphonuclear white blood cells) increases the risk of infection, thrombocytopenia increases the risk of bleeding, and anaemia may be severe. Causes include ionizing radiation, previous cytotoxic chemotherapy, retroviruses (e.g. human T-cell lymphotropic virus), chemicals, such as benzene, and genetic anomalies (e.g. Down's syndrome). The classification is according to cell type—lymphocytic or myelocytic—and the course is acute or chronic. Acute leukaemias have a rapid onset and early immature cells are produced (blast cells), commonly of the lymphoid and myeloid series. The acute leukaemias include acute lymphoblastic leukaemia (ALL) in children and acute myeloblastic leukaemia (AML) in adults. Chronic leukaemias have an insidious onset and the cells produced are more mature, commonly lymphocytes and granulocytes. Chronic forms can become acute with blast cell proliferation. Chronic leukaemias include chronic lymphocytic leukaemia (CLL) and chronic myeloid (granulocytic) leukaemia (CML), both of which affect adults. The chronic leukaemias may enter a 'blast crisis' or acute phase. Less common leukaemias include: monocytic, eosinophilic, basophilic and hairy cell. The management of leukaemia depends upon the cell type, whether acute or chronic, and the aim of treatment—remission or palliation. Therapeutic options include chemotherapy, radiotherapy, interferon-alpha, monoclonal antibodies and haemopoietic stem cell transplantation, either autologous or allograft, plus supportive measures that include antimicrobial drugs, blood components transfusion and protective isolation. ⇒ myeloproliferative disorders.

**leukocidins** *npl* exotoxins produced by streptococci and staphylococci. They cause white blood cell lysis and death. ⇒ Panton–Valentine leukocidin.

**leukoplakia** *n* white, thickened patch occurring on mucous membranes. Occurs on lips, inside mouth or on genitalia. Usually patchy and often premalignant. ⇒ kraurosis vulvae.

**leukotrienes** *npl* regulatory lipids derived from arachidonic acid (fatty acid). They function as signalling molecules in the inflammatory response and in some allergic responses.

**leukotriene receptor antagonists** drugs such as montelukast and zafirlukast that block the effects of leukotrienes in the airways by blocking the leukotriene receptors. Used in the management of asthma. ⇒ Appendix 5.

**levator** *n* **1.** a muscle which acts by raising a part. *levator scapulae*. ⇒ Appendix 1, Figure 5. **2.** an instrument for lifting a depressed part.

**Levin tube** (A Levin, American physician, 1880–1940) a plastic catheter used for gastric intubation; it has a closed weighted tip and an opening on the side.

**Lewy bodies** (F Lewy, German neurologist, 1885–1950) inclusion bodies found in damaged and dying nerve cells in the brain that is the pathological hallmark of Parkinson's disease. Also present in Lewy-body dementia, Alzheimer's disease and other neurodegenerative disease.

**Leydig cells** (F von Leydig, German anatomist, 1821–1908) ⇒ interstitial cells.

**LGVCFT** *abbr* lymphogranuloma venereum complement fixation test.

**LH** *abbr* luteinizing hormone.

**Lhermitte's sign** (J Lhermitte, French neurologist, 1877–1959) sudden electric shock-like sensations moving down the body when the head is flexed. It is indicative of compression of the cervical spinal cord or multiple sclerosis.

**libido** *n* Freud's term for the urge to obtain sensual satisfaction. Sometimes used to mean the sexual urge. Freud's meaning was satisfaction through all the senses.

**lice** *n* ⇒ pediculus.

**lichen** *n* aggregations of papular skin lesions— **lichenoid** *adj*.

**lichenification** *n* thickening of the skin, usually secondary to scratching. Skin markings become more prominent and the affected area appears to be composed of small, shiny rhomboids. ⇒ neurodermatitis.

**lichen nitidus** skin disorder characterized by minute, shiny, flat-topped, pink papules of pin-head size.

**lichen planus** a skin eruption of unknown cause showing purplish, angulated, shiny, flat-topped papules. ⊙ DVD

**lichen scrofulosorum** a form of tuberculide.

**lichen simplex** ⇒ neurodermatitis.

**Lieberkühn's glands** (J Lieberkühn, German anatomist, 1711–1756) also called crypts of Lieberkühn. Tubular intestinal glands.

**lien** *n* the spleen.

**lienculus** *n* a small accessory spleen.

**lienorenal** *adj* pertaining to the spleen and kidney. ⇒ splenorenal.

**life crisis** describes an unforeseen unpleasant occurrence, such as becoming the victim of a violent crime, sudden and severe ill health or a life event, e.g. marriage or divorce, becoming unemployed, retirement.

**life event** in sociology a term describing the major occurrences occurring during the lifespan, such as starting school, getting married or ending a relationship, changing job, moving house, or suffering a bereavement.

**life expectancy** the average age at which death occurs. Influenced by health/illness and by social factors such as level of education; and environmental factors such as housing, sanitation and the supply of clean water.

**lifelong learning** learning throughout the person's lifespan. Particularly important for health professionals who are required to update their knowledge and skills in order to fulfil the conditions set for periodic registration and licence to practise by their statutory regulation body.

**life-years gained** the average years of life gained per patient from a particular health care intervention. ⇒ quality-adjusted life years.

**lifestyle planning** techniques used in occupational therapy practice that enable an individual to achieve a balance between occupational roles in order to reduce stress, improve quality of life, develop potentials and attain relevant personal goals. Activity analysis is used to determine the occupational performance skills required and activities are recommended that are consistent with the individual's priorities and anticipated abilities.

**LFTs** *abbr* liver function tests.

**Li–Fraumeni syndrome** (F Li, American epidemiologist, 20th century; J Fraumeni, American epidemiologist, 20th century) also known by other names, for example, sarcoma, breast, leukaemia and adrenal gland (SBLA) syndrome. A very rare inherited condition that significantly increases the risk of developing several different cancers during childhood and early adulthood. These include cancers of the breast, brain, adrenal gland, osteosarcoma, soft-tissue sarcoma and leukaemia. It is inherited as an autosomal dominant condition and many of those affected inherit a mutation of the TP53 gene, which normally acts as a tumour suppressor gene. Mutations of the CHEK2 gene, another tumour suppressor gene, may be associated with an increased risk of a certain cancer, such as breast cancer.

**ligament** *n* a strong band of fibrous tissue serving to bind bones or other parts together, or to support an organ—**ligamentous** *adj*.

**ligand** *n* signalling chemicals that include cytokines, hormones or neurotransmitters. They can affect cell function by binding to specific cell membrane receptors. Many drugs cause their effects by being able to imitate the natural ligand.

**ligate** *vt* to tie off blood vessels, etc., at operation—**ligation** *n*.

**ligation** *n* tying off; usually reserved for *ligation of the uterine (fallopian) tubes*, a method of sterilization.

**ligature** *n* the material used for tying vessels or stitching the tissues. ⇒ suture.

**light adaptation** adjustments made by the eye in bright light. The pupils constrict, rhodopsin breakdown reduces retinal sensitivity and cone activity increases. ⇒ dark adaptation.

**lightening** *n* an informal term used to denote the relief of pressure on the diaphragm by the abdominal viscera, when the presenting part of the fetus descends into the pelvis in the last 3 weeks of a primigravida's pregnancy.

**lightning pains** symptomatic of tabes dorsalis. Occur as paroxysms of swift-cutting (lightning) stabs in the lower limbs.

**lignans** *npl* compounds present in various foods. They display both oestrogenic and anti-oestrogenic properties. ⇒ phyto-oestrogens.

**lignin** *n* lignocellulose. The indigestible part of the plant cell wall.

**Likert scale** (described by R Likert in 1932) a scale used in questionnaire surveys. Participants are asked to specify their degree of agreement with a particular statement, i.e. strongly agree, agree, unsure, disagree and strongly disagree.

**limbic system** a diffuse collection of nuclei and nerve fibres in an area within the cerebral hemispheres. Its structures include the hippocampus, hypothalamus, amygdala and part of the thalamus. It is part of the 'primitive' brain, formed from evolutionarily older cortex. Concerned with autonomic functions, feelings and emotions such as anger, rage, sadness, sexual arousal and pleasure. Also associated with the sense of smell and memories associated with a particular smell, motivation and memory.

**limbus** *n* in ophthalmology the circumference of the cornea at which it joins the sclera.

**liminal** *adj* of a stimulus, of the lowest intensity that can be perceived by human sense organs. ⇒ subliminal.

**liminality** *n* a transitional period between culturally defined life crises or social states.

**limits of stability** the range within which a person can move in any direction without a postural change or loss of balance.

**limosis** *n* abnormal appetite.

**linctus** *n* a sweet, syrupy liquid, usually given to relieve a cough.

**linea** *n* a line. *linea alba* the white line visible after removal of the skin in the centre of the abdomen, stretching from the ensiform cartilage to the pubis, its position on the surface being indicated by a slight depression. *lineae albicantes* white lines which appear on the abdomen after reduction of tension as after childbirth, drainage of ascites from the abdomen, etc. ⇒ striae gravidarum. *linea nigra* pigmented line from umbilicus to pubis which appears in pregnancy.

**linear accelerator** a mega-voltage machine which accelerates electrons and produces high-energy X-rays which are used in the treatment of various cancers.

**lingua** *n* the tongue—**lingual** *adj*.

**liniment** *n* a liquid applied to the skin using gentle friction.

**linitis plastica** also known as leather-bottle stomach. A form of gastric cancer which infiltrates throughout the gastric wall. This leads to diffuse thickening and failure to inflate at endoscopy and barium examinations.

**linkage** *n* in genetics, a state in which two or more genes are close together on a chromosome and so do not segregate independently during meiosis. This means that they are usually inherited together and are associated with a particular inherited characteristic. Genes located at more distant loci are more likely to cross over and become separated during meiosis.

**L**

**linoleic acid** an omega-6, polyunsaturated, essential fatty acid. It is found in vegetable seed oils, such as sunflower, corn and soya bean. ⇒ essential fatty acids.

**linolenic acids** polyunsaturated, essential fatty acids found in vegetable oils. There are two types: (a) alpha (α)-linolenic acid (ALA), an omega-3 fatty acid, which is found in flax (linseed) oil and soya bean oil. ALA is used by the body to produce docosahexaenoic acid (DHA) and eicosapentaenoic acid (EPA); and (b) gamma (γ)-linolenic acid (GLA), which is an omega-6 fatty acid found in evening primrose oil. GLA is important in the formation of prostaglandins. ⇒ essential fatty acids.

**lipaemia** n increased lipids (especially cholesterol) in the blood—**lipaemic** adj.

**lipase** n any fat-splitting enzyme, such as pancreatic lipase. They convert fats into fatty acids and glycerol.

**lipectomy** n surgical removal of subcutaneous fat, such as from the abdominal wall.

**lipid peroxidation** the oxidation of fatty acids in cell membranes by free radicals.

**lipids** npl large group of fat-like organic molecules which include: neutral fats, such as triglycerides (triacylglycerols), phospholipids, lipoproteins, fat-soluble vitamins, steroids, prostaglandins, leukotrienes and thromboxanes. They consist of carbon, oxygen and hydrogen, and some contain phosphorus and nitrogen. They are insoluble in water, but they can be dissolved in organic solvents such as alcohol. Lipids are important in the body both structurally and functionally. Fat deposits provide an energy store, insulate and offer some physical protection. Other lipids are important constituents of cell membranes, are precursors for steroid hormones, act as regulatory molecules, e.g. prostaglandins, and transport fats around the body, and the fat-soluble vitamins are concerned with blood clotting, vision and antioxidant functions.

**lipoatrophy** n breakdown of fat cells at sites used for repeated insulin injections. There is a hollowed appearance. Compare lipohypertrophy.

**lipochondrodystrophy** n ⇒ Hurler's syndrome.

**lipodystrophy** n a disorder of fat metabolism or the deposition of fat within the tissues. There is loss of fat tissue. It may be congenital or acquired.

**lipoedema** n the accumulation of fat in the lower extremities (hips down to ankles) with associated tenderness.

**lipofuscins** npl pigments formed mainly from the oxidation of fats that are deposited in a variety of body tissues, particularly the myocardium and liver in adults. Lipofuscins accumulate in the lysosomes during ageing.

**lipogenesis** n a metabolic process where amino acids and glucose are converted to triglycerides (triacylglycerols) prior to storage in adipose tissue. It is stimulated by insulin.

**lipohypertrophy** n an increase in subcutaneous fat at sites used for repeated insulin injections. Compare lipoatrophy.

**lipoid** adj, n (a substance) resembling fats or oil.

**lipoidosis/lipidosis** n disease due to disorder of fat metabolism—**lipoidoses** pl.

**lipolysis** n the chemical breakdown of fat; stored triglycerides (triacylglycerols) are released for energy. Stimulated by glucocorticoid hormones—**lipolytic** adj.

**lipoma** n a benign tumour of fatty tissue—**lipomata** pl, **lipomatous** adj.

**lipopolysaccharide** n a molecule containing lipids and polysaccharides found as a component of the cell wall in some bacteria.

**lipoprotein** n lipids combined with a protein that transport triglycerides (triacylglycerols) and cholesterol around the body in the blood. They are classified as: high-density lipoproteins (HDLs), low-density lipoproteins (LDLs) or very-low-density lipoproteins (VLDLs). A high level of LDL in the blood is associated with arterial disease whereas HDLs are considered to be protective and are associated with a decreased risk of arterial disease. ⇒ hyperlipidaemia, lipids.

**liposarcoma** n a malignant growth of fat cells—**liposarcomas, liposarcomata** pl.

**liposome** n a spherical body comprising a phospholipid bilayer enclosing an aqueous solution.

**liposome drug delivery** drug administration using drugs enclosed in vesicles. Drug release occurs when the liposome is broken down in the liver by cells of the monocyte–macrophage (reticuloendothelial) system.

**liposuction** n in cosmetic surgery a technique of vacuum extraction of subcutaneous fat using cannulae.

**lipotrophic substances** factors which cause the removal of fat from the liver by transmethylation.

**lipotrophin** n hormone secreted by the anterior pituitary gland that is involved in releasing fat from the stores in adipose tissue. It has two forms: beta (β)-lipotrophin; and gamma (γ)-lipotrophin. Lipotrophins are structurally similar to adrenocorticotrophic hormone, endorphins and melanocyte-stimulating hormones. ⇒ pro-opiomelanocortin.

**lipping** *n* abnormal bone growth adjacent to the margin of a joint. It is demonstrated radiographically and is a feature of degenerative conditions that include osteoarthritis.

**lipuria** *n* (*syn* adiposuria) fat in the urine—**lipuric** *adj*.

**liquid-based cytology (LBC)** a newer technology used in cervical screening for abnormal cells. It produces better specimens for cytological examination and early evidence suggests that sensitivity and specificity are improved. May also be used to detect infections such as the human papillomavirus.

**liquor** *n* a solution. *liquor amnii* fluid surrounding the fetus.

**Lisch nodules** (K Lisch, Austrian ophthalmologist, 1907–1999) small circular pigmented hamartomas present in the iris in neurofibromatosis.

**lissencephaly** *n* a rare chromosomal disorder in which the brain is malformed. The brain surface is smooth and has no sulci or gyri. The affected infant has other brain malformations and microcephaly. It is associated with abnormalities occurring in many body systems. The effects include abnormal facial appearance, failure to thrive, feeding difficulties, dysphagia, severe developmental problems, deformity of the hands and feet, muscle hypertonia and seizures. Various types exist and it may be associated with other syndromes, such as Miller–Dieker syndrome. The prognosis for affected infants is very variable and depends on the severity of the brain malformation, but many die during the first 2 years.

**listening** *n* a group of complex skills used in communication; health professionals should give their whole attention to what is being said, how it is being said, and whether or not it matches the non-verbal signals.

**Listeria** *n* a genus of bacteria present in animal faeces and soil. *Listeria monocytogenes* causes meningitis, septicaemia, and intrauterine or perinatal infections. ⇒ listeriosis.

**listeriosis** *n* infection caused by *Listeria*. Transmitted via contaminated soil, contact with infected animals and by eating unpasteurized foods, such as soft cheeses, that may be infected. Infection may lead to a flu-like illness but serious consequences may occur in infants, older people, debilitated or immunocompromised individuals and pregnant women. Infection

during pregnancy may lead to miscarriage, stillbirth, preterm labour and septicaemia and neonatal meningitis.

**literature review** the process of locating and appraising relevant information, usually from a range of sources. It involves a methodical and wide-ranging examination of the papers relevant to a topic. Research methods and results are analysed and presented critically. The literature review includes how the search was carried out, e.g. bibliographical databases such as Allied and Complementary Medicine Database (AMED), MEDLINE.

**lithiasis** *n* any condition in which there are calculi.

**lithium (Li)** *n* a metallic element. Lithium salts are used therapeutically in some mental health problems.

**litholapaxy** *n* (*syn* lithopaxy) crushing a stone within the urinary bladder and removing the fragments by irrigation.

**lithopaedion** *n* a dead fetus retained in the uterus, e.g. one of a pair of twins which dies and becomes mummified and sometimes impregnated with lime salts.

**lithotomy** *n* general term for the surgical incision of a duct or organ for the removal of calculi, especially one from the urinary tract.

**lithotomy position** with the patient lying down, the buttocks are drawn to the end of the table to which a stirrup is attached on either side. Each foot is placed in a sling attached to the top of the stirrup so that the perineum is exposed for genitourinary procedures.

**lithotripsy** *n* destruction or elimination of calculi in the urinary tract or gallbladder. It may be achieved either by surgical intervention to crush the calculus, or by non-invasive means such as the use of shock waves. ⇒ extracorporeal shock-wave lithotripsy.

**lithotriptor** *n* a machine which sends shock waves through calculi, causing them to fragment. The fragments are washed out, or in the case of renal calculi, they are passed naturally in the urine.

**lithotrite** *n* an instrument for crushing a stone in the urinary bladder.

**litmus** *n* a vegetable pigment used as an indicator of alkalinity (blue) or acidity (red). Often stored as paper strips: red litmus paper turns blue when exposed to an alkali; blue litmus paper turns red with an acid.

**Little's area** the area on the anterior nasal septum that contains Kiesselbach's plexus.

A common site for epistaxis (bleeding from the nose).

**Little's disease** a type of cerebral palsy. There is diplegia of spastic type causing 'scissor leg' deformity. ⇒ cerebral palsy.

**livedo** *n* mottling and discoloration of the skin, especially in cold weather.

**liver** *n* the largest gland and solid organ in the body, the weight in adults is within the range 1.2–1.5 kg. The liver is situated in the right upper part of the abdominal cavity. Functionally, it is divided into two parts (left and right) but it is still described as having four lobes— right, left, caudate and quadrate (Figure L.3). It receives blood from two sources—the hepatic artery and the hepatic portal vein. Blood leaves the liver via the hepatic vein. It is vital to homeostasis and its functions include: breakdown of red blood cells with the production of bile; detoxification of drugs, chemicals and hormones; the metabolism of proteins, fats and carbohydrates, the liver being central to blood glucose homeostasis; protein synthesis, e.g. blood coagulation factors; the storage of energy as glycogen; storage of vitamins and minerals; and it generates a considerable amount of heat.

**liver function tests (LFTs)** blood tests used to assess liver function, including: alanine aminotransferase (ALT), alkaline phosphatase, aspartate aminotransferase (AST), coagulation tests, gamma-glutamyltransferase (GGT, gamma-GT, γ-GT), serum bilirubin and serum proteins. ⇒ aminotransferases.

**liver transplant** surgical transplantation of a liver from a suitable donor or a segment from the liver of a living donor. May be used for individuals with end-stage liver failure such as that caused by congenital abnormalities of the liver and bile ducts or cirrhosis from long-term alcohol misuse.

**livid** *adj* showing blue discoloration due to bruising, congestion or insufficient oxygenation.

**living will** ⇒ advance directive.

**LMA** *abbr* laryngeal mask airway.

**LMP** *abbr* last menstrual period.

**LOA** *abbr* left occipitoanterior; used to describe the position of the fetal occiput in relation to the maternal pelvis.

***Loa loa*** a parasitic nematode causing loiasis (filariasis).

**lobe** *n* a rounded section of an organ, separated from neighbouring sections by a fissure or septum, etc.—**lobar** *adj*.

**lobectomy** *n* removal of a lobe, for example lung, or liver.

**lobotomy/prefrontal leucotomy** a seldom-performed procedure in which nerve pathways in the frontal lobe of the brain are cut.

**lobule** *n* a small lobe or a subdivision of a lobe—**lobular, lobulated** *adj*.

**local anaesthetic** ⇒ anaesthetic.

**local authority** in the UK, local government, e.g. regional councils, county councils, unitary authorities, city councils, district and town councils and parish councils. The levels of local government vary between the countries of the UK. All have powers to raise taxes and some have a statutory duty to provide services within a locality, such as environmental health, social services, education and policing.

**localize** *vt* **1.** to limit the spread. **2.** to determine the site of a lesion—**localization** *n*.

**local muscle endurance** a person's ability to sustain a physical activity that relates to a particular muscle or group of muscles; for example, the number of press-ups possible in a given time gives an indication of upper-arm and shoulder muscle endurance.

**lochia** *n* the vaginal discharge which occurs during the puerperium or following miscarriage. At first pure blood (lochia rubra), then more pink (lochia serosa) and later becomes paler (lochia alba), diminishes in quantity and finally ceases—**lochial** *adj*.

**locked-in syndrome** a paralytic condition in which there is normally critical neurological damage such that the patient is unable to move but is conscious and alert. The individual retains eye movement and blinking and may be able to use these in communication.

**lockjaw** *n* ⇒ tetanus.

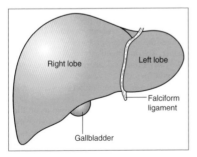

Right lobe

Left lobe

Falciform ligament

Gallbladder

**Figure L.3** Liver—general appearance *(reproduced from Watson 2000 with permission)*.

**locomotor** *adj* can be applied to any tissue or system used in movement. Most usually refers to nerves and muscles. Sometimes includes the skeletal system. *locomotor ataxia* the disordered gait and loss of sense of position (proprioception) in the lower limbs, which occurs in tabes dorsalis. ⇒ syphilis.

**loculated** *adj* divided into numerous cavities.

**locus of control** concept in health psychology. A behaviourist theory to describe individual differences in perceived control over events in people's lives. Some people feel that events in their lives are beyond their control, a belief in an external locus of control. This would consequently determine their response to stress and health-seeking (illness) behaviour, with an over-reliance on medical intervention for improving health. Others may feel that they do exercise a degree of control over events, a belief in an internal locus of control. This is more likely to lead to self-help: altered behaviour to reduce the risk of ill health, adoption of healthier lifestyles, adherence to medical advice.

**logopaedics** *n* study of speech disorders and their treatment.

**logorrhoea** *n* rapid speech that may be incoherent.

**loiasis** *n* special form of filariasis (caused by the worm *Loa loa*) which occurs in West Africa. The vector, a large horsefly, *Chrysops*, bites in the daytime. Larvae take 2–3 years to develop and may live in humans for 15 years. There is eosinophilia. The worms move about the subcutaneous tissues causing irritation and localized swellings, and sometimes a worm crosses the eye.

**loin** *n* that part of the back between the lower ribs and the iliac crest; the area immediately above the buttocks.

**longitudinal study** research study where data are collected on more than one occasion, such as the study of a cohort of people over time. ⇒ cohort study.

**long Q-T syndrome** an inherited condition with an extended Q-T interval; it predisposes to life-threatening ventricular arrhythmias, leading to sudden death, often during exertion, in otherwise healthy young people.

**longsighted** *adj* ⇒ hypermetropia.

**long slow distance training** training performed at low intensity (less than 70% $VO_{2max}$) but over time periods in excess of those during a race or other sporting competition.

**long-term memory (LTM)** the part of memory responsible for the retention of information for longer periods. Potentially permanent and has a much greater capacity than short-term memory.

**long-term oxygen therapy (LTOT)** controlled flow rate oxygen, provided for at least 15 hours per day, usually via an oxygen concentrator. Shown to prolong survival in those with severe hypoxaemia ($PaO_2$ <7.3 kPa with an $FEV_1$ <1.5 L) secondary to obstructive lung disease with concurrent right heart failure.

**loop diuretics** a group of drugs, e.g. furosemide, that make a diuretic effect by preventing the reabsorption of sodium, chloride and potassium in the thick part of the ascending limb of the loop of Henle. ⇒ Appendix 5.

**loose body** a fragment of loose material within a body cavity, such as in the knee joint, where it can lead to joint locking.

**LOP** *acron* **l**eft **o**ccipito**p**osterior; used to describe the position of the fetal occiput in relation to the maternal pelvis.

**lordoscoliosis** *n* lordosis complicated by the presence of scoliosis.

**lordosis** *n* an exaggerated forward convex curve of the lumbar spine—**lordotic** *adj*.

**lotion** *n* a fluid preparation for application to the skin or a wound, for example, an antiseptic or a treatment for a skin condition.

**Lou Gehrig's disease** ⇒ amyotrophic lateral sclerosis.

**loupe** *n* a magnifying lens, often attached to spectacles.

**louse** *n* ⇒ *Pediculus*—**lice** *pl*.

**Løvset's manoeuvre** (J Løvset, Norwegian obstetrician, 20th century) a manoeuvre used to deliver the shoulders and arms in breech presentation complicated by the arms being extended or displaced behind the neck.

**low-back pain** the commonest cause seems to be posterolateral prolapse of the intervertebral disc, putting pressure on the dura and cauda equina and causing the localized pain of lumbago. It can progress to trap the spinal nerve root, causing the nerve distribution pain of sciatica.

**low birth weight (LBW)** defined as a weight of less than 2500 g at birth, whether or not gestation was below 37 weeks. Very low birth weight is defined as less than 1500 g at birth, and extremely low birth weight is less than 1000 g at birth. ⇒ small for gestational age. Low birth weight can result from preterm birth or from intrauterine growth restriction/retardation (IUGR).

**low-density lipoprotein (LDL)** ⇒ lipoprotein.

L

**lower reference nutrient intake (LRNI)** one of the UK dietary reference values. The amount of a nutrient that will be enough for that small group within a population (2.5%) who have a low requirement. ⇒ dietary reference values.

**lower respiratory tract infection (LRTI)** ⇒ pneumonia.

**lower urinary tract symptoms (LUTS)** include dribbling, dysuria, frequency, hesitancy, incontinence, intermittency, nocturia, poor urinary flow rate, urgency. They are indicative of pathology affecting the bladder and urethra, such as outflow obstruction due to an enlarged prostate gland, or detrusor instability.

**lower uterine segment** the thinner, less vascular lower part of the uterus that is formed from the isthmus and cervix during pregnancy. The uterine isthmus is a narrow area between the cavity and cervix in the non-pregnant uterus. The lower segment thins and dilates during labour as it is stretched by the powerful contractions of the upper uterine segment.

**LP** *abbr* lumbar puncture.

**LRNI** *abbr* lower reference nutrient intake.

**LRTI** *abbr* lower respiratory tract infection.

**LS** *abbr* lecithin–sphingomyelin ratio.

**LSD** *abbr* lysergic acid diethylamide.

**LTM** *abbr* long-term memory.

**LTOT** *abbr* long-term oxygen therapy.

**lubb-dupp** *n* words descriptive of the heart sounds as heard on auscultation.

**lubricants** *npl* faecal softeners, e.g. arachis oil, that also lubricate and facilitate easy and painless defecation. ⇒ laxatives.

**lucid** *adj* clear; describing mental clarity. *lucid interval* a period of mental clarity which can be of variable length, occurring in people with organic mental disorder such as dementia or delirium. Importantly, a lucid interval is also a feature of extradural (epidural) haemorrhage. Bleeding is usually from the high-pressure, middle meningeal artery and follows head trauma. There is initial loss of consciousness, then a variable period of lucidity, which is followed by a sudden and rapid worsening in conscious level.

**Ludwig's angina** ⇒ cellulitis.

**lues** *n* obsolete term for syphilis.

**lumbago** *n* incapacitating pain low down in the back.

**lumbar** *adj* pertaining to the loin. *lumbar nerves* five pairs of spinal nerves (L1–L5). *lumbar*

*plexus* a network of nerves comprises the spinal nerves L1–L3 and part of L4. The lumbar plexus gives rise to nerves that innervate the muscles and skin of the lower abdomen, inguinal area, thigh and lower leg and foot, including the ilioinguinal, femoral and obturator nerves. ⇒ Appendix 1, Figure 11.

**lumbar puncture (LP)** the withdrawal of cerebrospinal fluid (CSF) through a hollow needle inserted into the subarachnoid space in the lumbar region of the spine (Figure L.4). The CSF obtained is examined for its chemical (e.g. glucose) and cellular (e.g. white blood cells) constituents and for the presence of microorganisms; CSF pressure can be measured by the attachment of a manometer.

**lumbar sympathectomy** surgical removal of the sympathetic chain in the lumbar region; used to improve the blood supply to the lower limbs by allowing vasodilation.

**lumbar vertebrae** five bones, the largest of the vertebrae reflecting their weight-bearing function. ⇒ Appendix 1, Figure 3.

**lumbocostal** *adj* pertaining to the loin and ribs.

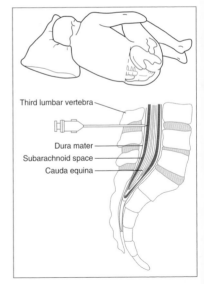

Third lumbar vertebra

Dura mater

Subarachnoid space

Cauda equina

**Figure L.4** Lumbar puncture *(reproduced from Walsh 2002 with permission).*

**lumbosacral** *adj* pertaining to the loin or lumbar vertebrae and the sacrum.

**Lumbricus** *n* a genus of earthworms. ⇒ ascarides, ascariasis.

**lumen** *n* the space inside a tubular structure—**lumina** *pl*, **luminal** *adj*.

**lumpectomy** *n* the surgical excision of a tumour with removal of minimal surrounding tissue. Increasingly used, with radiotherapy and chemotherapy, for treatment of breast cancer.

**lunate** *n* one of the carpal bones of the wrist. It articulates with the radius and other carpal bones scaphoid, triquetral, hamate and capitate.

**Lund and Browder's charts** used to calculate more accurately a burn area and illustrate the depth of area burnt, giving a calculation of burn severity. ⇒ rule of nines, total burn surface area.

**lungs** *npl* the two main organs of respiration which occupy the greater part of the thoracic cavity; they are separated from each other by the heart and other contents of the mediastinum (⇒ Appendix 1, Figures 6 and 7). Arranged in lobes, they receive air during inspiration from the trachea, main bronchi and smaller airways which communicate with the alveoli, the site of gaseous exchange. The lungs are concerned with gaseous exchange—the oxygenation of blood and excretion of carbon dioxide during expiration.

**lung transplantation** may be single, double, heart–lung transplants, or sometimes, in the case of child recipients, live-related lobar transplants.

**lunula** *n* the semilunar pale area at the root of the nail.

**lupus** *n* several destructive skin conditions, with different causes. ⇒ collagen diseases.

**lupus erythematosus (LE)** ⇒ systemic lupus erythematosus (SLE).

**lupus pernio** a form of sarcoidosis affecting the skin.

**lupus vulgaris** the commonest variety of skin tuberculosis; ulceration occurs over cartilage (nose or ear) with necrosis and facial disfigurement.

**lutein** *n* a naturally occurring yellow-red carotenoid pigment present in green leafy vegetables such as spinach and in some fruits.

**luteinizing hormone (LH)** a gonadotrophin secreted by the anterior pituitary gland. In females high levels in mid menstrual cycle stimulate ovulation and formation of the corpus luteum. The same hormone in males is called interstitial cell-stimulating hormone (ICSH); it stimulates the production of testosterone by the testes.

**luteotrophin/luteotrophic hormone** ⇒ prolactin.

**LUTS** *abbr* lower urinary tract symptoms.

**luxation** *n* partial dislocation.

**LVAD** *abbr* left ventricular assist device.

**Lyell's syndrome** (A Lyell, British dermatologist, 20/21st century). ⇒ toxic epidermal necrolysis.

**Lyme disease** an infection caused by the spirochaete *Borrelia burgdorferi*. It is transmitted to humans by the bites of infected ticks of the genus *Ixodes*. It is characterized by fatigue, skin rash, lymphadenopathy, joint pains, headache, pyrexia and occasionally arthritis, meningitis and cardiac arrhythmias. First identified in Lyme, Connecticut, USA. ⇒ Borrelia, relapsing fever.

**lymph** *n* the fluid contained in the lymphatic vessels. It is formed from interstitial (tissue) fluid and is similar in composition to plasma. Unlike blood, lymph contains only one type of cell, the lymphocyte. *lymph circulation* that of lymph collected from the tissue spaces; it then passes via lymph capillaries, vessels, nodes and ducts to be returned to the blood. *lymph nodes* accumulations of lymphatic tissue at intervals along lymphatic vessels. Sometimes erroneously referred to as lymph glands. They mainly act as filters in removing extraneous particles, including micro-organisms and cancer cells, and provide a site for B- and T-lymphocyte/cell proliferation and the production of immunoglobulins.

**lymphadenectomy** *n* excision of one or more lymph nodes.

**lymphadenitis** *n* inflammation of a lymph node.

**lymphadenopathy** *n* any disease of the lymph nodes—**lymphadenopathic** *adj*.

**lymphangiectasis** *n* dilatation of the lymph vessels—**lymphangiectatic** *adj*.

**lymphangiography** *n* ⇒ lymphography.

**lymphangioma** *n* a simple tumour of lymph vessels, frequently associated with similar formations of blood vessels—**lymphangiomata** *pl*, **lymphangiomatous** *adj*.

**lymphangioplasty** *n* any plastic surgery on lymph vessels, such as those used to improve drainage. ⇒ lymphoedema—**lymphangioplastic** *adj*.

**lymphangiosarcoma** *n* rare malignancy of lymph vessels.

**lymphangitis** *n* inflammation of a lymph vessel.

**lymphatic** *adj* pertaining to, conveying or containing lymph.

**lymphatic system** comprises a network of lymph capillaries, vessels and the two large ducts—the thoracic duct and the right lymphatic duct—that empty lymph into the subclavian veins; lymph nodes; the lymph fluid; lymph/lymphoid organs, e.g. spleen and thymus; and the diffuse lymphoid tissue or mucosa-associated lymphoid tissue (MALT), e.g. tonsils, Peyer's patches (lymphoid tissue in the small intestine) and also in the bone marrow. ⇒ thoracic duct.

**lymphoblast** *n* an immature lymphocyte. Present in the blood and bone marrow in conditions such as acute lymphoblastic leukaemia (ALL).

**lymphocele** *n* a collection of lymph in the tissues or a tumour, caused by leakage from damaged lymph vessels.

**lymphocyte** *n* one variety of white blood cell (leucocyte). The lymphocytic stem cells undergo transformation to T lymphocytes/cells (in the thymus), which provide cell-mediated immunity involved in destroying cancer cells, virus-infected cells and transplanted cells (graft), or B lymphocytes/cells, which form immunoglobulins (antibodies) and provide humoral immunity. The transformation is usually complete a few months after birth—**lymphocytic** *adj*.

**lymphocytopenia** *n* a decrease in the number of lymphocytes in the blood.

**lymphocytosis** *n* an increase in lymphocytes in the blood.

**lymphoedema** *n* excess fluid in the tissues from abnormality or obstruction of lymph vessels that blocks or interrupts lymph drainage. There is swelling of (usually) a limb and increased risk of cellulitis. It may be primary, such as with congenital abnormalities of the lymph vessels, or secondary, for example, after lymph node resection and/or radiotherapy; most common in breast cancer, or the blockage of lymph vessels caused by filarial worms. Its effects may be minimized by careful skin care to prevent injury and infection, exercises, specific massage and containment hosiery or bandaging. ⇒ elephantiasis, filariasis.

**lymphoepithelioma** *n* rapidly growing malignant pharyngeal tumour. May involve the tonsil. Often has metastases in cervical lymph nodes—**lymphoepitheliomata** *pl*.

**lymphogranuloma venereum** a sexually transmitted infection caused by *Chlamydia trachomatis*. There are ulcers on the genitalia and local lymph node enlargement. Occurs mainly in the tropics.

**lymphography** *n* X-ray examination of the lymphatic system after it has been rendered radiopaque. Generally replaced by computed tomography scanning—**lymphographical** *adj*, **lymphogram** *n*, **lymphograph** *n*, **lymphographically** *adv*.

**lymphoid** *adj* pertaining to lymph. *lymphoid tissue* (reticular tissue) tissue similar to lymph nodes, situated in a variety of locations, bone marrow, gut, liver, spleen, thymus and tonsils.

**lymphokine-activated killer cells (LAK)** cytotoxic cells that have been activated by the lymphokine interleukin-2. They do not require the presence of an antigen. LAK cells are able to destroy cancer cells that are not destroyed by natural killer cells. Used in immunotherapy for some cancers.

**lymphokines** *npl* a term applied to cytokines produced by stimulated T lymphocytes (e.g. interleukin-2). They function during the immune response as intercellular chemical mediators.

**lymphoma** *n* a group of neoplastic diseases developing in lymphoid tissue. Lymphoma is characterized by lymph node enlargement, night sweats/swinging pyrexia, pain from splenic enlargement/infarction, hepatomegaly, weight loss, malaise or recurrent infection. Causes include viral infections but most are idiopathic. Classified according to histological appearances to either Hodgkin's lymphoma or non-Hodgkin's lymphoma (NHL). Staging depends on sites involved—location and number, as well as associated 'secondary' symptoms. Therapy may be radiotherapy alone for the earliest stages, and/or chemotherapy. Bone marrow transplantation may also be necessary. ⇒ Burkitt's lymphoma.

**lymphopoiesis** *n* the production of lymphocytes in the bone marrow and other lymphoid tissues.

**lymphorrhagia** *n* an outpouring of lymph from a severed lymphatic vessel.

**lymphosarcoma** *n* obsolete term for some types of lymphoma.

**lyophilization** *n* freeze drying. Used to preserve biological substances such as plasma, tissue, etc.

**lyophilized skin** skin which has been subjected to lyophilization. It is reconstituted and used for temporary skin replacement.

**lymphuria** *n* the presence of lymph in the urine.

**Lyon hypothesis** (M Lyon, British geneticist, b. 1925) states that in females only one of the two female sex chromosomes (XX) is functional. The non-functional X chromosome becomes a Barr body. Either the paternal- or maternal-derived one may be non-functioning, which explains why an X-linked characteristic is expressed in some cells but not in others. ⇒ sex chromatin.

**lysergic acid diethylamide (LSD)** a potent hallucinogenic agent.

**lysin** *n* a substance present in blood that dissolves cells. ⇒ bacteriolysin, haemolysin.

**lysine** *n* an essential (indispensable) amino acid necessary for growth.

**lysis** *n* **1.** a gradual return to normal, used especially in relation to pyrexia. ⇒ crisis *opp.* **2.** disintegration of the membrane of cells or bacteria.

**lysosome** *n* a subcellular organelle that contains lytic enzymes.

**lysozyme** *n* an antibacterial enzyme present in many body fluids such as tears and saliva.

L

# M

MAb *abbr* monoclonal antibody.

maceration *n* softening of the horny layer of the skin by moisture, e.g. in and below the toes (in tinea pedis), or in perianal area (in pruritus ani). Maceration reduces the protective properties of the integument and so predisposes to penetration by bacteria or fungi.

Mackenrodt's ligaments also known as the transverse cervical ligaments or cardinal ligaments. ⇒ uterine supports.

Macleod's syndrome (W Macleod, British physician, 1911–1977) pathological changes in one lung that resemble those in emphysema. It follows respiratory infections, e.g. bronchiolitis, in childhood and may progress to bronchiectasis.

macrocephaly *n* large head, not caused by hydrocephalus—**macrocephalic** *adj*.

macrocheilia *n* excessive development of the lips.

macrocyte *n* a large red blood cell. Occurs in megaloblastic anaemia due to lack of vitamin $B_{12}$ and/or folic acid, either because of deficient intake or poor absorption in pernicious anaemia. Macrocytes are also associated with excess alcohol intake, liver disease and hypothyroidism—**macrocytic** *adj*.

macrocytosis *n* an increased number of macrocytes.

macrodactyly *n* excessive development of the fingers or toes.

macrodontian *n* unusually large teeth.

macroglia *n* a class of supporting, non-nervous tissue within the nervous system. They include astrocytes, ependymal cells, oligodendrocytes, satellite cells, Schwann cells. ⇒ microglia.

macroglobulin *n* a high-molecular-weight globulin protein. A term used to describe monoclonal immunoglobulin (IgM) molecules when excessive amounts are present in the blood, such as in conditions characterized by the production of abnormal IgM, for example in multiple myeloma. ⇒ paraprotein.

macroglobulinaemia *n* excessive amounts of monoclonal macroglobulins (IgM) present in the blood. The IgM is overproduced by plasma cells, and this is a feature of multiple myeloma and certain lymphomas such as Waldenström's macroglobulinaemia. The effects include increased blood viscosity with circulatory problems, fatigue and neurological symptoms. Moreover, normal immunoglobulin production is impaired and the person is at increased risk of serious infection. ⇒ Bence Jones protein, multiple myeloma.

macroglossia *n* an abnormally large tongue.

macrognathia *n* unusually large jaw.

macrolides *npl* a group of antibiotics (e.g. erythromycin) that may be prescribed for people with penicillin hypersensitivity. ⇒ Appendix 5.

macromastia *n* an abnormally large breast.

macronutrient *n* term used to describe the energy-yielding nutrients required in large quantities: carbohydrate, fat and protein.

macrophages *npl* mononuclear cells present in the tissues. They are derived from monocytes (a type of white blood cell). Some macrophages are able to move between sites as required, whilst others, such as those in the liver, alveoli, connective tissue, spleen and neural tissue, are fixed in position. They function as part of the non-specific (innate) body defences by destroying foreign bodies and cell debris by phagocytosis. Macrocytes also have roles in specific (adaptive) defences in stimulating various immune cells, secreting regulatory chemicals (e.g. interleukin-1) and by acting as antigen-presenting cells. They form part of the monocyte–macrophage (reticuloendothelial) system. ⇒ histiocytes, Kupffer cells, microglia.

macropsia *n* a visual defect in which objects are seen as much larger than they are in reality.

macroscopic *adj* visible to the unaided eye; gross. ⇒ microscopic *opp*.

macrosomia *n* in obstetrics, a large baby (birth weight in excess of 4000 g; some authorities define as over 4500 g). It is associated with maternal diabetes and hyperglycaemia, which leads to fetal hyperinsulinaemia and an increase in body fat and enlargement of organs. Macrosomia can be a cause of cephalopelvic disproportion and difficulties during delivery such as shoulder dystocia.

macrotia *n* congenital abnormality in which the outer/external ear is enlarged.

macrotrauma *n* a single force resulting in trauma to body tissues.

macula *n* a spot—**macular** *adj*.

macula densa specialized cells of the distal convoluted tubule (DCT) of the nephron. Forms part of the juxtaglomerular apparatus (JGA). The osmoreceptor/chemoreceptor cells of the macula densa monitor the level of sodium and chloride ions and fluid in the filtrate within the DCT and cause other cells of the JGA to secrete renin. ⇒ juxtaglomerular apparatus, renin, renin–angiotensin–aldosterone response.

**macula lutea** yellow spot situated close to the centre of the posterior part of the retina. A small depression in its centre (fovea centralis) which contains mostly cones is responsible for sharp central vision needed for tasks such as reading and colour vision. ⇒ Appendix 1, Figure 15.

**macular degeneration** *n* ⇒ age-related macular degeneration.

**macule** *n* a non-palpable localized area of change in skin colour—**macular** *adj*.

**maculopapular** *adj* the presence of macules and raised palpable spots (papules) on the skin.

**maculopathy** *n* a degenerative condition affecting the macula lutea.

**madarosis** *n* absence or loss of the eyelashes. It may be associated with blepharitis, alopecia or repeated trauma from rubbing.

**madura foot** ⇒ mycetoma.

**MAG3** *abbr* mercaptoacetyltriglycine. Used with technetium ($^{99m}$Tc) as a tracer in radio-isotope (radionuclide) imaging of the kidneys and in blood flow studies.

**maggots** *npl* the larvae of flies. Used in the management of some chronic wounds. ⇒ larval therapy.

**magnesium (Mg)** *n* a metallic element needed in the body for many enzyme-catalysed reactions. Magnesium is an intracellular cation and is present in bone, and its metabolism is linked to that of calcium. Many salts of magnesium are used therapeutically.

**magnesium carbonate and trisilicate** both used as an antacid to relieve dyspepsia.

**magnesium chloride** used intravenously for magnesium deficiency (hypomagnesaemia).

**magnesium hydroxide** an antacid and osmotic laxative.

**magnesium sulphate** (*syn* Epsom salts) an effective rapid-acting osmotic laxative. It is used topically as a paste with glycerin for the treatment of boils. Used parenterally in the treatment of eclampsia and magnesium deficiency.

**magnetic resonance imaging (MRI)** (*syn* nuclear magnetic resonance [NMR]) a non-invasive imaging technique that does not use ionizing radiation. Instead it uses a powerful magnetic field combined with radiofrequency pulses to excite hydrogen nuclei in the body. When the hydrogen nuclei settle the signal from the body is measured and reconstructed, using computer software, into two-dimensional or three-dimensional images. MRI can demon-strate anatomy and pathology in any plane, providing superior soft-tissue contrast and functional information (some procedures require the injection of contrast media). It is an established method of imaging the central nervous and musculoskeletal systems and increasingly for investigations of the cardiovascular system, liver and breast. MRI is also used to facilitate various therapeutic interventions. There are no known harmful biological effects, and MRI scanning is non-invasive, painless and safe (no ionizing radiation is used). However, there are still major safety issues to consider. Contraindications to the use of MRI include: heart pacemakers, intra-cerebral aneurysm clips, other metallic implants and metallic foreign objects such as coins.

**magnum** *adj* large or great, such as the fora-men magnum in the occipital bone through which the spinal cord passes into the cranial cavity.

**MAI** *abbr Mycobacterium avium intracellulare.*

**major histocompatibility complex (MHC)** both MHC class I and class II glycoproteins are members of the immunoglobulin superfam-ily, and present peptide antigens to the immune system to generate an immune response. The MHC genes are encoded on human chromo-some 6. Class I MHC genes encode proteins that are expressed on all nucleated cells and present self antigens to CD8+ T cells. Class II MHC genes encode proteins that are present on antigen-presenting cells (dendritic cells, macrophages and B cells) that present antigens to CD4+ T cells. Class III MHC genes encode a variety of molecules, including cytokines, com-plement components and other molecules essential for antigen presentation.

**Makaton** *n* a form of sign language. It is more basic than some other languages.

**mal** *n* disease. *mal de mer* seasickness. *grand mal* major epilepsy. *petit mal* minor epilepsy.

**malabsorption** *n* defective absorption of nutrients from the digestive tract.

**malabsorption syndrome** an inability to absorb nutrients in sufficient quantities for health, from the small bowel. There is loss of weight, abdominal bloating and pain and steatorrhoea, varying in severity. Caused by: (a) disease of the small intestine, such as coeliac disease, Crohn's disease; (b) lack of digestive enzymes or bile salts, e.g. cystic fibro-sis, pancreatitis; (c) surgical operations, e.g. extensive small-bowel resection. Leads to anaemia, fatigue, vitamin deficiencies and chronic ill health.

M

**malacia** *n* softening of a part. ⇒ keratomalacia, osteomalacia.

**maladaptation** *n* an abnormal or maladaptive response to a situation or change. It may relate to personal relationships, or to a stress response that leads to poor health, e.g. headaches, adverse changes in body chemistry.

**maladjustment** *n* bad or poor adaptation to environment. It may have social, mental or physical components.

**malaise** *n* a feeling of illness and discomfort.

**malalignment** *n* faulty alignment—as of bones after a fracture.

**malar** *adj* relating to the cheek. ⇒ zygomatic bone.

**malaria** *n* a serious infection caused by protozoa of the genus *Plasmodium* and carried by infected mosquitoes of the genus *Anopheles*. It occurs in tropical and subtropical regions and is seen in travellers returning from malarial areas. The parasite causes haemolysis during a complex life cycle. *Plasmodium falciparum* causes the most severe disease (malignant tertian malaria). *P. malariae* causes quartan malaria. *P. ovale* and *P. vivax* cause tertian malaria. The signs and symptoms depend on the type of malaria, but include: bouts of fever, rigors, headache, cough, vomiting, anaemia, jaundice and hepatosplenomegaly. Relapses are common in malaria. Various antimalarial drugs are available for both chemoprophylaxis and treatment. Elimination of the mosquito and its habitat are important in prevention—**malarial** *adj*.

**Malassezia** *n* (L Malassez, French physiologist, 1842–1909) previously known as *Pityrosporum*. A genus of fungi (yeasts) found normally on the skin surface. However, it is responsible for skin diseases, including many cases of dandruff. *Malassezia furfur* is associated with tinea (pityriasis) versicolor, which in many cases represents a change in the relationship between the host and resident yeast flora. Tinea versicolor is characterized by scaly macules with changes in pigmentation, mainly on the upper trunk and arms. The altered pigmentation can persist for several months.

**malathion** *n* it is an organophosphorus insecticide, which acts by binding irreversibly to the enzyme cholinesterase. It is used in suitable dilution for the topical treatment of infestations with scabies, head lice and body lice.

**malformation** *n* abnormal shape or structure; deformity.

**malignant** *adj* virulent and dangerous—**malignancy** *n*. *malignant growth* or *tumour* one that demonstrates the capacity to invade adjacent tissues/organs and spread (metastasize) to distant sites; often rapidly growing and with a fatal outcome. ⇒ cancer, carcinoma, sarcoma. *malignant melanoma* ⇒ melanoma. *malignant pustule* ⇒ anthrax.

**malignant hyperthermia** a rare inherited condition; transmitted as an autosomal dominant trait. It occurs as an abnormal response to volatile anaesthetic drugs, e.g. halothane, or depolarizing neuromuscular blocking muscle relaxants, e.g. suxamethonium. There is a rapid increase in body temperature, tachycardia, muscle rigidity and acidosis, which, if untreated, may be fatal. Treatment is with intravenous dantrolene. ⇒ neuroleptic malignant syndrome.

**malingering** *n* the deliberate simulation of physical or psychological illness motivated by external incentives or stressors.

**malleolus** *n* a part or process of a bone shaped like a hammer. *external malleolus* at the lower end of the fibula. *internal malleolus* situated at the lower end of the tibia—**malleoli** *pl*, **malleolar** *adj*.

**mallet finger** (*syn* hammer finger) the rupture of the extensor digitorum longus tendon from the distal phalanx (Figure M.1). Known as baseball finger in the USA.

**malleus** *n* the hammer-shaped lateral ossicle of the middle ear. It transmits sound waves from the tympanic membrane to the incus. (⇒ Appendix 1, Figure 13). ⇒ incus, stapes.

**Mallory bodies** (F Mallory, American pathologist, 1862–1941) abnormal inclusions present in hepatocytes in alcohol-induced liver injury, Wilson's disease, primary biliary cirrhosis, long-term cholestasis and liver cancer.

**Mallory–Weiss syndrome** (G Mallory, American pathologist, 20th century; S Weiss, American physician, 1898–1942) massive bleeding from a tear in the mucosa at the

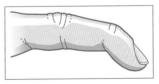

**Figure M.1** Mallet finger *(reproduced from Porter 2005 with permission).*

junction between the oesophagus and the stomach. It is caused by the straining associated with protracted vomiting. An uncommon cause of haematemesis.

**malnutrition** *n* the state of being poorly nourished due to the diet containing the incorrect amount of a micro- or macronutrient. Can result in disease, such as scurvy—malnutrition due to inadequate dietary intake of vitamin C, or obesity—malnutrition due to excessive energy intake. ⇒ chronic energy deficiency, eating disorders, obesity, protein–energy malnutrition.

**malocclusion** *n* any deviation from the normal occlusion of the teeth, often associated with an abnormal jaw relationship. ⇒ orthodontics.

**malposition** *n* any abnormal position of a part. In obstetrics, a cephalic presentation other than one where the fetal head is well flexed with the occiput in an anterior position relative to the maternal pelvis, such as a posterior position.

**malpractice** *n* improper or injurious medical or nursing treatment or other health care intervention. Professional practice that falls below accepted standards and causes harm. It may be negligence, unethical behaviour or abuse or involve criminal activities.

**malpresentation** *n* any presentation in which the fetus is not in the normal vertex position before or during labour, i.e. brow, face, shoulder or breech.

**MALT** *acron* **m**ucosa-**a**ssociated **l**ymphoid **t**issue.

**Malta fever** ⇒ brucellosis.

**maltase** *n* (*syn* α-glucosidase) an enzyme found in intestinal juice. It converts the disaccharide maltose to glucose.

**maltodextrin** *n* a polymer of glucose produced from starch.

**MALToma** *n* low-grade B-cell lymphoma of the mucosa-associated lymphoid tissue. It may be related to *Helicobacter pylori* infection which, when eradicated, may lead to disease regression.

**maltose** *n* malt sugar. A disaccharide produced by the hydrolysis of starch by amylase during digestion. Also manufactured commercially.

**malunion** *n* the union of a fracture in a bad position.

**mamma** *n* the breast—**mammae** *pl*, **mammary** *adj*.

**mammaplasty, mammoplasty** *n* any plastic operation on the breast—**mammaplastic** *adj*. ⇒ augmentation, implant, reduction.

**mammary glands** the breasts. Milk-secreting glands.

**mammilla** *n* **1.** the nipple. **2.** a small papilla—**mammillae** *pl*.

**mammogram** *n* a radiograph of breast tissue.

**mammography** *n* radiographic techniques used for the demonstration of the breast, which use specially low-penetration (long-wavelength) X-rays. Used in the diagnosis of or routine screening for breast conditions including cancer—**mammographic** *adj*, **mammographically** *adv*. ⇒ screening.

**Manchester operation** (*syn* Fothergill's operation) anterior colporrhaphy, amputation of part of the cervix and posterior colpoperineorrhaphy, performed for genital prolapse.

**mandible** *n* the large bone of the lower jaw. It is U-shaped and has a horizontal body, which contains the lower teeth, and two vertical rami. The condyle of each ramus articulates with the temporal bone at the temporomandibular joint—**mandibular** *adj*.

**mandibular advancement splint** a splint used to correct some jaw and dental problems. It is also used to reduce snoring and to alleviate some types of sleep apnoea. A mandibular advancement splint, which is worn in the mouth, may obviate the need for therapy with a continuous positive airway pressure mask.

**manganese (Mn)** *n* a metallic element needed by the body for many enzyme-catalysed reactions.

**mania** *n* a mood disorder characterized by elation, increased energy, overactivity, pressured speech, decreased need for sleep, irritability, grandiosity, distractibility and overspending. May be accompanied by psychotic symptoms, typically grandiose/religiose/persecutory delusions and hallucinations—**maniac** *adj*.

**manic depressive illness** ⇒ bipolar affective disorder.

**manipulation** *n* using the hands skilfully as in reducing a fracture or hernia, or changing an abnormal fetal position to facilitate a vaginal delivery.

**mannitol** *n* a sugar that is not metabolized in the body and acts as an osmotic diuretic. ⇒ Appendix 5.

**mannose** *n* a hexose (6-carbon) sugar present in legumes.

**Mann–Whitney *U*-test** a non-parametric substitute for Student's t-test for independent groups.

**manometer** *n* an instrument for measuring the pressure exerted by liquids or gases. Used for example for measuring the pressure exerted

M

by the cerebrospinal fluid during lumbar puncture, or sometimes for measuring central venous pressure.

**Mantoux reaction** (C Mantoux, French physician, 1877–1947) a skin test for tuberculosis. Tuberculin purified protein derivative is injected intradermally in the forearm. After 2–4 days, if induration is greater than or equal to 5 mm, the test is positive.

**manual hyperinflation** a technique in which the chest is hyperinflated in order to remove pulmonary secretions and to reinflate areas of collapsed lung in patients who are intubated. Hyperinflation is usually achieved by use of a hand-bagging circuit.

**manual muscle testing** a specific procedure used to evaluate the functional status of a muscle's innervation and contractile tissues; uses a graded strength test performed by applying manual resistance to a body segment in order to evaluate a particular muscle or group of muscles.

**manual removal of the placenta** a procedure, whereby a hand inserted into the uterus is used to remove an adherent placenta from the uterine wall when other methods have failed. It is usually undertaken by a doctor using strict aseptic technique and only after vascular access has been secured by siting an intravenous infusion. Effective anaesthesia is required, either by topping up an existing epidural anaesthetic, or by spinal or general anaesthetic.

**manubrium** *n* a handle-shaped structure; the upper part of the sternum.

**MAOI** *abbr* monoamine oxidase inhibitor.

**maple syrup urine disease** an aminoacidopathy, also known as branched-chain ketoaciduria. A genetic disorder transmitted as an autosomal recessive trait. The enzyme required for the metabolism of leucine, isoleucine and valine is missing. This results in high levels of the three amino acids in blood and their excretion in the urine, which has an odour similar to that of maple syrup. Symptoms vary according to the type and severity of the disease, but include poor feeding, vomiting, hypertonicity, respiratory difficulties; convulsions and severe damage to the central nervous system may occur, leading to learning disability. A diet low in the three amino acids may be effective if started sufficiently early; without treatment the disorder is rapidly fatal. Genetic counselling may be indicated.

**marasmic kwashiorkor** severe form of protein–energy malnutrition in children, accompanied by signs and symptoms of kwashiorkor.

**marasmus** *n* severe protein–energy malnutrition. Wasting away of the body, especially that of a baby. ⇒ failure to thrive, kwashiorkor—**marasmic** *adj*.

**marble bones** ⇒ osteopetrosis.

**Marburg disease** (*syn* green-monkey disease) a highly infectious viral haemorrhagic fever characterized by a sudden onset of fever, severe headache and malaise, vomiting, diarrhoea, pharyngitis and mucosal bleeding. Between days 5 and 7 a rash appears. Virus can persist in the body for 2–3 months after the initial attack. Cross-infection probably occurs by the aerosol route. Incubation period is believed to be 4–9 days. Treatment is symptomatic only and mortality rate in previous outbreaks has been as high as 90%.

**march fracture** a type of stress fracture caused by an increase in physical activity which may so stress a metatarsal (usually the second) as to produce an undisplaced self-healing fracture. There is local pain, tenderness and radiographic changes. Management usually involves moderate rest with supportive padding and strapping for a few weeks but sometimes a walking plaster is required.

**Marcus Gunn's syndrome** (R Marcus Gunn, British ophthalmologist, 1850–1909). ⇒ jaw-winking.

**Marfan's syndrome** (A Marfan, French paediatrician, 1858–1942) a genetic disorder of connective tissue that mainly affects the musculoskeletal system, the cardiovascular system and the eyes. It is inherited as an autosomal dominant trait. There is arachnodactyly, excessively long limbs, poorly developed and hypotonic musculature, lax ligaments with joint hypermobility and excessive height (adult height usually over 1.8 metres). Cardiovascular defects include mitral valve prolapse and defective structure of the aorta, which leads to aneurysm formation. There is dislocation of the lens and abnormalities of the iris.

**marginal cost** the cost of providing the extra resources required to carry out activity, such as a medical intervention, above a baseline number.

**marihuana, marijuana** *n* ⇒ cannabis.

**Marjolin's ulcer** (J Marjolin, French surgeon, 1780–1850) a squamous cell cancer that develops on damaged or chronically inflamed tissue, such as at the edge of a burn injury or a venous leg ulcer.

**marrow** *n* ⇒ bone marrow.

**Marshall–Marchetti–Krantz operation** (V Marshall, American urologist, b. 1913;

A Marchetti, American obstetrician, 1901–1970; K Krantz, American gynaecologist/obstetrician, 1923–2007) surgical procedure for stress incontinence. A form of abdominal cystourethropexy usually undertaken in patients whose loss of continence has not been controlled by a colporrhaphy.

**marsupialization** *n* an operation for cystic swellings, which entails stitching the margins of an opening made into the cyst to the edges of the wound, thus forming a pouch.

**masculinization** *n* the development of male secondary sexual characteristics. ⇒ virilism.

**Maslow's hierarchy of needs** (A Maslow, American psychologist, 1908–1970) a hierarchy of needs based on the humanistic approach. Generally shown as having five levels represented as a pyramid—commencing at the base with physiological needs required for survival; safety and security needs; love and belonging needs; self-esteem needs; and ending at the apex with self-actualization needs. A further two levels have since been added: cognitive needs and aesthetic needs, which are slotted in between self-esteem and self-actualization.

**masochism** *n* the deriving of pleasure from pain inflicted by others or occasionally by oneself. It may be a conscious or unconscious process and is frequently of a sexual nature. ⇒ sadism.

**mass number** the total mass of neutrons and protons within an atom.

**massage** *n* **1.** several different soft-tissue manipulations (kneading, stroking, rubbing, tapping, etc.). They are used at different depths and rates for various purposes: to improve circulation, metabolism and muscle tone, to break down adhesions, to expel gases, and either to relax or stimulate the patient. **2.** a complementary therapy that involves the conscious use of gentle muscle manipulation, using stroking or light kneading, to promote relaxation.

**masseter** *n* a cheek muscle, one of the muscles of mastication. Its origin is on the zygomatic arch and it inserts on to the ramus of the mandible.

**MAST** *acron* **m**ilitary **anti**shock **t**rousers.

**mast cells** cells produced in the bone marrow and present in connective tissues, which have similarities with basophils (a type of leucocyte). They have granules containing various chemicals that include heparin and histamine and other chemical mediators. They are generally located around small blood vessels in the skin, respiratory mucosa, gastrointestinal mucosa, the eyes, nose and mouth. They have an important role in body defences and function in the inflammatory response, allergic conditions, anaphylaxis and wound healing. Mast cells are activated to degranulate and release their chemicals in situations that include chemical or physical injury, or immunoglobulin E (IgE) binding to their receptors.

**mastalgia** *n* pain in the breast.

**mastectomy** *n* surgical removal of the breast. ⇒ lumpectomy. *simple mastectomy* removal of the breast with the overlying skin. *modified radical mastectomy* removal of the entire breast and division or excision of the pectoralis minor muscle with axillary lymph node clearance. *radical mastectomy* rarely performed operation that involves removal of the breast, pectoralis major muscle and clearance of the axillary lymph nodes.

**mastication** *n* chewing.

**mastitis** *n* inflammation of the breast. *chronic mastitis* the name formerly applied to the nodular changes in the breasts, now usually called fibrocystic disease.

**mastoid** *adj* nipple-shaped.

**mastoid air cells** extend in a backward and downward direction from the antrum.

**mastoid antrum** the air space within the mastoid process, lined by mucous membrane continuous with that of the tympanum and mastoid air cells.

**mastoid process** the prominence of the mastoid portion of the temporal bone just behind the ear.

**mastoidectomy** *n* drainage of the mastoid air cells and excision of diseased tissue. *cortical mastoidectomy* all the mastoid cells are removed, making one cavity which drains through an opening (aditus) into the middle ear. The external meatus and middle ear are untouched. *radical mastoidectomy* the mastoid antrum and middle ear are made into one continuous cavity for drainage of infection. Loss of hearing is inevitable.

**mastoiditis** *n* inflammation of the mastoid air cells.

**mastopexy** *n* surgical fixation of a pendulous breast.

**masturbation** *n* non-coital sexual arousal and orgasm by stimulation of the genitalia.

**materia medica** the science dealing with the origin, action and dosage of drugs.

**maternal mortality** death of a woman due to the complications of pregnancy. In the UK the rate is calculated as the number of deaths

**M**

per 100 000 births (including stillbirths) plus deaths due to abortion. The Confidential Enquiries into Maternal Deaths divides deaths into four groups: (a) direct, i.e. due to complications of the pregnancy, most commonly thromboembolic conditions; (b) indirect, i.e. from an existing disease that was worsened by pregnancy; (c) coincidental, i.e. deaths unrelated to the pregnancy; and (d) late deaths that occur between 42 days and 12 months after a miscarriage, an abortion or delivery.

**matriarchy** *n* describes a situation where a female (wife, mother or daughter) inherits, dominates and controls within a social structure.

**matrix** *n* the foundation substance in which the tissue cells are embedded.

**matrix band** in restorative dentistry, a band placed over a tooth to allow the use of restorative materials, e.g. to fill a cavity. It provides a retaining wall around a tooth that is missing some part.

**maturation** *n* the process of attaining full development. Describes the final stage in wound healing, during which the wound is strengthened and the scar gradually fades and shrinks.

**maturity-onset diabetes of the young (MODY)** an uncommon subtype of type 2 diabetes caused by a single gene defect. Accounts for <5% of cases of type 2 diabetes.

**Mauriceau–Smellie–Veit manoeuvre** (F Mauriceau, French obstetrician, 1637–1709; W Smellie, British obstetrician, 1697–1763; A Veit, German obstetrician, 1824–1903) a manoeuvre used during a breech delivery. The infant's jaw is flexed and traction applied to the shoulders.

**maxilla** *n* the jawbone; in particular the upper jaw—**maxillary** *adj*.

**maxillary sinus/antrum** one of two large paranasal air sinuses situated in the maxilla. It is lined with mucosa that is continuous with that lining the nasal cavity.

**maxillofacial** *adj* pertaining to the maxilla and face.

**maxillofacial surgery** branch of surgery concerned with the surgical management of developmental disorders and diseases or trauma of the facial structures.

**maxillotomy** *n* cutting through the maxilla in order to move all or some parts to a better position.

**maximal breathing capacity (MBC)** the maximum volume of air that can be inhaled and exhaled in a given time (e.g. 12 or 15 seconds) when the person is breathing as deeply and quickly as possible.

**maximal-intensity exercise** exercise that needs the person to make a maximum effort, and where most of the energy needed for the exercise is produced from anaerobic metabolism.

**maximal lactate steady state** the greatest intensity of exercise that can be sustained without a progressive increase in the amount of lactate in the blood.

**maximal oxygen consumption/uptake ($VO_{2max}$)** the highest rate at which a person can extract, transport and consume oxygen during exercise.

**maximum expiratory pressure (MEP)** a test used to assess global muscle strength. It is the highest pressure achieved during expiration after a full inspiration.

**maximum heart rate ($HR_{max}$)** a term used in sports medicine to describe an individual's maximum heart rate. $HR_{max}$ is calculated by subtracting the person's age in years from 220 ($HR_{max} = 220 -$ age in years).

**maximum inspiratory pressure (MIP)** a test used to assess global muscle strength. The highest pressure reached in the alveoli during a full inspiration.

**Mayer–Rokitansky–Küster–Hauser syndrome** (P Mayer, German gynaecologist, 1795–1868; C von Rokitansky, Austrian pathologist, 1804–1878; H Küster, German gynaecologist, 1879–1964; G Hauser, German gynaecologist, 20th century) müllerian agenesis. Congenital absence of the vagina and usually absence of the uterus and uterine tubes. There is normal ovarian development and function.

**MBC** *abbr* maximal breathing capacity. ⇒ respiratory function tests.

**MCA** *abbr* Medicines Control Agency. ⇒ Medicines and Healthcare products Regulatory Agency (MHRA).

**MCADD** *abbr* medium-chain acyl-CoA dehydrogenase deficiency.

**McArdle's disease** (B McArdle, British neurologist, 1911–2002) a glycogen storage disease.

**McBurney's point** (C McBurney, American surgeon, 1845–1913) a point one-third of the way between the anterior superior iliac spine and the umbilicus, the site of maximum tenderness in cases of acute appendicitis.

**McCune–Albright syndrome** ⇒ Albright's syndrome.

**MCH** *abbr* mean cell haemoglobin.

**MCHC** *abbr* mean cell haemoglobin concentration.

**McKenzie approach** an approach to mechanical diagnosis and therapy developed by R McKenzie (New Zealand physiotherapist). It is widely used in the management of both spinal and non-spinal problems affecting the musculoskeletal system.

**McMurray's osteotomy** (T McMurray, British orthopaedic surgeon, 1887–1949) division of femur between lesser and greater trochanter. Shaft displaced inwards beneath the head and abducted. This position maintained by a nail plate. Restores painless weight-bearing. In developmental dysplasia of the hip, deliberate pelvic osteotomy renders the outer part of the socket (acetabulum) more horizontal.

**MCP** *abbr* multiple cosmetic phlebectomy.

**McRoberts manoeuvre** a manoeuvre used to release the impacted anterior shoulder in shoulder dystocia, whereby the woman lies flat and bends her knees up to her chest.

**MCU** *abbr* micturating cystourethrogram.

**MCV** *abbr* mean cell volume.

**MDA** *abbr* Medical Devices Agency. ⇒ Medicines and Healthcare products Regulatory Agency.

**MDM** *abbr* mental defence mechanism. ⇒ defence mechanisms.

**MDR-TB** *abbr* multidrug-resistant tuberculosis.

**MDT** *abbr* multidisciplinary team.

**ME** *abbr* myalgic encephalomyelitis. ⇒ chronic fatigue syndrome.

**mean** *n* the average. *arithmetic mean* a figure arrived at by dividing the sum of a set of values by the number of items in the set. ⇒ central tendency statistic, median, mode.

**mean cell (corpuscular) haemoglobin (MCH)** *n* a red cell parameter estimated during a full blood count. It is the amount of haemoglobin in an average red blood cell.

**mean cell (corpuscular) haemoglobin concentration (MCHC)** *n* a red cell parameter measured during a full blood count. It is the weight (in grams) of haemoglobin in 100 mL of packed red blood cells.

**mean cell volume (MCV)** *n* a red cell parameter measured during a full blood count. It is the mean volume of red cells, which provides information about cell size. It is used to determine whether anaemia is macrocytic (MCV above normal) or microcytic (MCV below normal).

**measles** *n* (*syn* morbilli, rubeola) a potentially serious acute infectious disease caused by a paramyxovirus. It is highly contagious and spreads via droplets. The incubation period is about 10 days. It starts with a cold-like illness, cough, high fever, sore and watery eyes, Koplik's spots and photophobia. After 3–4 days a maculopapular rash appears. Complications include secondary bacterial infections such as pneumonia or otitis media, corneal ulceration and encephalitis. A rare late complication is subacute sclerosing panencephalitis (SSPE). Active immunization is offered as part of routine programmes during childhood. Endemic and worldwide in distribution, it is a cause of childhood mortality in developing countries and occasionally in economically developed counties. ⇒ Koplik's spots. ⊙ DVD

**meatotomy** *n* surgery to the urinary meatus for meatal stricture in men.

**meatus** *n* an opening or channel—**meatal** *adj*.

**mechanical ventilation** ⇒ intermittent positive-pressure ventilation.

**mechanism of labour** the series of passive movements of the baby as it descends through the birth canal propelled by the uterine contractions.

**mechanoreceptor** *n* sensory receptors that are responsive to mechanical forces or distortion. They include touch and pressure receptors in the skin; proprioceptors in tendons, muscles and joints; stretch receptors in the lung, bladder and gastrointestinal tract; baroreceptors in blood vessels; and receptors in the ear that respond to sound waves and changes in position.

**Meckel's diverticulum** (J Meckel, German anatomist, 1781–1833) a blind, pouch-like sac sometimes arising from the free border of the lower ileum. Occurs in 2% of the population: usually symptomless. May cause gastrointestinal bleeding or intussusception.

**meconium** *n* the discharge from the bowel of a neonate, the first stools. It is a greenish-black, viscid substance.

**meconium aspiration** inhalation by the fetus of meconium-stained amniotic fluid during labour/delivery. It can cause serious respiratory distress in the newborn.

**meconium ileus** impaction of meconium in bowel causing bowel obstruction. It is one presentation of cystic fibrosis.

**media 1.** *n* the middle coat of a vessel. **2.** *pl* nutritive jellies used for culturing microorganisms in the laboratory. ⇒ medium.

**medial** *adj* pertaining to or near the midline, or to the middle layer of a structure—**medially** *adv*.

**M**

**median** *adj* **1.** the middle. **2.** a central tendency statistic; the midway or middle value in a set of scores when placed in increasing order. ⇒ mean, mode.

**median line** an imaginary line passing through the centre of the body from a point between the eyes to between the closed feet.

**median nerve** a nerve arising from the brachial plexus, which supplies some muscles of the forearm and the skin and muscles of the thumb and fingers. ⇒ Appendix 1, Figure 11.

**median plane** a vertical plane that divides the body into right and left halves (Figure M.2). Also called the midsagittal plane.

**median vein** a superficial vein, which, if present, carries venous blood from part of the hand and forearm to the basilic vein or the median cubital vein. ⇒ Appendix 1, Figure 10.

**mediastinoscopy** *n* a minor endoscopic surgical procedure for visual inspection of the mediastinum. May be combined with biopsy of the lymph nodes for histological examination, and diagnosis or staging in the case of cancer.

**mediastinotomy** *n* incision of the mediastinum.

**mediastinum** *n* the space between the lungs. Contains the heart, great vessels and the oesophagus—**mediastinal** *adj*.

**medical** *adj* relating to medicine (the profession), or to conditions and treatment that are undertaken by physicians rather than surgeons.

**Medical Devices Agency (MDA)** ⇒ Medicines and Healthcare products Regulatory Agency (MHRA).

**medical emergency team** ⇒ critical care team.

**medical jurisprudence** ⇒ forensic medicine.

**medicament** *n* a medicine or remedy. ⇒ drug.

**medicated** *adj* impregnated with a medicine or drug.

**medication** *n* a therapeutic substance or drug, administered orally or by injection intra-arterially, subcutaneously, intramuscularly, intravenously, intraosseously, or into a body cavity (e.g. the bladder), or rectally, topically, transdermally, buccal or sublingual administration.

**medicinal** *adj* pertaining to a medicine.

**medicine** *n* **1.** science or art of healing, especially as distinguished from surgery and obstetrics. **2.** a therapeutic substance. ⇒ drug.

**Medicines and Healthcare products Regulatory Agency (MHRA)** an agency in the UK formed from a merger between the Medicines Control Agency (MCA) and the

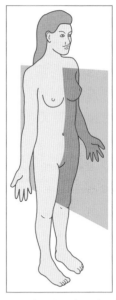

**Figure M.2** Median plane *(reproduced from Hinchliff et al. 1996 with permission).*

Medical Devices Agency (MDA). Its main function is to promote and protect public health and the safety of patients by ensuring that all medicines, health care products and medical devices/equipment meet suitable standards of safety, quality, performance and efficacy, and are used in a safe manner. ⇒ European Medicines Agency, National Patient Safety Agency.

**Medicines Commission** ⇒ Commission on Human Medicines.

**Medicines Control Agency (MCA)** ⇒ Medicines and Healthcare products Regulatory Agency (MHRA).

**medicochirurgical** *adj* pertaining to both medicine and surgery.

**medicosocial** *adj* pertaining to medicine and sociology.

**mediolateral** *adj* pertaining to the middle and one side.

**meditation** *n* an altered state achieved by rituals and exercises. It aims to produce relaxation (physical and mental). Various forms may be used as in relaxation as part of stress management strategies.

**Mediterranean spotted fever** ⇒ boutonneuse fever.

**medium** *n* a substance used in bacteriology for the growth of micro-organisms—**media** *pl*.

**medium-chain acyl-CoA dehydrogenase deficiency (MCADD)** a genetic metabolic disorder which is inherited as an autosomal recessive trait. The enzyme deficiency leads to faulty nutrient metabolism. It is known to be one cause of sudden infant death syndrome (SIDS). Infants/children may have a history of altered consciousness, especially if they miss a feed or meal. The previously asymptomatic disorder may become evident during an intercurrent illness such as an infection. The disorder can lead to seizures and liver failure. ⇒ genetic screening, neonatal screening.

**medium-chain triacylglycerols** triacylglycerols (trigylcerides) containing medium-chain (8–12 carbon atoms) fatty acids.

**MEDLARS** *abbr* medical literature analysis retrieval system. A computerized service provided by the United States National Library of Medicine. It contains references to medical journals and books published since 1966. It contains several databases, including MEDLINE.

**MEDLINE** *n* a US National Library of Medicine computerized database of medical science and associated literature.

**medulla** *n* **1.** the marrow in the centre of a long bone. **2.** the internal part of organs, e.g. kidneys, adrenals and lymph nodes, etc.

**medulla oblongata** the lowest part of the brainstem where it passes through the foramen magnum to become the spinal cord. It contains the nerve centres controlling various vital functions, e.g. cardiac centres. ⇒ Appendix 1, Figure 1.

**medullary** *adj* pertaining to the medulla. *medullary carcinoma* a malignant tumour with a soft consistency. May occur in the calcitonin-producing cells of the thyroid gland as part of some types of multiple endocrine neoplasia (MEN). ⇒ Sipple's syndrome.

**medullated** *adj* containing or surrounded by a medulla or marrow, particularly referring to myelinated nerve fibres.

**medulloblastoma** *n* malignant, rapidly growing tumour occurring in children; usually in the midline of the cerebellum. It generally occurs between 5 and 9 years of age and is more common in boys.

**medulloepithelioma** *n* also called neuroepithelioma. A malignant tumour of neuroepithelial tissue, affecting the brain or the retina.

**megacephalic** *adj* (*syn* macrocephalic, megalocephalic) large-headed.

**megacolon** *n* dilatation of the colon. *acquired megacolon* associated with chronic constipation of any cause, or may occur in acute severe colitis of any cause (toxic megacolon). *congenital megacolon (Hirschsprung's disease)* due to absence of ganglionic cells in a distal segment of the colon with loss of relaxation, resulting in dilatation of the normal proximal colon.

**megakaryoblast** *n* a large nucleated cell of the bone marrow. An early precursor cell in the development of megakaryocytes, which are involved in the production of platelets (thrombocytes).

**megakaryocyte** *n* large multinucleated cell of the bone marrow that gives rise to platelets (thrombocytes). The non-nucleated platelets form from fragments of the megakaryocytes during a process termed thrombopoiesis.

**megaloblast** *n* a large, nucleated, primitive red blood cell formed where there is a deficiency of vitamin $B_{12}$, folic acid or the intrinsic factor—**megaloblastic** *adj*.

**megaloblastic anaemia** an anaemia caused by a deficiency of vitamin $B_{12}$ or folic acid. It results in the formation of large red blood cells called megaloblasts. ⇒ anaemia.

**megalocephalic** *adj* ⇒ megacephalic.

**megalomania** *n* delusion of grandeur, characteristic of general paralysis of the insane.

**megaureter** *n* dilatation of one or both ureters caused by an obstruction to the flow of urine. It may be associated with vesicoureteric reflux of urine, or defective peristaltic action of the muscle layer of the ureter.

**meglitinides** *npl* a group of oral hypoglycaemic drugs, e.g. repaglinide, used for people with type 2 diabetes. ⇒ Appendix 5.

**megophthalmia** *n* a large eyeball.

**meibomian cyst** ⇒ chalazion.

**meibomian glands** (H Meibom, German anatomist and physician, 1638–1700) also known as the tarsal glands. Modified sebaceous glands lying in grooves on the inner surface of the eyelids, their ducts opening on the free margins of the lids.

**Meigs' syndrome** (J Meigs, American gynaecologist and obstetrician, 1892–1963) a benign, solid ovarian fibroma associated with ascites and hydrothorax.

**meiosis** *n* also called a reduction division. The process which, through two successive cell divisions, results in the production of mature gametes—oocytes or spermatozoa. There is pairing of the partner chromosomes, which

**M**

separate from each other at the meiotic divisions, so that the diploid (2n) chromosome number (i.e. 23 pairs) is reduced by half to 23 chromosomes, only one chromosome of each original pair, this set being the haploid (n) complement (Figure M.3). ⇒ mitosis, gamete.

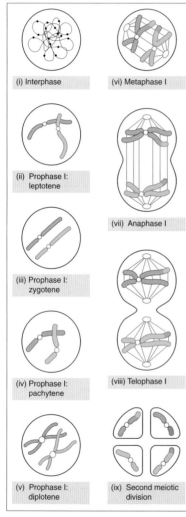

(i) Interphase

(vi) Metaphase I

(ii) Prophase I: leptotene

(vii) Anaphase I

(iii) Prophase I: zygotene

(iv) Prophase I: pachytene

(viii) Telophase I

(v) Prophase I: diplotene

(ix) Second meiotic division

**Figure M.3** Meiosis (reproduced from Hinchliff et al. 1996 with permission).

**Meissner's corpuscles** (G Meissner, German anatomist, 1829–1905) light-pressure sensory receptors in the skin.

**Meissner's plexus** (G Meissner) ⇒ submucosal plexus.

**melaena** n black, tar-like stools. Contains digested blood and has a distinctive odour. Evidence of upper gastrointestinal bleeding, such as from a peptic ulcer, gastric cancer, oesophageal varices, small-bowel disease, or as a drug side-effect.

**melancholia** n depression—from the Latin for black bile—**melancholic** adj.

**melanin** n a brown/black pigment found in hair, skin and the choroid of the eye.

**melanocytes** npl cells in the skin that produce melanin.

**melanocyte-stimulating hormones (MSH)** peptide hormones produced by many species in which it is important in changing skin colour. It is produced from a large precursor molecule in the pituitary gland, and is also present in the brain where it may act as a signalling molecule.

**melanoma** n a malignant tumour arising from the pigment-producing cells (melanocytes) of the skin, or of the eye. malignant melanoma malignant cutaneous mole or freckle (usually), it is the most dangerous of all skin cancers. Related to overexposure to ultraviolet radiation (sunburn); most common in fair-skinned, blond/red-haired people. It is characterized by change in colour, shape, size of mole or with bleeding or itching in a mole. The prognosis depends on Breslow's depth (thickness); staging involves lymph node status, with sentinel node biopsy (SNB) now becoming an integral part, along with computed tomography (CT) scan. Surgery is the only curative treatment: chemotherapy and radiotherapy are of limited effectiveness—**melanomatous** adj. ⇒ Breslow's depth, Clark's level. ⊙ DVD

**melanosis** n dark pigmentation of surfaces as in Addison's disease, etc.

**melanosis coli** brown pigmentation of the colonic mucosa associated with long-term misuse of stimulant laxative drugs—**melanotic** adj.

**melanoplakia** n pigmented patches on the oral mucosa.

**MELAS syndrome** abbr **m**itochondrial **e**ncephalopathy **l**actic **a**cidosis and **s**troke-like episodes. ⇒ mitochondrial genes and disorders.

**melasma** n (syn chloasma) hypermelanosis of the face, usually in women. Known as *melasma gravidarum* when it occurs during pregnancy.

**melatonin** *n* a hormone produced by the pineal body (gland) in response to the amount of light entering the eye. Influences sexual development and is involved in reproductive function. Also influences mood and various circadian rhythms, such as body temperature and sleep.

**Meleney's gangrene** (F Meleney, American surgeon, 1889–1963) gangrene affecting the skin and subcutaneous tissues postoperatively. A synergistic bacterial gangrene that involves a non-haemolytic streptococcus and *Staphylococcus aureus*.

**melioidosis** *n* caused by the bacterium *Burkholderia pseudomallei*. It occurs in tropical areas and is endemic in South-East Asia and northern Australia. In addition there are cases in Africa, India and the Middle East. It affects humans and many other animals, including cattle, pigs, sheep, goats, dogs, cats and horses. The disease is transmitted by direct contact with contaminated water and soil. The bacterium enters the body by inhalation or ingestion or through breaks in the skin. Melioidosis may be acute, when it causes pneumonia and septicaemia, or chronic, when it is characterized by abscess formation in many organs with the development of fistulas.

**melitensis** *n* ⇒ brucellosis.

**Melkersson–Rosenthal syndrome** (E Melkersson, Swedish physician, 1898–1932; C Rosenthal, German neurologist, 1892–1937) a syndrome usually commencing during childhood or adolescence. There is chronic facial swelling, facial nerve palsy and furrowing /fissuring of the tongue.

**membrane** *n* a thin lining or covering substance—**membranous** *adj*. *basement membrane* a thin layer beneath the epithelium of mucous surfaces. *hyaloid membrane* the transparent capsule surrounding the vitreous body (humour) of the eye. *mucous membrane* contains glands which secrete mucus. It lines the cavities and passages that communicate with the exterior of the body. *serous membrane* a lubricating membrane lining the closed cavities, and reflected over their enclosed organs. *synovial membrane* the membrane lining the intra-articular parts of bones and ligaments. It does not cover the articular surfaces. *tympanic membrane* the eardrum (⇒ Appendix 1, Figure 13).

**memory lapses** many adults have episodes of memory loss and some time later retrieve the appropriate information. The lapses often occur when individuals are under stress and typically increase with age. ⇒ Alzheimer's disease, dementia.

**memory** *n* the ability to retain and recall prior learning (information and events). It is a very complex process and includes different types of memory. ⇒ episodic memory, long-term memory, procedural memory, semantic memory, short-term memory.

**MEN** *acron* **m**ultiple **e**ndocrine **n**eoplasia.

**menaquinones** *npl* a form of vitamin K produced by bacteria in the gastrointestinal tract.

**menarche** *n* the first menstruation or menstrual bleed. In the vast majority of girls this usually occurs between 11 and 13 years of age but the timing depends on environment, genetics and achieving a particular body mass and percentage of body fat. The commencement of menstrual cycles is not usually accompanied by ovulation for several months.

**Mendel's law** (G Mendel, Austrian geneticist, 1822–1884) the fundamental theory of heredity and its laws, evolved by Mendel's work with peas. The laws determine the inheritance of different characters, and particularly the interaction of dominant and recessive traits in cross-breeding, the maintenance of the purity of such characters during hereditary transmission and the independent segregation of genetically different characteristics, such as the size of pea plants.

**Mendelson syndrome** (C Mendelson, American obstetrician, b. 1913) the aspiration (inhalation) of regurgitated acid stomach contents, which can cause immediate death from anoxia, or it may produce extensive lung damage or pulmonary oedema with severe bronchospasm. It may happen during the administration of a general anaesthesic to women in labour, or in situations where an unconscious person vomits (e.g. inebriation caused by an excessive intake of alcohol).

**Ménétrier's disease** (P Ménétrier, French physician, 1859–1935) also called giant hypertrophic gastritis or hypertrophic gastropathy. A rare condition characterized by the growth of tissue within the stomach, inflammation, possible ulceration and loss of albumen. There is pain, nausea, vomiting, haematemesis, anorexia and diarrhoea. It is associated with an increased risk of stomach cancer.

**Ménière's disease** (P Ménière, French physician, 1799–1862) distension of membranous labyrinth of inner ear from excess fluid. Pressure causes failure of function of the cranial

**M**

nerve responsible for balance and hearing (vestibulocochlear); thus there is fluctuating deafness, tinnitus and repeated attacks of vertigo.

**meninges** *npl* three membranes that surround the brain and spinal cord. From outside in they are the dura mater, a double layer of fibrous tissue (outer); the fibrous arachnoid membrane (middle) is separated from the dura mater by a subdural space and from the pia mater by the subarachnoid space, which contains cerebrospinal fluid; and the fragile pia mater (inner), containing many small blood vessels. It adheres to the brain and spinal cord, and follows every convolution (gyrus) and fissure (sulcus) of the brain (Figure M.4). ⇒ meningitis—**meninx** *sing*, **meningeal** *adj*. ⇒ falx cerebri, falx cerebelli, tentorium cerebelli.

**meningioma** *n* a slowly growing fibrous tumour arising in the meninges—**meningiomata** *pl*, **meningiomatous** *adj*.

**meningism** *n* (*syn* meningismus) a condition describing irritation and inflammation of the meninges due normally to infection or haemorrhage and consisting of neck stiffness and photophobia.

**meningitis** *n* inflammation of the meninges covering the brain and spinal cord due to infection by micro-organisms. It may be viral or bacterial. Viral meningitis is the more common cause, e.g. coxsackievirus, echovirus and mumps virus. It is usually a mild illness. Bacterial meningitis is a much more severe illness with considerable morbidity and a high mortality rate. It may be caused by *Haemophilus influenzae*, *Streptococcus pneumoniae*, *Neisseria meningitidis* (meningococcal), group B streptococci, Gram-negative bacilli and, less commonly, *Listeria monocytogenes*, *Cryptococcus neoformans*, *Staphylococcus aureus* and *Mycobacterium tuberculosis* (where the onset is insidious). Acute infections are characterized by a vague flu-like illness, headache, fever, neck stiffness, photophobia, vomiting, altered consciousness, convulsions, a positive Kernig's sign and changes in the cerebrospinal fluid on lumbar puncture. In infants and small children the signs may be less specific, with irritability and poor feeding. Patients with meningococcal septicaemia will also have a dark purple/red petechial rash that does not disappear when pressure is applied. Management involves the immediate administration of the appropriate antimicrobial drugs, supportive treatment, such as mechanical ventilation, and skilled nursing care and observation. ⇒ group C meningococcal disease.

**meningocele** *n* a protrusion of the meninges through a bony defect of the skull or vertebral column. It forms a cyst filled with cerebrospinal fluid but with no neural tissue. ⇒ neural tube defect, spina bifida.

**meningococcus** *n* the bacterium *Neisseria meningitidis*. A Gram-negative diplococcus that causes life-threatening meningococcal meningitis and septicaemia—**meningococcal** *adj*.

**meningoencephalitis** *n* inflammation of the brain and the meninges—**meningoencephalitic** *adj*.

**meningoencephalocele** *n* also known as encephalomeningocele. A sac containing cerebrospinal fluid, brain tissue and meninges that protrudes through a congenital defect in the skull. ⇒ neural tube defect.

**meningomyelocele** *n* (*syn* myelomeningocele) protrusion of a portion of the spinal cord,

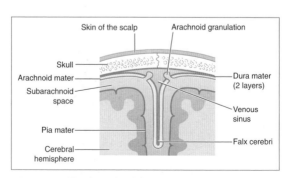

Skin of the scalp    Arachnoid granulation

Skull

Arachnoid mater

Subarachnoid space

Dura mater (2 layers)

Venous sinus

Pia mater

Falx cerebri

Cerebral hemisphere

**Figure M.4** Meninges—simplified (*reproduced from Brooker & Nicol 2003 with permission*).

its enclosing meningeal membranes and cerebrospinal fluid through a bony defect in the vertebral column. It differs from a meningocele in being covered with a thin, transparent membrane which may be granular and moist. ⇒ neural tube defect.

**meniscectomy** *n* the removal of a meniscus (semilunar cartilage) of the knee joint, following injury and displacement. The medial cartilage is torn most commonly and occurs in excessive twisting movements of the knee. Usually an endoscopic removal of damaged fragments is undertaken when there is pain and in locking or instability of the knee. ⇒ arthroscopy.

**meniscus** *n* **1.** semilunar cartilage, particularly those that deepen and stabilize the knee joint. **2.** the curved upper surface of a column of liquid—**menisci** *pl*.

**Menkes' disease** (J Menkes, American neurologist, b. 1928) an inherited disease of copper metabolism. The defective gene is transmitted on the X chromosome and mainly affects boys. The disease presents during infancy. Development may be normal or near normal for the first 3 months, after which there is marked developmental delay and loss of existing developmental skills. Affected infants fail to thrive, have seizures and have low body temperature and hair that is kinky, colourless and very fragile. There is serious neurodegeneration. Although treatment with subcutaneous or intravenous copper supplements may help, most children die before the age of 10 years.

**menopause** *n* the ending of menstruation. It is a single event occurring during the climacteric but is commonly used, erroneously, to describe all the changes occurring during the female climacteric. It normally occurs between the ages of 45 and 55 years. *artificial menopause* an earlier menopause caused by surgery or radiotherapy—**menopausal** *adj*. ⇒ climacteric.

**menorrhagia** *n* an excessive regular menstrual flow. The gynaecological causes include fibroids, endometrial polyps, endometrial hyperplasia, pelvic inflammatory disease, endometriosis, cancers of the endometrium and cervix, and intrauterine contraceptive devices. Menorrhagia may also be caused by thyroid dysfunction, coagulation disorders such as von Willebrand's disease, or with anticoagulant drugs.

**menses** *n* bloody fluid and tissue debris discharged from the uterus during menstruation; menstrual flow.

**menstrual** *adj* relating to the menses.

**menstrual or uterine cycle** the cyclical changes that occur as the endometrium responds to ovarian hormones. There are three phases: proliferative, secretory and menstrual, in which bleeding occurs for around 5 days. The cycle is repeated approximately every 28 days (21–35), except during pregnancy, from the menarche to the menopause.

**menstruation** *n* the flow of bloody fluid and tissue debris from the uterus once a month, or so, in the female. It usually starts at the age of 11–13 years in developed countries, and ceases around 50 years of age. ⇒ menarche, menopause.

**mental** *adj* **1.** pertaining to the mind. **2.** pertaining to the chin.

**mental aberration** a pathological deviation from normal thinking.

**mental age** the age of a person with regard to intellectual development, which can be determined by intelligence tests.

**mental defence mechanism (MDM)** unconscious defence mechanism by which individuals attempt to cope with stressful, difficult or threatening emotions. ⇒ defence mechanisms.

**mental disorder** mental illness, arrested or incomplete development of the mind, psychopathic disorder and any other disorder or disability of the mind, as defined by relevant legislation such as the Mental Health Act 1983. ⇒ mental health legislation.

**Mental Health Act Commission** in England and Wales the body that has the responsibility to review how the Mental Health (MH) Act 1983 is being applied in practice, and in particular to safeguard the interests of all patients detained under the MH Act 1983 and those patients who are liable to be detained. At the time of writing the government is planning to merge the Mental Health Act Commission with the Healthcare Commission and the Commission for Social Care Inspection in 2008 to create a single regulator.

**Mental Health Review Tribunal** in England and Wales a body with responsibility for hearing applications from or about people detained under the provisions of the Mental Health Act 1983. In Scotland the *Mental Health Tribunal* was created as part of the Mental Health (Care and Treatment) (Scotland) Act 2003 in order to decide issues concerning the compulsory care and treatment of patients suffering from a mental disorder.

M

**mental health legislation** law pertaining to mental disorder. For example, in England and Wales the main body of mental health legislation is the Mental Health Act 1983, which currently makes provision for the compulsory detention and treatment in hospital of those with a mental disorder. The Mental Health (Patients in the Community) Act 1995 amended the 1983 Act by providing for the 'supervised discharge' of those detained patients requiring a 'high degree' of supervision on discharge from hospital. However, many people with mental health problems are in hospital as voluntary (informal) patients. At the time of writing there are plans to amend the Mental Health Act 1983. The Mental Health (Care and Treatment) (Scotland) Act 2003 is the legal authority for mental health services in Scotland. This Act is rights-based and underpinned by a set of guiding principles.

**mentoanterior** *adj* forward position of the fetal chin in the maternal pelvis in a face presentation.

**mentoposterior** *adj* backward position of the fetal chin in the maternal pelvis in a face presentation.

**mentum** *n* the chin.

**MEP** *abbr* maximum expiratory pressure.

**meralgia paraesthetica** pain, tingling and numbness felt over the lateral surface of the thigh. It is caused by the entrapment of the lateral cutaneous nerve of the thigh as it passes through the inguinal ligament.

**mercurialism** *n* chronic poisoning with mercury. It may occur in individuals who are exposed to mercury at work, or it may be ingested in food, such as fish in some areas of the world, which may contain high levels. The effects of poisoning include loose teeth, stomatitis, gastrointestinal effects, renal problems, paraesthesia, ataxia, and visual and hearing problems.

**mercury (Hg)** *n* metallic element that is liquid at room temperature. Previously used in thermometers and sphygmomanometers. Toxicity means that local safety protocols should be followed in situations involving accidental spillage and contamination. Forms two series of salts: univalent mercurous salts and bivalent mercuric. ⇒ mercurialism.

**meridians** *npl* in complementary therapy the conceptual channels in which Qi energy flows. ⇒ acupuncture, shiatsu.

**merocrine (eccrine) gland** a type of exocrine gland in which the secretion is released by exocytosis into the lumen of the gland from

vesicles. The gland remains intact. ⇒ apocrine gland, holocrine gland.

**MESA** *acron* **m**icrosurgical **e**pididymal **s**perm **a**spiration.

**mesarteritis** *n* inflammation of the middle coat of an artery.

**mesencephalon** *n* midbrain. One of the three primary vesicles formed during embryonic development of the brain. It becomes the midbrain.

**mesenchyme** *n* embryonic connective tissue derived from mesoderm (one of the primary germ layers). It comprises cells embedded in a gelatinous matrix and eventually forms connective tissue.

**mesentery** *n* a double fan-shaped fold of peritoneum that attaches the jejunum and ileum to the posterior abdominal wall. Contains nerves, lymphatics and blood vessels—**mesenteric** *adj*.

**MESH, MeSH** *acron* **Me**dical **S**ubject **H**eadings. ⇒ indexing term.

**mesial** *adj* medial. Relating to or located in the median (midsagittal) plane or line; situated in the middle. Also describes the tooth surface closest to the midline of the face.

**mesiodens** *n* an unerupted or erupted supernumerary tooth between the central incisors of the upper jaw.

**mesocolon** *n* folds of peritoneum that attach the transverse colon (transverse mesocolon) to the abdominal wall, and the sigmoid colon (sigmoid mesocolon) to the pelvic wall. Contains nerves, lymphatics and blood vessels.

**mesoderm** *n* middle layer of the three primary germ layers of the early embryo. It gives rise to the cardiovascular system, lymphatic system, bone, muscles, blood, the dermis, pericardium, pleura, peritoneum, urogenital tract, gonads and the adrenal cortex. ⇒ ectoderm, endoderm, mesenchyme.

**mesometrium** *n* a double fold of peritoneum either side of the uterus that hangs down from the uterine tubes. Usually known as the broad ligaments.

**mesomorph** *n* a body type (physique) characterized by a well-covered person who has a well-developed musculature—**mesomorphic** *adj*. ⇒ ectomorph, endomorph.

**mesonephric duct** also known as the wolffian duct. The primitive embryonic duct that under the influence of testosterone becomes the internal genitalia (epididymis, deferent duct [vas deferens], seminal vesicles and ejaculatory ducts) in a genetically male embryo. ⇒ paramesonephric duct.

**M**

**mesonephros** *n* the wolffian body. An excretory organ that forms in early embryonic development. It is short-lived but the duct becomes part of the structures that later develop into the male reproductive structures. ⇒ metanephros, pronephros.

**mesophile** *n* a bacterium that thrives within the range 25–40°C. Most human pathogens thrive best at body temperature (37°C)—**mesophilic** *adj*.

**mesosalpinx** *n* the upper part of the broad ligament that encloses the uterine tubes.

**mesothelioma** *n* neoplasm of the pleura (commonly), pericardium or peritoneum; usually associated with asbestos exposure at least 20 years previously. Industrially related, therefore compensation is usually appropriate as few are operable and the median survival postdiagnosis is around 8 months. Therapy is almost universally palliative, as mesothelioma is generally chemo- and radioresistant.

**mesothelium** *n* a layer of flat cells that line the body cavity in the embryo. They are derived from the mesoderm layer. They continue as the layer of simple squamous epithelium that covers the serous membranes (pericardium, peritoneum, pleura) in adults.

**mesovarium** *n* a double fold of peritoneum that attaches the ovary to the broad ligament.

**messenger RNA (mRNA)** ⇒ ribonucleic acid.

**meta-analysis** *n* a statistical summary of several research studies using complex quantitative analysis of the primary data.

**metabolic** *adj* pertaining to metabolism—**metabolically** *adv*. ⇒ basal metabolic rate (BMR).

**metabolic equivalents (METS)** a unit of measurement of heat production by the body in a given time. It is expressed as multiples of basal (resting) metabolic rate. Used in sports medicine to estimate the intensity of exercise.

**metabolic syndrome** also known as metabolic syndrome X, syndrome X, insulin resistance syndrome. A group of risk factors for cardiovascular disease and type 2 diabetes. They include the degree of obesity—using waist measurement, waist:hip ratio and body mass index; insulin resistance—impaired fasting glucose/glycaemia, impaired glucose tolerance; cardiovascular risks—high blood pressure, low levels of high-density cholesterol, raised triglyceride and the presence of microalbuminuria.

**metabolic water** the water produced by the cells during the oxidation of nutrients.

**metabolism** *n* the continuous series of biochemical processes in the living body by which life is maintained. Nutrients and tissues are broken down (catabolism), new substances are created for growth and rebuilding (anabolism) and energy is released in catabolism and utilized in anabolism and heat production ⇒ adenosine diphosphate, adenosine triphosphate—**metabolic** *adj*. *basal metabolism* the minimum energy expended in the maintenance of essential physiological processes such as respiration.

**metabolite** *n* any product of or substance taking part in metabolism. *essential metabolite* one that is necessary for normal metabolism, e.g. B vitamins required for the synthesis of the coenzymes needed for many biochemical reactions.

**metacarpal 1.** *n* any one of the five slender bones forming the metacarpus. They articulate proximally with the carpal bones, and distally with the phalanges. **2.** *adj* relating to the metacarpus.

**metacarpophalangeal** *adj* pertaining to the metacarpus and the phalanges.

**metacarpus** *n* the five bones which form that part of the hand between the wrist and fingers (palm of the hand). They are numbered 1 to 5, starting at the thumb. ⇒ Appendix 1, Figure 2—**metacarpal** *adj*.

*Metagonimus n* a genus of minute intestinal flukes. *Metagonimus yokogawai* may infect humans who eat undercooked fish. Infestation known as metagonimiasis causes diarrhoea and abdominal colic. It occurs in the Balkans, Far East, Siberia and Spain.

**metalloenzyme** *n* an enzyme that contains metal ions, such as copper or zinc, as its prosthetic group. For example, carbonic anhydrase, the enzyme that catalyses the rapid reversible reactions that facilitate the transport of carbon dioxide from the tissues to the lungs, contains zinc.

**metalloprotein** *n* a protein that contains one or more metal ions as a cofactor. For example, iron in haemoglobin.

**metamorphopsia** *n* an abnormality of vision in which objects appear distorted. It results from retinal diseases such as macular degeneration.

**metamyelocyte** *n* an immature cell with a large kidney-shaped nucleus formed in the bone marrow during the development of the granulocyte series of white blood cells (leucocytes). Its presence in the blood is abnormal.

M

**metanephros** *n* the final fetal excretory organ with a complex tubular structure that will develop further to become a functioning kidney. ⇒ mesonephros, pronephros.

**metaphase** *n* the second stage of nuclear division in mitosis (see Figure M.6, p. 308) and both divisions in meiosis (see Figure M.3, p. 296). The chromosomes move to the middle of the cell and become arranged in the equatorial plane of the spindle. The centromeres attach to the spindle in preparation for separation. ⇒ anaphase, prophase, telophase.

**metaphysis** *n* in children the area of a growing long bone situated between each epiphysis (the end) and diaphysis (shaft).

**metaplasia** *n* process of substituting one type of mature epithelium for a different type of mature epithelium (usually less specialized) that is better suited to cope with the adverse environment which triggered the process. For example, the change from ciliated columnar epithelium to squamous epithelium in the respiratory mucosa of cigarette smokers. Metaplasia may occur in response to chronic inflammation; it is generally reversible if the cause is removed but may progress through dysplasia to malignant changes.

**metastasis** *n* the secondary spread of malignant tumour cells from one part of the body to another, either by the lymphatic route to the lymph nodes or to distant organs via the haematogenous (blood) route. Some cancers also spread across body cavities. Most solid tumours are not curable if metastasis has occurred—**metastases** *pl*, **metastatic** *adj*, **metastasize** *vi*.

**metatarsal 1.** *n* any one of the five bones forming the metatarsus. They articulate proximally with the tarsal bones, and distally with the phalanges. **2.** *adj* relating to the metatarsus.

**metatarsalgia** *n* pain under the metatarsal heads. ⇒ Morton's metatarsalgia. **metatarsophalangeal** *adj* pertaining to the metatarsus and the phalanges.

**metatarsus** *n* the five bones of the foot between the ankle and the toes. They are numbered 1 to 5 from medial to lateral aspects. ⇒ Appendix 1, Figure 2—**metatarsal** *adj*.

**metatarsus valgus** a congenital deformity where the forefoot is deviated outwards away from the midline of the body in relation to the hindfoot.

**metatarsus varus** also known as metatarsus adductus. A congenital deformity where the forefoot is deviated inwards towards the midline of the body in relation to the hindfoot.

**metencephalon** *n* one of the secondary enlargements during embryonic development of the brain. It becomes part of the hindbrain—the cerebellum and the pons.

**meteorism** *n* ⇒ tympanites.

**metered-dose inhaler** a device designed to deliver a dose of medication and a dry powder into the lungs (Figure M.5). It is frequently used by people with asthma to administer their medication. The inhaler can be used with a cone-shaped spacer device for small children and other people who are able to co-ordinate the action required to use the inhaler.

**methadone** *n* a synthetic opioid analgesic. It is used as part of a heroin withdrawal programme.

**methaemalbumin** *n* abnormal compound formed in blood from combination of haem with plasma albumin, under conditions of grossly accelerated red cell breakdown (haemolysis), such as the intravascular haemolysis that occurs as a complication of malaria (blackwater fever).

**methaemoglobin** *n* a form of haemoglobin consisting of a combination of globin with an oxidized haem, containing ferric iron. This pigment is unable to transport oxygen. Small amounts can be detected in the blood after smoking. It may be formed in babies after exposure to environmental chemicals such

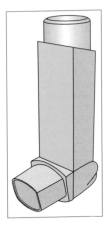

**Figure M.5** Metered-dose inhaler *(reproduced from Brooker & Waugh 2007 with permission).*

as the nitrates found in drinking water and some vegetables. It may form following the administration of a wide variety of drugs, including the sulphonamides. It may also be present in the blood as a result of an inherited deficiency of enzymes or in conditions where the haemoglobin is abnormal.

**methaemoglobinaemia** *n* methaemoglobin in the blood. If large quantities are present, individuals may show cyanosis, but otherwise no abnormality except, in severe cases, breathlessness on exertion, because the methaemoglobin cannot transport oxygen—**methaemoglobinaemic** *adj.*

**methane** *n* $CH_4$ a colourless, odourless, inflammable gas that results from the decomposition of organic matter.

**methanol** *n* methyl alcohol. Also known as wood alcohol or wood spirits, it is used as a solvent, fuel and antifreeze. Its ingestion, absorption or inhalation has very serious effects. It intoxicates; its breakdown product formaldehyde is toxic and causes blindness, by damaging the optic nerves; depression of the nervous system; and in severe cases metabolic acidosis, respiratory failure and death.

**meticillin (methicillin)-resistant *Staphylococcus aureus* (MRSA)** *n* strains of *Staphylococcus aureus* that are resistant to meticillin (not used clinically) and flucloxacillin. Causes serious and sometimes fatal infections in hospitals, and patients with MRSA are frequently encountered in community settings. Treatment depends on the sensitivity of the particular strain of MRSA to antibacterial drugs and on the site of infection. Drugs used include vancomycin, teicoplanin, combinations of rifampicin and sodium fusidate with each other or with a glycopeptide antibacterial, the streptogramin antibacterials quinupristin and dalfopristin combined, or linezolid, an oxazolidinone antibacterial. Topical mupirocin is used to eliminate nasal or skin carriage. Infection prevention and control measures that include strict adherence to hand-washing, proper environmental cleaning and isolation, or if single rooms are not available, patient cohorting are vital in controlling MRSA. Epidemic strains (EMRSA) have developed resistance to most antibiotics. ⇒ Panton–Valentine leukocidin, *Staphylococcus*, vancomycin-resistant *Staphylococcus aureus.*

**methionine** *n* one of the essential (indispensable) sulphur-containing amino acids. May be used in the treatment of hepatitis, paracetamol overdose and other conditions associated with liver damage.

**methylcellulose** *n* a bulk-forming laxative. ⇒ Appendix 5.

**methylmalonic acid** an intermediate formed during the metabolism of succinic acid. It tends to accumulate when there is a deficiency of vitamin $B_{12}$. Measuring the level in urine or serum provides information about vitamin $B_{12}$ status.

**metre (m)** *n* one of the seven base units of the International System of Units (SI). A measurement of length. ⇒ Appendix 2.

**metritis** *n* inflammation of the uterus.

**metropathia haemorrhagica** a term sometimes applied to irregular, prolonged and heavy menstrual bleeding. It is associated with the persistent production of high levels of oestrogen, which causes cystic glandular hyperplasia of the endometrium. It usually occurs in women nearing the menopause.

**metrorrhagia** *n* uterine bleeding between the menstrual periods such as after intercourse or examination.

**METS** *abbr* metabolic equivalents.

**MHC** *abbr* major histocompatibility complex.

**MHRA** *abbr* Medicines and Healthcare products Regulatory Agency.

**micelle** *n* tiny globules of fat and bile salts formed during fat digestion. Fatty acids and glycerol are transported into the intestinal cells (enterocytes) in this form, leaving the bile salts behind in the lumen of the bowel.

**microalbuminuria** *n* the presence of small amounts of albumen (within a range of 20–200 μg/min) in the urine, not revealed using a standard routine dipstick urinalysis. There are commercial dipsticks that will detect this lower level. The presence of microalbuminuria is an indication that early nephropathy is occurring in people who have diabetes for a number of years. It may also occur in people with hypertension and those with subclinical cardiac conditions. ⇒ diabetic nephropathy.

**microaneurysm** *n* dilatation of retinal blood vessels. May bleed or leak. Commonly present in diabetic retinopathy.

**microangiopathy** *n* small-vessel disease, with basement membrane thickening and endothelial dysfunction, usually in association with diabetes mellitus, but also seen in patients with connective tissue disease, infection and malignancy; results in retinopathy and nephropathy in patients with diabetes. ⇒ diabetic nephropathy, diabetic retinopathy.

**microbe** *n* ⇒ micro-organism—**microbial**, **microbic** *adj*.

**microbiological assay** a way of measuring substances such as amino acids and vitamins, using micro-organisms. The micro-organisms are introduced into a medium containing all the nutrients needed for growth except the one being investigated. The rate of microbial growth is then proportional to the amount of the missing nutrient subsequently introduced into the medium.

**microbiology** *n* the science of micro-organisms—**microbiological** *adj*.

**microcephaly** *n* an abnormally small head.

**microcirculation** *n* blood flow through the arterioles, capillaries and venules. Damage caused by prolonged compression to these vessels predisposes to the formation of pressure ulcers.

*Micrococcus n* a genus of Gram-positive bacteria. Found in soil and fresh water. Generally non-pathogenic, they are part of the skin flora. It can, however, cause opportunistic infections in immunocompromised individuals.

**microcyte** *n* an abnormally undersized red blood cell found, for example, in iron-deficiency anaemia, or in anaemia caused by chronic bleeding.

**microcytosis** *n* an increased number of microcytes in the circulating blood, such as in iron-deficiency anaemia—**microcytic** *adj*.

**microdiscectomy** *n* a minimally invasive surgical procedure using an operating microscope, undertaken for some patients with back pain caused by a prolapsed intervertebral disc. It is performed through a small laminectomy (surgical procedure, which includes removal of a portion of the lamina, to provide more room in the vertebral canal). A small part of the prolapsed disc is removed to relieve the pressure on the spinal cord or the spinal nerve roots.

**microdissection** *n* dissection of tissue or cells under the microscope.

**microdochectomy** *n* a surgical procedure used in the management of intraductal papillomas of the breast, in which the affected segment of breast is excised.

**microdontia** *n* a condition in which the teeth are abnormally small. It may affect some or all the teeth.

**microenvironment** *n* the environment at the microscopic or cellular level immediately surrounding the body.

**microfilaria** *n* immature filaria. ⇒ filariasis.

**microglia** *n* non-neural cells, a type of macrophage present in the central nervous system. They are phagocytic and are able to deal with cell debris. ⇒ macroglia.

**microglossia** *n* an abnormally small tongue.

**micrognathia** *n* small jaw, especially the lower one. May cause problems with feeding and with the eruption of the teeth. It is a feature of the chromosomal condition Edwards' syndrome, and Pierre–Robin syndrome, which is due to a developmental anomaly.

**microgram** (μg) *n* one millionth of a gram.

**micrometre** (μm) *n* also still called a micron. One millionth of a metre.

**micron** *n* ⇒ micrometre.

**micronutrients** *npl* nutrients needed by the body in relatively small amounts, such as vitamins and minerals. They are vital for the biochemical processes of the body. ⇒ macronutrients, trace elements.

**micro-organism** *n* (*syn* microbe) a microscopic cell. Often synonymous with bacterium but includes virus, protozoon, rickettsia, chlamydia and fungus.

**microphthalmos** *n* a congenital condition in which one or both eyes are abnormally small.

**micropsia** *n* a visual defect in which objects are seen as much smaller than they are in reality.

**microscopic** *adj* extremely small; visible only with the aid of a microscope. ⇒ macroscopic *opp*.

**microscopy** *n* the various techniques that utilize a microscope to view minute objects, such as body tissues, cells and cell organelles, or bacteria and viruses.

**microsome** *n* a minute fragment of endoplasmic reticulum and associated ribosomes. They result from cell breakdown during homogenization. The microsome fragments can be sorted from other subcellular organelles during centrifugation.

*Microsporum n* a genus of fungi. Parasitic, living in keratin-containing tissues of humans and animals. *Microsporum audouini* is the commonest cause of scalp ringworm. ⇒ dermatophytes, tinea.

**microsurgery** *n* use of the binocular operating microscope during the performance of operations that require delicate procedures involving small structures, such as repairing blood vessels and nerves following a traumatic amputation. Also increases access to areas such as the brain, spinal cord and the inner ear for operative procedures—**microsurgical** *adj*.

**microsurgical epididymal sperm aspiration (MESA)** a technique used in assisted conception. Spermatozoa are aspirated directly from the epididymis in men who have azoospermia caused by a permanent obstruction in the duct system, such as may follow infection or vasectomy. The spermatozoa, which can be frozen and stored, are used for repeated attempts to achieve in vitro fertilization, including using intracytoplasmic sperm injection. ⇒ intracytoplasmic sperm injection (ICSI).

**microtia** *n* a small ear. A congenital abnormality that may affect one or both ears. It is graded from a small, deformed pinna with a functional meatus/canal; through deformities that include a blocked or absent external auditory meatus/canal and absence of the tympanic membrane and conductive deafness; to complete absence of the ear (anotia).

**microtome** *n* an instrument used for cutting tissue sections for microscopic study, usually in the order of 4–6 μm in thickness.

**microtrauma** *n* injury to a small number of cells due to the cumulative effect of repetitive forces.

**microvascular surgery** surgery carried out on blood vessels using a binocular operating microscope. ⇒ microsurgery.

**microvilli** *npl* microscopic projections from the free surface of cell membranes whose role is to increase the exposed surface of the cell for absorption, e.g. intestinal epithelium.

**microwave** *n* electromagnetic radiation which has a frequency between 2,450 and 433 MHz. Therapeutic uses include electrotherapy techniques in physiotherapy, treatment of benign prostatic enlargement, and subjecting accessible tumour cells to hyperthermia.

**micturating cystourethrogram (MCU)** radiographic examination that can be used to investigate urinary incontinence. Following intravenous injection of a contrast medium or, more commonly, after contrast is introduced into the bladder via a urinary catheter until micturating begins. A series of X-rays are taken during the act of passing urine.

**micturition** *n* (*syn* urination) passing urine.

**midbrain** *n* the mesencephalon. The most anterior part of the brainstem that surrounds the cerebral aqueduct. It is situated between the cerebrum above and the pons below. It contains important nuclei and nerve tracts that connect the cerebrum with the brainstem and spinal cord. The nuclei include those of two cranial nerves (oculomotor and troch-

lear), the substantia nigra, the red nucleus. ⇒ Appendix 1, Figure 1.

**middle ear** *n* also called the tympanum. The tympanic cavity, situated in the temporal bone. The tympanic membrane separates it from the outer ear. It is an air-filled cavity containing the three tiny bones or ossicles: malleus, incus and stapes. The ossicles transmit the sound waves to the inner ear via the oval window. The middle ear communicates with the nasopharynx via the pharyngotympanic (eustachian or auditory) tube.

**midgut** *n* the middle part of the embryonic alimentary tract between the foregut and the hindgut. It is endodermal tissue and will form some of the small intestine and part of the large intestine. ⇒ foregut, hindgut.

**midriff** *n* the diaphragm.

**midsagittal plane** ⇒ median plane.

**midstream specimen of urine (MSU)** a specimen of urine obtained from the middle part of voiding. The first and last parts of the flow of urine are discarded. It is usually collected for microbiological examination to confirm the presence of a urinary tract infection, therefore it is collected in a sterile container and the risk of contamination is reduced by the person cleaning around the external urethral opening with the warm soapy water. Women and girls should clean from front to back. In older boys and adult males, the foreskin (if present) should be retracted, and the glans cleaned.

**mid-upper-arm circumference (MUAC)** an anthropometric test that assesses the amount of muscle tissue in the upper arm. The arm circumference is measured midway between the top of the acromion of the shoulder and the olecranon process of the elbow. Used as part of nutritional assessment. ⇒ anthropometry.

**midwife** *n* in the UK midwives are responsible for providing care to mothers and babies in accordance with the Nursing and Midwifery Council's current *Midwives' Rules and Code of Practice*. The care provided covers prenatal (antenatal), intranatal and postnatal periods. Midwives may practise in the woman's home, general practitioner's surgery, at a health centre or within a hospital. The practice of midwifery includes providing family planning advice; making a diagnosis of pregnancy; providing prenatal care and parenthood classes; care during labour and conducting deliveries; recognizing problems and abnormalities affecting mother or baby; and the care of both mother and child in the postnatal period. As midwives are members of a multiprofessional team, these activities are not pursued in isolation and midwives work with doctors, specialist community public health nurses and other professionals to provide high standards of care.

**migraine** *n* a condition characterized by paroxysmal headache, vomiting and focal neurological symptoms (usually visual). The presence of all three is classical migraine, whereas common migraine is defined as paroxysmal headache with or without vomiting but no focal neurological symptoms. Migraine sufferers also experience photophobia and phonophobia. The aura of migraine most often takes the form of shimmering zigzag lines that move across the visual field. Migraine attacks may be triggered by certain foods and beverages such as chocolate, cheese and red wine; hormonal changes during the menstrual cycle; and bright lights, and may occur during the time after stresses and strains such as weekends or holiday time—**migrainous** *adj*.

**Mikulicz's disease/syndrome** (J von Mikulicz-Radecki, Polish surgeon, 1850–1905) chronic hypertrophic enlargement of the lacrimal and salivary glands. It may be associated with other conditions, e.g. leukaemia, sarcoidosis.

**miliaria** *n* (*syn* strophulus) prickly heat common in the tropics, and affects waistline, cubital fossae and chest. Vesicular and erythematous eruption, caused by blocking of sweat ducts and their subsequent rupture, or their infection by fungi or bacteria.

**miliary** *adj* resembling a millet seed. *miliary tuberculosis* ⇒ tuberculosis.

**military antishock trousers (MAST)** an inflatable garment used to apply pressure to the abdomen and legs to minimize the pooling of blood in the lower body, thereby redistributing the available circulating volume to increase the perfusion of vital organs.

**milium** *n* condition in which tiny, white, cystic excrescences appear on the face, especially about the eyelids; the cysts contain keratin—**milia** *pl*.

**milk** *n* secretion of the mammary glands. Provided that the woman is taking an adequate diet, breast milk provides the perfect nutrition for healthy infants. It contains all the essential nutrients in proportions that meet growth and development needs of infants during the first 6 months of life. Moreover, breast milk contains maternal immunoglobulins and these help to protect infants while their own immune systems develop. In addition, there are advantages to the mother that include special contact with her infant and ready availability of feeds. ⇒ colostrum.

**milk sugar** lactose.

**milk teeth** the 20 deciduous teeth of the primary dentition.

**Miller–Abbott tube** (T Miller, American physician, 1886–1981; W Abbott, American physician, 1902–1943) double-lumen tube used for intestinal suction. The second channel leads to a balloon near the tip of the tube.

**Miller–Dieker syndrome** (J Miller, American physician, b. 1926; H Dieker, American geneticist, 20th century) ⇒ lissencephaly.

**milliampere (mA)** *n* a measurement of electrical current. One thousandth part of an ampere.

**milligram (mg)** *n* one thousandth part of a gram.

**millilitre (mL)** *n* one thousandth part of a litre. Equal to a cubic centimetre.

**millimetre (mm)** *n* one thousandth part of a metre.

**millimole (mmol)** *n* one thousandth part of a mole.

**Milroy's disease** (W Milroy, American physician, 1855–1942) a congenital condition in which there is lymphoedema caused by lymphatic obstruction. Usually affects the legs but other areas may be involved. ⇒ lymphoedema.

**Milwaukee brace** an orthotic device used in the corrective treatment of spinal curvature (scoliosis). It applies fixed traction between the occiput and the pelvis.

**Minamata disease** a severe neurological condition caused by mercury poisoning. It is named from the place in Japan where mercury released from a factory polluted the sea and the fish, which were eaten by the inhabitants. It is characterized by ataxia, dysarthria and visual impairment.

**mineralocorticoid** *n* a group of corticosteroid hormones produced by the adrenal cortex. Involved in the regulation of electrolyte and water balance. ⇒ aldosterone.

**minerals** *npl* inorganic elements required in the diet. They perform a vital role in body structure and functions. They are: calcium, chloride, iron, magnesium, phosphorus, potassium, sodium and zinc, and the trace elements cobalt, chromium, copper, fluoride, iodine, manganese, molybdenum and selenium, some of which are required in extremely minute amounts. ⇒ trace elements.

M

**Mini Mental State Examination (MMSE)** a test of cognitive function used to screen for dementia or delirium. It tests five areas including orientation, recall, language, etc.

**minimally invasive surgery (MIS)** known colloquially as 'keyhole surgery'. Surgical techniques that only require minimal access; the procedure is performed through very small incisions using endoscopic instruments. An increasing variety of procedures which cover a range of complexity are undertaken, e.g. female sterilization, cholecystectomy, vascular surgery. ⇒ laparoscopy.

**minitracheostomy** *n* cricothyroidotomy. The insertion of a fine-bore minitracheostomy tube to treat or prevent the retention of sputum in a variety of conditions and situations, such as following chest surgery. ⇒ tracheostomy.

**minute ventilation** also known as pulmonary ventilation. The volume of air moved into and out of the lungs in 1 minute. It is tidal volume × respiratory rate.

**miosis (myosis)** *n* constriction of the pupil of the eye.

**miotic (myotic)** *adj* an agent that causes miosis such as the drug pilocarpine. ⇒ Appendix 5.

**MIP** *abbr* maximum inspiratory pressure.

**MIS** *abbr* minimally invasive surgery.

**miscarriage** *n* spontaneous loss of pregnancy before 24 completed weeks of gestation (also referred to as abortion). *complete miscarriage* the entire contents of the uterus are expelled. *incomplete miscarriage* part of the fetus or placenta is retained in the uterus. ⇒ evacuation of retained products of conception. *inevitable miscarriage* loss of the pregnancy cannot be prevented. *missed miscarriage* the early signs and symptoms of pregnancy disappear and the fetus dies but is not expelled for some time. ⇒ carneous mole. *recurrent or habitual miscarriage* when miscarriage occurs in three successive pregnancies. *septic miscarriage* one associated with uterine infection. *spontaneous miscarriage* one which occurs naturally without intervention. *threatened miscarriage* characterized by slight vaginal bleeding whilst the cervix remains closed. *tubal miscarriage* an ectopic pregnancy in which the embryo dies and is expelled from the fimbriated end of the uterine (fallopian) tube.

**missed abortion** ⇒ miscarriage.

**Misuse of Drugs Act (1971, Regulations 1985)** in UK. Controls the manufacture, sale, possession, supply, storage, prescribing, dispensing and administration of certain groups of habit-forming drugs that are liable to misuse and dependence. They are called controlled drugs and are available to the public by prescription only. Drugs subject to the Act include the opioids, synthetic narcotics, cocaine, hallucinogens and barbiturates (with exceptions). The individual drugs include cocaine, diamorphine (heroin), methadone and pethidine. ⇒ Appendix 5.

**Mitchell's osteotomy** a surgical procedure involving a distal osteotomy of the first metatarsal. Used for hallux valgus.

**mite** *n* a minute arachnid related to ticks and spiders. Several species are parasitic, including *Sarcoptes scabiei*, which causes scabies. Some are responsible for spreading scrub typhus. ⇒ Trombiculidae. The house dust mite of the genus *Dermatophagoiges* is an important cause of allergic asthma. ⇒ house dust mite.

**mitochondrial genes and disorders** there are a number of genes present in the mitochondria; they encode several proteins. Mitochondrial genes are inherited from the woman and mutations do occur. *Mitochondrial disorders* result from the inheritance of faulty mitochondrial DNA. The effects of the disorders can be very variable and occur at any age. Examples include diabetes mellitus with deafness, Leber hereditary optic neuropathy, Leigh's disease and mitochondrial encephalopathy lactic acidosis and stroke-like episodes (MELAS).

**mitochondrion** *n* a membrane-bound subcellular organelle situated in the cytoplasm. They are the principal sites of adenosine triphosphate production from the oxidation of fuel molecules. They contain nucleic acids (DNA and RNA) and ribosomes, replicate independently, and synthesize some of their own proteins. They are particularly numerous in metabolically active cells, such as skeletal muscle and liver.

**mitosis** *n* nuclear (and usually cell) division, in which somatic cells divide. It involves the exact replication of chromosomes, which results in two 'daughter' cells that are genetically identical to the cell of origin, i.e. they have the diploid (2n) chromosome number, 46 in humans (Figure M.6). ⇒ meiosis— **mitoses** *pl*. **mitotic** *adj*.

**mitotic index** the ratio between the number of cells undergoing mitosis and the number of cells in total. It provides an indication of the rate of cell proliferation.

M

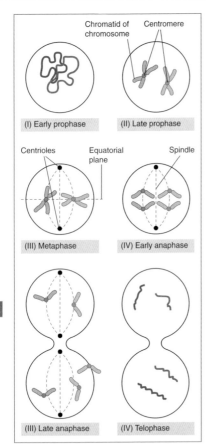

**Figure M.6** Mitosis *(reproduced from Hinchliff et al. 1996 with permission).*

**mitral** *adj* mitre-shaped, such as the valve between the left atrium and ventricle of the heart (bicuspid valve).

**mitral regurgitation (incompetence)** a defect in the closure of the mitral valve whereby blood tends to flow backwards into the left atrium from the left ventricle.

**mitral stenosis** narrowing of the mitral orifice, usually due to rheumatic fever.

**mitral valvulotomy (valvotomy)** an operation to correct a stenosed mitral valve.

**mittelschmerz** *n* abdominal pain midway between menstrual periods, at the time of ovulation.

**mixed venous oxygen saturation (S$\bar{v}$O$_2$)** percentage of oxygenated haemoglobin in venous blood returning to the lungs, measured in blood taken from the pulmonary artery.

**MLC** *abbr* multileaf collimation.

**MLNS** *abbr* mucocutaneous lymph node syndrome.

**MMR** *abbr* measles, mumps and rubella (vaccine).

**MMSE** *abbr* Mini Mental State Examination.

**MND** *abbr* motor neuron disease.

**mobilizations** *npl* the manual manipulations of spinal and peripheral (limb) joints in order to free them to move more normally. Physiotherapists use several methods named for their developers, e.g. Maitland mobilizations. Whereas osteopaths and chiropractors mobilize joints with the aim of restoring function, physiotherapists also mobilize muscles, nerves and other soft tissues in order to relieve pain and restore freedom of movement.

**mobilize** *v* to make ready for movement. *mobilizing a patient* locomotion. *mobilize joints and soft tissues* free them to move more normally.

**Mobitz type I heart block** (W Mobitz, German physician, 1889–1951) a type of second-degree atrioventricular (AV) block in which the P-R interval becomes progressively longer. Also known as Wenckebach heart block or phenomenon.

**Mobitz type II heart block** (W Mobitz) a rarer type of second-degree atrioventricular (AV) block in which there is a sudden failure to conduct the atrial impulse through the atrioventricular node to the ventricle, without any lengthening of the P-R interval.

**mode** *n* the most frequent (common) value in a series of scores. ⇒ central tendency statistic, mean, median.

**modality** *n* **1.** a sensation, such as the sense of hearing, smell, taste, touch, vision. **2.** the form or method of treatment or therapy. For example, cognitive therapies, medication, occupational therapy, physiotherapy, radiotherapy, speech and language therapy, surgery.

**modelling** *n* a psychological term describing the way people learn from watching and copying the behaviour of others. Often utilized in behavioural therapies.

**modiolus** *n* the bony central pillar of the cochlea. ⇒ cochlea, ear.

**MODS** *abbr* multiple-organ dysfunction syndrome.

**MODY** *abbr* maturity-onset diabetes of the young.

**Mohs' micrographic surgery** a surgical technique developed by F Mohs in the 1930s. It is a microscopically controlled excision usually of a malignant skin tumour. In particular basal cell carcinoma, squamous cell carcinoma and malignant melanoma.

**moist wound healing** achieved by application of an occlusive, semipermeable dressing which permits enough exudate to collect under the film to carry out its bactericidal functions and maintain wound hydration.

**molality** *n* the concentration of a solution expressed as the number of moles of solute (substance) per kilogram of water or other solvent.

**molar** *adj* describes a solution containing 1 mol of solute (substance) per litre of solution.

**molar tooth** multicuspid posterior grinding tooth (see Figure T.4B, p. 482), placed fourth and fifth from the midline in the primary dentition, and sixth, seventh and eighth in the secondary dentition.

**molarity** *n* the concentration of a solution expressed as the number of moles of solute (substance) per litre of solution (mol/L).

**mole** *n* **1.** one of the seven base units of the International System of Units (SI). The measurement of amount of substance (*abbr* mol). ⇒ Appendix 2. A mole of any substance is the amount that will contain the same number of elementary particles (e.g. atoms or molecules) as there are atoms contained within 12 g of carbon-12 ($6.02 \times 10^{23}$). This number is known as Avogadro's number. **2.** a pigmented area on the skin, usually brown. They may be flat, some are raised and occasionally have hairs growing from them. Alterations in shape, colour, size or bleeding may be indicative of malignant changes.

**molecule** *n* a combination of two or more atoms to form a specific chemical substance—**molecular** *adj*.

**molecular weight** the sum of the atomic weights of atoms in a molecule.

**mollities** *n* softness. *mollities ossium* osteomalacia.

**molluscum** *n* soft swellings, masses, nodules or tumour.

**molluscum contagiosum** an infectious condition common in children, caused by a poxvirus. It is characterized by the formation of tiny translucent papules with a central depression.

**molluscum fibrosum** the superficial tumours of von Recklinghausen's disease.

**monarticular** *adj* relating to one joint.

**Mönckeberg's sclerosis** (J Mönckeberg, German pathologist, 1877–1925) degenerative change resulting in calcification of the median muscular layer in arteries, especially of the limbs; leads to intermittent claudication and rarely to gangrene, if atherosclerosis coexists.

**Mongolian blue spot** a bluish-black area of skin on the sacral area of some neonates. It is commoner in infants with darker skins and usually disappears during childhood.

**Monilia** *n* ⇒ *Candida.*

**moniliasis** *n* ⇒ candidiasis.

**Monitor** *n* an anglicized version of the Rush Medicus quality assurance programme for use in hospitals.

**monitoring** *n* sequential recording. Term usually reserved for automatic visual display of such measurements as temperature, pulse, respiration and blood pressure.

**monoamine** *n* organic molecules with one amine ($NH_2$) group. Examples include adrenaline (epinephrine), dopamine, histamine, 5-hydroxytryptamine (serotonin), melatonin, noradrenaline (norepinephrine). ⇒ amines.

**monoamine oxidase** an enzyme that breaks down monoamines, such as dopamine, 5-hydroxytryptamine (serotonin) and noradrenaline (norepinephrine) in the brain.

**monoamine oxidase inhibitors (MAOIs)** a group of antidepressant drugs that inhibit the action of monoamine oxidase, thereby preventing the breakdown of 5-hydroxytryptamine and other monoamines, e.g. phenelzine. ⇒ Appendix 5.

**monoarthritis** *n* arthritis affecting a single joint.

**monoamniotic twins** monozygotic twins who develop within a single amnion.

**monoblast** *n* an immature cell formed in the bone marrow during the development of the monocytes (white blood cells). Its presence in the blood is abnormal and is indicative of some types of leukaemia.

**monochorionic twins** monozygotic twins who develop within a single chorion.

**monochromat** *n* an individual who is totally colour-blind.

**monoclonal** *adj* arising from a single B lymphocyte/cell and its subsequent clones, e.g. *monoclonal antibodies* (MAb), these identical specific antibodies are increasingly used in research, and for diagnostic assays and in treatment of cancers and other diseases. For example, bevacizumab and cetuximab for metastatic colorectal cancers; trastuzumab for

M

some early-stage breast cancers, and metastatic breast cancer; omalizumab for asthma; and infliximab, which is used for several diseases, including rheumatoid arthritis, inflammatory bowel disease and ankylosing spondylitis.

**monocular** *adj* pertaining to one eye.

**monocyte** *n* a phagocytic white blood cell that has a kidney-shaped nucleus. Monocytes migrate to the tissues to become macrophages—**monocytic** *adj*. ⇒ macrophages.

**monocyte–macrophage system** (*syn* reticuloendothelial system, mononuclear–phagocytic system) a widely disseminated system of specialized phagocytic cells in the bone marrow, alveoli, liver, lymph nodes, spleen, connective issue, neural tissue, and other tissues. Its functions include blood cell and haemoglobin breakdown, formation of bile pigments, removal of cell breakdown products and as part of the defences against microorganisms. ⇒ macrophages.

**monocytopenia** *n* a deficiency of monocytes in the peripheral blood.

**monocytosis** *n* an increase in the number of monocytes in the peripheral blood. The causes include some types of leukaemia and lymphomas, chronic inflammation, such as with tuberculosis, and autoimmune conditions.

**monodactylism** *n* a congenital deformity in which there is a single digit on a hand or foot.

**monomania** *n* obsession with a single idea.

**mononeuropathy** *n* a disorder that affects a single nerve. Includes entrapment, compression from a cast or splint, the effects of radiation, or trauma.

**mononuclear** *adj* describes a cell with a single nucleus such as a monocyte.

**mononucleosis** *n* an increase in the number of circulating monocytes (mononuclear cells) in the blood. ⇒ infectious mononucleosis.

**monoplegia** *n* paralysis of only one limb—**monoplegic** *adj*.

**monorchism** *n* also called monorchidism. The presence of a single testis in the scrotum due to the failure of the other testis to descend from the abdomen.

**monosaccharide** *n* a single-sugar carbohydrate with the general formula $(CH_2O)_n$. They may have between 3 and 9 carbon atoms, for instance ribose is a pentose sugar with 5-carbon atoms, and glucose, fructose and galactose are hexoses with 6-carbon atoms. They are the basic unit from which other carbohydrates are formed. Monosaccharide units link together to produce disaccharides and polysaccharides.

**monounsaturated fatty acid** a fatty acid that has one double bond in its structure, such as oleic acid. They are present in olive oil, avocados, canola (rapeseed oil), peanuts, etc. ⇒ fatty acids, oleic oil.

**monosodium glutamate** a sodium salt used as a flavour enhancer in savoury foods, such as soups.

**monosomy** *n* a type of aneuploidy. The absence of a chromosome from the normal diploid chromosome complement, resulting in 45 chromosomes rather than 46. For example, in Turner's syndrome where the female has XO instead of XX. ⇒ aneuploidy, polyploidy, trisomy.

**monovular** *adj* ⇒ uniovular.

**monozygotic** *adj* relating to one zygote. Describes identical twins that develop from a single zygote that splits into two embryos. ⇒ dizygotic *opp*. monoamniotic twins, monochorionic twins.

**mons veneris** also called mons pubis. The eminence formed by the pad of fat which lies over the pubic bone in the female.

**Monteggia's fracture** (G Monteggia, Italian physician, 1762–1815) an angular fracture of the ulna with associated dislocation of the head of the radius.

**Montgomery's glands** (W Montgomery, Irish obstetrician, 1797–1859) also known as areolar glands. Sebaceous glands in the areola surrounding the breast.

**mood** *n* an involuntary state of mind or feeling. Mood variations are normal, but frequent swings from depression to overexcitement may be considered abnormal. ⇒ bipolar affective disorder, cyclothymia, depression, mania.

**Mooren's ulcer** (A Mooren, German ophthalmologist, 1829–1899) peripheral ulcerative keratitis.

**Moraxella** *n* a genus of Gram-negative, non-motile bacteria. They are present as commensals and pathogens on the mucosal surfaces. *Moraxella catarrhalis* causes respiratory tract infections and otitis media. *M. lacunata* causes conjunctivitis.

**morbidity** *n* the state of being diseased. *standardized morbidity ratio (SMBR)* the degree of self-reported limiting long-term illness indirectly standardized for variations in age and gender.

**morbilli** *n* ⇒ measles.

**morbilliform** *adj* describes a rash resembling that of measles.

**moribund** *adj* in a dying state.

**Moro reflex** (E Moro, German paediatrician, 1874–1951) also called the startle reflex.

M

A normal reflex observed in infants from birth to the age of 3–4 months, whereby, on being startled, the legs are flexed and the infant throws out its arms, then brings them together in an embracing movement (Figure M.7).

**morphoea** *n* ⇒ scleroderma.

**morphogenesis** *n* the formation and differentiation of the body structures and form. Especially applied to that occurring during embryonic development.

**morphology** *n* the study of the form and structure of living things—**morphological** *adj*, **morphologically** *adv*.

**Morquio–Brailsford disease** (L Morquio, Uruguayan paediatrician, 1867–1935; J Brailsford, British radiologist, 1888–1961) a mucopolysaccharidosis. An inherited disease of mucopolysaccharide storage. It is transmitted as an autosomal recessive trait. The condition is characterized by faulty musculoskeletal development leading to short stature, macrocephaly with coarse facial features and widely spaced teeth, abnormal sternum, knock knees and spinal curvature. In addition there is corneal clouding, hepatomegaly, aortic valve regurgitation and neurological problems. ⇒ mucopolysaccharidoses.

**mortality** *n* **1.** being subject to death. **2.** number or frequency of deaths.

**mortality rate** *n* the death rate; the ratio of the total number of deaths to the total population. There are several specialized mortality rates and ratios, including: childhood mortality (children aged 1–14 years), infant mortality (first year of life), maternal mortality (deaths associated with pregnancy and childbirth), neonatal mortality (first 4 weeks of life), perinatal mortality (stillbirths plus deaths in the first week of life), stillbirth rate. ⇒ standardized mortality rate, standardized mortality ratio.

**mortification** *n* death of tissue. ⇒ gangrene.

**Morton's metatarsalgia** (T Morton, American surgeon, 1835–1903) also called Morton's disease, Morton's neuroma. Neuralgia caused by a neuroma on the digital branches of the plantar nerves, most commonly that supplying the third toe cleft. ⇒ metatarsalgia.

**morula** *n* a mass of cells formed from the cleavage (by mitosis) of the zygote prior to its implantation into the hormone-prepared uterine lining.

**mosaicism** *n* in genetics, a state in which an individual who develops from a single zygote has two or more cell populations that are genetically different. This may be seen as differences in the number of chromosomes in the cells. For example, those affecting the sex chromosomes in Klinefelter's syndrome and Turner's syndrome, or those affecting an autosomal chromosome such as in Down's syndrome.

**mosquito** *n* a blood-sucking arthropod of the family Culicidae. They are important vectors of serious human diseases through their bite, for example malaria. ⇒ *Aedes*, anopheles, filariasis, malaria, mosquito-transmitted haemorrhagic fevers.

**mosquito-transmitted haemorrhagic fevers** infections mainly occurring in tropical regions. The important ones are chikungunya, dengue, Rift Valley fever and yellow fever. ⇒ viral haemorrhagic fevers.

**motile** *adj* able to move spontaneously, such as certain bacteria and spermatozoa—**motility** *n*.

**motilin** *n* a peptide hormone secreted by cells of the small intestine. It is concerned with gastrointestinal contraction and motility.

**motion sickness** nausea and vomiting associated with any form of motion such as during journeys by car or plane.

**motivation** *n* in psychology, the underlying causes of action. Without motivation an individual would not function. It is what impels or drives individuals and is intimately related to their needs and influenced by their emotions, values, beliefs and goals. Motivation provides people with the focus and stamina needed to undertake activities.

**motor** *adj* pertaining to action.

**motor assessment scale** an outcome measure, used by physiotherapists, in the assessment of gross motor function.

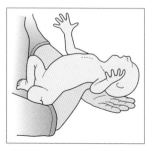

**Figure M.7** Moro or startle reflex *(reproduced from Brooker 2006A with permission)*.

M

**motor cortex** that part of the cerebral cortex that controls voluntary skeletal muscle movement. It includes the primary motor area, motor speech area (Broca's area) and the premotor area which co-ordinates movements stimulated by the primary motor area.

**motor end-plate** the tiny pads that form the communication between the axon terminal filaments and the muscle fibre (the motor unit) that it supplies (Figure M.8). ⇒ neuromuscular junction.

**motor neuron(e)** the nerve cell (or neuron) that supplies the electrical input to effector structures, such as skeletal muscles. The upper motor neurons arise in the primary motor area of the cortex or the brainstem and directly or indirectly affect the functioning of the lower motor neurons. The lower motor neuron directly innervates the muscle fibres or gland and originates in the brainstem or the spinal cord. ⇒ synapse.

**motor neuron disease (MND)** a group of neurodegenerative disorders affecting the nerves that supply the muscles, leading to weakness, muscle wasting, dysphagia, speech problems, difficulty breathing and eventually death. ⇒ amyotrophic lateral sclerosis.

**motor skill** the ability to perform a particular task which involves significant movement of one or more joints of the body, e.g. as part of a sports skill.

**motor unit** a lower motor neuron and all of the muscle fibres it innervates.

**motoricity index** a measure of limb function used in neurological rehabilitation.

**mould** n a multicellular fungus. Often used synonymously with fungus (excluding the yeasts). It consists of filaments or hyphae, which aggregate into a mycelium. Propagates by means of spores. Occurs in infinite variety, as common saprophytes contaminating foodstuffs, and more rarely as pathogens.

**moulding** n the compression of the fetal head during its passage through the genital tract in labour (Figure M.9).

**mountain sickness** ⇒ altitude sickness.

**mouth guard** an intraoral appliance worn during contact sports to prevent or minimize damage to the teeth or other oral structures.

**moving and handling** manual handling. All the activities including moving, lifting or supporting a load, and are subject to health and safety regulations.

**moxibustion** n the use of burning mugwort (the aromatic herb *Artemisia vulgaris*, also known as moxa) to heat the needles during acupuncture. ⇒ acupuncture.

**MRI** *abbr* magnetic resonance imaging.

**MRSA** *abbr* meticillin (methicillin)-resistant *Staphylococcus aureus*.

**MS** *abbr* multiple sclerosis.

**MSA** *abbr* multiple systems atrophy.

**MSH** *abbr* melanocyte-stimulating hormones.

**MSP** *abbr* Munchausen syndrome by proxy.

**MSU/MSSU** *abbr* midstream specimen of urine.

**MUAC** *abbr* mid-upper-arm circumference.

**mucilage** n the solution of a gum in water—**mucilaginous** *adj*.

**mucin** n viscous, glycoprotein (mucoprotein) constituent of mucus—**mucinous** *adj*.

**mucinase** n a specific mucin-dissolving enzyme.

**mucinolysis** n breakdown of mucin—**mucinolytic** *adj*.

**mucocele** n distension of a cavity with mucus.

**mucociliary escalator/transport** the synchronized process occurring in the respiratory

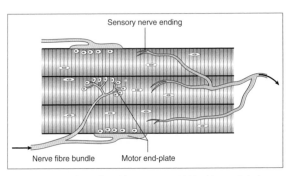

Sensory nerve ending

Nerve fibre bundle    Motor end-plate

**Figure M.8** Motor end-plates *(reproduced from Watson 2000 with permission).*

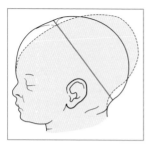

**Figure M.9** Moulding denoted by dotted line—vertex presentation, well-flexed head (*reproduced from Fraser & Cooper 2003 with permission*).

tract, whereby the mucus with any trapped foreign particles such as micro-organisms is moved upwards and out of the lungs.

**mucocutaneous** *adj* pertaining to mucous membrane and skin.

**mucocutaneous lymph node syndrome (MLNS)** a disease affecting mainly babies and children. It is an inflammatory vasculitis characterized by fever, dry lips, red mouth and strawberry-like tongue. There is a rash on the trunk, and erythema with desquamation affecting the extremities. There is cervical lymphadenopathy, polymorphonuclear leucocytosis and a raised erythrocyte sedimentation rate (ESR). Also known as Kawasaki disease.

**mucoid** *adj* resembling mucus.

**mucolytics** *npl* drugs which reduce the viscosity of respiratory secretions, e.g. dornase alpha. ⇒ Appendix 5.

**mucopolysaccharide** *n* complex polysaccharides containing hexosamine (amino sugar formed from hexoses). They are present as a constituent of the mucoproteins in connective tissue, e.g. chondroitin in cartilage, tendons.

**mucopolysaccharidoses** *npl* a group of inherited metabolic disorders in which the lack of specific enzymes causes the abnormal build-up of mucopolysaccharides. ⇒ gargoylism, Hunter's syndrome, Hurler's syndrome, Morquio–Brailsford disease.

**mucoprotein** *n* a substance containing protein and polysaccharides with several hexosamine residues. ⇒ glycoproteins.

**mucopurulent** *adj* containing mucus and pus.

**mucopus** *n* mucus containing pus.

**mucosa** *n* a mucous membrane—**mucosae** *pl*, **mucosal** *adj*.

**mucosa-associated lymphoid tissue (MALT)** collections of lymphoid tissue in the gastrointestinal tract, the respiratory tract and in the genitourinary tract. They are located in areas that are exposed to the outside environment and are important in the early detection of invading pathogens. Examples include Peyer's patches and the tonsils.

**mucositis** *n* inflammation of a mucous membrane such as the mouth, throat or gastrointestinal tract. It occurs after cytotoxic chemotherapy, radiotherapy and immunosuppression in preparation for a haemopoietic stem cell transplant. Mucositis affecting the gastrointestinal tract compromises the integrity of the mucosa and increases the risk of micro-organisms entering the blood. This is a particular problem for neutropenic patients.

**mucous** *adj* pertaining to or containing mucus. *mucous membrane* ⇒ membrane.

**mucous polyp** a growth (adenoma) of mucous membrane which becomes pedunculated.

**mucoviscidosis** *n* cystic fibrosis.

**mucus** *n* viscid secretion of mucous glands. It contains water, mucin, salts and cell debris—**mucous**, **mucoid** *adj*.

**müllerian duct** (J Müller, German physiologist, 1801–1858) ⇒ Mayer–Rokitansky–Küster–Hauser syndrome, paramesonephric duct.

**multiagency team** a team that involves practitioners from a range of different backgrounds or professions, such as health, social care and education, who work together with clients to achieve results that could not be achieved by any one agency working in isolation.

**multicellular** *adj* having many cells.

**multidisciplinary teams (MDT)** a team comprising different health care professionals working together to plan and deliver care for clients. The team may include specialist physicians and surgeons, general practitioners, physiotherapists, occupational therapists, dietitians, speech and language therapists, nurses and midwives.

**multigravida** *n* a woman who has had more than one pregnancy regardless of the outcome—**multigravidae** *pl*. ⇒ multipara.

**multi-infarct dementia** cerebrovascular dementia. A condition arising from progressive occlusion of the blood supply to regions of the brain.

**multileaf collimation (MLC)** a method of customized beam shaping in radiotherapy without the use of lead blocks.

**M**

**multilobular** *adj* possessing many lobes.

**multilocular** *adj* possessing many small cysts, loculi or pockets.

**multinuclear** *adj* possessing many nuclei, such as skeletal muscle cells—**multinucleate** *adj*.

**multipara** *n* a woman who has given birth to a viable infant (live or stillborn) on more than one occasion—**multiparae** *pl.* ⇒ **multigravida**.

**multiple endocrine neoplasia (MEN)** also known as multiple endocrine adenomas. A group of inherited autosomal dominant syndromes that are characterized by the presence of neoplasias in the endocrine glands that secrete amines or peptide hormones. Often the neoplasias are benign but some can be malignant; they may occur in the parathyroid glands, the pituitary gland, the islet cells of the pancreas (gastrinoma, insulinoma), the adrenal gland (phaeochromocytoma), gastrointestinal mucosal neuromas and the thyroid gland (medullary carcinoma). Each MEN syndrome has a typical pattern of sites of neoplasia formation. ⇒ Sipple's syndrome, Wermer's syndrome.

**multiple myeloma** a form of bone marrow cancer resulting from the accumulation of malignant plasma cells—**myelomata** *pl*, **myelomatous** *adj*. ⇒ Bence Jones protein.

**multiple-organ dysfunction syndrome (MODS)** syndrome in critically ill patients in which more than one organ system (e.g. kidneys, coagulation, gastrointestinal and respiratory) fails to function normally, may progress to multiple-organ failure. It requires appropriate organ support such as mechanical ventilation and haemofiltration. ⇒ acute respiratory distress syndrome, disseminated intravascular coagulation, renal failure, systemic inflammatory response syndrome.

**multiple sclerosis (MS)** (*syn* disseminated sclerosis) a variably progressive inflammatory demyelinating disease of the central nervous system. It is possibly triggered by infection by one or more viruses and most commonly affects young adults in whom patchy, degenerative changes occur in nerve sheaths in the brain, spinal cord and optic nerves, followed by sclerosis. The presenting symptoms can be diverse, ranging from diplopia to weakness or unsteadiness of a limb, pain; disturbances of micturition are common.

**multiple systems atrophy (MSA)** a condition characterized by rigidity and poverty of movement. It may be confused with parkinsonism or Parkinson's disease.

**multiprofessional** *adj* relating to teamwork among practitioners from different health care professions working side by side. ⇒ interprofessional.

**multivariate statistics** analysis of three or more variables simultaneously. Used to clarify the association of two variables after allowing for other variables.

**mumps** *n* (*syn* infectious parotitis) an acute, specific inflammation of the parotid glands, caused by a paramyxovirus. Spread is by droplets and the incubation period is around 18 days. There is fever, malaise, parotid salivary gland swelling and pain. Complications include pancreatitis, orchitis, oophoritis and meningitis. Active immunization is offered as part of routine programmes.

**Munchausen syndrome** (K von Münchausen, German officer and story teller, 1720–1797) ⇒ factitious disorder. *Munchausen syndrome by proxy (MSP)* the production of factitious disorders in a child by an adult, usually a parent or caregiver.

**mural** *adj* pertaining to the wall of a structure.

**murmur** *n* (*syn* bruit) abnormal sound heard on auscultation of heart or great vessels. *presystolic murmur* characteristic of mitral stenosis.

**Murphy's sign** (J Murphy, American surgeon, 1857–1916) a physical sign that may be present in acute inflammation of the gallbladder. Continuous pressure over the gallbladder during a deep inspiration will cause individuals to 'catch' their breath at the point of maximum inspiration.

*Musca* *n* genus of the common housefly, capable of transmitting many enteric infections.

**muscae volitantes** black dots or floaters seen before the eyes.

**muscarinic** *adj* a type of cholinergic receptor where muscarine would, if present, bind in place of acetylcholine. ⇒ nicotinic.

**muscarinic agonists** (*syn* parasympathomimetic) a group of drugs that stimulate or mimic parasympathetic activity. They have structural similarities with the neurotransmitter acetylcholine. ⇒ Appendix 5.

**muscarinic antagonists (antimuscarinic drugs)** (*syn* parasympatholytic) a group of drugs that prevent the action of acetylcholine at the muscarinic receptors ($ACh_m$), thereby inhibiting cholinergic nerve transmission, e.g. hyoscine hydrobromide. ⇒ Appendix 5.

**muscle** *n* one of the four basic tissues. Composed of specialized contractile tissue formed from excitable cells. (⇒Appendix 1, Figures

4 and 5)—**muscular** *adj*. There are three types: cardiac muscle, skeletal muscle and smooth muscle. ⇒ cardiac muscle, muscle fibre, red muscle, skeletal muscle, smooth muscle, white muscle.

**muscle fibre** a muscle cell. Skeletal muscle fibres are classified according to type of action and metabolism. ⇒ muscle fibre type—I, IIa, IIb, IIc.

**muscle fibre type I (slow-twitch oxidative)** fibres are characterized by relatively slow contraction time and high aerobic capacity. They are well suited to long-duration activities.

**muscle fibre type IIa (fast oxidative glycolytic)** fibres that are classed as fast-twitch but have some of the aerobic characteristics of slow-twitch fibres.

**muscle fibre type IIb (fast-twitch glycolytic)** fibres characterized by very fast contraction time and high anaerobic capacity. They are well suited to high explosive activities.

**muscle fibre type IIc** fibres thought to be changing from type II to type I, and are uncommon except in muscle undergoing intensive training.

**muscle pump** the muscular contraction in the calf that aids venous return to the heart by squeezing the blood from one valve to the next in the leg veins (Figure M.10).

**muscle relaxant** drug used during general anaesthesia to produce muscle paralysis.

**muscle spasm** involuntary muscle contraction involving the entire muscle; may occur secondary to injury, fatigue or pain.

**muscular dystrophies** a group of genetically transmitted diseases; they are all characterized by progressive atrophy of different groups of muscles with loss of strength and increasing disability and deformity. Pseudohypertrophic or Duchenne type is the most severe. Presents in early childhood. ⇒ Duchenne muscular dystrophy.

**muscular endurance** the ability of a muscle or group of muscles to produce force over an extended period of time, i.e. to perform repeated contractions against a submaximal load.

**muscular power** the ability of a muscle(s) to produce a force at a given time.

**muscular strength** the amount of force a muscle or group of muscles can exert. The ability to resist or produce a force.

**musculature** *n* the muscular system, or any part of it.

**musculocutaneous** *adj* pertaining to muscle and skin.

**musculocutaneous nerve** a nerve arising from the brachial plexus, which innervates the muscles of the upper arm and the skin of the forearm.

**musculoskeletal** *adj* pertaining to the muscular and skeletal systems.

**mutagen** *n* any agent that causes a gene or chromosome mutation.

**mutagenesis** *n* the creation of mutations—**mutagenic, mutagenetic** *adj*, **mutagenetically** *adv*.

**mutagenicity** *n* the capacity to produce gene mutations or chromosome aberrations.

M

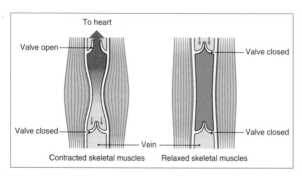

**Figure M.10** Muscle pump *(reproduced from Porter 2005 with permission).*

**mutant** *n* a cell (or organism) that has a genetic change or mutation.

**mutation** *n* a gene or chromosome alteration that results in genetic changes that alter the characteristics of the affected cell. The change is transmitted through succeeding generations. Mutations may be spontaneous, or induced by agents such as ionizing radiation that alter the chromosomal DNA.

**mute 1.** *adj* unable to speak. **2.** *n* a person who is unable to speak.

**mutilation** *n* the condition resulting from the removal of a limb or other part of the body. It results in a change of body image, to which there has to be considerable physical, psychological and social adjustment for a successful outcome.

**mutism** *n* (*syn* dumbness) inability or refusal to speak. It may be due to congenital causes, the most common being deafness; it may be the result of physical disease, such as a stroke, and it can be a manifestation of mental health problems.

**myalgia** *n* pain in the muscles—**myalgic** *adj.* epidemic myalgia ⇒ Bornholm disease.

**myalgic encephalomyelitis (ME)** ⇒ chronic fatigue syndrome/ME.

**myasthenia** *n* muscular weakness—**myasthenic** *adj.*

**myasthenia gravis** an autoimmune disorder in which an antibody reduces the efficiency of transmission between the motor neuron and muscle. The antibody blocks receptor sites at the neuromuscular junctions and prevents the normal action of acetylcholine and nerve impulse transmission. In many cases there is a disorder of the thymus gland. It is characterized by marked fatigue affecting the voluntary muscles, especially following exercise. Other muscles involved include those of the eye and shoulder girdle and those required for speaking, swallowing, chewing and breathing.

**myasthenic crisis** a sudden deterioration with weakness of respiratory muscles due to an increase in severity of myasthenia. It is distinguished from cholinergic crisis by giving edrophonium chloride intravenously. Marked improvement confirms myasthenic crisis. ⇒ edrophonium test.

**mycelium** *n* a mass of branching filaments (hyphae) of moulds or fungi—**mycelial** *adj.*

**mycetoma** *n* (*syn* Madura foot) chronic fungal disease affecting soft tissues and bones of the limbs (usually the foot), but it may occur in other sites. It causes swelling, nodules and sinus formation.

**Mycobacterium** *n* a genus of Gram-positive acid-fast bacteria. *Mycobacterium avium intracellulare (MAI)* atypical mycobacterium that causes infection in humans. *Mycobacterium bovis* causes tuberculosis in cattle. It can be transmitted to humans. *Mycobacterium leprae* causes leprosy and *Mycobacterium tuberculosis* causes tuberculosis.

**mycologist** *n* an expert in mycology.

**mycology** *n* the study of fungi—**mycological** *adj*, **mycologically** *adv.*

**Mycoplasma** *n* a genus of very small microorganisms. They have features in common with bacteria, but lack a cell wall. Some are parasites, some are saprophytes and others are pathogens; for example *Mycoplasma pneumoniae* causes primary atypical pneumonia.

**mycosis fungoides** a T-cell lymphomatous condition that initially may present as scaly patches on the skin. In later stages, large tumours may develop.

**mycosis** *n* disease caused by any fungus—**mycotic** *adj.*

**mycotoxins** *npl* the secondary metabolites of moulds or microfungi. Many chemical substances have been identified as mycotoxins, some of which are carcinogenic as well as causing other diseases—**mycotoxic** *adj.*

**mydriasis** *n* dilatation of the pupil of the eye.

**mydriatics** *npl* drugs which dilate the pupil (mydriasis), e.g. tropicamide. ⇒ Appendix 5.

**myelencephalon** *n* one of the secondary enlargements occurring during embryonic development of the brain. Part of the embryonic hindbrain, which becomes the medulla oblongata.

**myelin** *n* the white, fatty substance that covers and insulates some nerve fibres. ⇒ white matter.

**myelination** *n* the process by which myelin is produced and forms the insulation around the axons of certain nerves.

**myelitis** *n* inflammation of the spinal cord.

**myeloablative** *adj* describes the therapy (e.g. radiotherapy, chemotherapy) given intentionally to 'knock out' the bone marrow completely. Used in leukaemia; often precedes a haemopoietic stem cell transplant.

**myeloblasts** *npl* the early precursor cells of the polymorphonuclear granulocytic white blood cells. The presence of myeloblasts in the blood is abnormal and occurs in acute myeloblastic leukaemia—**myeloblastic** *adj.*

**myelocele** *n* a neural tube defect. Occurs with spina bifida wherein development of the spinal cord itself has been arrested, and the central canal of the cord opens on the skin surface, discharging cerebrospinal fluid.

**myelocytes** *npl* precursor cells of polymorpho-nuclear granulocytic white blood cells. The presence of myelocytes in the blood is abnormal and occurs in some leukaemias—**myelocytic** *adj*.

**myelofibrosis** *n* a myeloproliferative disorder characterized by the formation of fibrous tissue within the bone marrow cavity. Interferes with the formation of blood cells.

**myelogenous** *adj* produced in or by the bone marrow.

**myelography** *n* radiographic examination of the spinal canal by injection of a contrast medium into the subarachnoid space. Superseded by computed tomography and magnetic resonance imaging—**myelographic** *adj*, **myelogram** *n*, **myelograph** *n*, **myelographically** *adv*.

**myeloid** *adj* **1.** pertaining to the bone marrow. **2.** pertaining to the granulocyte precursor cells in the bone marrow. **3.** pertaining to the spinal cord.

**myeloma** *n* ⇒ multiple myeloma.

**myelomatosis** *n* ⇒ multiple myeloma, Bence Jones protein.

**myelomeningocele** *n* ⇒ meningomyelocele.

**myelopathy** *n* disease of the spinal cord. Can be a serious complication of cervical spondylosis—**myelopathic** *adj*.

**myeloproliferative disorders** condition where there is proliferation of one or more of the cellular components of the bone marrow such as myelofibrosis, primary proliferative polycythaemia and thrombocythaemia. ⇒ leukaemia, polycythaemia.

**myenteric plexus** Auerbach's plexus. A plexus of autonomic (sympathetic and parasympathetic) nerves that innervate the smooth-muscle layer and the associated blood vessels in the gastrointestinal tract.

**myiasis** *n* infestation of tissues or organs with fly larvae (maggots).

**myocardial infarction** part of the spectrum of acute coronary syndromes. Death of a part of the myocardium (heart muscle) from deprivation of blood following occlusion of a coronary artery, for example from thrombosis (Figure M.11). The patient experiences a 'heart attack' with sudden intense chest pain which may radiate to the arms (especially the left), abdomen, back and lower jaw. Management includes: aspirin, thrombolytic therapy, pain relief, antiemetics, oxygen therapy, bed rest, observations, including continuous

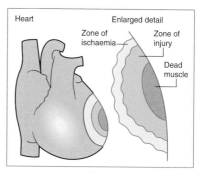

**Figure M.11** Myocardial infarction—grades of muscle damage *(reproduced from Hinchliff et al. 1996 with permission)*.

electrocardiograph and later mobilization and cardiac rehabilitation. Patients should be cared for in a coronary care unit for 12–24 hours because of the risk of life-threatening arrhythmias such as ventricular fibrillation, and the need for skilled staff to monitor the effects of thrombolytic therapy. ⇒ angina pectoris, cardiac enzymes, coronary heart disease.

**myocarditis** *n* inflammation of the myocardium.

**myocardium** *n* the middle layer of the heart wall. Formed from highly specialized cardiac muscle. ⇒ muscle—**myocardial** *adj*.

**myocele** *n* protrusion of a muscle through its ruptured sheath.

**myoclonus** *n* clonic contractions of individual or groups of muscles. Normal individuals occasionally experience an isolated myoclonic jerk or two during drowsiness or light sleep. ⇒ clonus.

**myoelectric** *adj* relating to the electrical properties of muscle.

**myoepithelium** *n* a type of specialized epithelium that has contractile properties. Located around the secretory system of certain glands, e.g. mammary glands, sweat glands, it assists with secretion discharge.

**myofascial pain dysfunction syndrome** persistent pain of soft tissue, characterized by taut fibrous bands and focal areas of hypersensitivity known as trigger points.

**myofibril** *n* bundle of fibres contained in a muscle fibre. Formed from filaments of contractile proteins. ⇒ actin, myosin, tropomyosin, troponin.

M

**myofibrosis** n excessive connective tissue in muscle. Leads to inadequate functioning of part—**myofibroses** pl.

**myogenic** adj originating in or starting from muscle.

**myoglobin** n (syn myohaemoglobin) a haem protein molecule of skeletal muscle. It is involved with the oxygen released by the red blood cells, which it stores and transports to muscle cell mitochondria where it is used to produce energy. Myoglobin escapes from damaged muscle and appears in the urine in crush syndrome.

**myoglobinuria** n (syn myohaemoglobinuria) excretion of myoglobin in the urine, as in crush syndrome.

**myohaemoglobin** n ⇒ myoglobin.

**myohaemoglobinuria** n ⇒ myoglobinuria.

**myokymia** n muscle twitching. In the lower eyelid it is benign. facial myokymia may result from long-term use of phenothiazines; has also been observed in patients with multiple sclerosis.

**myoma** n a tumour of muscle tissue—**myomata** pl, **myomatous** adj.

**myomectomy** n enucleation of uterine fibroid(s).

**myometrium** n the specialized muscular wall of the uterus.

**myoneural** adj pertaining to muscle and nerve.

**myopathy** n disease of muscle (usually applied to non-inflammatory conditions)—**myopathic** adj.

**myope** n a shortsighted person—**myopic** adj.

**myopia** n shortsightedness caused by high refractive power or increased axial length of the eye, with the result that the light rays are focused in front of, instead of on, the retina—**myopic** adj.

**myoplasty** n plastic surgery of muscles—**myoplastic** adj.

**myosarcoma** n a malignant tumour derived from muscle—**myosarcomata** pl, **myosarcomatous** adj.

**myosin** n a contractile protein, one of the filaments of a myofibril; reacts with actin in the muscle cell to cause contraction.

**myosis (miosis)** n constriction of the pupil of the eye—**myotic** adj.

**myositis** n inflammation of a muscle or its connective tissue. ⇒ connective tissue diseases. myositis ossificans deposition of active bone cells in muscle, resulting in hard swellings.

**myotatic on-stretch reflex** a reflex that involves the lengthening of a muscle followed by sudden shortening to generate power. ⇒ plyometric exercise.

**myotome** n the muscles supplied by a single spinal nerve (Table M.1).

**myotomy** n cutting or dissection of muscle tissue.

**myotonia** n an increase in muscle tone at rest—**myotonic** adj.

**myotonia congenita** a genetically determined form of congenital muscular spasticity, usually presenting in infancy and due to degeneration of anterior horn cells in the spinal cord. Fibrillation of affected muscles is characteristic. It is inherited as either an autosomal dominant or autosomal recessive trait.

**myringitis** n inflammation of the eardrum (tympanic membrane).

**myringoplasty** n operation designed to close a defect in the tympanic membrane with a graft—**myringoplastic** adj.

**myringotome** n a delicate instrument for incising the eardrum (tympanic membrane).

**myringotomy** n incision into the eardrum (tympanic membrane). Performed for the drainage of pus or fluid from the middle ear. Middle-ear ventilation is maintained by insertion of a grommet or tube.

**myxoedema** n ⇒ hypothyroidism.

**myxoedema coma** rare but serious event characterized by alterations in consciousness and hypothermia, usually in an older person

**Table M.1** Myotomes

| Myotome | Function |
|---------|----------|
| C1 | Upper cervical flexion |
| C2 | Upper cervical extension |
| C3 | Cervical side flexion |
| C4 | Shoulder shrug |
| C5 | Shoulder abduction, external rotation |
| C6 | Elbow flexion, wrist extension |
| C7 | Elbow extension, wrist flexion |
| C8 | Thumb extension, finger flexion |
| T1 | Finger ab/adduction |
| L2 | Hip flexion |
| L3 | Knee extension |
| L4 | Ankle dorsiflexion |
| L5 | Great toe dorsiflexion (extension) |
| S1–2 | Ankle plantar flexion, knee flexion |
| S3–4 | Rectal sphincter |

C, cervical; T, thoracic; L, lumbar; S, sacral. Reproduced from Porter (2005) with permission.

with hypothyroidism. There is a high mortality, and treatment involves parenteral thyroid hormone and supportive measures.

**myxoma** *n* a connective tissue tumour composed largely of mucoid material—**myxomata** *pl*, **myxomatous** *adj*.

**myxosarcoma** *n* a malignant tumour of connective tissue with a soft, mucoid consistency—**myxosarcomata** *pl*, **myxosarcomatous** *adj*.

**myxoviruses** *npl* ⇒ orthomyxoviruses and paramyxoviruses.

M

# N

**nabothian cyst/follicle** (M Naboth, German physician, anatomist and chemist, 1675–1721) cystic distension of chronically inflamed Naboth's glands (mucus-secreting glands of the uterine cervix), where the duct of the gland has become obliterated by a healing epithelial covering and the normal mucus cannot escape.

**NAD/NADH** *abbr* nicotinamide adenine dinucleotide (oxidized and reduced forms respectively).

**NADP/NADPH** *abbr* nicotinamide adenine dinucleotide phosphate (oxidized and reduced forms respectively).

**Nägele's obliquity** (F Nägele, German obstetrician, 1777–1851) tilting of the fetal head to one or other side to decrease the transverse diameter presented to the pelvic brim. ⇒ asynclitism.

**Nägele's rule** (F Nägele) a method of calculating the expected date of delivery—3 calendar months are subtracted from the date of the first day of the woman's last menstrual period and 7 days are added. It is based on a standard gestation period of 280 days and takes no account of variation in the length of calendar months. Accuracy is affected by the length of a woman's menstrual cycle and whether or not the bleeding is true menstrual bleeding.

**naevoid amentia** ⇒ Sturge–Weber syndrome.

**naevus** *n* a general term for a congenital or acquired skin lesion, including a variety of pigmented birthmarks. There is a circumscribed lesion of the skin arising from pigment-producing naevus cells or due to a developmental abnormality of blood vessels (angioma). Naevi are usually benign and only rarely undergo malignant changes—**naevi** *pl*. **naevoid** *adj*.

**NAI** *abbr* non-accidental injury.

**nail** *n* unguis. The keratinized plates of stratified squamous epithelial tissue covering and protecting the ends of the digits. Similar to the claws and hooves of other species. The exposed portion of a nail (nail plate) grows out from a germinative zone of epithelial cells known as the nail bed. A nail comprises a root, nail body/plate and a free edge. At its proximal edge the nail is thickened to form the white lunula, which is covered by eponychium (cuticle). *nail involution* a nail condition in which the transverse curvature increases along its longitudinal axis, reaching its maximum at the distal part. Often causes onychophosis. *pincer nail* the lateral edges of the nail practically meet. Lateral compression of the nail may cause damage to the soft tissues and reduce circulation to the nail bed. Subungual ulceration can result.

**nail blanch test** a test of capillary refill time used to assess the amount of blood passing through the skin (skin perfusion). Light pressure is applied to the nail bed for 5 seconds; when the pressure is released the normal nail colour should return within 2 seconds.

**nanogram (ng)** *n* one-thousandth part of a microgram. $10^{-9}$ of a gram.

**nanometre (nm)** *n* one-thousandth part of a micrometre. $10^{-9}$ of a metre.

**nanophthalmos** *n* congenital disorder in which the eyes are small but without other defects.

**nape** *n* the nucha; back of the neck.

**napkin rash** erythema of the napkin area. Causes include contact with ammonia formed from the decomposition of urine, candidiasis, infantile psoriasis, allergy to detergents, excoriation from diarrhoea.

**narcissism** *n* self-love. In psychoanalysis the narcissistic type of personality is one where the love object is the self.

**narcoanalysis** *n* controversial method of analysing mental content using medication—**narcoanalytic** *adj*, **narcoanalytically** *adv*.

**narcolepsy** *n* excessive somnolence. A condition occurring in around 0.05% of the population, commonly presenting in teenagers and young adults. Characterized by an irresistible urge to sleep, excessive daytime sleepiness, sleep paralysis and hallucinations at the onset of sleep (hypnogogic stage) or during the stage between sleep and waking (hypnopompic stage) and cataplexy (loss of muscle tone)—**narcoleptic** *adj*.

**narcosis** *n* drug-induced unconsciousness. ⇒ narcotic. *carbon dioxide narcosis* full bounding pulse, muscular twitchings, confusion and eventual unconsciousness due to increased $PaCO_2$. ⇒ hypercapnia.

**narcosynthesis** *n* the building up of a clearer mental picture of an incident involving the client by reviving memories of it, using medication, so that both the client and the therapist can examine the incident in clearer perspective.

**narcotic** *n, adj* (describes) a drug causing abnormally deep sleep. Strong analgesic narcotics, such as the opioids that include morphine, may cause respiratory depression which is reversible by the use of narcotic antagonists.

**nares** *n* (*syn* choanae) the nostrils—**naris** *sing.* *anterior nares* the pair of openings from the exterior into the nasal cavities. *posterior nares* the pair of openings from the nasal cavities into the nasopharynx.

**nasal** *adj* pertaining to the nose.

**nasal bone** *n* one of two facial bones that form the superior and lateral surfaces of the nasal bridge.

**nasal cavity** *n* an irregular cavity divided by the nasal septum. It is lined with ciliated epithelium containing numerous mucus-producing glands. This lining is continuous with that of the paranasal sinuses. The nasal cavity is the main entry for air during inspiration. Air enters via the anterior nares and passes through the posterior nares to the nasopharynx. Nerve endings in the roof of the nose are concerned with the sense of smell (olfaction).

**nasal conchae** *npl* also called the turbinate bones: three thin bones (superior, middle, inferior) that project into the nasal cavity, increasing the mucosal surface area and causing air turbulence.

**nasal flaring** enlargement of the anterior nares (nostrils) during inspiration. It is usually observed in infants and young children and can be a sign that breathing is difficult and needs more effort. Nasal flaring can be indicative of respiratory distress caused by a variety of conditions, including croup, bronchiolitis, pneumonia and asthma. It may be accompanied by head bobbing as the infant or child breathes in.

**nasal septum** *n* a partition that divides the nasal cavity into two. The posterior bony part is formed by the ethmoid bone and the anterior part is formed from hyaline cartilage.

**nasoduodenal** *adj* pertaining to the nose and duodenum, as passing a *nasoduodenal tube* via this route, for feeding. ⇒ enteral.

**nasogastric (NG)** *adj* pertaining to the nose and stomach, as passing a *nasogastric tube* via this route, usually for aspiration, or feeding.

**nasojejunal** *adj* pertaining to the nose and jejunum, usually referring to a tube passed via the nose into the jejunum for feeding.

**nasolacrimal** *adj* pertaining to the nose and lacrimal apparatus.

**naso-oesophageal** *adj* pertaining to the nose and the oesophagus.

**nasopharyngeal** *adj* pertaining to the nose and the pharynx, or to the nasopharynx. ⇒ airway.

**nasopharyngitis** *n* inflammation of the nasopharynx.

**nasopharyngoscope** *n* an endoscope for viewing the nasal passages and postnasal space—**nasopharyngoscopic** *adj*.

**nasopharynx** *n* the portion of the pharynx behind the nose and above the soft palate. The posterior nares open into the nasopharynx. The nasopharynx communicates with the middle ear via the pharyngotympanic (eustachian or auditory) tube. The nasopharyngeal tonsils are present on the posterior wall; these are known as adenoids when enlarged. Air passes through the nasopharynx, making it exclusively respiratory in function, unlike the oral and laryngeal parts of the pharynx—**nasopharyngeal** *adj*. ⇒ Waldeyer's ring.

**natal teeth** teeth present at birth. They may be extra teeth or may be due to the early eruption of primary teeth.

**nates** *npl* the buttocks. Formed from the bulk of the gluteal muscles and fatty tissue—**natis** *sing.*

**National Confidential Enquiries** four national enquiries that investigate clinical practice in specific areas: Confidential Enquiry into Maternal Deaths (CEMD); National Confidential Enquiry into Perioperative Deaths (NCEPOD); Confidential Enquiries into Stillbirths and Deaths in Infancy (CESDI); and Confidential Inquiry into Suicide and Homicide by people with mental illness (CISH).

**National Health Service (NHS)** the three-layer system of preventive and therapeutic health care services and facilities available within the UK. Care and treatment are delivered by primary (e.g. general practitioners), secondary (e.g. local hospitals) and tertiary (regional and supraregional specialist hospitals) providers. It is financed by central government through money raised by taxation.

**National Institute for Health and Clinical Excellence (NICE)** an independent body that generates and distributes clinical guidance based on evidence of clinical and cost-effectiveness for England and Wales. For example, the cost-effectiveness of new drugs and treatments or the management of a particular condition. It merged with the Health Development Agency in 2005.

**National Patient Safety Agency (NPSA)** an agency set up to improve patient safety within the NHS. All NHS staff are encouraged to report patient safety incidents without fear of blame, and for colleagues to learn from

**N**

such incidents (actual and near misses). The NPSA assesses reports from all areas and introduces preventive measures as necessary. For example, increased safety measures to ensure that patients receive the correct blood for transfusion, the use of the standard internal telephone number (2222) in NHS trusts in England and Wales to summon the 'crash' team to an in-hospital cardiac arrest.

**National Service Frameworks (NSFs)** evidence-based frameworks for major care areas and particular groups of disease, e.g. diabetes, older people, mental health, cancer, renal services, etc., that state what patients/clients can presume to receive from the NHS. Forthcoming NSFs include one for chronic obstructive pulmonary disease.

**natriuresis** *n* the excretion of larger amounts than normal of sodium in the urine.

**natural family planning** methods that do not make use of appliances or drugs. Family planning that is based on an awareness of the naturally occurring fertile and non-fertile phases of the female's menstrual cycle. Couples may use one or a combination of: a commercially produced system for measuring urinary hormone levels to predict the fertile phase; basal body temperature recorded daily may give an indication of progesterone secretion from the ovary and thus, by observing when the basal body temperature rises, gives an approximate guide to the timing of ovulation; menstrual cycle calendar (rhythm method); or changes in the amount and consistency of cervical mucus. ⇒ Billing's method, coitus interruptus.

**natural killer (NK) cells** non-phagocytic cytotoxic cells belonging to a group of large granular lymphocytes. They function as part of the non-specific (innate) body defences. NK cells kill virus-infected cells and cancer cells. They become active in response to various substances, including interferons and other cytokines. They may have a surveillance role in detecting cells with malignant changes. ⇒ interferons.

**natural killer cytotoxic activity** the ability of natural killer cells to kill virus-infected cells and cancer cells.

**naturopathy** *n* a multidisciplinary approach to health care that includes all aspects of one's lifestyle, e.g. natural foods grown without chemicals and medicines based on plants. It is founded upon the belief of the body's power

to heal itself given an optimal environment for healing—**naturopathic** *adj*.

**nausea** *n* a feeling of impending vomiting. May be accompanied by an unpleasant feeling in the abdomen and throat with a gagging sensation, the production of excessive watery saliva, increased swallowing, sweating and pallor. Vomiting does not always occur—**nauseate** *vt*.

**navel** *n* ⇒ umbilicus.

**navicular 1.** *adj* shaped like a boat, such as the bone in the ankle. **2.** *n* one of the tarsal bones of the ankle (also known as the scaphoid bone). It articulates with the talus, the cuboid and the three cuneiform bones.

**nebula** *n* a cloud-like corneal opacity.

**nebulizer** *n* an apparatus for converting a liquid into a fine spray. It is used to deliver medicaments for application to the respiratory tract or the skin. A very common method of drug delivery used in the management of asthma (Figure N.1).

**NEC** *abbr* necrotizing enterocolitis.

***Necator*** *n* a genus of parasitic nematode hookworms that includes *Necator americanus*. ⇒ *Ancylostoma*.

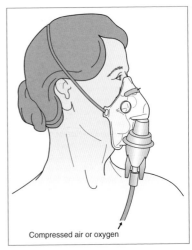

Compressed air or oxygen

**Figure N.1** Nebulizer *(adapted from Nicol et al. 2004 with permission).*

**necatoriasis** *n* infestation with the hookworm *Necator americanus*, which is found in the New World and tropical Africa. The larvae are present in the soil and gain access to the body through the skin of the lower limbs and feet, or contaminated water or food. Many infestations are asymptomatic but can cause abdominal pain, diarrhoea and iron-deficiency anaemia. Infestation is prevented by wearing shoes and effective sanitation to prevent contamination of soil with human faeces.

**neck** *n* **1.** the narrow, constricted part of an organ or other structure. For example, the neck of the femur and the humerus, and the neck (cervix) of the uterus. **2.** the narrow area between the head and the body.

**necrobiosis** *n* tissue changes characterized by swelling, the presence of basophils and the deformation of collagen in the dermis. There may be loss of normal tissue structure but with cell necrosis. *necrobiosis lipoidica* a form of necrobiosis that may be associated with diabetes. It mainly affects women and is characterized by yellow-brown plaques on the skin of the shins and arms.

**necrophilia** *n* **1.** an abnormal liking for dead bodies. **2.** the perversion of being sexually attracted to dead bodies. It may involve sexual gratification in the presence of a dead body, or sexual contact with the dead body, usually a man having sexual intercourse with a dead woman.

**necropsy** *n* the examination of a dead body.

**necrosectomy** *n* removal of necrotic tissue, e.g. necrotic pancreas, as a consequence of severe acute pancreatitis.

**necrosis** *n* localized death of tissue—**necrotic** *adj*.

**necrotizing enterocolitis (NEC)** a condition occurring primarily in preterm or low-birth-weight neonates. Parts of the gut wall become necrotic, leading to intestinal obstruction and peritonitis. Probably caused by a combination of ischaemia, hypoxia and bacterial infection.

**necrotizing fasciitis** rare infection caused by some strains of group A *Streptococcus pyogenes*. There is very severe inflammation of the muscle sheath and massive soft-tissue destruction. The mortality rate is high.

**necrotizing ulcerative periodontitis** acute periodontal disease in which there is redness of the gingival and alveolar mucosa. There is interdental ulceration and loss of interdental soft tissue and bone, leading to loss of periodontal attachments.

**needlestick injury** a particular hazard for health care workers and other groups, where accidental injury is sustained when skin or mucosa is penetrated by contaminated needles or other items. There is a risk of infection with various hepatitis viruses (e.g. hepatitis B or C) or, more rarely, the human immunodeficiency virus (HIV). All health care facilities or services should have a risk assessment, staff training, and policies and procedures in place for protective clothing, safer needles, proper disposal of equipment and action to be taken should injury occur. Postexposure prophylaxis with antiretroviral drugs may be indicated. The person should obtain immediate expert advice.

**needling** *n* procedure for removal of congenital cataract, now superseded.

**needs assessment** estimating the need (quantifying) for services in a population. Normative, or assessed, need defined by the expert or professional in any given situation; felt need, or want, perceived by the individual; expressed need, or operationalized felt need; comparative need, using the characteristics of a population receiving a service to define those with similar characteristics as in need. Needs assessment uses broad, non-specific indicators of need obtained through repeated health surveys of the general population (e.g. General Household Survey, Health Survey for England) and more specific indicators based on surveys of particular groups (e.g. survey of people with disabilities, loss of urinary continence). The weighted capitation formula for resource allocation is based on the characteristics of populations using hospital services as indicators of need.

**Neer classification** a classification used for fractures affecting the proximal humerus. There are six groups, ranging from group 1, minimal displacement, to group 6, fracture and dislocations.

**negative feedback** in physiology, a homeostatic mechanism, whereby high levels, for example, of a particular hormone in the blood 'turn off' or negate the stimulus that causes the hormone secretion (see Figure F.1, p. 179). Once hormone levels fall below the normal range, the stimulus is activated and again causes the hormone to be secreted. ⇒ feedback, homeostasis, positive feedback.

**negativism** *n* active refusal by the patient to co-operate, usually shown by the patient consistently doing the exact opposite of what is asked. Seen in catatonic schizophrenia.

**negligence** *n* a form of professional malpractice which includes the omission of acts that a prudent health professional would have done or the commission of acts that a prudent health professional would not do. It is a professional duty to avoid patient/client injury or suffering caused in this way. It can become the basis of litigation for damages. ⇒ Bolam test, duty of care.

**Neisseria** *n* (A Neisser, German dermatologist, bacteriologist, 1855–1916) a genus of aerobic and facultatively anaerobic, Gram-negative bacteria. They belong to the family Neisseriaceae. Some are commensals found in the pharynx and genitourinary tact and on the skin in humans, but others are pathogens. *N. gonorrhoeae* causes gonorrhoea and *N. meningitidis* causes life-threatening meningitis and meningococcal septicaemia.

**Nélaton's line** (A Nélaton, French physician and surgeon, 1807–1873) an imaginary line joining the anterior superior iliac spine to the ischial tuberosity. The great trochanter of the femur normally lies on or below this line.

**Nelson syndrome** (D Nelson, American physician, b. 1925) hyperpigmentation, including marked darkening of fair skin, as a result of uncontrolled adrenocorticotrophic hormone (ACTH) secretion from a pituitary adenoma, usually after treatment of the associated Cushing's disease by bilateral adrenalectomy.

**nematodes** *npl* parasitic worms that can be divided into three groups: (a) those that mainly live in the intestine, e.g. *Ancylostoma duodenale* (hookworm), *Ascaris lumbricoides* (roundworm), *Enterobius vermicularis* (threadworm), *Necator americanus*, *Strongyloides stercoralis* and *Trichuris trichiura* (whipworm); (b) those that are mainly in the tissues, e.g. *Dracunculus medinensis* (guinea worm) and the filarial worms that include *Loa loa*; (c) those from other species (zoonotic), e.g. *Toxocara canis*, *Trichinella spiralis*.

**neoadjuvant therapy** in cancer treatment the use of preliminary chemotherapy or radiotherapy to reduce tumour size before further treatment such as surgery. Aims to improve the outcome of surgery and to reduce the risk of metastatic spread.

**neologism** *n* the creation of a new word. A type of thought disorder seen in schizophrenia, mania and other psychotic illnesses.

**neonatal** *adj* relating to the first 28 days of life.

**neonatal hearing screening** hearing screening can be performed in small babies by use of computer-linked otoacoustic emission (OAE) testing or automated auditory brainstem response (AABR) testing. Where the two screening test are unavailable, a less reliable distraction test using simple sounds can be performed in infants.

**neonatal herpes** acquired during vaginal delivery from a mother actively shedding herpes simplex virus. It is a devastating illness with a 75% mortality rate and a high incidence of severe neurological sequelae among survivors.

**neonatal mortality** the death rate of babies in the first 28 days of life.

**neonatal respiratory distress syndrome (NRDS)** respiratory failure due to surfactant deficiency in the newborn. Most commonly affects premature infants.

**neonatal screening** screening tests undertaken soon after birth to detect diseases and abnormalities. Screening involves a thorough physical (head-to-toe) examination, which includes checking for congenital cataracts, developmental hip dysplasia, congenital heart defects and undescended testes; a blood spot test for various conditions, including phenylketonuria, cystic fibrosis, hypothyroidism, galactosaemia (in some countries), sickle-cell diseases and thalassaemia, medium-chain acyl-CoA dehydrogenase deficiency (MCADD); and a hearing test.

**neonatal unit (NNU/NICU/SCBU)** usually reserved for preterm and small-for-dates babies between 700 and 2000 g in weight, mostly requiring the use of high technology which is available in these units.

**neonate** *n* a newborn baby up to 28 days old.

**neonatology** *n* the scientific study of the newborn.

**neonatorum** *adj* pertaining to the newborn.

**neoplasia** *n* literally, the formation of new tissue. Customarily refers to the pathological process in the growth of a benign or malignant tumour—**neoplastic** *adj*.

**neoplasm** *n* a new growth; a tumour that is either cancerous or non-cancerous.

**neovascularization** *n* the formation of new abnormal blood vessels. A feature of the proliferative stage of diabetic retinopathy.

**nephralgia** *n* pain in the kidney.

**nephrectomy** *n* surgical removal of a kidney.

**nephritis** *n* non-specific term for inflammation within the kidney—**nephritic** *adj*.

**nephroblastoma** *n* the most common solid tumour of the kidney. Usually presents as an abdominal mass. Also known as Wilms' tumour. ⇒ Wilms' tumour.

**nephrocalcinosis** *n* the deposition of calcium salts within the renal tubules (the substance of the kidneys). It results from hyperparathyroidism and high levels of calcium in the blood, or disorders of the kidney, such as some types of renal tubular acidosis. It may lead to nephrolithiasis (the formation of renal calculi) and possible renal failure.

**nephrogenic** *adj* coming from or produced by the kidney.

**nephrolithiasis** *n* **1.** the formation of calculi in the kidney (kidney stones or renal calculi). **2.** the presence of calculi in the kidney(s).

**nephrolithotomy** *n* removal of a stone from the kidney by an incision through the kidney substance. ⇒ percutaneous nephrolithotomy.

**nephrology** *n* study of diseases of the kidney.

**nephron** *n* the functional unit of the kidney, comprising a glomerulus (a knot of capillaries) and a renal tubule with the associated peritubular capillary network. The tubule has a Bowman's capsule, proximal and distal convoluted tubules, loop of Henle and a collecting tubule that drains urine from many nephrons to the renal pelvis (Figure N.2).

**nephronophthisis** *n* rare disorder involving the growth of many small cysts in the medulla of the kidney; often leads to renal failure.

**nephropathy** *n* any disease of the kidney in which inflammation is not a major component. ⇒ diabetic nephropathy—**nephropathic** *adj*.

**nephropexy** *n* surgical fixation of a floating kidney.

**nephroptosis** *n* downward displacement of the kidney. The word is sometimes used for a floating kidney.

**nephrosclerosis** *n* a hardening or sclerosis of the kidney. There are changes in the renal arterioles leading to ischaemia. Commonly caused by hypertension, or associated with general arteriosclerosis in older people.

**nephroscope** *n* an endoscope for viewing kidney tissue. It can be designed to create a continuous flow of irrigating fluid and provide an exit for the fluid and accompanying debris—**nephroscopic** *adj*.

**nephrosis** *n* nephropathy. Any degenerative disease of the renal tubules. ⇒ nephrotic syndrome.

**nephrostomy** *n* a surgically established fistula from the pelvis of the kidney to the body surface.

**nephrotic syndrome** disease characterized by heavy proteinuria, low serum albumin (hypoalbuminaemia) and oedema formation; there are a wide range of causes.

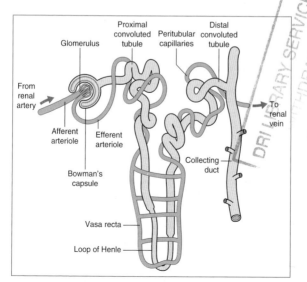

**Figure N.2** Nephron—simplified (*reproduced from Brooker & Waugh 2007 with permission*).

**nephrotoxic** *adj* describes any substance or process that is injurious to renal tissue or function, for example, the aminoglycoside antibiotics (e.g. gentamicin)—**nephrotoxin** *n*.

**nephroureterectomy** *n* removal of the kidney along with a part or the whole of the ureter. Also known as ureteronephrectomy.

**nerve** *n* an elongated bundle of fibres which serves for the transmission of impulses between the periphery and the nerve centres. *afferent nerve* one conveying impulses from the tissues to the nerve centres; also known as sensory nerves. *efferent nerve* one which conveys impulses outwards from the central nervous system to the muscles and glands; also known as motor nerves.

**nerve block anaesthesia** regional anaesthesia. The injection of a local anaesthetic (e.g. lidocaine) into an area close to a nerve, thus blocking the conduction in the nerve and producing anaesthesia in the structures supplied by that nerve.

**nerve conduction test** an electrical test used to ascertain whether nerve impulse transmission is occurring in the peripheral nerves. The nerve is electrically stimulated and a distal electrode records the impulse. Used in the diagnosis of polyneuropathies and in nerve entrapment.

**nerve entrapment syndrome** a type of mononeuropathy in which a nerve is trapped and compressed, for example as it passes through a bony canal or through fascia, such as carpal tunnel syndrome or meralgia paraesthetica. It is characterized by abnormal sensation, pain, muscle weakness and muscle wastage.

**nerve growth factor (NGF)** *n* protein growth factor required for nerve differentiation and growth during embryonic development and for later nerve maintenance.

**nerve impulse** the transmission of electrochemical energy occurring along a nerve fibre as electrical and concentration gradients across the excitable cell membrane are caused by ion (sodium and potassium) movement (Figure N.3). ⇒ action potential, depolarization, polarized, repolarization.

**nerve stimulator** apparatus used to stimulate electronically peripheral nerves to locate them and test nerve blockade. ⇒ nerve conduction test.

**nervous** *adj* **1.** relating to nerves or nerve tissue. **2.** referring to a state of restlessness or timidity.

**nervous system** the structures controlling the actions and functions of the body; it comprises

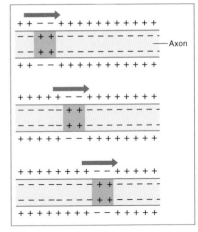

**Figure N.3** Propagation of a nerve impulse—simplified *(reproduced from Waugh & Grant 2006 with permission)*.

the brain and spinal cord (central nervous system [CNS]), and all the peripheral nerve fibres and ganglia that are outside the brain and spinal cord. The peripheral nervous system can be further subdivided into the sensory division and the motor division. The latter is in turn divided into the voluntary somatic nervous system and the involuntary autonomic system, which is divided into the sympathetic and parasympathetic nervous systems. ⇒ Appendix 1, Figures 1 and 11, autonomic nervous system, peripheral nervous system, parasympathetic nervous system, sympathetic nervous system.

**Nesbit's operation** (R Nesbit, American surgeon, 20th century) an operative procedure undertaken to relieve the curvature of the penis, such as that occurring in Peyronie's disease.

**net oxygen cost** the oxygen used during physical activity in excess of that required at rest.

**nettlerash** *n* ⇒ urticaria.

**neural** *adj* pertaining to nerves.

**neural arch** ⇒ vertebral arch.

**neural canal** ⇒ vertebral canal.

**neural crest** *n* the ectodermal cells present on the outer aspects of both sides of the neural tube during early embryonic development. The ectodermal cells migrate through the developing embryo where they will eventually form cells of the peripheral nervous system—neurons and supporting neuroglia, pigment cells, hormone-producing cells (e.g. in adrenal gland) and other cell types. ⇒ neural tube.

**neural fold** *n* one of two folds that form during invagination of the neural plate. They come together to form the neural tube.

**neural plate** *n* the plate of ectodermal cells that forms in week 2 of embryonic development. It grows and folds in on itself (invaginates) to form the neural folds and then the neural tube, the structure which, after many changes in shape, forms the structures of the central nervous system. ⇒ neural tube.

**neuralgia** *n* pain in the distribution of a nerve—**neuralgic** *adj*.

**neural tube** *n* the longitudinal ectodermal structure formed from the fusion of the neural folds. It gives rise to the brain and spinal cord.

**neural tube defect (NTD)** any of a group of congenital abnormalities where there are defects in the skull and/or the vertebral column. It is caused by the failure of the neural tube to close during the first 30 days of embryonic development. NTDs include anencephaly, encephalocele, hydrocephalus, meningocele, meningoencephalocele, meningomyelocele, myelocele and spina bifida. The developing nervous system is particularly susceptible to maternal deficiency of folate (folic acid) during early pregnancy. Adequate intake of folate before conception and for the first few weeks of pregnancy is important in reducing the incidence of NTDs. ⇒ alphafetoprotein, folate.

**neurapraxia** *n* temporary loss of function in peripheral nerve fibres. Most commonly due to crushing or prolonged pressure. ⇒ axonotmesis.

**neurasthenia** *n* historically described as a form of 'nervous exhaustion'. Now regarded as an anxiety disorder characterized by persistent fatigue together with poor appetite, irritability, insomnia, headache and poor concentration—**neurasthenic** *adj*.

**neurectasis** *n* ⇒ neurotony.

**neurectomy** *n* excision of part of a nerve.

**neurilemma (neurolemma)** *n* the thin membranous covering of a nerve fibre surrounding the myelin sheath.

**neurilemmoma** *n* also known as Schwann cell tumour or schwannoma. A benign tumour growing on the neurilemma of peripheral nerves.

**neuritis** *n* inflammation of a nerve—**neuritic** *adj*.

**neuroblast** *n* a primitive embryonic nerve cell.

**neuroblastoma** *n* a rare malignant tumour of primitive ectodermal cells arising in the adrenal medulla or any tissue of the sympathetic nervous system. Neuroblastomas metastasize to bone, liver, lungs or lymph nodes. It occurs in infants and children—**neuroblastomata** *pl*, **neuroblastomatous** *adj*.

**neurodermatitis** *n* (*syn* lichen simplex) leathery, thickened patches of skin secondary to pruritus and scratching. As the skin thickens, irritation increases, scratching causes further thickening and so a vicious circle is set up.

**neurodevelopmental therapy** in physiotherapy, an approach to neurological rehabilitation that is based on knowledge of motor development and neurophysiology.

**neuroendocrine** *adj* relating to the close relationship between the nervous system and endocrine structures. For example, *neuroendocrine cells* (specialized neurons), which secrete neurohormones including some types of gastrin and vasopressin (or arginine vasopressin [AVP]).

**neuroepithelioma** *n* ⇒ medulloepithelioma.

**neuroepithelium** *n* specialized epithelial tissue present as sensory cells, for example, of the tongue, the olfactory epithelium of the nose and the vestibule and cochlea of the inner ear.

**neurofibrils** *npl* microscopic threads found in the cytoplasm of neurons, they may extend into the axon.

**neurofibrillary tangles** a pathological change occurring in the brain of people with Alzheimer's disease. There are tangled clumps of neurofibrils within the neurons. ⇒ Alzheimer's disease.

**neurofibroma** *n* a tumour arising from the connective tissue of peripheral nerves. A proliferation of Schwann cells—**neurofibromata** *pl*, **neurofibromatous** *adj*.

**neurofibromatosis** *n* a genetically determined condition in which there are many fibromata. ⇒ von Recklinghausen's disease.

**neurogenesis** *n* the development of nervous tissue.

**neurogenic** *adj* originating within or forming nervous tissue.

**neurogenic bladder** interference with the nerve control of the urinary bladder causing either retention of urine, which presents as incontinence, or continuous dribbling without retention. When necessary the bladder is emptied by exerting manual pressure on the anterior abdominal wall. ⇒ incontinence.

**neuroglia** *n* (*syn* glia) the non-excitable supporting tissue of the central nervous system (brain and spinal cord). ⇒ astrocytes, ependymal cells, macroglia, microglia, oligodendrocytes—**neuroglial** *adj*.

**neurohormone** *n* hormones and related chemicals produced by specialized neurons (neurosecretory neuroendocrine cells) present in areas that include the hypothalamus, adrenal medulla and some nerve fibres. The hormones, which include vasopressin (or arginine vasopressin [AVP]) and gastrin, are released into the blood or cerebrospinal fluid or directly into the spaces between cells. ⇒ neuropeptides, neuromodulators, neurotransmitters.

**neurohypophysis** *n* the posterior lobe of the pituitary gland. The neural part of the gland that develops from a portion of diencephalon. It stores two hormones—oxytocin and antidiuretic hormone (vasopressin or arginine vasopressin [AVP]). ⇒ pituitary gland.

**neurokinin receptor antagonist** a class of antiemetic drug, e.g. aprepitant. It is used with other drugs to control the nausea and vomiting associated with cisplatin chemotherapy.

**neuroleptic malignant syndrome** a rare but potentially life-threatening side-effect of neuroleptics (antipsychotic drugs). ⇒ Appendix 5. It is characterized by increased temperature (hyperthermia), tachycardia, hypotension, confusion and delirium, urinary incontinence, altered consciousness, muscle tremors and rigidity, and metabolic acidosis. There is no specific treatment but the antipsychotic drug should be discontinued and appropriate supportive treatment provided.

**neuroleptics** *npl* usually known as antipsychotics. Drugs acting on the nervous system. ⇒ antipsychotic drugs, Appendix 5.

**neurolinguistic programming (NLP)** communication-based techniques that seek to improve a person's awareness of his or her experiences and levels of 'self'. It incorporates the use of verbal and non-verbal communication, sensory events and particular patterns of behaviour.

**neurologist** *n* a specialist in neurology or a medically qualified person who specializes in diagnosing and treating diseases of the nervous system.

**neurology** *n* **1.** the science and study of nerves—their structure, function and pathology. **2.** the branch of medicine dealing with diseases of the nervous system—**neurological** *adj*.

**neuroma** *n* a tumour of nervous tissue.

**neuromuscular** *adj* pertaining to nerves and muscles.

**neuromuscular electrical stimulation** various devices are used to administer electrical stimulation to nerves and muscle. It is used in a variety of clinical situations, which include reducing spasticity, to enhance wound healing, to strengthen muscles, increase muscle function and to prevent muscle atrophy. For example, it may be used to strengthen the pelvic floor in the management of urinary incontinence and to improve motor recovery following a stroke.

**neuromuscular junction** the communication between the axon of a myelinated nerve and the muscle fibre. ⇒ motor end-plate, neurotransmitters, synapse.

**neuron(e)** *n* a nerve cell. The basic unit of the nervous system comprising fibres (dendrites) which convey impulses to the nerve cell, the nerve cell body itself, and the fibres (axons) which convey impulses from the cell body (Figure N.4). They are specialized excitable cells that are able to transmit an action potential. ⇒ motor neuron disease—**neuronal, neural** *adj*. *lower motor neuron* the cell body is in the anterior horn of the spinal cord and the axon passes to skeletal muscle; *upper motor neuron* the cell body is in the motor cortex and the axon terminates in the anterior horn of the spinal cord.

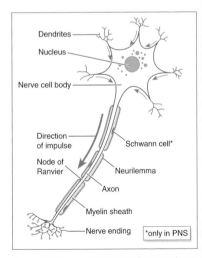

**Figure N.4** Neuron *(reproduced from Brooker & Nicol 2003 with permission).*

**neuronoplasty** *n* any restorative operation to repair a nerve.

**neuropathic** *adj* relating to disease of the nervous system.

**neuropathic pain** pain experienced without any identifiable tissue damage. It is caused by faulty processing of sensory inputs by the nervous system and is associated with chronic non-malignant pain. Examples include neuralgia following an attack of herpes zoster (shingles) and phantom limb pain/syndrome.

**neuropathology** *n* a branch of medicine dealing with diseases of the nervous system—**neuropathological** *adj*.

**neuropathy** *n* inflammation or degeneration leading to loss of function of peripheral nerves. It may be focal (e.g. carpal tunnel syndrome), known as a mononeuropathy, or generalized, as in polyneuropathy.

**neuropeptides** *npl* a group of peptides found in the brain, including endorphins, vasopressin (or arginine vasopressin [AVP]). They act as neurotransmitters and as hormones. *neuropeptide Y* a neurotransmitter that is believed to be involved in appetite control and feeding in conjunction with leptin. ⇒ neurohormones, neurotransmitters.

**neuropharmacology** *n* the branch of pharmacology dealing with drugs that act on the nervous system—**neuropharmacological** *adj*.

**neurophysiology** *n* the study of the functioning of nervous tissue and the nervous system.

**neuroplasticity** *n* the ability of nerve cells to regenerate.

**neuroplasty** *n* surgical repair of nerves—**neuroplastic** *adj*.

**neuropsychiatry** *n* a subspecialty of psychiatry dealing with mental disorder and its relationship to brain/central nervous system (dys)function—**neuropsychiatric** *adj*.

**neuroretinitis** *n* inflammation affecting the optic nerve and the retina.

**neurorrhaphy** *n* suturing the ends of a divided nerve.

**neurosis** *n* an outdated term. The traditional division between psychosis and neurosis has fallen out of favour. However, the term 'neurotic disorders' is a grouping term for anxiety disorders, phobias and obsessive-compulsive disorder—**neurotic** *adj*.

**neurosurgery** *n* surgery of the nervous system—**neurosurgical** *adj*.

**neurosyphilis** *n* infection of brain or spinal cord, or both, by *Treponema pallidum*. The variety of clinical pictures produced is large, but the two common syndromes encountered are tabes dorsalis and general paralysis of the insane (GPI). Very often symptoms of the disease do not arise until 20 years or more after the date of primary infection—**neurosyphilitic** *adj*.

**neurotmesis** *n* damage to a peripheral nerve, usually through transection, in which there is disruption of the axon and damage to the covering connective tissue layer. Microsurgical techniques may improve function.

**neurotomy** *n* surgical cutting of a nerve.

**neurotony** *n* also called neurectasis. The stretching of a nerve or nerve trunk.

**neurotoxic** *adj* poisonous or destructive to nervous tissue—**neurotoxin** *n*.

**neurotransmitters** *npl* a large group of chemicals released by nerve endings. They modify or facilitate the passage of a nerve impulse across a synapse. Examples include: acetylcholine, adrenaline (epinephrine), dopamine, endorphins, enkephalins, gamma-aminobutyrate, glutamic acid, glycine, 5-hydroxytryptamine (serotonin), noradrenaline (norepinephrine) and substance P.

**neurotropic** *adj* with predilection for the nervous system. *Treponema pallidum* produces neurosyphilitic complications. Neurotropic viruses (e.g. rabies, poliomyelitis) attack nerve cells.

**neutron** *n* the subatomic particle that has no electrical charge.

**neutropenia** *n* reduction in the number of circulating neutrophils to less than $1.0 \times 10^9$/L, but not sufficiently reduced to warrant the description of agranulocytosis. It may occur as a side-effect of cancer treatment with chemotherapy and/or radiotherapy, which cause depression of the haemopoietic bone marrow. Because neutrophils are responsible for phagocytosis, patients with neutropenia are at high risk of serious and potentially fatal infection. Potential sites of infection include the blood, respiratory system, urinary tract and the skin, especially when vascular access devices are in situ, such as an intravenous cannula, or a central line for the administration of drugs, or nutrition—**neutropenic** *adj*.

**neutrophil** *n* the most numerous white blood cell (leucocyte). It is a phagocytic polymorphonuclear cell with granules (Figure N.5). A vital component of non-specific (innate) defence mechanisms.

**New Ballard Score** (J Ballard, American paediatrician, 20th–21st century) a system of assessing gestational age in preterm neonates. It has 12 criteria in two categories: neuromuscular,

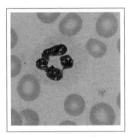

**Figure N.5** Neutrophil *(reproduced from Boon et al. 2006 with permission).*

e.g. posture, popliteal angle, arm recoil; and physical, e.g. skin, lanugo, eye and ear development and genitalia. ⇒ Dubowitz score.

**newborn life support** the basic life support measures used immediately after birth. Some infants, who breathe spontaneously, may only require drying and warmth, whereas other infants will need airway clearance, oxygen therapy or even cardiopulmonary resuscitation. ⊙DVD

**newton (N)** *n* (I Newton, British scientist, 1642–1727) a unit of force. Derived SI unit (International System of Units). ⇒ Appendix 2.

**NG** *abbr* nasogastric.

**NGF** *abbr* nerve growth factor.

**NGU** *abbr* non-gonococcal urethritis.

**NHL** *abbr* non-Hodgkin's lymphoma.

**NHS** *abbr* National Health Service.

**NHS Direct/NHS 24** telephone services—NHS Direct in England and NHS 24 in Scotland—which offer 24-hour nurse-led health information and advice services. These organizations are increasingly people's first contact with the NHS, especially out of hours. They also provide a comprehensive online health information service.

**NHSLA** *abbr* NHS Litigation Authority.

**NHS Litigation Authority (NHSLA)** a special health authority in England, which deals with claims of negligence against NHS bodies. The NHSLA remit also extends to risk management, directed at raising standards of care and reducing claims of negligence.

**NHS Trusts** public accountable bodies that provide NHS health care to the population in England, either in hospital or the community.

**niacin** *n* a generic term that includes nicotinamide and nicotinic acid.

**NICE** *acron* **N**ational **I**nstitute for Health and Clinical **E**xcellence.

**nicotinamide** *n* the amide of nicotinic acid, a member of the vitamin B complex. It is part of the coenzymes *nicotinamide adenine dinucleotide (NAD/NADH)* and *nicotinamide adenine dinucleotide phosphate (NADP/NADPH)*, essential in metabolism. It is obtained from meat, pulses and wholegrain cereals in the diet, and it is formed from nicotinic acid or synthesized in the liver from the amino acid tryptophan. ⇒ niacin, pellagra.

**nicotinamide adenine dinucleotide (NAD/ NADH)** a coenzyme synthesized from nicotinamide. It is a major electron carrier in the oxidation of fuel molecules.

**nicotinamide adenine dinucleotide phosphate (NADP/NADPH)** a coenzyme synthesized from nicotinamide. It is an important electron carrier in the synthesis of molecules that include fatty acids.

**nicotine** *n* a poisonous alkaloid present in tobacco.

**nicotinic** *adj* a type of cholinergic receptor where nicotine would, if present, bind in place of acetylcholine. ⇒ muscarinic.

**nicotinic acid** a member of the vitamin B complex, which has antipellagra properties and occurs in the diet. Has a direct vasodilatory action and is used in the management of peripheral vascular disease. ⇒ niacin, nicotinamide, pellagra.

**nictitation** *n* rapid and involuntary blinking of the eyelids.

**NICU** *abbr* neonatal intensive care unit.

**nidation** *n* implantation of the early embryo in the decidua.

**NIDDM** *abbr* non-insulin-dependent diabetes mellitus. ⇒ diabetes mellitus type 2.

**nidus** *n* any structure resembling a nest in appearance or function.

**nidus of infection** a breeding place where bacteria and other pathological agents lodge and form a focus.

**Niemann–Pick disease** (A Niemann, German paediatrician, 1880–1921; L Pick, German pathologist, 1868–1944) an inherited lipid metabolic disturbance, chiefly in female Jewish infants. There are several types which are classified by age of onset and the effects on the central nervous system. Now thought to be due to absence or inadequacy of the enzyme sphingomyelinase. There is enlargement of the liver, spleen and lymph nodes caused by fat accumulation and learning disability. Now classified as a lipid reticulosis.

**night blindness** (*syn* nyctalopia) maladaptation of vision to darkness; may occur in vitamin A deficiency or genetic disorders of the retina.

**night cry** a shrill noise, made during sleep. May be of significance in hip disease when pain occurs in the relaxed joint.

**night splinting** the passive nighttime use of orthoses such as splints to maintain corrected deformities produced dynamically during walking. This may be an additional silicone digital device to maintain correction in bed, or a night splint to maintain ankle extension at 90° where there is tightening of the Achilles tendon. Night splints for the management of hallux valgus are often used as the only corrective measure.

**night sweat** profuse sweating, usually during sleep; typical of tuberculosis or lymphoma.

**night terror** ⇒ sleep terror.

**nihilistic** *adj* the belief that nothing is real. Nihilistic delusions.

**Nikolsky's sign** (P Nikolsky, Russian dermatologist, 1858–1940) slight pressure on the skin causes 'slipping' of apparently normal skin typically adjacent to a blister. Characteristic of pemphigus and other bullous conditions.

**nine-hole peg test** a test of manual dexterity and hand and arm speed, in which a person is timed whilst placing nine pegs in holes on a base.

**nipple** *n* the conical eminence in the centre of each breast, containing the outlets of the milk ducts.

**NIPPV** *abbr* non-invasive intermittent positive-pressure ventilation.

**Nissl body/granule** (F Nissl, German neurologist, 1860–1919) one of the basic-staining granular structures formed from rough endoplasmic reticulum and ribosomes, present in the cytoplasm of neurons.

**nit** *n* the egg of the head louse (*Pediculus capitis*). It is firmly attached to the hair.

**nitrates** *npl* a group of drugs that act as coronary vasodilators, e.g. glyceryl trinitrate. There is a reduction in venous return to the heart and the work of the left ventricle. ⇒ Appendix 5.

**nitric oxide (NO)** an endogenous neuromodulator. It is involved with processes that include neurotransmission, memory, learning, gastric emptying, smooth muscle relaxation, nociception and penile erection. May be used therapeutically for patients with acute respiratory distress syndrome.

**nitrogen (N)** *n* **1.** an almost inert gaseous element; the chief constituent of the atmosphere (78–79%), but it cannot be utilized directly by humans. However, certain organisms in the soil and roots of legumes are capable of nitrogen fixation. It is a vital constituent of many complements of living cells, e.g. proteins. **2.** the essential constituent of protein foods—**nitrogenous** *adj*.

**nitrogen balance** the situation when a person's daily intake of nitrogen from proteins equals the daily excretion of nitrogen. Nitrogen is excreted mainly as urea in the urine; ammonia, creatinine and uric acid account for a further small amount. Less than 10% total nitrogen is excreted in faeces. A *positive nitrogen balance* occurs during pregnancy and in growing children. A *negative nitrogen balance* occurs when excretion of nitrogen exceeds the daily intake. This occurs in inadequate protein intake, starvation or a debilitating illness (e.g. cancer), with glucocorticoid therapy, and after major surgery, trauma and sepsis when protein utilization increases.

**nitrous oxide (N$_2$O)** gas used widely as an adjuvant for general anaesthesia and for analgesia. Known colloquially as laughing gas.

**NK cell** *abbr* natural killer cell.

**NLP** *abbr* neurolinguistic programming.

**NMR** *abbr* nuclear magnetic resonance.

**NNU** *abbr* neonatal unit.

**nociceptors** *npl* receptors that respond to harmful stimuli that cause pain, such as trauma and inflammation.

**nociceptive** *adj* relating to nerve endings that respond to harmful stimuli.

**nociceptive pain** acute pain. It is associated with tissue injury, such as a cut or burn. Uusually of brief duration and subsides as healing occurs.

**nocturia** *n* passing urine at night.

**nocturnal** *adj* nightly; during the night.

**node** *n* a protuberance or swelling. A constriction.

**node of Ranvier** (L Ranvier, French pathologist, 1835–1922) the regular gaps in the myelin sheaf of a myelinated nerve axon. There is a concentration of voltage-gated sodium/potassium ion channels at the gap where the action potential is regenerated, thus facilitating the transmission of the nerve impulse from node to node. ⇒ salutatory conduction.

**nodule** *n* a small node—**nodular** *adj*.

**no-fault liability** acknowledgement that compensation is payable without the requirement to prove a failure in fulfilling the duty of care.

**noma** *n* also called cancrum oris and gangrenous stomatitis. An acute necrotizing ulceration with gangrene affecting cheek mucosa. Various micro-organisms may be involved, for example *Treponema vincentii*. It can, in severe cases, also involve the gingiva and jaw bone. In some forms the genitalia are also affected. It usually occurs in malnourished or debilitated children.

**nominal data** categorical data where the classes have no particular value or order, such as road names or colours. ⇒ ordinal data.

**nomogram** *n* graph with several variables used to determine another related variable, such as body surface area from weight and height.

**non-accidental injury (NAI)** physical maltreatment, usually of children by their parents, carers, other adults, or even other children. The injuries cannot be attributed to natural disease processes or simple accident. The injuries are often multiple and typically include bruising with finger marks, shaking injuries, fractures and burns, and involve the head, soft tissues, long bones and the thoracic cage. There may be evidence of neglect and usually there is associated psychological harm. ⇒ abuse.

**non-compliance** *n* a term used when patients who understand their drug regimen do not comply with it.

**non compos mentis** not mentally competent.

**non-disjunction** *n* the failure of homologous chromosomes to separate during the first meiotic division, or the chromatids of a chromosome do not separate during mitosis or the second meiotic division. It results in 'daughter' cells with too many or too few chromosomes. ⇒ monosomy, trisomy.

**non-gonococcal urethritis (NGU)** (*syn* non-specific urethritis—NSU) a common sexually transmitted disease in men. At least half of cases are caused by *Chlamydia trachomatis*. Uncommonly caused by *Trichomonas vaginalis* or herpes simplex virus. Aetiology in remaining cases is uncertain, but the bacteria *Ureaplasma urealyticum* and *Mycoplasma genitalium* may be causes.

**non-Hodgkin's lymphoma (NHL)** tumour of lymphoid tissue. More common in older people. The cure rate is less good than Hodgkin's disease. ⇒ lymphoma.

**non-insulin-dependent diabetes mellitus (NIDDM)** ⇒ diabetes mellitus type 2.

**non-invasive** *adj* describes any diagnostic or therapeutic technique that does not require penetration of the skin or of any cavity or organ.

**non-invasive intermittent positive-pressure ventilation (NIPPV)** a type of respiratory support that uses a nasal or full-face mask rather than an endotracheal or tracheostomy tube.

**non-maleficence** *n* ethical principle of doing no harm. ⇒ beneficence.

**non-milk extrinsic sugars** extrinsic sugars except that found in milk (lactose).

**non-nucleoside reverse transcriptase inhibitor** a class of antiviral drugs, e.g. efavirenz, used for human immunodeficiency virus (HIV) and acquired immunodeficiency syndrome (AIDS).

**non-occlusion** *n* the tooth/teeth in one arch do not make contact with those in the other arch.

**non-parametric test** statistical test that makes no presupposition about the distribution of data. When data are not normally distributed a non-parametric test, such as the Mann–Whitney *U*-test, which does not assume a normal distribution is the preferred option. Non-parametric tests are less powerful than the equivalent parametric test. ⇒ parametric tests.

**non-protein nitrogen (NPN)** nitrogen from nitrogenous substances other than protein, i.e. urea, uric acid, creatinine, creatine and ammonia.

**non-rapid eye movement sleep (NREM)** ⇒ sleep.

**non-secretor** *n* a person who does not secrete ABO blood antigens in saliva or gastric juice. ⇒ secretor.

**non-small cell lung carcinoma (NSCLC)** commonest type of lung cancer, accounting for approximately 80% of tumours. The histological subtypes include squamous, adenocarcinoma and large cell. The doubling time is approximately 130 days. Clinical presentation may be with cough, haemoptysis, recurrent pneumonia, increasing breathlessness, weight loss, or may be an incidental finding on chest X-ray. Therapy may include surgery (in approximately 20%), chemotherapy and/or radiotherapy.

**non-specific urethritis (NSU)** ⇒ non-gonococcal urethritis.

**non-staphylococcal scalded-skin syndrome** ⇒ toxic epidermal necrolysis.

**non-starch polysaccharides (NSP)** polysaccharides other than starch that occur in plant material that is not digested in the human gastrointestinal tract. Can be divided into two types: non-soluble, e.g. cellulose, and soluble, e.g. pectins and mucilages. An important component of the diet to prevent constipation, diverticular disease and colorectal cancer. They provide most dietary fibre in the diet.

**non-steroidal anti-inflammatory drugs (NSAIDs)** a large group of drugs with varying degrees of anti-inflammatory, antipyretic and analgesic action, e.g. diclofenac. They inhibit enzymes needed for the synthesis of prostaglandins and thromboxanes. ⇒ fenamates, oxicams, propionic acids, pyrazolones, salicylates. ⇒ Appendix 5.

**Noonan's syndrome** (J Noonan, American paediatric cardiologist, b. 1921) occurs in either males or females, with eyes set apart (hypertelorism) and other ocular and facial abnormalities; cardiac abnormalities, short stature, cryptorchidism, sometimes with neck webbing (and other Turner-like features). Generally not chromosomal; most cases sporadic; a few either dominantly or recessively inherited. ⇒ Turner's syndrome.

**noradrenaline (norepinephrine)** *n* a catecholamine neurohumoral transmitter released from adrenergic nerve endings and in small amounts from the adrenal medulla. Its physiological effects include vasoconstriction and a rise in blood pressure. ⇒ adrenaline (epinephrine).

**norm** *n* a measure of a phenomenon generally accepted as an ideal against which all other measures of the phenomenon can be measured, i.e. the standard against which values are measured.

**normal distribution curve** in statistics, when scores are plotted they form a symmetrical bell-shaped curve that has the mean, median and mode in the centre (Figure N.6). ⇒ skewed distribution.

**normal flora** ⇒ flora.

**normalization** *n* also called social role valorization. Philosophy underpinning learning disability service provision. Individualized programmes of learning and goal setting are provided, which will facilitate the acquisition of the skills of daily living and maximum levels of independence.

**normal movement** the coordinated, smooth, effective, efficient, effortless and appropriate response of the nervous system for achieving the sensorimotor goal.

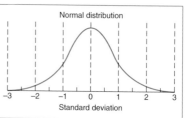

**Figure N.6** Normal distribution curve *(reproduced from Gunn 2001 with permission).*

**normative play** child-led play that aims to set up rules and norms. It is the type of play most often used and includes others and toys. It can assist in bringing normality to very strange and unfamiliar situations, such as when a child or a sibling is hospitalized. ⇒ therapeutic play.

**normoblast** *n* a normal-sized nucleated red blood cell, the precursor of the mature erythrocyte—**normoblastic** *adj.*

**normocyte** *n* a red blood cell of normal size—**normocytic** *adj.*

**normoglycaemic** *adj* a normal amount of glucose in the blood—**normoglycaemia** *n.*

**normotension** *n* normal tension, by custom alluding to blood pressure—**normotensive** *adj.*

**normothermia** *n* normal body temperature, as opposed to hyperthermia and hypothermia—**normothermic** *adj.*

**normotonic** *adj* normal strength, tension, tone, by convention referring to muscle tissue. Spasmolytic drugs induce normotonicity in muscle, and can be used before radiography—**normotonicity** *n.*

**Noroviruses (Norwalk-like viruses)** *npl* a group of viruses that cause outbreaks of winter gastroenteritis—'winter vomiting disease'. Transmission is via the faecal–oral route, by aerosols from vomit, enviromental contamination and contaminated food and water. It spreads rapidly in semiclosed institutions such as care homes, hospitals and schools.

**Northern blot technique** an electrophoretic technique used to identify the presence or absence of specific messenger ribonucleic acid (mRNA). ⇒ Southern blot technique.

**nose** *n* the organ of smell. It is part of the respiratory tract and the nasal mucosa warms, moistens and filters inspired air. ⇒ nares, nasal cavity, nasal conchae, nasal septum.

**nosocomial** *adj* pertaining to a hospital. ⇒ infection.

**nosology** *n* the science concerned with the classification of disease.

**Nosopsyllus** *n* genus of fleas. *Nosopsylla fasiatus* is the common rat flea in Europe and North America. Transmits murine typhus and probably the plague bacteria.

**nostalgia** *n* homesickness; a longing to return to a place to which, and where, one may have emotional bonds—**nostalgic** *adj*.

**nostrils** *npl* the anterior openings into the nose; the anterior nares; choanae.

**notochord** *n* the body of tissue comprising mesodermal cells, which forms the primitive axis in the early embryo.

**notifiable** *adj* describes incidents or occurrences and diseases that must by law be made known to the appropriate agency. For example, diseases such as tuberculosis, food poisoning and measles must be reported to the relevant department.

**NPN** *abbr* non-protein nitrogen.

**NPSA** *abbr* National Patient Safety Agency.

**NRDS** *abbr* neonatal respiratory distress syndrome.

**NREM** *abbr* non-rapid eye movement (sleep). ⇒ sleep.

**NSAIDs** *abbr* non-steroidal anti-inflammatory drugs.

**NSCLC** *abbr* non-small cell lung carcinoma.

**NSFs** *abbr* National Service Frameworks.

**NSP** *abbr* non-starch polysaccharide.

**NSU** *abbr* non-specific urethritis. ⇒ non-gonococcal urethritis.

**NTD** *abbr* neural tube defect.

**nucha** *n* the nape of the neck—**nuchal** *adj*.

**nuchal thickness scanning** *n* a specific fetal ultrasound scan performed to measure the fluid located in a temporary swelling in the neck, and whether or not the nasal bone is present. It is used with maternal age and the gestation period to estimate the risk of chromosomal abnormalities, including Down's syndrome.

**nuclear family** in western societies the conventional family group of two married parents and their dependant children.

**nuclear magnetic resonance (NMR)** ⇒ magnetic resonance imaging.

**nuclear medicine** the use of radioisotope (radionuclide) techniques for the diagnosis, treatment and study of disease.

**nuclease** *n* an enzyme that breaks the bonds between nucleotides in nucleic acids.

**nucleated** *adj* possessing one or more nuclei.

**nucleic acids** biological macromolecules comprising many subunits called nucleotides. ⇒ deoxyribonucleic acid, ribonucleic acid.

**nucleic acid synthesis inhibitor** antiviral drugs, such as aciclovir, that are used for herpes simplex and varicella-zoster infections.

**nucleolus** *n* structures (usually two) involved in nuclear division. They are within the nuclear membrane and contain both DNA and RNA.

**nucleoplasm** *n* the protoplasm within the nuclear envelope.

**nucleoproteins** *npl* proteins conjugated with nucleic acids found in the cell nucleus. Uric acid is an end-product of nucleoprotein metabolism, which is normally excreted in the urine. ⇒ gout.

**nucleoside** *n* a compound of a sugar and a nitrogenous base, either a pyrimidine or a purine.

**nucleoside reverse transcriptase inhibitor** a class of antiviral drugs, e.g. zidovudine, used for human immunodeficiency virus (HIV) disease. ⇒ Appendix 5.

**nucleotides** *npl* the subunits from which nucleic acids are formed. Consist of sugars and nitrogenous bases (nucleosides) and phosphate groups.

**nucleotoxic** *adj* toxic to the cell nucleus, e.g. some chemicals and viruses—**nucleotoxin** *n*.

**nucleus** *n* **1.** the membrane-bound cellular structure which contains the genetic material (chromosomes). **2.** a confined accumulation of nerve cells in the central nervous system associated with a particular function—**nuclei** *pl*, **nuclear** *adj*.

**nucleus pulposus** *n* the soft, elastic core of an intervertebral disc which can prolapse into the spinal cord and cause back pain or sciatica (Figure N.7).

**null hypothesis** a statement that asserts there to be no relationship between the dependent and independent variables.

**nullipara** *n* a woman who has not borne a child—**nulliparous** *adj*, **nulliparity** *n*.

**numbers needed to treat** a method of stating the benefits of a therapeutic intervention. The number of subjects who need to receive treatment before one subject has a positive outcome.

**nummular** *adj* coin-shaped; resembling rolls of coins, such as the sputum in tuberculosis.

**nurse anaesthetist** a nurse trained to administer general anaesthesia.

**nurse practitioner** a nurse who has undertaken specific role preparation in order to

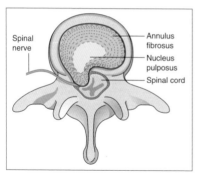

Spinal nerve

Annulus fibrosus

Nucleus pulposus

Spinal cord

**Figure N.7** Prolapsed intervertebral disc showing nucleus pulposus *(reproduced from Waugh & Grant 2006 with permission)*.

practise at an advanced level within a particular setting. For example, this may be within primary care, in an emergency department or with a specific client group, e.g. clients with mental health problems. Nurse practitioners can offer a nurse-led service.

**nursing home** an institution where nursing care is delivered by the independent sector, charitable organizations, social services or, rarely, the NHS.

**nutation** *n* nodding; applied to uncontrollable head shaking.

**nutraceuticals** *npl* non-nutrient substances present in some foods, which may have potential benefits.

**nutrient** *n, adj* a chemical substance (e.g. protein, vitamin C) found in food that can be digested and absorbed and used to promote body function. ⇒ macronutrient, micronutrients.

**nutrient artery** *n* one which enters a long bone.

**nutrient foramen** *n* hole in a long bone which admits the nutrient artery.

**nutrition** *n* the sum total of the processes by which the living organism receives and utilizes the materials necessary for survival, growth and repair of worn-out tissues.

**nutrition surveillance** the process of monitoring health status, nutrition, eating behaviour and the nutritional knowledge of the public in order to plan and evaluate nutritional policy. Particularly important in developing countries where monitoring can provide an early warning of emergencies, such as impending famine.

**nutritional** *adj* pertaining to nutrition.

**nutritional assessment** the assessment of an individual's nutritional status used to identify those who are malnourished and those who are at risk of becoming malnourished. Factors included in the assessment are dietary intake, nutritional requirements, clinical condition, physical appearance, anthropometric and biochemical measurements.

**nutritional support** intervention to improve nutrient intake. Interventions include increasing the number of meals and amounts of food provided, fortifying food with additional nutrients, sip feeds, enteral and parenteral nutrition.

**nyctalgia** *n* pain occurring during the night.

**nyctalopia** *n* night blindness.

**nyctophobia** *n* abnormal fear of the night and darkness.

**nymphae** *npl* the labia minora.

**nymphomania** *n* excessive sexual desire in women—**nymphomaniac** *adj*. compare ⇒ satyriasis.

**nystagmus** *n* jerky, involuntary and repetitive movement of the eyeball(s). It can occur under physiological situations but can also indicate diseases, especially of the cerebellum or the inner ear.

**N**

## O

**OAE** *abbr* otoacoustic emission.

**oat cell carcinoma** histological subtype of small cell cancer, most commonly of bronchogenic epithelium. It accounts for approximately 20% of all lung cancers and is characterized by rapid growth (doubling time approximately 29 days). The highest incidence is in smokers. The lung primary may present with cough, haemoptysis, recurrent pneumonia, increasing breathlessness and weight loss or may be an incidental finding on chest X-ray. Therapy generally does not include surgery, but 90% are sensitive to chemotherapy, which is usually the treatment of choice.

**obesity** *n* the deposition of excessive fat around the body, particularly in the subcutaneous tissue, internal organs and within the abdominal cavity. Develops when the intake of food is in excess of the body's energy requirements—the most common nutritional disorder worldwide; incidence is increasing. Obesity is linked with a variety of conditions that include: hypertension, cardiovascular disease (coronary heart disease and strokes), type 2 diabetes, sleep apnoea syndromes, osteoarthritis and some cancers. It is categorized by body mass index (BMI). Most authorities define obesity in adults as a BMI 30–34.9; morbid obesity as a BMI 35–39.9; and extreme obesity as BMI greater than 40. Waist circumference and waist:hip ratio are also used as indicators of the amount of fat present in the abdomen. ⇒ body mass index.

**objective** *adj* pertaining to things external to oneself. ⇒ subjective *opp*. *objective signs* those which the observer notes, as distinct from the symptoms of which the patient complains.

**OBLA** *abbr* onset of blood lactate accumulation.

**obligate** *adj* distinguished by the ability to survive only in a particular set of environmental conditions, such as a micro-organism.

**OBS** *abbr* organic brain syndrome. ⇒ dementia.

**observational study** research in which the researcher observes, listens and records the events of concern. Where the researcher participates and has a role, it is termed a *participant observational study*. May be used in qualitative social science research.

**obsessive-compulsive disorder (OCD)** recurrent obsessional thoughts and/or compulsive acts occurring on most days for at least 2 weeks. The thoughts are usually distressing and are therefore (often unsuccessfully) resisted by the sufferer.

**obstetrician** *n* a qualified doctor who practises the science and art of obstetrics.

**obstetrics** *n* the science dealing with the care of the pregnant woman during the antenatal, parturient and puerperal stages; midwifery.

**obstructive sleep apnoea (hypopnoea) syndrome (OSAS; OSAHS)** sometimes referred to as sleep apnoea syndrome. A condition characterized by irregular breathing during sleep, episodes of apnoea/hypopnoea during sleep, snoring and feeling tired and sleepy during the day, with poor concentration and irritability. As the person falls asleep the muscles in the pharynx relax, causing the airway to narrow or close, thus reducing the airflow. The reduction in airflow and apnoea/hypopnoea means that inspiratory effort is increased and the person moves to a lighter level of sleep or to full wakefulness. The pattern is repeated throughout the night with poor-quality sleep. ⇒ apnoea hypopnoea index (AHI), continuous positive airways pressure (CPAP), laser-assisted uvulopalatoplasty, uvulopalatopharyngoplasty.

**obturator** *n* that which closes an aperture.

**obturator foramen** the opening in the innominate bone which is closed by muscles and fascia.

**occipital** *adj* pertaining to the back of the head.

**occipital bone** the cranial bone forming the back and part of the base of the skull. It has a large opening, the foramen magnum, through which the spinal cord passes out of the skull.

**occipital lobe** a small lobe of the cerebrum lying beneath the occipital bone. It has the primary visual cortex and the visual association area.

**occipitoanterior** *adj* describes a presentation when the fetal occiput lies in the anterior half of the maternal pelvis.

**occipitofrontal** *adj* pertaining to the occiput and the frontal bone (forehead).

**occipitoposterior** *adj* describes a presentation when the fetal occiput is in the posterior half of the maternal pelvis.

**occiput** *n* the posterior region of the skull.

**occlusal** *adj* in dentistry, relating to the contacting surfaces of the teeth in the upper arch and those in the lower arch.

**occlusion** *n* **1.** the closure of an opening, especially of ducts or blood vessels. **2.** in dentistry, the contact of the upper and lower teeth in any jaw position. *centric occlusion* contact of the upper and lower teeth with maximum interdigitation of the cusps. *traumatic occlusion* any malocclusion resulting in damage to the teeth or periodontal tissues—**occlusal** *adj.*

**occult** *adj* concealed.

**occult blood** minute amount of blood present in, for example, faeces, that is not visible and can only be detected by chemical tests, or microscopic or spectroscopic examination. ⇒ faecal occult blood.

**occupation** *n* the purposeful, functional, productive, playful or creative activities of daily living performed by an individual throughout his or her life.

**occupational asthma** asthma caused by inhalation of specific agents in the workplace that leads to sensitization of the individual following an immune response. Symptoms do not occur on first exposure but a pattern emerges as symptoms are provoked by work exposure and relieved when away from work. Treatment is by prevention and control of exposure. Untreated the condition can become persistent and chronic.

**occupational behaviour** interaction with the social, temporal and physical environments in a variety of activities of daily living, throughout an individual's life. These activities should be consistent with a person's occupational role, involve achievement, and address the financial realities of life.

**occupational competency** being able to perform at the level required to fulfil occupational identity.

**occupational deprivation** a situation in which the person has few occupations or lacks the opportunity to engage in the range of occupations which would normally be expected of people at a certain age, in their culture.

**occupational disease** ⇒ industrial disease.

**occupational dysfunction** temporary or permanent inability to engage in a range of relationships, roles and occupations usually needed in daily life.

**occupational health** the active and proactive management of health in the workplace. Achieved through an occupational health department and the employment of occupational health doctors and/or nurses, and other health professionals as appropriate.

**occupational identity** how a person perceives him- or herself in terms of the names of occupations which he or she feels apply to them. Having occupational identity is part of personal identity, sense of self and gives meaning to daily living.

**occupational performance** the skills and actions that result in the ability to perform functional, purposeful activities of daily living in a variety of associated occupational roles and environments.

**occupational role** the expression of an individual's occupational behaviour through various activities of daily living that identifies his or her place in society.

**occupational therapy (OT)** the use of purposeful activity and meaningful occupation for people with physical and psychosocial dysfunction and disability to enable them to regain, or maintain, their health, well-being and optimal level of functional independence in all aspects of life. Occupational therapists help people, through the analysis and application of specific, selected activities, to develop the occupational performance skills and roles required to perform consistently and competently activities of daily living in a variety of physical, temporal and social environments.

**occupational therapy assessment** the use of both formal and informal screening and evaluation methods, including medical records, interview, observation, standardized and non-standardized tests, to assess occupational performance areas, performance components and occupational role performance. This provides the occupational therapist with the means to develop treatment objectives and methods to remediate, or compensate for, any problems identified. Assessment can also be used to determine the effectiveness of treatment and any modifications that might be needed.

**occupational therapy process** a systematic approach of enquiry and action used to structure occupational therapy interventions. It involves information gathering, setting goals, implementation, evaluation and review.

**OCD** *abbr* obsessive-compulsive disorder.

**ochronosis** *n* greyish discoloration of connective tissue, such as occurs in alkaptonuria.

**ocular** *adj* pertaining to the eye.

**oculogyric** *adj* referring to movements of the eyeball. *oculogyric crisis* an attack in which the eyes stay in a fixed position for minutes or even hours. Usually the eyes are positioned up and to the side, but in some cases they are fixed to the side or down.

**oculomotor** *n* the third pair of cranial nerves which innervate four of the extraocular/extrinsic muscles that move the eyeball, and the upper eyelid. They also alter the shape of the lens and control pupil size.

**ODD** *acron* **o**ppositional **d**efiant **d**isorder.

**odds ratio** in statistics, the odds of a disease occurring in a person exposed to the risk factor divided by the odds of a disease occurring in a person who has not been exposed to the risk factor.

**odontalgia** *n* toothache.

**odontoblasts** *npl* the dentine-forming cells in teeth.

**odontoclasts** *npl* cells in the teeth that are responsible for the resorption of dentine and cementum.

**odontodysplasia** *n* abnormal development of the teeth, with deficient formation of enamel and dentine. The teeth have a characteristic radiographic appearance and are known as *ghost teeth*.

**odontogenesis** *n* the formation of the teeth. *odontogenesis imperfecta* a general term that includes defects in both the epithelial and mesenchymal tissue components needed for tooth formation.

**odontogenic tumours** several types of neoplasms arising in tooth-forming tissues. They may be benign (e.g. odontogenic fibroma) or malignant (e.g. odontogenic fibrosarcoma).

**odontoid** *adj* resembling a tooth.

**odontoid process** also known as the dens. A peg-like projection of the axis (second cervical vertebra) that fits into the posterior part of the vertebral foramen of the atlas (first cervical vertebra). The atlas rotates around the odontoid process, which acts as a pivot during movement of the head.

**odontology** *n* the scientific study of the development, structure and function of the teeth and associated oral structures.

**odontolysis** *n* resorption of a tooth root.

**odontoma** *n* a tumour-like anomaly of the hard tissue of teeth (e.g. dens in dente). It comprises cementum, dentine, enamel and pulp that may be ordered in the form of teeth.

**odynophagia** *n* intense pain and burning sensation during swallowing. It results from irritation of the oesophageal mucosa caused by certain foods, gastro-oesophageal reflux disease, infection, cancer, or from muscular problems such as achalasia.

**oedema** *n* abnormal collection of fluid in the tissues such as around the ankles, lower leg or sacral area. Fluid may also collect in the pleural cavity, pericardial sac and within the abdominal cavity. The formation of oedema can be caused by: reduced blood albumin, such as may occur in some kidney diseases, liver disease or when protein intake is insufficient; increased hydrostatic pressure leading to venous congestion, as in chronic heart failure; 'leaky' capillaries during the inflammatory response; and when lymphatic drainage is impaired, e.g. cancer affecting the lymph nodes. ⇒ angioedema, ascites, pleural effusion, pulmonary oedema—**oedematous** *adj*.

**Oedipus complex** an unconscious attachment of a son to his mother, resulting in a feeling of jealousy towards the father and then guilt, producing emotional conflict.

**oesophageal** *adj* pertaining to the oesophagus.

**oesophageal ulcer** ulceration of the oesophagus due to gastro-oesophageal reflux disease caused by hiatus hernia.

**oesophageal varices** varicosity of the veins at the gastro-oesophageal junction due to hepatic portal hypertension, often caused by alcohol-related cirrhosis or chronic hepatitis. These varices can bleed and may cause a massive haematemesis. Management of bleeding includes endoscopic banding, sclerotherapy or use of tissue adhesives, which are often combined with a vasoactive drug such as octreotide. Use of temporary tamponade with a Sengstaken–Blakemore tube; transjugular intrahepatic portosystemic stent shunting (TIPSS); surgery, including ligation of the varices, transection of the oesophagus and various portosystemic shunts to divert blood away from the hepatic portal circulation. ⇒ Sengstaken–Blakemore tube, transjugular intrahepatic portosystemic stent shunting.

**oesophagectomy** *n* excision of part or the whole of the oesophagus.

**oesophagitis** *n* inflammation of the oesophagus.

**oesophagogastroduodenoscopy (OGD)** fibreoptic endoscopic examination of the oesophagus, stomach and duodenum. Used to obtain tissue samples and for treatments, which include banding of varices, coagulation of bleeding ulcers and dilatation of the stomach prior to the insertion of a percutaneous gastrostomy tube.

**oesophagoscope** *n* an endoscope for passage into the oesophagus—**oesophagoscopy** *n*, **oesophagoscopic** *adj*.

**oesophagostomy** *n* a surgically established fistula between the oesophagus and the skin in the root of the neck. May be used temporarily for feeding after excision of the pharynx for malignant disease.

**oesophagotomy** *n* an incision into the oesophagus.

O

**oesophagus** *n* the musculomembranous canal, around 23 cm in length in adults, extending from the pharynx to the stomach (⇒ Appendix 1, Figure 18B)—**oesophageal** *adj*.

**oestradiol (estradiol)** *n* an endogenous oestrogen secreted by the corpus luteum.

**oestriol (estriol)** *n* an endogenous oestrogen. Produced by the fetus and placenta. Oestriol levels in maternal blood or urine can be used to assess fetal well-being and placental function.

**oestrogen receptor** surface receptors expressed in some cells. The receptors are ligand-activated and regulate the cellular response to oestrogens in both sexes. ⇒ anti-oestrogens, selective (o)estrogen receptor modulators (SERMS).

**oestrogens (estrogens)** *npl* a generic term referring to a group of steroid hormones, oestradiol, oestriol and oestrone. Produced by the ovaries, placenta, testes and, in smaller amounts, the adrenal cortex in both sexes. Oestrogens are responsible for female secondary sexual characteristics and the development and proper functioning of the female genital organs. Used in the combined oral contraceptive and as hormone replacement—**oestrogenic** *adj*.

**oestrone (estrone)** *n* an endogenous oestrogen.

**OGD** *abbr* oesophagogastroduodenoscopy.

**ointment** *n* a semisolid preparation, usually greasy, for application to the skin.

**olecranon process** the large process at the upper end of the ulna; it forms the point of the elbow when the arm is flexed. *olecranon bursitis* ⇒ bursitis.

**oleic acid** an omega-9 monounsaturated fatty acid, an abundant fatty acid in olive oil.

**olfactory** *adj* pertaining to the sense of smell—**olfaction** *n* the sense of smell.

**olfactory nerve** the first pair of cranial nerves. They carry sensory impulses from the olfactory epithelium of the upper part of the nasal cavity, through the cribriform plate of the ethmoid bone to the temporal lobe of the cerebrum, where smell is perceived.

**olfactory organ** the nose. ⇒ Appendix 1, Figure 14.

**oligaemia** *n* ⇒ hypovolaemia.

**oligoclonal bands** a marker of inflammation that is found on electrophoresis of cerebrospinal fluid (CSF) in some conditions such as multiple sclerosis.

**oligodactyly** *n* a developmental absence of one or more digits (fingers or toes). There is total absence of all parts of the digit, e.g. metatarsal parts and all phalanges.

**oligodendrocyte** *n* part of the macroglia. A neuroglial cell of the central nervous system.

**oligodendroglioma** *n* a tumour of glial cells (neuroglial tissue) of the brain.

**oligodipsia** *n* diminished sense of thirst.

**oligodontia** *n* partial anodontia. A condition in which some teeth develop, but not all.

**oligohydramnios** *n* lack of amniotic fluid. The volume, which is normally around 1 L at 38 weeks' gestation, may be between 300 and 500 mL, but can be less. Oligohydramnios is associated with fetal urinary tract abnormalities such as absence of the kidneys (renal agenesis). There is less room for fetal movement and the cramped position can lead to talipes and other defects that include facial abnormalities, and dry leathery skin. Oligohydramnios may also occur in post-term pregnancies. ⇒ amniotic fluid, polyhydramnios, Potter's syndrome.

**oligomenorrhoea** *n* infrequent menstruation; the normal cycle is prolonged beyond 35 days.

**oligopeptides** *npl* peptides containing four or more amino acids, but not as many as 20.

**oligosaccharides** *npl* carbohydrates containing between 3 and 10 monosaccharide units.

**oligospermia** *n* reduction in number of spermatozoa in the semen. ⇒ azoospermia.

**oliguria** *n* reduced urine output. Usually considered to be a volume of less than 0.5 millilitres per kilogram body weight per hour (mL/kg per h)—**oliguric** *adj*.

**Ollier's dyschondrosis** (L Ollier, French surgeon, 1830–1900) a rare disorder of bone in which deposits of cartilage occur in the metaphysis (area of growing long bone between each epiphysis and the diaphysis). The cartilage remains unossified and affects the epiphyseal plate, which results in abnormal bone growth and deformity.

**omega-3 fatty acids** *npl* essential polyunsaturated fatty acids which have one of their carbon-carbon (C=C) double bonds at the third carbon atom from the omega end of the molecule. They include docosahexaenoic acid (DHA), eicosapentaenoic acid (EPA) and α-linolenic acid (ALA). Present in fish oils, flax oil, soya bean oil, eggs from certain hens, etc. ⇒ essential fatty acids.

**omega-6 fatty acids** *npl* essential polyunsaturated fatty acids which have one of their carbon-carbon (C=C) double bonds at the sixth carbon atom from the omega end of the

O

molecule. They include linoleic acid and γ-linolenic acid. Present in most vegetable and seed oils, e.g. corn oil, sunflower oil, and also present in evening primrose.

**omega-9 fatty acids** *npl* monounsaturated fatty acids which have a single carbon-carbon (C=C) double bond. They include oleic oil and erucic oil. Present in avocados, nuts, olives, olive oil, sesame oil, canola (rapeseed) oil.

**omentectomy** *n* the excision of all or part of the omentum.

**omentum** *n* a sling-like fold of peritoneum— **omental** *adj*. The functions of the omentum are support and protection, limiting infection and fat storage. *greater omentum* the fold which hangs from the lower border of the stomach and covers the front of the intestines. *lesser omentum* a smaller fold, passing between the transverse fissure of the liver and the lesser curvature of the stomach.

**Ommaya reservoir** a special reservoir implanted under the scalp used in specialist centres to administer drugs, e.g. anticancer chemotherapy, into the cerebrospinal fluid (CSF), and to obtain samples of CSF for testing. It is used in the management of some types of leukaemia, for example acute lymphoblastic. One advantage is that it avoids the need for repeated lumbar puncture.

**omophagia** *n* the consumption of uncooked or raw food.

**omphalitis** *n* inflammation of the umbilicus.

**omphalocele** *n* a congenital defect in the abdominal wall resulting from abnormal development of the abdominal muscles in the fetus. Normally the developing intestine protrudes into the umbilical cord until week 10 of gestation, when it returns to the abdominal cavity. In omphalocele this fails to happen and loops of intestine, the liver and sometimes other structures are outside the abdomen at birth. The defect is closed surgically very soon after birth. ⇒ exomphalos, hernia.

**omphalus** *n* the umbilicus.

**Onchocerca** *n* a genus of filarial worms such as *Onchocerca volvulus*.

**onchocerciasis** *n* infestation of the soft tissues, skin and eye with *Onchocerca volvulus*. Adult worms encapsulated in subcutaneous connective tissue. Larval migration to the eyes leads to partial or total visual impairment— 'river blindness'.

**oncofetal antigens** *npl* proteins normally produced during fetal development. They include alphafetoprotein (AFP), carcinoembryonic antigen (CEA) and pancreatic

oncofetal antigen (POA). The gene that produces the antigen is normally not active in adults, but may be expressed in certain cancers, such as AFP in liver cancer, or in non-malignant diseases, e.g. CEA in pancreatitis.

**oncogene** *n* a gene that may be activated by physical factors, carcinogenic chemicals, radiation or oncogenic viruses to induce cancer in the host cell.

**oncogenesis** *n* the cause and process that produce tumours, either benign or malignant.

**oncogenic** *adj* capable of tumour production. *oncogenic viruses* viruses that activate an oncogene to cause tumour formation. Examples include Epstein–Barr virus and the human papillomavirus.

**oncology** *n* the scientific study and therapy of neoplastic growths—**oncological** *adj*, **oncologically** *adv*.

**oncolysis** *n* **1.** the destruction of cancer cells and tumours. **2.** the reduction in size of a mass or swelling.

**oncotic** *adj* relating to or caused by swelling.

**oncotic pressure** also called colloid osmotic pressure. The osmotic pressure exerted by the colloids in the blood. It is vital in maintaining the fluid balance between the blood and the interstitial spaces.

**onomatomania** *n* an obsession with particular names or words.

**onset of blood lactate accumulation (OBLA)** (*syn* lactate threshold) the point during the build-up of lactic acid caused by physical activity when the blood lactate level exceeds the resting level.

**onychatrophia** *n* (*syn* anonychia) a nail that has reached mature size and then undergoes partial or total regression.

**onychauxis** *n* uniform thickening of the nail. It increases from the nail base to the free edge, and is often brownish in colour.

**onychia** *n* acute inflammation of the matrix and nail bed; suppuration may spread beneath the nail, causing it to become detached and fall off. Frequently originates from paronychia.

**onychocryptosis** *n* (*syn* ingrowing nail) occurs when a spike, shoulder or serrated edge of the nail pierces the epidermis of the sulcus and penetrates the dermal tissues, most frequently in the hallux of male adolescents. The portion of nail penetrates further into the tissues, producing acute inflammation in the surrounding soft tissues, often becoming infected (paronychia) and resulting in excess granulation tissue.

**onychogryphosis, oncogryposis** *n* (*syn* ostler's toe, ram's horn) a ridged, thickened deformity of the nails, common in older people. There is hypertrophy, and gross deformity of the nail, which develops into a curved or 'ram's horn' shape. The nail is usually dark brown or yellowish in colour, with both longitudinal and transverse ridges on its surface.

**onycholysis** *n* separation of the nail from the bed at the distal end and/or the lateral margins—**onycholytic** *adj*. It may be idiopathic or secondary to systemic and cutaneous diseases, or may result from local causes such as harsh manicuring. It is more common in fingernails than toenails and affects women more frequently than men.

**onychomadesis** *n* (*syn* onychoptosis, aplastic anonychia) the spontaneous separation of the nail, beginning at the matrix area and quickly reaching the free edge. It is often accompanied by transient arrest of nail growth, which is characterized by a Beau's line.

**onychomycosis** *n* (*syn* tinea unguium) a fungal infection of the nail bed and plate. The nail plate becomes thickened, brittle and yellowish-brown in colour. Eventually it develops a porous appearance.

**onychophosis** *n* a condition where a callus and/or a corn forms in the nail sulcus. It causes pain and inflammation.

**onychorrhexis** *n* (*syn* reed nail) a brittle nail with a series of narrow, parallel longitudinal superficial ridges.

**O'nyong-nyong fever** (*syn* joint-breaker fever) caused by a togavirus transmitted primarily by infected anopheline mosquitoes in East Africa. It is characterized by high temperature, arthritis affecting several joints with effusion, a maculopapular rash, lymphadenitis, painful red eyes and chest pain.

**oocyte** *n* an immature ovum.

**oocyte donation** 'egg' donation. Part of some assisted conception techniques in which a woman donates oocytes to another woman who cannot produce her own, such as following cytotoxic drugs for cancer, early ovarian failure, or because her oocytes have a genetic defect. The donated oocytes are fertilized in the laboratory using her partner's sperm. Some couples who are undergoing an in vitro fertilization (IVF) fertility cycle agree to donate surplus oocytes to another infertile couple who cannot produce their own.

**oogenesis** *n* the formation of oocytes ('eggs') in the ovary (Figure O.1). During fetal life primordial germ cells differentiate to become

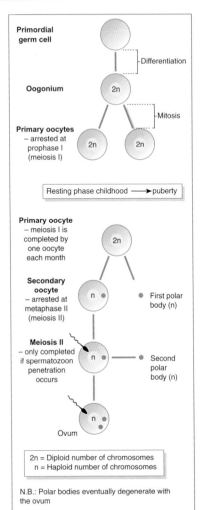

**Figure O.1** Oogenesis *(reproduced from Brooker & Nicol 2003 with permission).*

diploid stem cells called oogonia (2n). The oogonia multiply by mitotic division to form many thousands of primary oocytes (2n). Mitosis is followed by growth and the formation of primordial follicles which surround the primary

341

oocytes. At this stage the first meiotic division commences in the primary oocyte, but is arrested at prophase I. The primary oocyte now commences a variable-length resting stage before meiosis is completed, in a few hundred cells, some time during the woman's life. At puberty several primary oocytes are activated during each ovarian cycle. The arrested meiosis I (started during fetal life) is restarted in several primary oocytes but usually only one completes the process. During meiosis I the diploid primary oocyte produces two very dissimilar haploid cells: the secondary oocyte (n) and a polar body (n). The secondary oocyte is released from the surface of the ovary at ovulation. Meiosis II starts in the secondary oocyte, only to be arrested, this time in metaphase II, and will only be completed if it is penetrated by a spermatozoon. If this occurs the secondary oocyte completes meiosis II with the production of two haploid cells, a viable ovum (n) and a second polar body (n). The first and second polar bodies will eventually degenerate—**oogenetic** *adj.* ⇒ gametogenesis, spermatogenesis.

**oogonium** *n* one of the diploid precursor cells that form in the ovary during fetal development. They are derived from primordial germ cells and eventually give rise to oocytes—**oogonia** *pl.* ⇒ oogenesis.

**oophorectomy** *n* (*syn* ovariectomy, ovariotomy) excision of an ovary, such as for a cyst or cancer.

**oophoritis** *n* (*syn* ovaritis) inflammation of an ovary. It may occur with salpingitis, generalized pelvic inflammatory disease, or secondary to infections such as mumps.

**oophoron** *n* an ovary.

**oophoropexy** *n* an operation to fix an ovary in position.

**oophorosalpingectomy** *n* ⇒ salpingo-oophorectomy.

**opacity** *n* non-transparency; cloudiness; an opaque spot, as on the cornea or lens.

**open-chain exercise** ⇒ open kinetic chain.

**open fracture** also known as compound fracture. ⇒ fracture.

**open kinetic chain** in sports medicine or physiotherapy describes a motion during which the distal segment of an extremity moves freely in space, i.e. is non-weight-bearing (Figure O.2). ⇒ closed kinetic chain, kinematic chain exercises.

**operant conditioning** ⇒ conditioning.

**operating microscope** an illuminated binocular microscope enabling surgery to be carried

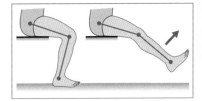

**Figure O.2** Open kinetic chain (*reproduced from Porter 2005 with permission*).

out on delicate tissues such as nerves and blood vessels, the brain and ear. Some models incorporate a beam splitter and a second set of eyepieces to enable a second person to view the operation site.

**operation** *n* surgical procedure upon a part of the body.

**operational management** the management of the day-to-day activities (operations) of an organization such as a general hospital. ⇒ strategic management.

**opercula** *npl* three areas of cerebral cortex (pars orbitalis, pars triangularis and pars basilaris), which are known collectively as the opercula of the frontal and parietal lobes. With the operculum of the temporal lobe they overlie the insula.

**operculum** *n* the plug of mucus that occludes the cervical canal during pregnancy. It protects against ascending infection. The operculum is discharged from the vagina as the 'show' of blood-stained mucus that may precede the onset of labour or once labour commences—**opercula** *pl.*

**ophthalmia** *n* (*syn* ophthalmitis) inflammation of the eye. *sympathetic ophthalmia* inflammation of one eye secondary to injury or disease of the other. Also known as sympathetic ophthalmitis.

**ophthalmia neonatorum** defined as a purulent discharge from the eyes of an infant commencing within 21 days of birth. A notifiable condition.

**ophthalmic** *adj* pertaining to the eye. *ophthalmic nerve* the first division of the trigeminal nerve. It innervates the skin of the forehead, eyelids, nose and scalp, the conjunctiva, the eyeball, the lacrimal glands, nasal septum and part of the nasal mucosa, the paranasal air sinuses and part of the dura mater (outer meningeal membrane).

**ophthalmitis** *n* ⇒ ophthalmia.

**ophthalmodynamometry** *n* an investigation used to determine the pressure of the blood in the vessels supplying the retina.

**ophthalmologist** *n* a medically qualified specialist in ophthalmology.

**ophthalmology** *n* the science that deals with the structure, function, diseases and treatment of the eye—**ophthalmological** *adj*.

**ophthalmoplegia** *n* paralysis of one or more extraocular/extrinsic muscles of the eye leading to an inability to move the eyes normally, or the internal muscles that control pupil size. Various causes include stroke, diabetes, brain tumours, trauma, multiple sclerosis, polyneuropathy, myasthenia gravis and exophthalmos associated with Graves' disease—**ophthalmoplegic** *adj*.

**ophthalmoscope** *n* an instrument for examining the interior of the eye. *direct ophthalmoscope* uses a perforated illuminated mirror to visualize eye structures directly. *indirect ophthalmoscope* forms an inverted image of the fundus of the eye using an illuminating lamp, usually worn on the examiner's head, and a convex lens, usually hand-held—**ophthalmoscopic** *adj*.

**ophthalmotomy** *n* an incision into the eyeball.

**opiate** *n* strictly speaking a drug derived from the opium poppy (*Papaver somniferum)*, which has analgesic and narcotic properties. Important alkaloids obtained from the poppy include codeine, morphine and papaverine. ⇒ opioids.

**opioids** *npl* **1.** endogenous chemicals with morphine-like effects, e.g. endorphins, enkephalins. **2.** a large group of exogenous substances that have morphine-like effects, which can be reversed by opioid receptor antagonists such as naloxone. Side-effects include constipation, dry mouth, nausea and vomiting, drowsiness and respiratory depression. They include the opiates, semisynthetic morphine analogues and synthetic analogues. This list includes alfentanil, buprenorphine (agonist and antagonist actions), codeine, dextropropoxyphene, diamorphine (heroin), dihydrocodeine, fentanyl, methadone, morphine sulphate, naloxone (an antagonist), pentazocine, pethidine. ⇒ opiate, Appendix 5.

**opisthorchiasis** *n* infestation with one of the species of *Opisthorchis* trematode liver flukes. It infests the liver and biliary tract and can lead to inflammation and cholangiocarcinoma (cancer of the gallbladder and/or bile ducts), which is an usual cancer. The fluke, which is common in South-East Asia, is associated with eating raw or inadequately cooked fish.

**Opisthorchis** *n* a genus of trematode liver flukes; it includes the species *Opisthorchis felineus* and *O. viverrini*.

**opisthotonos** *n* extreme extension of the body, occurring in tetanic spasm. In extreme cases the patient may be resting on heels and head alone—**opisthotonic** *adj*.

**opium** *n* the dried juice of the opium poppy (*Papaver somniferum)*. It contains morphine and other related alkaloids. ⇒ opiate, opioids.

**opportunistic infection** ⇒ infection.

**opportunity cost** when a resource is used in a particular way, the opportunity to use it for another purpose is lost. This includes money, time and the activities which cannot be undertaken. An example in health care would be the decision to use money for an expensive cancer drug leading to a lost opportunity to spend the money for another service such as cataract surgery.

**opposition** *n* describes the position of the thumb and fingers when objects are picked up or grasped between thumb and fingers.

**oppositional defiant disorder (ODD)** a pattern of behaviour lasting longer than 6 months in which the child is abnormally defiant, hostile and disobedient to parents and other people in authority. The features include temper tantrums, argumentative, negativism, spiteful behaviour, anger, blaming others, vindictiveness, difficulty in making or keeping friends.

**opsoclonus** *n* rapid, erratic movements of the eyeballs in several different directions. It may occur with neurological disorders.

**opsomania** *n* intense desire to consume special foodstuffs.

**opsins** *npl* protein part of visual pigments, which combine with retinal in the cones and rods of the retina. Found in the cones as iodopsins and in the rods as rhodopsin (visual). There are three iodopsins in different types of cones; they form the pigments known as chlorolabe, cyanolabe and erythrolabe.

**opsonic index** a measurement that indicates the ability of phagocytes to ingest foreign bodies such as bacteria.

**opsonin** *n* complement protein or an antibody which coats an antigen. ⇒ opsoninization—**opsonic** *adj*.

**opsonization** *n* a process where antigens are coated with opsonins, thereby increasing their susceptibility to phagocytosis.

**optic** *adj* pertaining to sight.

**optic atrophy** pathological whitening of the optic nerve head with loss of nerve axons.

O

**optic chiasma** the meeting of the two optic nerves; where the fibres from the medial or nasal half of each retina (supplying half the visual field in either eye) cross the middle line to join the optic tract of the opposite side (Figure O.3). ⇒ chiasma.

**optic disc** the point on the retina at which the optic nerve leaves the eyeball. There are no light-sensitive receptors at this point and it is called the blind spot ⇒ Appendix 1, Figure 15.

**optic foramen** one of two openings in the sphenoid bone that give passage to the optic nerve and the ophthalmic artery.

**optic nerves** second pair of cranial nerves. They convey impulses from the rods and cones in the retina to the visual area of the cerebral cortex in the occipital lobes of the cerebral hemispheres. ⇒ Figure O.3 and Appendix 1, Figure 15.

**optic neuritis** also called retrobulbar neuritis. Inflammation, swelling and/or demyelination affecting an optic nerve. It leads to loss of vision; it may be an early and sometimes the single sign of multiple sclerosis. Other causes include infection, vasculitis and autoimmune disorders.

**optic neuropathy** disease of the optic nerve resulting in destruction of the nerve or loss of function. Causes include lack of blood supply caused by compression or an aneurysm; toxic chemicals such as methanol; and brain/head injury.

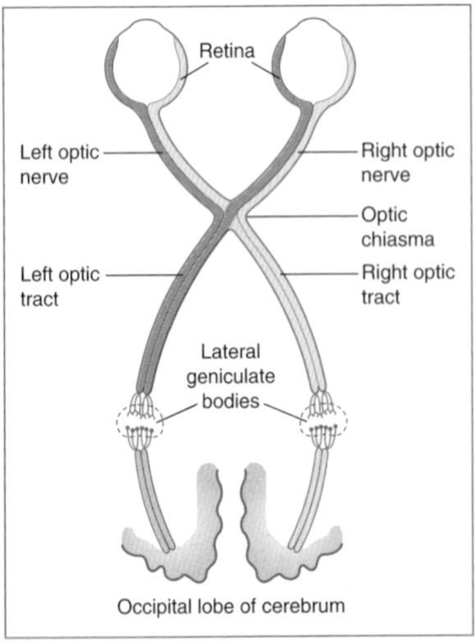

**optical** *adj* relating to sight. *optical aberration* any imperfection in the focus of light rays by a lens. *optical density* the light absorbed by a solution. Can be used to determine substance concentration.

**optician** *n* a person qualified and registered to make and fit spectacles/contact lenses (dispensing optician), or test visual acuity, prescribe and dispense spectacles or contact lenses (ophthalmic optician, now known as optometrist) to correct refractive errors. ⇒ optometrist.

**opticokinetic** *adj* also called optokinetic. Relating to the movement of the eyes in response to objects moving in the visual field.

**optics** *n* the scientific study of the properties of light.

**optimum** *adj* most favourable. *optimum position* that which will be most useful and cause the least problems should a limb remain permanently paralysed, such as following a stroke.

**optometer** *n* ⇒ refractometer.

**optometrist** *n* previously known as ophthalmic optician. A person qualified and registered to practise optometry. They are involved in primary health eye care, eye examination, testing visual acuity and early disease detection, optical dispensing and fitting of contact lenses.

**optometry** *n* the study of visual sciences and the management of human eye optics. ⇒ optometrist.

**oral** *adj* pertaining to the mouth—**orally** *adv*.

**oral contraceptive** commonly referred to as 'the pill'. *combined oral contraceptive* contains varying amounts of the two hormones, oestrogen and progestogen. ⇒ contraceptive, progestogen-only pill.

**oral medicine** branch of dentistry concerned with the management of diseases of the oral mucosa and related structures, including oral manifestations of systemic diseases.

**oral rehydration solution (ORS)** an oral solution for the replacement of fluids and electrolytes lost in diarrhoea. The World Health Organization (WHO) advocates a single solution, which is used flexibly depending on the specific situation. The WHO solution contains more sodium than the one used in the UK, but both provide sodium, potassium, chloride, citrate and glucose.

**oral rehydration therapy (ORT)** administration of oral rehydration solution by mouth to correct dehydration.

**Figure O.3** Optic chiasma *(reproduced from Brooker 2006A with permission).*

**oral surgery** branch of dentistry concerned with minor surgery to the teeth and jaws.

**orbicular** *adj* resembling a globe; spherical or circular.

**orbicularis** *n* a muscle that encircles an orifice. *orbicularis oculi* the muscle around the eyeball, eyelid and the orbit. It contracts to close the eye and when necessary contracts strongly to 'screw' the eyes shut, such as in very bright sunlight. *orbicularis oris* the muscle around the mouth. It shuts the lips and allows activities that include whistling.

**orbit** *n* the bony socket containing the eyeball and its appendages. It is formed from parts of the sphenoid, frontal, zygomatic, maxilla, orbital plate of the ethmoid, lacrimal and palatine bones—**orbital** *adj*.

**orchidalgia** *n* pain felt in a testis. The pain may arise from testicular problems such as inflammation (orchitis) or torsion, but may be caused by a hernia or associated with renal colic.

**orchidectomy** *n* excision of a testis, such as following injury or to remove a cancer.

**orchidometer** *n* an instrument for assessing the volume of a testis. *Prader orchidometer* (A Prader, Swiss paediatrician/endocrinologist, 1919–2001) a series of beads of different volumes (1 to 25 mL) used as a comparison for assessing the volume of the patient's testes. Provides information about testicular growth and development, onset of puberty, reasons for early puberty, hypogonadism or abnormally large testes.

**orchidopexy** *n* surgical procedure of bringing an undescended testis into its correct location in the scrotum, and fixing it in this position.

**orchiotomy** *n* an incision into a testis.

**orchis** *n* the testis.

**orchitis** *n* inflammation of a testis usually caused by a viral infection, particularly mumps. The testes are swollen and painful and the patient has a fever. Orchitis may occur with inflammation of the epididymis (epididymo-orchitis).

**ordinal data** categorical data that can be ordered or ranked, e.g. general condition—good, fair or bad—or size in general terms, as in 'smaller than'. ⇒ nominal data.

**orexigenic** *adj* stimulating or increasing appetite.

**orexins** *npl* also known as hypocretin. Two excitatory neuropeptides produced by nerve cells in the hypothalamus. With other substances, they function in the regulation of wakefulness and appetite. ⇒ hypocretin.

**orf** *n* purulent skin lesions caused by a type of poxvirus normally affecting sheep and goats.

**organ** *n* an assembly of different tissues to form a distinct functional unit, e.g. liver, uterus, able to perform specialized functions. Organs may be hollow, such as the stomach, or compact, e.g. liver.

**organelle** *n* subcellular structures, such as mitochondria, the endoplasmic reticulum and the Golgi apparatus, which perform specialized functions in the cell.

**organic** *adj* pertaining to an organ. Associated with life. *organic brain syndrome* ⇒ dementia.

**organic compounds** chemical compounds containing carbon and hydrogen in their structure, e.g. glucose. They include the large biological molecules (macromolecules), such as lipids and proteins.

**organic disease** one in which there is structural change.

**organism** *n* a living cell or group of cells differentiated into functionally distinct parts which are interdependent.

**organ of Corti** (A Corti, Italian anatomist, 1822–1888) the spiral organ sited in the cochlea of the inner ear, it contains the auditory receptors (hair cells) which convert sound vibrations to nerve impulses. The nerve impulses are transmitted to the brain via the cochlear branch of the vestibulocochlear nerve.

**organogenesis** *n* the process whereby the body organs develop from embryonic tissue. It commences at about 2 weeks' gestation and is complete by week 8. The developing embryo is particularly vulnerable during this period to factors such as micro-organisms, e.g. rubella virus, that can seriously disrupt organ development.

**organophosphorus compounds** several highly toxic anticholinesterase compounds usually used as commercial insecticides. They cause irreversible inhibition of cholinesterase.

**orgasm** *n* the climax of sexual excitement.

**oriental sore** (*syn* Delhi boil) a form of cutaneous leishmaniasis producing papular, crusted, granulomatous skin eruptions. Occurs in tropical and subtropical regions (Old World).

**orientation** *n* clear awareness of one's position relative to the environment. In mental conditions orientation 'to people, space and time' means that the patient knows who people are, where he or she is and is aware of the passage of time, i.e. can give the correct date. Disorientation means the reverse. ⇒ delirium, dementia, reality orientation.

**orifice** *n* a mouth or opening.

O

**origin** *n* the commencement or source of anything. *origin of a muscle* the end that remains relatively fixed during contraction of the muscle.

**ornithine** *n* an amino acid, produced from arginine during the urea cycle.

**ornithine cycle** ⇒ urea cycle.

*Ornithodoros n* a genus of ticks; some act as vectors for the bacteria causing relapsing fevers.

**ornithosis** *n* human illness resulting from disease of birds. ⇒ *Chlamydia*, psittacosis.

**orogenital** *adj* pertaining to the mouth and the external genital area.

**oropharyngeal** *adj* pertaining to the mouth and pharynx, or to the oropharynx. ⇒ airway.

**oropharynx** *n* that portion of the pharynx which is below the level of the soft palate and above the level of the hyoid bone. The palatine tonsils are present in folds on the lateral walls. Air, food and fluid pass through the oropharynx. ⇒ fauces, Waldeyer's ring.

**orotic acid** intermediate substance formed during the synthesis of pyrimidines.

**Oroya fever** ⇒ bartonellosis.

**ORS** *abbr* oral rehydration solution.

**ORT** *abbr* oral rehydration therapy.

**orthodontic device** *n* device used to move teeth by the controlled application of force. May be removable, myofunctional (functional) or fixed.

**orthodontics** *n* a branch of dentistry concerned with the prevention and correction of irregularities and malocclusion of the teeth.

**orthodontist** *n* a dentist with specialist qualifications who diagnoses, prevents and treats malocclusion and other dental irregularities.

**orthodox sleep** *n* (*syn* non-rapid eye movement [NREM] sleep) ⇒ sleep.

**orthognathic surgery** *n* surgery aimed at correcting abnormalities in position of the jaw to improve function and appearance.

**orthomyxovirus** *n* a family of RNA viruses that cause influenza in humans.

**orthopaedics** *n* formerly a specialty devoted to the correction of deformities in children. It is now a branch of surgery dealing with all conditions affecting the locomotor system.

**orthopnoea** *n* breathlessness that occurs when the person lies flat. It occurs because this position results in the redistribution of blood, leading to an increased central and pulmonary blood volume and fluid accumulation in the lungs—**orthopnoeic** *adj*.

**orthoptics** *n* the study and treatment of eye movement disorders.

**orthoptist** *n* one who specializes in the assessment and treatment of eye movement disorders.

**orthoptoscope** *n* ⇒ amblyoscope.

**orthosis** *n* external device utilized to correct, control or counteract the effect of an actual or developing deformity. They include braces, callipers and splints. ⇒ night splint, prosthesis—**orthoses** *pl*, **orthotic** *adj*.

**orthostatic** *adj* caused by the upright stance. *orthostatic albuminuria* occurs in some healthy subjects only when they stand upright.

**orthotics** *n* the scientific study and manufacture of devices which can be applied to or around the body in the care of physical impairment or disability. ⇒ prosthesis.

**orthotist** *n* a person who practises orthotics.

**orthotopic transplant** ⇒ transplant.

**orthotopic bladder substitution** surgical technique of bladder reconstruction using the site of the excised native bladder with an anastomosis to the native urethra.

**Ortolani's sign/test** (M Ortolanli, Italian surgeon, 20th century) a test performed shortly after birth for the diagnosis of developmental dysplasia of the hip (congenital dislocation of the hip). It should always be undertaken by an experienced clinician. Often used in conjunction with Barlow's sign/test. ⇒ developmental dysplasia of the hip.

**os** *n* a mouth. *external os* the opening of the cervix into the vagina (⇒ Appendix 1, Figure 17). *internal os* the opening of the cervix into the uterine cavity—**ora** *pl*.

**OSAS** *abbr* obstructive sleep apnoea (hypopnoea) syndrome.

**OSAHS** *abbr* obstructive sleep apnoea hypopnoea syndrome.

**oscillometry** *n* measurement of vibration, using a special device (oscillometer).

**oscilloscope** *n* a device that uses a fluorescent screen to display various electrical waveforms such as that produced by the heart.

**Osgood–Schlatter disease** (R Osgood, American surgeon, 1873–1956; C Schlatter, Swiss surgeon, 1864–1934). ⇒ Schlatter's disease.

**Osler's nodes** (W Osler, Canadian/British physician, 1849–1919) small painful areas in pulp of fingers or toes, or palms and soles, caused by emboli. Occurs in infective endocarditis.

**osmolality** *n* the number of osmoles per kilogram of solution. An expression of osmotic pressure.

O

**osmolarity** *n* the osmotic pressure exerted by a given concentration of osmotically active solute in aqueous solution, defined in terms of the number of active particles per unit volume (osmoles or milliosmoles per litre).

**osmole** *n* the standard unit of osmotic pressure which is equal to the gram molecular weight of a solute divided by the number of particles or ions into which it dissociates in solution.

**osmophiles** *npl* micro-organisms that can thrive in a high-osmotic-pressure environment, e.g. in jam, honey or pickles; the mould (yeasts) found on the surface of homemade jam.

**osmoreceptors** *npl* specialized neurons in the hypothalamus that respond to the osmotic pressure, i.e. the relative concentration of water and solutes, of blood and extracellular fluid. They deal with changes through thirst mechanisms and the amount of antidiuretic hormone (vasopressin, or arginine vasopressin [AVP]) released.

**osmosis** *n* the passage of pure solvent across a semipermeable membrane under the influence of osmotic pressure. It is the movement of a dilute solution into a more concentrated solution. ⇒ active transport, diffusion, filtration.

**osmotic diuretics** inert substances such as mannitol that exert a diuretic effect. They cause an osmotic 'pull' as they are excreted by the kidney where they are filtered but not reabsorbed. ⇒ Appendix 5.

**osmotic laxatives** ⇒ laxatives. ⇒ Appendix 5.

**osmotic pressure** the pressure with which solvent molecules are drawn across a semipermeable membrane separating different concentrations of solute (such as sugars) dissolved in the same solvent, when the membrane is permeable to the solvent but impermeable to the solute.

**osseointegration** *n* the growth in bone, as it integrates with biocompatible materials, such as titanium, to form a strong and secure anchor for a dental implant or a prosthesis such as a bone-anchored hearing aid.

**osseous** *adj* relating to or resembling bone.

**ossicles** *npl* small bones, particularly those within the tympanic cavity of the middle ear; the malleus, incus and stapes. ⇒ Appendix 1, Figure 13.

**ossification** *n* the conversion of cartilage, etc. into bone. Also known as osteogenesis—**ossify** *vt, vi*.

**osteitis** *n* inflammation of bone. *osteitis deformans* ⇒ Paget's disease.

**osteitis fibrosa** cavities form in the interior of bone. The cysts may be solitary or the disease may be generalized. This second condition may be the result of excessive parathyroid gland secretion and absorption of calcium from bone.

**osteoarthritis** *n* sometimes termed degenerative arthritis, although the disease process is much more than simply 'wear and tear'; may be primary, or may follow injury or disease involving the articular surfaces of synovial joints. The articular cartilage becomes worn, osteophytes form at the periphery of the joint surface and loose bodies may result. ⇒ arthropathy—**osteoarthritic** *adj*.

**osteoarthrosis** *n* ⇒ osteoarthritis.

**osteoblast** *n* a bone-forming cell derived from embryonic mesenchyme. It produces the materials required for the osteoid matrix—**osteoblastic** *adj*.

**osteocalcin** *n* a protein required for the mineralization of bone.

**osteochondritis** *n* originally an inflammation of bone cartilage. Usually applied to non-septic conditions, especially avascular necrosis involving joint surfaces, e.g. *osteochondritis dissecans*, in which a portion of joint surface may separate to form a loose body in the joint. ⇒ Legg–Calvé–Perthes disease, Köhler's disease, Scheuermann's disease, Schlatter's disease, Sever's disease.

**osteochondroma** *n* a benign bony and cartilaginous tumour.

**osteochondrosis** *n* an idiopathic disease characterized by a disorder of the ossification of hyaline cartilage (endochondral). It encompasses a group of syndromes classified on the basis of their anatomical location. **1.** primary articular epiphysis—Freiberg's disease and Köhler's disease. **2.** secondary articular epiphysis—osteochondritis dissecans of the talus. **3.** non-articular epiphysis (apophyseal injury)— Sever's disease. The osteochondroses occur during the years of rapid growth. Aetiology has been linked to hereditary factors, trauma, nutritional factors and ischaemia. The articular osteochondroses such as Freiberg's, Köhler's and osteochondritis dissecans are characterized by fragmentation with a centre of ossification.

**osteoclasis** *n* the therapeutic fracture of a bone.

**osteoclast** *n* **1.** a large multinucleated bone cell that resorbs bone. **2.** an instrument used for osteoclasis (therapeutic fracture).

**osteoclastoma** *n* a tumour of the osteoclasts. May be benign, locally recurrent or frankly malignant. The usual site is near the end of a long bone.

**O**

347

**osteocyte** *n* a bone cell, a mature osteoblast.

**osteodystrophy** *n* any generalized faulty growth of bone, usually caused by abnormal metabolism of calcium and phosphorus. It occurs in chronic renal failure—renal osteodystrophy.

**osteogenesis** *n* bone formation. ⇒ ossification.

**osteogenesis imperfecta** a hereditary disorder usually caused by an autosomal dominant gene. It may be present at birth or develop during childhood. The congenital form is much more severe and may lead to early death. The bones are extremely fragile and may fracture following minimal trauma.

**osteogenic** *adj* bone-producing.

**osteogenic sarcoma** *n* malignant tumour that originates from bone-producing cells.

**osteology** *n* the scientific study of the development, structure and function of bones and associated structures.

**osteolysis** *n* pathological dissolution of bone, such as following infection or where the blood supply is impaired.

**osteolytic** *adj* destructive of bone, e.g. osteolytic malignant deposits in bone.

**osteoma** *n* a benign tumour of bone which may arise in the compact tissue (*ivory osteoma*) or in the cancellous tissue. May be single or multiple.

**osteomalacia** *n* demineralization of the mature skeleton, with softening and bone pain. It is commonly caused by insufficient dietary intake of vitamin D or lack of sunshine, or both.

**osteomyelitis** *n* inflammation commencing in the marrow of bone—**osteomyelitic** *adj*.

**osteon** *n* a haversian system, the basic structural unit of bone (see Figure B.6, p. 66).

**osteopath** *n* a person qualified and registered to practise osteopathy.

**osteopathy** *n* an established clinical discipline. It is concerned with the inter-relationship between structure and function of the body. Osteopathy may be effective for the relief or improvement of a wide variety of conditions, e.g. digestive disorders, as well as mechanical problems. Osteopathy is subject to statutory self-regulation and registration on a par with more established health care professions such as medicine—**osteopathic** *adj*.

**osteopenia** *n* decrease in the mineralization of bone or bone density.

**osteopetrosis** *n* (*syn* Albers–Schönberg disease, marble bones) a congenital abnormality giving rise to very dense bones which fracture easily.

**osteophyte** *n* a bony outgrowth or spur, usually at the margins of joint surfaces, e.g. in osteoarthritis—**osteophytic** *adj*.

**osteoplasty** *n* reconstructive operation on bone—**osteoplastic** *adj*.

**osteoporosis** *n* loss of bone density caused by excessive absorption of calcium and phosphorus from the bone, due to progressive loss of the protein matrix of bone which normally carries the calcium deposits. Associated with ageing in both men and women. Common cause of fractures, particularly fractures of the wrist, crush fractures of the spine and neck of femur fractures—**osteoporotic** *adj*.

**osteosarcoma/osteogenic sarcoma** *n* a malignant tumour growing from bone cells (osteoblasts)—**osteosarcomata** *pl*, **osteosarcomatous** *adj*.

**osteosclerosis** *n* increased density or hardness of bone—**osteosclerotic** *adj*.

**osteotome** *n* an instrument for cutting bone; it is similar to a chisel, but it is bevelled on both sides of its cutting edge.

**osteotomy** *n* division of bone followed by realignment of the ends to encourage union by healing. ⇒ McMurray's osteotomy.

**ostium** *n* the opening or mouth of any tubular structure—**ostia** *pl*, **ostial** *adj*.

**OT** *abbr* occupational therapy/therapist.

**otalgia** *n* earache.

**otalgia dentalis** *n* pain felt in the ear; caused by dental disease.

**OTC** *abbr* over-the-counter (medicines).

**otic** *adj* relating to the ear.

**otitis** *n* inflammation of the ear. *otitis externa* inflammation of the skin of the external auditory meatus/canal. *otitis media* inflammation of the middle-ear cavity. The effusion can be serous, mucoid or purulent. Non-purulent effusions in children are often called glue ear. ⇒ acute suppurative otitis media, chronic suppurative otitis media, grommet.

**otoacoustic emission (OAE) testing** a computer-linked hearing test used for screening babies soon after birth. It depends on the sound normally emitted by the outer hair cells of the inner ear. A microphone placed in the external auditory meatus/canal picks up the emissions. Used to determine whether the inner ear is functioning. ⇒ neonatal hearing screening.

**otolaryngology** *n* ⇒ otorhinolaryngology.

**otoliths** *npl* tiny calcareous (calcium) deposits within the utricle and saccule of the inner ear.

**otologist** *n* a person who specializes in otology.

**otology** *n* the science which deals with structure, function and disorders of the ear.

**otomycosis** *n* a fungal (e.g. *Aspergillus, Candida*) infection of the external auditory meatus/canal—**otomycotic** *adj*.

**otoplasty** *n* plastic operation to correct ear deformities.

**otorhinolaryngology** *n* the science that deals with the structure, function and disorders of the ear, nose and throat; each of these three may be considered a specialty. ⇒ laryngology, otology, rhinology.

**otorrhoea** *n* a discharge from the ear. It may be serous, sanguineous (bloody) or purulent. The discharge may be crystal-clear cerebrospinal fluid; this can occur in fractures of the base of skull.

**otosclerosis** *n* abnormal bone formation affecting primarily the footplate of the stapes. A common cause of progressive conductive deafness—**otosclerotic** *adj*.

**otoscope** *n* an instrument for examining the ear, usually incorporating both magnification and illumination. Also called an auriscope.

**ototoxic** *adj* having a toxic action on the ear. For example, the aminoglycosides, antibiotics (e.g. gentamicin), platinum-based chemotherapy (e.g. cisplatin), and aspirin.

**outcome measures** scales developed to measure health outcome from clinical interventions: generic measures encompassing dimensions of physical, mental and social health; disease-specific scales detecting the effects of treatment of specific conditions. ⇒ quality-adjusted life years.

**outer ear** also known as external ear. Comprises the auricle and the external auditory meatus/canal. ⇒ ear.

**ova** *npl* the female gametes (reproductive cells). More correctly known as a secondary oocyte until penetration by a spermatozoon—**ovum** *sing*.

**oval window** fenestra ovalis. The oval opening between the middle and inner ear. The stapes vibrates in it to transmit sound waves to the inner ear.

**ovarian** *adj* relating to the ovaries.

**ovarian cancer** a common gynaecological cancer: many women present with advanced disease. Predominantly occurs in older postmenopausal women. Risk factors include childlessness, genetic factors and late menopause. Carcinomas are the most common type and the International Federation of Gynecologists and Obstetricians (FIGO) has provided a classification of the stages of ovarian cancer linked to the locality and extent of the disease. Symptoms are often vague, but can include abnormal vaginal bleeding, gastrointestinal symptoms, distended abdomen, pressure symptoms, such as urinary frequency and ascites in advanced disease. Surgery involves removal of the uterus, both tubes and ovaries, part of the omentum and biopsies to ascertain the degree of spread. Chemotherapy is used after surgery, e.g. platinum-based carboplatin alone or with paclitaxel.

**ovarian cycle** the changes occurring in the ovary during the development of the follicle and oogenesis. It has two phases: follicular (days 1–14), when ovulation occurs, and luteal (days 15–28), when the corpus luteum develops. The cycle is controlled by follicle-stimulating hormone and luteinizing hormone.

**ovarian cyst** a tumour of the ovary, usually containing fluid—may be benign or malignant.

**ovarian hyperstimulation syndrome** a side-effect associated with the use of gonadotrophins during an in vitro fertilization (IVF) cycle. Milder cases are characterized by enlargement of the ovaries, gastrointestinal symptoms, abdominal pain and weight gain. In more severe cases it is associated with fluid and electrolyte imbalance, ascites, pleural effusion, hypovolaemia, coagulation disorders and impaired renal function.

**ovariectomy** *n* ⇒ oophorectomy.

**ovariotomy** *n* ⇒ oophorectomy.

**ovaritis** *n* ⇒ oophoritis.

**ovary** *n* a female gonad. One of two small oval bodies situated on either side of the uterus on the posterior surface of the broad ligament (⇒ Appendix 1, Figure 17). Controlled by pituitary hormones, they produce oocytes and oestrogen and progesterones—**ovarian** *adj*. *polycystic ovaries* ⇒ polycystic ovary syndrome.

**overbite** *n* a bite in which the upper teeth vertically overlap the lower teeth.

**overcompensation** *n* a term that describes any type of behaviour which a person adopts in order to disguise a deficiency. Thus a person who is afraid may react by becoming arrogant or boastful or aggressive.

**overheads** *npl* the cost of services that contribute to the general upkeep and running of the organization, e.g. grounds maintenance, that cannot be linked directly to the core activity of a department.

**overload principle** the use of physiological overload in order to produce physiological improvements, i.e. when an individual physically demands more of the muscles than is normally required.

O

**over-the-counter (OTC) medicines** describes those medicines on sale to the public without a prescription. ⇒ general sales list, pharmacy-only medicine.

**overuse injury** an injury that is caused by excessive repetitive movement of a body part. Often occurs following periods of inadequate rest or recovery, overactivity or repetitive overloading of a part or structure.

**overuse syndrome** injury caused by accumulated microtraumatic stress placed on a structure or body area.

**oviduct** *n* uterine or fallopian tubes.

**ovulation** *n* the maturation and rupture of a Graafian follicle with the discharge of an oocyte.

**ovum** *n* **1.** an egg. **2.** a female gamete. ⇒ ova.

**oxalic acid** toxic organic acid found in plants, e.g. rhubarb leaves.

**oxalosis** *n* a condition in which crystals of calcium oxalates are deposited in the kidney and in other organs.

**oxaluria** *n* excretion of oxalates (salts of oxalic acid) in the urine.

**oxazolidones** *npl* a class of antibacterial drugs, e.g. linezolid, which can be used to treat infections caused by meticillin (methicillin)-resistant *Staphylococcus aureus* (MRSA) and vancomycin-resistant enterococci (VRE).

**oxicams** *npl* a group of non-steroidal anti-inflammatory drugs. ⇒ Appendix 5.

**oxidase (oxygenases)** *n* any enzyme that catalyses biological oxidation reactions.

**oxidation** *n* the act of oxidizing or state of being oxidized. It involves the addition of oxygen, e.g. formation of oxides, or the loss of electrons or the removal of hydrogen. A part of metabolism, whereby energy is released from fuel molecules. ⇒ reduction.

**oxidative phosphorylation** a mitochondrial energy-producing metabolic process, whereby adenosine diphosphate (ADP) is converted to adenosine triphosphate (ATP) by the addition of a phosphate group.

**oxidoreductase** *n* an enzyme that catalyses a reaction in which one substance is oxidized and another is reduced (e.g. dehydrogenases).

**oximetry** *n* ⇒ pulse oximeter.

**oxygen (O)** *n* a colourless, odourless, gaseous element, necessary for life and combustion. Constitutes 20% of atmospheric air. Used therapeutically as an inhalation to increase blood oxygenation. Delivered as part of a general anaesthetic to maintain life. ⇒ hyperbaric oxygen therapy. *oxygen concentrator* a device

for removing nitrogen from the air to provide a high concentration of oxygen for use by patients with chronic respiratory diseases requiring at least 15 hours of oxygen therapy each day at home. ⇒ long-term oxygen therapy.

**oxygenation** *n* the saturation of a substance (particularly blood) with oxygen. Arterial oxygen tension ($PaO_2$) indicates degree of oxgygenation (normally more than 97% saturated)—**oxygenated** *adj.* ⇒ pulse oximeter.

**oxygenator** *n* apparatus used to oxygenate the patient's blood during open-heart surgery, or to support critically ill patients. ⇒ cardiopulmonary bypass, extracorporeal membrane oxygenator.

**oxygen consumption/uptake ($VO_2$)** amount of oxygen consumed by the body per minute, typically 250 mL/min. ⇒ peak oxygen consumption/uptake.

**oxygen debt/deficit** (*syn* excess postexercise oxygen consumption, oxygen recovery) the total amount of oxygen needed to replace adenosine triphosphate (ATP), restore creatine phosphate (phosphocreatine) and remove lactic acid in active tissue during the recovery process following exercise. ⇒ alactacid oxygen debt component, lactacid oxygen debt component.

**oxygen delivery ($DO_2$)** amount of oxygen delivered to the tissues per minute; product of cardiac output and arterial oxygen content, typically 1000 mL/min.

**oxygen dissociation curve** sigmoid-shaped curve showing the different affinity each haem group of the haemoglobin molecule has for oxygen. It indicates the ease with which the oxygen dissociates and the haem groups give up the oxygen to the tissues. This also depends on temperature, pH and carbon dioxide tension (Figure O.4). ⇒ Bohr effect.

**oxygen saturation** percentage of oxygenated haemoglobin present in the blood. ⇒ pulse oximeter.

**oxyhaemoglobin** *n* oxygenated haemoglobin, an unstable compound formed from haemoglobin on contact with air in the alveoli.

**oxyntic** *adj* producing acid. *oxyntic cells* the cells in the gastric mucosa which produce hydrochloric acid. Also known as parietal cells.

**oxyntomodulin** *n* a form of enteroglucagon.

**oxytocic** *adj, n* hastening parturition; an agent that stimulates uterine contractions. ⇒ Appendix 5.

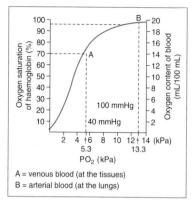

A = venous blood (at the tissues)
B = arterial blood (at the lungs)

**Figure O.4** Oxygen dissociation curve (at 37°C, pH 7.4, Hb 15 g/dL) *(reproduced from Brooker 2006A with permission).*

**oxytocin** *n* a hormone released from the posterior pituitary. It contracts the uterine muscle and milk ducts and is involved in reflex milk ejection.

**oxyuriasis** *n* ⇒ enterobiasis.

***Oxyuris*** *n* ⇒ *Enterobius*.

**ozaena** *n* atrophic rhinitis.

**ozone** *n* a form of oxygen. $O_3$. Has powerful oxidizing properties and is therefore antiseptic and disinfectant. It is both irritating and toxic to the pulmonary system.

O

# P

³²P *abbr* radioactive isotope of phosphorus.

**P₄₅₀ enzymes** *npl* the cytochrome P₄₅₀ proteins that include an important group of drug-metabolizing enzymes and those that metabolize some endogenous substances, for example thromboxanes, prostacyclins, cholesterol and vitamins A and D. ⇒ cytochromes.

**PA** *abbr* pernicious anaemia.

**pacchionian granulations/bodies** (A Pacchioni, Italian anatomist, 1665–1720) the arachnoid villi/granulations through which cerebrospinal fluid returns to the blood. ⇒ cerebrospinal fluid.

**pacemaker** *n* the region of the heart that initiates atrial contraction and thus controls heart rate. The natural pacemaker is the sinus node (sinoatrial node) which is situated at the junction of the superior vena cava and the right atrium; the wave of contraction begins here, then spreads over the heart. *artificial pacemaker* ⇒ cardiac pacemaker.

**pachycheilia** *n* abnormally thick or swollen lips.

**pachydactyly** *n* abnormally thickened fingers and toes.

**pachyderma** *n* thick skin. ⇒ elephantiasis.

**pachyglossia** *n* abnormally thickened tongue.

**pachymeningitis** *n* inflammation of the dura mater, the outer meningeal membrane.

**pachymeninx** *n* dura mater.

**pachyonychia congenita** a congenital condition in which the nails are very thick with thickening of the skin on the palms and soles.

**pacing** *n* compensatory techniques used by occupational therapists that enable an individual to perform activities of daily living in a planned, balanced, continuous manner by strictly adhering to measurable, personal goals. It involves the use of activity analysis, timing, resting and alternating movements in order to maximize optimal performance and minimize pain, stress and fatigue by expending effort consistently over a period of time.

**pacinian corpuscles** (F Pacini, Italian anatomist, 1812–1883) deep-pressure sensory receptors in the skin.

**packed cell volume (PCV)** volume of red cells (erythrocytes) in the blood, expressed as a percentage of the total blood volume. Also called the haematocrit.

**PaCO₂** *abbr* the partial pressure or tension of carbon dioxide in arterial blood.

**PACO₂** *abbr* the partial pressure or tension of carbon dioxide in alveolar air.

**PACS** *abbr* picture archiving communication system.

**PADL** *abbr* personal activities of daily living.

**paediatric advanced life support (PALS)** ⇒ advanced life support (ALS).

**paediatric basic life support** the basic life support measures used for children from 1 year of age until puberty. Artificial respiration, usually by rescue breaths (mouth-to-mouth/nose breathing) and chest compressions (external cardiac massage) to save life without the use of artificial aids or equipment in the case of cardiac or respiratory arrest. ⊙ DVD

**paediatrician** *n* a doctor who is a specialist in children's diseases.

**paediatrics** *n* the branch of medicine dealing with children and their diseases—**paediatric** *adj*.

**paedophilia** *n* the sexual attraction to children.

**PAFC** *abbr* pulmonary artery flotation catheter.

**Paget's disease** (J Paget, British surgeon, 1814–1899) **1.** (*syn* osteitis deformans) excess of the enzyme alkaline phosphatase causes too rapid bone formation; consequently bone is thin. There is loss of stature, crippling deformity, enlarged head and collapse of vertebrae, and neurological complications can result. Sufferers are particularly susceptible to sarcoma of bone. If the vestibulocochlear (auditory) nerve is involved, there is impairment of hearing. Calcitonin is the drug of choice. **2.** erosion of the nipple caused by invasion of the dermis by intraduct carcinoma of the breast.

**Paget–Schröetter syndrome** (J Paget; L von Schröetter, Austrian laryngologist/physician, 1837–1908) axillary or subclavian vein thrombosis, often associated with effort in fit young persons.

**pain** *n* unpleasant sensation experienced when nociceptors are stimulated. It is individual and subjective with a physiological, emotional and social component. Pain ranges from mild to agonizing, but individual responses are influenced by factors which include: information about cause, age, whether acute or chronic and pain tolerance. ⇒ acute pain, chronic pain, neuropathic pain, nociceptive pain, phantom-limb pain, referred pain.

**pain management** involves a holistic multidisciplinary approach, and in many health care settings there is a designated pain team or nurse specialist.

**pain threshold** the lowest intensity at which a stimulus is felt as pain. There is very little difference between people.

**pain tolerance** the greatest intensity of pain that the individual is prepared to endure or put up with. There is substantial variation between people.

**PAL** *abbr* physical activity level.

**palate** *n* the roof of the mouth. ⇒ Appendix 1, Figure 18B—**palatal, palatine** *adj. cleft palate* ⇒ cleft palate. *hard palate* the front part of the roof of the mouth formed by the two palatine bones and the maxilla. *soft palate* situated at the posterior end of the palate and consisting of muscle covered by mucous membrane.

**palatine** *adj* pertaining to the palate.

**palatine arches** *npl* the bilateral double pillars or arch-like folds formed by the descent of the soft palate as it meets the pharynx.

**palatine bones** *npl* two small L-shaped bones of the face. They form part of the hard palate, the orbital cavities and the lateral part of the nasal cavities.

**palatopharyngoplasty** *n* ⇒ uvulopalato-pharyngoplasty.

**palatoplasty** *n* plastic surgery to repair defects in the palate.

**palatoplegia** *n* paralysis of the soft palate—**palatoplegic** *adj.*

**palatorrhaphy** *n* also called staphylorrhaphy. An operation to repair a cleft palate.

**palilalia** *n* a speech disorder characterized by rapid repetition of words or phrases.

**palindromic** *adj* relating to symptoms or disease that worsens or recurs.

**palliate** *v* relieve symptoms. Often refers to the option where a patient's condition is no longer curable and is fit only for treatment to prevent or reduce distress from symptoms. It may involve surgery (e.g. stent insertion into a bile duct, stoma formation to relieve obstruction), chemotherapy, radiotherapy (e.g. to relieve pain), nerve block and drugs (typically opioids) to relieve pain, or other symptoms.

**palliative** *adj, n* (describes) anything that serves to alleviate but cannot cure a disease.

**palliative care** the multidisciplinary specialty of symptom relief, and the care and support of the patient, family and friends—**palliation** *n.*

**pallidectomy** *n* destruction of a predetermined section of globus pallidus. ⇒ chemopallidectomy, stereotactic surgery.

**pallidotomy** *n* surgical severance of the fibres from the cerebral cortex to the corpus striatum. Previously used for relief of tremor in Parkinson's disease.

**pallor** *n* extreme paleness of the skin, such as in anaemia, or after blood loss. It may also be due to lack of natural skin pigment, for instance in individuals who are not exposed to sunlight, or those with conditions that include albinism and phenylketonuria.

**palm** *n* the anterior or flexor surface of the hand.

**palmar** *adj* pertaining to the palm of the hand.

**palmar arches** superficial and deep, are formed by the anastomosis of the radial and ulnar arteries. Smaller arteries arise from the arches to supply blood to the fingers. ⇒ Appendix 1, Figure 9.

**palmar grasp reflex** a primitive reflex present in newborns whereby they will flex their fingers to grasp a finger placed on the palm. ⇒ grasp reflex.

**palpable** *adj* capable of being palpated (felt).

**palpation** *n* the act of manual examination—**palpate** *vt.*

**palpebra** *n* an eyelid—**palpebrae** *pl,* **palpebral** *adj.*

**palpitation** *n* rapid, pounding beating of the heart of which the person is often aware. It can be caused by emotions and exertion, but may be indicative of heart disease.

**PALS** *abbr* **1.** paediatric advanced life support. **2.** patient advocacy liaison service.

**palsy** *n* paralysis. An obsolete word that is only retained in compound forms—Bell's palsy, cerebral palsy and Erb's palsy.

**panacea** *n* a medicine, remedy or treatment that claims to cure all diseases.

**panarthritis** *n* inflammation involving all of the structures of a joint.

**pancarditis** *n* inflammation involving all of the structures of the heart.

**Pancoast's syndrome** (H Pancoast, American radiologist, 1875–1939) shoulder pain and pain down the inner aspect of the arm caused by pressure on the lower brachial plexus. It is associated with bronchial cancer situated in the apex of the lung (superior sulcus tumour) and may be accompanied by Horner's syndrome.

**pancreas** *n* a tongue-shaped, mixed endocrine and exocrine gland lying below and behind the stomach (⇒ Appendix 1, Figure 18B). Its head is encircled by the duodenum and its tail touches the spleen. It is about 20 cm long and weighs about 100 g. The endocrine islet cells secrete hormones that include insulin and glucagon. Exocrine glands in lobules secrete alkaline pancreatic juice which contains digestive enzymes involved in the digestion of

P

fats, carbohydrates and proteins in the small intestine. The pancreatic juice leaves the pancreas through the pancreatic duct, which unites with the common bile duct before entering the duodenum at the hepatopancreatic ampulla. ⇒ pancreatic hormones, pancreatic juice.

**pancreas divisum** a developmental anomaly in which parts of the pancreas fail to fuse during embryonic development. Most people are asymptomatic, but it may be associated with abdominal pain, acute pancreatitis or chronic pancreatitis in some cases.

**pancreatectomy** *n* excision of part or the whole of the pancreas. It may be undertaken for cancer, cysts, or sometimes for pancreatitis. Patients in whom a large amount of pancreas has been resected will need insulin therapy, oral replacement of digestive enzymes and nutritional advice and support as necessary. ⇒ Whipple's operation.

**pancreatic function tests** indirect tests involve measurement of pancreatic enzyme metabolites in faeces, urine, plasma or breath. Estimation of serum amylase is undertaken when acute pancreatitis is suspected. Less often, pancreatic function tests involve intubation tests, in which pancreatic juice is collected from the duodenum and measured for enzyme activity and bicarbonate after endocrine or meal stimulation.

**pancreatic hormones** the islet cells secrete several hormones: the alpha ($\alpha$) cells produce glucagon; insulin and amylin are secreted from the beta ($\beta$) cells; the delta ($\delta$) cells secrete somatostatin (growth hormone release-inhibiting hormone); and other cells produce pancreatic polypeptide which inhibits exocrine pancreatic function.

**pancreatic juice** the secretion from the exocrine cells of the pancreas is stimulated by the hormones secretin and cholecystokinin (CCK) produced by duodenal cells. The juice contains water and electrolytes, including bicarbonate ions, enzymes and inactive enzymes. The bicarbonate ions ensure an alkaline (pH 8) environment in the duodenum by neutralizing the acidic chyme from the stomach. The enzymes are: amylase (carbohydrate digestion) and lipase (fat digestion) and the inactive proteolytic enzyme precursors chymotrypsinogen, trypsinogen, and procarboxypeptidase. Trypsinogen is converted to active trypsin by the enzyme enterokinase in the duodenum, and in turn it produces active chymotrypsin and carboxypeptidase. They

are not activated until they reach the duodenum so as to avoid damage to the pancreas by autodigestion.

**pancreaticoduodenectomy** *n* surgical excision of the duodenum and head of the pancreas, carried out in cases of cancer arising in the region of the head of the pancreas.

**pancreaticojejunostomy** *n* surgical procedure to establish an anastomosis between the pancreatic duct and the jejunum.

**pancreatic oncofetal antigen (POA)** an oncofetal antigen. Its presence in the serum of adults can be a tumour marker for pancreatic cancer. Lower levels may be indicative of other cancers elsewhere. ⇒ oncofetal antigens.

**pancreatic polypeptide** a polypeptide secreted by the islet cells of the pancreas, exocrine cells of the pancreas and intestinal cells. It inhibits the production of pancreatic enzymes.

**pancreatin** *n* an oral supplement of digestive enzymes obtained from animal sources. They are used for people with cystic fibrosis, after pancreatectomy or in chronic pancreatitis. In order to reduce the effects of stomach acid on the enzymes they are taken just before food, with food or immediately after eating. Capsules are swallowed whole or the contents are mixed with fluid or food and taken at once. Some preparations are enteric-coated; these too are swallowed whole.

**pancreatitis** *n* inflammation of the pancreas which may be acute or chronic. *acute pancreatitis* usually associated with gallstones or alcohol misuse. It is a serious condition and can be life-threatening with enzyme autodigestion of the pancreas leading to peritonitis, hypovolaemia, shock and multiple-organ dysfunction syndrome. Depending on severity it is characterized by severe abdominal and back pain, abdominal/flank skin discoloration, nausea and vomiting, jaundice, tachycardia, hypotension, tachypnoea, hypoxia, oliguria, an elevated serum amylase, hypocalcaemia and hyperglycaemia. Management is supportive with pain relief (not morphine), intravenous fluid replacement, antibiotics and organ support as required. Longer-term complications, which include the formation of pseudocysts, pancreatic abscess and pancreatic necrosis, may require surgical intervention. ⇒ Cullen's sign, Grey Turner's sign. *chronic pancreatitis* is most often caused by alcohol misuse and may occur after acute pancreatitis. There is permanent pancreatic damage and both endocrine and exocrine functions are affected.

Pancreatic failure leads to diabetes mellitus and pancreatic enzyme insufficiency. It is characterized by abdominal pain, anorexia, malabsorption and steatorrhoea, weight loss, obstructive jaundice, hypocalcaemia and impaired glucose tolerance. Management includes pain relief, pancreatic enzyme replacement, low-fat diet and insulin therapy for diabetes.

**pancreatography** *n* radiographic investigation, in which contrast medium is introduced into the pancreatic duct during endoscopic retrograde cholangiopancreatography, or directly at operation in order to obtain an image of the pancreas and the ducts.

**pancreozymin** *n* intestinal hormone identical to cholecystokinin (CCK). Previously both names were used.

**pancytopenia** *n* describes a peripheral blood picture when red cells, granular white cells and platelets are reduced, as occurs when bone marrow function is suppressed. Causes include aplastic anaemia, drug side-effects and following chemotherapy or radiotherapy.

**pandemic** *n* an infection spreading over a whole country or the world. For example, the influenza pandemic between 1917 and 1928, or the plague (black death) during the 14th century.

**panhypopituitarism** *n* Simmonds' disease. Deficient secretion of the hormones from the anterior lobe of the pituitary gland. ⇒ hypopituitarism.

**panic attack** ⇒ anxiety.

**panniculitis** *n* also known as Weber–Christian disease. An inflammation of the subcutaneous fat with tender nodules.

**panniculus** *n* a sheet of membranous tissue, layers of fascia.

**pannus** *n* fibrovascular membrane, usually within the anterior stroma of the cornea.

**panophthalmitis** *n* a serious condition involving inflammation of all the tissues of the eyeball. ⇒ endophthalmitis.

**panosteitis** *n* inflammation of all constituents of a bone—medulla, bony tissue and periosteum.

**panretinal photocoagulation (PRP)** treatment of the mid-peripheral retina with laser burns to reduce proliferative retinopathy, for example in diabetes.

**pantomography** *n* a panoramic radiographic technique that produces simultaneous images of the maxillary and mandibular dental arches.

**Panton–Valentine leukocidin (PVL)** a toxin produced by certain strains of the bacterium *Staphylococcus aureus*. The toxin affects white blood cells. Although PVL has been detected in meticillin (methicillin)-susceptible *Staphylococcus aureus*, the majority of strains are meticillin-resistant *S. aureus*. The PVL-producing strains of *S. aureus* have a different epidemiology and pathogenesis with increased virulence. PVL causes a variety of infections, including boils and cellulitis, septicaemia and a community-acquired necrotizing pneumonia, with a high mortality, which affects previously healthy young people.

**pantothenic acid** a member of the vitamin B complex. It is part of acetyl coenzyme A (acetyl CoA) and is involved in the metabolism of macronutrients and alcohol. It is so widely distributed in food that dietary deficiency is very rare; if it develops it will be in association with other deficiency disorders.

**PAO** *abbr* peak acid output. ⇒ pentagastrin.

**PaO₂** *abbr* partial pressure or tension of oxygen in arterial blood.

**PAO₂** *abbr* partial pressure or tension of oxygen in alveolar air.

**PAOP** *abbr* pulmonary artery occlusion pressure.

**papain** *n* a proteolyic enzyme (proteose) obtained from the papaya tree *(Carica papaya)*. It is prescribed in some countries for enzymatic wound débridement.

**Papanicolaou test** (G Papanicolaou, Greek/American cytologist and pathologist, 1883–1962) also known as a Pap smear. A smear of epithelial cells taken from the cervix using a special brush or spatula is stained and examined under the microscope for detection of the early stages of cancer. ⇒ cervical intraepithelial neoplasia.

**papilla** *n* a minute nipple-shaped eminence—**papillae** *pl*, **papillary** *adj*. renal papilla ⇒ Appendix 1, Figure 20.

**papillary muscle** the small muscles which help to stabilize the atrioventricular valves of the heart. They are attached to the chordae tendineae in the cardiac ventricles. ⇒ Appendix 1, Figure 8.

**papillary necrosis** infarction and necrosis of the renal papillae.

**papillectomy** *n* excision of a papilla.

**papillitis** *n* **1.** inflammation of the optic nerve head (disc). **2.** inflammation of a renal papilla.

**papilloedema** *n* swelling of the optic nerve head (disc), seen during examination of the fundus of the eye using an ophthalmoscope. It is usually bilateral, caused by raised intracranial pressure, such as that present in cerebral oedema, expanding lesions in the

P

skull (e.g. bleeding, tumours), hydrocephalus. ⇒ Glasgow Coma Scale, head injury.

**papilloma** *n* a simple tumour arising from a non-glandular epithelial surface—**papillomata** *pl*, **papillomatous** *adj*.

**papillomatosis** *n* the growth of benign papillomata on the skin or a mucous membrane. Removal by laser means fewer recurrences.

**papillomavirus** *n* a DNA-containing virus that causes warts. Many papillomaviruses are oncogenic and initiate malignant changes in cells. ⇒ human papillomavirus.

**papillotomy** *n* incision of a papilla, e.g. duodenal papilla for endoscopic extraction of ductal calculi.

**Pappataci fever** also called sandfly fever. ⇒ phlebotomus fever.

**papule** *n* (*syn* pimple) a small circumscribed elevation of the skin—**papular** *adj*.

**papulopustular** *adj* pertaining to a skin eruption with both papules and pustules.

**papulosquamous** *adj* pertaining to skin eruptions with both papules and scales.

**PAR** *abbr* physical activity ratio.

**para-aortic** *adj* near the aorta.

**paracentesis** *n* usually applied to the surgical puncture of the peritoneal cavity (paracentesis abdominis or abdominocentesis) for the aspiration of fluid. Either a catheter is inserted into the abdominal cavity through a small incision or a trocar and cannula are used to drain ascitic fluid. *paracentesis thoracis* (thoracentesis) draining fluid from the pleural cavity. ⇒ aspiration—**paracenteses** *pl*.

**paracetamol** *n* known as acetaminophen in North America. A non-opioid analgesic drug which has antipyretic properties. It is effective in mild to moderate pain, and having no anti-inflammatory action it is less likely to irritate the stomach. It is present in many over-the-counter medicines and in combination with other analgesic drugs. *paracetamol poisoning* paracetamol is toxic at relatively low levels, for example the ingestion of 10–15 g can damage liver cells (hepatocellular necrosis), and less often damage the kidneys (tubular necrosis). Paracetamol depletes the amount of glutathione in the liver and in appropriate cases the administration of acetylcysteine or methionine following paracetamol overdose helps to replenish glutathione levels and protect the liver. The decision to administer acetylcysteine or methionine depends on factors that include the time since ingestion and the

concentration of paracetamol in the plasma. ⇒ Appendix 5.

**parachute reflex** a reflex that appears between 7 and 9 months of age (i.e. before walking) in which the infant will, if held upright and suddenly moved to a horizontal prone position, extend the arms as if trying to break a fall. Persists into adulthood.

**paracrine** *adj* denoting a hormone, which has a localized action. Its effects are confined to adjacent cells or those in the immediate vicinity. ⇒ autocrine, endocrine.

**paracusis** *n* a disorder of hearing.

**paradigm** *n* an example, model or set of ideas or assumptions. *paradigm shift* the changes that occur as the build-up of evidence causes a paradigm to be questioned and eventually replaced by a new set of ideas.

**paradoxical respiration** associated with injuries that result in the ribs on one side being fractured in two places, such as in flail chest. The injured side of the chest moves in (deflates) on inspiration and vice versa. ⇒ flail chest.

**paradoxical sleep** (*syn* rapid eye movement [REM] sleep) ⇒ sleep.

**paraesthesia** *n* any subjective abnormality of sensation such as tingling, 'pins and needles', a feeling of tightness, swelling or numbness. A feature of many neurological disorders, including polyneuropathy and some spinal cord lesions. Also occurs in electrolyte and pH disturbances, such as with hypocalcaemia, or in the respiratory alkalosis caused by hyperventilation. ⇒ tetany.

**paraffin** *n* medicinal paraffins are: *hard paraffin*, used in wax baths for rheumatic conditions; *liquid paraffin*, previously used as a lubricant/softener laxative; and *soft paraffin*, used as an ointment base.

**paraganglioma** *n* phaeochromocytoma occurring outside the adrenal medulla.

**paraganglion** *n* any one of the small collections of chromaffin cells around the sympathetic ganglia. The paraganglia secrete the catecholamine hormones adrenaline (epinephrine) and noradrenaline (norepinephrine).

**parageusia** *n* an abnormality of the sense of taste (gustation).

**paragonimiasis** *n* endemic haemoptysis. Infestation with the lung fluke *Paragonimus westermani*. It occurs mainly in the Far East but is also present in other areas, including South America and India. It is acquired by eating raw or inadequately cooked shellfish, such as fresh-water crabs and crayfish. Symptoms are similar to chronic bronchitis, including cough, haemoptysis and breathlessness. Can also cause diarrhoea and abdominal pain, or problems in the central nervous system, such as encephalitis.

***Paragonimus*** *n* a genus of trematode flukes. For example, *Paragonimus westermani*.

**parainfluenza virus** a paramyxovirus causing acute upper respiratory infection, mainly in infants and children. Its various serotypes may cause croup, bronchiolitis, laryngotracheobronchitis, bronchopneumonia and tracheobronchitis.

**paralysis** *n* complete or incomplete loss of nervous function to a part of the body. This may be sensory or motor or both. Paralysis may be flaccid or spastic. ⇒ hemiplegia, monoplegia, paraplegia, quadriplegia, tetraplegia. *paralysis agitans* ⇒ parkinsonism.

**paralytic** *adj* pertaining to paralysis.

**paralytic ileus** paralysis of the intestinal muscle leading to a decrease or complete cessation of peristalsis. Thus the bowel content cannot pass onwards even though there is no mechanical obstruction. It may occur after abdominal surgery, especially gastrointestinal surgery; in peritonitis; ischaemic bowel; injury; drugs such as opiates; hypokalaemia; spinal cord injury; and hypothyroidism. ⇒ aperistalsis, ileus, intestinal obstruction, meconium ileus.

**paramedian** *adj* near the middle, such as the position of an abdominal incision.

**paramedical** *adj* allied to medicine. Relating to the health professions closely linked to the medical profession, e.g. physiotherapy, occupational therapy, emergency paramedic, speech and language therapist. ⇒ professions allied to medicine.

**paramesonephric duct** also known as müllerian duct. One of the paired primitive embryonic ducts that become the internal genitalia (uterine tubes, uterus) in a genetically female embryo. ⇒ mesonephric duct, müllerian duct.

**parameter** *n* **1.** a numerically measured property such as blood pressure. A constant or value used in the measurement of data relating to a physiological function, for example blood chemistry, haematological indices, which are used in the assessment of health status. **2.** in statistics, a measurement or value of a population characteristic, such as mean or standard deviation. **3.** general term meaning boundaries or limits.

**parametric tests** statistical tests that presuppose the data are from a sample from a population that has a normal distribution curve, i.e. a histogram of values shows a bell-shaped curve, with most values lying close to the middle of the distribution, and increasingly extreme values seen with increasingly lower frequency. Parametric tests, which include Student's t-test for independent groups, are more powerful than the equivalent non-parametric tests. ⇒ non-parametric tests.

**parametritis** *n* inflammation of the structures around the uterus, the parametrium. ⇒ cellulitis, pelvic inflammatory disease.

**parametrium** *n* the connective tissues immediately surrounding the uterus—**parametrial** *adj*.

**paramnesia** *n* **1.** a distortion of memory whereby individuals believe that they remember a set of circumstances that did not occur. They are unable to differentiate between reality and fantasy. **2.** the use of remembered words without having any understanding of what they mean. ⇒ confabulation, déjà vu phenomenon.

**paramyotonia** *n* a condition characterized by muscle spasms resulting from an abnormality of muscle tone. *myotonia congenita* a genetically determined disorder of muscle contraction inherited as an autosomal dominant trait. Affected individuals experience prolonged muscle contraction, particularly when exposed to cold. It is made worse by exercise.

**paramyxovirus** *n* a family of RNA viruses that include the measles virus, mumps virus, parainfluenza virus and the respiratory syncytial virus.

**paranasal** *adj* near the nasal cavities, such as the various sinuses. *paranasal sinuses* the air-filled sinuses in the bones around the nasal cavity. There are ethmoidal air cells and frontal, maxillary and sphenoidal sinuses (Figure P.1). They are lined with ciliated mucous membrane, which is continuous with that lining the nasal cavity. The sinuses lighten the skull and give the voice resonance.

**paraneoplastic syndromes** *npl* the indirect symptoms or signs associated with the presence of a cancer, but which occur away from the primary cancer or any metastatic sites. They are caused by the production of hormones, other chemicals and immune responses. They may be haematological, endocrine or neurological or affect the skin and muscles. Examples include dermatomyositis; hypercalcaemia caused by production of parathyroid hormone (PTH) in breast cancer; ectopic production of adrenocorticotrophic

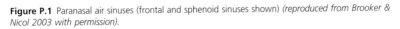

**Figure P.1** Paranasal air sinuses (frontal and sphenoid sinuses shown) *(reproduced from Brooker & Nicol 2003 with permission).*

hormone (ACTH) in some lung cancers; myasthenia gravis associated with thymic cancers; and cerebellar degeneration associated with cancers of the ovary, breast, lung, etc.

**paranoia** *n* an abnormal tendency to mistrust or suspect others—**paranoid** *adj.*

**paranoid behaviour** acts denoting suspicion of others.

**paranoid schizophrenia** a form of schizophrenia characterized by (often persecutory) delusions and hallucinations.

**paraoesophageal** *adj.* near the oesophagus.

**paraparesis** *n* loss of power in the legs.

**paraphasia** *n* a disorder of language in which the person uses meaningless words or uses words in the wrong sense, speech is unintelligible and incoherent.

**paraphimosis** *n* retraction of the prepuce (foreskin) behind the glans penis so that a tight ring of skin produces oedema of the preputial skin. Thus the prepuce cannot be returned to its normal position. ⇒ circumcision, phimosis.

**paraphrenia** *n* a persistent delusional disorder with onset in later life—**paraphrenic** *adj.*

**paraplegia** *n* paralysis of the lower limbs, usually affecting the nerves that control bowel and bladder function. Often the result of traumatic spinal cord damage, but also caused by multiple sclerosis or tumours—**paraplegic** *adj.* ⇒ hemiplegia, monoplegia, spinal cord compression (SCC), tetraplegia.

**paraprax** *n* known as a 'Freudian slip'. A verbal error caused by unconscious conflicts.

**paraprotein** *n* an abnormal protein including the abnormal monoclonal immunoglobulins produced in plasma cell disorders.

**parapsychology** *n* the study of extrasensory perception, telepathy and other psychic phenomena.

**paraquat dichloride** widely used as a herbicide. Exposure leads to local effects depending on the route, but include: oral/oesophageal damage, skin blisters, epistaxis or severe inflammation of the conjunctiva or cornea. Systemic effects that may be delayed are usually associated with ingestion and include damage to the myocardium, lungs, liver and kidneys.

**pararectal** *adj* near the rectum.

**parasitaemia** *n* parasites in the blood—**parasitaemic** *adj*.

**parasite** *n* an organism that obtains nutrients or shelter from another organism, the host—**parasitic** *adj*.

**parasiticide** *n* an agent that will kill parasites.

**parasomnias** *npl* a broad class of sleep-associated disturbances; it includes sleepwalking, nightmares and bruxism.

**parasternal** *adj* near the sternum.

**parasuicide** *n* a suicidal gesture: drug overdose or a self-mutilating act which may or may not be provoked by a real wish to die. Commonly seen in young people who are distressed but not mentally ill. May be linked to low self-esteem. ⇒ deliberate self-harm, Samaritans.

**parasympathetic nervous system** *n* the part of the autonomic nervous system having craniosacral outflow. It is concerned with the normal at-rest body processes, such as digestion, and opposes the action of the sympathetic nervous system.

**parasympatholytic** *adj* usually describes a drug that reduces or eradicates the effects of parasympathetic stimulation. ⇒ muscarinic antagonist.

**parasympathomimetic** *adj* describes an agent, usually a drug, that causes similar effects as or stimulates parasympathetic activity. ⇒ muscarinic agonist.

**parathormone** *n* parathyroid hormone. ⇒ parathyroid hormone.

**parathyroid glands** four small endocrine glands usually lying close to or embedded in the posterior surface of the thyroid gland (Figure P.2). They may, however, be located at other sites in the neck, thorax and mediastinum. They secrete parathyroid hormone.

**parathyroid hormone (PTH)** parathormone. A polypeptide hormone secreted by the parathyroid glands. It regulates calcium and phosphate homeostasis and is released when calcium concentration in serum is decreased. Parathyroid hormone indirectly increases calcium by absorbing more from food in the intestine, reducing the amount excreted by the kidneys and, if necessary, by stimulating the reabsorption of calcium from bone. ⇒ calcitonin.

**parathyroidectomy** *n* excision of one or more parathyroid glands.

**paratope** *n* the antigen-binding site of an antibody molecule. ⇒ epitope.

**paratyphoid fever** a variety of enteric fever, less severe and prolonged than typhoid fever. Caused by *Salmonella paratyphi* A and B, and more rarely C.

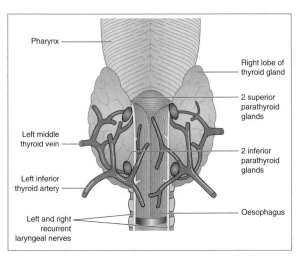

**Figure P.2** Position of parathyroid glands and related structures *(reproduced from Waugh & Grant 2006 with permission)*.

**paraurethral** *adj* near the urethra.

**paravaginal** *adj* near the vagina.

**paravertebral** *adj* near the spinal column. *paravertebral block anaesthesia* (more correctly, analgesia) is induced by infiltration of local anaesthetic around the spinal nerve roots as they emerge from the intervertebral foramina. *paravertebral injection* of local anaesthetic into sympathetic chain can be used as a test in ischaemic limbs to see if sympathectomy is indicated.

**pareidolic image** a sensory deception. A vivid perception of visual images in response to an indistinct stimulus. The image and the percept coexist, and the image is normally accepted as being 'unreal'. For instance, faces or objects seen in a cloud formation. An example of an illusion. ⇒ eidetic, illusion.

**parenchyma** *n* the tissues and cells of an organ which, in contradistinction to its supporting interstitial tissue, are concerned with its function—**parenchymal, parenchymatous** *adj*.

**parenteral** *adj* not via the alimentary tract. Therapy such as fluid, drugs or nutrition administered by a route other than the alimentary tract.

**parenteral nutrition** a method of providing nutrition by administering nutrients directly into the circulatory system via a venous catheter. It can be given temporarily in hospital, or permanently at home (home parenteral nutrition) in the treatment of intestinal failure. A special intravenous catheter is used to infuse various nutrient solutions into a central vein. Usually the catheter is sited centrally, through the subclavian vein into the superior vena cava. Sometimes it is possible to use peripherally inserted central catheters (PICC) which are inserted through the basilic vein (of the arm) to the superior vena cava via the right subclavian vein. Parenteral nutrition is used for patients whose gastrointestinal tract is not functioning. It should only be used if nutritional needs cannot be met via the enteral route. The term 'total parenteral nutrition' is used in some countries—**parenterally** *adv*.

**paresis** *n* partial or slight paralysis; weakness of a limb—**paretic** *adj*.

**pareunia** *n* coitus.

**pareve (parve)** *n* a Jewish word for dishes that do not contain meat or milk. Orthodox Jews are prohibited from combining meat or milk foods or eating or drinking milk products for 3 hours following a meal with meat. ⇒ kosher, traife.

**paries** *n* a wall, such as that of a body cavity or a hollow organ—**parietes** *pl*.

**parietal** *adj* **1.** pertaining to an outer wall, such as the parietal pleura or parietal peritoneum. **2.** pertaining to the parietal lobes of the cerebrum and the parietal bones of the skull.

**parietal bone** one of two bones which form the sides and vault of the skull.

**parietal cells** ⇒ oxyntic.

**parietal lobe** the part of each cerebral hemisphere underlying the parietal bone. The parietal lobe contains the somatosensory area of the cerebral cortex and the large parieto-occipitotemporal area, which are concerned with the integration of incoming sensory impulses from receptors in the skin, those in skeletal muscle and joints. The areas in the parietal lobe are concerned with the perception of sensations of pain, pressure, touch, temperature and the awareness of muscle and joint action; and functions that include the manipulation and identification of objects, remembering the names of objects and spatial awareness.

**parity** *n* status of a woman with regard to the number of children she has borne.

**Parkinson's disease** (J Parkinson, British physician, 1755–1824) an idiopathic incurable neurodegenerative condition in which there are changes in the substantia nigra and a relatively selective loss of dopamine nerve cells in the brain causing a resting tremor, bradykinesia (slowness of movement) and rigidity in the limbs. Some people differentiate between idiopathic Parkinson's disease and parkinsonism, the causes of which are multiple and include repeated brain trauma (as in boxing), stroke, atherosclerosis, brain cancers, Wilson's disease, various toxic agents, viral encephalitis, carbon monoxide poisoning and as a side-effect of typical antipsychotic drugs (neuroleptics). ⇒ tardive dyskinesia.

**parkinsonism** *n* a condition resembling Parkinson's disease clinically.

**Parliamentary and Health Service Ombudsman** an organization that independently investigates complaints from the public about the actions of the NHS in England, government departments and many public bodies in the UK, and the service they received from them.

**PARNUTS** *abbr* foods for particular nutritional purposes. The term used by the European Union for the dietetic foods for people with metabolic disorders (e.g. phenylketonuria) or certain physiological conditions (e.g. coeliac disease) or for infants and young children.

**paronychia** *n* (*syn* whitlow) inflammation of the tissue around a nail plate, which may be bacterial or fungal. It frequently occurs with onychia.

**paroophoron** *n* vestigial remains of the embryonic mesonephros located in the broad ligament between the epoophoron and the uterus. ⇒ epoophoron.

**parosmia** *n* altered, dysfunctional sense of smell, usually of unpleasant hallucinatory nature.

**parotid gland** the large salivary gland situated in front of and below the ear on either side. The parotid duct (Stenson's duct) opens on to the inner surface of the cheek at the level of the second upper molar tooth.

**parotidectomy** *n* excision of a parotid (salivary) gland, such as for removal of a tumour.

**parotitis** *n* inflammation of a parotid salivary gland. *infectious parotitis* ⇒ mumps. *septic parotitis* refers to ascending infection from the mouth via the parotid duct, when a parotid abscess may result.

**parous** *adj* having borne a child or children.

**paroxysm** *n* a sudden, temporary attack.

**paroxysmal** *adj* coming on in attacks or paroxysms.

**paroxysmal fibrillation** occurs in the atrium of the heart and is associated with a ventricular tachycardia and total irregularity of the pulse rhythm.

**paroxysmal nocturnal dyspnoea (PND)** sudden bouts of dyspnoea occurring mostly at night in patients with cardiac disease, usually left ventricular failure. It awakens the person, following some hours of sleep. It is often accompanied by feelings of panic, respiratory distress, sweating, tachycardia and coughing up frothy sputum.

**paroxysmal tachycardia** may result from ectopic impulses arising in the atrium or in the ventricle itself.

**parrot disease** ⇒ psittacosis.

**Parrot's nodes** (J Parrot, French physician, 1829–1883) bossing of frontal bones and parietal bones of the skull in congenital syphilis.

**pars flaccida** *n* the upper part of the tympanic membrane.

**pars tensa** *n* the lower four-fifths of the tympanic membrane.

**partial agonist** a drug that only has a partial physiological effect, having reduced efficacy compared with a full agonist.

**partial pressure** pressure exerted by a gas in a mixture of different gases. It is directly related to its concentration and the pressure exerted by the total mixture.

**partnership working** in the UK a working relationship between central government, local NHS services, local government authorities, and local communities. It should enable greater co-ordination and co-operative multi-agency/multiprofessional working that aim to improve health and well-being.

**partogram/partograph** *n* a chart that provides a graphic record of progress during labour. Information recorded includes fetal heart, maternal vital signs, contraction frequency and strengths, cervical dilatation and descent of presenting part, drugs administered, etc. and allows for the prompt identification of departures from normal.

**parturient** *adj* pertaining to childbirth.

**parturition** *n* ⇒ labour.

**pascal (Pa)** *n* derived SI unit (International System of Units) for pressure. The kilopascal (kPa) is now frequently used for measuring blood gases. It would be used for measuring blood pressure instead of millimetres of mercury pressure (mmHg) if the change was ever made. ⇒ Appendix 2.

**passive** *adj* inactive. ⇒ active *opp*. *passive hyperaemia* ⇒ hyperaemia. *passive immunity* ⇒ immunity.

**passive movement** performed by a health care professional or carer, the patient being relaxed.

**passive stretching** stretching of a body part by use of a force other than tension in the antagonist muscles, e.g. by an examiner without assistance from the athlete.

*Pasteurella* *n* (L Pasteur, French chemist, pathologist, 1822–1895) a genus of Gram-negative, facultative anaerobic bacteria that causes infection in humans and domestic animals. Humans may be infected through animal bites and scratches. ⇒ *Francisella*, *Yersinia*.

**pasteurization** *n* a process whereby pathogenic organisms in fluid (especially milk) are killed by heat. *flash method of pasteurization* (HT, ST—high-temperature, short-time), the fluid is heated to 72°C, maintained at this temperature for 15 s, then rapidly cooled. *holder method of pasteurization* the fluid is heated to 63–65.5°C, maintained at this temperature for 30 min, then rapidly cooled.

**Patau's syndrome** (K Patau, German/American geneticist, 20th century) trisomy 13. An autosomal trisomy of chromosomes in group D (13–15) but usually chromosome 13. Closely

**P**

associated with severe learning disability. Numerous physical defects include microcephaly, neural tube defect, coloboma, cleft lip and palate, polydactyly, cardiac defects and abnormalities of the genitalia. Most infants die during the first few months of life.

**patch test** a skin test for type IV (delayed-type) hypersensitivity to allergens, which are incorporated into an adhesive patch applied to the skin. Forty-eight hours after application the skin under the patch is examined for signs of redness and swelling. Comparison is made against a negative control containing a neutral non-allergenic compound.

**patella** *n* a triangular, sesamoid bone present in the patellar tendon of the quadriceps femoris muscle; the kneecap (⇒ Appendix 1, Figure 2)—**patellae** *pl*, **patellar** *adj*.

**patellar reflex** a deep tendon reflex. Also called the knee jerk reflex. ⇒ knee.

**patellectomy** *n* excision of the patella.

**patent** *adj* open; not closed or occluded—**patency** *n*.

**patent ductus arteriosus** failure of the ductus arteriosus to close soon after birth, so that an abnormal shunt between the pulmonary artery and the aorta is preserved. If spontaneous closure does not occur, surgical correction is undertaken. Minimally invasive surgical techniques are increasingly used to close the defect.

**patent interventricular communication** a congenital defect in the dividing wall between the right and left ventricle of the heart. ⇒ ventricular septal defect.

**paternalism** *n* overprotective or restricting, such as withholding information about potential risks of health care interventions, or well-meaning rules and regulations that reduce individual autonomy.

**pathogen** *n* a disease-producing agent, usually applied to a living agent, such as a bacterium—**pathogenic** *adj*, **pathogenicity** *n*.

**pathogenesis** *n* the origin and development of disease—**pathogenetic** *adj*.

**pathogenicity** *n* the capacity to cause disease.

**pathognomonic** *adj* characteristic of or peculiar to a disease.

**pathological fracture** ⇒ fracture.

**pathology** *n* the science which deals with the cause and nature of disease—**pathological** *adj*, **pathologically** *adv*.

**pathophobia** *n* a morbid dread of disease—**pathophobic** *adj*.

**pathophysiology** *n* the science that deals with abnormal functioning of the human being—**pathophysiological** *adj*, **pathophysiologically** *adv*.

**patient advocacy liaison service (PALS)** an advocacy service to patients in NHS and Primary Care Trusts, representing their concerns and complaints to the relevant department within the Trust.

**patient compliance** a term used when a patient takes the prescribed drug, in the prescribed dose, at the prescribed time and by the prescribed route. ⇒ concordance, non-compliance *opp*.

**patient-controlled analgesia (PCA)** equipment that enables patients to control the delivery of analgesic drugs (within prescribed limits). Usually via an intravenous line, but patient-controlled epidural analgesia (PCEA) may be suitable in some situations. ⇒ analgesia, epidural.

**patriarchy** *n* a community or family where the oldest male (father) dominates, controls and is the highest authority.

**patulous** *adj* opened out; expanded.

**Paul–Bunnell test** (J Paul, American physician, 1893–1971; W Bunnell, American pathologist, 1895–1979) a serological test used in the diagnosis of infectious mononucleosis.

**pavementation** *n* the process in which white blood cells (leucocytes) adhere to the endothelial lining of blood vessels when blood flow slows during the inflammatory response.

**Pawlik's manoeuvre** a rarely used single-hand palpation method that determines the size of the fetal head, the degree of flexion and mobility.

**PBD** *abbr* peak bone density.

**PBM** *abbr* peak bone mass.

**PBMC** *abbr* peripheral blood mononuclear cells.

**PCAG** *abbr* primary closed-angle glaucoma.

**PCA(S)** *abbr* patient-controlled analgesia (system).

**PCEA** *abbr* patient-controlled epidural analgesia.

**PCI** *abbr* percutaneous coronary intervention.

**PCM** *abbr* protein–calorie malnutrition.

**PCO₂** *abbr* the partial pressure of carbon dioxide, for example in atmospheric or expired air.

**PCOS** *abbr* polycystic ovary syndrome.

**PCP** *abbr* pneumocystis pneumonia.

**PCR** *abbr* polymerase chain reaction.

**PCT** *abbr* Primary Care Trust.

**PCV** *abbr* packed cell volume.

**PDGF** *abbr* platelet-derived growth factor.

**PDT** *abbr* photodynamic therapy.

**PE** *abbr* pulmonary embolism.

**PEA** *acron* **p**ulseless **e**lectrical **a**ctivity.

**peak bone density (PBD) or mass (PBM)** the greatest bone density achieved by an individual, usually achieved in the late 20s or early 30s. ⇒ bone mineral density (BMD).

**peak expiratory flow rate (PEFR)** the greatest flow of air during a forced expiration, measured with a peak flow meter (Figure P.3). Usually three measurements are taken and the best of these is recorded. Used to monitor various respiratory diseases, particularly asthma, and to assess the effects of drug therapy.

**peak mucus day** during the menstrual cycle the last day when the cervical mucus is clear, thin, slippery and elastic. This is characteristic of the time around ovulation and can be used retrospectively in some natural family planning methods to identify the period of peak fertility. ⇒ Billings' method, spinnbarkeit.

**peak oxygen consumption/uptake (peak VO₂)** the highest oxygen consumption/uptake measured during a test of physical activity to the point of exhaustion.

**peak postexercise lactate** the highest concentration of lactate in the blood reached during or just after a period of exercise.

**peau d'orange** appearance of (usually) the breast when a cancer results in lymphatic obstruction and dimpling at the hair follicles, causing the breast to look (literally) like orange skin; usually a sign of locally advanced disease.

**pectoral** *adj* pertaining to the chest.

**pectoral girdle** the shoulder girdle.

**pectoral muscles** two muscles of the upper anterior chest (⇒ Appendix 1, Figure 4): the *pectoralis major*, a large fan-shaped muscle. Its origin is on the clavicle, sternum, costal cartilages (1–6) and the aponeurosis of the abdominal external oblique muscle and it inserts on to the greater tubercle of the humerus. It is a prime mover of arm flexion, medial rotation of the arm and arm adduction; and the *pectoralis minor* a thin, flat muscle under the *p. major*. Its origin is on the ribs (3–5) and it inserts on to the coracoid process of the scapula. Contraction draws the scapula down and forwards, and ribcage upwards during a forced inspiration.

**pectus** *n* the chest. *pectus carinatum* ⇒ pigeon chest. *pectus excavatum* ⇒ funnel chest.

**pedal** *adj* pertaining to the foot.

**pedal pulse** the dorsalis pedis artery palpated on the dorsum of the foot. Used to check circulation to the foot in peripheral vascular disease, leg trauma and following vascular surgery.

**pedicle** *n* a stalk, e.g. the narrow part by which a tumour is attached to the surrounding structures.

**pediculosis** *n* infestation with lice (pediculi).

**Pediculus** *n* a genus of parasitic insects (lice) important as vectors of disease. *Pediculus humanus capitis* the head louse. ⊙DVD *Pediculus corporis* the body louse. *Pediculus* (more correctly, *Phthirus*) *pubis* the crab or pubic louse. In some regions of the world body lice are responsible for the transmission of typhus and other diseases.

**pedometer** *n* a small device, usually worn on the waistband or belt, which counts the number of steps taken.

**pedopompholyx** *n* ⇒ cheiropompholyx.

**peduncle** *n* a stalk-like structure, such as the *cerebral peduncles* and *cerebellar peduncles*, which are bands of nerves fibres that connect different parts of the brain—**peduncular, pedunculated** *adj*.

**peeling** *n* desquamation.

**PEEP** *acron* **p**ositive **e**nd-**e**xpiratory **p**ressure.

**peer review** the process whereby clinicians of equal status review the practice and actions of each other. Also part of the academic process in which research and other material

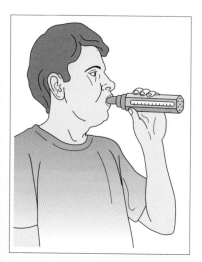

**Figure P.3** Peak flow meter *(reproduced from Nicol et al. 2004 with permission).*

for publication are scrutinized by a group of eminent members of the same profession who judge whether the material is worthy of publication.

**peer support** support from other members of a group to which one belongs. For example, new patients perceive established patients as providing support. Likewise, health professionals use their peer groups to gain and provide support, particularly in stressful circumstances.

**PEFR** *abbr* peak expiratory flow rate.

**PEG** *acron* **p**ercutaneous **e**ndoscopic **g**astrostomy.

**Pel–Ebstein fever** (P Pel, Dutch physician, 1852–1919; W Ebstein, German physician, 1836–1912) recurring bouts of pyrexia in regular sequence found in Hodgkin's disease. A less frequent manifestation with improving treatment.

**pellagra** *n* a deficiency disease caused by lack of the B-vitamin niacin and/or the amino acid tryptophan. Syndrome includes glossitis; dermatitis, especially in skin exposed to sunlight; diarrhoea; mental confusion, depression and eventually dementia; and peripheral neuritis and spinal cord changes (even producing ataxia).

**pellet** *n* a small pill. ⇒ implant.

**pelvic** *adj* relating to the pelvis.

**pelvic floor** a mainly muscular partition with some fascia situated between the pelvic cavity above and the perineum below. The pelvic floor comprises two halves that unite along the midline. It is perforated by the urethra, vagina and anus in females, and the urethra and anus in males. The two muscles are the levator ani and the coccygeus. It supports the pelvic structures and maintains continence. In the female, weakening of the pelvic floor during childbirth can contribute to urinary incontinence and uterine prolapse.

**pelvic floor exercises** ⇒ Kegel exercises.

**pelvic floor repair** operation performed to correct genital prolapse. ⇒ Manchester repair.

**pelvic girdle** the bony pelvis comprising two innominate bones, the sacrum and coccyx.

**pelvic inflammatory disease (PID)** acute or chronic inflammation of the ovaries, uterine (fallopian) tube and uterus. Infection may spread from adjacent pelvic structures, including the bowel or appendix or through the cervix from the vagina and may be sexually transmitted. It is characterized by lower abdominal pain, and urgent antibiotic treatment is essential if tubal occlusion and infertility are to be prevented.

**pelvic pain syndrome (PPS)** pelvic pain which occurs in women but for which no pathological cause is evident.

**pelvimeter** *n* an instrument especially devised to measure the pelvic diameters for obstetric purposes.

**pelvimetry** *n* the measurement of the dimensions of the pelvis—**pelvimetric** *adj*.

**pelvis** *n* **1.** a basin-shaped cavity, e.g. pelvis of the kidney (⇒ Appendix 1, Figure 20). **2.** the large bony basin-shaped cavity formed by the innominate bones and sacrum, containing and protecting the bladder, rectum and, in the female, the organs of generation—**pelvic** *adj*. *contracted pelvis* one in which one or more diameters are smaller than normal; this may result in difficulties in childbirth. *false pelvis* the wide expanded part of the pelvis above the brim. *true pelvis* that part of the pelvis below the brim.

**pelviureteric junction (PUJ) obstruction** a condition, often congenital, resulting in obstruction at the junction of the renal pelvis and proximal ureter.

**PEM** *abbr* protein–energy malnutrition.

**pemphigoid** *n* a bullous eruption, usually in the latter half of life, which is of autoimmune cause. Histological examination of a blister differentiates it from pemphigus. Treated by systemic corticosteroids.

**pemphigus** *n* a group of rare but serious diseases called pemphigus vulgaris, pemphigus vegetans and pemphigus erythematosus. *pemphigus vulgaris* a bullous disease, mostly of middle age, of autoimmune aetiology. Blister formation occurs in the epidermis, with resulting secondary infection and rupture, so that large raw areas develop. Bullae develop also on mucous membranes. The condition is treated by systemic corticosteroids and immunosuppressive drugs.

**Pendred's syndrome** (V Pendred, British physician, 1869–1946) congenital bilateral sensorineural deafness associated with the later development of goitre. There is defective synthesis of thyroxine due to deficiency of an enzyme. Inherited as an autosomal recessive trait.

**pendular response** a pathological response to the stretch reflex commonly seen in cerebellar disease. When a muscle is stretched by distortion of its tendon, the stretch reflex response is sluggish and is not checked by a reciprocal response in the antagonist muscle; e.g. if the knee jerk is invoked, there will not be one sharp jerk but the leg will swing like a pendulum.

**pendulous** *adj* hanging down. *pendulous abdomen* a relaxed condition of the anterior wall, allowing it to hang down over the pubis. May require plastic surgery to improve the person's self-esteem and to prevent excoriation between the skin surfaces.

**penetrance** *n* in genetics, the frequency in which an allele is expressed in the individual who has it. If the trait is expressed in the phenotype in 100% of cases it is termed fully penetrant. When expression of the trait is less than 100% it is termed reduced or incomplete penetrance. This can lead to inherited disorders missing or skipping a generation. When a person who has the allele, which generally leads to an abnormal phenotype, has a normal phenotype the allele is described as non-penetrant.

**penetrating ulcer** an ulcer that is locally invasive.

**penetrating wound** (*syn* puncture wound) caused by a sharp, usually slim object, or a missile, which passes through the skin into the tissues beneath.

**penicillinase** *n* ⇒ beta (β)-lactamase.

**penicillins** *npl* a large group of β-lactam antibiotics. Many have activity against a broad range of bacteria (known as broad-spectrum antibiotics) but they produce hypersensitivity reactions and many micro-organisms have developed resistance. Some penicillins are β-lactamase resistant. ⇒ Appendix 5.

*Penicillium* *n* a genus of moulds. The hyphae bear spores characteristically arranged like a brush. A common contaminant of food. The species *Penicillium notatum* was shown by Fleming (in 1928) to produce penicillin.

**penis** *n* the male organ of copulation, it is homologous with the female clitoris. The urethra runs through the penis to the outside and provides passage for both urine and semen. The penis has a root embedded in the perineum and a shaft which terminates at the expanded glans penis. The glans is normally covered with the prepuce (foreskin), a loose double fold of skin. The penis comprises three columns of erectile tissue containing vascular spaces, connective tissue and involuntary muscle. There are two lateral columns, the corpora cavernosa (*sing.* corpus cavernosum) and the ventral corpus spongiosum, surrounding the urethra. Normally the penis is

flaccid but during sexual arousal the vascular spaces fill with blood which causes it to become erect. (⇒ Appendix 1, Figure 16)—**penile** *adj*.

**pentagastrin** *n* a synthetic pentapeptide hormone used in gastric function tests to produce maximal gastric acid secretion. *pentagastrin test* measures gastric acid secretion by oxyntic (parietal) cells in the stomach.

**pentose** *n* a five-carbon monosaccharide (sugar) such as ribose.

**pentosuria** *n* excretion of pentose sugars in the urine. It may occur after consuming fruits such as pears. Pentosuria also occurs in an inherited metabolic disorder seen in Ashkenazi Jews; it causes no ill effects.

**pepsin** *n* a proteolytic enzyme secreted by the stomach, as the precursor pepsinogen, which hydrolyses proteins to polypeptides. Pepsin activity has an optimum pH of 1.5–2.0.

**pepsinogen** *n* an inactive proenzyme secreted mainly by the chief cells in the gastric mucosa and converted to pepsin in the acidic environment created by hydrochloric acid secretion in the stomach, or existing pepsin.

**peptic** *adj* pertaining to pepsin or to digestion generally.

**peptic ulcer** a non-malignant ulcer in those parts of the digestive tract that are exposed to the gastric secretions; hence usually in the stomach or duodenum but sometimes in the lower oesophagus, in the jejunum following surgical anastomosis to the stomach, or with a Meckel's diverticulum. ⇒ duodenal ulcer, gastric ulcer.

**peptidase** *n* an enzyme that breaks down proteins by splitting peptides into amino acids. ⇒ aminopeptidases, carboxypeptidases, dipeptidases.

**peptides** *npl* organic compounds that yield two or more amino acids on hydrolysis; e.g. dipeptides and polypeptides. *peptide bond* a chemical bond formed during a dehydration synthesis reaction when two amino acids form peptides.

**peptone** *n* a mixture of protein fragments produced by the partial breakdown of a native protein by acid or enzyme.

**percept** *n* the mental product of a sensation; a sensation plus memories of similar sensations and their relationships.

**perception** *n* the reception of a conscious impression through the sensory organs by which individuals differentiate objects one from another and recognize their qualities according to the different sensations they produce.

**percussion** *n* tapping to determine the resonance or dullness of the area examined. Normally a finger of the left hand is laid on the patient's skin and the middle finger of the right hand (plexor) is used to strike the left finger.

**percutaneous** *adj* through the skin.

**percutaneous coronary interventions (PCI)** interventions used to reopen coronary arteries stenosed by the build-up of atheromatous plaques. It is used in the treatment of patients with stable angina and unstable angina and recent myocardial infarction. The term generally refers to balloon angioplasty, which is often combined with stent insertion, but other interventions include the use of lasers and other treatments to reduce risk of vessel restenosis. ⇒ percutaneous transluminal coronary angioplasty.

**percutaneous endoscopic gastrostomy (PEG)** gastrostomy tube inserted through the abdominal wall after the stomach has been distended endoscopically (Figure P.4). Used for long-term enteral feeding.

**percutaneous epididymal sperm aspiration (PESA)** technique used in assisted conception. ⇒ microsurgical epididymal sperm aspiration (MESA).

**percutaneous myocardial revascularization** a treatment for angina. A catheter with laser energy source is introduced into the heart via the femoral artery. The laser is used to produce channels through to the myocardium, thus allowing more oxygenated blood to reach the myocardium.

**percutaneous nephrolithotomy** a minimally invasive technique where the kidney pelvis is punctured using X-ray control. A guidewire is inserted through which the stone is removed using a nephroscope (endoscope). ⇒ nephrolithotomy.

**percutaneous transhepatic cholangiography (PTC)** a radiographic image of the biliary tree achieved by injecting contrast medium though the abdominal wall directly into a small hepatic bile duct. ⇒ cholangiography.

**percutaneous transluminal coronary angioplasty (PTCA)** a procedure used in the treatment of coronary artery disease. A balloon-tipped catheter is used to dilate a stenosed coronary artery. The balloon is inflated several times to compress atheromatous plaques against the walls of the vessel. Stent insertion to prevent restenosis is normally performed, but not in all cases.

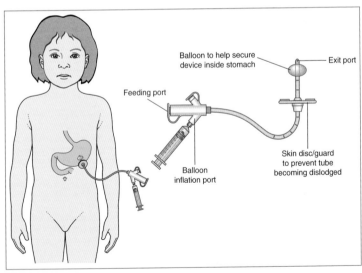

Balloon to help secure device inside stomach

Exit port

Feeding port

Skin disc/guard to prevent tube becoming dislodged

Balloon inflation port

**Figure P.4** Percutaneous endoscopic gastrostomy *(adapted from Huband & Trigg 2000 with permission).*

**perforation** *n* a hole in a previously intact sheet of tissue. Used in reference to perforation of the tympanic membrane, or the wall of the stomach or gut, constituting a surgical emergency.

**perforin** *n* a protein produced by cytotoxic T cells (CD8 cells) and natural killer (NK) cells. It forms a pore in the membrane of targeted cells, leading to lysis and apoptosis (cell death).

**performance components** the basic skills required to perform activities of daily living, including sensorimotor, cognitive, psychosocial, psychological and spiritual skills.

**performance indicators (PIs)** quantitative measures of the activities and resources used in health care delivery.

**perfusion** *n* **1.** the flow of blood through tissues and organs, such as the skin, kidney or lung. **2.** fluid and/or drugs intended for a specific organ are injected into the blood stream.

**perfusion scan** a radiographic technique used to assess the blood flow (perfusion) through an organ. It involves the injection of radioactive tracers. It is commonly performed to detect areas in the lung with reduced perfusion, such as caused by pulmonary emboli. A perfusion scan may be combined with a ventilation scan in which the radioactive tracer is inhaled to identify areas of the lung that are not inflated, and to calculate the ventilation–perfusion ratio. ⇒ ventilation–perfusion (*V/Q*) ratio, ventilation–perfusion scanning.

**perfusionist** *n* a health professional qualified and registered to assist in procedures that involve extracorporeal circulation techniques, such as during cardiac bypass surgery or extracorporeal membrane oxygenation in critically ill patients.

**perianal** *adj* surrounding the anus. *perianal abscess* also known as anorectal abscess. A cavity containing pus, which may be caused when micro-organisms infect the anal gland or enter a tear in the anal mucosa. Abscess formation may also be associated with Crohn's disease. The abscess can track further into the perianal region or into the ischiorectal fossae. It may be associated with fistulae formation. Patients report extreme pain in the perianal region, especially on sitting and during defecation.

**periapical** *adj* surrounding an apex. Relating to the tissues and structures around the apex of a tooth root, including the connective tissue and alveolar bone. *periapical abscess* acute or chronic infection of the periapical tissues. There is pus formation at the tooth apex, and it generally results from death of the pulp tissue. The abscess may discharge into the mouth or into a maxillary air sinus; cause cellulitis of the face; or spread to alveolar bone.

**periarterial** *adj* surrounding an artery.

**periarteritis** *n* inflammation of the outer sheath of an artery and the periarterial tissue. *periarteritis nodosa* ⇒ polyarteritis.

**periarthritis** *n* inflammation of the tissues and structures surrounding a joint. Sometimes applied to frozen shoulder.

**periarticular** *adj* surrounding a joint.

**peribulbar** *adj* around the eyeball inside the orbit.

**pericardectomy** *n* surgical removal of the pericardium, thickened from chronic inflammation (pericarditis) and restricting the pumping action of the heart.

**pericardiocentesis** *n* aspiration of fluid from the pericardial sac.

**pericardiorrhaphy** *n* surgical repair of the pericardium; includes traumatic wounds and incisions made during planned surgery.

**pericardiotomy** *n* an incision into the pericardium.

**pericarditis** *n* inflammation of the pericardial covering of the heart; it may be acute or chronic. It may or may not be accompanied by an effusion, which in extreme cases can cause tamponade, a pericardial friction rub, or the formation of adhesions between the two layers. Causes of acute pericarditis include injury, viral infection, myocardial infarction, uraemia, malignant disease and connective tissue diseases (e.g. systemic lupus erythematosus). Chronic pericarditis is associated with bacterial infections, including tuberculosis, with rheumatoid arthritis, or may follow viral pericarditis. ⇒ pericardectomy.

**pericardium** *n* comprises two sacs—the outer fibrous sac and an inner double serous membranous sac which envelops the heart. The fibrous sac is formed from the same tissue as the tunica adventitia of the great vessels and it is attached to the diaphragm. The fibrous sac stops overdistension as the heart fills with blood. The inner layer of the serous membrane in contact with the heart is called visceral pericardium (or epicardium); that reflected to form the outer serous membrane, which lines the fibrous sac, is called the parietal pericardium. Between the two serous membranes is a potential space, the pericardial cavity, which normally contains a thin film of serous fluid, which allows the two membranes to move easily when the heart beats—**pericardial** *adj*.

**perichondritis** n inflammation of the fibrous connective tissue surrounding cartilage (the perichondrium). It usually refers to that affecting the outer/external ear. Trauma to the ear leading to haematoma formation can cause perichondritis and this can result in a 'cauliflower-ear' deformity.

**perichondrium** n the fibrous tissue covering of cartilage (except articular cartilage in synovial joints)—**perichondrial** adj.

**pericolic** adj around the colon, such as a *pericolic abscess* that can occur in diverticulitis.

**pericranium** n the periosteal covering of the cranium—**pericranial** adj.

**pericystitis** n inflammation involving the tissues surrounding the bladder. ⇒ pelvic inflammatory disease.

**perifollicular** adj around a follicle.

**perihepatitis** n inflammation involving the capsule of the liver and surrounding tissues.

**perilymph** n the fluid contained in the inner ear, between the membranous and bony labyrinth. ⇒ endolymph.

**perimenopause** n the period of time, characterized by increasing irregularity of the menstrual cycle and menopausal symptoms such as hot flushes, that occurs before the menopause (the last menstrual period), and the year following the last menstrual period.

**perimetritis** n inflammation of the outer layer of the uterus—the perimetrium.

**perimetrium** n the peritoneal covering of the uterus—**perimetrial** adj.

**perimetry** n measurement and documentation of the field of vision.

**perimolysis** n the mechanical wearing down of tooth enamel, or the damage caused by chemicals. For instance, the frequent vomiting and exposure to acid vomit in eating disorders.

**perimysium** n the fibrous connective tissue that covers a bundle of muscle fibres. ⇒ endomysium, epimysium.

**perinatal** adj pertaining to the period around birth. The weeks before a birth, the birth and the week following. ⇒ mortality.

**perineal body** the wedge-shaped mass of muscle and fascia situated between the scrotum and rectum in males and between the vagina and rectum in females. ⇒ perineum.

**perineal tear** a spontaneous tear occurring in the perineum during childbirth. They are classified in degrees. *first-degree tear* a tear that only affects the fourchette; *second-degree tear* one that involves the fourchette and the superficial muscles of the perineum (e.g. transverse perineal muscles); *third-degree tear* more extensive, with damage as before plus damage to the anal sphincter; and *fourth-degree tear* one in which the tear involves all the structures as before but extends to involve the rectal mucosa.

**perineometer** n a pressure gauge inserted into the vagina to register the strength of contraction in the pelvic floor muscles.

**perineoplasty** n a plastic operation to enlarge the vaginal introitus.

**perineorrhaphy** n a surgical procedure for the suture of a perineal tear, an incision or defect.

**perineotomy** n episiotomy.

**perinephric** adj surrounding the kidney. *perinephric abscess* an abscess in the fat around the kidney; it is usually secondary to an abscess within the kidney tissue.

**perineum** n the area of the body, which extends backwards from the pubic arch to the end of the coccyx and is bounded laterally by the ischial tuberosities. It is formed from the muscles and fascia situated at the pelvic outlet, and can be divided into the anterior urogenital triangle and the posterior anal triangle. It overlies the levator ani and coccygeus muscles of the pelvic floor and helps to support the pelvic structures—**perineal** adj. ⇒ perineal body.

**perineurium** n connective tissue enclosing a bundle of nerve fibres. ⇒ endoneurium, epineurium.

**periodic breathing** a period of apnoea in a newborn baby of 5–10 s followed by a period of hyperventilation at a rate of 50–60 breaths/min, for a period of 10–15 s. The overall respiratory rate remains between 30 and 40 breaths/min.

**periodization** n a planned variation to a training programme over a period of time, so that the athlete/sportsperson achieves optimal adaptive potential just before the race, game or other event.

**periodontal disease** ⇒ periodontitis.

**periodontal ligament** the system of connective tissue fibres that attach the root of the tooth to the alveolar bone.

**periodontal pockets** an abnormal deepening of the gingival sulcus as supporting tissues are lost.

**periodontics** n branch of dentistry concerned with prevention and treatment of diseases of the supporting tissues of the teeth.

**periodontitis** n inflammatory disease of the periodontium, resulting in destruction of the periodontal ligament.

**periodontium** *n* collective name given to the tissues supporting a tooth and comprising the gingivae, periodontal ligament, cementum and surrounding alveolar bone.

**periodontometer** *n* an instrument used to measure the degree of movement in a tooth.

**perioperative** *adj* refers to the period during which a surgical operation is carried out, as well as to the pre- and postoperative periods.

**perioral** *adj* around the mouth.

**periosteum** *n* the membrane which covers a bone. In long bones only the shaft as far as the epiphysis is covered. It protects and allows regeneration—**periosteal** *adj*. ⇒ endosteum.

**periostitis** *n* inflammation of the periosteum. *diffuse periostitis* that involving the periosteum of long bones. *haemorrhagic periostitis* that accompanied by bleeding between the periosteum and the bone.

**peripartum** *n* at the time of delivery. A precise word for what is more commonly called perinatal.

**peripheral** *adj* relating to the outer parts of any structure.

**peripheral blood mononuclear cells (PBMC)** the group of leucocytes that includes all the monocytes and lymphocytes, but excludes granulocytes.

**peripheral nervous system (PNS)** that part of the nervous system outside the central nervous system. It includes all the motor and sensory peripheral nerve fibres and ganglia that are outside the brain and spinal cord. The PNS comprises 12 pairs of cranial nerves and 33 pairs of spinal nerves. The PNS can be further subdivided into the sensory division and the motor division. The latter is in turn divided into the voluntary somatic nervous system and the involuntary autonomic system, which is divided into the sympathetic and parasympathetic nervous systems. Sometimes the term PNS is applied to those nerves that supply the musculoskeletal system and surrounding tissues, to differentiate it from the autonomic nervous system.

**peripheral neuropathy** a disease affecting the peripheral nerves. Also called polyneuropathy or multiple neuropathy. ⇒ neuropathy, polyneuropathy.

**peripheral resistance (PR)** the resistance to blood flow exerted by the arteriolar walls; it is an important factor in the control of normal blood pressure.

**peripheral vascular disease (PVD)** any abnormal condition arising in the blood vessels outside the heart, the main one being atherosclerosis. Associated with smoking, diabetes and hypertension. It is characterized by aching in the calf or buttock during exercise, eventual rest pain, numbness, diminished or absent pulses distal to the diseased area, pallor and cooling of the skin and areas with no hair growth. It can lead to thrombosis and occlusion of the vessel that can result in gangrene and the need for amputation. ⇒ claudication.

**peripheral vision** being able to see objects at the outer edge of the visual field, that area surrounding the central field of vision.

**periphlebitis** *n* inflammation around a vein.

**periportal** *adj* surrounding the hepatic portal vein.

**perirenal** *adj* around the kidney.

**perisplenitis** *n* inflammation of the peritoneal coat of the spleen and of the adjacent structures.

**peristalsis** *n* a rhythmic wave-like contraction and dilatation occurring in the smooth (involuntary) muscle of a hollow structure, e.g. ureter, gastrointestinal tract. In the intestine it is the movement by which the contents (food and waste) are propelled along the lumen. It consists of a wave of contraction preceded by a wave of relaxation—**peristaltic** *adj*.

**peritomy** *n* incision of the conjunctiva around the corneal limbus.

**peritoneal dialysis** a form of dialysis in which the peritoneum is the diffusible semipermeable membrane, and synthetic fluid is inserted into, and removed along with toxins, nitrogenous waste, excess fluid and electrolytes from, the peritoneal cavity via a catheter. Different techniques exist, such as automated peritoneal dialysis and continuous ambulatory peritoneal dialysis.

**peritoneal lavage** irrigation of the peritoneal cavity for diagnosis, such as obtaining cells for examination; or as treatment for infection.

**peritoneoscopy** *n* ⇒ laparoscopy.

**peritoneum** *n* the delicate serous membrane which lines the abdominal and pelvic cavities (parietal layer) and also covers some of the organs (visceral layer) contained in them (Figure P.5)—**peritoneal** *adj*. ⇒ mesentery, omentum.

**peritonitis** *n* inflammation of the peritoneum, usually secondary to disease of one of the abdominal or pelvic organs but it may be caused by blood-borne micro-organisms, such as tubercular peritonitis. It may be bacterial (e.g. following perforation of the bowel) or chemical (e.g. in pancreatitis or a perforated peptic ulcer) in nature.

P

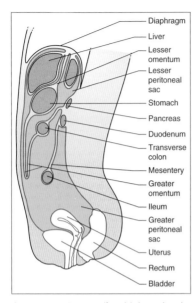

**Figure P.5** Peritoneum (female) *(reproduced from Watson 2000 with permission).*

**peritonsillar abscess (quinsy)** abscess formation in the loose tissue around the palatine tonsil, it may occur as a complication of tonsillitis. It is characterized by a very sore throat, high temperature, dysphagia, otalgia, voice changes and sometimes trismus (unable to open the mouth). Management includes incision and drainage or aspiration of the abscess, which will relieve the pressure and pain but vitally reduces the risk that the airway will become blocked, and intravenous antibiotics. It may also involve the immediate removal of the acutely infected tonsils, but usually tonsillectomy is undertaken when the infection has subsided.

**peritrichous** *adj* applied to a bacterium that has flagella on all sides of the cell. ⇒ *Bacillus*.

**periumbilical** *adj* surrounding the umbilicus.

**periurethral** *adj* surrounding the urethra, such as a periurethral abscess.

**perivascular** *adj* around a blood vessel.

**perlèche** *n* lip licking. An intertrigo at the angles of the mouth with maceration, fissuring or crust formation. May result from use of poorly fitting dentures, bacterial and fungal

infection, vitamin deficiency, drooling or thumb sucking.

**permeability** *n* in physiology, the extent to which substances dissolved in the body fluids are able to move through cell membranes or layers of cells (e.g. the walls of capillaries or absorptive tissues).

**pernicious** *adj* highly destructive, tending to a fatal outcome without effective treatment. *Addisonian pernicious anaemia* (PA) a type of megaloblastic, macrocytic anaemia specifically caused by a deficiency of gastric intrinsic factor required for the absorption of vitamin $B_{12}$. It is characterized by the signs of anaemia, mild jaundice, glossitis, paraesthesia, weakness and in severe cases the development of subacute combined degeneration of the (spinal) cord. ⇒ anaemia.

**perniosis** *n* chronic chilblains.

**peromelia** *n* a teratogenic malformation of a limb.

**peroneal nerve** the common peroneal nerve is a branch of the sciatic nerve. It divides into the superficial peroneal (musculocutaneous) and the deep peroneal (anterior tibial) nerves, which innervate the muscles and skin of the front of the leg and dorsum of the foot and toes. ⇒ Appendix 1, Figure 11.

**peroneus longus** superficial lateral muscle of the leg. Its origin is on the upper fibula and it inserts with a long tendon on to the first metatarsal and the medial cuneiform bones. Contraction of the muscle plantar flexes and everts the foot. ⇒ Appendix 1, Figures 4 and 5.

**peroneus muscles** muscles of the lateral compartment of the leg. *peroneus brevis* muscle under the *p. longus*. Its origin is on the shaft of the fibula and it inserts with a tendon on to the fifth metatarsal bone. Contraction of the muscle plantar flexes and everts the foot.

**peroral** *adj* through the mouth.

**peroxisome** *n* minute bodies present in kidney and liver cells. They contain several enzymes, including peroxidase, catalase and oxidases. They may be involved in oxidation reactions involving hydrogen peroxide, and in gluconeogenesis and in lipid and purine metabolism.

**PERRLA** *abbr* pupils equal, round, react to light, accommodation.

**perseveration** *n* constant repetition of words or phrases. Seen in organic brain disease. ⇒ delirium, dementia.

**persistent vegetative state (PVS)** a completely dependent state caused by irreparable damage to the cerebral cortex, but in which the vital functions of the brainstem continue. The person, who appears to be awake, neither responds nor is able to initiate any voluntary action.

**personal activities of daily living (PADL)** include activities such as washing and dressing.

**personality** *n* the various mental attitudes, traits and characteristics which distinguish a person. The sum total of the mental make-up. ⇒ psychopathic personality.

**personality disorder** a disturbance of personality together with deeply ingrained maladaptive behavioural patterns established by late adolescence/early adulthood resulting in personal and social difficulties.

**personal protective equipment (PPE)** equipment, such as eye protection, masks, gloves and aprons, used in standard precautions. ⇒ standard precautions.

**perspiration** *n* the excretion from the sweat glands through the skin pores. *insensible perspiration* the water lost by evaporation through the skin surface other than by sweating. It is significantly increased in inflamed skin. *sensible perspiration* the term used when there are visible drops of sweat on the skin.

**Perthes' disease** (*syn* pseudocoxalgia) ⇒ Legg–Calvé–Perthes disease.

**pertussis** *n* (*syn* whooping cough) a serious infectious respiratory disease caused by the bacterium *Bordetella pertussis*. It is spread by droplets and has an incubation period of 7–14 days. It is characterized by conjunctivitis, rhinitis, dry cough and later bouts of paroxysmal coughing with a 'whoop' and vomiting. Complications may include pneumonia, bronchiectasis and convulsions. Active immunization is available as part of the routine programme in infancy.

**pes** *n* a foot or foot-like structure.

**PESA** *abbr* percutaneous epididymal sperm aspiration.

**pes cavus (high arched foot)** (*syn* clawfoot) a pathological elevation of the longitudinal arch caused by plantar flexion of the forefoot relative to the rearfoot. The medial longitudinal arch is most affected but the lateral longitudinal arch can also be elevated. There is dorsal humping of the midfoot and associated forefoot and rearfoot deformities. These may include clawing or retraction of the lesser toes, a trigger first toe, and a depressed first metatarsal with either heel varus or equinus. It may be congenital or acquired.

**pes planus** (*syn* flat-foot) a generic term for a foot with an abnormally low arch. The medial longitudinal arch is depressed or absent, and the foot has an increased contact area with the ground. During weight-bearing the foot appears to have no longitudinal arch. It may be congenital or acquired. When young children first stand the feet appear to be flat, as adipose tissue under the medial longitudinal arch is pressed close to the ground. Older children very frequently have flattening of the medial longitudinal arch on standing but the arch reappears on standing on tiptoe (a mobile flat foot). *flexible pes planus* generally asymptomatic in children but may become a semirigid condition in adulthood. It has been linked with excess laxity of the joint capsule and the ligaments supporting the arch, which allows it to collapse when weight is applied. *rigid pes planus* in adults may be a progression from flexible to semirigid to rigid as part of the ageing process. Structural changes due to the existing abnormal position become fixed, as soft and osseous tissues adapt. Rigidity is increased where there are significant osteoarthritic changes or inflammatory arthritic destruction.

**pessary** *n* **1.** a device inserted into the vagina to correct uterine displacements. A *ring* or *shelf pessary* is used to support a prolapse. A *Hodge pessary* is used to correct a retroverted uterus. **2.** a suppository containing a medication inserted into the vagina.

**PET** *acron* **p**ositron **e**mission **t**omography.

**petechia** *n* a small, haemorrhagic spot—**petechiae** *pl*, **petechial** *adj*.

**petit mal** minor epilepsy. ⇒ epilepsy.

**pétrissage** *n* rhythmical massage manipulations of muscle and other soft tissues where pressure is used to help venous and lymphatic drainage and to mobilize skin and connective tissue. It may be slow and deep to produce relaxation and reduce spasm, or brisk to invigorate. The manipulation may be performed with one hand alone, or with both hands working alternately.

**petrositis** *n* inflammation involving the petrous portion of the temporal bone.

**petrous** *adj* resembling stone.

**Peutz–Jeghers syndrome** (J Peutz, Dutch physician, 1886–1957; H Jeghers, American physician, 1904–1990) a type of familial adenomatous polyposis inherited as an autosomal dominant trait. It is characterized by excessive melanin production and pigmentation in the skin and mucosa (typically in the mouth)

**P**

and the presence of many hamartomas, usually in the small bowel, but they also occur in the colon. It is associated with intussusception and bleeding into the bowel. People with the syndrome may have gastrointestinal cancers, and also have a tendency to develop cancers elsewhere, such as the pancreas, lung, testes, ovaries and breast. ⊙DVD

**Peyer's patches** (J Peyer, Swiss anatomist, 1653–1712) part of mucosa-associated lymphoid tissue. Aggregates of lymphatic tissue situated in the ileum. Function to prevent micro-organisms entering the blood. Site of infection in typhoid fever.

**Peyronie's disease** (F de la Peyronie, French surgeon, 1678–1747) deformity and painful erection of penis due to fibrous tissue formation from unknown cause. Can be associated with Dupuytren's contracture. ⇒ Nesbit's operation.

**PFI** *abbr* private finance initiative.

**PGD** *abbr* preimplantation genetic diagnosis.

**PGDRS** *abbr* psychogeriatric dependency rating scale.

**PGH** *abbr* preimplantation genetic haplotyping.

**pH** *abbr* hydrogen ion concentration, expressed as a negative logarithm. A neutral solution has a pH 7.0. With increasing acidity the pH falls and with increasing alkalinity it rises.

**phacoemulsification** *n* (*syn* pakoemulsification) ultrasonic vibration is used to liquefy nuclear lens fibres. The liquid lens matter is then sucked out in an action similar to that of a vacuum cleaner.

**phaeochromocytoma** *n* (*syn* paraganglioma) a condition in which there is a tumour of the adrenal medulla, or of the structurally similar tissues associated with the sympathetic chain. It secretes adrenaline (epinephrine) and allied hormones and the symptoms are due to the excess of these substances. Results in hypertensive crises, with associated headache, flushing and tachycardia.

**phage typing** identifying bacterial strains by their bacteriophages.

**phagocyte** *n* a cell capable of engulfing bacteria and other particulate material such as cell debris Examples of phagocytic cells include neutrophils and macrophages—**phagocytic** *adj.*

**phagocytosis** *n* the process by which phagocytic cells engulf particles such as bacteria (Figure P.6).

**phagomania** *n* also called sitomania. An abnormal obsession with food.

**phagophobia** *n* also called sitophobia. An abnormal fear of food.

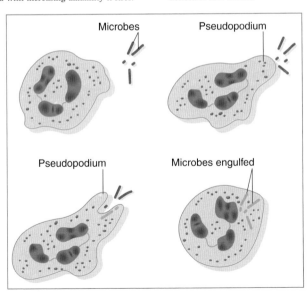

Microbes    Pseudopodium

Pseudopodium    Microbes engulfed

**Figure P.6** Phagocytosis *(reproduced from Waugh & Grant 2006 with permission).*

**phalanges** *n* the 14 small bones that form the fingers on each hand or the toes on each foot. (⇒ Appendix 1, Figures 2 and 3)—**phalanx** *sing*, **phalangeal** *adj*.

**phalloplasty** *n* plastic operation on the penis. Undertaken to correct congenital defects, such as hypospadias, or after injury.

**phallus** *n* the penis—**phallic** *adj*.

**phantasy** *n* ⇒ fantasy.

**phantom limb pain/syndrome** the sensation that a limb is still attached to the body after it has been amputated. Pain may seem to come from the amputated limb. It is neuropathic pain, a type of chronic non-malignant pain. The pain is experienced because of altered pain processing by the nervous system, possibly caused by previous tissue or nerve damage. Effective pain relief before amputation is important in minimizing the risk of developing phantom limb pain. ⇒ chronic pain, neuropathic pain.

**phantom pregnancy** (*syn* pseudocyesis) signs and symptoms simulating those of early pregnancy; it may occur in a childless woman who has an overwhelming desire to have a child.

**pharmaceutical** *adj* relating to drugs.

**pharmacist** *n* a person who is qualified and registered to dispense drugs. Pharmacists also provide advice and information for other health professionals and the public.

**pharmacodynamics** *n* the study of how a drug acts in a living system and how it alters cell metabolism to exert its effects. This includes how the drug binds to cell receptor proteins: the specificity of the receptor for the drug; and its affinity for the drug, which influences the dose required to have an effect.

**pharmacokinetics** *n* the study of the way the body deals with a drug over time. It considers drug absorption, distribution around the body, metabolism and excretion. Each of these processes occurs at a specific rate characteristic for that drug, and the overall action of the drug (be it therapeutic or toxic) will be dependent on these processes. A number of factors can influence the pharmacokinetics of a drug and so alter its effect on the body. For example, drug absorption is affected by the formulation of the drug, the gastrointestinal contents and motility. Drug distribution depends on blood flow to the tissues, obstacles such as the blood–brain barrier that make it difficult for drugs to enter the central nervous system and plasma protein binding. Enzymes within the liver carry out drug metabolism, and as there is considerable genetic variation in liver enzymes, the ability to metabolize drugs can vary significantly from one person to another. The presence of other drugs can also affect the rate of metabolism, either speeding it up or slowing it down. Drugs are mainly eliminated by the kidneys and are particularly affected by glomerular filtration rate, which decreases with age and disease.

**pharmacology** *n* the science dealing with drugs, their properties, uses and effects at their cell receptor proteins—**pharmacological** *adj*, **pharmacologically** *adv*.

**pharmacopoeia** *n* an authorized book detailing drugs available for prescribing in a specific country, such as the British Pharmacopoeia (BP) or United States Pharmacopoeia.

**pharmacy** *n* **1.** the place where drugs are prepared and dispensed. **2.** the science of preparing drugs.

**pharmacy-only medicine (P)** in the UK, medicines that may be bought by the public from a pharmacy but only when a pharmacist is in attendance.

**pharmafoods** *npl* ⇒ functional foods.

**pharyngeal pouch** pathological dilatation of the lower part of the pharynx.

**pharyngeal reflex** ⇒ gag.

**pharyngectomy** *n* surgical removal of the pharynx (partial or total), such as for cancer.

**pharyngismus** *n* spasm of the pharynx.

**pharyngitis** *n* inflammation of the pharynx, which may be acute or chronic. Acute pharyngitis leads to a sore, dry throat and pain on swallowing. Causes include tonsillitis, streptococcal infections, herpes and diphtheria.

**pharyngolaryngeal** *adj* pertaining to the pharynx and larynx.

**pharyngolaryngectomy** *n* surgical removal of the pharynx and larynx, such as for laryngeal cancer.

**pharyngoplasty** *n* any plastic operation to the pharynx.

**pharyngoscope** *n* an endoscope used to examine the pharynx.

**pharyngotomy** *n* a surgical opening into the pharynx.

**pharyngotympanic tube** (*syn* eustachian or auditory tube) a canal, partly bony, partly cartilaginous, connecting the pharynx with the tympanic cavity (⇒ Appendix 1, Figure 13). It allows air to pass into the middle ear, so that the air pressure is kept even on both sides of the eardrum.

**pharynx** *n* the cavity at the back of the mouth (⇒ Appendix 1, Figures 6 and 14).

**P**

It is cone-shaped and is lined with mucous membrane; at the lower end it opens into the oesophagus. The pharyngotympanic (eustachian or auditory) tubes pierce its lateral walls and the posterior nares pierce its anterior wall. The larynx lies immediately below it and in front of the oesophagus—**pharyngeal** *adj*.

**PHC** *abbr* primary health care.

**phenol** *n* (*syn* carbolic acid) a powerful disinfectant. Phenolic disinfectants are used in suitable dilution for environmental use. They are toxic and corrosive.

**phenothiazines** *npl* a group of typical antipsychotic drugs (neuroleptics), e.g. chlorpromazine. ⇒ tardive dyskinesia. ⇒ Appendix 5.

**phenotype** *n* the observable physical characteristics of an organism that result from the interaction between its genotype (genetic make-up) and environment. ⇒ genotype.

**phenylalanine** *n* an essential (indispensable) amino acid required for growth and development during infancy and childhood, and for cell repair and growth during adulthood. Individuals who lack the enzyme required for its metabolism develop phenylketonuria.

**phenylketonuria (PKU)** *n* metabolites of phenylalanine (e.g. phenylketones) excreted in the urine. Occurs in hyperphenylalaninaemia, owing to the lack of, or inactivity of, the liver enzyme phenylalanine hydroxylase that normally converts dietary phenylalanine into tyrosine (a non-essential [dispensable] amino acid). The enzyme defect is inherited as an autosomal recessive disease. The presence of high levels of phenylalanine are especially toxic to the developing brain. In the absence of treatment individuals will have a learning disability, eczema, their urine and skin will have a 'mousy' odour, and, because they lack tyrosine, which is needed for pigmentation, they will have very fair hair. Thus routine screening for phenylketonuria is undertaken in newborns, as early detection allows for the introduction of a modified formula milk that is low in phenylalanine to prevent damage to the brain. The diet, low in phenylalanine, and regular monitoring of phenylketone levels in the blood were previously continued until brain development was complete, but many physicians recommend that a low-phenylalanine diet be followed for life. Whichever regimen is followed, women with phenylketonuria planning to become pregnant are advised to recommence the low-phenylalanine diet prior to conception and during pregnancy to protect the developing fetus—**phenylketonuric** *adj*.

**pheromones** *npl* chemicals with a specific odour. They are present in the sweat produced by the apocrine sweat glands. They are involved in communication and influence sexual behaviour.

**Philadelphia chromosome (Ph[1])** an anomaly of chromosome number 22. It is found in the blood cells of most people with chronic myeloid leukaemia.

**philtrum** *n* the vertical indentation present at the midline of the upper lip.

**phimosis** *n* tightness of the prepuce so that it cannot be retracted over the glans penis.

**phlebectomy** *n* excision of a vein. *multiple cosmetic phlebectomy (MCP)* removal of varicose veins through little stab incisions which heal without scarring.

**phlebitis** *n* inflammation of a vein—**phlebitic** *adj*. ⇒ thrombophlebitis.

**phlebography** *n* ⇒ venography.

**phlebolith** *n* a concretion that forms in a vein.

**phlebothrombosis** *n* a blood clot or thrombus in a vein. ⇒ deep-vein thrombosis, embolism, pulmonary embolus.

**phlebotomist** *n* a technician who is trained to take blood samples from patients.

*Phlebotomus* *n* a genus of sandfly. They transmit the parasite of leishmaniasis in old-world countries. Some species of *Phlebotomus* are vectors for the arboviruses that cause a variety of diseases including phlebotomus fever (sandfly fever) and the bacterium that causes bartonellosis.

**phlebotomus fever** also called Pappataci fever or sandfly fever. An acute viral infection caused by several arboviruses, it occurs in hot regions that include Central Asia, Central and South America and some areas around the Mediterranean. Humans become infected by a bite from an infected sandfly. It is characterized by pyrexia, headache, conjunctivitis, muscle pain and sometimes a rash. The disease is self-limiting and treatment is symptomatic only, such as fluids and mild analgesics.

**phlebotomy** *n* ⇒ venesection, venotomy.

**phlegm** *n* lay term for sputum. Mucus expectorated (coughed up) from the bronchi.

**phlegmasia alba dolans** also known as white leg or milk leg. Phlebitis affecting the femoral vein that leads to a swollen, white and painful leg. Sometimes occurs after childbirth or an acute illness with high temperature.

**phlegmatic** *adj* describes a person who is emotionally stable.

**phlyctenule** *n* a small inflammatory nodule which occurs on conjunctiva or cornea close to the corneal limbus.

**phlyctenulosis** *n* eye disease characterized by phlyctenules.

**phobia** *n* a morbid fear. An irrational, focused fear of an object, state or event, which causes the person to feel anxious. Specific phobias include those in respect of spiders or mice, acrophobia, agoraphobia, claustrophobia, dysmorphophobia, nyctophobia, etc.—**phobic** *adj*.

**phocomelia** *n* teratogenic malformation. Arms and feet attached directly to trunk giving a seal-like appearance. Many cases in the 1960s were associated with the use of the drug thalidomide during pregnancy.

**phonation** *n* voice production by vibration of the vocal cords.

**phonocardiography** *n* the graphic recording of heart sounds and murmurs by electric reproduction. The fetal heart rate and its relation to uterine contraction can be measured continuously. ⇒ cardiotocography—**phonocardiographic** *adj*, **phonocardiogram** *n*, **phonocardiograph** *n*, **phonocardiographically** *adv*.

**phonophobia** *n* a dislike of noise in general such as during an attack of migraine, or a dislike or hypersensitivity to certain sounds.

**phoria** *n* latent strabismus. May be used as a suffix.

**phosphatases** *npl* enzymes needed to catalyse the reactions concerning phosphate esters, e.g. nucleotides, carbohydrate metabolism, phospholipids. Phosphatases are present in a variety of tissues, including the blood, bone, liver, kidney, prostate gland and semen. ⇒ acid phosphatase, alkaline phosphatase.

**phosphates** *npl* salts or esters of phosphoric acid. A component of food, such as some proteins. Phosphates are present in various tissues (e.g. bone). They are vital in physiological processes, including: adenosine diphosphate (ADP) and adenosine triphosphate (ATP) that function in the reactions that produce and store energy; and in the nucleotides that are part of the nucleic acids.

**phosphatidylcholines** *npl* phospholipids, also known as lecithins.

**phosphatidylserine** *n* a phospholipid found in the brain.

**phosphaturia** *n* excess phosphates in the urine—**phosphaturic** *adj*.

**phosphocreatine** *n* creatine phosphate. ⇒ creatine.

**phosphofructokinase** *n* 6-phosphofructokinase. An important phosphorylase enzyme, which catalyses the phosphorylation of fructose-6-phosphate to fructose-1,6-diphosphate by adenosine triphosphate (ATP). The reaction, which is irreversible, is a key stage during glycolysis. The enzyme controls the rate of glycolysis.

**phospholipids** *npl* organic molecules comprising a lipid plus nitrogen and phosphate groups, vital in the formation of the cell (plasma) membrane.

**phosphonecrosis** *n* tissue destruction, usually involving the jaw bone ('phossy jaw'). It is caused by exposure to phosphorus, such as may occur during an industrial process and is designated as an industrial disease. It was a problem for people working without proper protection in the match industry during the 19th century and early 20th century. The phosphorus toxicity eventually caused organ failure and death.

**phosphoproteins** *npl* proteins that contain phosphates in their structure.

**phosphorus (P)** *n* a poisonous element. Forms an important constituent (as phosphates) of nucleic acids, bone and all cells. *phosphorus-32 ($^{32}$P)* radioactive phosphorus used in the treatment of thrombocythaemia.

**phosphorylases** *npl* a group of enzymes needed for the addition of phosphate groups to other molecules, e.g. phosphofructokinase concerned with glucose metabolism.

**phosphorylation** *n* the metabolic process of introducing a phosphate group into an organic molecule.

**photalgia** *n* pain in the eyes caused by bright light, such as the effect of sunlight on snow.

**photoablation** *n* the destruction of tissue achieved by the use of light, including laser. It can be used in the surgical correction of refractive errors and in some corneal conditions. It is one method used for endometrial ablation in which a laser is used to destroy the basal layer of the endometrium.

**photochemical** *adj* chemically reactive in the presence of light.

**photochemotherapy** *n* ⇒ photodynamic therapy.

**photocoagulation** *n* burning of the tissues with a powerful, focused light source. It may be used in the treatment of retinopathies where leaky vessels can be sealed and diseased areas on the retina destroyed, and to seal a detached retina.

**photodermatosis** *n* a skin condition caused by exposure to light.

**photodynamic therapy (PDT)** sometimes called photochemotherapy. It is a treatment that utilizes a photosensitizer drug or agent, which, when activated by a specific wavelength of light, produces a type of oxygen that is capable of killing nearby cells. It is used to destroy cancer cells in conditions that include: basal cell carcinoma of the skin, bladder cancer, oesophageal cancer and some types of lung cancer. PDT is used in both curative and palliative treatments. The photosensitizer is injected intravenously and is taken up by cells, but remains in cancerous cells longer than normal cells. In the next step the cancer cells are exposed to the specific wavelength of light often by use of a laser. The photosensitizer produces the form of oxygen which destroys the cancer cells. The light source may be directed at the surface of the body for some cancers, or laser light is applied using an endoscope in other cancers, such as bladder or lung cancer. The use of PDT causes photosensitivity in the skin and eyes for around 6 weeks after treatment and patients are advised to avoid exposure to sunlight or bright lights during this time. Research continues into further applications for PDT.

**photoendoscope** *n* an endoscope incorporating a camera, thus allowing a permanent record of clinical findings to be made—**photoendoscopic** *adj*, **photoendoscopy** *n*, **photoendoscopically** *adv*.

**photomicrograph** *n* a photographic image of an object viewed with an electron microscope.

**photophobia** *n* dislike of bright light, usually associated with eye pain, such as in migraine and meningism—**photophobic** *adj*.

**photophthalmia** *n* inflammation of the eye caused by exposure to excessively bright light.

**photopic vision** vision in bright light. That occurring in daylight involving the retinal cone photoreceptor cells.

**photopsia** *n* the perception of flashes of light. Associated with retinal tears or detachment, migraine aura and vitreous body detachment.

**photoretinitis** *n* inflammation of the retina caused by exposure to intense light, such as looking directly at the sun. It can cause permanent damage and impaired vision.

**photosensitive** *adj* reactive to light.

**photosensitivity** *n* an exaggerated inflammatory reaction of the skin in response to light.

**phototherapy** *n* literally any treatment that involves the use of light, such as exposure to white light for seasonal affective disorder, or ultraviolet light for psoriasis. Generally refers to exposure to artificial blue light, most commonly for treatment of jaundice in neonates. Effectiveness most likely due to its ability to convert bilirubin to water-soluble forms that are easily excreted.

**phren** *n* the diaphragm—**phrenic** *adj*.

**phrenic nerve** a mixed nerve that arises from the cervical nerve roots 3–5. It supplies motor fibres to the diaphragm which stimulate contraction during inspiration, and also innervates the pleura and pericardium.

**phrenicotomy** *n* division of the phrenic nerve to paralyse one-half of the diaphragm.

**phrenoplegia** *n* paralysis of the diaphragm—**phrenoplegic** *adj*.

**phrynoderma** *n* 'toad skin'. Hyperkeratosis of the hair follicles that leads to rough, raised papules on the skin. It is possible that a deficiency of vitamins and fatty acids is responsible, but it also occurs in the absence of nutritional deficiencies.

**phthiriasis** *n* infestation with the pubic louse, *Phthirus pubis*. Most commonly transmitted by sexual contact, but non-sexual acquisition of the insect is also possible.

**phylloquinone** *n* a member of the vitamin K family of compounds found in green vegetables.

**physical abuse** ⇒ abuse, non-accidental injury.

**physical activity level (PAL)** the ratio of daily physical energy expenditure to basal metabolic rate (BMR). This factor reflects the average activity both at work and at leisure and is used to estimate average energy requirement. Average energy requirement = PAL × BMR. Examples of PALs for population groups are estimated to be: 1.4 for inactive men and women, 1.6 for moderately active women, and 1.7 for moderately active men.

**physical activity ratio (PAR)** the ratio of the energy cost of a specific activity to the basal metabolic rate (BMR). Factors range from 1 for complete rest to 9 for very vigorous sporting activities, and are used to estimate the energy requirement of a specific activity.

**physician** *n* a qualified and registered medical practitioner who practises medicine rather than surgery.

**physicochemical** *adj* relating to physics and chemistry, or to physical and chemical properties or characteristics.

**physiological** *adj* often used to describe a normal process or structure, to distinguish it from an abnormal or pathological feature (e.g. the physiological level of glucose in the blood).

**physiological advantage** a muscle's ability to shorten. Its greatest physiological advantage is when a muscle is at rest.

**physiological solution** a fluid isotonic with the body fluids and containing similar salts. ⇒ hypertonic, hypotonic, isotonic.

**physiology** *n* the science dealing with normal functioning of the body—**physiological** *adj*, **physiologically** *adv*.

**physiotherapy** *n* traditionally describes treatment to improve, restore and sometimes cure, using manipulation, electrotherapy, and exercise therapy and rehabilitation following injury or disease, e.g. stroke. Contemporarily, it also includes assessment and diagnosis, health promotion and education, and prevention of disability. ⇒ extended-scope physiotherapy practitioners.

**phytase** *n* a phosphatase enzyme that catalyses the hydrolysis of phytate to inositol and phosphate.

**phytate inositol polyphosphate** a substance present in plants which binds some metal ions such as ferrous iron, zinc, etc., thus reducing the bioavailability of these ions for intestinal absorption from the food. This may be a problem in certain groups, such as strict vegetarians and vegans, who may become deficient in minerals leading to iron-deficiency anaemia and other problems.

**phytates, phytic acid** chemicals present in wholegrain cereals. They can decrease intestinal absorption of some minerals, e.g. calcium, zinc and iron.

**phytoagglutinins** *npl* ⇒ lectins.

**phyto-oestrogens** *npl* chemicals with oestrogen-like effects (oestrogenic) and antioestrogenic effects that originate in plants that include soya beans, soya products such as tofu and flax seed. Phyto-oestrogens comprise mainly flavonoids, e.g. isoflavones, with some non-flavonoids such as lignans.

**phytophotodermatitis** *n* a type of contact dermatitis that is caused by exposure to a phototoxin present in certain plants such as members of the Umbelliferae family (e.g. cow parsley and the wild parsnip). The phototoxin results from a reaction between light-sensitive chemicals, such as psoralens, in the plant and ultraviolet light. The dermatitis is characterized by burning rather than itching, redness, possible blistering and secondary areas of hyperpigmentation.

**phytotherapy** *n* phytomedicine, herbal medicine. The use of plant material or plant extracts as remedies that promote health, prevent disorders and in the treatment of disorders. In addition, there are numerous examples of the use of medicines from plant sources in conventional western medical practice, such as taxanes (cytotoxic drugs derived from the yew tree) in some countries St John's wort is prescribed by conventionally qualified doctors for depressive illness. ⇒ herbalism.

**phytotoxin** *n* toxic substances present in plants, including those used for food, wild plants and those cultivated in gardens. Examples include oxalic acid and oxalates in rhubarb leaves, cardiac glycosides in foxgloves, ricin in the castor oil plant and hemlock.

**PIs** *abbr* performance indicators.

**pia mater** the innermost of the meninges; the delicate, vascular membrane which lies in close contact with the brain and spinal cord.

**pica** *n* a desire for extraordinary or abnormal types of food. Seen in pregnancy. Also known as allotriophagy, cissa and cittosis.

**PICC** *abbr* peripherally inserted central catheter.

**Pick's disease 1.** (A Pick, Czech neurologist/ psychiatrist, 1851–1924) a type of cerebral atrophy producing dementia during midlife (between 40 and 60 years of age). There is degeneration in the frontal and temporal lobes of the cerebrum. It is characterized by changes in and eventual disintegration of personality and emotions, disinhibited behaviour and changes in attitudes; impaired speech and language deficits, poor concentration, loss of motivation, poor memory and deterioration in cognitive skills and intellect, There is considerable overlap with Alzheimer's disease. **2.** (F Pick, Czech physician, 1867–1926) syndrome of ascites, hepatomegaly, oedema and pleural effusion that occurs with constrictive pericarditis.

**picornavirus** *n* derived from pico (very small) and RNA (ribonucleic acid). Small RNA viruses. Includes the enteroviruses (polio, coxsackie, hepatitis A and echovirus) and the rhinoviruses. They cause diverse diseases that include poliomyelitis, common cold, aseptic meningitis, gastroenteritis, hepatitis A, herpangina, etc. ⇒ virus.

**picture archiving communications system (PACS)** in radiography. A networked system of viewing monitors connected to a central image database that allows integration of image and demographic information.

**PID** *abbr* **1.** pelvic inflammatory disease. **2.** prolapse of an intervertebral disc. ⇒ prolapse.

**piedra** *n* a fungal disease affecting hair. It is characterized by black or white nodules on

**P**

377

the hair. Black piedra affects the scalp hair and is caused by *Piedraia hortae*, a species of the genus *Piedraia*. Species of the genus *Trichosporon* are responsible for white piedra which involves the beard, pubic hair and axillary hair.

**Pierre Robin syndrome** (Pierre Robin, French dental surgeon, 1867–1950) a syndrome of congenital anomalies inherited as an autosomal recessive disorder. Affected infants have micrognathia and a cleft palate, often associated with abnormality of the tongue and larynx. There are feeding difficulties and some infants are at risk of inhaling fluid into the respiratory tract. Management involves protecting the airway, the selection of safe and effective feeding methods, plastic surgery to repair the cleft palate and possibly surgery to enlarge the lower jaw, speech and language therapy and specialist orthodontic treatment.

**pigeon chest** (*syn* pectus carinatum) a narrow chest, bulging anteriorly in the breast bone region.

**piggyback port** a special coupling device in a primary intravenous administration set, which is used for the intermittent administration of a supplementary (piggyback) intravenous solution containing a drug into the primary line.

**pigment** *n* any colouring matter of the body. For example, the visual pigment rhodopsin; melanin in hair, iris, choroid and skin; haemoglobin; stercobilin in faeces; and the bile pigments biliverdin and bilirubin.

**pigmentation** *n* the deposit of pigment, especially when abnormal or excessive, such as the pigmentation associated with Addison's disease, arsenic poisoning, haemochromatosis, melanoma, melanosis coli, naevus, Nelson syndrome, etc.

**Pilates method** (J Pilates, German/American exercise therapist, 1880–1967) a low-impact system of focused body–mind exercises. They aim to tone, stretch, strengthen, improve exercise efficiency and breathing and increase body awareness.

**piles** *npl* ⇒ haemorrhoids.

**pili** *npl* hair-like appendages of many bacteria, and used for the transfer of genetic material—**pilus** *sing*.

**pilomotor nerves** tiny nerves that innervate the arrectores pilorum muscles of the hair follicles, causing the hairs to become erect and give the appearance of 'gooseflesh'.

**pilomotor reflex** the erection of the hairs on the skin causing 'gooseflesh'. It is due to the contraction of the arrectores pilorum muscles in response to cold, emotional arousal and fear.

**pilonidal** *adj* hair-containing.

**pilonidal sinus** an abnormal tract or sinus containing hairs, which is usually found in hirsute people in the cleft between the buttocks, most often situated close to the tip of the coccyx. There is constant irritation and in this situation it is liable to infection and abscess formation. Initial management includes pain relief and antibiotics before wide surgical excision and drainage. The wound is not closed and is allowed to heal by secondary intention using appropriate dressing products, thereby ensuring that the infection is eliminated and recurrence does not occur. ⇒ wound healing.

**pilosebaceous** *adj* pertaining to the hair follicle and the sebaceous gland opening into it. *pilosebaceous unit* comprises the hair follicle, the hair and the associated sebaceous gland.

**pilot study** an early smaller-scale study carried out before the main research project to evaluate viability and to identify problems with the research methodology.

**pimple** *n* ⇒ papule.

**pin index** system designed to prevent the wrong connection of a gas cylinder to an anaesthetic machine.

**pineal body (gland)** also known as the epiphysis cerebri. A tiny reddish-grey conical structure situated above the third ventricle of the brain and attached to it by a stalk. It secretes various substances which include 5-hydroxytryptamine and melatonin. The release of melatonin is influenced by the amount of light entering the eye and varies with the seasons as daylight hours change. Melatonin levels fluctuate during the 24 hours; it is at its highest level during darkness and at its lowest level around midday. Melatonin appears to influence gonadotrophin secretion, diurnal rhythms such as sleep, and mood. ⇒ depression, seasonal affective disorder.

**pinguecula** *n* a yellowish, slightly elevated thickening of the bulbar conjunctiva between the eyelids. Associated with the ageing eye.

**pink disease** ⇒ erythroedema polyneuropathy.

**pink eye** ⇒ conjunctivitis.

**pinna** *n* the auricle. That part of the ear which is external to the head. ⇒ Appendix 1, Figure 13.

**pinnaplasty** *n* a plastic operation on the pinna, such as for the correction of 'bat ears'.

**pinocytosis** *n* the process whereby the plasma membrane engulfs a minute water droplet within a vesicle or vacuole, which is taken into the cell.

**pinta** *n* a mild contagious disease, caused by *Treponema pallidum* (ssp. *carateum*), similar to yaws but confined to Central and South America. It occurs following prolonged and close contact. It is characterized by the formation of a large papule and enlarged lymph nodes; later there is a macular rash and eventually loss of skin pigment. ⇒ bejel, yaws.

**pinworm** *n* threadworm. ⇒ enterobiasis (oxyuriasis), *Enterobius*.

**piriformis** *n* a pyramidal muscle on the posterior part of the hip, situated under the gluteus minimus muscle of the buttock. Its origin is on the anterolateral part of the sacrum and it inserts on the greater trochanter of the femur. Contraction of the muscle laterally rotates the thigh. ⇒ Appendix 1, Figure 5.

**pisiform** *adj* pea-shaped. One of the carpal bones of the wrist. It articulates with the triquetral bone, another carpal. ⇒ Appendix 1, Figure 2.

**pitting** *n* making an indentation, e.g. in the nails as in psoriasis, or in oedematous tissues.

**pituicyte** *n* a type of cell of the posterior lobe of the pituitary gland.

**pituitary gland** (*syn* hypophysis cerebri) a small oval endocrine gland lying in the pituitary fossa of the sphenoid bone (Figure P.7). The anterior lobe (adenohypophysis) produces and secretes several hormones: growth hormone (GH), adrenocorticotrophic hormone (ACTH), thyroid-stimulating hormone (TSH), luteinizing hormone (LH), follicle-stimulating hormone (FSH) and prolactin (PRL), the lactogenic hormone. The posterior lobe (neurohy-

pophysis) stores and secretes oxytocin and antidiuretic hormone (vasopressin or arginine vasopressin [AVP]). These hormones are made by nerve fibres in the hypothalamus.

**pityriasis** *n* scaly (branny) eruption of the skin. *pityriasis alba* a common eruption in children characterized by scaly hypopigmented macules on the cheeks and upper arms. *pityriasis capitis* dandruff. *pityriasis rosea* a slightly scaly eruption of ovoid erythematous lesions which are widespread over the trunk and proximal parts of the limbs. It is a self-limiting condition. *pityriasis rubra pilaris* a chronic skin disease characterized by coalescing red papules of perifollicular distribution. *pityriasis versicolor*, also called 'tinea versicolor', is a yeast infection which causes the appearance of buff-coloured patches on the trunk.

***Pityrosporum*** *n* ⇒ *Malassezia*.

**pivot joint** also known as a trochoid joint. A type of synovial joint in which rotation is the only movement possible. The joint comprises a pivot-like bony process that fits into a ring formed from ligament and bone, and rotates within the ring. Examples include the proximal radioulnar joint, and the joint formed by the peg-like dens of the axis (second cervical vertebra) fitting into the ring formed by part of the atlas (first cervical vertebra) and the transverse ligament.

**PKU** *abbr* phenylketonuria.

**placebo** *n* a harmless substance given as medicine. In a randomized placebo-controlled trial, an inert substance, identical in appearance with the material being tested. When neither the researcher nor the subject knows which is which, the trial is said to be double-blind.

**P**

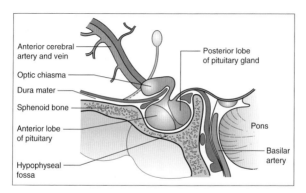

**Figure P.7** Pituitary gland *(reproduced from Watson 2000 with permission).*

*placebo effect* a therapeutic effect which is observed after the administration of a placebo.

**placenta** *n* the afterbirth, a hormone-secreting vascular structure developed and functioning by about the third month of pregnancy and attached to the inner wall of the uterus. It is normally sited in the upper segment of the uterus. The placental hormones include human chorionic gonadotrophin (hCG), human placental lactogen (HPL), oestrogens and progesterone. The maternal surface of the placenta is dark red in colour and lobulated. The fetal surface is covered by amnion; it is white and shiny and it is has branches of the umbilical vessels (Figure P.8). The amnion-covered umbilical vessels (two arteries and a vein) eventually leave the placenta as the umbilical cord, which links the fetus and the placenta. The placenta ensures that the fetus is supplied with nourishment and oxygen and through it the fetus gets rid of waste carbon dioxide and nitrogenous waste products. In normal labour it is expelled, with the fetal membranes, during the third stage of labour. When this does not occur it is termed a *retained placenta* and may be an *adherent placenta*.

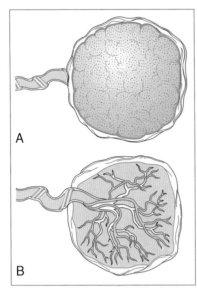

**Figure P.8** Placenta at term: (A) maternal surface; (B) fetal surface *(reproduced from Fraser & Cooper 2003 with permission).*

An abnormally adherent placenta may be: a *placenta accreta* (into the myometrium); a *placenta increta* (into the perimetrium); a *placenta percreta* (through the myometrium)— **placental** *adj*.

**placenta praevia** the placenta is usually attached to the upper segment of the uterus; where part or all of it lies in the lower uterine segment it is called a *placenta praevia*. It may cause placental abruption with painless antepartum vaginal bleeding. A placenta praevia should be considered if there is an unstable lie, non-engagement of the presenting part in a primigravida after 36 weeks' gestation or an abnormal presentation.

**placental abruption** premature placental separation from the uterine wall prior to the delivery of the fetus resulting in haemorrhage.

**placental insufficiency** inefficiency of the placenta. Can occur due to maternal disease or postmaturity of fetus, giving rise to a 'small for dates' baby. ⇒ intrauterine growth restriction/retardation.

**placentography** *n* X-ray examination of the placenta, now superseded by ultrasound.

**plagiocephaly** *n* a congenital anomaly whereby the skull shape is distorted and asymmetrical. It is caused by abnormally early or irregular closure of the skull sutures.

**plague** *n* very contagious epidemic disease caused by the bacterium *Yersinia pestis*, and spread by infected rats. Transfer of infection from rat to human is through bites from rat fleas, but droplet spread may occur between humans. The main clinical types are bubonic, pneumonic or septicaemic. It is endemic in areas of Asia and Africa. There are also small scattered outbreaks in rural areas of the western USA, where the disease is highly prevalent in wild rodents.

**plane** *n* in anatomy, it describes a hypothetical surface, which divides part of the body. Used to describe the position of various body structures in relation to that surface. ⇒ frontal (coronal) plane, median (midsagittal) plane, transverse (horizontal) plane.

**plantar** *adj* pertaining to the sole of the foot.

**plantar arch** the union of the plantar and dorsalis pedis arteries in the sole of the foot.

**plantar flexion** downward movement of the big toe. ⇒ Babinski's reflex or sign.

**planteris** *n* a small superficial muscle of the posterior compartment of the leg. Its origin is on the posterior distal femur and its long, thin tendon inserts into the calcaneus. Contraction of the muscle assists with flexion of the knee and plantar flexion. ⇒ Appendix 1, Figure 5.

**plaque** *n* **1.** an elevated area on the skin or internal organ. **2.** a deposit of atheroma on a vessel wall. ⇒ dental calculus, dental plaque.

**plasma** *n* the pale yellow fluid part of blood, in which the cellular components are suspended: red blood cells (erythrocytes), white blood cells (leucocytes) and blood platelets (thrombocytes). Plasma is mainly water (90–92%) and contains a variety of substances, including: plasma proteins such as albumin and the clotting factors, inorganic ions (e.g. sodium, calcium, bicarbonate), amino acids, glucose, lipids, vitamins, enzymes, hormones, gases, drugs and metabolic waste. Plasma forms around 55% of blood volume.

**plasma cell** an immune cell that produces antibodies (immunoglobulins). It is derived from B-lymphocytes/cells and is involved in humoral immunity.

**plasmacytoma** *n* a malignant tumour of plasma cells, it may be within the bone marrow, such as in multiple myeloma, or in other tissues—**plasmacytomas, plasmocytomata** *pl.* ⇒ multiple myeloma.

**plasmapheresis** *n* taking blood from a donor, removing some desired fraction, then returning the red cells and repeating the whole process. Donated plasma is used to produce fresh frozen plasma and a variety of specific components such as individual coagulation factors. Plasmapheresis is also used in the treatment of some diseases which are caused by antibodies or immune complexes circulating in a patient's plasma, e.g. myasthenia gravis, Guillain–Barré syndrome. Removing the plasma and replacing it with donated plasma or a plasma substitute can improve the prognosis of the disease and prevent or delay the onset of renal failure. ⇒ apheresis.

**plasma thromboplastin antecedent** factor XI of blood coagulation. It is produced in the liver and is required for the formation of prothrombin activator. A very rare inherited autosomal deficiency leads to a bleeding disorder.

**plasmid** *n* DNA present in some bacteria. The transfer of this genetic material between bacteria during sexual reproduction allows the exchange of genes for antibiotic resistance.

**plasmin** *n* proteolytic enzyme produced when plasminogen is activated. It breaks down fibrin clots when healing is complete. Also called fibrinolysin. ⇒ fibrinolysis.

**plasminogen** *n* inactive precursor of plasmin. Release of activators, e.g. tissue plasminogen activator (t-PA), from damaged tissue promotes the conversion of plasminogen into plasmin.

**plasminogen activators** a group of endopeptidase enzymes that convert inactive plasminogen into the active form plasmin, which is fibrinolytic. They include tissue plasminogen activator (t-PA) and urinary plasminogen activator (urokinase).

*Plasmodium* *n* a genus of protozoa. Parasites in the blood of warm-blooded animals which complete their sexual cycle in blood-sucking arthropods such as mosquitoes. Malaria is caused by four species of *Plasmodium*—**plasmodial** *adj*.

**plaster model** in dentistry, a cast of the teeth and jaw made for diagnostic purposes, such as prior to orthodontic treatment, or to produce a very precise appliance. e.g. the retainer to be bonded on to the teeth following orthodontic treatment.

**plaster of Paris (POP)** ⇒ gypsum.

**plastic** *adj* capable of taking a form or mould.

**plastic surgery** transfer of healthy tissue to repair damaged area and the use of implants to restore form and function, or alter size or shape. Some procedures are undertaken for cosmetic reasons.

**platelet** *n* (*syn* thrombocyte). Cellular fragments without a nucleus that are mainly concerned with blood coagulation. They are formed in the bone marrow by the megakaryoctes and released into the blood. ⇒ platelet plug.

**platelet-derived growth factor (PDGF)** a peptide growth factor important during embryonic development; after birth it stimulates cell growth, cell differentiation, cell migration and the development of new blood vessels (angiogenesis). It is present in granules in platelets and is released when platelets are in contact with damaged tissue. PDGF stimulates the proliferation of fibroblasts and angiogenesis during wound healing.

**platelet plug** one of the four overlapping stages of haemostasis. Platelets aggregate and adhere to form a temporary plug at the site of blood vessel damage (Figure P.9). ⇒ coagulation, fibrinolysis, vasoconstriction.

**platyhelminth** *n* flat worm; cestodes (tapeworms) and trematodes (flukes). ⇒ *Echinococcus*, schistosomiasis, *Taenia*.

**platyopnoea** *n* breathlessness experienced in an upright position.

**platysma** *n* a superficial muscle of the neck. Its origin is on the fascia overlying the pectoral and deltoid muscles and it inserts into the lower edge of the mandible. It is involved in

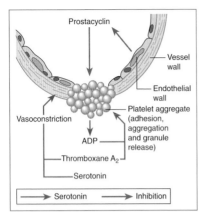

**Figure P.9** Platelet plug formation *(reproduced from Hinchliff et al. 1996 with permission).*

depressing the mandible and pulling the lower lip down and back. ⇒ Appendix 1, Figure 4.

**play** *n* ⇒ normative play, therapeutic play.

**play therapist** a person who uses play constructively to help children come to terms with having to be in hospital.

**pleiotropy** *n* the capacity of a single gene to have multiple effects on the phenotype. For example, the diverse characteristics of an inherited disease.

**pleocytosis** *n* the presence of an abnormal number of cells in cerebrospinal fluid.

**pleomastia** *n* also known as polymastia. The presence of supernumerary breasts or nipples, usually occurring on the nipple line, i.e. on a line stretching from the midclavicular point to the pelvic girdle.

**pleomorphism** *n* denotes a wide range in shape and size of individuals in a bacterial population—**pleomorphic** *adj.*

**plethora** *n* fullness; overloading. Previously applied to an excess of blood causing a red face—**plethoric** *adj.*

**plethysmograph** *n* an instrument which accurately measures blood flow. Used to measure and record changes in the volume and size of organs or an extremity—**plethysmographic** *adj.*

**pleura** *n* the serous membrane covering the surface of the lung, including the fissures between the lobes of the lungs (visceral pleura), the diaphragm, the mediastinum and the chest wall (parietal pleura). A potential space exists between the visceral and parietal

layers. A thin film of serous fluid present in the space provides the lubrication that prevents friction when the two layers glide effortlessly over each other when the volume of the lungs changes during breathing. The integrity of both pleural layers is essential to keeping the underlying lung inflated—**pleural** *adj,* **pleurae** *pl.* ⇒ pneumothorax.

**pleural cavity** the potential space between the visceral and parietal layers of the pleura. ⇒ pleura.

**pleural effusion** also known as hydrothorax. A collection of excess fluid in the pleural cavity, which may be an exudate or a transudate. It can be associated with inflammation, pleurisy, pneumonia, tuberculosis, lung cancer, mesothelioma, pulmonary infarction, abdominal disorders such as pancreatitis, cardiac failure, post myocardial infarction, hypoproteinaemia, renal failure and connective tissue diseases.

**pleurectomy** *n* surgical stripping of the pleura to achieve a surgical pleurodesis.

**pleurisy, pleuritis** *n* inflammation of the pleura. May be fibrinous (dry), associated with an effusion (wet), or complicated by empyema—**pleuritic** *adj.*

**pleurocentesis** *n* also known as paracentesis thoracis or thoracentesis. Aspiration or drainage of fluid from the pleural cavity.

**pleurodesis** *n* adherence of the visceral to the parietal pleura. Used therapeutically to prevent recurrence of metastatic pleural effusions, or recurrent pneumothoraces. Achieved by the use of sclerosing agents such as talc. ⇒ pleurectomy.

**pleurodynia** *n* intercostal myalgia or muscular rheumatism (fibrositis). ⇒ Bornholm disease.

**pleurolysis** *n* surgical separation of the pleura from its attachments.

**pleuropneumonia-like organisms (PPLO)** ⇒ *Mycoplasma.*

**pleuropulmonary** *adj* relating to the pleura and lung.

**pleurotomy** *n* incision of the pleura.

**plexus** *n* a network of vessels or nerves. For example, choroid plexus, cervical plexus, etc. ⇒ Appendix 1, Figure 11.

**plication** *n* a surgical procedure of making tucks or folds to decrease the size of an organ, such as reducing the size of the stomach in the management of morbid obesity—**plica** *sing,* **plicae** *pl,* **plicate** *adj, vt.*

**plombage** *n* extrapleural compression of a tuberculous lung cavity to deprive tubercle of oxygen. Widely used surgical technique before the introduction of antibiotic therapy for tuberculosis. Now sometimes used in multidrug-resistant tuberculosis.

**plumbism** *n* ⇒ lead poisoning.

**Plummer's disease** (H Plummer, American physician, 1874–1937) also called toxic nodular goitre. Hyperthyroidism caused by a solitary toxic adenoma in the thyroid gland. Most often affects females over the age of 40 years.

**Plummer–Vinson syndrome** (*syn* Kelly–Paterson, Paterson–Brown–Kelly syndrome) (H Plummer, American physician, 1874–1937; P Vinson, American surgeon, 1890–1959) sideropenic dysphagia. A combination of chronic iron-deficiency anaemia, glossitis, fissuring in the corners of the mouth (angular stomatitis) and dysphagia caused by the development of a postcricoid web. A rare condition occurring mainly in middle-aged females.

**pluriglandular** *adj* pertaining to several glands, as in cystic fibrosis.

**plyometric exercise** explosive exercise that maximizes the myotactic on-stretch reflex, i.e. a lengthening of a muscle followed by a sudden shortening in order to produce power.

**PMB** *abbr* postmenopausal bleeding.

**PMI** *abbr* point of maximum impulse.

**PMS** *abbr* premenstrual syndrome.

**PND** *abbr* paroxysmal nocturnal dyspnoea.

**pneumatocele** *n* **1.** a sac or swelling that contains air. **2.** a hernia of lung tissue.

**pneumaturia** *n* bubbles of air or other gases in the urine. It may be the passage of flatus with urine, usually as a result of a vesicocolic (bladder–colon) fistula, such as that caused by diverticular disease when a segment of diseased bowel adheres to the bladder.

**pneumococcus** *n Streptococcus pneumoniae*. A Gram-positive diplococcus. Causes lobar pneumonia and other infections, e.g. meningitis—**pneumococcal** *adj*.

**pneumoconiosis** *n* (*syn* dust disease) fibrosis of the lung caused by long-continued inhalation of dust in industrial occupations. There is breathlessness, chronic bronchitis and a gradual decline in gaseous exchange and respiratory function with right heart failure. The most important complication is the occasional superinfection with tuberculosis—**pneumoconioses** *pl. rheumatoid pneumoconiosis* fibrosing alveolitis occurring in patients suffering from rheumatoid arthritis. ⇒ anthracosis, asbestosis, byssinosis, siderosis, silicosis.

*Pneumocystis jirovecii* formerly known as *Pneumocystis carinii*. An opportunistic micro-

organism that causes pneumonia in immunocompromised individuals, such as infants, debilitated and immunosuppressed patients and those with human immunodeficiency virus (HIV) disease; mortality is high.

**pneumocystis pneumonia (PCP)** pneumonia caused by a fungal species of the genus *Pneumocystis.* ⇒ *Pneumocystis jirovecii.*

**pneumocytes** *npl* cells lining the alveolar walls in the lungs. Type I are flat cells; type II are cuboidal and secrete surfactant.

**pneumoencephalography** *n* radiographic examination of the cerebral ventricles after injection of air by means of a lumbar or cisternal puncture—**pneumoencephalogram** *n*.

**pneumolysis** *n* separation of the two pleural layers, or the outer pleural layer from the chest wall, to collapse the lung.

**pneumomycosis** *n* fungal infection affecting the lung, e.g. actinomycosis, aspergillosis, candidiasis—**pneumomycotic** *adj*.

**pneumonectomy** *n* excision of a lung.

**pneumonia** *n* a lower respiratory tract infection. Acute infection of the lung by an invading organism associated with new pulmonary shadowing on a radiograph. Can be subdivided into community-acquired, hospital-acquired, and pneumonia associated with profound immunosuppression. Types include atypical pneumonia, aspiration pneumonia, bacterial pneumonia, bronchopneumonia, fungal pneumonia, lobar pneumonia, mycoplasma pneumonia, pneumocystis pneumonia, viral pneumonia.

**pneumonic plague** ⇒ plague.

**pneumonitis** *n* inflammation of lung tissue.

**pneumoperitoneum** *n* air or gas in the peritoneal cavity. It may result from the perforation of the stomach or intestine. Can be introduced for diagnostic or therapeutic purposes such as during laparoscopic examination and operative procedures.

**pneumotaxic centre** a respiratory control centre in the pons, which has an inhibitory effect on the nerves controlling inspiration and helps to ensure a smooth respiratory rhythm. If it is damaged the unopposed action of the apneustic centre leads to prolonged gasping inspiration with only infrequent expiration. ⇒ apneustic centre.

**pneumothorax** *n* air or gas in the pleural cavity separating the visceral from the parietal pleura so that underlying lung tissue collapses. Occurs spontaneously when an overdilated pulmonary air sac ruptures, permitting communication of respiratory passages with

P

the pleural cavity. Associated with many lung diseases, including asthma, bronchial cancer, chronic obstructive pulmonary disease, congenital cysts and tuberculosis. Also caused by trauma, and can occur during positive-pressure ventilation. *tension pneumothorax* a valve-like wound or tear in the lung allows air to enter the pleural cavity with each inspiration, but not to escape on expiration, thus progressively increasing intrathoracic pressure and constituting an acute medical emergency. Signs are of hyperinflation, midline shift and increasing respiratory distress.

**PNF** *abbr* proprioceptive neuromuscular facilitation.

**PNI** *abbr* psychoneuroimmunology.

**PNS** *abbr* peripheral nervous system.

**PO₂** *abbr* the partial pressure of oxygen, for example in atmospheric or expired air.

**POA** *abbr* pancreatic oncofetal antigen.

**POAG** *abbr* primary open-angle glaucoma.

**pockmark** *n* pitted scar left on the skin at the site of a healed pustule of chickenpox or smallpox.

**podalic version** ⇒ version.

**podiatrist** *n* a primary health care professional responsible for the assessment, diagnosis and management of conditions affecting the foot and lower limb without referral from medical practitioners. Podiatrists adopt holistic approaches to the assessment and treatment of individuals and utilize a wide range of treatment modalities, many of which are performed under local anaesthesia.

**podiatry** *n* a term that is generally used in western Europe and the rest of the English-speaking countries to describe chiropody. The practice of podiatry involves maintaining the feet in a healthy condition. It recognizes the interdependence of the health of the foot with the rest of the body.

**podopompholyx** *n* pompholyx on the feet.

**POEMS syndrome** also called Crow–Fukase syndrome. A syndrome comprising polyneuropathy, organomegaly, endocrinopathy, M component and skin involvement. It may be associated with the presence of unusual proteins.

**poikilocyte** *n* red blood cell (erythrocyte) of abnormal shape, e.g. elliptical or spherical.

**poikilocytosis** *n* an abnormal variation in the shape of the red blood cells (erythrocytes) in the blood, such as in elliptocytosis or spherocytosis.

**poikilothermic** *adj* describes an animal that is unable to maintain a constant body temperature. Its body temperature varies throughout the 24-hour period and is influenced by environmental conditions. Cold-blooded. Compare homoeothermic.

**point of maximum impulse (PMI)** the point at which the apical beat is palpated or seen at its strongest, usually just medial to the left midclavicular line, at the level of the fifth intercostal space (see Figure A.10, p. 36).

**polar body** one of two small haploid structures produced during the two meiotic divisions of oogenesis, in which the secondary oocyte is formed. They are non-functional and will eventually undergo disintegration. ⇒ oogenesis.

**polarized** *adj* describes the resting state of the plasma membrane of an excitable cell where there is no impulse transmission. The inside of the membrane is electrically negative relative to the outside. ⇒ depolarization.

**polioencephalitis** *n* inflammation of the grey matter of the brain. It is caused by infection with one of the polioviruses.

**polioencephalomyelitis** *n* inflammation of the grey matter of the brain and that of the spinal cord. It is caused by infection with one of the polioviruses.

**poliomyelitis** *n* (*syn* infantile paralysis) an epidemic infection caused by one of three polioviruses which attack the motor neurons of the anterior horns in the brainstem (*bulbar poliomyelitis*) and spinal cord. An attack may be asymptomatic, mild without paralysis, or the paralytic form. The latter leads to paralysis of the lower motor neuron type with loss of muscular power and flaccidity. Immunization is available as part of routine programmes during infancy with booster doses before starting school, and again before leaving school.

**polioviruses** *npl* three enteroviruses that cause poliomyelitis. ⇒ virus.

**pollenosis** *n* an allergic condition arising from sensitization to pollen.

**pollex** *n* the thumb.

**pollicization** *n* a surgical procedure whereby the index finger is rotated and shortened to produce apposition as a thumb.

**polyarteritis** *n* inflammation of many arteries. In *polyarteritis nodosa* (*syn* periarteritis nodosa) aneurysmal swellings and thrombosis occur in the affected vessels. Further damage may lead to haemorrhage and the clinical picture presented depends upon the site affected. ⇒ collagen, connective tissue diseases.

**polyarthralgia** *n* pain in several joints.

**polyarthritis** *n* inflammation of several joints.

**polycoria** *n* **1.** a rare anomaly in which the eye has more than one pupil or opening. **2.** additional reserve material within tissues, which is used for enlargement.

**polycystic** *adj* composed of many cysts.

**polycystic kidney diseases** a number of conditions which have variable effects on kidney function. *adult polycystic kidney disease* (APKD) is a multisystem condition in which there is multiple cyst formation in the kidneys and other body sites, including the meninges and the liver. It is inherited as an autosomal dominant trait. The condition is characterized by flank or abdominal pain, bleeding into the cysts that may cause haematuria, recurrent urinary tract infection, the formation of renal calculi and hypertension. There may also be manifestations linked to cyst formation in the liver and elsewhere. Eventually there is a decline in renal function, which may lead to end-stage renal failure and the need for dialysis or renal transplantation.

**polycystic ovary syndrome (PCOS)** sometimes called Stein–Leventhal syndrome. A complex syndrome of amenorrhoea or oligomenorrhoea, infertility, hirsutism, acne and occasionally obesity. The ovaries contain multiple follicular cysts. In PCOS the normal feedback mechanisms do not occur, resulting in increased levels of luteinizing hormone (LH) and decreased levels of follicle-stimulating hormone (FSH). Oestrogen levels are similar to those early in the menstrual cycle and as a result women do not ovulate. There are problems associated with androgen hormone (testosterone) production. Women with PCOS also have reduced sensitivity to insulin and therefore insulin levels in the blood are raised (hyperinsulinaemia), leading to an increased risk of developing type 2 diabetes. Management includes relief of symptoms, increasing fertility if desired and preventing long-term complications such as type 2 diabetes mellitus. Ovulation may be stimulated with clomiphene, and other infertility treatment offered as appropriate. Metformin may be used to increase the chances of conception. Previously, wedge resection of ovarian tissue was undertaken to induce ovulation; this has since been replaced by a laparoscopic procedure whereby laser or diathermy is used on the surface of the ovary. A reduction in weight can improve symptoms and reduce hirsutism, but cosmetic therapies such as depilatory treatments may be needed.

**polycythaemia** *n* increase in the number of circulating red blood cells. This may result from dehydration or be a compensatory phenomenon to increase the oxygen-carrying capacity, as in congenital heart disease, chronic lung disease and living at high altitudes. *primary proliferative polycythaemia (polycythaemia vera)* also known as Vaquez–Osler disease. It is an idiopathic, myeloproliferative condition in which the red cell count is very high, thus increasing blood viscosity. The patient may complain of headache and lassitude, and there is danger of thrombosis and haemorrhage.

**polydactyly, polydactylism** *n* having more than the normal number of fingers or toes. On the foot the extra digits may develop from one metatarsal or there may be duplication of metatarsal segments. Sometimes selective amputation at an early age is indicated. This ensures optimum foot function, thus facilitating shoe fitting in childhood and adult life.

**polydipsia** *n* excessive thirst, such as occurs in diabetes mellitus and diabetes insipidus.

**polygene inheritance** describes physical characteristics such as hair colour that are determined by the combined effects of several paired genes at different loci.

**polygraph** *n* instrument which records several variables simultaneously.

**polyhydramnios** *n* often referred to as hydramnios. An excessive amount of amniotic fluid, usually referring to volumes over 1.5 L. It is associated with fetal abnormality, including oesophageal atresia and some neural tube defects, maternal diabetes and multiple pregnancy. Polyhydramnios can lead to serious complication such as unstable fetal lie and malpresentation (e.g. shoulder, face), presentation of or prolapse of the umbilical cord, preterm labour, increased perinatal mortality and postpartum haemorrhage. ⇒ amniotic fluid, oligohydramnios.

**polymer** *n* a molecule made up of many smaller molecules or subunits, such as glycogen; a polymer of glucose molecules.

**polymerase chain reaction (PCR)** an in vitro method for the enzymic synthesis of specific DNA sequences and hence the capacity to amplify these segments of DNA. A modification of the method also allows the rapid detection and analysis of RNA.

**polymorph** *n* a shortened term for a polymorphonuclear white blood cell; includes neutrophil, eosinophil and basophil.

**polymorphism** *n* existing in several different forms, for example, different forms of haemoglobin.

**polymorphonuclear** *adj* having a many-shaped or lobulated nucleus, usually applied to the phagocytic leucocytes (granulocytes), neutrophils, basophils and eosinophils.

**polymyalgia rheumatica** a syndrome occurring in older people comprising a sometimes crippling ache in the shoulders, pelvic girdle muscles and spine, with pronounced morning stiffness and a raised erythrocyte sedimentation rate. There is an association with temporal arteritis. Clinically different from rheumatoid arthritis. ⇒ arthritis.

**polymyositis** *n* manifests as muscle weakness, most commonly in middle age. Microscopic examination of muscle reveals inflammatory changes that respond to corticosteroids. ⇒ dermatomyositis.

**polyneuritis** *n* multiple neuritis, affecting many nerves—**polyneuritic** *adj*.

**polyneuropathy** *n* also known as multiple neuropathy and peripheral neuropathy. It is a disorder that affects many peripheral nerves simultaneously. The types and causes are varied and include: diabetes, associated with an acute infection, Guillain–Barré syndrome, toxins and poisons such as arsenic, chronic uraemia, vitamin deficiencies and paraneoplastic syndromes.

**polyopia** *n* seeing many images of a single object.

**polyp, polypus** *n* a pedunculated tumour arising from any epithelial surface, e.g. cervical, uterine, nasal, intestinal. Usually benign but may be malignant. Adenomatous polyps are premalignant. ⇒ polyposis. Tissue overgrowth underlying the epithelium may also be the cause of polyp formation—**polypous** *adj*.

**polypectomy** *n* surgical removal of a polyp such as from the bowel or nose.

**polypeptides** *npl* molecules comprising several amino acids joined by peptide bonds. They are between peptides and proteins in size.

**polyphagia** *n* also called hyperphagia. Excessive and abnormal eating. ⇒ Prader–Willi syndrome.

**polypharmacy** *n* describes a situation when many drugs are prescribed for the same person, usually defined as four or more. It increases the risk of adverse drug reactions, non-compliance and readmissions to hospital. It is a particular problem in older people who are likely to be taking prescription drugs, with as many as a third of people aged 75 years or over taking more that four drugs. The problems are compounded by the use of over-the-counter medicines, or herbal medicines that the person may not mention to the prescriber.

**polyphenols** *npl* several groups of organic molecules, which can inhibit iron absorption from the intestine.

**polyploidy** *n* a multiple of the normal haploid (n) chromosome number of 23, other than the normal diploid (2n) number of 46, e.g. 69. This state is not compatible with life. ⇒ aneuploidy, mononsomy, polysomy, triploid, trisomy.

**polypoid** *adj* resembling a polyp.

**polyposis** *n* a condition in which there are numerous intestinal polyps. ⇒ familial adenomatous polyposis.

**polyradiculitis** *n* also called polyradiculopathy. Inflammation of many nerve roots. It may occur as part of a polyneuropathy.

**polysaccharide** *n* complex carbohydrates that contain a large number of monosaccharide units. Starch, inulin, glycogen, dextrin and cellulose are examples. Important as structural compounds and as energy storage. ⇒ non-starch polysaccharides, polymer.

**polyserositis** *n* inflammation of several serous membranes. A genetic type is called familial Mediterranean fever. ⇒ amyloidosis.

**polysome** *n* also known as polyribosome. A structure free in the cytoplasm of the cell comprising a group of ribosomes bound to a strand of messenger ribonucleic acid (mRNA). The ribosomes 'read' the code on the mRNA and add amino acids to the growing polypeptide during the synthesis of proteins.

**polysomnography** *n* a graphical recording of the changes occurring in several biophysiological parameters during sleep, such as eye movement, heart rate and rhythm, brain wave pattern, muscle contraction, oxygen saturation levels and nasal airflow. Used in the investigation of some sleep disorders.

**polysomy** *n* the occurrence of more than two copies of a chromosome in a diploid cell that would otherwise be normal. An example of polysomy is a male with Klinefelter's syndrome who has three copies (trisomy) of the X chromosome (XXXY) or four copies (a tetrasomy) (XXXXY); caused by non-disjunction of the chromosome during meiotic division.

**polyunsaturated fatty acid (PUFA)** a fatty acid with two or more double bonds in its structure. Examples include sunflower oil and fish oils. ⇒ arachidonic acid, essential fatty acids, linoleic acid, linolenic acids, monounsaturated fatty acids, omega-3 fatty acids, omega-6 fatty acids.

**polyuria** *n* excretion of an excessive volume of urine. Causes include an abnormally large fluid intake that can occur with some mental health disorders, diabetes mellitus, diabetes insipidus, some renal diseases, with diuretic drugs and hypercalcaemia—**polyuric** *adj*.

**POM** *abbr* prescription-only medicine.

**POMC** *abbr* pro-opiomelanocortin.

**pompholyx** *n* vesicular skin eruption on the skin associated with itching or burning. ⇒ cheiropompholyx, podopompholyx.

**POMR** *abbr* problem-oriented medical record.

**pons** *n* a bridge; a process of tissue joining two sections of an organ. *pons varolii* part of the brainstem between the midbrain and the medulla. It comprises mainly nerve fibres (white matter) which connect the various lobes of the brain. Also contains several nuclei, including those of some cranial nerves (trigeminal, abducens, facial) and the apneustic and pneumotaxic respiratory centres. (⇒ Appendix 1, Figure 1)—**pontine** *adj*.

**Pontiac fever** a flu-like illness with little or no pulmonary involvement and no mortality, caused by *Legionella pneumophila*. ⇒ legionnaires' disease.

**POP** *acron* **1.** progestogen-only pill. **2.** plaster of Paris.

**popliteal** *adj* pertaining to the popliteus. *popliteal artery* formed from the femoral artery as it enters the popliteal fossa, it supplies arterial blood to the knee and surrounding structures. *popliteal fossa/space* the diamond-shaped depression behind the knee, bounded by muscles and containing nerves and the popliteal vessels (artery and vein). *popliteal vein* a deep vein that receives venous blood carried by the superficial saphenous veins from the lower leg. ⇒ Appendix 1, Figures 9 and 10.

**popliteus** *n* a deep, triangular muscle of the posterior compartment of the leg. It is situated behind the knee in the popliteal space. Its origin is on the lateral condyle of the femur and it inserts into the proximal tibia. Contraction of the muscle flexes and rotates the leg.

**population-attributable risk** the rate of a condition in a population minus the rate that would occur if everyone in the population were unexposed to the risk factor. It can be expressed as the attributable risk multiplied by the prevalence of risk factor exposure in the population. Used to inform decisions about public health policies and their impact on a population. ⇒ risk.

**pore** *n* a minute surface opening. One of the mouths of the ducts (leading from the sweat glands) on the skin surface; they are controlled by fine papillary muscles, closing in the cold and opening in the presence of heat.

**pores of Kohn** alveolar pores. Tiny ventilation channels which allow the movement of air between adjacent alveoli.

**porphyria** *n* a group of inborn errors of haem biosynthesis caused by enzyme deficiencies, usually hereditary, causing pathological changes in nervous and muscular tissue in some varieties and photosensitivity in others, depending on the level of the metabolic block involved. Excess porphyrins or precursors, produced either by the haemopoietic bone marrow or the liver, are found in the urine or stools or both. Those affected may present with bouts of abdominal pain, peripheral neuropathy, skin blistering, ⊙**DVD** confusion, hypertension, tachycardia and mental health problems. In acute porphyria a porphyric crisis can be precipitated by alcohol; hormones; and certain drugs, which include some antidepressants, barbiturates, some hormones, sulphonamides, etc.

**porphyrins** *npl* group of organic compounds that form the basis of respiratory pigments, including the haem of haemoglobin. Naturally occurring porphyrins are uroporphyrin and coproporphyrin. ⇒ porphyria.

**porphyrinuria** *n* excretion of porphyrins in the urine. Such pigments are produced as a result of an inborn error of metabolism. The urine may change colour and darken on standing. ⇒ porphyria.

**porta** *n* the depression (hilum) of an organ at which the vessels enter and leave—**portal** *adj*. *porta hepatis* the transverse fissure through which the hepatic portal vein, hepatic artery and bile ducts pass on the undersurface of the liver.

**portacaval, portocaval** *adj* relating to the hepatic portal vein and inferior vena cava. *portacaval anastomosis* the hepatic portal vein is joined to the inferior vena cava with the object of reducing the pressure within the hepatic portal vein in cases of hepatic portal hypertension.

**portal circulation** ⇒ hepatic portal circulation.

**portal hypertension** ⇒ hepatic portal hypertension.

**portal vein** ⇒ hepatic portal vein.

**positive end-expiratory pressure (PEEP)** the maintenance of positive pressure in the airway of a ventilated patient at the end of expiration. Analogous to continuous positive airway pressure in a spontaneously breathing patient.

**positive feedback** the mechanism through which a few homeostatic regulation processes work. An amplifier or cascade system in which an increase in the level of product from the process stimulates the process still further. Positive feedback usually functions in processes that occur relatively infrequently, such as parturition (labour) and normal blood clotting, which are not everyday events requiring constant regulation. For example, the events of labour are stimulated as the presenting part moves down the birth canal to exert pressure on the cervix. This pressure leads to the release of the hormone oxytocin from the pituitary gland, which in turn increases the rate and intensity of uterine muscle contractions, causing the cervix to dilate and the birth of the infant. ⇒ feedback, homeostasis, negative feedback.

**positive-pressure ventilation (PPV)** positive-pressure inflation of lungs to produce inspiration via endotracheal tube, tracheostomy or a nasal mask. ⇒ intermittent positive-pressure ventilation.

**positive regard** also termed unconditional positive regard. A concept of client-centred therapy. It is the ability to hold and convey feelings for other people that are not based on negative beliefs about the person. Having positive regard for clients and patients enables the health professional to approach others with positive intentions towards them. Positive regard, along with rapport, trust, empathy, genuineness and warmth are prerequisites for a successful therapeutic relationship.

**positivism** *n* the assertion that there is an absolute reality, which is capable of being measured, studied and understood.

**positron emission tomography (PET)** an imaging technique used in nuclear medicine to produce three-dimensional images showing metabolic activity in specific areas of the body. A cyclotron is used to produce radioactive isotopes of extremely short half-life that emit positrons; when positrons react with electrons in the body gamma rays are emitted. The radioactive isotopes are linked to molecules, such as glucose, that are active in metabolism (e.g. fluorodeoxyglucose) and administered to the patient, usually intravenously. The scan takes place after a suitable period to allow time for the radioactive isotope to build up in the cells. PET scanning is used in research; to evaluate the metabolic activity of organs and structures including the brain and heart; and in the detection of primary cancers and the presence of metastases.

**positrons** *npl* positively charged particles that combine with electrons (negative charge), causing gamma rays to be emitted.

**posseting** *n* regurgitation of small amounts of curdled milk in infants.

**Possum** *acron* derived from patient-operated selector mechanism, a device used by individuals with paralysis to achieve maximum independence by being able to operate equipment or devices that include computers, telephone and other communications systems.

**postabsorptive state** the metabolic state existing between meals, such as before lunch, late afternoon and at night. Fuel molecules for immediate energy use are in short supply and the body uses catabolic processes, e.g. glycogenolysis, lipolysis, to break down complex substances to provide energy. ⇒ absorptive state.

**postanaesthetic** *adj* after anaesthesia.

**postanal** *adj* behind the anus.

**postcibal** *adj* postprandial. Relating to an event that occurs after eating, such as pain or vomiting. ⇒ 'dumping syndrome'.

**postcoital** *adj* after sexual intercourse. *postcoital contraception* ⇒ emergency contraception. *postcoital test* used during the investigation of infertility to determine spermatozoa survival in ovulatory cervical mucus. A sample of endocervical mucus is obtained around 6 hours after sexual intercourse at the likely time of ovulation. The presence of sufficient numbers of healthy motile spermatozoa indicates that there is no incompatibility between the cervical mucus and the spermatozoa.

**postconcussional syndrome 1.** the association of headaches, giddiness and a feeling of faintness, which may persist for a considerable time after a head injury. **2.** a term used in sports medicine to describe a progressive deterioration of cognitive function following repeated brain trauma such as that caused during boxing.

**postdiphtheritic** *adj* following an attack of diphtheria. Refers especially to the paralysis of limbs and palate.

**postepileptic** *adj* following an epileptic seizure. *postepileptic automatism* is a fugue state, following a seizure (fit), when the patient may undertake a course of action, even involving violence, without having any memory of this (amnesia).

P

**posterior** *adj* situated at the back. ⇒ anterior *opp*. *posterior chamber of the eye* situated between the anterior surface of the lens and the posterior surface of the iris. ⇒ aqueous—**posteriorly** *adv*.

**posterior cruciate ligament** a major stabilizing ligament of the knee, it limits backward movement of the tibia (Figure A.9, p. 31). Also involved in proprioception. A site of sports injury, e.g. a tear, which may occur during hockey or rugby football, or in conjunction with an anterior cruciate ligament injury.

**posteroanterior** *adj* from back to front.

**postganglionic** *adj* situated distal to a collection of nerve cells (ganglion), as a postganglionic nerve fibre.

**postgastrectomy syndrome** covers two sets of symptoms, those of hypoglycaemia when the patient is hungry, and those of a vasovagal attack immediately after a meal.

**posthepatic** *adj* behind the liver.

**postherpetic** *adj* after herpes infection such as *postherpetic neuralgia* following an attack of herpes zoster (shingles). The pain is particularly difficult to treat. ⇒ neuropathic pain.

**posthitis** *adj* inflammation of the prepuce.

**posthumous** *adj* occurring after death. *posthumous birth* **1.** delivery of a baby by caesarean section after the mother's death, or **2.** birth occurring after the father's death.

**postmature** *adj* past the expected date of delivery. A baby is postmature when labour is delayed beyond the usual 40 weeks—**postmaturity** *n*.

**postmenopausal** *adj* occurring after the menopause has been established. *postmenopausal bleeding (PMB)* vaginal bleeding occurring after the menopause. Investigation is essential to exclude malignancy.

**postmortem** *adj* after death, usually implying dissection of the body. ⇒ antemortem *opp*, autopsy.

**postmyocardial infarction syndrome** Dressler's syndrome. A late complication presenting as pericarditis developing from 2 weeks to a few months after myocardial infarction. Due to an autoimmune response to products released from dead muscle.

**postnasal** *adj* behind the nose and in the nasopharynx—**postnasally** *adv*.

**postnatal** *adj* after delivery. ⇒ antenatal *opp*. *postnatal depression* describes a low mood experienced by some mothers for a few days following the birth of a baby; sometimes called 'four-day blues'. Less severe than puerperal

psychosis. *postnatal examination* routine examination 6 weeks after delivery—**postnatally** *adv*.

**postoperative** *adj* after surgical operation—**postoperatively** *adv*.

**postpartum** *adj* after a birth (parturition). *postpartum haemorrhage* excessive bleeding after delivery of the infant. It may be due to incomplete placental separation during the third stage of labour. Secondary postpartum haemorrhage is excessive uterine bleeding occurring more than 24 h after delivery. It is usually caused by infection associated with the retention of placental tissue.

**postprandial** *adj* following a meal. *postprandial lipaemia* the increase in blood level of triacylglycerols (triglycerides) after eating a fatty meal.

**post-traumatic amnesia** the period of time between a brain injury and the point when the functions involved in memory are judged to be restored.

**post-traumatic stress disorder (PTSD)** a mixed emotional disorder arising in response to an exceptional trauma, such as witnessing or being a victim of violent crime, war, natural disaster. Symptoms include autonomic arousal, intrusive images ('flashbacks' or nightmares), emotional numbness, anhedonia and avoidance of reminders of the trauma.

**postural** *adj* relating to posture. *postural albuminuria* ⇒ orthostatic albuminuria.

**postural adjustments/background movements** the spontaneous body adjustments occurring in response to information from proprioceptors and the vestibular apparatus, in order to maintain body alignment, centre of gravity and stability. For example, the adjustments of the trunk when reaching for a distant object.

**postural drainage** techniques that use gravity and position to drain respiratory secretions. The airways of infected lung lobes or segments are positioned as vertically as possible. Also known as tipping because the lower lobes need to be raised higher than the mouth for secretions to drain into the trachea to stimulate the cough reflex. Apical segments of the upper lobe drain in sitting. The chest is percussed with clapping and vibrated and sputum coughed into a suitable disposable container or removed by suctioning. Children with cystic fibrosis must have this treatment at home and family members learn the techniques required. Small children are usually tipped across an adult's thighs but bigger children

P

and adults can be tipped by raising the foot end of the bed, or over a roll or special frame. ⇒ tapôtement.

**postural hypotension** orthostatic hypotension. A reduction in blood pressure when a person stands up from lying or sitting. It may occur in older people, or as a side-effect of some drugs, such as alpha-adrenoceptor antagonists (alpha blockers). ⇒ Appendix 5.

**postural muscles** those muscles, mostly extensors, which counter the downward pull of gravity to maintain the body in an upright posture.

**postural reflex** describes any of the reflexes concerned with establishing or maintaining an individual's posture, particularly against the downward pull of gravity.

**posture** *n* the manner in which the body is held in lying, sitting, standing and walking; a particular position or attitude of the body. *hemiplegic posture* the position of the head, neck, trunk and limbs after a stroke. *opisthotonic posture* characterized by the arched position of complete extension of the head, spine and limbs typically in severe meningeal irritation and other serious neurological conditions. ⇒ opisthotonos.

**postviral fatigue** ⇒ chronic fatigue syndrome/myalgic encephalomyelitis.

**potassium (K)** *n* a metallic element. A major intracellular cation essential for proper neuromuscular conduction. ⇒ hyperkalaemia, hypokalaemia.

**potassium channel activator** a class of drug, e.g. nicorandil. It causes vasodilation in both arteries and veins and is used in the prophylaxis and treatment of angina.

**potassium chlorate** a mild antiseptic used in mouthwashes and gargles.

**potassium chloride** used to correct hypokalaemia, and as a supplement with some diuretic drugs.

**potassium citrate** alkalinizes urine; still used in cystitis to minimize discomfort.

**potassium deficiency** ⇒ hypokalaemia.

**potassium permanganate** used in solution for some skin conditions for its cleansing and deodorizing properties.

**potassium-sparing diuretics** a group of diuretic drugs that act to retain potassium and increase loss of sodium and water, or by reducing potassium loss and sodium reabsorption. ⇒ Appendix 5.

**Pott's disease** (P Pott, British surgeon, 1714–1788) spondylitis; spinal caries; spinal tuberculosis. The resultant necrosis of the vertebrae causes kyphosis.

**Pott's fracture** (P Pott) a fracture-dislocation of the ankle joint. A fracture of the lower end of the tibia and fibula, 75 mm above the ankle joint, and a fracture of the medial malleolus of the tibia.

**potter's rot** one of many lay terms for silicosis arising in workers in the pottery industry.

**Potter's syndrome** (E Potter, American pathologist, 1901–1993) a syndrome that includes renal agenesis (absence of kidneys) and a typical flattened face associated with accompanying oligohydramnios. It is not compatible with life.

**pouch** *n* a pocket or recess. *pouch of Douglas* the rectouterine pouch.

**poultice** *n* fomentation. Local application of heat, such as with warmed kaolin spread between two layers of gauze, used to relieve pain, act as a counterirritant or increase blood flow.

**Poupart's ligament** (F Poupart, French physician, 1616–1708) ⇒ inguinal ligament.

**poverty** *n* may be *absolute poverty* where people have insufficient resources to maintain physical health, such as not having food, shelter or the means to keep warm, or *relative poverty* when an individual's living standards are less than those that generally exist in a particular population. Definitions of what constitutes relative poverty show considerable variation between different communities and the same community over time.

**povidone iodine** ⇒ iodine.

**power calculation** in research, a measure of statistical power. The likelihood of the research study to generate statistically significant results.

**powerlessness** *n* a feeling of being trapped and unable to control or influence the situation. People may feel powerless in their dealings with health care professionals and health care systems.

**pox** *n* a slang name for syphilis.

**poxvirus** *n* viruses belonging to the family Poxviridae. Those affecting humans are the virus causing molluscum contagiosum, smallpox virus and vaccinia virus. The pox viruses are responsible for many animal diseases, e.g. orf in sheep and goats.

**PPE** *abbr* personal protective equipment.

**PPLO** *abbr* pleuropneumonia-like organism. ⇒ *Mycoplasma*.

**PPS** *abbr* pelvic pain syndrome.

**PPV** *abbr* positive-pressure ventilation.

**P-QRS-T complex** the letters used to denote the five deflection waves of the electrocardio-

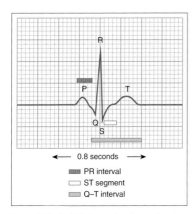

R

P      T

Q

S

◄— 0.8 seconds —►

▨▨ PR interval
▭ ST segment
▨ Q–T interval

**Figure P.10** P–QRS–T complex *(reproduced from Brooker 2006A with permission).*

graph (ECG) waveform (Figure P.10). The deflection waves represent the electrical activity in the heart and correspond to the events occurring during a cardiac cycle. The dome-shaped P-wave represents atrial depolarization as the impulse is conducted across the atria, resulting in atrial systole (contraction). The PR interval represents the time taken for the impulse to be conducted from the sinus node, across the atria to the atrioventricular node and hence to the ventricles. The three waves that form the large narrow QRS complex represent depolarization of the ventricles that occurs just before contraction (ventricular systole). The gently rounded T-wave represents repolarization of the ventricles (ventricular diastole). The QT interval is the time between the start of ventricular depolarization, through contraction to repolarization of the ventricles. The ST segment represents the short period of inactivity and repolarization of the ventricles that follows the QRS complex. Importantly, the coronary arteries receive blood during the ST segment when the heart is relaxed.

**PR** *abbr* **1.** per rectum: describes the route used for examination of the rectum, or introduction of drugs or fluids into the body. **2.** peripheral resistance.

**P-R interval** ⇒ P-QRS-T complex.

**Prader–Willi syndrome** (A Prader, Swiss paediatrician/endocrinologist, 1919–2001; H Willi, Swiss paediatrician, 1900–1971) an inherited condition that arises from mutations in the paternal chromosome 15 during the formation of the gamete. There is learning disability, hypotonia, short stature, hyperphagia and morbid obesity. ⇒ Angelman syndrome.

**praecordial** *adj* ⇒ precordial.

**preagonal** *adj* pertaining to the events that may occur just before death. ⇒ agonal.

**preanaesthetic** *adj* before an anaesthetic.

**prebiotics** *npl* oligosaccharides present in food that are not digested and support the growth of potentially beneficial colonic bacteria. ⇒ probiotics.

**precancerous** *adj* outdated term. ⇒ carcinoma in situ.

**precipitate labour** a labour of very short duration, perhaps as short as 1 hour. There are very strong contractions from the onset. The fetus may be hypoxic. There is increased risk of damage to the cervix and perineal tears. Retained placenta or postpartum haemorrhage can occur because the uterine muscle does not function normally during the third stage of labour.

**precipitin** *n* an antibody that is capable of forming an immune complex with an antigen and becoming an insoluble precipitate, which can be detected in laboratory assays. This reaction forms the basis of many delicate diagnostic serological tests for the identification of antigens in serum and other fluids. ⇒ immunoglobulins.

**precocious puberty** the early appearance of signs of sexual development, such as breast development in girls, or the enlargement of the external genitalia in boys. It may be due to an endocrine disorder such as an ovarian tumour, or congenital adrenal hyperplasia.

**preconceptual** *adj* before conception. Preconception care refers to the physical and mental preparation for childbearing of both parents before pregnancy. Health-promoting activity focuses on measures aimed at reducing the risk of fetal problems and maternal complications during pregnancy and labour. The measures include the importance of an adequate diet, such as the provision of sufficient folic acid in the diet of women of childbearing age, and the avoidance of alcohol, drugs (prescribed, over-the-counter and illegal) and smoking in the months before a couple decide to have a baby.

**preconscious** *adj* information in the subconscious mind that can be evaluated and allowed to enter the conscious mind if we so wish.

**precordial, praecordial** *adj* relating to the area of the chest immediately over the heart.

P

*precordial thump* some authorities advocate the delivery of a sharp blow to the victim's mid-sternum during the first few seconds of ventricular fibrillation or pulseless ventricular tachycardia, i.e. a monitored or witnessed cardiac arrest, where there is no access to a defibrillator.

**precursor** *n* forerunner. For example, an inactive hormone or enzyme.

**prediabetes** *n* ⇒ impaired fasting glucose, impaired glucose tolerance.

**predisposition** *n* a natural tendency to develop or contract certain diseases.

**pre-eclampsia** *n* a serious hypertensive disorder of pregnancy. It is characterized by proteinuria and hypertension, with oedema, arising usually in the latter part of pregnancy. The incidence increases with maternal age. It may be suspected without proteinuria if the woman's blood pressure is raised and she complains of visual problems such as blurred vision, headache and abdominal pain. There may also be abnormal blood test results, specifically a low platelet count (thrombocytopenia) and abnormal liver enzyme levels. ⇒ eclampsia, HELLP syndrome.

**prefrontal** *adj* situated in the anterior portion of the frontal lobe of the cerebrum.

**preganglionic** *adj* proximal to a collection of nerve cells (ganglion), as a preganglionic nerve fibre.

**pregnancy** *n* being with child, i.e. gestation from the first day of the last menstrual period to parturition, normally 40 weeks or 280 days. ⇒ ectopic pregnancy, phantom pregnancy.

**pregnancy test** based on the presence of beta-human chorionic gonadotrophin (hCG) in the woman's urine or serum. Commercially produced urine test kits are available for home-testing.

**preimplantation genetic diagnosis (PGD)** a technique used in in vitro fertilization (IVF) assisted conception to determine the genetic constitution of an embryo prior to implantation in the uterus.

**preimplantation genetic haplotyping (PGH)** a recently developed technique that can be used to check embryos produced for in vitro fertilization (IVF) for several inherited conditions prior to implantation. A cell is extracted from the early embryo, the genetic material is replicated many times and the DNA is examined for the presence of chromosomes with the faulty genes that cause conditions including cystic fibrosis and sex-linked conditions such as Duchenne muscular dys-

trophy. In sex-linked conditions it will be possible to distinguish between healthy male embryos and those with the faulty genes, thus allowing a male embryo to be implanted where previously only female embryos were used.

**prejudice** *n* a preconceived opinion or bias which can be negative or positive. It can be for or against members of particular groups and may lead to discrimination, racism, sexism or intolerance.

**preload** *n* the degree of stretch present in the myocardial muscle fibres at the end of diastole. It is determined by the pressure and volume of blood in the ventricles at the end of diastole (end-diastolic volume [EDV]). Thus, in situations in which venous return to the heart is decreased the preload will be reduced. ⇒ afterload, Starling's law of the heart, stroke volume.

**premature** *adj* occurring before the proper time. *premature beat* ⇒ extrasystole. *premature birth* ⇒ preterm birth.

**premedication** *n* drugs given before the administration of another drug, e.g. those given before a general anaesthesia to reduce anxiety.

**premenstrual** *adj* preceding menstruation. *premenstrual (cyclical) syndrome (PMS)* a group of physical and mental changes occurring any time between 2 and 14 days before menstruation. They are relieved almost immediately when menstruation starts.

**premenstruum** *n* that part of the menstrual cycle immediately before bleeding commences.

**premolar tooth** permanent tooth with two cusps (bicuspid) (see Figure T.4B, p. 482), placed fourth and fifth from the midline. They succeed the primary molars.

**prenatal** *adj* antenatal. Pertaining to the period between the last menstrual period and birth of the child, normally 40 weeks or 280 days—**prenatally** *adv*.

**preoperative** *adj* before operation—**preoperatively** *adv*.

**preparalytic** *adj* before the onset of paralysis, usually referring to the early stage of poliomyelitis.

**prepatellar** *adj* in front of the patella, as applied to a large bursa. ⇒ bursitis.

**prepubertal** *adj* before puberty.

**prepuce** *n* the foreskin of the penis. The loose fold of skin that covers the glans penis, or the clitoris. In males the prepuce may be removed for cultural or religious reasons, or for the treatment of phimosis and paraphimo-

P

sis—**preputial** *adj.* (⇒ Appendix 1, Figure 16), ⇒ circumcision.

**prerenal** *adj* literally, before or in front of the kidney, but usually refers to perfusion of the kidneys.

**presbycusis** *n* idiopathic sensorineural hearing loss caused by or associated with age changes.

**presbyopia** *n* failure of accommodation in those of 45 years and onwards—**presbyopic** *adj*, **presbyope** *n*.

**prescribed diseases** a list of diseases which can be linked to occupation. They can be classified by the cause—physical, biological, chemical and other. Physical causes and diseases include: radiation (e.g. leukaemia and certain other cancers); vibration (e.g. blanching of fingers); noise (e.g. sensorineural deafness); and heat (e.g. cataract). Biological causes can result in a number of infections, such as tuberculosis, Weil's disease, orf, etc. Exposure to toxic chemicals cause a range of diseases that include anaemia from exposure to lead; cadmium exposure leading to the development of emphysema; a form of leukaemia following exposure to benzene; and cirrhosis of the liver after working with chlorinated naphthalenes. The last category of other causes includes pneumoconiosis, mesothelioma, dermatitis, etc.

**prescribing analysis and costs** the information supplied to prescribers about their prescribing.

**prescription** *n* a written or computer-generated formula, signed by the authorized prescriber, instructing the pharmacist to supply the required drugs. *prescription-only medicine* a drug that requires a written/computer-generated prescription, except in an emergency when the pharmacist may dispense the drug if certain criteria are met.

**presenile dementia** ⇒ dementia.

**presenility** *n* a condition occurring before senility is established. ⇒ dementia—**presenile** *adj*.

**presentation** *n* the part of the fetus which first enters the pelvic brim and will be felt by the examining finger through the cervix in labour. May be vertex, face, brow, shoulder or various types of breech.

**pressor** *n* a substance which raises the blood pressure.

**pressure areas** any body area subjected to pressure sufficient to compress the capillaries and disrupt the microcirculation. Usually occurs where tissues are compressed between a bone and a hard surface, e.g. theatre table, trolley, bed, chair, splint, or pressure damage caused by equipment such as oxygen tubing. Areas at risk of pressure damage include: head, ears, spine, sacral area, shoulders, elbows, hips, area over ischial tuberosities, heels and ankles. The most common site for pressure damage is the tissues over the sacral area, followed by the heels. The area over the ischial tuberosities is most at risk in people who sit for long periods. The head in infants is the most common site due to the differences in body proportions. ⇒ pressure ulcer.

**pressure garment** a skin-coloured, Lycra garment used to exert firm, even pressure to a specific part of the body. Often used in the treatment of varicose veins and burns and scalds to prevent keloid scarring.

**pressure groups** organizations formed to exert pressure on government (central and local) in order to further the interests of certain groups, such as older people.

**pressure point** a place at which an artery passes over a bone, against which it can be compressed, to stop bleeding (Figure P.11).

**pressure sore** ⇒ pressure ulcer.

**pressure support** mode of positive-pressure ventilation, which augments the size of a patient's spontaneous breaths.

**pressure transducer** device that converts pressure into calibrated electrical signals which can be displayed on a monitor.

**pressure ulcer** (*syn* decubitus ulcer, pressure sore) previously called a bedsore. Defined by the European Pressure Ulcer Advisory Panel (EPUAP) as an area of localized damage to the skin and underlying tissue caused by pressure, shear, friction or a combination of these factors. There are several grading scales, but the EPUAP advocates the use of a four-point grading scale. Pressure ulcers develop when any area of the body is subjected to unrelieved pressure that leads to local hypoxia, ischaemia and necrosis, with inflammation and ulcer formation (Figure P.12). Shearing forces also disrupt the microcirculation when they cause the skin layers to move against one another. Shearing damages the deeper tissues and can lead to an extensive pressure ulcer. Friction from continual rubbing leads to blisters, abrasions and superficial pressure ulcers, and is made worse by moisture such as urine or sweat. Factors that increase the risk of pressure ulcer formation include: poor oxygenation, incontinence, age over 65–70, immobility, altered consciousness, dehydration and malnutrition.

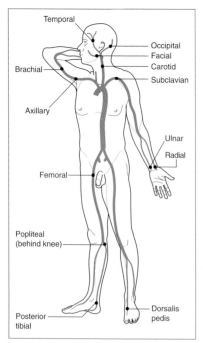

Temporal

Occipital
Facial
Carotid
Subclavian

Brachial

Axillary

Ulnar

Radial

Femoral

Popliteal
(behind knee)

Dorsalis
pedis

Posterior
tibial

**Figure P.11** Pressure points for arresting hae-morrhage *(reproduced from Brooker 2006A with permission).*

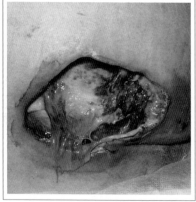

**Figure P.12** Pressure ulcer *(reproduced from Brooker & Nicol 2003 with permission).*

**presystole** *n* the period preceding the systole or contraction of the heart muscle—**presysto-lic** *adj.*

**preterm birth** the birth of a baby before the 37th completed week of gestation, regardless of the infant's birth weight. In the UK it is a birth after 24 weeks' gestation and before 37 weeks. If a fetus is delivered before 24 weeks and shows no signs of life it is termed a mis-carriage. ⇒ low birth weight.

**pretibial laceration** injury on the front of the shin; especially common in older adults.

**pretibial myxoedema** purple/pink indurated areas of skin, usually on the anterior aspect of the leg and dorsum of the foot. It is a feature of Graves' disease. The skin may be itchy and coarse hair is present.

**prevalence** *n* total number of cases of a dis-ease existing in a population at a single point in time. *prevalence ratio* the prevalence of a dis-ease, expressed as a ratio of population size. ⇒ incidence.

**priapism** *n* prolonged penile erection of 4–6 hours, in the absence of sexual stimulation. It is associated with spinal cord injuries and lesions, some types of leukaemia, sickle-cell disease, thalassaemia and drugs, e.g. alprosta-dil, used to treat erectile dysfunction. It requires urgent decompression, initially by aspirating blood from one corpus cavernosum or both in order to prevent damage to penile tissues. This may include thrombosis or ischaemia and can lead to erectile dysfunc-tion.

**prickle cell** a cell of the stratum spinosum layer of the epidermis.

**prickly heat** ⇒ miliaria.

**prima facie** 'at first sight', or sufficient evi-dence brought by one party to require the other party to provide a defence.

**primary** *adj* first in order. *primary tumour* the neoplasm at the site of origin.

**Primary Care Trust (PCT)** in England a stat-utory body that has three core functions: (a) to work with local government departments and the voluntary sector to improve health; (b) to reduce inequalities in health and improve access to services for the local population and commission appropriate health services for the local population, including those provided by general practitioners, pharmacists, optome-trists and dental surgeons in the community, secondary hospital services and services for people with mental health care needs; and (c) directly to provide community services that include district nursing, specialist community public health nursing (health visiting), rehabilitation, dental services, children's health, etc. ⇒ Strategic Health Authority.

**primary complex** (*syn* Ghon focus) the initial tuberculous infection in a person, usually in the lung, manifesting as a small focus of infection in the lung tissue and enlarged caseous, hilar lymph nodes. It usually heals spontaneously.

**primary health care (PHC) 1.** the first-level contact with the health care system. For example, general practitioner or practice nurse. Health care provided in the community by general practitioners and the practice team and other health professionals. Other services include NHS and private walk-in centres; nurse-led 24-hour telephone health information and advice services. ⇒ NHS Direct/NHS 24, primary health care team. **2.** defined by World Health Organization (WHO)–United Nations Children's Fund (UNICEF) declaration (Alma-Ata, 1978) as 'essential health care based on practical, scientifically sound and socially acceptable methods and technology, made universally available to individuals and families in the community through their full participation and at a cost that the community and the country can afford, to maintain every stage of their development in the spirit of self-reliance and self-determination'. In its original and narrowest sense, primary health care refers to first-contact care where patients contact health care workers directly. Principles on which effective primary health care is based are education about diseases, health care problems and their control; safe water and sanitation; maternal and child health, including family planning; immunization against major infectious diseases; appropriate treatment of common diseases and injuries; providing essential drugs.

**primary health care team** in the UK an interdependent multiprofessional group of individuals with a common purpose and responsibility, each member clearly understanding his or her own role, and those of other team members, in offering an equitable, efficient and effective primary health care service. The health professionals involved may include: community nurses, counsellors, general practitioners, specialist community public health nurses (health visitors), midwives, occupational therapists, physiotherapists, podiatrists, practice nurses, speech and language therapists, pharmacists and dental surgeons and optometrists working in the community.

**primary-intention healing** also known as first-intention. Uncomplicated wound healing that occurs where there is little tissue loss and it is possible to draw the wound edges together, such as in a surgical incision. ⇒ secondary-intention healing, wound healing.

**primary prevention** ⇒ disease prevention.

**primary teeth** ⇒ deciduous.

**primigravida** *n* a woman who is pregnant for the first time—**primigravidae** *pl*.

**primipara** *n* a woman who has given birth to a child for the first time—**primiparous** *adj*.

**primitive streak** an area at the posterior (caudal) end of the embryonic disc. It develops during the proliferation and movement of cells and produces the mesoderm layer.

**primordial** *adj* primitive, original; applied to the ovarian follicles present at birth.

**prion** *n* an infectious agent consisting of protein, similar to viruses but containing no nucleic acids.

**prion disease** a range of disorders in which there is an abnormal deposition of prion protein in the brain, of which the most common example is Creutzfeldt–Jakob disease.

**private finance initiative (PFI)** a joint venture between private and public sector to build a facility, e.g. a hospital, using private finance. The health authority then leases the building. Some non-clinical services may also be provided under the lease agreement.

**PRL** *abbr* prolactin.

**proband** *n* in the genetically inherited diseases, the first family member to present for investigation.

**probiotics** *npl* the addition of live microorganisms to human food, or used as animal feed. They include species of the genera *Bifidobacterium* and *Lactobacillus*. It is thought that they may provide health benefits by re-establishing the microbial balance in the colon. ⇒ prebiotics.

**problem-oriented medical record** a multiprofessional system of keeping patient records. Entries are made using the SOAP formula: S = subjective, O = objective, A = assessment, P = plan.

**procarcinogen** *n* a substance that is not carcinogenic, but during metabolism in the body it produces a carcinogen.

**procedural memory** that part of memory that stores information needed to do things, e.g. take a venous blood sample or record a television programme.

**process** *n* a prominence or outgrowth of any part.

**procidentia** *n* complete prolapse of the uterus, so that it lies within the vaginal sac but outside the contour of the body.

**proctalgia** *n* pain in the anal or rectal region. *proctalgia fugax* severe but intermittent pain in the rectum. May be caused by muscle spasm.

**proctectasia** *n* abnormal dilatation of the rectum and anus.

**proctectomy** *n* surgical excision of the rectum.

**proctitis** *n* inflammation of the rectum.

**proctocele** *n* ⇒ rectocele.

**proctoclysis** *n* introduction of fluid into the rectum for absorption. ⇒ enteroclysis.

**proctocolectomy** *n* surgical excision of the rectum and colon. Performed for severe ulcerative colitis or Crohn's disease and for familial polyposis coli. Requires a permanent ileostomy or some type of restorative procedure such as an ileoanal reservoir.

**proctocolitis** *n* inflammation of the rectum and colon.

**proctodynia** *n* pain in the anal and rectal region.

**proctology** *n* the branch of medicine that involves the study of diseases of the anus and rectum and their treatment.

**proctorrhaphy** *n* repair of a tear in the anus or rectum.

**proctoscope** *n* a speculum or rigid tubular instrument for examining the anal canal and rectum. ⇒ endoscope—**proctoscopic** *adj*.

**proctoscopy** *n* inspection of the anal canal and rectum using a rigid instrument.

**proctosigmoiditis** *n* inflammation of the rectum and sigmoid colon.

**proctotomy** *n* surgery opening into the anus and rectum.

**prodromal** *adj* preceding, such as the transitory rash before the true rash of an infectious disease.

**prodrug** *n* a drug administered as an inactive form that may be activated in a number of ways, e.g. by bowel bacteria, in the brain or by liver enzymes. Used for a variety of reasons such as avoiding gastrointestinal side-effects, or crossing the blood–brain barrier.

**proenzyme** *n* the inactive (or precursor) form of a proteolytic enzyme, such as pepsinogen or trypsinogen. Also called a zymogen.

**professional self-regulation** the professional quality and continuing professional development standards set by various professional regulatory bodies for health professionals, e.g. General Medical Council, for professional practice, discipline and conduct.

**professional socialization** tertiary socialization involves the acquisition of knowledge, skills and attitudes required in performing high-level occupations such as medicine, nursing and allied health professions.

**professions allied to medicine** ⇒ allied health professions.

**profiling (community)** *n* process of producing a profile of a specific community. It includes demographic information such as the age profile, social and economic makeup, existing facilities, networks and services. The profile may be produced by people living in the community with varying degrees of support from the local authority, development agencies or health services.

**profunda** *adj* relating to blood vessels and other structures that are deeply enclosed within the tissues.

**progeria** *n* a rare congenital condition in which the person ages prematurely. It is characterized by the appearance of the signs of ageing, such as skin wrinkling and grey hair, in prepubertal children. Death frequently occurs before the teenage years from coronary artery disease.

**progestational** *adj* before pregnancy. Favouring pregnancy—**progestation** *n*.

**progesterone** *n* a steroid hormone secreted by the corpus luteum, placenta and, in limited amounts, by the adrenal glands. Progesterone acts on the endometrium, myometrium, cervical mucus and breasts. It is important in the preparation for and maintenance of pregnancy.

**progestogen** *n* any natural or synthetic progestational hormone, including progesterone. *progestogen-only contraceptives* available in several formulations: as an oral contraceptive, the progestogen-only pill (POP) that is taken continuously and at regular time intervals to provide effective contraception; for parenteral administration as an intramuscular injection, or a subdermal implant that releases hormone to provide contraception for up to 3 years; and as an intrauterine device that contains progestogen. This device is also used in the management of menorrhagia and to provide progestogen where oestrogen-only hormone replacement is prescribed for a woman with an intact uterus.

**proglottis** *n* a sexually mature segment of tapeworm—**proglottides** *pl*.

**prognathism** *n* an anomaly in which one or both upper and lower jaw bones projects forward.

**prognosis** *n* a forecast of the probable course and termination of a disease—**prognostic** *adj*.

P

**projection** *n* a defence mechanism occurring in normal people unconsciously, and in exaggerated form in some mental health problems, whereby the person fails to recognize certain motives and feelings in himself or herself but attributes them to other people.

**projective techniques** the therapeutic use of creative media such as art and music to encourage individuals to express themselves and to explore and interpret their thoughts and feelings.

**prolactin (PRL)** *n* a hormone secreted by the anterior pituitary, which initiates milk production. It suppresses ovulation naturally during lactation; however, this does not always happen and pregnancies may occur. Excessive secretion of prolactin can be a cause of infertility. ⇒ hyperprolactinaemia.

**prolactinoma** *n* prolactin-secreting pituitary adenoma. ⇒ hyperprolactinaemia.

**prolapse** *n* descent; the falling of a structure. *prolapse of an intervertebral disc (PID)* protrusion of the disc nucleus into the spinal canal. Most common in the lumbar region, where it causes low-back pain and/or sciatica. *prolapse of the iris* iridocele. *prolapse of the rectum* the lower portion of the intestinal tract descends outside the external anal sphincter. The rectal mucosa may be visible outside the anus. May be associated with chronic constipation with straining. *prolapse of the uterus* the uterus descends into the vagina and may be visible at the vaginal orifice. ⇒ procidentia.

**prolapsed umbilical cord** ⇒ cord prolapse.

**proliferate** *vi* increase by cell division—**proliferation** *n*, **proliferative** *adj*.

**prolific** *adj* fruitful, multiplying abundantly.

**proline** *n* a conditionally essential (indispensable) amino acid.

**promontory** *n* a projection; a prominent part.

**promoter** *n* **1.** a sequence of deoxyribonucleic acid (DNA) that controls the start of transcription. **2.** a substance that acts with another carcinogen to stimulate cells to divide more rapidly than usual, thereby increasing the risk of malignant changes.

**pronate** *vt* to place ventral surface downward, e.g. on the face; to turn (the palm of the hand) downwards. ⇒ supinate *opp*—**pronation** *n*.

**pronator** *n* that which pronates, usually applied to a muscle. For example, the two-headed *pronator teres*, a superficial muscle of the forearm. Its origin is on the medial epicondyle of the humerus and on the coronoid process of the ulna; its common tendon inserts on

to the shaft of the radius. Contraction of the muscle pronates the forearm and hand. ⇒ supinator *opp*. ⇒ Appendix 1, Figure 4.

**prone** *adj*. **1.** lying on the anterior surface of the body with the face turned to the side. **2.** of the hand, with the palm downwards. ⇒ supine *opp*.

**pronephros** *n* the earliest non-functional kidney tissue that forms in the embryo. ⇒ mesonephros, metanephros.

**pronucleus** *n* the nuclear material of the ovum and spermatozoon following the penetration of the oocyte by the spermatozoon. Each contains the haploid (n) number of chromosomes, but before fusion to create the nucleus of the zygote with the diploid (2n) number of chromosomes.

**pro-opiomelanocortin (POMC)** *n* a large protein prohormone which is produced in the anterior lobe of the pituitary gland and found in other tissues. It gives rise to adrenocorticotrophic hormone (ACTH), endorphins, enkephalins, lipotrophins and melanocyte-stimulating hormones.

**properdin** *n* a globulin involved in the alternative pathway of complement activation.

**prophase** *n* the first stage in both mitosis (see Figure M.6, p. 308) and meiosis (see Figure M.3, p. 296). In mitosis the chromatin condenses and shortens to form a visible double set of chromosomes (from DNA replication during interphase). The double chromosomes are joined by the centromeres; each half of the chromosome is known as a chromatid. The nucleoli start to break down and the nuclear membrane disappears. Each pair of centrioles moves to opposite poles of the cell where they commence the formation of the mitotic spindle which eventually reaches from one pair of centrioles to the other. Prophase I in meiosis takes longer than in mitosis. Unique to meiosis, there is pairing or synapsis of homologous chromosomes to form a bivalent, comprising two chromosomes, which coil around each other. The chromosome pairs undergo incomplete separation and each chromosome now has two chromatids; now each unit has four strands (quadrivalents). Several 'crossover' points or chiasmata form between the chromatids. This facilitates the exchange of genetic material between the chromosomes of the homologous pair and the production of gametes of infinite genetic variability. Separation of the two bivalents continues and the nucleolus and nuclear membrane disappear. Prophase II in the second meiotic division

**P**

follows the same steps but this time with only 23 chromosomes, rather than homologous pairs. ⇒ anaphase, metaphase, telophase.

**prophylaxis** *n* (attempted) prevention, e.g. immunization—**prophylactic** *adj*, **prophylactically** *adv*.

**propionic acids** a group of non-steroidal anti-inflammatory drugs, e.g. ibuprofen. ⇒ Appendix 5.

**proprietary name** (*syn* brand name) the name given to e.g. a drug by the pharmaceutical company which developed it. It should always be spelt with a capital letter to distinguish it from the approved (generic) name, which can be used by other companies.

**proprioception** *n* appreciation of balance and the position of the body and individual body parts in relation to each other, especially as they change during movement.

**proprioceptive neuromuscular facilitation (PNF)** exercises that stimulate proprioceptors in muscles, tendons and joints in order to improve strength and flexibility.

**proprioceptor** *n* a sensory receptor located in a muscle, tendon, ligament or vestibular apparatus of the ears whose reflex function is locomotor or postural.

**proptosis** *n* forward protrusion, especially of the eyeball.

**prosencephalon** *n* forebrain. One of the three primary vesicles formed during early embryonic development of the brain. It becomes the diencephalon and the telencephalon.

**prosody** *n* describes the phonological features of speech that include rate, rhythm, stress, loudness and pitch.

**prospective study** research that deals with future data, moving forward in time. ⇒ retrospective study.

**prostacyclin** *n* a substance derived from prostaglandins. Produced by endothelial cells lining blood vessels. It inhibits platelet aggregation and is concerned with preventing intravascular clotting.

**prostaglandins** *npl* a large group of potent regulatory lipids derived from arachidonic acid. They have a short duration of action and modulate the action of several hormones. Found in most body tissues where they regulate physiological functions, including: smooth muscle contraction, inflammation, gastric secretion and blood clotting. Used therapeutically to terminate pregnancy, induce labour, and for the treatment of asthma, erectile dysfunction and gastric hyperacidity. ⇒ Appendix 5.

**prostate** *n* a small conical gland at the base of the male bladder and surrounding the first part of the urethra. Adds alkaline fluid containing enzymes into the semen (⇒ Appendix 1, Figure 16)—**prostatic** *adj*.

**prostate cancer** a common cancer in men over the age of 50 years. It is characterized by dysuria, prostatis/cystitis, frequency, poor urine stream, hesitancy, dribbling, etc. Management may include careful monitoring, radiotherapy, hormone therapy or surgery. ⇒ prostate-specific antigen.

**prostate-specific antigen (PSA)** protein secreted by prostatic tissue. Acts as a tumour marker for prostate cancer, and its detection in the blood forms the basis for a screening test. Conditions other than prostate cancer can cause an increase in PSA level.

**prostatectomy** *n* surgical removal of the prostate gland. *retropubic prostatectomy* the prostate is reached through a lower abdominal (suprapubic) incision, the bladder being retracted upwards to expose the prostate behind the pubis. *transurethral prostatectomy* ⇒ transurethral resection of prostate (TUR/ TURP). *transvesical prostatectomy* the operation in which the prostate is approached through the bladder, using a lower abdominal (suprapubic) incision.

**prostatic** *adj* relating to the prostate. *benign prostatic hyperplasia* (BPH) ⇒ benign prostatic enlargement. *prostatic acid phosphatase* ⇒ acid phosphatase.

**prostatism** *n* term used to describe the symptom complex associated with bladder outflow obstruction.

**prostatitis** *n* inflammation of the prostate gland.

**prosthesis** *n* an artificial substitute for a missing part—**prostheses** *pl*, **prosthetic** *adj*.

**prosthetic group** a non-protein coenzyme or metal ion which must attach to an enzyme protein in order for enzyme activity to occur. ⇒ apoenzyme.

**prosthetics** *n* the branch of surgery which deals with prostheses.

**protanopia** *n* a severe type of colour blindness in which the person has no retinal photoreceptors for red light. ⇒ daltonism, deuteranopia.

**protease** *n* an enzyme which digests protein (proteolytic). *protease enzymes*, e.g. streptokinase, are used in the management of leg ulcers to remove slough and facilitate healing.

**protease inhibitor** a class of antiviral drugs, e.g. ritonavir, used in the treatment of human immunodeficiency virus (HIV) disease and acquired immunodeficiency syndrome (AIDS).

**protective isolation** reverse barrier nursing. Involves separating patients who are immunocompromised and susceptible to infection, either by disease or treatment. The type of patients needing protection from infection include those with leukaemia and those having immunosuppressant treatment for organ transplantation, chemotherapy or radiation or neutropenic patients. ⇒ containment isolation, source isolation.

**proteinase** *n* proteolytic enzyme that hydrolyses protein.

**protein-bound iodine** a former test of thyroid function superseded by tests that directly measure the thyroid hormone levels.

**protein–energy malnutrition (PEM)** previously known as protein–calorie malnutrition (PCM). Describes a condition in which individuals have depleted body fat and protein resulting from a diet that is deficient in both protein and energy. It develops during famine, during illness and during childhood due to inappropriate weaning. ⇒ chronic energy deficiency, kwashiorkor, marasmus.

**proteins** *npl* highly complex nitrogenous compounds found in all animal and vegetable tissues. They are built up of amino acids and are essential for growth and repair of the body. Those from animal sources are of high biological value since they contain the essential amino acids. Those from vegetable sources contain not all, but some, of the essential amino acids. Proteins are hydrolysed in the body to produce amino acids, which are then used to build up new body proteins.

**proteinuria** *n* excretion of abnormally high levels of protein in the urine. ⇒ albuminuria.

**proteolysis** *n* the hydrolysis of the peptide bonds of proteins with the formation of smaller polypeptides by the action of enzymes, alkalis or acids —**proteolytic** *adj*.

*Proteus* *n* a bacterial genus of Gram-negative motile rods of the family Enterobacteriaceae. Found in damp surroundings and is a commensal of the intestinal tract. Species including *Proteus mirabilis* and *P. vulgaris* cause urinary tract infections and wound infections.

**prothrombin** *n* inactive precursor of the enzyme thrombin produced in the liver. Factor II in blood coagulation.

**prothrombin time** assesses the activity of the extrinsic coagulation pathway. It is the time taken for plasma to clot in vitro following the introduction of thromboplastin in the presence of calcium. It is inversely proportional to the amount of prothrombin present; a normal person's plasma is used as a standard of comparison. The prothrombin time is extended in people taking anticoagulant drugs and in some haemorrhagic conditions.

**proton** *n* subatomic particle having a positive charge.

**proton pump** $H^+/K^+$-ATPase, an enzyme concerned with the production of gastric acid. An adenosine triphosphate (ATP)-powered pump by which hydrogen ions enter the lumen of the stomach and potassium ions move into the parietal cell in the production of hydrochloric acid.

**proton pump inhibitors** a group of drugs, e.g. omeprazole, that decrease gastric acid secretion by irreversibly blocking the proton pump ($H^+/K^+$-ATPase). ⇒ Appendix 5.

**proto-oncogene** *n* a gene with the potential to become a cancer-causing oncogene if stimulated by mutagenic carcinogens. ⇒ oncogene.

**protopathic** *adj* the term applied to the somatic sensations of fast localized pain; slow, poorly localized pain; and temperature. ⇒ epicritic *opp*.

**protoplasm** *n* ⇒ cytoplasm.

**protoporphyrin** *n* a porphyrin produced during the synthesis of haem, it combines with ferrous iron to form haem. Excess amounts are present in the faeces in some types of porphyria. Measuring the level of protoporphyrin in the red blood cells (erythrocytes) is used as a test for iron deficiency and other states where iron is not incorporated within haem, such as in lead poisoning.

**protozoa** *npl* unicellular microscopic animals. Some are pathogenic. Includes the genera *Plasmodium*, *Leishmania* and *Entamoeba*—**protozoon** *sing*, **protozoal** *adj*. ⇒ amoebiasis, giardiasis, leishmaniasis, malaria, toxoplasmosis, trichomoniasis.

**protraction** *n* a forward movement such as thrusting out the jaw. ⇒ retraction *opp*.

**proud flesh** excessive granulation tissue.

**provitamin** *n* a vitamin precursor, e.g. β-carotene that is converted into vitamin A, or 7-dehydrocholesterol in the skin that is converted into vitamin D.

**proximal** *adj* nearest to the head or source. ⇒ distal *opp*—**proximally** *adv*.

**PRP** *abbr* panretinal photocoagulation.

**prune-belly syndrome (Eagle–Barrett syndrome)** a condition found in male infants with obstructive uropathy and atrophy

P

of the abdominal musculature. The term is descriptive.

**prurigo** *n* a chronic itching disease often associated with skin lichenification.

**pruritus** *n* itching. *pruritus ani* and *pruritus vulvae* may be due to a number of causes, e.g. vaginitis. Generalized pruritus may be a symptom of systemic disease, as in renal failure, Hodgkin's disease, cancer or jaundice—**pruritic** *adj*.

**PSA** *abbr* prostate-specific antigen.

**pseudoangina** *n* false angina. Sometimes referred to as 'left mammary pain', it occurs in anxious individuals. Usually there is no cardiac disease present. May be part of effort syndrome.

**pseudoarthrosis** *n* a false joint, e.g. due to ununited fracture; also congenital, e.g. in tibia.

**pseudobulbar paralysis** there is disturbance in the higher control of the tongue and pharynx, typically with cognitive and limb abnormalities, and found most often in the context of amyotrophic lateral sclerosis (ALS) or a succession of 'strokes'.

**pseudocoxalgia** *n* ⇒ Legg–Calvé–Perthes disease.

**pseudocrisis** *n* a rapid reduction of body temperature resembling a crisis, followed by further fever.

**pseudocyesis** *n* ⇒ phantom pregnancy.

**pseudocyst** *n* a collection of fluid or gas, which lacks a containing membrane. A feature of pancreatitis.

**pseudogout** *n* an arthritis (usually monoarthritis) caused by crystals of calcium pyrophosphate dihydrate within the joint.

**pseudohermaphrodite** *n* a person in whom the gonads of one sex are present, whilst the external genitalia comprise those of the opposite sex.

**pseudologia fantastica** a tendency to tell, and defend, fantastic lies plausibly.

**pseudomembranous colitis** inflammation of the colon coated in pale plaques (pseudomembranes). Usually caused by superinfection with *Clostridium difficile*. Recent antibiotic usage predisposes.

*Pseudomonas* *n* a bacterial genus. Gram-negative motile rods. Found in water and decomposing vegetable matter. Some are pathogenic to plants and animals and *Pseudomonas aeruginosa* is a cause of urinary, wound and respiratory infection in humans. It can cause superinfection where the normal commensals have been eliminated by antibiotic usage.

Produces blue-green exudate or pus with a characteristic musty odour.

**pseudomucin** *n* a gelatinous substance (not mucin) found in some ovarian cysts.

**pseudophakia** *n* presence of an artificial lens. Describes an eye after cataract surgery with intraocular lens implantation.

**pseudopolyposis** *n* widely scattered polyps, usually the result of previous inflammation—sometimes ulcerative colitis.

**pseudoseizures** *npl* attacks that can look like epileptic seizures but which have no electrical basis and are normally related to mental health problems.

**psittacosis** *n* disease of parrots, pigeons and budgerigars which is occasionally responsible for atypical pneumonia in humans. Caused by *Chlamydia psittaci*.

**psoas** *n* two muscles of the loin. *psoas major* ⇒ iliopsoas (⇒ Appendix 1, Figure 4). *Psoas minor* long slender muscle, which, if present is adjacent to the psoas major.

**psoas abscess** a cold abscess in the psoas muscle, resulting from tuberculosis of the vertebrae. The abscess appears as a firm smooth swelling which does not show signs of inflammation—hence the adjective 'cold'.

**psoralen** *n* a naturally occurring photosensitive compound, used in psoralen with ultraviolet A (PUVA) treatment.

**psoriasis** *n* a genetically determined chronic skin disease in which erythematous scaly plaques characteristically occur on the elbows, knees and scalp—**psoriatic** *adj*.

**psoriatic arthritis** arthritis occurring in association with psoriasis.

**psyche** *n* Greek term for 'life force', used to describe that which makes up the mind and all its processes, and sometimes used to describe 'self'.

**psychiatrist** *n* a doctor with additional qualifications in the diagnosis and treatment of mental health disorders.

**psychiatry** *n* the branch of medicine that addresses the diagnosis and treatment of mental health disorders—**psychiatric** *adj*.

**psychic** *adj* of the mind.

**psychoactive** *adj* substances and drugs that may alter mental processes.

**psychoanalysis** *n* a specialized branch founded by Freud. It is a method of diagnosis and treatment of some mental health problems. Briefly the method is to revive past forgotten experiences and effect a cure by helping the patient readjust his or her attitudes to those experiences—**psychoanalytic** *adj*.

P

**psychodrama** n a psychotherapy technique whereby patients act out their personal problems by adopting roles in spontaneous dramatic performances. Group discussion aims at giving the patients a greater awareness of the problems presented and possible strategies for dealing with them.

**psychodynamics** n the science of the mental processes, especially of the factors causing mental activity.

**psychogenesis** n the development of the mind.

**psychogenic** adj arising from the mind. *psychogenic symptom* originates in the mind.

**psychogeriatric** adj outdated term, relating to the application of psychology to geriatrics. The phrase 'elderly mentally ill' (EMI) has also been used. *psychogeriatric dependency rating scales* (PGDRS) construction of these scales was based on three basic dimensions—psychological deterioration, physical infirmity and psychological agitation.

**psychologist** n a person who specializes in psychology: development, processes of the mind and behaviour. *clinical psychologist* a suitably qualified person who provides professional services for people with emotional problems in a variety of settings.

**psychology** n the study of behaviour and mental processes.

**psychometry** n the science involved with mental testing.

**psychomotor** adj pertaining to the motor effects of mental activity.

**psychoneuroimmunology (PNI)** n study of the integration of neural and immune responses in relation to psychological state. Psychological distress/stress is associated with the impairment of immune system function.

**psychoneurosis** n outdated term. ⇒ neurosis.

**psychopath** n one who is morally irresponsible and intent on instant gratification—**psychopathic** adj.

**psychopathic personality** a persistent disorder of the mind (whether or not including learning disability) which results in abnormally aggressive or seriously irresponsible behaviour that requires, or is susceptible to, medical treatment. ⇒ mental health legislation.

**psychopathology** n the pathology of abnormal mental states—**psychopathological** adj, **psychopathologically** adv.

**psychopharmacology** n the study and use of drugs which influence the affective and emotional state—**psychopharmacological** adj, **psychopharmacologically** adv.

**psychophysics** n a branch of experimental psychology concerned with stimuli and sensations—**psychophysical** adj.

**psychoprophylactic** adj that which aims at preventing mental health problems.

**psychosexual** adj pertaining to the mental aspects of sexuality.

**psychosexual counselling** usually sought by one or both members of a partnership because one or both is unable to obtain emotional and sexual satisfaction within the relationship. Psychosexual counselling of otherwise 'healthy' people is provided by specialists and is rarely provided by the NHS in the UK. Health care professionals need to be aware that any health disturbance may create actual or potential psychosexual problems.

**psychosexual development** according to Freud's theory, development occurs through five stages (oral, anal, phallic, latent and genital). Each stage is characterized by a different area of pleasurable stimulation.

**psychosis** n the term 'psychotic' is used as a grouping term for disorders where a lack of contact with reality occurs, e.g. by hallucinations or delusions—**psychoses** pl, **psychotic** adj.

**psychosomatic** adj pertaining to the mind and body. *psychosomatic disorder* a term previously used to describe a physical condition where psychological factors such as stress may be involved in the cause, such as some types of peptic ulcer.

**psychotherapy** n treatment of emotional and psychological problems by individual or group interaction, usually by talking, but many other approaches exist—**psychotherapeutic** adj. *group psychotherapy or group therapy* a therapist enables and encourages people to understand and analyse their own problems and those of other group members.

**psychotropic** adj that which exerts its specific effect upon the brain cells.

**psychrophiles** npl micro-organisms that grow and divide at low temperature. Usually within a range 15–20°C, but they will grow at lower temperatures.

**PTA** abbr percutaneous transluminal angioplasty.

**PTC** abbr percutaneous transhepatic cholangiography.

**PTCA** abbr percutaneous transluminal coronary angioplasty.

**pteroylglutamic acid** ⇒ folic acid.

**pterygium** n **1.** a wing-shaped degenerative condition of the conjunctiva which encroaches on the cornea. **2.** adhesion of the eponychium (cuticle) to the nail bed. It follows destruction of the matrix due to diminished circulation or some systemic diseases. The entire nail plate is eventually shed.

**PTH** *abbr* parathyroid hormone.

**ptosis** *n* a drooping, particularly that of the upper eyelid. Common in old age—**ptotic** *adj*.

**PTSD** *abbr* post-traumatic stress disorder.

**ptyalin** *n* ⇒ amylase.

**puberty** *n* the period during which the reproductive organs become functionally active and the secondary sexual characteristics develop—**pubertal** *adj*.

**pubes** *n* the hair-covered area over the pubic bone.

**pubiotomy** *n* rarely performed surgery that involves cutting the pubic bone to facilitate delivery of an infant.

**pubis** *n* the pubic bone or os pubis. The two bones that meet at the symphysis pubis—**pubic** *adj*.

**public health** broadly defined as health activity for populations in small areas, regions, nations and worldwide. In the UK public health involves the following functions: (a) health surveillance, monitoring and analysis; (b) investigation of disease outbreaks, epidemics and risks to health; (c) establishing, designing and managing health promotion and disease prevention programmes; (d) enabling and empowering communities and citizens to promote health and reduce inequalities; (e) creating and sustaining cross-governmental and intersectoral partnerships to improve health and reduce inequalities; (f) ensuring compliance with regulations and laws to protect and promote health; (g) developing and maintaining a well-educated and trained, multidisciplinary public health workforce; (h) ensuring the effective performance of the NHS services to meet goals in improving health, preventing disease and reducing inequalities; (i) research, development, evaluation and innovation; and (j) quality-assuring the public health function.

**pudendal block** the rendering insensitive of the pudendum by the injection of local anaesthetic. Used mainly for episiotomy and forceps delivery. ⇒ transvaginal.

**pudendum** *n* the external reproductive organs, especially of the female—**pudenda** *pl*, **pudendal** *adj*.

**puerperal** *adj* pertaining to childbirth. *puerperal psychosis* a serious mental illness (psychosis) occurring in the puerperium. ⇒ postnatal depression. *puerperal sepsis* infection of the genital tract occurring within 21 days of abortion or childbirth.

**puerperium** *n* the period immediately following childbirth to the time when involution is completed, usually 6–8 weeks—**puerperia** *pl*.

**PUFA** *abbr* polyunsaturated fatty acid.

**PUJ** *abbr* pelviureteric junction.

***Pulex irritans*** the human flea.

**pulmonary** *adj* pertaining to the lungs. *pulmonary tuberculosis* ⇒ tuberculosis.

**pulmonary artery** the large artery that carries deoxygenated blood from the right ventricle to the lungs. It divides into two to form a right and left pulmonary artery, one to each lung. ⇒ Appendix 1, Figures 7 and 8.

**pulmonary artery flotation catheter (PAFC)** specialized balloon-tipped catheter which is 'floated' from the central veins, through the heart and into the pulmonary artery (Figure P.13). Allows measurement of pulmonary artery occlusion pressure. More specialized PAFCs can measure cardiac output, and from it calculate the cardiac index, stroke volume, pulmonary vascular resistance and systemic vascular resistance.

**pulmonary artery occlusion pressure (PAOP)** pressure in the left atrium measured by inflating a balloon on the tip of a pulmonary artery catheter, thereby temporarily occluding the pulmonary artery; also known as wedge pressure.

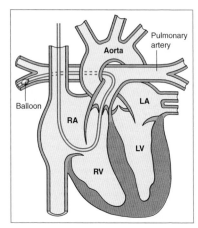

**Figure P.13** Pulmonary artery flotation catheter *(reproduced from Boon et al. 2006 with permission)*.

**pulmonary artery pressure** blood pressure in the pulmonary artery, usually measured using a pulmonary artery catheter.

**pulmonary circulation** deoxygenated blood leaves the right ventricle, flows through the lungs where it loses carbon dioxide, becomes oxygenated and returns to the left atrium of the heart. ⇒ circulation.

**pulmonary embolus (PE)** an embolism which occurs in the pulmonary arterial system, most commonly as a result of deep-vein thrombosis in the leg or pelvic veins. Prophylaxis includes deep breathing and foot exercises, early mobilization, antithromboembolic stockings with the administration of heparin in at-risk groups.

**pulmonary emphysema** overdistension and subsequent destruction of alveoli and reduced gas exchange in the lungs. Associated with tobacco smoking, it is a form of chronic obstructive pulmonary disease (COPD). ⇒ bronchitis.

**pulmonary hypertension** raised blood pressure within the pulmonary circulation, due to increased resistance to blood flow within the pulmonary vessels. It may be primary (genetic) or secondary due to chronic lung disease or chronic pulmonary embolism.

**pulmonary infarction** necrosis of lung tissue resulting from an embolism.

**pulmonary oedema** fluid within the alveoli. The lungs are 'waterlogged' and gas exchange is reduced, such as in left ventricular failure, mitral stenosis or fluid excess in renal failure.

**pulmonary rehabilitation** combination of graded physical exertion, educational, psychological and behavioural interventions designed to improve symptoms in those with chronic lung disease.

**pulmonary valve** semilunar valve situated between the pulmonary artery and right cardiac ventricle. *pulmonary stenosis* narrowing of the pulmonary valve.

**pulmonary vascular resistance (PVR)** *n* the resistance in the pulmonary vascular bed which the right ventricle must overcome in order to pump blood into the pulmonary circulation.

**pulmonary veins** four veins, two from each lung, which convey oxygenated blood from the lungs to the left atrium. ⇒ Appendix 1, Figures 7 and 8.

**pulmonary ventilation** or minute volume. The amount of air moved in and out of the lungs in 1 minute.

**pulp** *n* the soft, interior part of some organs and structures. *digital pulp* the tissue pad of the finger tip. ⇒ dental pulp.

**pulsatile** *adj* beating, throbbing.

**pulsation** *n* beating or throbbing, as of the arteries or heart.

**pulse** *n* the impulse transmitted to arteries by contraction of the left ventricle, and customarily palpated in the radial artery at the wrist. The *pulse rate* is the number of beats or impulses per minute and is about 130 in the newborn infant, 70–80 in the adult and 60–70 in old age. The *pulse rhythm* is its regularity—and can be regular or irregular; the *pulse volume* is the amplitude of expansion of the arterial wall during the passage of the wave; the *pulse force* or tension is its strength, estimated by the force needed to obliterate it by pressure of the finger.

**pulse deficit** the difference between heart rate (counted by stethoscope) and pulse rate (counted at the wrist), as seen in atrial fibrillation.

**pulse oximeter** an instrument attached to the finger, ear or nose to 'sense' the oxygen saturation of arterial blood (Figure P.14). An accurate non-invasive technique.

**pulse pressure** the difference between the systolic and diastolic blood pressures.

**pulseless disease (Takayasu's disease)** progressive obliterative arteritis of the vessels arising from the aortic arch, resulting in diminished or absent pulse in the neck and arms. Thromboendarterectomy or a bypass procedure may prevent blindness by improving the carotid blood flow at its commencement in the aortic arch.

**pulseless electrical activity (PEA)** a type of cardiac arrest where there is a normal or nearly normal electrical activity without an effective cardiac output. Also known as electromechanical dissociation.

**pulseless ventricular tachycardia** a form of cardiac arrest. ⇒ ventricular tachycardia.

**pulsus alternans** a regular pulse with alternate beats of weak and strong amplitude; associated with left ventricular heart failure.

**pulsus bigeminus** double pulse wave produced by interpolation of extrasystoles. A coupled beat.

**pulsus paradoxus** arterial pulsus paradoxus is alteration of the volume of the arterial pulse sometimes found in pericarditis. The volume becomes greater with expiration. Venous pulsus paradoxus (Kusman's sign) is an increase in the height of the venous pressure with inspiration,

**P**

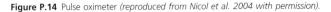

**Figure P.14** Pulse oximeter *(reproduced from Nicol et al. 2004 with permission)*.

the reverse of normal. Sometimes found in pericardial or right ventricular disease.

**pulvis** *n* a powder.

**punctate** *adj* dotted or spotted, e.g. punctate
basophilia describes red cells in which there
are droplets of blue-staining material in the
cytoplasm.

**punctum** *n* entrance to lacrimal drainage system on eyelid margin—**puncta** *pl.*

**puncture** *n* a stab; a wound made with a sharp
pointed hollow instrument for withdrawal or
injection of fluid or other substance. ⇒ cisternal puncture, lumbar puncture, penetrating
wound.

**PUO** *abbr* pyrexia of unknown origin.

**pupil** *n* the opening in the iris of the eye, which
allows the passage of light—**pupillary** *adj.*

**pupillary** *adj* relating to the pupil.

**pupillary light reflex** the reflex dilatation
and constriction of the pupil in response
to the amount of light entering the eye.

Controlled by the oculomotor nerves (third
pair of cranial nerves).

**purgative** *n* a drug that causes the evacuation
of fluid faeces.

**purines** *npl* nitrogenous base, such as adenine
and guanine, needed as constituents of nucleosides, nucleotides and nucleic acids. Uric acid
is produced when purines are broken down.
Increased uric acid in the blood is associated
with disorders of metabolism and excretion of
uric acid, and leads to the development of gout.

**purpura** *n* superficial haemorrhage, less than
1 cm, into the skin. A disorder characterized
by extravasation of blood from the capillaries
into the skin, or into or from the mucous membranes. May be small red spots (petechiae) or
large bruises (ecchymoses) or by oozing from
minor wounds confined to the mucous membranes. It may be due to impaired integrity
of the capillary walls, or defective quality or
quantity of platelets. Purpura can be caused by

many different conditions, e.g. infective, toxic, allergic, etc. ⇒ Henoch–Schönlein purpura.

**purulent** *adj* pertaining to or resembling pus.

**pus** *n* a liquid, usually yellowish in colour, formed in certain infections and composed of tissue fluid containing bacteria and leucocytes. Various types of bacteria are associated with pus having distinctive features, e.g. the faecal smell of pus due to *Escherichia coli*; the green colour of pus due to *Pseudomonas aeruginosa*.

**pustule** *n* a visible collection of free pus in a blister usually indicates an infection (e.g. furuncle) but not always (e.g. pustular psoriasis)—**pustular** *adj*. malignant pustule ⇒ anthrax.

**putrefaction** *n* rotting; bacterial destruction of organic material.

**putrescine** *n* a molecule produced when protein breaks down during the putrefaction of animal tissue. It results from the breakdown of ornithine, an amino acid, and has an extremely foul odour. ⇒ cadaverine.

**PUVA** *abbr* psoralen with ultraviolet radiation of a long wavelength used for the treatment of skin diseases, particularly psoriasis.

**PV** *abbr* per vaginam: describes the route used for examination of the vagina, or the administration of drugs.

**P-value** in all inferential statistics a P-value is given. This is the probability that the results found have occurred by chance alone. The probability is measured on a scale of 0–1—a P-value of $P = 0.05$ means 5% or a 1 in 20 chance, and $P = 0.01$ means a 1% or 1 in 100 chance. A common error is to assume a high P-value means the result is significant: a low value shows significance. So the probability of a test result occurring by chance is the P-value. Lower-case *p* is used for proportions.

**PVD** *abbr* peripheral vascular disease.

**PVL** *abbr* Panton–Valentine leukocidin.

**PVR** *abbr* pulmonary vascular resistance.

**PVS** *abbr* persistent vegetative state.

**pyaemia** *n* the presence of septic emboli in the circulation. They can lodge in organs such as the liver, brain, kidneys and lungs, to form multiple abscesses—**pyaemic** *adj*.

**pyarthrosis** *n* pus in a joint cavity.

**pyelitis** *n* obsolete term. ⇒ pyelonephritis.

**pyelography** *n* ⇒ urography.

**pyelolithotomy** *n* the operation for removal of a stone from the renal pelvis.

**pyelonephritis** *n* acute infection within the substance of the kidney, often derived either from the urine or from the blood—**pyelonephritic** *adj*.

**pyeloplasty** *n* a reconstructive operation on the kidney pelvis. ⇒ hydronephrosis.

**pyelostomy** *n* surgical formation of an opening into the kidney pelvis.

**Pyemotes** *n* previously called *Pediculoides*. A genus of mites found in grain straw and hay. The species *Pyemotes ventricosus* causes an allergic dermatitis ('grain itch').

**pyknosis** *n* darkening and condensation of nuclear chromatin.

**pylethrombophlebitis** *n* inflammation and thrombus in the hepatic portal vein.

**pyloric stenosis 1.** narrowing of the pylorus due to scar tissue formed during the healing of a peptic ulcer. **2.** congenital hypertrophic pyloric stenosis due to a thickened pyloric sphincter muscle. ⇒ pyloromyotomy.

**pyloroduodenal** *adj* pertaining to the pylorus and the duodenum.

**pyloromyotomy** *n* (*syn* Ramstedt's operation) incision of the pyloric sphincter muscle as in pyloroplasty.

**pyloroplasty** *n* a plastic operation on the pylorus designed to widen the passage.

**pylorospasm** *n* spasm of the pylorus, usually due to the presence of a duodenal ulcer.

**pylorus** *n* region containing the opening of the stomach into the duodenum, controlled by a sphincter muscle—**pyloric** *adj*.

**pyocolpos** *n* pus in the vagina.

**pyodermia, pyoderma** *n* any purulent condition of the skin—**pyodermic** *adj*.

**pyogenic** *adj* relating to pus formation.

**pyometra** *n* pus retained in the uterus and unable to escape through the cervix—**pyometric** *adj*.

**pyonephrosis** *n* distension of the renal pelvis with pus—**pyonephrotic** *adj*.

**pyopericarditis** *n* pericarditis with purulent effusion.

**pyopneumothorax** *n* pus and gas or air within the pleural sac.

**pyorrhoea** *n* a flow of pus.

**pyosalpinx** *n* a uterine (fallopian) tube containing pus.

**pyothorax** *n* pus in the pleural cavity.

**pyramidal** *adj* applied to some conical eminences in the body. *pyramidal cells (Betz cells)* nerve cells in the precentral motor area of the cerebral cortex, from which originate impulses to voluntary muscles. *pyramidal tracts* main motor tracts in the brain and spinal cord, which transmit impulses arising from the pyramidal cells. Most decussate (cross over) in the medulla.

**P**

**pyrazolones** *npl* a group of non-steroidal anti-inflammatory drugs. ⇒ Appendix 5.

**pyrexia** *n* body temperature above normal, usually between 37°C and 40/41°C. *pyrexia of unknown origin* (PUO) where the reason for the raised body temperature is not known. ⇒ fever, hyperpyrexia—**pyrexial** *adj*.

**pyridoxal phosphate** the major form of vitamin $B_6$ in the body.

**pyridoxine** *n* vitamin $B_6$, a mixture of the phosphates of pyridoxine, pyridoxal and pyridoxamine; important as a cofactor in glycogen and amino acid metabolism. Deficiency may lead to dermatitis and neuritic pains. Used in nausea of pregnancy and radiation sickness, muscular dystrophy, pellagra, the premenstrual syndrome, etc.

**pyrimidines** *npl* nitrogenous bases, such as cytosine, thymine and uracil, needed as constituents of nucleic acids.

**pyrogen** *n* a substance producing fever—**pyrogenic** *adj*.

**pyrosis** *n* (*syn* heartburn, waterbrash) eructation of acid gastric contents into the mouth, accompanied by a burning sensation felt behind the sternum.

**pyrotherapy** *n* production of fever by artificial means. ⇒ hyperthermia.

**pyrroles** *npl* substances that form part of porphyrin and haem.

**pyruvic acid** pyruvate. An important metabolic molecule. Converted to acetyl coenzyme A, which is used in the Krebs' cycle, or forms lactic acid during anaerobic glucose metabolism.

**pyuria** *n* pus in the urine (more than three leucocytes per high-power field)—**pyuric** *adj*.

P

## Q

**QALYs** *abbr* quality-adjusted life years.

**Q fever** a febrile disease caused by the Gram-negative bacterium *Coxiella burnetii*. It is transmitted to humans from sheep, cattle or in unpasteurized milk and from domestic animals. Pasteurization of milk kills *C. burnetii*.

**Qi energy** also known as chi, yin/yang. In complementary medicine, the person's inborn energy focused on maintaining health and well-being. The concept of Qi energy is fundamental to therapies such as acupuncture where the energy is believed to flow through meridians.

**Q–T interval** ⇒ P-QRS-T complex.

**quadrantanopia** *n* loss of vision in one quadrant of the visual field.

**quadratus** *adj* having four sides. *quadratus femoris* a short muscle with its origin on the ischial tuberosity and its insertion on the greater trochanter on the femur. It is a lateral rotator of the thigh and stabilizes the hip. *quadratus lumborum* a muscle of the posterior abdominal wall. Its origin is on the iliac crest and it inserts on to the upper lumbar vertebrae and the last rib. If one side contracts it flexes the spine laterally, or both sides work together to maintain the upright position.

**quadriceps femoris** *n* large four-part extensor muscle of the anterior and lateral thigh, comprising the rectus femoris, vastus medialis, vastus lateralis and vastus intermedius. The origins depend on the individual muscles, but are either on the ilium or the upper end of the femur. All four parts insert via a common tendon on to the tibial tuberosity and the patella. Its main action is to extend the knee. ⇒ rectus femoris, vastus. ⇒ Appendix 1, Figure 4.

**quadriparesis** *n* weakness of all four limbs.

**quadriplegia** *n* ⇒ tetraplegia—**quadriplegic** *adj*.

**qualitative** *adj* relating to quality.

**qualitative research** research study based on observation and/or interviews to ascertain people's opinions, feelings or beliefs. Non-statistical methods often used in analysis. ⇒ quantitative research.

**quality-adjusted life years (QALYs)** measure of years of life gained through a health intervention adjusted for the quality of life. For example, if an intervention prolongs life by 5 years, but at only half the quality of normal life, this produces 2.5 QALYs. Quality of life (QoL) is a patient-centred subjective outcome measure to complement clinical outcomes. Usually measures the presence or absence of symptoms (e.g. pain), side-effects of treatment (e.g. tiredness, loss of hair), feelings of well-being, impact on income, family, work and social life.

**quality assurance** systematic monitoring and evaluation of agreed levels of service provision which are followed by modifications in the light of the evaluation and/or audit. ⇒ benchmarking, clinical audit, performance indicators.

**quality circles** an initiative to improve the quality of care in a specific area. The health professionals in a clinical area investigate a health care intervention systematically and relate it to good standards of practice.

**quantitative** *adj* relating to quantity.

**quantitative research** research study based on the measurement and analysis of observations using statistical methods. ⇒ qualitative research.

**quarantine** *n* a period of isolation of infected people or those suspected of having an infectious disease with the objective of preventing spread to others. For contacts it is usually the same period as the longest incubation period for the specific disease.

**quartan** *adj* recurring every 72 hours (fourth day), such as the fever of quartan malaria.

**Queckenstedt's test** (H Queckenstedt, German physician, 1876–1918) during lumbar puncture compression on the internal jugular vein normally produces a rise in cerebrospinal fluid (CSF) pressure if there is no obstruction to circulation of fluid.

**quellung reaction** swelling of the capsule of a bacterium when exposed to specific antisera. It allows the identification of bacteria causing a disease.

**Quetelet's index** (A Quetelet, Belgian mathematician/sociologist, 1796–1874) an index of body mass. ⇒ body mass index.

**quickening** *n* the first perceptible fetal movements felt by the mother, usually at 16–18 weeks' gestation.

**quiescent** *adj* becoming quiet or inactive.

**quinine** *n* an alkaloid of cinchona, previously standard treatment for malaria. Use is increasing in regions where resistance to newer antimalarials is a problem.

**quininism** *n* toxic effects such as headache, tinnitus and partial deafness, disturbed vision and nausea arising from an overdose or long-term use of quinine.

**quinsy** *n* ⇒ peritonsillar abscess.

**quotient** *n* a number obtained by division. ⇒ respiratory quotient. *intelligence quotient* ⇒ intelligence.

**R**

**RA latex test** used in rheumatoid arthritis. A blood test used to detect the presence of the rheumatoid factor. ⇒ sheep cell agglutination test (SCAT).

**rabbit fever** ⇒ tularaemia.

**rabid** *adj* infected with rabies.

**rabies** *n* (*syn* hydrophobia) fatal infection of the central nervous system caused by a virus; infection follows the bite of a rabid animal, e.g. dog, cat, fox, vampire bat. It is distributed worldwide apart from a few areas; human and animal vaccines are available—**rabid** *adj*.

**race** *n* often mistakenly linked to ethnicity. However, race only applies to biological characteristics such as facial features, skin colour or hair type that distinguish a specific group. ⇒ ethnic.

**racemose** *adj* resembling a bunch of grapes, such as the alveoli that cluster around the terminal airways, or certain exocrine glands.

**rachitic** *adj* relating to rickets, or resembling or affected by rickets.

**racism** *n* an opinion of particular groups that is founded on race alone. It results in negative stereotyping, prejudice and discrimination. Racism may be overt, where individuals are subjected to oppressive acts, or covert, where a climate of institutional racism permits one section of society to oppress and subordinate other groups.

**rad** *n* obsolete term. ⇒ gray (Gy).

**radial** *adj* pertaining to the radius. *radial artery* the artery running down the lateral aspect of the forearm to the wrist, where it is easily felt and is used to count the pulse rate. *radial nerve* a branch of the brachial plexus, it innervates the triceps muscle at the back of the arm, the extensor muscles of the wrist and hand and some of the skin of the digits. *radial vein* one of the deep veins of the forearm. ⇒ Appendix 1, Figures 9 and 10.

**radiation** *n* emanation of radiant energy in the form of electromagnetic waves including: gamma rays, infrared, ultraviolet rays, X-rays and visible light rays. Subatomic particles, such as neutrons or electrons, may also be radiated. Radiation may be non-ionizing or ionizing and has many diagnostic and therapeutic uses. ⇒ ionizing radiation.

**radiation oncologist** medical specialist in the treatment of disease by X-rays and other forms of radiation.

**radiation sickness** tissue damage from exposure to ionizing radiation leading to diarrhoea, vomiting, anorexia, and later, alopecia, bleeding and bone marrow failure. Other longerterm effects include fetal damage and birth defects, sterility, eye damage, leukaemia and other cancers.

**radical** *adj* pertaining to the root of a thing. *radical surgery* usually extensive and aims to be curative, not palliative, such as a Whipple's operation for cancer of the head of pancreas.

**radiculitis** *n* inflammation affecting a nerve root.

**radiculography** *n* X-ray of the spinal nerve roots after rendering them radiopaque to locate the site and size of a prolapsed intervertebral disc. Superseded by computed tomography and magnetic resonance imaging—**radiculogram** *n*.

**radiculopathy** *n* entrapment of the nerve as it passes out from the spinal cord to the arm or leg, and usually occurs as a result of intervertebral disc prolapse and degenerative disease in the facet joints of the spine.

**radioactive** *adj* exhibiting radioactivity. Describes an unstable atomic nucleus which emits charged particles as it disintegrates. ⇒ radioisotope. *radioactive decay* the spontaneous disintegration of radioactive atoms within a radioactive substance. ⇒ half-life. *radioactive fallout* release of radioactive particles into the atmosphere. Results from industrial processes or accidents, and the testing or use of nuclear weapons.

**radioallergosorbent test (RAST)** an obsolete test for immunoglobulin E (IgE) antibodies against specific allergens. Now largely replaced by non-radioactive enzyme-based assays.

**radiobiology** *n* the study of the effects of radiation on living tissue—**radiobiological** *adj*, **radiobiologically** *adv*.

**radiocarbon** *n* a radioactive form of the element carbon, such as carbon-14 ($^{14}$C), used for investigations, e.g. absorption tests and research.

**radiodermatitis** *n* the skin changes caused by exposure to ionizing radiation, such as during radiotherapy for cancer, or occupational exposure. The affected skin is red and sore with blister formation and weeping. There may be lasting effects that include fibrosis, scarring and loss of skin pigment.

**radiograph** *n* a photographic image formed by exposure to X-rays; the correct term for an 'X-ray'—**radiographic** *adj*.

**radiographer** *n* there are two distinct professional disciplines within radiography, diagnostic and therapeutic; they are registered health professionals qualified in the use of ionizing radiation and other techniques, either in diagnostic imaging or radiotherapy.

**radiography** *n* the use of X-radiation: (a) to create images of the body from which medical diagnosis can be made (diagnostic radiography); or (b) to treat a person suffering from a (malignant) disease, according to a medically prescribed regimen (therapeutic radiography). ⇒ radiotherapy.

**radioimmunoassay** *n* the use of radioactive substances to measure substances such as hormones and drugs in the blood.

**radioiodinated human serum albumin (RIHSA)** used for detection and localization of brain lesions, determination of blood and plasma volumes, circulation time and cardiac output.

**radioisotope** *n* (*syn* radionuclide) forms of an element which have the same atomic number but different mass numbers, exhibiting the property of spontaneous nuclear disintegration. Different radioisotopes are used in diagnosis, treatment and research. Examples of radioisotopes include iodine-131 ($^{131}$I), strontium-90 ($^{90}$Sr), technetium ($^{99m}$Tc). *radioisotope scan* pictorial representation of the amount and distribution of radioactive isotope present in a particular organ. When administered orally, by injection, or inhaled, they can be traced using a gamma camera. They are also used in types of tomography, such as positron emission tomography.

**radiologist** *n* a medical specialist in diagnosis by using X-rays and other allied imaging techniques.

**radiology** *n* the study of the diagnosis of disease by using X-rays and other allied imaging techniques—**radiological** *adj*, **radiologically** *adv*.

**radiolucent** *adj* relating to substances that permit X-rays and other types of radiant energy to pass through with minimum loss through absorption; appearing as dark images on exposed film.

**radiomimetic** *adj* exerting effects similar to those of ionizing radiation.

**radionuclide** *n* ⇒ radioisotope.

**radiopaque** *adj* having the property of significantly absorbing X-rays, thus becoming visible on a radiograph. Barium and iodine compounds are used, as contrast media, to produce artificial radiopacity—**radiopacity** *n*.

**radioresistance** *n* the ability of tissues, both normal and some cancers, to withstand the effects of ionizing radiation.

**radiosensitive** *adj* applied to tissues, normal and some cancers, which are sensitive to the killing effects of ionizing radiation. Radiosensitizer drugs are used in some cases to increase the sensitivity of some cancers.

**radiosurgery** *n* (*syn* stereotactic radiotherapy) a radiotherapy treatment based on a three-dimensional co-ordinate system designed to achieve a high concentration of absorbed dose to an intracranial target.

**radiotherapist** *n* ⇒ radiation oncologist.

**radiotherapy** *n* the use of ionizing radiation in the treatment of proliferative disease, especially cancer, and certain non-malignant diseases, such as the use of a precisely focused radiation for the relief of pain in trigeminal neuralgia. Radiotherapy may be used alone but is more often used in combination with surgery, chemotherapy, or hormone therapy and other biological treatment modalities. It may be used as a curative treatment or as palliative treatment to reduce symptoms of advanced disease, such as pain. Total body irradiation is used to prepare patients with haemopoietic cancers for a haemopoietic stem cell transplant (bone marrow transplant). Ionizing radiation interrupts deoxyribonucleic acid (DNA) synthesis or decreases the rate of mitotic divisions. Thus cell replication is prevented, although several cell divisions may need to occur before cell death eventually occurs. The therapy may be applied by external-beam methods (teletherapy) by employing a unit which emits megavoltage radiation in order to treat cancers deep within the body, and lower-energy units such as orthovoltage or kilovoltage units for more superficial cancers. A course of radiotherapy usually takes a few minutes each day, but is spread over a number of weeks. Brachytherapy describes radiotherapeutic modalities in which sealed (removed after treatment) or unsealed radiactive sources are delivered close to the cancer, such as a radioactive source placed into the body for some gynaecological cancers. In systemic therapy, radioactive isotopes (radionuclides), (e.g. yttrium-90 [$^{90}$Y] for neuroendocrine cancers and iodine–131 [$^{131}$I] for thyroid cancer) are administered orally or intravenously and are preferentially taken up by the cancerous tissue. Radiotherapy aims to deliver a homogeneous cancer-killing dose to a precisely localized area of the body, to avoid as much normal tissue as possible

**R**

without compromising the treatment outcome and to avoid any critical structures such as the gonads, kidney or spinal cord, which may be particularly sensitive to radiation. Although radiation is unable to discriminate between normal and malignant tissues, there is a differential effect and cancer cells are more sensitive to the effects of treatment.

**radioulnar joint** one of two joints between the radius and ulna. *proximal radioulnar joint* a pivot joint in which the rim of the head of the radius articulates in the radial notch of the ulna at the elbow joint. *distal radioulnar joint* a pivot joint in which the distal extremity of the radius articulates with the head of the ulna.

**radium (Ra)** *n* a radioactive element occurring in nature, historically a mainstay of radiotherapy. However, it has been largely replaced by radioisotopes of caesium and cobalt.

**radius** *n* outer bone of the forearm, it articulates with the humerus at the elbow, the carpal bones at the wrist, and with the ulna at the proximal and distal radioulnar joints. ⇒ Appendix 1, Figures 2 and 3.

**radon seeds** capsules containing radon—a radioactive gas produced by the disintegration of radium atoms. Historically used in radiotherapy.

**raised intracranial pressure (RIP)** an elevation in intracranial pressure is a serious situation. Causes include: tumours, intracranial haemorrhage, brain injury causing oedema or haematoma and obstruction to the flow of cerebrospinal fluid. The features depend on the cause, but there may be headache, vomiting, papilloedema, seizures (fits), bradycardia, arterial hypertension and changes in the level of consciousness. ⇒ benign intracranial hypertension.

**râle** *n* abnormal sound heard on auscultation of lungs when fluid is present in bronchi.

**Ramsay Hunt syndrome** (J Ramsay Hunt, American neurologist, 1872–1937) herpes zoster causing vesicles on the ear lobe with pain, vertigo, impaired hearing, facial paralysis and loss of taste.

**Ramstedt's operation** (C Ramstedt, German surgeon, 1867–1972) ⇒ pyloromyotomy.

**random sampling** in research. The selection process whereby every person in the population has an equal chance of being selected.

**randomized controlled trial (RCT)** research study using two or more randomly selected groups: experimental and control. It produces high-level evidence for practice.

**range** *n* describes the span of values (lowest–highest) observed in a sample.

**range of motion (ROM)** the movements possible at a joint.

**ranula** *n* a cystic swelling beneath the tongue due to blockage of a duct—**ranular** *adj*.

**rape** *n* unlawful sexual intercourse without consent which is achieved by force or deception. Full penetration of the vagina (or other orifice) by the penis and ejaculation of semen is not necessary to constitute rape. Many rapes include force and violence, but acquiescence because of verbal threats should not be interpreted as consent. Where women are admitted to hospital, a police surgeon will perform an examination to obtain the necessary specimens for forensic examination in the presence of specially trained female police officers who then support the victim throughout the interviews and subsequent investigation and possible prosecution of the alleged perpetrator. Male rape, the rape of a male by another male, is increasingly recognized.

**raphe** *n* a seam, suture, ridge or crease.

**rapid eye movement sleep (REM)** also known as paradoxical sleep. ⇒ sleep.

**rapid plasma reagin test (RPR)** a non-specific serological test for syphilis.

**rarefaction** *n* becoming less dense, as applied to diseased bone—**rarefied** *adj*.

**RAS** *abbr* reticular activating system.

**rash** *n* skin eruption. It may be described in several ways: cause, e.g. napkin rash, nettlerash; colour, e.g. rose-coloured; distribution or shape, e.g. centripetal, butterfly-shaped; and by type of lesion, e.g. macular, maculopapular, papular, papulopustular, papulosquamous, petechial, pustular. ⇒ urticaria.

**Rasmussen's aneurysm** (F Rasmussen, Danish physician, 1837–1877) an aneurysm of a pulmonary artery within a tuberculous cavity.

**Rasmussen's encephalitis (disease or syndrome)** (T Rasmussen, American neurologist, 1910–2002) a rare, progressive brain disorder, in which there is chronic inflammation of one side of the brain; possibly caused by an autoimmune process. It mainly affects children under 10 years of age and is characterized by a deterioration in motor skills and speech, seizures, hemiparesis and a decline in mental abilities. Frequent seizures cause brain damage, which results in permanent neurological deficits.

**RAST** *abbr* radioallergosorbent test.

**rat-bite fever** *n* a relapsing fever caused by the Gram-negative bacterium *Streptobacillus moniliformis* or the spirochaete *Spirillum minus*. Usually transmitted by rat bites or, less often, by other rodents. There is fever, joint and muscle pain and a rash; also causes local inflammation, splenomegaly and lymphadenitis.

**ratio data** measurement data with a numerical score, e.g. height, that has a true zero of 0. It is interval data with an absolute zero. ⇒ interval data.

**rationalization** *n* a defence mechanism whereby a person justifies his or her actions following the event, so it looks more rational or socially acceptable.

**Raynaud's disease** (M Raynaud, French physician, 1834–1881) paroxysmal spasm of the digital arteries producing pallor or cyanosis of fingers or toes, and occasionally resulting in gangrene. The form of the disease most often affects young women aged 18–30 years.

**Raynaud's phenomenon** episodic discoloration of the fingers and sometimes the toes (classically the fingers turn white, then blue, then red), tingling, burning and pain usually in response to temperature change or stress. ⇒ CREST syndrome, hand–arm vibration syndrome.

**RBC** *abbr* red blood cell. ⇒ blood.

**RCT** *abbr* randomized controlled trial.

**RDA** *abbr* recommended daily allowance.

**RDI** *abbr* recommended daily intake.

**RDS** *abbr* respiratory distress syndrome.

**reaction** *n* **1.** response to a stimulus. **2.** a chemical change. *allergic reaction* ⇒ allergy.

**reaction formation** a defence mechanism in which attitudes completely opposite to those unconsciously held are expressed, or the person behaves in a way that is completely contrary to what would normally be anticipated.

**reactive arthritis** (*syn* Reiter's syndrome) arthritis that develops in response to infection, usually urogenital, gastrointestinal or throat infection. ⇒ sexually acquired reactive arthritis.

**reactive oxygen species (ROS)** free radicals and other highly reactive molecules formed from molecular oxygen during normal cell metabolism; also formed in response to insults caused by chemicals, smoking or infection, for example. They include superoxide radical ($O_2^-$), hydroxyl radical ($OH^-$) and hydrogen peroxide ($H_2O_2$).

**reagent** *n* a substance that participates in a chemical reaction, in order to detect, measure or produce other substances.

**reagin** *n* an antibody (immunoglobulin) of the immunoglobulin E (IgE) class that mediates the type I hypersensitivity reactions occurring, for example, in allergies to foodstuffs and atopic conditions such as asthma or hayfever.

**reality orientation (RO)** *n* a form of therapy useful for withdrawn, confused and depressed patients: they are frequently reminded of their name, the time, place, date and so on. Reinforcement is provided by clocks, calendars and signs prominently displayed in the environment.

**real-time imaging** the use of specialized recording equipment to produce images almost instantaneously, such as ultrasound scanning and other imaging techniques, particularly during interventional radiology.

**reasonable doubt** to secure a conviction in criminal proceedings, the prosecution must establish beyond reasonable doubt the guilt of the accused.

**rebore** *n* ⇒ disobliteration.

**recalcitrant** *adj* refractory. Describes medical conditions that are resistant to treatment.

**recall** *n* part of the process of memory. Memory consists of memorizing, retention and recall.

**recannulation** *n* re-establishment of the patency of a vessel.

**receptaculum** *n* receptacle, often forms a reservoir.

**receptive aphasia** a type of aphasia where there are problems of varying severity with language comprehension. Those affected may also have expressive aphasia.

**receptor** *n* **1.** sensory afferent nerve ending capable of receiving and transmitting stimuli. **2.** a protein situated on or inside a cell membrane, or within the cytoplasm. They act as binding sites for various endogenous molecules such as hormones, neurotransmitters or cell mediators. Drugs exert their effects by binding to receptor proteins and interacting in one of two main ways: they may act as an agonist or an antagonist. Those that act as agonists bind to the receptor and imitate the response of the naturally occurring ligand (the endogenous chemical). Drugs can also act as antagonists and bind to receptors, preventing endogenous agonists from binding.

**recessive** *adj* receding; having a tendency to disappear. *recessive trait* a genetic character or trait that is expressed when the determining allele is present at both paired chromosomal loci (i.e. homozygous or 'in double dose'), for example in the inheritance of cystic fibrosis. When the specific allele is present in

R

411

single dose the characteristic is not expressed as it is overpowered by the dominant allele at the other locus, but the person having the single allele is a carrier. However, recessive X-linked genes in males will be expressed in a single dose, such as haemophilia and red–green colour blindness. ⇒ dominant.

**recipient** *n* the individual who receives something from a donor such as blood, an organ such as a kidney or bone marrow. ⇒ blood groups.

**reciprocal inhibition** a technique in which an active contraction of the agonist muscle is used to produce a reflex relaxation of the antagonist, thereby allowing the antagonist muscle to be stretched.

**reciprocal innervation** the interaction between opposing muscle groups that facilitates the contraction needed for controlled movements and stability.

**reciprocal lengthening** when muscles work concentrically, the opposite muscles lengthen to permit movement. ⇒ concentric muscle work.

**reciprocal ponderal index** a way of expressing adiposity. It is the person's height divided by the cube root of his or her weight.

**reciprocal shortening** when muscles work eccentrically, the opposite muscles take up the slack. ⇒ eccentric muscle work.

**Recklinghausen's disease** ⇒ von Recklinghausen's disease.

**recombinant DNA** deoxyribonucleic acid (DNA) produced by recombining chemically the DNA of two different organisms. Used for the study of both normal and abnormal genes and so, for example, of genetic disorders. The practical applications include diagnosis (including prenatal diagnosis) and in the manufacture of therapeutic products, e.g. human insulin, human erythropoietin.

**recommended daily allowance (RDA)** (*syn* recommended daily intake—RDI) refers to national and international standards that recommend the intake level of a particular nutrient for specific groups of people. The term is used in some countries but in the UK dietary reference values (DRVs) are also used. ⇒ dietary reference values.

**recommended International Nonproprietary Name (rINN)** the system of non-proprietary drug names in use internationally.

**reconstituted family** a family with step-parents resulting from divorce or remarriage.

**recovery** *n* a return to a normal state of health. It may be total or only partial.

**recovery position** a first-aid measure where a person with altered level of consciousness is positioned so as to maintain the airway and prevent aspiration of secretions or vomit into the airway (Figure R.1).

**recrudescence** *n* the return of symptoms.

**recruitment** *n* **1.** occurs in sensorineural deafness, where it describes a situation in which the person perceives a rapid increase in loudness of a sound when the increase was only very small. **2.** skeletal muscle is able to 'recruit' more active motor units to increase the strength of muscle contraction.

**rectal varices** haemorrhoids.

**rectocele** *n* prolapse of the rectum, so that it lies outside the anus. Usually used to describe the herniation of the anterior rectal wall into the posterior vaginal wall, caused by injury to the levator ani muscles during childbirth (Figure R.2). Repaired by a posterior colporrhaphy. ⇒ cystocele, procidentia.

**rectosigmoid** *adj* pertaining to the rectum and sigmoid colon.

**rectouterine** *adj* pertaining to the rectum and uterus, such as the rectouterine pouch (pouch of Douglas).

**rectovaginal** *adj* pertaining to the rectum and vagina.

**rectovesical** *adj* pertaining to the rectum and bladder.

**rectum** *n* the slightly dilated, lower part of the large intestine between the sigmoid colon and anal canal. It is about 13 cm in length in adults. The rectum is normally empty until faeces move down from the colon just before defecation. (⇒ Appendix 1, Figure 18B)—**rectal** *adj*, **rectally** *adv*.

**rectus** *n* a straight muscle, such as the four extraocular rectus muscles of the eye, or the rectus femoris of the thigh. ⇒ extraocular, rectus femoris.

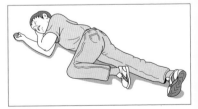

**Figure R.1** Recovery position—adult *(reproduced from Nicol et al. 2004 with permission).*

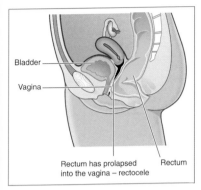

Bladder

Vagina

Rectum has prolapsed into the vagina – rectocele

Rectum

**Figure R.2** Rectocele *(reproduced from Brooker & Nicol 2003 with permission).*

**rectus abdominis** one of a pair of superficial, medial abdominal muscles. It extends from the pubis to the ribs and is covered by the aponeuroses of the other three pairs of abdominal muscles (internal and external obliques and the transversus abdominis). The two muscles are separated by the linea alba formed from the aponeuroses. Its origin is on the crest of the pubis and it inserts on to the costal cartilages of ribs 5–7 and the xiphoid process of the sternum. The rectus abdominis flexes the lower vertebral column, provides pelvic stability during movement and increases intra-abdominal pressure, such as during defecation. ⇒ Appendix 1, Figure 4.

**rectus femoris** one of the four-part quadriceps femoris muscle. A superficial muscle of the anterior aspect of the thigh. Its origin is on anterior superior iliac spine being it inserts via a common tendon on to the tibial tuberosity and the patella. ⇒ quadriceps femoris.

**recumbent** *adj* lying or reclining—**recumbency** *n. recumbent position* lying on the back with the head supported on a pillow.

**recurrent (habitual) abortion** ⇒ miscarriage.

**recurring costs** regular and ongoing costs, such as planned maintenance and staff salaries.

**red blood cell (RBC)** *n* ⇒ erythrocytes.

**red muscle** describes muscle consisting mainly of slow-twitch fibres. The red colour is derived from the plentiful blood supply and myoglobin.

**reducing sugars** sugars that are reducing agents, such as glucose, lactose and fructose.

**reduction** *n* **1.** the process of reducing or state of being reduced. It is the removal of oxygen or the addition of hydrogen or electrons to a substance. ⇒ oxidation. **2.** making smaller. Commonly applied to plastic surgical procedures used to decrease the size of structures, for example the nose or breast. **3.** returning to the normal position, e.g. a hernia or after dislocation or fracture.

**reduction division** the first division occurring during meiosis in which the chromosome numbers are halved from the diploid (2n) number to produce the haploid gametes (n). ⇒ meiosis.

**Reed–Sternberg cell** (D Reed, American pathologist, 1874–1964; K Sternberg, Austrian pathologist, 1872–1935) a large, abnormal multinucleated cell found in the lymphatic system in Hodgkin's disease.

**reference nutrient intake (RNI)** one of the UK dietary reference values. The amount of a nutrient required to make sure that the needs of most people in a group (97.5%) are met. Commonly used as an estimate of the micronutrient, e.g. specific vitamins, requirement of a population. ⇒ dietary reference values, Appendix 4.

**referred pain** pain arising in the viscera but occurring at a distance from its source, e.g. pain felt in the arms, neck or jaw in angina pectoris or myocardial infarction despite there being no tissue injury at those locations. It occurs because sensory impulses from the left arm and heart enter the spinal cord at the same level and the person perceives the pain as coming from the arm. Other examples of referred pain include that from the gallbladder felt in the scapular region or the initial pain of acute appendicitis, which may be experienced in the umbilical region despite the appendix being sited in the right, lower part of the abdomen.

**reflective practice** the conscious and systematic process in which a health professional reflects on personal actions, aspects of practice and evaluates the outcomes. The ability to review, analyse and evaluate situations, during or after events in order to develop professionally and improve practice.

**reflex 1.** *adj* literally, reflected or thrown back; involuntary, not controlled by will. **2.** *n* a reflex action. Examples include abdominal reflex, accommodation reflex, anal reflex, asymmetric tonic neck reflex, conditioned reflex, corneal reflex, cough reflex, doll's-eye reflex, gag reflex, grasp reflex, knee jerk reflex,

**R**

Moro (startle) reflex, parachute reflex, pupillary light reflex, rooting reflex, stepping reflex.

**reflex action** an involuntary motor or secretory response by tissue to a sensory stimulus, e.g. tendon stretch, sneezing, blinking, coughing. Reflexes may be postural or protective. Testing reflexes provides valuable information in the localization and diagnosis of neurological diseases.

**reflex arc** the basic neurological components that facilitate a simple reflex action—a sensory neuron, which synapses with a motor neuron in the spinal cord or brain. In some reflexes a connector neuron(s), also known as an interneuron(s), provides the connection between sensory and motor neurons via several synapses (Figure R.3).

**reflex sympathetic dystrophy** rare chronic pain syndrome. It is now more correctly termed 'complex regional pain syndrome' as the pathophysiology is more complex and varied than first thought. ⇒ complex regional pain syndrome.

**reflexology** *n* a complementary therapy based upon the assertion that the internal body

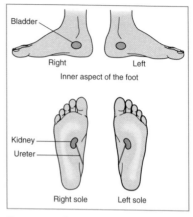

**Figure R.4** Reflexology pressure points on the feet *(reproduced from Brooker & Waugh 2007 with permission).*

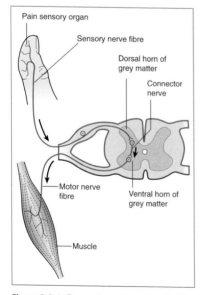

**Figure R.3** Reflex arc *(reproduced from Brooker 2006A with permission).*

structures are 'mapped out' on the soles and palms (Figure R.4). It is thought that gentle pressure upon the areas corresponding to specific structures can lead to a therapeutic response. ⇒ zones.

**reflux** *n* backward flow. ⇒ gastro-oesophageal reflux disease.

**reflux nephropathy** *n* previously known as chronic pyelonephritis. Caused by failure of the one-way valve system where the ureters enter the bladder. This allows urine to reflux up the ureters when pressure increases in the bladder during voiding. This urine later returns to the bladder and is not immediately voided, thus leading to urine stasis, which in turn predisposes to infection. The constant reflux of infected urine up the ureters results in damage to the renal tissue that can, without effective treatment with antibiotics and/or surgical reimplantation of the ureters, lead to renal failure. ⇒ vesicoureteric reflux.

**refraction** *n* the bending of light rays as they pass through media of different densities. In normal vision, this occurs so that the image is focused on the retina—**refractive** *adj*.

**refractive error** a condition in which the refractive power of the eye is unable to focus an image on the retina. ⇒ astigmatism, hypermetropia, myopia.

**refractory** *adj* resistant to treatment or unmanageable.

**refractory period** the period of time during which a nerve or muscle fibre is not able to respond to a stimulus. It may be an *absolute refractory period* in which the production of another action potential is impossible, regardless of the nature of the stimulus, or a *relative refractory period* when an action potential may be elicited if the stimulus is sufficiently strong.

**regeneration** *n* renewal of tissue. Some very superficial wounds may heal by regeneration to leave no visible signs. Damage to fetal tissue also heals by regeneration; healing is characterized by minimal inflammation, fibrosis or scar formation.

**regional ileitis** ⇒ Crohn's disease.

**regression** *n* **1.** reversion to an earlier stage of development, becoming more childish. Occurs in dementia, especially in older people, and more normally, as a defence mechanism, for instance, in a young child reacting to the birth of a sibling. **2.** in genetics, the tendency for physical characteristics in successive generations to move toward the mean for the population rather than being representative of the parents. For instance, a child who has a very tall parent or very short parent is likely to be of average height for the population. **3.** describes the recovery from, or lessening of, signs and symptoms of, a disease, for example a patient with leukaemia following a course of treatment with cytotoxic drugs.

**regression techniques** in statistics, various analytical methods used in multivariate statistics. Used to predict dependent variable(s) from independent variable(s).

**regurgitation** *n* backward flow, e.g. of stomach contents into, or through, the mouth, or blood through an incompetent (regurgitant) heart valve.

**rehabilitation** *n* a planned programme in which convalescents or people with disabilities progress towards, or maintain, the maximum degree of physical and psychological independence of which they are capable. Planned rehabilitation programmes are provided for a variety of conditions that include acute myocardial infarction, cardiac failure, chronic respiratory diseases, musculoskeletal injuries, amputations, stroke, spinal cord injury and brain injury. ⇒ cardiac rehabilitation, Functional Independence Measure, pulmonary rehabilitation.

**rehabilitation clinician** in sports medicine a medical professional who is responsible for the design, progression, supervision and administration of a rehabilitation programme for an injured athlete or sports participant.

**rehearsal in memory** memory processing depends on two forms of rehearsal of facts: *maintenance rehearsal* where information re-enters short-term memory (STM) by repetition (such as repeating the names of a new group); each time the information enters STM appears to enhance its chance of storage in long-term memory (LTM); and *elaborative rehearsal* processing information in STM so that it can be coded for storage in LTM. It may use sensory factors, such as sound, or focus on the meaning of the information.

**Reifenstein's syndrome** (E Reifenstein, American physician/endocrinologist, 1908-1975) an inherited syndrome characterized by hypogonadism, gynaecomastia and azoospermia due to a partial resistance to androgen hormones.

**reiki therapy** a complementary therapy whereby a reiki practitioner positions the hands on a part of the body or in close proximity to the part so that 'universal life force' is transferred to the client. The therapy claims to supply the necessary harmony that benefits various health problems.

**reinforcement** *n* a psychological term that describes the methods employed during conditioning to increase the probability and strength of a response.

**Reissner's membrane** (E Reissner, German anatomist, 1824–1878) the membrane separating the scala vestibuli and scala media in the cochlea of the inner ear. ⇒ basilar membrane.

**Reiter's syndrome** (H Reiter, German physician, 1881–1969) ⇒ reactive arthritis, sexually acquired reactive arthritis.

**rejection** *n* **1.** the act of excluding or denying affection to another person. **2.** the process which leads to the destruction of grafted tissues.

**relapsing fever** louse-borne or tick-borne infection caused by spirochaetes of the genus *Borrelia*. Characterized by a febrile period of a week or so, with apparent recovery, followed by a further bout of fever.

**relative risk** ⇒ risk.

**relaxant** *n* a drug or technique that reduces tension. ⇒ muscle.

**relaxation** *n* a state of consciousness where individuals feel calm and peaceful. Muscle tension, anxiety and stress are all released.

**relaxation techniques** often used in health care and health promotion activities such as stress management. They include meditation,

R

progressive muscle relaxation, visual guided imagery and yoga. ⇒ biofeedback, hypnosis.

**relaxin** *n* polypeptide hormone secreted by the placenta and ovaries. It is considered to have a role in softening the cervix, relaxing myometrial cells and in loosening the ligaments of the pelvic girdle in preparation for labour.

**releaser/releasing mechanism** a stimulus that launches a cycle of instinctive behaviour.

**reliability** *n* in research, a term meaning consistency of results. The likelihood of achieving the same findings using the same research conditions over a period of time or when conducted by different researchers or observers.

**REM sleep** *abbr* rapid eye movement sleep. ⇒ sleep.

**remedial** *adj* describes a therapy or treatment intended to cure or improve a condition or deficit.

**reminiscence therapy** a technique, also known as nostalgia therapy, that provides older persons and others with the opportunity to reflect on, and validate, their memories of the past through the use of old pictures, music and objects. These are used to prompt shared discussion of personal experiences.

**remission** *n* the period of abatement of a fever or other disease.

**remittent** *adj* increasing and decreasing at periodic intervals.

**renal** *adj* relating to the kidney. *renal capsule* ⇒ Appendix 1, Figure 20. *renal function tests* ⇒ kidney function tests. *renal rickets* ⇒ rickets.

**renal artery** paired visceral arteries that branch from the abdominal aorta to supply around 25% of the resting cardiac output to the kidneys each minute. ⇒ Appendix 1, Figures 19 and 20.

**renal calculus** stone in the kidney.

**renal colic** extremely severe loin pain caused by the movement of stones within the ureter or kidney. Pain may also be felt in the labia or testes, or the groin. It is characterized by nausea and vomiting, tachycardia and fever if infection is present. Patients are sweaty and may thrash about in an effort to find a position that gives relief.

**renal failure** can be described as acute or chronic. Acute renal failure (ARF) occurs when previously healthy kidneys suddenly fail because of a variety of problems affecting the kidney and its perfusion with blood. This condition is potentially reversible. ARF is treated by haemofiltration or haemodiafiltration until kidney function improves. Chronic renal failure (CRF) occurs when irreversible and

progressive pathological destruction of the kidney leads to end-stage renal disease/failure (ESRD). This process usually takes several years, but once ESRD is reached, death will follow unless the patient is treated with some type of renal replacement therapy such as dialysis or renal transplant. ⇒ acute tubular necrosis, crush syndrome, uraemia.

**renal glycosuria** occurs in patients with a normal blood glucose (sugar) and a lowered renal threshold for glucose.

**renal threshold** the level of a substance (e.g. glucose) in the blood at which it is excreted into the urine.

**renal transplant** kidney transplant. The transplantation of a single well-matched kidney from a living or cadaveric donor to a recipient with end-stage renal failure. The donated kidney is usually sited in the iliac fossa, rather than in its normal anatomical position, i.e. a heterotopic transplant.

**renal tubule** the tubular component of the nephron. It comprises Bowman's capsule, proximal convoluted tubule, the loop of Henle, distal convoluted tubule and the collecting tubule. ⇒ nephron.

**renal vein** paired veins that convey venous blood from the kidney to the inferior vena cava (IVC). The left vein is longer and receives blood from the left suprarenal and gonadal (ovarian or testicular) vein before draining into the IVC. ⇒ Appendix 1, Figures 19 and 20.

**renin** *n* a proteolytic enzyme produced and released by the kidney (juxtaglomerular apparatus) in response to low serum sodium or low blood pressure.

**renin–angiotensin–aldosterone response** a mechanism initiated by renin that is involved with the regulation of fluid balance, sodium level and blood pressure. A plasma protein (angiotensinogen) is activated to produce angiotensin I, which in turn is converted into the powerful vasocontrictor angiotensin II. This also causes aldosterone to be secreted, leading to sodium reabsorption with water, thus further raising blood pressure. ⇒ aldosterone, angiotensin.

**rennin** *n* milk-curdling enzyme found in the gastric juice of human infants and ruminants. It converts caseinogen into casein.

**renography** *n* radioisotope study of the kidney.

**reovirus** *n* a group of RNA viruses that includes the rotavirus, which causes gastroenteritis.

**repetitive strain injury (RSI)** a misleading term used to describe diffuse pain and inflammation randomly occurring in the hand and forearm arising from repetitive activities in the workplace, aggravated by static posture. ⇒ work-related upper-limb disorder.

**repolarization** *n* the process whereby the membrane potential of an excitable cell returns from the depolarized state to its polarized resting (negative) state.

**repression** *n* a mental defence mechanism whereby painful events, unacceptable thoughts and impulses are impelled into, and remain in, the unconscious mind.

**reproductive system** the structures necessary for reproduction. In the male it includes the testes, deferent ducts (vas deferens), prostate gland, seminal vesicles, urethra and penis (⇒ Appendix 1, Figure 16). In the female it includes the ovaries, uterine tubes, uterus, vagina and vulva (⇒ Appendix 1, Figure 17).

**RES** *abbr* reticuloendethelial system. ⇒ monocyte–macrophage system.

**rescue breaths** artificial respiration used in first-aid situations to oxygenate the blood when the casualty is not breathing or has suffered a cardiac arrest. Depending on the age of the casualty, mouth-to-mouth or mouth-to-mouth/nose rescue breaths are used (Figure R.5). ⊙DVD

**research** *n* systematic investigation of data, etc., and observations to establish facts or principles, so as to produce organized scientific knowledge. Research may be quantitative or qualitative. Quantitative research defines variables to be collected and converted into numerical values. The data are analysed either to describe the data using descriptive statistics, or to test whether there are relationships between the data using inferential statistics. On the other hand, in qualitative research typically there is uncertainty about the relevance of data, so predefining the data to collect is not useful. Qualitative research studies typically use small samples, but collect more data on each subject, usually by observation or interview. *research design* how a research study is to be undertaken, such as data collection method, statistical analysis, etc.

**resection** *n* surgical excision.

**resectoscope** *n* an instrument passed along the urethra; it permits resection of tissue from the base of the bladder and prostate under direct vision, and for other treatments for benign enlargement of the prostate. ⇒ transurethral resection of prostate.

**reservoirs of infection** the skin, respiratory tract and bowel are colonized by bacteria and fungi which form the normal flora in humans. The normal flora may become pathogenic under certain circumstances.

**resident flora** normal flora. ⇒ transient flora.

**residential home** the premises where residential care is delivered by the independent sector, social services or voluntary organizations.

**residual** *adj* remaining.

**residual air** the air remaining in the lung after forced expiration.

**residual urine** the volume of urine remaining in the bladder after micturition.

**resistance** *n* power of resisting. In psychology, describes the force which prevents repressed thoughts from re-entering the conscious mind from the unconscious. *resistance to infection* the capacity to withstand infection. ⇒ immunity. *peripheral resistance* ⇒ peripheral.

**resistance training** strength training. In sports medicine, the training activities that increase muscle size and strength by working against resistance.

**resisted range of movement** a range of movement that occurs with resistance being applied.

**resolution** *n* the subsidence of inflammation; describes the earliest indications of a return to normal, as when, in lobar pneumonia, the consolidation begins to liquefy.

**resonance** *n* the musical quality elicited on percussing a cavity which contains air. *vocal resonance* is the reverberating note heard through the stethoscope when the patient is asked to say 'one, one, one' or '99'.

**resorption** *n* the act of absorbing again, e.g. absorption of (a) callus following bone

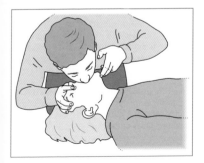

**Figure R.5** Rescue breaths—adult *(reproduced from Brooker & Waugh 2007 with permission).*

R

fracture; (b) roots of the deciduous teeth; and (c) blood from a haematoma.

**respiration** *n* the gaseous exchange between a cell and its environment—**respiratory** *adj. external respiration* is the exchange of gases between alveolar air and pulmonary capillary blood. Oxygen in the alveolar air moves into the blood, and carbon dioxide moves from the blood into the air in the lungs for excretion. *internal* or *tissue respiration* is the reverse process, involving gaseous exchange between the cells and blood. Oxygen moves from the blood, via the tissue fluid, to the cells, and waste cellular carbon dioxide moves into the blood for onward transport to the lungs. ⇒ abdominal breathing, Cheyne–Stokes respiration, Kussmaul respiration, paradoxical respiration.

**respirator** *n* an apparatus worn over the nose and mouth and designed to purify the air breathed through it.

**respiratory distress syndrome (RDS)** ⇒ acute/adult respiratory distress syndrome, multiple-organ dysfunction syndrome, neonatal respiratory distress syndrome.

**respiratory failure** failure of the lungs to oxygenate the blood adequately or remove waste carbon dioxide ($CO_2$). The management depends on the type, cause and severity, but includes: oxygen therapy, mechanical ventilation, tracheostomy, supportive measures and treatment of the underlying cause. It may be classified into two broad types: *type I respiratory failure*, which is usually acute but may be chronic. It is characterized by hypoxia without hypercapnia. The blood gases show hypoxaemia – $PaO_2$ is low (<8.0 kPa) without hypercapnia and the $PaCO_2$ is normal or reduced (<6.6 kPa). It occurs in conditions that damage lung tissue. Acute causes include acute/adult respiratory distress syndrome (ARDS), asthma, pneumonia, pulmonary oedema, pulmonary embolus, pneumothorax, etc. Chronic type I failure may occur in pulmonary fibrosis, severe anaemia, etc. *type II respiratory failure* is more often chronic but can be acute, when it is called asphyxia. Type II is characterized by hypoxia and hypercapnia. The blood gases show hypoxaemia – $PaO_2$ is low (<8.0 kPa) and there is hypercapnia—$PaCO_2$ is high (>6.6 kPa). It occurs in situations where alveolar ventilation is inadequate to excrete the waste carbon dioxide generated by cell metabolism. Acute causes include acute epiglottitis, foreign body in the airway, flail chest, severe acute asthma, paralysis of respiratory muscles, injury to brainstem, narcotic drugs, etc. Chronic type II failure occurs in chronic obstructive pulmonary disease.

**respiratory function tests** tests available for assessing respiratory function and aiding in diagnosis of respiratory disease. Includes spirometry to measure forced expiratory volume in 1 second ($FEV_1$) and forced vital capacity (FVC), and in more specialized laboratories measurements of total lung volume and gas transfer factor.

**respiratory quotient** the ratio between inspired oxygen and expired carbon dioxide during a specified time.

**respiratory syncytial virus (RSV)** a paramyxovirus that causes bronchiolitis and pneumonia in infants and small children. Infants under 6 months may be severely affected.

**respiratory system** deals with gaseous exchange. Comprises the nose, nasopharynx, larynx, trachea, bronchi and lungs. ⇒ Appendix 1, Figures 6 and 7.

**respite care** short-term or temporary care provided within a health or social care facility to allow relief for family and other home carers. May be residential or on a daily basis.

**resting cell** describes a cell that is between mitotic divisions. ⇒ cell cycle.

**restless-leg syndrome** restless legs characterized by paraesthesiae-like creeping, crawling, itching and prickling.

**restorative dentistry** the branch of dentistry that specializes in restoring the hard tissues of teeth that have been damaged or become diseased. Includes the use of fillings, caps, inlays, crowns, bridges, dentures and implants.

**rest pain** pain in the legs and feet caused by ischaemia. The pain occurs when the patient lies down and is relieved by sitting or standing up. ⇒ peripheral vascular disease.

**rest reinjury cycle** a pattern of injury that occurs when an athlete returns to activity after an injury and subsequently aggravates that injury due to inadequate recovery.

**restrictive lung disease** conditions that limit lung and chest wall expansion, thereby reducing lung capacity. They include pulmonary fibrosis, muscular dystrophies, bony abnormalities of the thoracic cage and spine.

**resuscitation** *n* restoration to life of one who is collapsed or apparently dead—**resuscitative** *adj.* ⇒ cardiopulmonary resuscitation.

**retainer** *n* various devices used in dentistry, such as the fixed or removable retainer used to maintain the position of the teeth following orthodontic treatment.

**retardation** *n* **1.** the slowing of a process which has already been carried out at a quicker rate or higher level. **2.** arrested growth or function from any cause.

**retching** *n* straining at vomiting.

**rete** *n* a network, especially of blood vessels.

**retention** *n* **1.** retaining of facts in the memory. **2.** accumulation of that which is normally excreted. *retention cyst* a cyst caused by the blocking of a duct. ⇒ ranula.

**retention of urine** accumulation of urine within the bladder due to interference of nerve supply, obstruction or psychological factors.

**reticular** *adj* resembling a net.

**reticular activating system (RAS)** a diffuse functional area in the reticular formation of the brainstem. It has connections with other parts of the brain, including the cerebral cortex, thalamus, hypothalamus and cerebellum; it is involved in the level of consciousness, sleep–wake cycles, the state of cortical arousal and some autonomic functions.

**reticular formation** the collection of neurons present in the brainstem that regulate the level of consciousness and some autonomic functions. ⇒ reticular activating system.

**reticulin** *n* the protein found in connective reticular fibres present in lymphoid tissue.

**reticulocyte** *n* an immature circulating red blood cell which still contains traces of the nucleus. Accounts for up to 2% of circulating red cells.

**reticulocytosis** *n* an increase in the number of reticulocytes in the blood, indicating active red blood cell formation in the marrow. ⇒ reticulocyte.

**reticuloendothelial system (RES)** ⇒ monocyte–macrophage system.

**reticulosis** *n* abnormal proliferation of cells of the reticuloendothelial system (monocyte–macrophage system) such as occurs in lymphomas and certain leukaemias.

**retina** *n* layer of tissue in the eye that converts light into electrical signals. Consists of a multiple-layer complex of neurosensory retina containing nerve cells that include photoreceptors (rods and cones) and a layer of pigmented cells beyond the neurosensory retina (Figure R.6). ⇒ Appendix 1, Figure 15—**retinal** *adj*.

**retinaculum** *n* tenaculum. A structure that keeps another body structure/organ in place, for example, the retinacula over the tendons of the hand—**retinacula** *pl*.

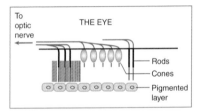

**Figure R.6** Layer of rods and cones on the outside of the retina—simplified *(reproduced from Watson 2000 with permission).*

**retinal** *n* also known as retinene or retinaldehyde. A light-sensitive molecule present in the photoreceptors of the retina. It is derived from retinol (vitamin A) and combines with an opsin to form rhodopsin.

**retinal detachment** occurs when the neural retina becomes separated from the pigmented epithelium. It is known as rhegmatogenous if a hole is present, and non-rhegmatogenous without a hole. Retinal detachment may be associated with myopia, head trauma, age-related retinal degeneration and following cataract surgery, tumours, inflammation and diabetes. It is characterized by the presence of dark spots (floaters) that move with the eye, a curtain or shadow in the field of vision, flashing lights and possibly visual distortions. Early treatment is essential to prevent blindness in the affected eye. Retinal detachment involving the area around the macula lutea is treated as an emergency. The hole or detachment may be sealed using techniques that include lasers, cryotherapy, injection of a gas bubble or bands.

**retinene** *n* ⇒ retinal.

**retinitis** *n* inflammation of the retina. *retinitis pigmentosa* an inherited non-inflammatory degenerative condition of the retina that leads to visual impairment and blindness.

**retinoblastoma** *n* a malignant tumour of the neuroglial element of the retina; occurs exclusively in children.

**retinochoroiditis** *n* ⇒ chorioretinitis.

**retinoids** *npl* a group of vitamin A derivatives. ⇒ Appendix 5.

**retinol** *n* various forms of vitamin A, which can be converted to metabolically active substances, such as retinal.

**retinopathy** *n* disease of the retina. Includes those caused by diabetes, abnormality of the retinal vessels and hypertension. *retinopathy of prematurity* previously called retrolental fibroplasia. A circulatory disorder occurring in preterm babies. ⇒ diabetic retinopathy.

**retinoschisis** *n* a split in the layers of the retina. A type of retinal detachment.

**retinoscope** *n* instrument for detection of refractive errors by illumination of retina using a mirror.

**retinotoxic** *adj* toxic to the retina.

**retractile** *adj* capable of being drawn back, i.e. retracted.

**retraction** *n* a backward movement. ⇒ protraction *opp*.

**retraction ring** the ridge or retraction ring that forms between the upper and lower uterine segments as the lower segment thins during labour, as the presenting part descends and the cervix dilates. ⇒ Bandl's ring.

**retractor** *n* a surgical instrument for holding apart the edges of a wound to reveal underlying structures.

**retrobulbar** *adj* pertaining to the back of the eyeball. *retrobulbar neuritis* inflammation of the optic nerve behind the eyeball.

**retrocaecal** *adj* behind the caecum.

**retroflexion** *n* the state of being bent backwards, such as of the uterus. ⇒ anteflexion *opp*.

**retrognathic** *adj* pertaining to a mandible that is posterior to its normal position in relation to other facial structures.

**retrograde** *adj* going backward. *retrograde amnesia* ⇒ amnesia. *retrograde ejaculation* ⇒ ejaculation. *retrograde urography/pyelography* ⇒ urography.

**retroperitoneal** *adj* behind the peritoneum, such as the kidneys and adrenal glands. *retroperitoneal abscess* pus in the space behind the peritoneum of the posterior abdominal wall. *retroperitoneal fibrosis* inflammation leading to the formation of fibrous tissue behind the peritoneum of the posterior abdominal wall. It may be idiopathic or associated with the use of certain drugs (e.g. methysergide used in migraine prophylaxis, pergolide used in Parkinson's disease).

**retropharyngeal** *adj* behind the pharynx, such as a retropharyngeal abscess.

**retroplacental** *adj* behind the placenta.

**retropubic** *adj* behind the pubis.

**retrospection** *n* morbid dwelling on the past.

**retrospective study** research that deals with past data, moving backwards in time. ⇒ prospective study.

**retrosternal** *adj* behind the sternum.

**retrotracheal** *adj* behind the trachea.

**retroversion** *n* turning backward. ⇒ anteversion *opp*. *retroversion of the uterus* tilting of the whole of the uterus backward with the cervix pointing forward—**retroverted** *adj*.

**retroviruses** *npl* family of ribonucleic acid (RNA) viruses that include the human immunodeficiency viruses (HIV 1 and 2) and the human T-cell lymphotropic viruses (HTLV 1 and 2).

**Rett's syndrome** (A Rett, Austrian paediatrician, 1924–1997) a neurodegenerative disorder occurring in girls. X-linked dominant inheritance. There is progressive neurological and developmental regression from early childhood. Death occurs by second or third decade.

**revascularization** *n* the regrowth of blood vessels into a tissue or organ after deprivation of its normal blood supply.

**revenue budget** the budget allocation for day-to-day running costs, e.g. salaries, telephone, electricity and drugs, etc. ⇒ capital budget.

**reverse barrier nursing** ⇒ protective isolation.

**reverse transcriptase inhibitors (nucleoside/non-nucleoside)** two groups of drugs that act by inhibiting the enzyme reverse transcriptase, required for viral replication, e.g. efavirenz, zidovudine. ⇒ Appendix 5.

**Reye syndrome** (R Reye, Australian pathologist, 1912–1977) 'wet brain and fatty liver' as described in 1963. There is cerebral oedema without cellular infiltration, and diffuse fatty infiltration of liver and other organs, including the kidney. The age range of recorded cases is 2 months–15 years. Presents with vomiting, hypoglycaemia and disturbed consciousness, jaundice being conspicuous. There is an association with aspirin administration and infections including chickenpox and influenza. Aspirin and aspirin-containing products should not be given to children and young people under the age of 16 years, except where it is specifically indicated.

**RF** *abbr* rheumatoid factor.

**Rh** *abbr* Rhesus factor. ⇒ blood groups.

**rhabdomyolysis** *n* disease of skeletal muscle where muscle injury leads to myoglobinuria. It may also be due to crush injury or compression, which can result in acute renal failure.

**rhabdomyoma** *n* a benign tumour of muscle, occurring in the heart or tongue and in other sites.

**rhabdomyosarcoma** *n* a rare malignancy of primitive striated muscle cells.

R

**rhagades** *npl* superficial elongated scars radiating from the nostrils or angles of the mouth and which are found in congenital syphilis. One of the stigmata of the disease.

**RHD** *abbr* rheumatic heart disease.

**rhegmatogenous** *adj* pertaining to a hole or tear. ⇒ retinal detachment.

**Rhesus factor (Rh)** ⇒ blood groups.

**Rhesus incompatibility, isoimmunization** this problem arises when a Rhesus-negative woman carries a Rhesus-positive fetus. During or before the birth there is mixing of fetal and maternal bloods. The woman's body then develops antibodies against the Rhesus-positive blood. If a subsequent fetus is also Rhesus-positive, then maternal antibodies will attack the fetal blood, causing severe haemolysis. ⇒ blood groups.

**rheumatic** *adj* pertaining to rheumatism, a non-specific term. *rheumatic diseases* a diverse group of diseases affecting connective tissue, joints and bones. They include: inflammatory joint disease, e.g. rheumatoid arthritis, septic arthritis and gout; connective tissue disease, e.g. systemic lupus erythematosus; osteoarthritis; non-articular/soft-tissue rheumatism, e.g. fibromyalgia. *rheumatic heart disease (RHD)* chronic cardiac disease with valve damage resulting from rheumatic fever.

**rheumatic fever** (*syn* acute rheumatism) a disorder, tending to recur but initially commonest in childhood, classically presenting as fleeting polyarthritis of the larger joints with swelling and pain, tachycardia, pyrexia, rash and pancarditis (involving all layers of the heart wall) of varying severity within 3 weeks following a streptococcal throat infection. Atypically, but not infrequently, the symptoms are trivial and ignored, but carditis may be severe and result in permanent cardiac damage, particularly of heart valves. It may also lead to neurological problems. ⇒ chorea.

**rheumatism** *n* a non-specific term embracing a diverse group of diseases and syndromes which have in common disorder or diseases of connective tissue and hence usually present with pain, or stiffness, or swelling of muscles and joints. Used colloquially to describe ill-defined aches and pains. ⇒ rheumatic diseases.

**rheumatoid arthritis** a disease of unknown aetiology, characterized by polyarthritis, usually affecting firstly the smaller peripheral joints, before extending to involve larger joints accompanied by general ill health, and eventually resulting in varying degrees of joint destruction and deformity with associated muscle wasting. Patients have fever, extreme fatigue and weight loss. It is not just a disease of joints; most body systems can be affected; there may be associated alveolitis, cardiovascular problems, anaemia, eye damage, peripheral nerve problems, etc. Many rheumatologists therefore prefer the term 'rheumatoid disease'. There is some question of it being an autoimmune process. ⇒ connective tissue diseases, Felty's syndrome, juvenile idiopathic arthritis. Management depends on severity and presentation but includes: rest, both general and for specific joints with splints; maintaining joint function with exercise, good positioning and posture with expert physiotherapy; warmth; drugs including non-steroidal anti-inflammatory drugs (NSAIDs), oral and intra-articular corticosteroids, antimalarial drugs, e.g. chloroquine, gold, cytotoxic drugs, and immunosuppressants; immunotherapy with cytokine inhibitors such as infliximab, which inhibit tumour necrosis factor-$\alpha$ (TNF); and surgery.

**rheumatoid factors (RFs)** autoantibodies found in most people with rheumatoid arthritis. It is not yet known whether they are the cause of, or the result of, arthritis.

**rheumatology** *n* the science or the study of the rheumatic diseases.

**rhinitis** *n* inflammation of the nasal mucous membrane. Several types exist including allergic or atrophic. ⇒ atopic syndrome, atropic rhinitis, hayfever.

**rhinology** *n* the study of disorders of the nose—**rhinologist** *n*.

**rhinomanometry** *n* a test used for assessment of the nasal airway and to measure the nasal airflow and pressure during respiration.

**rhinomycosis** *n* a fungal infection affecting the nasal mucosa.

**rhinophyma** *n* nodular enlargement of the skin of the nose.

**rhinoplasty** *n* plastic surgery of the nasal framework.

**rhinorrhoea** *n* nasal discharge. Usually describes a thin watery fluid, but also includes the discharge of cerebrospinal fluid from the nose following a fracture of the base of the skull.

**rhinoscopy** *n* inspection of the nose using a nasal speculum or a flexible endoscope designed for the nasal cavity—**rhinoscopic** *adj*.

**rhinosinusitis** *n* inflammation of the nose and paranasal sinuses.

R

**rhinoscleroma** *n* a granulomatous disease characterized by the formation of nodules in the nasal passages and nasopharynx. It may be caused by the bacterium *Klebsiella rhinoscleromatis*.

**rhinosporidiosis** *n* a fungal condition affecting the mucosa of the nose, eyes, ears, larynx and occasionally the genitalia.

*Rhinosporidium* *n* a genus of fungi parasitic to humans.

**rhinovirus** *n* group of picornaviruses responsible for the common cold (coryza).

**rhizotomy** *n* surgical division of a root; usually the posterior root of a spinal nerve. *chemical rhizotomy* accomplished by injection of a chemical, often phenol.

**rhodopsin** *n* the visual purple (pigment) found in the rods of the retina. It comprises a protein, opsin and retinal derived from retinol (a form of vitamin A). Thus vitamin A is needed for its formation. Rhodopsin is required for vision in low-intensity light. Its colour is maintained in darkness; bleached by daylight.

**rhombencephalon** *n* hindbrain. One of the three primary vesicles formed during embryonic development of the brain. It becomes the pons, medulla oblongata and cerebellum.

**rhomboid** *adj* diamond-shaped.

**rhonchus** *n* an adventitious sound heard on auscultation of the lung. Passage of air through bronchi obstructed by oedema or exudate produces a musical note.

**rhythm method** also known as the calendar method. ⇒ natural family planning.

**riboflavin(e)** *n* vitamin B$_2$, part of the large group of water-soluble B vitamins. Used therapeutically to treat angular stomatitis and other effects of riboflavin(e) deficiency, and for neonatal hyperbilirubinaemia. ⇒ ariboflavinosis, Appendix 4.

**ribonuclease** *n* an enzyme that breaks down ribonucleic acid.

**ribonucleic acid (RNA)** nucleic acids present in all living cells. Composed of a single chain of nucleotides formed from ribose (a 5-carbon sugar), phosphates and the nitrogenous bases: adenine (A), guanine (G), cytosine (C) and uracil (U). There are three forms: messenger (mRNA), ribosomal (rRNA) and transfer (tRNA), which have specific functions during protein synthesis. ⇒ deoxyribonucleic acid, transcription, translation.

**ribose** *n* a 5-carbon (pentose) sugar; required for the formation of the nucleic acids and several coenzymes.

**ribosomal RNA (rRNA)** ⇒ ribonucleic acid.

**ribosomes** *npl* submicroscopic structures inside all cells. They are formed from ribonucleic acid and proteins. They are concerned with the synthesis of new proteins for cell use. They may be present on the rough endoplasmic reticulum, or free within the cytoplasm as single units, or in groups known as polysomes.

**ribs** *npl* the 12 pairs of bones which articulate with the 12 dorsal vertebrae posteriorly and form the walls of the thorax (⇒ Appendix 1, Figures 2, 3 and 6). The upper seven pairs are *true ribs* and are attached to the sternum anteriorly by costal cartilage. The remaining five pairs are the *false ribs*; the first three pairs of these do not have an attachment to the sternum but are bound to each other by costal cartilage. The lower two pairs are the *floating ribs* which have no anterior articulation. *cervical ribs* are an extension of the transverse process of the seventh cervical vertebra in the form of bone or fibrous tissue; this causes an upward displacement of the subclavian artery.

**RICE** *acron* **r**est, **i**ce, **c**ompression and **e**levation. Used in the management of acute injuries to minimize the inflammatory process and to accelerate the recovery process by eliminating swelling.

**rice-water stool** the stool of cholera. The 'rice grains' are desquamated intestinal epithelium.

**ricin** *n* an extremely toxic substance obtained from the castor oil plant (*Ricinus communis*).

**rickets** *n* bone disease caused by vitamin D deficiency during infancy and childhood (prior to ossification of the epiphyses) which results from poor dietary intake or insufficient exposure to sunlight. There is abnormal metabolism of calcium and phosphate with poor ossification and bone growth. There is muscle weakness, anaemia, respiratory infections, bone tenderness and pain, hypocalcaemia and seizures. Delays occur in motor development such as with walking, eruption of teeth and closure of the fontanelles. Later there may be bony deformities, e.g. bow legs. ⇒ rickety rosary. Rickets may be secondary to vitamin D malabsorption, or impaired metabolism, such as with chronic renal failure (*renal rickets*). The same condition in adults is known as osteomalacia.

*Rickettsia* *n* (H Ricketts, American pathologist, 1871–1910) small pleomorphic parasitic Gram-negative micro-organisms that have similarities with both viruses and bacteria. Like viruses, they are obligate intracellular parasites. *Rickettsia* are intestinal parasites of arthropods such as fleas, lice, mites and ticks;

transmission to humans is by bites from these arthropods and contact with their faeces, which may be rubbed in the eyes, or it can be airborne transmission. They cause various types of the typhus group of diseases and Rocky Mountain spotted fever. ⇒ rickettsial fevers, spotted fever.

**rickettsial fevers** a group of rickettsial diseases that include epidemic typhus caused by *Rickettsia prowazekii*; endemic typhus caused by *R. mooseri*; scrub typhus caused by *Orientia tsutsugamushi* (formally known as *R. tsutsugamushi*); and Rocky Mountain spotted fever caused by *R. rickettsii*. They are transmitted by ticks, fleas, lice and mites and are associated with overcrowding and poor hygiene (e.g. after natural disasters, during war, or in refugee camps). ⇒ typhus.

**rickety rosary** a series of protuberances (bossing) at junction of ribs and costal cartilages in children suffering from rickets.

**rider's bone** a bony mass in the origin of the adductor muscles of the thigh, from repeated minor trauma in horse riding.

**Riedel's thyroiditis** (B Riedel, German surgeon, 1846–1916) a chronic fibrosis of the thyroid gland; ligneous goitre.

**Rift Valley fever** one of the mosquito-transmitted haemorrhagic fevers.

**rights** *npl* the recognition in law that certain inalienable rights should be respected, such as Article 2, 'The right to life', of the Human Rights Act 1998.

**rigidity** *n* (*syn* lead-pipe rigidity, parkinsonian rigidity) increased tension or tone of muscle (hypertonia) with increased resistance to passive stretch in any direction that is uniform throughout the whole movement. ⇒ cogwheel rigidity.

**rigor** *n* a sudden chill, accompanied by severe shivering. The body temperature rises rapidly and remains high until perspiration ensues and causes a gradual fall in temperature.

**rigor mortis** the stiffening of the body after death. It commences within a few hours of death because muscle cells have insufficient energy (adenosine triphosphate [ATP]) and intracellular calcium levels rise, causing the binding together of the muscle proteins, actin and myosin. The maximum degree of rigor will develop between 12 and 48 hours after death depending on environmental conditions. Rigor wears off as enzymic tissue decomposition begins and proteins are digested.

**RIHSA** *abbr* radioiodinated human serum albumin.

**rima** *n* a fissure or cleft. *rima glottidis* the glottis. An opening between the abducted vocal folds in the larynx.

**Ringer's solution** (S Ringer, British physician/physiologist, 1835–1910) an intravenous infusion solution containing sodium chloride with potassium chloride and calcium chloride. *lactated Ringer's solution (Ringer lactate or Hartmann's solution)* one that also contains sodium lactate.

**ringworm** *n* (*syn* tinea) generic term used to describe contagious fungal infection of the skin, because of the common circular (circinate) scaly patches. ⇒ dermatophytes.

**rINN** *abbr* recommended International Non-proprietary Name.

**Rinne's test** (H Rinne, German otologist, 1819–1868) a tuning fork test used to distinguish between conductive and sensorineural deafness. ⇒ Weber's test.

**RIP** *abbr* raised intracranial pressure.

**risk** *n* a potential hazard. *attributable risk* the disease rate in people exposed to the risk factor minus the occurrence in unexposed people. *relative risk* the ratio of disease rate in people exposed to the risk factor to those not exposed. It is related to the odds ratio, which is the odds (as in betting) of disease occurring in an exposed person divided by the odds of the disease occurring in an unexposed person.

**risk assessment** a structured and methodical assessment of risk carried out for a particular area or activity. For example, moving and handling patients in the operating theatre.

**risk factors** factors associated with an increase in the likelihood of ill health, disease, handicap or disability. Demonstration of the association has to fulfil Sir Austin Bradford Hill's eight criteria (e.g. smoking and lung cancer): (a) biological plausibility—tobacco tar contains known carcinogens, the stages of tumour development following exposure are clearly demonstrated; (b) reversibility—smoking cessation reduces subsequent increase in risk of lung cancer by half in the first year, to nil after 10 years; (c) animal demonstration—model of beagles in laboratory experiments; (d) dose–response—risk of lung cancer in smokers shown to increase progressively with the number of cigarettes smoked per day; (e) follows exposure—temporal relationship demonstrated, lung cancer always follows exposure to cigarettes with a time lag of 20–30 years; (f) over time and overseas—relationship consistent between different case series and different places (in the world);

**R**

(g) experimental design—must be reliable. Randomized controlled trials most convincing, but may be unethical. Observational studies (case control, cohort) useful if correctly carried out; and (h) strength of the effect—the larger the increase in risk, the more likely the causal relationship.

**risk management** managing risk in health care settings involves identification of the risk, analysis of the risk and controlling the risk.

**risus sardonicus** the spastic 'grin' of tetanus; caused by facial muscle spasm.

**Ritter's disease** (G Ritter von Rittershain, German physician, 1820–1883) ⇒ staphylococcal scalded-skin syndrome.

**river blindness** ⇒ onchocerciasis.

**Rivermead motor assessment** a scale originally designed to test motor function in people who had suffered a stroke. It tests overall function and mobility by separately testing three areas: gross function, leg and trunk, and arm. It has a hierarchical structure that assumes that recovery of function has a pattern, and if a person is unable to perform a task, no more tasks are attempted on that sub-area.

**RNA** *abbr* ribonucleic acid.

**RNA viruses** viruses that contain RNA as their nucleic acid, such as picornavirus, retrovirus.

**RNI** *abbr* reference nutrient intake.

**RO** *abbr* reality orientation.

**ROA** *abbr* right occipitoanterior; used to describe the position of the fetal occiput in relation to the maternal pelvis.

**Rocky Mountain spotted fever** a tick-borne rickettsial infection. Characterized by fever, myalgia, headache and petechial rash. Occurs in the USA. ⇒ rickettsial fevers.

**rodent ulcer** ⇒ basal cell carcinoma.

**rods** *npl* photoreceptors in the retina for appreciation of coarse detail vision in low light conditions. They contain the visual pigment rhodopsin.

**role** *n* the characteristic social behaviour of a person in relation to others in the group, for example that of a physiotherapist vis-à-vis that of the doctor. *role model* an individual who acts as a model for another individual's behaviour in a particular role. Important for development during childhood, and also as part of professional education and development. *role playing* may be used during professional education when a student assumes the role of a patient/client so that other students may practise a particular skill, such as communication. Also used in therapeutic situations, e.g. patients with mental health problems.

**rollator frame** a mobility aid; a Zimmer-type walking frame which incorporates wheels at the front, thus allowing it to be pushed forward rather than lifted during walking.

**ROM** *abbr* **1.** range of motion. **2.** resisted range of movement.

**Romberg's sign** a sign of impaired balance. Inability to stand erect (without swaying) when the eyes are closed and the feet together. Also called 'Rombergism'.

**root canal treatment/filling** also called pulp canal treatment. An endodontic treatment, in which the canal in a tooth root is cleared of diseased pulp tissue, cleaned and prepared, prior to filling the cavity with a non-irritant material.

**rooting reflex** a primitive reflex present in newborns. The infant will turn his or her head to that side when the cheek is touched. The reflex normally disappears between 3 and 4 months of age.

**ROP** *abbr* right occipitoposterior; used to describe the position of the fetal occiput in relation to the maternal pelvis.

**ROS** *abbr* reactive oxygen species.

**rosacea** *n* a skin disease which shows on flush areas of the face. In affected areas there is chronic dilatation of superficial capillaries and hypertrophy of sebaceous follicles, often complicated by a papulopustular eruption. ⊙ DVD

**rose Bengal** a staining agent used to detect diseased corneal and conjunctival epithelium.

**roseola** *n* a rose-coloured rash.

**Ross River virus disease/fever** a disease caused by an alphavirus. It is transmitted by mosquitoes and is found in Australia, Papua New Guinea and other areas in the Pacific region. It is characterized by polyarthritis and a rash.

**rotation** *n* a limb movement around the axis down the centre of a long bone.

**rotator** *n* a muscle that acts to turn a part. *rotator cuff* four muscles: subscapularis, supraspinatus, infraspinatus and teres minor. Their insertional tendons converge to form a cuff over the shoulder joint. Controls and produces rotation of the shoulder.

**rotaviruses** *npl* viruses belonging to the reovirus group, mainly associated with gastroenteritis in children and infants. It is a very common cause worldwide of severe diarrhoeal disease in children.

**Roth spots** (M Roth, Swiss pathologist, 1839–1914) pale, round spots in the retina in some cases of infective endocarditis; thought to be of embolic origin.

**R**

**roughage** *n* an outdated term. ⇒ non-starch polysaccharides.

**rouleau** *n* a stack of red blood cells, resembling a roll of coins.

**round ligaments** uterine supports that run from the uterus, through the inguinal canal, to the labia majora. ⇒ Appendix 1, Figure 17.

**round window** a round opening between the middle and inner ear. It is situated on the medial wall of the middle ear and is covered by fibrous tissue. It is in contact with the cochlea.

**roundworm** *n* (*Ascaris lumbricoides*) intestinal nematodes with worldwide distribution. Parasitic to humans. Eggs passed in stools; ingested; hatch in bowel; migrate through tissues, lungs and bronchi before returning to the bowel as mature worms. During migration worms can be coughed up. Heavy infections can produce pneumonia. They cause abdominal discomfort and may be vomited or passed per rectum. A tangled mass can cause intestinal obstruction or appendicitis. Adult worms can obstruct pancreatic and bile ducts. ⇒ *Toxocara*.

**Roux-en-Y operation** (C Roux, Swiss surgeon, 1857–1934) originally the distal end of divided jejunum was anastomosed to the stomach, and the proximal jejunum containing the duodenal and pancreatic digestive juices was anastomosed to the jejunum about 75 mm below the first anastomosis. The term is now used to include joining of the distal jejunum to a divided bile duct, oesophagus or pancreas, in major surgery of these structures.

**Rovsing's sign** (N Rovsing, Danish surgeon, 1862–1927) pressure in the left iliac fossa (see Appendix 1, Figure 18A) causes pain in the right iliac fossa in appendicitis.

**RPR** *abbr* rapid plasma reagin (test).

**RSI** *abbr* repetitive strain injury.

**RSV** *abbr* respiratory syncytial virus.

**rubefacients** *npl* substances which, when applied to the skin, cause redness (hyperaemia).

**rubella** *n* (*syn* German measles) an acute, infectious, eruptive fever (exanthema) caused by a virus and spread by droplet infection. There is mild fever, a scaly, pink, macular rash and enlarged occipital and posterior cervical lymph nodes. Complications are rare, except when contracted in the first trimester of pregnancy, when it may produce fetal deformities, such as heart abnormalities, cataracts, deafness and brain damage. Immunization is available as part of routine programmes during childhood and to non-pregnant woman of childbearing age with insufficient immunity.

**rubeola** *n* measles.

**rubeosis iritis** *n* neovascularization (growth of new, abnormal blood vessels) of the iris.

**rubidium (Rb)** *n* a metallic element. Emits some radioactivity and is used in radioisotope scanning.

**Rubin's manoeuvre** an invasive procedure that can be used in shoulder dystocia.

**Rubinstein–Taybi syndrome** (J Rubinstein, American paediatrician, 1925–2006; H Taybi, Iranian/American paediatric radiologist, b. 1919) includes mental and motor retardation, broad thumbs and toes, growth retardation, susceptibility to infection in the early years and characteristic facial features.

**rubor** *n* redness; usually used in the context of being one of the five classical signs and symptoms of inflammation—the others being calor, dolor, loss of function and tumor.

**rugae** *npl* folds present in the gastric mucosa, and the ridges present in the mucosa of the vagina. They facilitate stretching of the stomach after a meal, and of the vagina during the birth of a baby—**ruga** *sing*.

**rule of nines** a method of calculating the percentage of body surface area affected by a burn injury, using standard body maps. For example, in an adult, a burn injury affecting the front of the leg would be approximately 9%, or a burn of the back of the head would be 4½% (Figure R.7). Modified charts are available for infants and children because they have proportionally larger heads; a burn affecting half the head in a newborn baby would be 9½%. ⇒ total burn surface area.

**runner's nipples** a colloquial expression used in sports medicine to describe irritation of the nipples due to friction caused by the runner's shirt rubbing over his or her nipples.

**rupture** *n* **1.** a bursting or tearing of a body structure, e.g. uterine tube due to ectopic pregnancy, a ruptured uterus during pregnancy/labour. Also describes the rupture of the fetal membranes. **2.** a lay term for hernia.

**Ryle's tube** (J Ryle, British physician, 1889–1950) a narrow-bore nasogastric tube, used mainly to aspirate gastric contents following abdominal surgery, when the bowel is obstructed or in paralytic ileus. Sometimes used for short-term enteral feeding.

**R**

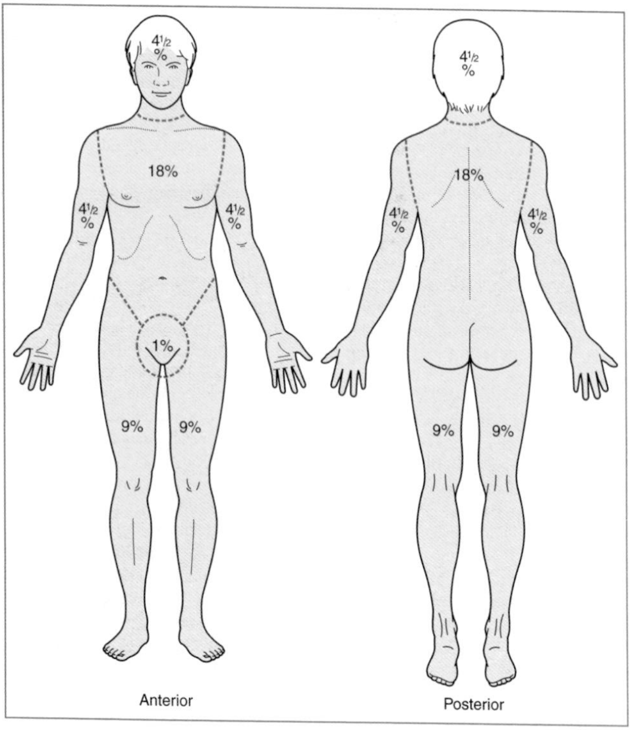

**Figure R.7** Rule of nines—adult *(reproduced from Brooker & Waugh 2007 with permission).*

# S

**Sabin vaccine** (A Sabin, Polish/American physician, 1906–1993) a live attenuated poliomyelitis vaccine given orally.

**sac** *n* any small pouch-like structure, such as the conjunctival sac.

**saccade** *n* abrupt, rapid involuntary movements, such as those of the eyes when scanning a page of print in a document—**saccades** *pl.*

**saccharide** *n* a series of carbohydrates. Includes monosaccharides, disaccharides and polysaccharides.

**saccharin(e)** *n* a synthetic substance with intense sweetness; used as a sweetening agent.

**sacculation** *n* appearance of several saccules.

**saccule** *n* a minute sac. A fluid-filled sac in the inner ear. Part of the vestibular apparatus concerned with static equilibrium; contains hair cells and otoliths—**saccular, sacculated** *adj.* ⇒ utricle.

**SACN** *abbr* Scientific Advisory Committee on Nutrition.

**sacral** *adj* pertaining to the sacrum. *sacral nerves* five pairs of nerves that leave the lower spinal cord. *sacral plexus* a nerve plexus formed by the anterior rami of the lumbosacral trunk (fourth and fifth lumbar nerves) and the sacral nerves 1 to 4. It includes the sciatic nerve and the pudendal nerve. *sacral vertebrae* ⇒ sacrum. ⇒ Appendix 1, Figure 11.

**sacroanterior** *adj* describes the position of a breech presentation in the pelvis when the fetal sacrum is in the anterior part of the maternal pelvis—**sacroanteriorly** *adv.*

**sacrococcygeal** *adj* pertaining to the sacrum and the coccyx.

**sacroiliac** *adj* pertaining to the sacrum and the ilium. For example, the sacroiliac joints in which each side of the sacrum articulates with the ilium.

**sacroiliitis** *n* inflammation of a sacroiliac joint. Involvement of both joints characterizes conditions such as ankylosing spondylitis, Reiter's syndrome and psoriatic arthritis.

**sacrolumbar** *adj* pertaining to the sacrum and the loins.

**sacroposterior** *adj* describes the position of a breech position in the pelvis when the fetal sacrum is in the posterior part of the maternal pelvis—**sacroposteriorly** *adv.*

**sacrum** *n* the triangular bone lying between the fifth lumbar vertebra and the coccyx. ⇒ Appendix 1, Figure 3. In adults, it comprises five vertebrae fused together, and it articulates on each side with the innominate bones of the pelvis, forming the synovial sacroiliac joints—**sacral** *adj.*

**SAD** *acron* **s**easonal **a**ffective **d**isorder.

**saddle embolism** a clot (thrombus) that straddles the bifurcation of the aorta where it divides to form the right and left common iliac arteries.

**saddle joint** a type of synovial joint in which bones with both concave and convex surfaces fit together. For example, the carpometacarpal joint of the thumb, which allows movement in two planes: flexion and extension, and adduction and abduction.

**saddle nose** one with a flattened bridge; may be a sign of congenital syphilis.

**sadism** *n* the obtaining of pleasure from inflicting pain, violence or degradation on another person. ⇒ masochism.

**SADS** *abbr* sudden adult/arrhythmia death syndrome. ⇒ long Q-T syndrome.

**sagittal** *adj* resembling an arrow.

**sagittal plane** the anteroposterior plane of the body.

**sagittal sinuses** two dural venous channels (sinuses) that drain blood from the brain.

**sagittal suture** the immovable joint between the two parietal bones.

**SAH** *abbr* subarachnoid haemorrhage.

**SAID** *acron* **s**pecific **a**daptation to **i**mposed **d**emands.

**Saint's triad** (C Saint, South African radiologist, 20th century) the presence of hiatus hernia, gallstones and diverticulosis.

**salicylates** *npl* a group of analgesic, antipyretic, non-steroidal anti-inflammatory drugs, such as aspirin. ⇒ Appendix 5.

**salicylic acid** used topically, it is keratolytic and has fungicidal and bacteriostatic properties. Used in a variety of hyperkeratotic skin conditions such as corns, and combined with other substances for the treatment of scalp psoriasis.

**saline** *n* a solution of sodium chloride and water. Normal or physiological saline is a 0.9% solution with the same osmotic pressure as that of plasma. ⇒ hypertonic, hypotonic, isotonic.

**saliva** *n* fluid secreted by the salivary glands. It contains water, salts, mucus and salivary amylase—**salivary** *adj.*

**salivary** *adj* pertaining to saliva.

**salivary calculus** a stone formed in the salivary ducts.

**salivary glands** the three pairs of glands that secrete saliva—the parotid, submandibular and sublingual glands (Figure S.1).

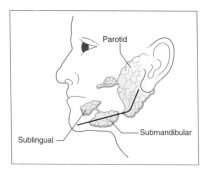

**Figure S.1** Salivary glands *(reproduced from Brooker 2006A with permission).*

**salivation** *n* an increased secretion of saliva.
**Salk vaccine** (J Salk, American virologist, 1914–1995) a preparation of killed poliomyelitis virus used as an antigen to produce active artificial immunity to poliomyelitis. It is given by injection.
***Salmonella*** *n* (D Salmon, American veterinary pathologist, 1850–1914) a genus of bacteria of the family Enterobacteriaceae. Gram-negative rods, which are parasitic in many animals and humans in whom they are often pathogenic. Some species, such as *Salmonella typhi*, are host-specific, infecting only humans, in whom they cause typhoid fever. Others, such as *S. typhimurium*, may infect a wide range of host species, usually through contaminated foods. *Salmonella enteritidis* a motile Gram-negative rod, widely distributed in domestic animals, particularly poultry, and in rodents, and sporadic in humans as a cause of food poisoning.
**salmonellosis** *n* infection caused by bacterial species of the genus *Salmonella*. For example, food poisoning. ⇒ food poisoning, gastroenteritis.
**salpingectomy** *n* excision of a uterine (fallopian) tube such as for a ruptured tubal (ectopic) pregnancy.
**salpingitis** *n* acute or chronic inflammation of the uterine (fallopian) tubes. ⇒ hydrosalpinx, pelvic inflammatory disease, pyosalpinx.
**salpingography** *n* radiological examination of tubal patency by retrograde introduction of opaque medium into the uterus and along the uterine tubes. Being superseded by ultrasound examination—**salpingographic** *adj*, **salpingography** *n*, **salpingographically** *adv*.

**salpingolysis** *n* a procedure to divide adhesions blocking the uterine tubes in order to restore patency and increase the chances of conception.
**salpingo-oophorectomy** *n* excision of a uterine (fallopian) tube and ovary.
**salpingo-oophoritis** *n* inflammation of the uterine tube and the ovary.
**salpingostomy** *n* an operation performed to restore the patency of the uterine tube. Or making an opening in the uterine tube.
**salpinx** *n* a tube, especially the uterine (fallopian) tube or the pharyngotympanic (eustachian or auditory) tube.
**salt** *n* a substance produced by the combination of an acid and an alkali (base), e.g. potassium chloride.
**saltatory conduction** the propagation of action potentials along a myelinated nerve in which the impulse jumps between the gaps in the myelin sheath, i.e. from one node of Ranvier to the next node. There is a concentration of voltage-gated sodium/potassium ion channels at the gap where the action potential is regenerated, thus explaining the rapid transmission of impulses in myelinated nerves.
**Samaritans** a voluntary befriending service available 24 hours/day to support suicidal and despairing people who make contact by telephone, e-mail or by visiting a local centre.
**sample** *n* the particular subset chosen from a population.
**sandfly** *n* an insect (*Phlebotomus*) responsible for transmitting viral sandfly fever and the protozoa that cause leishmaniasis.
**sandfly fever** ⇒ phlebotomus fever.
**sanguineous** *adj* pertaining to or containing blood.
**SaO₂** *abbr* arterial oxygen saturation. ⇒ pulse oximeter.
**saphenous** *adj* apparent; manifest. The name given to two superficial veins in the leg. *Great (long) saphenous vein*, which is the longest vein in the body, carries blood from the foot, leg and thigh to the femoral vein; and the *small (short) saphenous vein*, which carries blood from the foot and leg to the popliteal vein (⇒ Appendix 1, Figure 10). The *saphenous nerve* is a branch of the femoral nerve, it innervates the medial aspects of the lower leg and the foot (⇒ Appendix 1, Figure 11).
**saprophyte** *n* free-living micro-organism obtaining nutrients from dead and decaying animal or plant tissue—**saprophytic** *adj*.
**SARA** *abbr* sexually acquired reactive arthritis.

**sarcoid** *adj* a term applied to a group of lesions in skin, lungs or other organs, which resemble tuberculous foci in structure, but the true nature of which is still uncertain.

**sarcoidosis** *n* also known as Boeck's disease. A granulomatous disease of unknown aetiology in which histological appearances resemble tuberculosis. May affect any organ of the body, but most commonly presents as a condition of the skin, lymph nodes or the bones of the hand.

**sarcolemma** *n* the plasma membrane that encloses the sarcoplasm (cytoplasm) of a muscle cell (fibre).

**sarcoma** *n* malignant tumour of connective tissue, such as bone, but the suffix is also applied to tumours of muscle, nervous or vascular tissue. Examples of sarcomas include chondrosarcoma, fibrosarcoma, myosarcoma, myxosarcoma, osteosarcoma and rhabdomyosarcoma. Treatment options include surgery, radiotherapy and chemotherapy, usually in combination. ⇒ Ewing's tumour—**sarcomata** *pl*, **sarcomatous** *adj*.

**sarcomatosis** *n* a condition in which sarcomata are widely spread throughout the body.

**sarcomere** *n* the segment of a myofibril that forms the smallest functional contractile unit in striated (skeletal) muscle.

**sarcoplasm** *n* the cytoplasm within a muscle cell (fibre).

**sarcoplasmic reticulum** *n* forms a set of tubules within the muscle cell. Functions with another set of tubules, the transverse (T) tubules, to maintain the correct concentration of intracellular calcium by releasing and storing calcium ions in order to transmit the action potential to the contractile units.

**Sarcoptes scabiei** *n* a species of itch mite responsible for scabies.

**SARS** *abbr* severe acute respiratory syndrome.

**sartorius** *n* the longest muscle in the body, it is known as the 'tailor's muscle', since it flexes one leg over the other. It is a strap-like muscle of the thigh, which crosses the hip and knee joints. Its origin is on the anterior superior iliac spine and it inserts on to the medial aspect of the tibia. It contracts to flex and laterally rotate the thigh. Also a weak flexor of the knee. ⇒ Appendix 1, Figures 4 and 5.

**satellite cell 1.** cells associated with muscle cells. Important for muscle growth and repair. **2.** neuroglial cells that surround some neurons.

**satiety** *n* being satisfied; the feeling of fullness after a meal.

**saturated fatty acids** those having no double bonds in their structure. Most, but not all, originate from animal sources. High dietary intake is associated with an unfavourable high-density lipoprotein (HDL):low-density lipoprotein (LDL) ratio and the development of arterial disease.

**satyriasis** *n* excessive, abnormal or uncontrolled sexual activity in males. Compare ⇒ nymphomania.

**SBLA syndrome** *abbr* sarcoma, breast, leukaemia and adrenal gland syndrome. ⇒ Li–Fraumeni syndrome.

**SBS** *abbr* short-bowel syndrome.

**scab** *n* a dried crust forming over an open wound.

**scabies** *n* a parasitic skin disease caused by the itch mite. Highly contagious. ⊙ DVD

**scala** *n* the fluid-filled structures in the cochlea; scala media (also known as the cochlear duct) containing endolymph, and the scala tympani and scala vestibuli that both contain perilymph.

**scald** *n* an injury caused by moist heat.

**scalded-skin syndrome** ⇒ toxic epidermal necrolysis.

**scale 1.** *v* to remove calculus from the teeth. **2.** *n* a flake of exfoliated epidermis.

**scalenus** *n* one of four paired muscles situated laterally on the neck—the scalenus anterior, medius, minimus (pleuralis) and posterior. Known collectively as the scalene muscles. The origins are on the transverse processes of the cervical vertebrae and they insert on to the first two ribs. They contract to raise the first two ribs during inspiration and may be involved in coughing; they also function to flex and rotate the neck.

**scalenus syndrome** pain in arm and fingers, often with wasting, because of compression of the lower trunk of the brachial plexus behind scalenus anterior muscle at the thoracic outlet.

**scalp** *n* the hair-bearing skin which covers the cranium. *scalp cooling* technique used to minimize or prevent alopecia associated with the administration of cytotoxic drugs such as doxorubicin.

**scalpel** *n* a surgeon's knife, which may or may not have detachable blades.

**scan** *n* an image built up by movement along or across the object scanned, either of the detector or of the imaging agent, to achieve complete coverage, e.g. ultrasound scan.

**scanning speech** an abnormal staccato speech pattern. The person hesitates between syllables, which are equally stressed. This produces words that sound clipped.

**scaphocephaly** *n* a congenital malformation that results in an abnormally long skull. It is caused by early closure of the sagittal suture.

**scaphoid** *n* boat-shaped, as a bone of the carpus and the tarsus (where it is called the navicular bone). *scaphoid bone* one of the carpal bones of the wrist. It articulates with the radius, and other carpal bones—lunate, capitate, trapezoid and trapezium.

**scaphoid fracture** commonly occurs as a result of compression of the scaphoid, when there is a fall on to the outstretched hand in hyperextension. Commonly, if the fracture involves the proximal third of the scaphoid, there is a high risk of non-union and threat of avascular necrosis, due to the poor blood supply.

**scapula** *n* the shoulder-blade—one of two large, flat triangular bones of the pectoral (shoulder) girdle. It is situated on the posterior thoracic wall with a layer of muscle separating it from the ribs. Each has two surfaces, three borders and three angles. The posterior surface is marked by a prominent ridge or spine which extends to the acromion process. The scapula articulates with the clavicle at the acromioclavicular joint. A shallow fossa, known as the glenoid cavity, situated at the lateral angle, accommodates the head of the humerus to form the ball-and-socket shoulder joint. The coracoid process provides attachment for muscles that include the biceps brachii and pectoralis minor. (⇒ Appendix 1, Figure 3)—**scapulae** *pl.* **scapular** *adj*.

**scar** *n* (*syn* cicatrix) the dense, avascular white fibrous tissue, formed as the end-result of healing, especially in the skin. ⇒ hypertrophic scar, keloid.

**scarification** *n* the making of a series of small, superficial incisions or punctures in the skin for the purpose of introducing a vaccine.

**scarlatina** *n* ⇒ scarlet fever.

**scarlet fever** *n* (*syn* scarlatina) infection by β-haemolytic streptococcus (Lancefield group A). Occurs mainly in children. Starts commonly with a throat infection, leading to fever, and a punctate erythematous rash on the skin of the trunk that is followed by desquamation. Characteristically the area around the mouth escapes (circumoral pallor).

**Scarpa's triangle** (A Scarpa, Italian anatomist/surgeon, 1752–1832) also known as the femoral triangle. ⇒ femoral.

**SCAT** *abbr* sheep cell agglutination test.

**SCBU** *abbr* special care baby unit. ⇒ neonatal unit.

**SCC** *abbr* **1**. spinal cord compression. **2**. squamous cell carcinoma.

**Scheuermann's disease** (H Scheuermann, Danish orthopaedic surgeon, 1877–1960) osteochondritis of the spine affecting the ring epiphyses of the vertebral bodies. Occurs during adolescence and can lead to kyphosis.

**Schick test** (B Schick, American physician, 1877–1967) a skin test used to determine susceptibility or immunity to diphtheria. It consists of the intradermal injection of diphtheria toxin. A positive reaction (susceptibility to diphtheria) is indicated by the appearance of a round red area within 24–48 hours. The absence of any skin reaction to the toxin indicates immunity to the disease.

**Schilder's disease** (P Schilder, Austrian neurologist, 1886–1940) a genetically determined degenerative disease associated with learning disability. ⇒ adrenoleucodystrophy.

**Schilling test** (R Schilling, American haematologist, b. 1919) estimation of absorption of radioactive vitamin $B_{12}$ for investigation of the cause of vitamin $B_{12}$ deficiency.

*Schistosoma* *n* (*syn* Bilharzia) a genus of blood flukes which require freshwater snails as an intermediate host before infesting humans. Includes: *S. haematobium* in Africa and the Middle East, *S. japonicum* in Japan, the Philippines and Eastern Asia and *S. mansoni* in the Middle East, Africa, South America and the Caribbean.

**schistosomiasis** *n* (*syn* bilharziasis) infestation by *Schistosoma* that enter via the skin or mucosae. A single fluke can live in one part of the body, depositing eggs over many years. Prevention is by water chlorination, safe disposal of human waste and eradication of freshwater snails. There may be irritation at the entry site and after 3–5 weeks signs of larval migration, e.g. fever, eosinophilia, pneumonitis and hepatitis. Later, effects depend on where the eggs are deposited and the type, e.g. hepatitis, colitis, skin lesions, cystitis and haematuria. Many years later there may be organ damage due to fibrosis such as hepatic fibrosis and hepatic portal hypertension, urinary tract damage and pulmonary hypertension.

**schistosomicide** *n* any agent lethal to *Schistosoma*—**schistosomicidal** *adj*.

**schizophrenia** *n* a group of psychotic disorders characterized by disturbances of thinking, perceiving and affect. The course can be at

S

times chronic, at times marked by acute episodes. Schizophrenia is one of the major diagnostic categories of mental illness. It may present with a variety of symptoms that include: thought echo, insertion, withdrawal or broadcasting; delusions; hallucinations; incoherence, irrelevant speech or neologisms; catatonic behaviour; and negative symptoms, including apathy, scantiness of speech and blunting of affect, usually resulting in social withdrawal. Symptoms can be classified as positive and negative. For example, positive symptoms may be hearing voices and/or having strange thoughts, whereas negative symptoms include withdrawal from social contact and severe lack of motivation. The causes of schizophrenia are not fully understood but a genetic link is clear. Management includes medication with atypical antipsychotic (neuroleptic) drugs and other non-drug therapies that include social skills training, cognitive-behavioural and psychosocial interventions—**schizophrenic** *adj.* ⇒ expressed emotion.

**Schlatter's disease** (*syn* Osgood–Schlatter disease) (C Schlatter, Swiss surgeon, 1864–1934) osteochondritis of the tibial tubercle.

**Schlemm's canal** (F Schlemm, German anatomist, 1795–1858) ⇒ glaucoma, scleral venous sinus.

**Schmidt's syndrome** (M Schmidt, German pathologist, 1863–1949) also known as polyglandular autoimmune syndrome type II. An autoimmune syndrome which may affect the function of more than one endocrine gland, including the endocrine pancreas, thyroid, parathyroids, adrenals and the ovaries or testes. This is accompanied by problems caused by autoimmune processes in non-endocrine structures, including alopecia and pernicious anaemia.

**Schönlein's disease** ⇒ Henoch–Schönlein purpura.

**Schultz–Charlton test** a blanching produced in the skin of a patient showing scarlet fever rash, around an injection of serum from a convalescent case, indicating neutralization of toxin by antitoxin.

**Schwann cells** (T Schwann, German anatomist, 1810–1882) part of macroglia. Neuroglial cells of the peripheral nervous system. They are concerned with the production of the myelin sheath that surrounds some nerve fibres.

**sciatica** *n* entrapment of the sciatic nerve during its course from the lower back to the leg causing pain that is felt down the back of the leg to the heel and which can lead on to weakness such as foot drop and sensory loss in the lower leg.

**sciatic nerve** the largest nerve in the body. The sciatic nerve arises from the sacral plexus and contains fibres from the fourth and fifth lumbar nerves and the first three sacral nerves. It passes into the buttock and down the posterior aspect of the thigh to supply the hamstring group of muscles. Halfway down the thigh it divides into the common peroneal and tibial nerves, which innervate the muscles and skin of the lower leg, ankle and foot.

**SCID** *abbr* severe combined immunodeficiency.

**Scientific Advisory Committee on Nutrition (SACN)** provides independent expert advice to the Food Standards Agency and government departments, including the Department of Health, on matters relating to nutrients present in foods, dietary advice and the nutritional status of specific groups of the population.

**scintillography** *n* (*syn* scintiscanning) visual recording of radioactivity over selected areas after administration of suitable radioisotope (radionuclide).

**scirrhous** *adj* relating to something that is hard. For example, a scirrhous cancer of the breast, which contains connective tissue and feels hard and gritty.

**scissor-leg deformity** the legs are crossed in walking—following bilateral hip joint disease, or as a manifestation of Little's disease (spastic cerebral diplegia).

**scissors gait** ⇒ gait.

**SCJ** *abbr* squamocolumnar junction.

**sclera** *n* the 'white' of the eye (⇒ Appendix 1, Figure 15); the opaque bluish-white fibrous outer coat of the eyeball covering the posterior five-sixths; it merges into the cornea at the front—**sclerae** *pl*, **scleral** *adj*.

**scleral venous sinus** canal of Schlemm. A canal in the inner part of the sclera, close to its junction with the cornea, which it encircles. It drains excess aqueous humour to maintain normal intraocular pressure (IOP). Impaired drainage results in raised IOP, leading to glaucoma and visual impairment in the absence of effective treatment. ⇒ Appendix 1, Figure 15. ⇒ glaucoma.

**sclerectomy** *n* an operation to remove part of the sclera.

**sclerema** *n* a rare disease in which hardening of the skin results from the deposition of mucinous material.

**scleritis** *n* inflammation of the sclera.

431

**sclerocorneal** *adj* pertaining to the sclera and the cornea, such as the circular junction of these two structures.

**sclerodactyly** *n* deformity affecting the fingers. There is fixed, partial flexion of the fingers with subcutaneous calcification. Ulceration of the finger tips may occur. Associated with scleroderma. ⇒ CREST syndrome.

**scleroderma** *n* a disease in which localized oedema of the skin is followed by hardening, atrophy, deformity and ulceration. Occasionally it becomes generalized, producing immobility of the face and contraction of the fingers; it can involve internal organs with diffuse fibrosis of the myocardium, kidneys, digestive tract and lungs (systemic sclerosis). When confined to the skin it is termed morphoea. ⇒ collagen, connective tissue diseases, CREST syndrome, dermatomyositis.

**scleromalacia** *n* softening and thinning of the sclera which results in the appearance of dark bluish-grey patches, as the pigmented layer of the eye is exposed. It occurs as a systemic effect of rheumatoid arthritis, when it is known as *scleromalacia perforans*.

**sclerosis** *n* a word used in pathology to describe abnormal hardening or fibrosis of a tissue. ⇒ amyotrophic lateral sclerosis, multiple sclerosis, tuberous sclerosis—**sclerotic** *adj*.

**sclerotherapy** *n* injection of a sclerosing agent for the treatment of varicose veins. When, after the injection, rubber pads are bandaged over the site to increase localized compression, the term *compression sclerotherapy* is used. Sclerotherapy is a treatment option for oesophageal varices in which the sclerosing agent is administered through an endoscope—**sclerotherapeutic** *adj*, **sclerotherapeutically** *adv*.

**sclerotomy** *n* incision into the sclera of the eye.

**scolex** *n* the head of the tapeworm which it uses to attach itself to the intestine, and from which the segments (proglottides) develop.

**scoliosis** *n* lateral curvature of the spine, which can be congenital or acquired and is due to abnormality of the vertebrae, muscles and nerves (Figure S.2). *idiopathic scoliosis* is characterized by a lateral curvature together with rotation and associated rib hump or flank recession. The treatment is by spinal brace or traction or internal fixation with accompanying spinal fusion. ⇒ halopelvic traction, Harrington rod, Milwaukee brace—**scoliotic** *adj*.

**scorbutic** *adj* relating to or affected with scurvy.

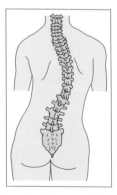

**Figure S.2** Scoliosis *(reproduced from Porter 2005 with permission)*.

**scotoma** *n* a blind spot in the field of vision. May be normal or abnormal. *arcuate scotoma* a visual field defect in the area extending from the normal blind spot in an arc either above or below the central field. *central scotoma* a defect affecting the central field of vision. *centrocaecal scotoma* a defect extending from the normal blind spot to the central field of vision—**scotomata** *pl*.

**scotopic vision** dark-adapted vision.

**scrapie** *n* a transmissible spongiform encephalopathy of sheep and goats caused by a prion. It is characterized by intense pruritus that leads to affected animals scraping themselves on fences (hence the name), etc., neuromuscular inco-ordination and eventual death. ⇒ bovine spongiform encephalopathy.

**screening** *n* a preventive measure to identify potential or incipient disease at an early stage when it may be more easily treated. It is carried out in a variety of settings, including primary care, hospitals and clinics for antenatal care, and well-baby, well-man and well-woman clinics. Screening checks include: mammography; cervical cytology; blood pressure checks; urine testing for diabetes mellitus; faecal occult blood for colorectal cancer; prostate-specific antigen test for prostate cancer; ultrasound and blood tests to detect fetal abnormalities during pregnancy; and the checks performed during neonatal screening such as tests for developmental hip dysplasia, hearing tests and blood tests. The screening process may cause anxiety even when no abnormality is found (negative result). ⇒ genetic screening, Guthrie test, neonatal screening, sensitivity, specificity.

**scrofula** *n* a form of tuberculosis that is characterized by tuberculous abscess formation affecting the lymph nodes, usually those in the cervical region. It is a rare condition but occurs in individuals who are immunocompromised, such as persons with human immunodeficiency virus (HIV) disease.

**scrotum** *n* the pouch of pigmented skin and fascia in the male, in which the testes are suspended outside the body. Each testis occupies a separate compartment within the scrotum. This arrangement helps to ensure that the testes are kept at optimum temperature for the production of healthy spermatozoa, i.e. 4–7°C below core body temperature. The scrotum also has numerous sweat glands, which assist in cooling the testes. In order to maintain a constant temperature the position of the scrotum can be changed by muscle contraction. This occurs in response to temperature changes: heat causes the scrotum to hang loosely away from the body, but it moves closer to the body when cold. (⇒ Appendix 1, Figure 16)—**scrotal** *adj*.

**scrub typhus** a mite-borne febrile disease caused by the micro-organism *Orientia tsutsugamushi* (formerly called *Rickettia tsutsugamushi*). It occurs in the Far East, India, Pakistan, Bangladesh, parts of Australia, Indonesia and the Pacific Islands. It is characterized by sudden onset of fever, headache, enlarged lymph nodes and cough, and later a maculopapular rash often appears. In severe cases it may be complicated by pneumonia and damage to other structures, such as the heart.

**scurf** *n* a lay term for dandruff.

**scurvy** *n* a deficiency disease caused by lack of vitamin C (ascorbic acid). Clinical features include fatigue and haemorrhage. The latter may take the form of oozing at the gums or large ecchymoses. Tiny bleeding spots on the skin around hair follicles are characteristic. In children painful subperiosteal haemorrhage (rather than other types of bleeding) is pathognomonic.

**scybala** *npl* rounded, hard, faecal lumps—**scybalum** *sing*.

**SD** *abbr* standard deviation.

**SDA** *abbr* specific dynamic action.

**SDH** *abbr* subdural haematoma.

**SE** *abbr* standard error.

**seasonal affective disorder (SAD)** a form of mood disorder (usually depression) with a strong association with the reduced day length and longer nights of autumn and winter. The lack of exposure to light that occurs affects the secretion of melatonin by the pineal body (gland). Presentation varies but can include sleep disturbances such as early-morning awakening, sleeping longer and daytime sleepiness; poor concentration; low mood or mood swings; feeling tired and lethargic; reduced libido; increased appetite, particularly for carbohydrate and sugary foods, leading to weight gain; and in severe cases stress and anxiety and depression. Symptoms abate as the day length increases during spring, but it can be successfully treated with exposure to white light with the use of a light box.

**sebaceous** *adj* literally, pertaining to fat; usually refers to sebum.

**sebaceous cyst** (*syn* wen) a cyst that actually contains keratin. Such cysts are most commonly found on the scalp, scrotum and vulva.

**sebaceous glands** the cutaneous glands which secrete an oily substance called sebum. The ducts of these glands are short and straight and open into the hair follicles (⇒ Appendix 1, Figure 12). ⇒ pilosebaceous unit.

**seborrhoea** *n* greasy condition of the scalp, face, sternal region and elsewhere due to overactivity of sebaceous glands.

**sebum** *n* the secretion of the sebaceous glands; it contains fatty acids, cholesterol and dead cells.

**secondary** *adj* second in order.

**secondary care** includes the inpatient and outpatient specialist medical and surgical services that are normally provided by district general hospitals. They include general medicine, surgery and specialist services, such as orthopaedics, midwifery, child health and some inpatient mental health services. Secondary care is indirectly accessed by referral from primary care practitioners, or directly as an emergency via emergency departments.

**secondary-intention healing** a type of wound healing that occurs when there is loss of tissue and it is neither possible nor desirable to pull the wound edges together. The healing process in wounds with considerable loss of tissue, such as traumatic wounds and pressure ulcers, usually involves granulation whereby new capillaries and healthy moist tissue form in the wound bed, wound contraction and epithelialization, where new epithelial cells migrate across the granulation tissue to cover the surface of the wound. ⇒ primary-intention healing, wound healing.

**secondary prevention** ⇒ disease prevention.

**secondary tumour** refers to a primary cancer that has spread to other distant sites in the body, such as colorectal cancer spreading to the liver, or breast cancer spreading to the brain or bone. ⇒ metastasis.

**second-degree tear** ⇒ perineal tear.

**second messenger** intracellular signalling molecules that include cyclic adenosine monophosphate (cAMP), calcium ions ($Ca^{2+}$) and inositol triphosphate ($IP_3$), which act between the hormones and neurotransmitters that act as first messengers, and the particular cellular regulation process. Particularly important in regulatory processes where many reactions are occurring simultaneously (enzyme cascade).

**secretin** *n* a hormone produced by cells in the duodenal mucosa, which causes the secretion of alkaline pancreatic juice that is low in enzymes, and with other regulatory peptides inhibits gastric secretion and motility.

**secretion** *n* a fluid or substance, formed or concentrated in a gland and passed into the gastrointestinal tract, the blood or to the exterior. ⇒ apocrine gland, holocrine gland, merocrine (eccrine) gland.

**secretor** *n* a person who secretes ABO blood group antigens in saliva or gastric juice. ⇒ non-secretor.

**secretory** *adj* involved in the process of secretion: describes a gland which secretes.

**secular** *adj* describes the civil, state or non-religious influences on society. *secular beliefs* those not overtly or specifically religious. The strong non-religious convictions/values that guide concepts of morality that affect everyday life. ⇒ spiritual beliefs.

**sedation** *n* the production of a state of lessened functional activity.

**sedative** *n* an agent which reduces functional activity by its action on the nervous system. ⇒ anxiolytic.

**sedimentation rate** ⇒ erythrocyte sedimentation rate.

**segment** *n* a part of an anatomical structure, such as a lung segment, or the upper and lower uterine segments.

**segregation** *n* a genetic term. The separation of the two alleles, each carried on one of a pair of chromosomes; this happens during meiosis when the haploid (n) gametes (spermatozoa, oocytes) are formed. ⇒ Mendel's law.

**seizures** *npl* result from abnormal electrical activity in the brain. They are associated with many disorders, and may take several forms, some with convulsions, including: absences, atonic, clonic, generalized tonic-clonic, myoclonic, partial or focal, tonic, etc. ⇒ convulsions, epilepsy, febrile seizures, pseudoseizure.

**Seldinger technique** a special, small catheter and guidewire for insertion into an artery, along which it is passed to, for example, the heart. Its guidewire is used to direct large-bore cannula insertion, thereby minimizing the risk of misplacement.

**selective movement** in physiotherapy, a purposeful movement that is co-ordinated and precise, and is based on a suitable level of stability.

**selective (o)estrogen receptor modulators (SERMs)** a group of tissue-specific drugs that modulate oestrogen receptors in some tissues but not others, e.g. raloxifene. They may have oestrogen-agonist or oestrogen-antagonist effects in different tissues. ⇒ Appendix 5.

**selective serotonin reuptake inhibitors (SSRIs)** a group of antidepressant drugs that act by preventing the reuptake of the neurotransmitter serotonin (5-hydroxytryptamine), e.g. fluoxetine. ⇒ Appendix 5.

**Selectron** *n* a proprietary device which stores sealed radioactive sources of caesium or iridium in a shielded container in readiness for intracavitary treatment in the uterus, cervix or vagina. In recent years extended to other body sites such as bronchus and oesophagus. ⊙DVD

**selenium (Se)** *n* an antioxidant. A trace element needed in the diet to facilitate reactions that protect cells from oxidative damage.

**self-actualization** *n* in humanistic psychology the fulfilment of one's potential. The highest level of human achievement in Maslow's hierarchy of needs. ⇒ Maslow's hierarchy.

**self-care** *n* **1.** the ability to perform activities, such as washing, dressing, eating, drinking, elimination needs, etc., without assistance. **2.** taking responsibility for one's own medical or treatment needs following suitable education. For example, self-administration of drug regimens, monitoring a medical condition, dialysis or enteral or parenteral feeding.

**self-catheterization** *n* ⇒ intermittent self-catheterization.

**self-concept** *n* the view that individuals have of their total characteristics, ideas, feelings, qualities and negative features.

**self-esteem** *n* the value or worth individuals place on themselves.

**self-fulfilling prophecy** a situation whereby people's expectations of another person cause them to behave in such a way as to cause the exact response that was anticipated.

**self-infection** *n* the unwitting transfer of micro-organisms from one part of the body to another, in which it produces an infection.

**self-inflating bag** a bag used for ventilation of a patient during anaesthesia or resuscitation.

**self-monitoring of blood glucose (SMBG)** use of capillary blood, usually obtained by a fingerprick, for glucose estimation by a hand-held meter, allowing people to monitor and manage their diabetes.

**sella turcica** a fossa located on sphenoid bone of the skull, which contains the pituitary gland.

**Sellick's manoeuvre** (B Sellick, British anaesthetist, 1918–1996) ⇒ cricoid pressure.

**semantic memory** that part of memory that stores general information about the world, e.g. where lions and tigers are found.

**semen** *n* seminal fluid. Thick, white fluid ejaculated during coitus. It comprises spermatozoa from the testes and the secretions from the: seminal vesicles—this fluid contains nutrients, prostaglandins and enzymes, and forms around 60% of semen volume; prostate gland, which contains enzymes such as acid phosphatase that activates the sperm, and forms around 30% of semen volume; and bulbourethral glands, that produce a fluid which helps to maintain the slightly alkaline pH of semen. A normal ejaculate is around 5 mL in volume and contains 50–150 million sperm/mL. *semen analysis* a test undertaken early during infertility investigations. A fresh sample of semen is analysed to check the number, morphology and motility of the sperm. The volume of the sample, number of sperm and their motility and the percentage of abnormal sperm are measured.

**semicircular canals** three fluid-filled canals contained within the bony labyrinth of the inner ear (⇒ Appendix 1, Figure 13). Oriented in the three planes of space, they are part of the vestibular apparatus concerned with dynamic equilibrium and balance.

**semicomatose** *adj* describes a condition bordering on the unconscious. ⇒ Glasgow Coma Scale (GCS).

**semilunar** *adj* shaped like a crescent or half-moon.

**semilunar cartilages** the two crescentic interarticular cartilages of the knee joint (menisci). They are situated between the femur and the tibia, and function to stabilize the knee joint. Very commonly damaged, especially during certain sports.

**semilunar valves** valves with cusps that are half-moon-shaped, such as those in the heart—the aortic valve between the aorta and the left ventricle and the pulmonary valve between the pulmonary artery and the right ventricle.

**semimembranosus** *n* one of the hamstring muscles. A muscle of the posterior thigh. Its origin is on the ischial tuberosity and it inserts on to the medial condyle of the tibia. It contracts to flex the knee, medially rotate the leg and extend the thigh. ⇒ biceps (femoris), semitendinosus.

**seminal** *adj* pertaining to semen.

**seminal vesicle** one of two tubular accessory glands behind the male bladder. They produce a thick alkaline fluid, which forms some 60% of semen volume. ⇒ semen. ⇒ Appendix 1, Figure 16.

**seminiferous** *adj* carrying or producing semen. *seminiferous tubules* coiled structures present in the lobules of the testis. They are formed from sperm-producing germinal epithelium and are involved in the production of immature spermatozoa (spermatogenesis). The spermatozoa leave the seminiferous tubules to enter the epididymis where they mature during a process called spermiogenesis.

**seminoma** *n* a neoplasm of the testis; subtype of germ cell tumour—**seminomata** *pl*, **seminomatous** *adj*.

**semipermeable** *adj* selectively permeable. Describes a membrane which is permeable to some substances in solutions, but not to others.

**semiprone** *adj* describes a position in which the person is partially prone, on the side with the face down, but with the knees flexed to one side. It can be used for nursing unconscious patients.

**semitendinosus** *n* one of the hamstring muscles. A muscle of the posterior thigh. Its origin is on the ischial tuberosity with the long head of the biceps femoris and it inserts on to the medial aspect of the shaft of the tibia. It contracts to flex the knee, medially rotate the leg and extend the thigh. ⇒ biceps (femoris), semimembranosus.

**senescence** *n* normal physical and mental changes in increasing age—**senescent** *adj*.

**Sengstaken–Blakemore tube** incorporates gastric and oesophageal balloons which when

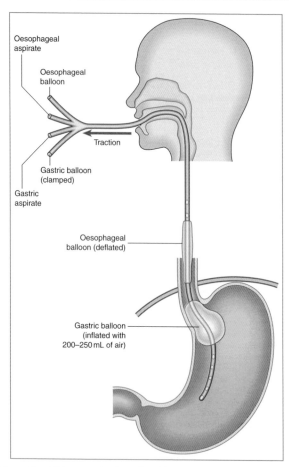

Oesophageal
aspirate

Oesophageal
balloon

Traction

Gastric balloon
(clamped)

Gastric
aspirate

Oesophageal
balloon (deflated)

Gastric balloon
(inflated with
200–250 mL of air)

**Figure S.3** Sengstaken–Blakemore tube *(reproduced from Boon et al. 2006 with permission).*

inflated apply pressure to bleeding oesophageal varices (Figure S.3).

**senile** *adj* suffering from senescence complicated by morbid processes, commonly called
degeneration—**senility** *n. s. dementia* ⇒
dementia.

**senna** *n* leaves and pods of a purgative
plant. Used as a stimulant laxative. ⇒
Appendix 5.

**sensation** *n* consciousness of a feeling that
results from nerve impulses from the sensory
organs reaching the brain.

**sensible** *adj* **1.** endowed with the sense of feeling. **2.** detectable by the senses.

**sensible perspiration** fluid loss through
sweating which is sufficient to be observed.
⇒ insensible (water loss).

**sensitive** *adj* **1.** capable of responding to stimuli. **2.** reacting adversely or being susceptible to an antigen, drug or other substance.
**3.** describes a micro-organism that is killed
or its growth is restricted by a particular antimicrobial drug. **4.** being perceptive in communication with others.

**sensitivity** *n* **1.** high sensitivity is the ability of a screening test to identify accurately affected individuals, such as mammography screening for breast cancer. Low sensitivity can lead to false negatives, i.e. the test fails to detect all abnormal cases. ⇒ specificity. **2.** the extent to which a micro-organism is likely to respond to treatment with a particular antimicrobial drug. Sensitivity testing is undertaken in the microbiological laboratory. A micro-organism may be described as sensitive if the antimicrobial drug is an effective treatment, or resistant if that antimicrobial drug is not effective in inhibiting microbial growth.

**sensitivity training group** individuals learn about what occurs during their interactions with other people within a supportive environment. They can test and refine different behavioural responses in the light of feedback, and are encouraged to try the positively modified behaviours in situations outside the group.

**sensitization** *n* rendering sensitive. Persons may become sensitive to a variety of substances, which may be food (e.g. shellfish), bacteria, plants, chemical substances, drugs, sera, etc. Liability is much greater in some persons than others. ⇒ allergy, anaphylaxis.

**sensorineural** *adj* pertaining to sensory neurons. *sensorineural deafness* a discriminating term for nerve deafness.

**sensory** *adj* pertaining to sensation.

**sensory cortex** that part of the cerebral cortex that receives sensory inputs and decodes them to facilitate perception. It includes the somatosensory area, which is concerned with sensations such as pressure, touch, pain and temperature and inputs from proprioceptors in muscles and joints. It also contains specialist areas—taste, auditory, olfactory, visual and association areas that include a sensory speech area (Wernicke's area).

**sensory deprivation** a situation in which the usual sensory stimuli are absent, such as for patients in intensive care units, or long periods of isolation, or loss of sight. It can lead to problems that include disruption to sleep–wake patterns, tiredness, increased irritability, poor concentration, anxiety, depression, delusions or hallucinations.

**sensory nerve** those which transmit impulses from peripheral receptors to the brain and spinal cord.

**sensory overload** a situation in which the person receives more sensory inputs (usually visual or auditory but can be other stimuli) than can be meaningfully processed. It may

occur in patients in hospital, particularly in critical care facilities where there is 24-hour activity involving bright light and the noise of equipment and staff talking, or in people who have difficulty processing stimuli (e.g. autistic spectrum disorders).

**sentinel node biopsy (SNB)** procedure used in staging (mainly) breast cancer and melanoma where (blue) dye is injected at the primary tumour site and traced to the nearest nodal basin where the first node involved with tumour will accumulate the dye; resection of that node may improve the cure rate.

**separation anxiety** feelings of apprehension, fear and distress caused by being separated from safe and familiar situations and significant individuals, such as the mother or other main carer. For example, that occurring in preschool children separated from their mothers through admission to hospital. There are three stages: characterized first by loud protest and then despair/depression and lastly detachment or denial, in which the child may appear to accept the situation. Regression to earlier behaviours may occur, such as loss of continence, clinging to parents or refusing to eat. The degree of the child's distress is influenced by factors that include the degree of parental involvement in the child's care, parenting styles, parent's response, etc. ⇒ attachment.

**sepsis** *n* the state of being infected with pyogenic (pus-forming) micro-organisms—**septic** *adj*.

**septal defects** congenital anomalies in which an opening exists between the right and left sides of the heart. The defect may be between the two atria or the two ventricles. ⇒ atrial septal defect, ventricular septal defect.

**septic abortion** ⇒ miscarriage.

**septicaemia** *n* the multiplication of living bacteria in the blood stream, causing infection—**septicaemic** *adj*.

**septicaemic plague** ⇒ plague.

**septic arthritis** arthritis caused by infection in the joint.

**septoplasty** *n* conservative operation to straighten the nasal septum, usually undertaken for deviations and dislocations of the quadrilateral cartilage. The nasal septum is repositioned in the midline with minimal removal of nasal cartilage.

**septum** *n* a partition between two cavities, e.g. between the nasal cavities and the cardiac septum, that separates the right and left sides of the heart—**septa** *pl*, **septal**, **septate** *adj*.

437

**sequela** *n* pathological consequence of a disease—**sequelae** *pl.*

**sequestrectomy** *n* excision of a sequestrum.

**sequestrum** *n* a piece of dead bone which separates from the healthy bone but remains within the tissues—**sequestra** *pl.*

**serine** *n* a conditionally essential (indispensable) amino acid.

**SERMs** *abbr* selective (o)estrogen receptor modulators.

**seroconversion** *n* a change from a negative serological test where specific antibodies are absent to a positive test in which the presence of antibodies in the serum confirms that a response to an antigen (vaccine or infection) has occurred.

**serofibrinous** *adj* relating to an exudate containing serum and fibrin.

**serology** *n* the study of blood serum and its reactions. Important in immunological diagnostic techniques involving the detection of antigen–antibody reactions.

**seropurulent** *adj* relating to exudate containing serum and pus.

**serosa** *n* a serous membrane, e.g. the peritoneal covering of the abdominal viscera—**serosal** *adj.*

**serositis** *n* inflammation of a serous membrane.

**serotonin** *n* also called 5-hydroxytryptamine (5-HT). A monoamine formed from tryptophan (amino acid). Liberated by blood platelets after injury and found in high concentrations in the central nervous system and gastrointestinal tract. It is a vasoconstrictor, inhibits gastric secretion, stimulates smooth muscle and acts as a central neurotransmitter. It is also involved in pain transmission and perception, and sleep–wake cycles.

**serotyping** *n* classification of micro-organisms based on specific antigenic features.

**serous** *adj* pertaining to serum. *serous membrane* ⇒ membrane.

**serpiginous** *adj* snakelike, coiled, irregular; used to describe the margins of skin lesions, especially ulcers and ringworm.

**Serratia** *n* a genus of Gram-negative bacteria of the family Enterobacteriaceae. Motile bacilli capable of causing infection in humans. The species *Serratia marcescens* is an endemic hospital resident and is an opportunistic pathogen that affects immunocompromised individuals. It causes urinary tract infection, pneumonia, bacteraemia and endocarditis.

**serration** *n* a saw-like notch—**serrated** *adj.*

**serratus anterior** *n* a muscle of the anterior chest wall located over the lateral ribs. It has a serrated appearance. It arises from the first eight or nine ribs and it inserts on to the scapula. It contracts to rotate the scapula and raise the shoulder. It is important in arm abduction and in horizontal pushing or punching movements.

**Sertoli cells** (E Sertoli, Italian physiologist/histologist, 1842–1910) cells associated with the seminiferous tubules. They are vital in nourishing and supporting the sperm-producing germ cells of the germinal epithelium.

**serum** *n* the clear fluid remaining after blood has clotted—**sera** *pl.*

**serum sickness** the allergic illness occurring 7–10 days following the injection of foreign serum for treatment or prophylaxis of infection. Rarely seen now that serum from other species has been replaced by the use of human immunoglobulins. ⇒ anaphylaxis.

**sesamoid bone** a small area of bone formation in muscle tendons such as the patella in the tendon of the quadriceps femoris.

**severe acute asthma** (*syn* status asthmaticus) severe life-threatening asthma attack. Typically there is respiratory distress, cyanosis (central), tachycardia, sweating, an unproductive cough, exhaustion and severe hypoxia. It is a medical emergency requiring immediate treatment with high-concentration oxygen, intravenous access, systemic corticosteroids and inhaled $\beta_2$-adrenoceptor agonists. Respiratory support may be necessary for patients who do not improve with this treatment regimen.

**severe acute respiratory syndrome (SARS)** an atypical viral pneumonia caused by the SARS coronavirus (SARS CoV) which emerged as a new infection in South-East Asia to cause a worldwide outbreak during 2003. It is characterized by fever, headache, dyspnoea, cough and typical changes on chest X-ray. To date there is neither specific treatment nor an effective vaccine.

**severe combined immunodeficiency (SCID)** a group of immunodeficiency disorders presenting in infancy, characterized by failure of cellular and humoral immunity due to a genetic defect in a critical immune system component. SCID is generally fatal unless successfully treated by bone marrow transplantation or gene therapy. Examples include adenosine deaminase (an enzyme) deficiency (ADA-SCID) and X-linked SCID, caused by a defective cytokine.

**Sever's disease** (J Sever, American orthopaedic surgeon, 20th century) calcaneal epiphysitis. Occurs in children and is caused by damage to the bone–cartilage layer in the heel, resulting in pain.

**sex chromatin** in females the chromatin in one of the sex chromosomes (pair of X chromosomes) is inactive and appears in a somatic cell nucleus as a densely staining mass called a Barr body.

**sex chromosomes** the two chromosomes that determine genetic sex; XX in females and XY in males.

**sex hormones** the steroid hormones that include the androgens, oestrogens and progesterone produced by the gonads (ovaries or testes) and to a lesser extent the adrenal glands.

**sexism** *n* a view that members of one sex are superior to the other. Leads to discrimination and may be a limiting influence in education, professional development, etc.

**sex-limited gene** *n* a gene (autosomal or sex-linked) that leads to the expression of a trait in one sex only.

**sex-linked** *adj* refers to genes located on the sex chromosomes or, more especially, on the X chromosome.

**sex-linked gene** a gene present on the X or the Y chromosome (the sex chromosomes). The genes for a number of important disorders, such as haemophilia, Duchenne muscular dystrophy and colour blindness, are carried on the X chromosome. By convention it is usual to refer to these genes (and the characters that they determine) as X-linked, whereas the genes on the Y chromosome are not known to cause any significant disorders.

**sexual abuse** performing a sexual act with a child or with an adult against the person's wishes. The commonest type is that occurring between a father (or father figure) and daughter. ⇒ abuse, incest.

**sexual deviation** sexual acts or behaviours that are considered to be abnormal by society. Examples include exhibitionism, fetishism, masochism, necrophilia, paedophilia, sadism, etc.

**sexual dysfunction** a lack of desire or the ability to achieve coitus in one or both partners. ⇒ dyspareunia, erectile dysfunction, frigidity, impotence, libido, vaginismus.

**sexual intercourse** coitus.

**sexuality** *n* the sum of the structural, functional and psychological characteristics as they are expressed by a person's gender identity and sexual behaviour.

**sexual orientation** describes an individual's sexual attraction: towards people of the same sex (homosexuality), the opposite sex (heterosexuality) or both sexes (bisexuality). The particular preference may be transitory or lifelong.

**sexually acquired reactive arthritis (SARA)** *n* (*syn* Reiter's disease) often caused by infection with *Chlamydia trachomatis*, but intestinal infections can also be the triggering event. Arthritis occurs together with conjunctivitis or uveitis, urethritis (or cervicitis in women) and sometimes psoriasis. ⇒ reactive arthritis.

**sexually transmitted disease (STD)** previously called venereal disease. ⇒ sexually transmitted infection.

**sexually transmitted infection (STI)** the infections, including those defined legally as venereal, which are usually transmitted through sexual contact, but not exclusively so. They include: gonorrhoea, syphilis, human immunodeficiency virus (HIV), candidiasis, chlamydial infection, genital herpes, genital warts and trichomoniasis.

**SFD** *abbr* small for dates.

**SFS** *abbr* Social Functioning Scale.

**SGA** *abbr* small for gestational age.

**SGOT** *abbr* serum glutamic oxaloacetic transaminase. ⇒ aminotransferase.

**SGPT** *abbr* serum glutamic pyruvic transaminase. ⇒ aminotransferase.

**shaping** *n* a technique used in behaviour therapy, whereby the therapist initially reinforces behaviour that only slightly resembles the desired goal; as the programme progresses the therapist only reinforces behaviour that is increasingly close to the desired behaviour until the goal is reached.

**shearing force** when any part of the supported body is on a gradient, the tissues nearest the bone 'slide' towards the lower gradient while the skin stays in contact with the supporting surface because of friction which is increased in the presence of moisture. The deep blood vessels are stretched and bent and the deeper tissues become ischaemic with consequent necrosis. ⇒ pressure ulcers.

**Sheehan's syndrome** (H Sheehan, British pathologist, 1900–1988) hypopituitarism caused by postpartum necrosis of the pituitary gland resulting from hypovolaemia such as that occurring with severe postpartum haemorrhage. A rare condition characterized by

**S**

the loss of pubic and axillary hair, possible failure of the establishment of lactation, continuing amenorrhoea as menstrual cycles do not return, symptoms of reduced cortisol secretion and secondary hypothyroidism. ⇒ hypopituitarism, Simmonds' syndrome.

**sheep cell agglutination test (SCAT)** a test for rheumatoid factor in the blood, detected by the sheep cell agglutination titre.

**shelf operation** an operation to deepen the acetabulum in some cases of developmental dysplasia of the hip (formally known as congenital dislocation of the hip), involving the use of a bone graft. Performed at 7–8 years of age after failure of conservative treatment.

**shiatsu** *n* a form of Japanese health care similar in principle to acupuncture. Specific points along the body surface are pressed using the thumbs, fingers or palms to stimulate energy flow and to start self-healing processes. The belief is that an imbalance in a person's energy may result in physical symptoms. The aims of shiatsu are to rebalance self-healing energy and so promote health and well-being.

**Shigella** *n* (K Shiga, Japanese bacteriologist, 1870–1957) a genus of Gram-negative, non-motile bacilli of the family Enterobacteriaceae. Several species cause dysentery: *Shigella boydii*, *S. dysenteriae* and *S. flexneri* in tropical and subtropical areas. *S. sonnei* causes dysentery in temperate regions and is the most common type in the UK. Commonly affects young children and is spread by the faecal–oral route. ⇒ dysentery.

**shin bone** ⇒ tibia.

**shingles** *n* herpes zoster. A condition arising when the infecting agent (varicella-zoster virus) attacks sensory nerves, causing severe pain and the appearance of vesicles along the nerve's distribution (usually unilateral). ⇒ herpes zoster. ⊙DVD

**Shirodkar's operation** (N Shirodkar, Indian obstetrician, 1900–1971) placing of a purse-string suture around an incompetent cervix during pregnancy. It is removed when labour starts.

**shock** *n* condition in which there is inadequate flow of oxygenated blood to the tissues. There is cell hypoxia and inadequate tissue perfusion. Causes include haemorrhage, fluid deficits (hypovolaemic shock), heart failure (cardiogenic shock), infection (septic shock) and allergic reaction (anaphylactic shock). ⇒ systemic inflammatory response syndrome, toxic shock syndrome.

**short-bowel syndrome (SBS)** a disorder characterized by malabsorption of nutrients which, in children, is commonly caused by congenital anomalies (e.g. small bowel atresia, gastroschisis), necrotizing enterocolitis and trauma or vascular injury, such as that caused by a volvulus. The medical management centres around maintaining nutrition through enteral feeding to ensure optimum growth and development while intestinal adaptation occurs. The initial phase of nutrition is via total parenteral nutrition (TPN), which helps to stimulate the adaptation response of the small intestine. In children, SBS results in a compensatory increase in the mucosal surface area, mostly by villus hyperplasia, and a small increase in the length and diameter of the small intestine. These changes enable a gradual increase in the absorption of nutrients.

**shortening fraction** in cardiology, the difference between ventricular diameter at the end of systole and its original diameter at the end of diastole, expressed as a percentage.

**Short Portable Mental State Questionnaire (SPMSQ)** an assessment of cognitive function used to screen for impairment and dementia. The areas assessed are orientation, mathematical ability, practical skills and memory (both short-term and long-term).

**short-sightedness** ⇒ myopia.

**short-term memory (STM)** working memory. The portion of memory that is responsible for the retention of information for a few seconds only. It can only be retained if it is rehearsed or moved to long-term memory (LTM). ⇒ chunking, rehearsal in memory.

**shoulder dystocia** impacted shoulders. The fetal shoulders do not spontaneously pass through the pelvis after the delivery of the head. The anterior shoulder is caught up behind or at the symphysis pubis. It is an obstetric emergency, which can result in perinatal morbidity or mortality. It can occur with a very large fetus (over 4000 g). Management may involve a change in maternal position or an invasive manipulative procedure. ⇒ macrosomia, McRobert's manoeuvre, Rubin's manoeuvre, Wood's manoeuvre, Zavanelli manoeuvre.

**shoulder girdle** pectoral girdle. Formed by the clavicle and scapula on either side.

**shoulder presentation** a presentation in which the fetus lies across the uterus, i.e. a transverse lie. It may be dorsoanterior or dorsoposterior (Figure S.4). A caesarean section will

S

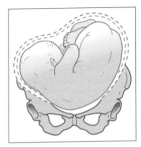

**Figure S.4** Shoulder presentation—dorsoanterior *(reproduced from Fraser & Cooper 2003 with permission).*

be necessary if the shoulder presentation continues in labour.

**'show'** *n* a popular term for the blood-stained vaginal discharge that occurs at the commencement of labour.

**shunt** *n* a term applied to the passage of fluid through other than the usual channel. This may refer to shunting of blood (e.g. some cardiac septal defects, arteriovenous shunt) or cerebrospinal fluid (e.g. ventriculoperitoneal shunt).

**SI** *abbr* Système International d'Unités.

**SIADH** *abbr* syndrome of inappropriate antidiuretic hormone secretion.

**sialadenitis** *n* inflammation of one or more salivary glands. Causes include surgery, infection (e.g. mumps), tumours and obstruction to salivary ducts (e.g. by calculi).

**sialagogue** *n* an agent which increases saliva production.

**sialogram** *n* radiographic image of the salivary glands and ducts, after injection of an opaque contrast medium—**sialography** *n*, **sialographic** *adj*, **sialographically** *adv*.

**sialolith** *n* a calculus (stone) in a salivary gland or duct.

**sialorrhoea** *n* hypersalivation. Excessive flow of saliva. It may be caused by teething, oral inflammation, poorly fitting dentures, neurological disorders and, more rarely, mercurialism.

**Siamese twins** ⇒ conjoined twins.

**sibilant** *adj, n* hissing or whistling sound.

**sickle-cell anaemia/disease** an inherited haemoglobinopathy; it is transmitted as an autosomal recessive condition. It is due to an abnormal haemoglobin (HbS) in which the beta-globin gene is faulty. Individuals who inherit one normal gene for adult haemoglobin (HbA) and one abnormal gene for sickle haemoglobin (HbS) will have sickle-cell trait; they are carriers of sickle-cell anaemia and can transmit the gene to their offspring, but they will not have clinical problems. The disease mainly affects people of African, African–Caribbean or African–American descent, but can also be found in those with Indian, Middle Eastern, Far Eastern and southern European ancestry. The disease is associated with regions of the world in which falciparum malaria is endemic. When HbS becomes deoxygenated, crystals form in the red cells, which become distorted and sickle-shaped. The red cells, once oxygenated again, can return to a normal shape, but over time the affected cells become increasingly rigid and are prematurely destroyed by the cells of the monocyte–macrophage system in the spleen and liver. The life span of these red cells is much less than the 120 days for a normal red cell. Sickle-cell disease is characterized by chronic haemolytic anaemia and intermittent painful crises. Affected individuals will often have a low haemoglobin level and will usually be mildly jaundiced and have splenomegaly. At-risk populations should be screened for the abnormal HbS. Affected individuals are also offered an immunization programme that includes protection against *Haemophilus influenzae* type b, influenza (annually), meningococcal C and pneumococcal infections. Sickle-cell crises occur when many red cells become sickle-shaped; the rigid cells are unable to pass through small blood vessels, the blood vessels are occluded and tissue ischaemia and infarction can result. These crises are associated with excruciating pain in the affected area of the body. Factors associated with triggering crises include: infection, reduced tissue oxygenation, general anaesthesia, dehydration, extremes of temperature, high altitude, excessive alcohol consumption, strenuous exercise, pregnancy and emotional stress. Severe crises can be life-threatening, particularly when they affect blood vessels in the brain or lungs. Management of sickle-cell crises will depend on the severity; a severe crisis will require admission to hospital for strong opioid analgesics, intravenous fluid replacement, oxygen therapy and close observation. Patients with chest pain, caused by a sickling crisis affecting the lungs ('chest crisis'), have a significant risk of mortality. Therefore, this

441

may be treated by an exchange transfusion in which some of the patient's blood is removed and replaced by donated blood transfused by apheresis. At present, there is no cure for sickle-cell disease apart from haemopoietic stem cell transplantation from a sibling donor. ⇒ malaria, thalassaemia.

**side-effect** n any physiological change other than the wanted one from a drug, e.g. oral iron causes the side-effect of black faeces. Also covers undesirable drug reactions. Some are predictable, being the result of a known metabolic action of the drug, e.g. hair loss with cytotoxic drugs. Unpredictable reactions can be: (a) immediate: anaphylaxis, angioedema; (b) erythematous: all forms of erythema, including nodosum and multiforme and purpuric rashes; (c) cellular eczematous rashes and contact dermatitis; and (d) specific, e.g. light-sensitive eruptions with griseofulvin (antifungal). ⇒ adverse drug reactions.

**sideroblast** n a nucleated red blood cell precursor, a normoblast present in the bone, which contains granules of iron. The presence of *ringed sideroblasts*, which have a ring of iron granules around the cell nucleus, is a feature of sideroblastic anaemia.

**sideroblastic anaemias** npl a group of rare anaemias caused by defective iron metabolism; they may be inherited or acquired.

**sideropenia** n abnormally low level of iron in the serum.

**siderosis** n excess of iron in the blood or tissues. Inhalation of iron oxide into the lungs can cause one form of pneumoconiosis. ⇒ haemochromatosis, haemosiderosis.

**SIDS** abbr sudden infant death syndrome.

**sievert (Sv)** n the SI unit (International System of Units) for radiation dose equivalent. It has replaced the rem. ⇒ Appendix 2.

**sigmoid** adj shaped like the letter S.

**sigmoid colon** the part of the descending colon after it enters the pelvis. The S-shaped bend (sigmoid flexure) at the lower end of the descending colon, which is continuous with the rectum below. ⇒ Appendix 1, Figure 18B.

**sigmoidectomy** n excision of the sigmoid colon. Most commonly undertaken for colorectal cancer, but also may be required for other conditions, such as diverticular disease.

**sigmoidoscope** n an instrument for visualizing the rectum and sigmoid colon. ⇒ endoscope—**sigmoidoscopic** adj.

**sigmoidoscopy** n endoscopic examination of the rectum and distal colon (sigmoid colon). ⇒ colonoscopy.

**sigmoidostomy** n the formation of a colostomy (stoma) in the sigmoid colon.

**sign** n any objective evidence of disease. For example, high temperature, a rash, swelling, abnormal breath sounds or vomiting blood.

**signal node** also known as Troisier's sign or Virchow's node. An enlarged supraclavicular lymph node, often on the left side, indicative of metastatic spread from an abdominal cancer, such as that of the stomach.

**significance** n ⇒ statistical significance.

**sign language** a form of non-verbal language using the hands and upper body to make signs, whereby hearing impaired people can communicate with each other and with family and friends. ⇒ British sign language, finger spelling, Makaton.

**silicone** n a water-repellent compound. Used in some types of wound dressings, such as sheets, foams and gels, where it fits exactly the contours of the granulating wound to provide an ideal environment for wound healing. Also used as implants in breast reconstruction.

**silicosis** n a form of pneumoconiosis or industrial dust disease found in metal grinders, stone-workers, etc.

**Silverman score** a method of rating respiratory distress by assessing movement of accessory muscles and degree of expiratory grunt.

**silver nitrate** used as a caustic for warts.

**SIMA** abbr system for identifying motivated abilities.

**Simmonds' disease** (M Simmonds, German physician, 1855–1925) panhypopituitarism. ⇒ hypopituitarism.

**simple fracture** ⇒ fracture.

**Sims' position** (J Sims, American gynaecologist, 1813–1883) an exaggerated left lateral position with the right knee well flexed and the left arm drawn back over the edge of the bed.

**Sims' speculum** (J Sims) a type of vaginal speculum.

**simulator** n computer-linked equipment that is used to calculate exact treatment location prior to commencing a course of radiotherapy.

**SIMV** abbr synchronized intermittent mandatory ventilation.

**single-cell protein** a term used to describe a biomass of yeast, bacteria or algae that may be of use as human or animal food.

**single-nucleotide polymorphism (SNP)** a type of genetic polymorphism occurring between two genomes in which the exchange, insertion or deletion of material involves a single nucleotide.

S

**single-photon emission computed tomography (SPECT)** an imaging technique that is a variation of computed tomography. It involves the administration of radioisotopes (radionuclides) that emit gamma radiation, which is detected by several gamma cameras that are arranged to rotate around the patient. A computer constructs a three-dimensional image.

**sinoatrial node** ⇒ sinus node.

**sinus** *n* **1.** a hollow or cavity, especially the paranasal air sinuses (Figure P.1, p. 358). ⇒ paranasal. **2.** a channel containing blood, especially venous blood, e.g. the dural sinuses draining venous blood from the brain. ⇒ cavernous sinus, dural sinuses. **3.** a recess or cavity within a bone. **4.** any abnormal blind tract or channel opening on to the skin or a mucous surface. ⇒ pilonidal sinus.

**sinus arrhythmia** an increase of heart rate on inspiration, decrease on expiration.

**sinusitis** *n* inflammation of a sinus, used exclusively for the paranasal sinuses.

**sinus node (sinoatrial node)** the pacemaker of the heart. Part of the specialized tissue that forms the conducting system of the heart. It is situated at the junction of the superior vena cava and the right atrium. It initiates the wave of cardiac contraction. ⇒ pacemaker.

**sinusoid** *n* a dilated channel into which arterioles or veins open in some organs, e.g. liver, and which act in place of the usual capillaries.

**sinus rhythm** normal rhythm of the heart. ⇒ P-QRS-T complex.

**Sipple's syndrome** (J Sipple, American physician, b. 1930) a type of multiple endocrine neoplasia (MEN) in which the inheritance is usually autosomal dominant. It is characterized by medullary cancer of the thyroid, parathyroid tumours or hyperplasia leading to overactivity and the presence of phaeochromocytoma. ⇒ Wermer's syndrome.

**SIRS** *abbr* systemic inflammatory response syndrome.

**sitapophasis** *n* refusal to eat in people with mental health problems.

**sitology** *n* the science dealing with the study of food.

**sitomania** *n* also called phagomania. An abnormal obsession with food and eating.

**sitophobia** *n* also called phagophobia. An abnormal fear of food.

**sitz bath** *n* a hip bath.

**Sjögren–Larsson syndrome** (K Sjögren, Swedish psychiatrist/physician, 1896–1974; T Larsson, Swedish statistician, 1905–1998) genetically determined congenital ectodermosis. Associated with learning disability.

**Sjögren syndrome** (H Sjögren, Swedish ophthalmologist, 1899–1986) deficient secretion from lacrimal, salivary and other glands, mostly in postmenopausal women. There is keratoconjunctivitis, dry tongue and hoarse voice. Thought to be due to an autoimmune process. Also called keratoconjunctivitis sicca. ⇒ connective tissue diseases.

**skatole** *n* 3-methylindole. A constituent of faeces, it contributes to the characteristic odour. It is produced in the intestine from the decomposition of proteins and from the amino acid tryptophan. Its oxidation product may appear in the urine.

**skeletal muscle** striated, voluntary muscle tissue. Forms the skeletal muscles that cover the bony skeleton and allow movement. The individual cells or fibres are multinucleate and form extended cylinders. Skeletal muscle is the only muscle tissue which may be controlled consciously. However, in many cases, this control operates through reflexes. Skeletal muscle is stimulated by the voluntary motor division (somatic) of the peripheral nervous system. ⇒ muscle.

**skeleton** *n* the bony framework of the body, supporting and protecting the soft tissues and organs and acting as attachments for muscles. (⇒ Appendix 1, Figures 2 and 3)—**skeletal** *adj*. *appendicular skeleton* the bones forming the pectoral (shoulder) girdle, upper limbs, pelvic girdle and lower limbs. *axial skeleton* the bones forming the head and trunk: skull, spinal column, hyoid bone, ribs and sternum.

**Skene's glands (**A Skene, American gynaecologist, 1839–1900) two small mucussecreting glands at the entrance to the female urethra; the lesser vestibular or paraurethral glands.

**skewed distribution** a statistical term that describes any distribution of scores where there are a greater number of values on one side of the mean than the other, i.e. not symmetrical. ⇒ normal distribution curve.

**skill** *n* the ability to perform a specific task competently and consistently with minimum effort and maximum effect.

**skill mix** the level, range and variety of skills of the staff in a department, unit or team which is needed to meet the organizational outcomes.

**skin** *n* the tissue which forms the outer covering of the body; it consists of two layers, the outer epidermis (cuticle), dermis (true skin) and the appendages; nails, hair follicles and sebaceous glands (pilosebaceous units) and sweat glands. The skin is concerned with a number of functions, including: sensation, protection, thermoregulation, excretion, absorption, storage, synthesis and communication. The epidermis contains several special cell types: keratinocytes (produce keratin); corneocytes (contain water-retaining substances and moisturizing factor); immune Langerhans' cells (dendritic cells); and melanocytes (produce melanin). The epidermis has several layers of stratified epithelium through which cells progress, losing water and protein as they go. The epidermis has an outer horny zone consisting of three layers—(a) stratum corneum (horny layer); (b) stratum lucidum (clear layer), which is not present in all areas; and (c) stratum granulosum (granular layer)—which overlay the germinative zone. The germinative zone has two layers: stratum spinosum (prickle layer) and the stratum basale (basal layer), which contains the melanocytes responsible for melanin production and skin pigmentation. The epidermis undergoes renewal as the stratum corneum is continually shed to be replaced by new cells formed in the stratum basale which move upwards through the layers over a period of around 35 days, depending on age and other factors. The continual shedding of the outer keratinized cells as flakes or scales poses a potential risk of infection in health care settings. The exfoliated flakes contain the micro-organisms normally resident on the skin, and these may cause infection in susceptible patients, such as those who are immunocompromised. Epidermal cohesion is maintained during the renewal by the desmosomes which bind the keratinocytes together and prevent structural disruption. As the cells migrate upwards there is nuclear disintegration, keratinization and flattening. The dermis is connective tissue containing collagen, elastin and reticular fibres, cells such as fibroblasts and macrophages, blood and lymph vessels and different types of nerve endings. ⇒ hair, nail, pilosebaceous, sebaceous glands, sweat glands. ⇒ Appendix 1, Figure 12.

**skin cancer** ⇒ basal cell carcinoma, melanoma, squamous cell carcinoma.

**skin expansion** a technique utilizing an inflatable prosthesis to distend and expand the skin and subcutaneous tissue.

**skin flap** ⇒ flap.

**skin flora** also called resident flora. The commensal micro-organisms normally present on the skin are part of the normal flora of the body. Micro-organisms forming the skin flora include *Candida*, corynebacteria, micrococci, *Neisseria*, staphylococci and streptococci. The type of micro-organism varies across body sites, and depends on factors that include humidity and temperature.

**skin fold thickness** an anthropometric measurement used as part of a holistic nutritional assessment. It measures subcutaneous fat in various sites, usually four, and is a guide to total body fat content. Special calipers are used to measure the fat at the following sites: the middle of the posterior aspect of the upper arm (triceps), middle of the anterior aspect of the upper arm (biceps), below the point of the scapula at an angle of 45° (subscapular) and above the iliac crest in the mid-axillary line (suprailiac). ⇒ anthropometry.

**skin graft** sheet of skin containing dermis and epidermis separated from its blood supply and applied to a raw surface. *full-thickness (Wolfe) graft* full-thickness skin graft that requires closure of the donor site. *split-thickness (Thiersch) graft* partial-thickness skin graft where the donor site heals spontaneously.

**skull** *n* the bony framework of the head, the face (13 bones) and the cranium (8 bones). ⇒ Appendix 1, Figure 2.

**SLE** *abbr* systemic lupus erythematosus.

**sleep** *n* a naturally altered state of consciousness occurring in humans in a 24-h biological rhythm. A *sleep cycle* consists of alternating cycles of non-rapid eye movement sleep (NREM) or orthodox sleep, which has four stages, and rapid eye movement sleep (REM) or paradoxical sleep (Figure S.5).

**sleep apnoea syndrome** recurrent periods of apnoea and hypopnoea while sleeping due to repeated upper-airway obstruction. Associated with transient hypoxaemia, severe headaches and daytime sleepiness (somnolence). More often seen in obese individuals, or those with soft palate abnormalities. ⇒ continuous positive airway pressure, obstructive sleep apnoea (hypopnoea) syndrome (OSAS/OSAHS).

**sleep deprivation** a cumulative condition arising when there is interference with a person's established rhythm of paradoxical sleep. It can result in tiredness, feeling cold, headaches, reduced appetite, slurred rambling speech, irritability, disorientation, confusion, slowed reaction time, poor co-ordination,

**S**

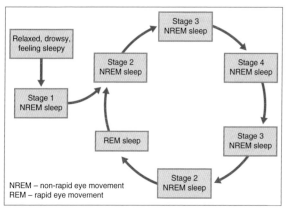

**Figure S.5** Sleep cycle—adults *(reproduced from Brooker & Waugh 2007 with permission).*

inability to perform skilled tasks, occurrence of 'microsleeps', increased risk of accidents, poor concentration, malaise, mood swings, increased aggression, progressing to illusions, delusions, hallucinations, paranoia and hyperactivity.

**sleep disorder** describes a change in normal sleep pattern or rhythm. Sleep disorders include bruxism, insomnia, narcolepsy, nightmares, sleep apnoea, sleep/night terrors and sleep walking. ⇒ parasomnias.

**sleep hygiene** describes the pre-sleep routines that relax, enhance settling and promote sleep. These may include going to bed and getting up at around the same time each day, and reducing activity during the evening before bedtime. Routines often include activities such as having a warm bath and changing into nightclothes, reading in bed or a bedtime story for children, a milky drink, teeth/denture cleaning and passing urine.

**sleeping sickness** a disease endemic in Africa; there is increasing somnolence caused by infection of the brain by trypanosomes. ⇒ trypanosomiasis.

**sleep study** tests and observations undertaken during sleep in a specialist centre. Used in the investigation of some sleep disorders and to diagnose nocturnal hypoxaemia and apnoeic episodes. ⇒ polysomnography.

**sleep terror** also called night terror. The person, usually a child, wakes suddenly during stage 3 or 4 of non-rapid eye movement sleep. It is characterized by episodes of sudden waking, screaming, intense fear, anxiety, agitation, confusion and disorientation. The child is sweaty and both heart rate and respiratory rate are increased.

**sleep walking** ⇒ somnambulism.

**slipped disc** *n* prolapsed intervertebral disc. ⇒ prolapse.

**slipped epiphysis** displacement of an epiphysis, especially the upper femoral one. ⇒ epiphysis.

**slit lamp** a device used in ophthalmology to carry out a very detailed examination of the eye. It is a binocular microscope mounted on a table, with a light source that is directed through a narrow slit. It is used to provide the examiner with a three-dimensional view of the external and internal structures of the eye. The magnification and the light source can be adjusted as necessary.

**slough** *n* soft, usually creamy yellow material, present at the surface of a wound. It is formed from cellular and fibrin debris, and may vary in colour as wound healing progresses.

**slow-release drugs** drug formulations which do not dissolve until they reach the small intestine, where the drug is slowly released and absorbed. Many slow-release preparations are now incorporated into transdermal patches.

**slow virus** an infective agent (prion) that only causes infection after a long latent period, perhaps many years. Many cases may never develop overt symptoms but may still be a link in the chain of infectivity. ⇒ Creutzfeldt–Jakob disease.

**SLT** *abbr* speech and language therapist/therapy.

**SMA** *abbr* spinal muscular atrophy.

**small-cell lung carcinoma** a type of lung cancer. ⇒ oat cell carcinoma.

**small for dates (SFD)** small for gestational age.

**small for gestational age (SGA)** babies who weigh less than expected for a given gestational age. They are either constitutionally small or suffer from intrauterine growth restriction/retardation. ⇒ low birth weight.

**smallpox** *n* (*syn* variola) caused by a virus: eradicated following a World Health Organization worldwide campaign. Vaccination may be required for laboratory staff working with pox viruses and others at risk of exposure. ⇒ vaccinia.

**SMART** *acron* a goal-setting acronym: **s**pecific **m**easurable **a**chievable **r**ealistic **t**ime-oriented.

**SMBG** *abbr* self-monitoring of blood glucose.

**smear** *n* a film of material spread out on a glass slide for microscopic examination. ⇒ carcinoma, cervical intraepithelial neoplasia (CIN), cervical smear, colposcope, cytology.

**smegma** *n* the sebaceous secretion which accumulates beneath the prepuce and clitoris.

**Smith-Petersen nail** (M Smith-Petersen, American orthopaedic surgeon, 1886–1953) a trifin, cannulated metal nail used to provide internal fixation for intracapsular fractures of the femoral neck.

**Smith's fracture** (R Smith, Irish surgeon, 1807–1873) a fracture of the distal radius with forward (volar) displacement of the distal fragment. Compare Colles' fracture.

**smoking (passive)** *n* passive smoking is described as the involuntary inhalation of smoke from burning tobacco generated by another person over a period of time. It is associated with an increased risk of smoking-related illnesses such as coronary heart disease, hypertension, bronchial cancer and chronic obstructive pulmonary disease and can also trigger an asthma attack, or lead to sudden unexpected deaths in infancy. Passive smoking is an occupational hazard, for example for those working in bars and clubs, and efforts to reduce the risk include the introduction of no-smoking legislation in the workplace in the UK and the Republic of Ireland and encouraging employers to support smoking cessation programmes. Babies and children are especially vulnerable and have little choice about exposure to tobacco smoke. ⇒ sudden unexpected deaths in infancy (sudden infant death syndrome).

**smooth muscle** unstriated, involuntary muscle tissue. Found in hollow organs, such as the gastrointestinal tract, ureter, bladder, the bronchi, blood vessels and the uterus. Spindle-shaped smooth muscle cells (fibres) have a single nucleus and form flat sheets of contractile units. Smooth muscle contraction is involuntary; stimulation occurs through the action of autonomic nerves and various hormones and regulatory peptides. It responds slowly, and the contraction, which is less intense than that in skeletal muscle, is usually more sustained. Contractions of smooth muscle are more widespread, with all the fibres within the sheet able to contract together. In addition some smooth muscle fibres act as 'pacemakers' which are capable of initiating inherent, rhythmic contractions that may be modified by neural or hormonal influences. ⇒ muscle.

**SMR** *abbr* **1.** standardized mortality ratio. **2.** submucous resection.

**snapping-hip syndrome** a snapping sensation either heard or felt in the hip during movement of the joint. The nature of the signs and symptoms will indicate whether the structure at fault is more likely to be the iliotibial band or the iliopsoas tendon.

**snare** *n* a surgical instrument with a wire loop at the end; used for removal of polypi.

**SNB** *abbr* sentinel node biopsy.

**Snellen test type chart** (H Snellen, Dutch ophthalmologist, 1834–1908) a series of charts used for testing visual acuity. They comprise a chart of different-sized letters arranged in lines that can be read by a normal (emmetropic) eye at 60, 36, 24, 18, 12, 9, 6, 5 and 4 metres. Acuity is checked, in good light, in each eye separately and expressed as 6 over the smallest line of letters that can be read. For example, being able to read the 6-metre line at 6 metres is described as visual acuity of 6/6. Special E test-type with different orientations of the letter E can be used to test young children and other groups unable to read the letters. Charts showing objects of decreasing size can be used to test prelingual children.

**Snoezelen** *n* a controllable multisensory stimulation environment that uses light, colour, sound, tactile surfaces and scents, including essential oils, to stimulate the senses in a relaxing and soothing way. It has been used with people with dementia and various learning disabilities, including autistic spectrum disorders.

S

**snoring** *n* a harsh breathing sound during sleep. It is caused by vibration of the soft palate and uvula ⇒ obstructive sleep apnoea (hypopnoea) syndrome.

**snow blindness** painful eyes and photophobia caused by overexposure to the glare from sunlight on snow. It can be accompanied by inflammation of the cornea (keratitis) and conjunctiva (conjunctivitis).

**SNP** *abbr* single-nucleotide polymorphism.

**snuffles** *n* a snorting inspiration due to congestion of nasal mucous membrane. It is a sign of early congenital (prenatal) syphilis, when the nasal discharge may be purulent or blood-stained.

**SOAP** *acron* **s**ubjective **o**bjective **a**ssessment **p**lan. ⇒ problem-oriented medical records.

**social class** the classification of people into social groups. Various classifications are used, and one such is a five-category socioeconomic classification based on the householder's occupation. I, professional, e.g. lawyer; II, intermediate, e.g. nurse; III, skilled (non-manual), e.g. secretary and (manual), e.g. carpenter; IV, semiskilled, e.g. agricultural worker; V, unskilled, e.g. cleaner.

**social deprivation measurement** composite index of deprivation (poverty) in a defined population based on census-derived social and economic variables. Geographically defined populations include residents within a Strategic Health Authority (population up to several million) or district (population 0.5–1 million), administrative (electoral) wards (several thousands) or enumerator districts (25 households). Deprivation indices may also be attributed to general practice populations based on the wards or enumerator districts from which the practice draws its registered patients.

**social exclusion** the lack of social connections, social support or access to social networks for particular groups in the population (community). Groups affected include rough sleepers, teenage mothers, refugees and many young people. Research has reported higher levels of ill health (illness, psychological ill health, disease, disability, mortality) in people with low levels of social support and integration, independent of physical health, socioeconomic status and lifestyle. Two main theories: social support affects health directly; social support protects against life stresses. Conversely, social exclusion increases the risk of physical and psychological ill health. ⇒ underclass.

**Social Functioning Scale (SFS)** a scale used to assess aspects of everyday social functioning which are negatively affected by mental health problems. There are seven main areas, for example, interpersonal behaviour, social engagement, etc.

**social isolation** a term that can be applied to an individual, a family or a group of individuals. Interaction with other people does not conform to the usual pattern, for reasons that may include immobility, poverty, etc.

**socialization** *n* the means by which individuals learn the social norms and the value of abiding by them. The process that facilitates the transmission of culture from one generation to another, ensuring its continuity, e.g. language, knowledge and way of life. It may occur informally in the family (primary socialization), and more formally when starting school and continuing throughout life (secondary socialization). Sometimes the term 'tertiary' or 'professional' socialization is applied to the acquisition of the knowledge, skills and attitude needed to perform high-level occupational roles such as medicine.

**social norms** describes socially acceptable behaviour. Norms may prescribe some forms of behaviour and prohibit others. ⇒ anomie.

**social role valorization** ⇒ normalization.

**social services** personal social services that include social work and social care carried out by, or on behalf of, local authority social services departments, other statutory organizations, private and voluntary agencies.

**social stratification** the means of dividing populations into unequal strata using different characteristics, for example, age, gender, income, ethnicity, etc.

**sociocultural** *adj* pertaining to culture in its sociological context.

**sociology** *n* the scientific study of societies and groups, and interpersonal and intergroup social relationships and interactions—**sociological** *adj*.

**sociology of sport** area of study concerned with the social structure, social patterns and social organization of groups and subcultures in sport.

**sociomedical** *adj* relating to sociology and medicine. For example, how social influences may predispose to diseases, e.g. sleeping rough may increase the risk for hypothermia, unemployment may increase the risk of mental health problems, such as depression, etc.

**sodium (Na)** *n* metallic element. A major extracellular cation concerned with the

**S**

447

composition of fluid compartments and neuro-muscular function.

**sodium bicarbonate (NaHCO₃)** also known as sodium hydrogen carbonate. It functions in the body as part of a buffer system to prevent pH changes in the blood. Administered intravenously to correct metabolic acidosis, such as in renal failure, or during cardiac arrest.

**sodium chloride** 'common salt'. Often used in intravenous fluids to replace fluids and correct electrolyte levels.

**sodium citrate** used as an in vitro anticoagulant, e.g. for stored blood.

**sodium hypochlorite** a powerful disinfectant used, in suitable dilutions, in many situations, such as dealing with environmental contamination with blood and other body fluids, and disinfection of infant feeding bottles. It is effective against many micro-organisms, including the hepatitis B virus and human immunodeficiency virus (HIV).

**sodium lactate** a sodium salt present in some intravenous infusion solutions, such as compound lactate solution (Hartmann's solution, Ringer lactate solution).

**sodium–potassium pump** a protein that facilitates the active transport mechanism (needing adenosine triphosphate) that pumps sodium and potassium ions through semipermeable cell membranes.

**sodomy** n **1.** anal intercourse between two men, or a man and a woman. **2.** can be used to describe intercourse between a human and an animal. This is also called bestiality or zoophilia. **3.** a more general term used to describe sexual acts or behaviours that are not acceptable to the majority in society.

**soft sore** chancroid.

**soft-tissue mobilization** physiotherapists and sports therapists use pétrissage or kneading techniques using the whole hand or the finger pads to stretch retracted muscles and tendons, relieve spasm and help to remove metabolic waste products from muscles. Kneading with the finger pads is also used during some natural childbirth methods. Physiotherapists use percussive manipulations, collectively called tapôtement, to move thick secretions from the respiratory tract and assist expectoration.

**solanine** n a very toxic compound that is naturally present in nightshade plants, such as tomatoes and potatoes. Most is ingested from eating potatoes, especially if the potatoes have turned green and sprouted, after being exposed to light. The toxin is not completely

destroyed by heat (heat-stable) and, if ingested, can lead to a variety of effects, mainly gastrointestinal or neurological. These include: nausea and vomiting, colicky abdominal pain and diarrhoea, low temperature, bradycardia, decreased respiratory rate, dilated pupils and visual disturbances, headache, altered sensation, delirium and hallucination. On rare occasions it results in death.

**solar plexus** a large network of sympathetic (autonomic) nerve ganglia and fibres in the upper abdomen. It supplies the abdominal organs. *solar plexus punch* a blow to the abdomen that results in an immediate inability to breathe freely.

**soleus** n a muscle of the posterior aspect of the lower leg. It is covered by the large gastrocnemius calf muscle. Its origin is on the superior part of the tibia and fibula and it inserts on to the calcaneus (os calcis) via the calcaneal tendon (Achilles tendon) of the gastrocnemius. Contracts to plantar flex the foot; important during walking and running. ⇒ Appendix 1, Figures 4 and 5.

**solute** n substance dissolved in a solvent.

**solution** n a fluid that contains a dissolved substance or substances. *saturated solution* one in which the maximum amount of a particular substance is dissolved.

**solvent** n an agent that is capable of dissolving other substances (solutes). The component of a solution that is present in excess.

**solvent misuse** the practice of inhaling volatile substances, such as those in some adhesives, solvents and fuels, to produce euphoria and intoxication. Characterized by odour on clothes and hair, redness and blistering around the nose and mouth, and behaviour changes. Dependence, local damage to the nasal mucosa and organ damage, e.g. the brain, may result. Death may be caused by asphyxia or toxicity. ⇒ drug misuse.

**soma** n **1.** the body as separate and distinct from the mind. **2.** the body excluding the gametes (germ cells).

**somatic** *adj* relating to the body such as somatic cells (body cells), as distinct from the gametes. *somatic nerves* nerves controlling the function of voluntary, skeletal muscle.

**somatization** n the presence of physical symptoms without organic pathology. A number of terms have, in the past, been used to describe such events, including psychosomatic illness, functional illness, hysteria/conversion disorder, etc. Somatization is encountered in all specialisms in medicine. For example, abdominal pain with intermittent constipation and diarrhoea (irritable bowel syndrome), chest pain without cardiac pathology and atypical face pain.

**somatoform disorders** the *International Classification of Diseases* (ICD-10) classifies somatoform disorders in seven categories: (a) hypochondriacal disorder; (b) persistent somatoform pain disorder; (c) somatoform autonomic dysfunction; (d) somatization disorder; (e) undiffentiated somatoform disorder; (f) other somatoform disorders; and (g) somatoform disorder unspecified. Of these, hypochondriacal disorder and somatization disorder are the most common. The disorders have overlapping characteristics and, in practice, it is often very hard to distinguish between them. The classification in the *Diagnostic and Statistical Manual of Mental Disorders* (DSM-IV) is more specific.

**somatomedin** *n* ⇒ insulin-like growth factor

**somatostatin** *n* growth hormone release-inhibiting hormone (GHRIH). ⇒ growth hormone.

**somatostatinoma** *n* a rare somatostatin-secreting tumour of the islet cells of the pancreas. Causes dyspepsia, reduced secretion of gastric acid, steatorrhoea, the formation of gallstones, impaired glucose tolerance or diabetes mellitus. They also occur in the duodenum. ⇒ islet cell tumours.

**somatotrophin** *n* ⇒ growth hormone.

**somatotyping** *n* a way of describing body type or physique using a classification that has three basic types: ectomorphic, endomorphic and mesomorphic.

**somite** *n* any of the segments (somites) that form in the paired blocks of mesoderm that develop either side of the neural tube during the early days of embryonic development. The ventromedial somites will give rise to ligaments, cartilage and bone, and the dorsolateral somites will form skeletal muscle and the dermis of the skin.

**somnambulism** *n* (*syn* sleepwalking) occurs during stage 4 non-rapid eye movement sleep and mostly affects children. Following a short sleep period, children sit up; their eyes are open, they leave the bed and walk about. During this period they may do unusual things, such as urinating in the bedroom. Afterwards they may proceed directly to bed and will have no recall of events when they wake normally in the morning. Adults can also be affected, particularly if anxious or stressed, and may resume sleepwalking as they once did as children.

**Somogyi phenomenon** (M Somogyi, American biochemist, 1883–1971) in diabetes mellitus, the rebound hyperglycaemia that occurs following hypoglycaemia. It is caused by the release of hormones that cause glycogenolysis, gluconeogenesis and lipolysis, thus raising blood glucose.

**sonography** *n* ultrasonography.

**soporific** *adj*, *n* (describes) an agent which induces deep sleep.

**souffle** *n* puffing or blowing sound. *funic souffle* auscultatory murmur of pregnancy. Synchronizes with the fetal heart beat and is caused by pressure on the umbilical cord. *uterine souffle* soft, blowing murmur which can be auscultated over the uterus after the fourth month of pregnancy.

**sound** *n* an instrument introduced into a hollow organ or duct to detect a stone or to dilate a stricture.

**source isolation** is used for patients who are sources of micro-organisms that may be transmitted from them to infect others. *strict source isolation* is for highly transmissible and dangerous diseases. *standard source isolation* is for other communicable diseases/infections.

**Southern blot technique** (E Southern, British biochemist, b. 1938) a technique used to analyse fragments of DNA and identify the genes present. ⇒ Northern blot technique.

**soya protein** a protein that is extracted from soya bean, a legume used in Asiatic countries in place of meat. It is useful in dietetic preparations for those people who are allergic to cows' milk. Soya protein is a constituent of soya milk used as a substitute for cows' milk by vegans.

**spansule** *n* a drug preparation designed to produce controlled release when given orally.

**spasm** *n* **1.** a sudden involuntary contraction of a muscle. **2.** sustained contraction of a muscle or group of muscles due to pain. **3.** a seizure or convulsion of the whole body.

**spasmodic dysmenorrhoea** ⇒ dysmenorrhoea.

**spasmolytic** *adj*, *n* ⇒ antispasmodic.

**spastic colon** ⇒ irritable bowel syndrome.

**spasticity** *n* increased tension or tone of muscle (hypertonia) with increased resistance to passive movement out of the tonic posture proportional to the rate of stretch and characterized by the clasp-knife phenomenon, exaggerated deep tendon reflexes, Babinski's sign and clonus. Spasticity of one side of the body following stroke (cerebrovascular accident) is accompanied by loss of voluntary movement

449

and postural reactions of one side of the body (spastic hemiplegia)—**spastic** *adj*.

**spatial awareness** a knowledge of where all parts of the body are in relation to the physical characteristics of the immediate environment. Important in judging distances, such as reaching for an object, or safely going up or down steps.

**spatial relations problems** a variety of problems (e.g. trips and falls, accidents involving hot liquids, etc.) caused when people are not able to work out how the position of several objects in the environment relates to them, or their own position in relation to each separate object.

**spatula** *n* a flat flexible instrument with blunt edges for spreading creams, ointment, etc. *tongue spatula* a rigid, blade-shaped instrument for depressing the tongue during physical examination.

**species** *n* a systematic category, subdivision of genus. Individuals within a species group have common characteristics and differ, fairly obviously, from a related species.

**specific** *adj* special; characteristic; peculiar to. *specific disease* one that is always caused by a specified organism, e.g. typhoid fever is caused by the bacterium *Salmonella typhi*.

**specific adaptation to imposed demands (SAID) principle** in sports medicine the principle of specificity of training. ⇒ training.

**specific dynamic action (SDA)** the increase in body temperature and metabolism that occurs when energy is used in the assimilation of ingested food. Protein foods in particular cause a sustained increase in basal metabolic rate that lasts for some hours.

**specific gravity** the weight of a substance, as compared with that of an equal volume of pure water, the latter being represented by 1000.

**specificity** *n* high specificity is the ability of a test to identify accurately non-affected individuals, such as faecal occult blood screening for colorectal cancer. Low specificity can lead to false positives, i.e. it detects disease in cases where it is not present. ⇒ sensitivity.

**SPECT** *abbr* single-photon emission computed tomography.

**spectrophotometer** *n* a spectroscope combined with a photometer for quantitatively measuring the relative intensity of different parts of a light spectrum—**spectrophotometric** *adj*.

**spectroscope** *n* an instrument for observing spectra of light.

**speculum** *n* an instrument used to hold the walls of a cavity apart, so that the interior of the cavity can be examined or treated—**specula** *pl*. *nasal speculum* used for examination of the nose and for treatments, such as nasal cautery and packing to stop bleeding. *vaginal speculum* used to examine the vagina and cervix, for taking high vaginal swabs and cervical smears and for some treatments. Types include Cusco's bivalve and Sims' speculum (Figure S.6).

**speech and language therapist** the health professional responsible for the assessment, diagnosis and treatment of speech and language disorders and disorders affecting swallowing in children and adults. In the USA and Australia they are known as speech–language pathologists.

**speech and language therapy (SLT)** one of the professions allied to medicine. Describes the therapy provided by a speech and language therapist to people with impaired communication, e.g. aphasia. Speech and language therapy is provided for people who are dysfluent (stammer), have impaired hearing, have language difficulties (grammar and vocabulary and the social use of language), have problems producing the correct sounds for speech so that they are difficult to understand, or have difficulties with their voice. Speech and language therapy referrals are also made for people who have dysphagia (difficulty in swallowing), particularly following a stroke or in other neurological conditions. Speech and language therapy includes assessment and treatment of these difficulties. In the UK therapy with adults is usually carried out

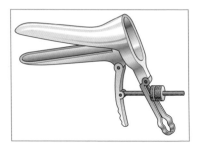

**Figure S.6** Cusco's vaginal speculum *(reproduced from Brooker & Nicol 2003 with permission).*

within an NHS setting, including hospitals and nursing homes. Children may be seen in health centres but increasingly speech and language therapy services are being offered in educational settings, including mainstream schools. Speech and language therapy aims to achieve the best level of communication possible for the person concerned. As well as being provided for individuals, speech and language therapy may be provided for small groups, such as in units dedicated to stroke care, or brain injury. Programmes may also be set up for other staff such as nurses to carry out. Speech and language therapists are a valuable resource for other members of the multidisciplinary team and can provide advice on how to achieve optimum communication with people with difficulties in communicating.

**speech mechanism** normal speech involves several processes: breathing, phonation, articulation, resonance and prosody. It is disturbed in various combinations and degrees in dysarthria and dysphasia.

**sperm** *n* an abbreviated form of the word spermatozoon or spermatozoa. *sperm count* a test undertaken as part of investigations for infertility, in which semen is examined for volume, sperm numbers, morphology, motility and chemical composition. ⇒ semen.

**spermatic** *adj* pertaining to or conveying semen.

**spermatic cord** suspends the testis in the scrotum and contains the testicular artery and vein and the deferent duct (vas deferens). ⇒ Appendix 1, Figure 16.

**spermatid** *n* the cells produced at the meiosis II stage of spermatocytogenesis from secondary spermatocytes. They change and mature to become functional spermatozoa during spermiogenesis. ⇒ spermatogenesis.

**spermatocele** *n* a swelling of the rete testis or epididymis that contains spermatozoa.

**spermatocyte** *n* the primary spermatocyte is a diploid cell, derived from the spermatogonium; it undergoes meiosis I to produce two haploid secondary spermatocytes. ⇒ spermatogenesis.

**spermatocytogenesis** *n* the stage of spermatogenesis during which the haploid spermatids are formed.

**spermatogenesis** *n* the formation and development of spermatozoa. It comprises the reduction division of meiosis in which the spermatids are formed in a stage known as spermatocytogenesis, and a further maturation stage, which is called spermiogenesis. The seminiferous tubules of the adult testis contain the diploid germ cells or spermatogonia and Sertoli cells. The germ cells, which are all at different stages of development, will eventually become spermatozoa; the supporting Sertoli cells help to nourish the germ cells, secrete hormones and provide the blood–testis barrier which prevents the immune system having contact with the spermatozoa antigens, which are formed long after immunocompetence is achieved. The diploid stem cells divide by mitosis to form primary spermatocytes, which in turn enter meiosis I to produce haploid secondary spermatocytes. The secondary spermatocytes then undergo the second meiotic division, which results in four haploid cells known as spermatids. Each spermatid still needs considerable modification during spermiogenesis, before it becomes a highly specialized motile spermatozoon with a head, midpiece and tail. These modifications, which occur in the epididymis, include nuclear changes, loss of excess cytoplasm and the formation of a tail (a flagellum).

**spermatogonium** *n* the undifferentiated, diploid germ cell in the male—**spermatogonia** *pl.* ⇒ spermatogenesis.

**spermatorrhoea** *n* involuntary discharge of semen without orgasm.

**spermatozoon** *n* a fully motile, mature, male gamete comprising a head, midpiece and tail (Figure S.7). The genetic material is condensed

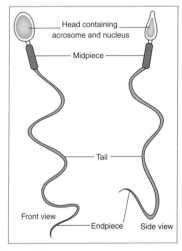

**Figure S.7** Spermatozoon *(reproduced from Brooker 2006A with permission).*

in the head, which is topped by an acrosome containing lytic enzymes. These enzymes allow the spermatozoa to pass through the cervical mucus and ultimately to penetrate the oocyte. The midpiece contains many mitochondria, arranged in a spiral, which produce the adenosine triphosphate (ATP) required to power the movements of the tail—**spermatozoa** *pl.*

**spermaturia** *n* seminuria. Spermatozoa in the urine; may be caused by retrograde ejaculation into the bladder, such as in diabetes mellitus or following prostate surgery.

**spermicide, spermatocide** *n* an agent that kills spermatozoa—**spermicidal** *adj.*

**spermiogenesis** *n* the maturation stage of spermatogenesis.

**sphenoid** *a* wedge-shaped bone at the base of the skull containing the sphenoidal sinus—**sphenoidal** *adj.*

**spherocyte** *n* round red blood cell, as opposed to biconcave—**spherocytic** *adj.*

**spherocytosis** *n* a hereditary disorder transmitted as a dominant gene. It is present at birth, but symptoms may vary from nonexistent to severe; thus it is sometimes discovered by 'accidental' examination of the blood, which reveals that the red cells are predominantly spherocytic. ⇒ jaundice.

**sphincter** *n* a circular muscle, contraction of which serves to close an orifice. For example, the anal, urethral and pyloric sphincters. ⇒ Appendix 1, Figure 19.

**sphincterectomy** *n* surgical excision of a sphincter.

**sphincteroplasty** *n* plastic surgical reconstruction of a sphincter.

**sphincterotomy** *n* surgical incision of a sphincter.

**sphingolipid** *n* sphingosine combined with a lipid. A constituent of biological membranes, especially in the brain.

**sphingomyelin** *n* a phospholipid formed from sphingosine found as part of biological membranes.

**sphingomyelinase** *n* an enzyme concerned with the metabolism and storage of lipids.

**sphingosine** *n* an amino alcohol constituent of sphingolipids and sphingomyelin.

**sphygmomanometer** *n* an instrument used for non-invasive measurement of arterial blood pressure. Some utilize a column of mercury, but are generally being replaced by aneroid (not containing a liquid) or electronic devices that contain no mercury (Figure S.8).

**spica** *n* a bandage applied in a figure-of-eight pattern.

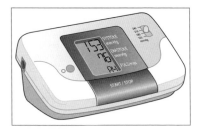

**Figure S.8** Electronic sphygomomanometer *(reproduced from Jamieson et al. 2002 with permission).*

**spicule** *n* a small, spike-like fragment, especially of bone.

**spigot** *n* plastic peg used to close a tube.

**spina bifida** a congenital defect in which there is incomplete closure of the neural canal, usually in the lumbosacral region. *spina bifida occulta* the defect does not affect the spinal cord or meninges. It is often marked externally by pigmentation, a haemangioma, a tuft of hair or a lipoma which may extend into the spinal canal. *spina bifida cystica* an externally protruding spinal lesion. It may vary in severity from meningocele to myelomeningocele. The condition can be detected during pregnancy by an increased concentration of alphafetoprotein in the amniotic fluid or by ultrasonography. ⇒ folate, neural tube defect.

**spinal** *n* pertaining to the spine. *spinal canal* ⇒ vertebral column. *spinal column* ⇒ vertebral column.

**spinal accessory nerve** ⇒ accessory nerve.

**spinal anaesthetic** a local anaesthetic solution injected into the subarachnoid space, so that it renders the area supplied by the selected spinal nerves insensitive.

**spinal cord** the continuation of nervous tissue of the brain down the spinal canal to the level of the first or second lumbar vertebra in adults. ⇒ Appendix 1, Figures 1 and 11.

**spinal cord compression (SCC)** pressure on the spinal cord. Often caused by tumour (which is commonly metastatic tumour from lung, breast or gastrointestinal cancers), but other causes include spinal fractures, swelling or haemorrhage affecting the spinal cord. Early diagnosis is vital to prevent permanent effects, including paralysis. Treatment usually involves corticosteroids and radiotherapy.

**spinal muscular atropy (SMA)** a group of genetic conditions, usually inherited as an

S

autosomal recessive trait. Degeneration of nerve cells, including those of anterior horn cells in the spinal cord, results in muscle atrophy and death from respiratory complications during childhood. In some types of SMA, individuals may survive into early adulthood.

**spinal nerves** 31 pairs of mixed nerves that leave the spinal cord and pass out of the spinal canal to supply the periphery. The nerves are named by the level at which they exit the spinal column. There are eight cervical nerves (C1–8), 12 thoracic nerves (T1–12), five lumbar (L1–5), five sacral (S1–5) and a single coccygeal nerve (Co).

**spinal shock** the initial, temporary loss of reflexes below the level of a spinal cord injury. It can last hours, weeks or months. There is flaccid paralysis and spinal reflexes are absent. When it subsides, reflexes show a vigorous response; there is muscle hypertonia, which can lead to spasticity and deformity.

**spinal stenosis** a bony narrowing of the spinal (vertebral) canal. Although it may be congenital, it is more commonly acquired. It may occur secondary to disc degeneration and subluxation of the posterior facet joints. Symptoms include pain that ranges from a dull backache to the more severe pain and paraesthesia felt in the buttock and leg, and leg weakness.

**spindle** *n* **1.** the structure that forms in the nucleus during cell division; it is involved in the movement of chromosomes or chromatids during mitosis and meiosis. **2.** the end-organ mechanoreceptors present in tendons and skeletal muscles. Those in skeletal muscles respond to passive stretch and are involved in the myotactic (stretch) reflex. ⇒ Golgi tendon organ. **3.** bursts of brain waves of a frequency of 14 per second that are recorded during light sleep.

**spine** *n* **1.** a popular term for the bony spinal or vertebral column. **2.** a sharp process of bone—**spinous, spinal** *adj*.

**spinhaler** *n* a nebulizer (atomizer) which delivers a preset drug dose.

**spinnbarkeit** *n* the cervical mucus characteristic of the time around ovulation. It is clear, thin, slippery and more elastic than usual. ⇒ Billings' method, peak mucus day.

**spinocerebellar** *adj* relating to the spinal cord and the cerebellum. For example, the *spinocerebellar tracts* that convey touch sensation and proprioceptor information to the cerebellum.

**spinocerebellar degeneration** a group of inherited conditions in which degenerative changes affect the cerebellum and the tracts in the spinal cord, resulting in ataxia.

**spiral computed tomography** a type of computed tomography which is capable of imaging a volume in a single breath-hold, thus reducing breathing artefacts and examination times. Patients pass through the scanner in a continuous movement, thereby ensuring that the path of the beam passing through them is a continuous spiral.

**Spirillum** *n* a genus of small spiral bacteria. *Spirillum minus* is found in rodents and causes one type of rat-bite fever—**spirilla** *pl*, **spirillary** *adj*.

**spiritual beliefs** may be a belief system ascribed by a particular religion; a modified version of these, reached following questioning, thinking and reasoning. Other people form a strong non-religious belief system to guide their concept of morality, and to find meaning in life. ⇒ secular beliefs.

**spiritual distress** may occur when a person's spiritual beliefs are derived from a particular religion, which requires the person to observe certain practices in everyday living activities, e.g. the preparation of food, types of food eaten, fasting, attending public worship, prayer, personal hygiene and type of clothing. Distress is likely if they are unable to conform to the teachings of their religious faith such as might occur during illness and hospitalization.

**spirochaetaemia** *n* spirochaetes in the blood stream such as occurs in the secondary stage of syphilis—**spirochaetaemic** *adj*.

**spirochaete** *n* an order of tiny spiral bacteria that includes the genera *Borrelia*, *Leptospira* and *Treponema* such as *Treponema pallidum*, the cause of syphilis—**spirochaetal** *adj*.

**spirograph** *n* an apparatus which records the movement of the lungs—**spirographic** *adj*, **spirography** *n*, **spirographically** *adv*.

**spirometer** *n* an instrument for measuring the volume of inhaled and exhaled air. Can be used to calculate various lung capacities and changes in volume—**spirometric** *adj*, **spirometry** *n*. ⇒ respiratory function tests.

**Spitz–Holter valve** a special valve used to drain excess cerebrospinal fluid in hydrocephalus.

**splanchnic** *adj* pertaining to or supplying the viscera.

**splanchnic nerves** sympathetic nerve fibres that supply the viscera and other structures.

S

453

**splanchnicectomy** *n* surgical removal of the splanchnic nerves, whereby certain viscera are deprived of sympathetic impulses; occasionally performed in the treatment of hypertension or for the relief of certain kinds of visceral pain.

**splanchnology** *n* the study of the structure and function of the viscera.

**spleen** *n* a lymphoid, vascular organ immediately below the diaphragm, at the tail of the pancreas, behind the stomach. It is part of the monocyte–macrophage (reticuloendothelial) system. Functions include the destruction of worn-out blood cells, filtering the blood of debris and providing a site for lymphocyte proliferation and antibody production, fetal production of red blood cells—**splenic** *adj*.

**splenectomy** *n* surgical removal of the spleen. Loss of the spleen reduces defences against infection and patients are advised to have immunizations that offer protection against pneumococcal infections and influenza and *Haemophilus influenzae* type b and meningococcal C, if not already protected. In elective splenectomy these should be given prior to surgery. Children up to the age of 16 years should be offered prophylactic antibiotic drugs during the 2 years following surgery.

**splenic flexure** the left colic flexure. The 90° angle in the colon adjacent to the spleen.

**splenitis** *n* inflammation of the spleen.

**splenocaval** *adj* pertaining to the spleen and inferior vena cava, usually referring to anastomosis of the splenic vein to the latter.

**splenomegaly** *n* enlargement of the spleen.

**splenoportal** *adj* pertaining to the spleen and hepatic portal vein.

**splenoportogram** *n* radiographic demonstration of the spleen and hepatic portal vein after injection of radiopaque contrast medium. Superseded by ultrasound examination.

**splenorenal** *adj* pertaining to the spleen and kidney, as anastomosis of the splenic vein to the renal vein; a procedure carried out in some cases of hepatic portal hypertension.

**splenunculus** *n* an accessory spleen.

**splint** *n* ⇒ orthosis.

**splinter haemorrhage** splinter-like haemorrhage under the finger or toe nails; may be caused by trauma or associated with infective endocarditis.

**splinting** *n* used by physiotherapists and others in preventive treatment; corrective treatments; and to maximize function.

**SPMSQ** *abbr* Short Portable Mental State Questionnaire.

**SPOD** *abbr* sexual problems of the disabled.

**spondyl(e)** *n* a vertebra.

**spondylitis** *n* inflammation of the spine—**spondylitic** *adj*. ⇒ ankylosing spondylitis.

**spondylography** *n* a method of measuring and studying the degree of kyphosis by directly tracing the line of the back.

**spondylolisthesis** *n* forward displacement of lumbar vertebra(e)—**spondylolisthetic** *adj*.

**spondylosis** *n* degenerative disease of the whole spine, with osteophyte formation on either side of the intervertebral disc. Often associated with osteoarthritis of the apophyseal (facet) joints.

**spondylosyndesis** *n* spinal fusion. Usually applies to surgical procedures to immobilize unstable vertebrae. It may be performed after surgery to deal with a prolapsed intervertebral disc, or as treatment for a spinal fracture.

**spongiform encephalopathy** one of a group of degenerative neurological diseases. In humans it is a progressive dementia. ⇒ bovine spongiform encephalopathy, Creutzfeldt–Jakob disease, kuru, scrapie.

**spontaneous abortion** ⇒ miscarriage.

**spontaneous fracture** ⇒ fracture.

**sporadic** *adj* scattered; occurring in isolated cases; not epidemic—**sporadically** *adv*.

**spore** *n* **1.** a phase in the life cycle of a limited number of bacterial genera (*Clostridium* and *Bacillus*) where the cell is encapsulated and metabolism almost ceases. Spores are highly resistant to adverse environmental conditions such as heat and desiccation. The spores are ubiquitous so that sterilization procedures must ensure their removal or death. ⇒ endospore. **2.** reproductive body produced by some plants, particularly fungi, and by protozoa.

**sporicidal** *adj* lethal to spores—**sporicide** *n*.

**sporotrichosis** *n* chronic infection of a wound by the fungus *Sporotrichum schenkii*. A sore, ulcer or abscess forms with lymphangitis and subcutaneous painless granulomata. Occurs amongst agricultural workers.

**sport biomechanics** the study of determining optimal techniques for sport performance, the design of sports equipment and investigation of the stresses placed upon the athlete's body during performance. ⇒ biomechanics.

**sport psychology** the study of human behaviour and mind in sport. Includes the areas of motor learning, sport skill acquisition and psychological skills training.

**sports medicine** branch of medicine concerned with the diagnosis, treatment,

S

rehabilitation and prevention of traumatic and non-traumatic injuries and disease affecting the athlete. May also be used to describe both medical and scientific aspects of sport and exercise. ⇒ sports science.

**sports science** a broad discipline that is mainly concerned with the processes that explain behaviour in sport and how athletic performance can be improved. Includes kinesiology, kinanthropometry, sport biomechanics, exercise physiology, sport psychology and sociology of sport.

**spotted fever** ⇒ Rocky Mountain spotted fever.

**sprain** *n* injury to the soft tissues surrounding a joint, resulting in discoloration, swelling and pain. There is stretching or tearing of a ligament or capsular structure of a joint.

**Sprengel's shoulder deformity** (O Sprengel, German surgeon, 1852–1915) congenital high scapula, a permanent elevation of the shoulder, often associated with other congenital deformities, e.g. the presence of a cervical rib or the absence of vertebrae.

**sprue** *n* a chronic malabsorption disorder. ⇒ coeliac, tropical sprue.

**SPSS** *abbr* Statistical Package for the Social Sciences.

**spur** *n* a small projection of bone.

**spurious** *adj* not genuine or what it appears to be.

**spurious diarrhoea** the leakage of fluid faeces past a solid impacted mass of faeces. More common in children and older people.

**sputum** *n* the mucus and other matter expectorated (coughed up) from the lower respiratory tract.

**squamocolumnar junction (SCJ)** also called the transformation zone. The variable region where the columnar epithelium lining the endocervical canal meets the stratified squamous epithelium of the ectocervix (vaginal portion). It is influenced by oestrogens, particularly at puberty and during pregnancy.

**squamous** *adj* scaly.

**squamous cell carcinoma (SCC)** a common type of skin cancer. Carcinoma arising in squamous epithelium; epithelioma. ⊙DVD

**squamous epithelium** the non-glandular epithelial covering of the external body surfaces.

**squint** *n* ⇒ strabismus.

**SSPE** *abbr* subacute sclerosing panencephalitis.

**SSRIs** *abbr* selective serotonin reuptake inhibitors.

**SSSS** *abbr* staphylococcal scalded-skin syndrome.

**stable factor (proconvertin)** *n* factor VII in the blood coagulation cascade. It is produced in the liver and requires vitamin K. It complexes with factor III (thromboplastin) to activate factor X (Stuart–Prower factor) in the extrinsic pathway. A very rare inherited (autosomal recessive) deficiency leads to a bleeding disorder.

**staghorn calculus** a large renal calculus that takes the shape of the calices and renal pelvis (Figure S.9).

**staging** *n* process of measuring how advanced a tumour is and to which sites it has spread; may be locally advanced or metastatic. Usually involves imaging with computed tomography, bone scan and often surgery. The TMN classification includes tumour (T) size, nodal (N) status and metastatic (M) sites present/absent.

**stagnant-loop syndrome** ⇒ blind-loop syndrome.

**stain 1.** *n* a dye used to colour micro-organisms or tissue prior to microscopic examination, e.g. Gram stain, or to elicit a reaction. **2.** *v* to apply a stain to tissue or micro-organisms. **3.** *n* a mark or area of discoloration.

**stammering** *vi* stuttering. A speech disorder in which the person hesitates, repeats syllables or words and pauses.

**standard** *n* a level or measure against which the performance of an activity can be monitored.

**standard deviation (SD)** in statistics, a measure of dispersion of scores around the mean value. It is the square root of variance.

**standard error (SE)** in statistics, a measure of variability of many mean values of different samples from a population. Used to calculate the chance of a sample mean being smaller or bigger than that for the population.

**standard precautions** sometimes referred to as universal precautions. A set of infection control guidelines recommended by the US Centers for Disease Control and Prevention (CDC). They should be used when dealing with all hospitalized patients at all times, whatever their diagnosis or presumed infection status. They involve the universal blood and body fluids precautions and body substance isolation, which are designed to reduce the risk of transmission of pathogens present in blood, body fluids, secretions and excretions (but not sweat), non-intact skin and the mucosae. They are also required to prevent the spread of diseases that are transmitted by airborne, droplet or contact routes.

**S**

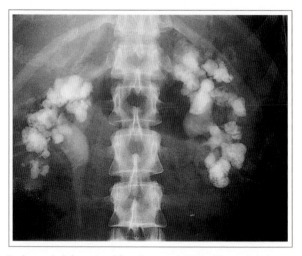

**Figure S.9** Staghorn calculi *(reproduced from Boon et al. 2006 with permission).*

These are the isolation precautions that are always used in conjunction with standard precautions. Standard precautions involve effective hand hygiene; appropriate use of personal protective equipment (PPE); safe use and disposal of sharps, such as needles or blades; effective domestic cleaning; proper decontamination, disinfection and sterilization of equipment; safe waste disposal; and safe management of linen. ⇒ containment isolation, protective isolation, source isolation.

**standardized mortality rate** the number of deaths per specific population standardized for age.

**standardized mortality ratio (SMR)** allows comparisons to be made between the death rates in populations with different demographic structures. It involves the application of national age-specific mortality rates to local populations so that a ratio of expected deaths to actual deaths can be calculated. The comparative national figure is, by convention, 100 and, for example, a local figure of 106 means that there is an increased risk of 6%, whereas a local figure of 94 indicates a risk 6% lower.

**Stanford Binet Intelligence Scale** a test adapted from Binet's test, used to test children in the United States. ⇒ Binet's test.

**stanols** *npl* plant substances that inhibit the absorption of cholesterol from the intestinal tract.

**St Anthony's fire** historical term for the mental abnormalities and painful vasoconstriction leading to gangrene of the extremities caused by ergot poisoning. Occurred through eating rye infested with a fungus containing alkaloids of ergot.

**stapedectomy** *n* surgical removal of stapes for otosclerosis. After stapedectomy, stapes can be replaced by a prosthesis. Normal hearing is restored in 90% of patients.

**stapedial mobilization, stapediolysis** release of a stapes rendered immobile by otosclerosis.

**stapedius** *n* a tiny muscle of the middle ear. It contracts reflexly (sound attenuation reflex) with another muscle, the tensor tympani, to protect the ear from very loud sounds by reducing conduction.

**stapes** *n* the stirrup-shaped medial ossicle (bone) of the middle ear. (⇒ Appendix 1, Figure 13). ⇒ incus, malleus.

**staphylectomy** *n* ⇒ uvulectomy.

**staphylococcal scalded-skin syndrome (SSSS)** Ritter's disease. A condition mainly occurring in infants. It is caused by certain strains of *Staphylococcus aureus* that produce toxins that affect the skin. It is characterized by the presence of vesicles and bullae, erythema, peeling and necrosis of the epidermis, creating the appearance of 'scalded' skin. Compare with toxic epidermal necrolysis.

*Staphylococcus* n a genus of Gram-positive bacteria occurring in clusters. Some types are commensal on the skin and may be found in the nasopharynx, axillae, groin and perineum of some individuals. They cause infections that include: boils, impetigo, wound infection, endocarditis, pneumonia, osteomyelitis, toxic shock syndrome and septicaemia. Staphylococci cause many health care-associated infections. The genus includes the major pathogen *Staphylococcus aureus*, which produces the enzyme coagulase; some strains produce a powerful exotoxin, and others are meticillin (methicillin)-resistant. *Staphylococcus epidermidis* is a skin commensal (non-coagulase producer). It infects wounds and increasingly causes infection involving intravascular devices, peritoneal dialysis catheters, valves, etc. Treatment is problematic as the micro-organism has a natural resistance to many antibiotics. ⇒ meticillin (methicillin)-resistant *Staphylococcus aureus*, Panton–Valentine leukocidin, vancomycin-resistant *Staphylococcus aureus*.

**staphyloma** n a protrusion of the cornea or sclera of the eye—**staphylomata** pl.

**staphylorrhaphy** n also called palatorrhaphy. Operation to repair a cleft palate.

**staple food** traditional food used as the main source of energy within a community. It varies between different communities and regions and includes maize, wheat, rice, potatoes, cassava, sago, pulses, etc.

**staples** npl pieces of wire sometimes used to close a surgical wound, or used in a special stapling device to form an anastomosis.

**starch** n a polysaccharide formed from glucose molecules, the carbohydrate present in potatoes, rice and maize.

**Starling's law of the heart** (E Starling, British physiologist, 1866–1927) also known as Frank–Starling law of the heart (E Starling; O Frank, German physiologist, 1865–1944) states that the force of myocardial contraction is proportional to the length (stretching) of the ventricular muscle fibres. Increased stretching results in the next contraction being more powerful.

**startle reflex** ⇒ Moro reflex.

**start-up costs** the costs, such as the purchase of equipment that occur at the start of a project.

**stasis** n stagnation; cessation of motion.

**static muscle actions** actions in which muscle fibres generate force without any change in muscle.

**static reflex** a reflex that maintains muscle tone and posture.

**static stretching** a technique of muscle stretching used to increase range of motion; the muscle/muscle group is held at the end of its range of movement, in a static position for a period of time.

**statins** npl colloquial expression for 3-hydroxy-3-methyl-glutaryl (HMG)-coenzyme A (CoA) reductase inhibitors.

**Statistical Package for the Social Sciences (SPSS)** software package often used in the analysis of quantitative data.

**statistical significance** in research, an expression of how likely it is that a set of results happened by chance, e.g. 0.05, 0.01 and 0.001 levels. ⇒ P-value.

**statistics** n scientific study of numerical data collection and its analysis and evaluation.

**status** n state; condition.

**status asthmaticus** ⇒ severe acute asthma.

**status epilepticus** describes epileptic seizures following each other almost continuously. It is a medical emergency and requires immediate treatment.

**statutory bodies** bodies such as Strategic Health Authorities, or the Health Professions Council, which are set up by legislation and provide a statutory service controlled by legislation.

**STD** abbr sexually transmitted disease.

**steatoma** n a fatty tumour, or a sebaceous cyst.

**steatopygia** n the deposition of excessive amounts of fat in the buttocks.

**steatorrhoea** n passage of pale, frothy, foul-smelling oily stool due to fat malabsorption. It floats and is difficult to flush away.

**steatosis** n fatty infiltration of hepatocytes; occurs in alcohol misuse and protein–energy malnutrition.

**Stein–Leventhal syndrome** (I Stein, American gynaecologist, 1887–1976; M Leventhal, American gynaecologist, 1901–1971) ⇒ polycystic ovary syndrome.

**Steinmann's pin** (F Steinmann, Swiss surgeon, 1872–1932) an alternative to the use of a Kirschner wire for applying skeletal traction to a limb. It has its own introducer and stirrup.

**stellate** adj star-shaped.

**stellate fracture** a star-shaped fracture with numerous cracks radiating from the point of impact.

**S**

**stellate ganglion** a large collection of nerve cells (ganglion) on the sympathetic chain in the root of the neck.

**stellate ganglionectomy** surgical removal of the stellate ganglion.

**Stellwag's sign** (C Stellwag, Austrian ophthalmologist, 1823–1904) occurs in Graves' disease: the person blinks infrequently and the eyelids are retracted. ⇒ exophthalmos.

**stem cell** an undifferentiated, pluripotent cell capable of giving rise to other types of cells. For example, the stem cells normally present in the bone marrow and umbilical cord blood that are capable of developing into any of a full range of mature blood cells. They are the 'active ingredient' of haemopoietic stem cell transplants.

**stenosis** *n* a narrowing—**stenoses** *pl*, **stenotic** *adj*.

**Stensen's duct** (N Stensen, Danish anatomist, 1638–1686) the duct of the parotid salivary gland.

**stent** *n* device used to provide a shunt or keep a tube or vessel open. For example, stent insertion into the bile duct to relieve obstructive jaundice, stenting the ureters to overcome urinary obstruction and stenting the oesophagus for palliation of dysphagia caused by oesophageal cancer. ⇒ transjugular intrahepatic portosystemic stent shunting.

**stepping reflex** also called step or dance reflex. A primitive reflex normally present in newborns; when infants are held upright over a flat surface so that their feet press on the surface they will make walking movements (reciprocal flexion and extension). The reflex normally disappears around 4–6 weeks of age.

**stercobilin** *n* the brown pigment of faeces; it is formed from stercobilinogen which is derived from the bile pigments.

**stercobilinogen** *n* faecal urobilinogen. It is formed by bacterial action on the bile pigment bilirubin. ⇒ urobilinogen.

**stercolith** *n* a hard stone-like mass of faeces.

**stereognosis** *n* the faculty of recognizing the shape of objects by the sense of touch.

**stereoisomer** *n* chemical compounds that comprise the same atoms with the same linkages, but the atoms have a different spatial arrangement. Some of these compounds are mirror images of each other.

**stereopsis** *n* ability to use both eyes together (binocular vision) for the perception of depth, distance and shape. Stereoscopic vision.

**stereotactic radiotherapy** ⇒ radiosurgery.

**stereotactic surgery** electrodes and cannulae are passed to a predetermined point in the brain for physiological observation or destruction of tissue—**stereotaxy** *n*.

**stereotype** *n* a generalization about a behaviour, individual or a group; can be the basis for prejudice.

**stereotypy** *n* inappropriate repetition of actions, postures or speech. It is a feature of some mental health disorders and autistic disorders and occurs with some types of learning disability.

**sterile** *adj* free from living micro-organisms, including bacterial spores—**sterility** *n*.

**sterility** *n* infertility. The inability to reproduce.

**sterilization** *n* **1.** activity that kills or removes all types of micro-organisms, including spores. It is accomplished by the use of heat, radiation, chemicals or filtration. **2.** rendering incapable of reproduction, such as following vasectomy.

**sternal puncture** insertion of a special guarded hollow needle with a stylet into the body of the sternum for aspiration of a bone marrow sample for examination.

**Sternberg–Reed cell** ⇒ Reed–Sternberg cell.

**sternoclavicular** *adj* pertaining to the sternum and the clavicle.

**sternocleidomastoid muscle** a strap-like, two-headed anterolateral neck muscle. Its origins are on the sternum and clavicle and it inserts on to the mastoid process of temporal bone. Contracts to flex the head. (⇒ Appendix 1, Figures 4 and 5). ⇒ torticollis.

**sternocostal** *adj* pertaining to the sternum and ribs.

**sternotomy** *n* surgical division of the sternum.

**sternum** *n* the breast bone—**sternal** *adj*. ⇒ Appendix 1, Figure 2.

**steroids** *npl* a large group of organic compounds (lipids) that have a common basic chemical structure: three 6-carbon rings and a 5-carbon ring. They include: bile salts, vitamin D precursors, sex hormones and the corticosteroid hormones.

**sterol** *n* chemicals with the basic steroid structure combined with an alcohol group such as cholesterol.

**stertor** *n* loud snoring; sonorous breathing—**stertorous** *adj*.

**stethoscope** *n* an instrument used for listening to the various body sounds, especially those of the heart and chest—**stethoscopic** *adj*, **stethoscopically** *adv*.

**Stevens–Johnson syndrome** (A Stevens, American paediatrician, 1884–1945; F Johnson, American physician, 1894–1934) severe variant of the allergic response—erythema multiforme. It is an acute hypersensitivity state and can follow a viral or bacterial infection, or drugs such as long-acting sulphonamides, some anticonvulsants and some antibiotics. In some cases no cause can be found. Lung complications during the acute phase can be fatal. Mostly it is a benign condition, and there is complete recovery.

**STI** *abbr* sexually transmitted infection.

**stigma** *n* a defining feature or characteristic of a person, or an action usually viewed in a negative way by others.

**stigmata** *npl* marks of disease, or congenital abnormalities, e.g. facies of congenital syphilis—**stigma** *sing*.

**stilet** *n* a wire or metal rod for maintaining patency of hollow instruments.

**stillbirth** *n* birth of a baby, after 24 weeks' gestation, that shows no sign of life.

**stillborn** *n* born dead.

**Still's disease** (G Still, British physician, 1868–1941) term seldom used, having been superseded by systemic-onset juvenile idiopathic arthritis. ⇒ juvenile idiopathic arthritis.

**stimulant** *adj, n* stimulating. An agent which excites or increases function.

**stimulant laxative** ⇒ laxatives. ⇒ Appendix 5.

**stimulus** *n* anything which excites functional activity in an organ or part.

**stitch** *n* **1.** a sudden, sharp darting pain or spasm in the chest wall or abdomen, usually on the lower right-hand side during exertion. **2.** a suture.

**STM** *abbr* short-term memory.

**Stokes–Adams syndrome** (W Stokes, Irish physician, 1804–1878; R Adams, Irish surgeon, 1791–1875) a fainting (syncopal) attack, commonly transient, which occurs in patients with heart block. If severe, may take the form of a convulsion, or patient may become unconscious.

**stoma** *n* the mouth; any opening. ⇒ colostomy, ileostomy, urostomy—**stomata** *pl*, **stomal** *adj*.

**stomach** *n* the most dilated part of the digestive tube, situated between the oesophagus and the duodenum (⇒ Appendix 1, Figure 18B); it lies in the epigastric, umbilical and left hypochondriac regions of the abdomen (⇒ Appendix 1, Figure 18A). The wall is composed of four coats: serous, muscular, submucous and mucous. It produces gastric juice containing digestive enzymes, hydrochloric acid and mucus.

**stomatitis** *n* inflammation of the mouth. *angular stomatitis* fissuring in the corners of the

mouth consequent upon riboflavin deficiency. Sometimes misapplied to: (a) the superficial maceration and fissuring at the labial commissures in perlèche; and (b) the chronic fissuring at the site in older people with loose lower lip or poorly fitting dentures. *aphthous stomatitis* recurring crops of small ulcers in the mouth. ⇒ aphthae. *gangrenous stomatitis* ⇒ cancrum oris—**stomal** *adj*.

**stomatodynia** *n* mouth soreness or pain.

**stomatology** *n* the study of the oral cavity; structure, function, diseases and treatment.

**stomodeum** *n* in the early embryo the depression in the ectoderm of the foregut, which becomes the mouth.

**stone** *n* calculus; a hardened mass of mineral matter.

**stone bruise** ⇒ heel bruise.

**stool** *n* faeces.

**stove-in chest** there may be multiple anterior or posterior fractures of the ribs (causing paradoxical respiration) and fractures of sternum, or a mixture of such fractures.

**strabismus** *n* (*syn* squint) abnormal position of the eyes relative to each other, such that the visual axes of the two eyes fail to meet at the object of regard. *comitant* (or *concomitant*) *strabismus* consistent deviation between the eyes in all positions of gaze. *convergent strabismus* when the eyes turn inwards. *divergent strabismus* when the eyes turn outwards. *latent strabismus* deviation only present when eyes are dissociated, e.g. by converging one eye. *manifest strabismus* deviation present without dissociation.

**strain** *n* **1.** group of micro-organisms within the same species but with different characteristics. **2.** injury to the musculotendinous (muscle and tendon) unit resulting from excessive stretch or tension during physical activity (Figure S.10).

**strangulated hernia** ⇒ hernia.

**strangulation** *n* constriction which impedes the circulation—**strangulated** *adj*.

**strangury** *n* a constant painful urge to micturate.

**Strassman operation** (P Strassman, German gynaecologist, 1866–1938) a plastic operation to make a bicornuate uterus a near-normal shape.

**Strategic Health Authority** a body responsible for strategic health planning for a geographical area with a population of many millions (e.g. the English counties of Cambridgeshire, Norfolk, Suffolk, Bedfordshire, Hertfordshire and Essex). They are also responsible

**S**

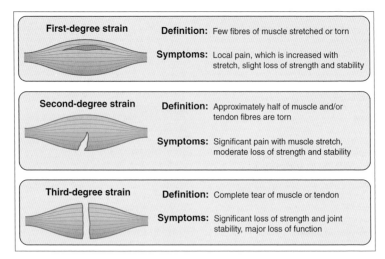

**Figure S.10** A classification of strains *(reproduced from Porter 2005 with permission)*.

for the performance management of the Primary Care Trusts within that area.

**strategic management** the management function concerned with longer-term future strategy. Financial and resource planning. ⇒ operational management.

**stratified** *adj* arranged in layers.

**stratum** *n* a layer or lamina, e.g. the various layers of the epithelium of the skin, i.e. stratum granulosum, stratum corneum.

**strawberry naevus** a red birthmark caused by a capillary haemangioma.

**strawberry tongue** the tongue is thickly furred with projecting red papillae. As the fur disappears the tongue is vividly red like an overripe strawberry. A characteristic of streptococcal scarlet fever. ⊙DVD

**strength** *n* the maximum force or torque that can be developed during maximal voluntary contraction of muscle(s).

***Streptobacillus*** *n* a genus of Gram-negative bacteria. *Streptobacillus moniliformis* causes a type of rat-bite fever in humans.

***Streptococcus*** *n* a genus of bacteria. Gram-positive cocci, often occurring in chains. They have varying haemolytic ability, α, β and non-haemolytic, and some types produce powerful toxins. Some streptococci are commensal in

the intestinal tract (*S. faecalis*) and respiratory tract (*S. viridans*). The commensal streptococci, together with the pathogens *S. pyogenes* and *S. pneumoniae*, cause serious infections that include: tonsillitis, scarlet fever, otitis media, erysipelas, endocarditis, wound infections, pneumonia, meningitis and urinary infection. Glomerulonephritis and rheumatic fever may follow some streptococcal infections. Group B streptococcus, an intestinal and vaginal commensal, may cause meningitis, pneumonia and septicaemia in neonates infected by bacteria present in the maternal genital tract. ⇒ Griffith's typing, Lancefield's groups, necrotizing fasciitis.

**streptodornase** *n* a proteolytic enzyme used with streptokinase to liquefy blood clot and pus.

**streptokinase** *n* a streptococcal enzyme. Used with streptodornase in wound management. Plasminogen activator. Used as a fibrinolytic drug in the management of several thromboembolic conditions, including acute myocardial infarction and pulmonary embolism.

**streptolysins** *npl* exotoxins produced by streptococci. Streptolysin antibody may be measured as an indicator of recent streptococcal infection.

***Streptothrix*** *n* a filamentous bacterium which shows true branching. ⇒ *Streptobacillus*.

**stress** *n* the response of an organism to any demand made upon it by agents threatening physical or emotional well-being. Hans Selye (⇒ general adaptation syndrome) described such agents as stressors, which could be physical, physiological, psychological or sociocultural. Stress may be either *distress*, a negative event which has long-term effects on health when it becomes chronic, or *eustress*, a more positive event that accompanies pleasurable excitement and euphoria.

**stress fracture** (*syn* fatigue fracture) a bone fracture resulting from repeated loading with relatively low-magnitude forces. Can be caused by a number of factors, including overtraining, incorrect biomechanics, fatigue, hormonal imbalance, poor nutrition and osteoporosis.

**stress incontinence** ⇒ incontinence.

**stress management** a range of measures that reduce the negative effects of stress, such as relaxation techniques, biofeedback, etc., or reducing stress, e.g. delegation. ⇒ general adaptation syndrome.

**stressors** *npl* factors that cause stress responses. They may be physical, physiological, psychological and sociocultural, and include: pain, cold, trauma and blood loss, heavy workload, a life crisis such as the death of a close relative, job loss, or serious illness. ⇒ burnout.

**stretching** *n* exercises that may involve static or dynamic stretching. Static stretching involves holding a position for a period of time; it requires the correct alignment of the body and awareness of posture and fine motor control. Dynamic stretching may be used in the management and rehabilitation of sporting injuries.

**stretch receptor** mechanoreceptors in muscle spindles and tendons that respond to stretch.

**stretch reflex** a short-latency reflex often used to examine spinal cord function. The stimulus is a rapid stretch of muscle and the response is a contraction of muscle that is checked by reciprocal stretch of antagonistic muscle, e.g. in the knee jerk, contraction of the quadriceps femoris muscles (agonists) is checked by contraction of the hamstring muscles (antagonists).

**striae** *npl* streaks; stripes; narrow bands. Occur when the abdomen enlarges, such as with obesity, ascites, tumours and pregnancy, when the marks are called *striae gravidarum*. They are red at first and then become sil-

very-white. Striae may also occur as a side-effect of corticosteroid therapy—**stria** *sing*, **striated** *adj*.

**striated muscle** ⇒ skeletal muscle.

**stricture** *n* a narrowing, especially of a tube or canal, due to scar tissue or tumour.

**stricturoplasty** *n* surgical reconstruction of a stricture by means of a longitudinal muscle-splitting incision and transverse suture repair, e.g. for the strictures of Crohn's disease.

**stridor** *n* a harsh breathing sound caused by turbulent airflow through constricted air passages—**stridulous** *adj*.

**strobila** *n* the term applied to all the segments (proglottides) of a tapeworm.

**stroke** *n* a popular term for cerebrovascular accident. Sudden loss of blood supply to a part of the brain leading to a neurological defect lasting more than 24 hours. ⇒ cerebrovascular accident, transient ischaemic attack.

**stroke unit** a dedicated unit for the management of stroke patients. A multidisciplinary team of specialist practitioners work collaboratively to improve patient outcomes.

**stroke volume (SV)** the volume of blood pumped out of the heart by each ventricular contraction. The difference between end-diastolic volume (EDV) and end-systolic volume (ESV).

**stroma** *n* the interstitial or foundation substance of a structure.

***Strongyloides*** *n* a genus of small intestinal nematode worms, e.g. *Strongyloides stercoralis*. They infest humans (natural host), but can infest dogs. ⇒ strongyloidiasis.

**strongyloidiasis** *n* infestation with the nematode *Strongyloides stercoralis*. It commonly occurs in the tropics and subtropics, but may also infest immunocompromised people, such as those with acquired immunodeficiency syndrome (AIDS). Infestation usually occurs through the skin from contaminated soil, but can be through the mucosae. There may be an itchy rash at the site of larval entry. The larvae migrate through the lungs and may cause respiratory symptoms as the larvae are coughed up in sputum. Some larvae are swallowed and lead to varying abdominal symptoms, e.g. pain, diarrhoea and malabsorption, as the female worm burrows into the intestinal mucosa and submucosa. Some individuals have allergic reactions such as wheezing.

**strontium (Sr)** *n* a metallic element present in bone. Isotopes of strontium are used in radioisotope (radionuclide) scanning of bone.

461

*Strontium-90* ($Sr^{90}$) a radioisotope with a half-life of 28 years, produced during atomic explosions. It is dangerous when it becomes integrated within bone tissue, where turnover is slow.

**Stuart–Prower factor** *n* factor X in the blood coagulation cascade. It is produced in the liver and requires vitamin K. Activation of factor X is needed for prothrombin activator through both the intrinsic and extrinsic pathways. A very rare inherited (autosomal recessive) deficiency leads to a bleeding disorder.

**struma** *n* a goitre.

**Stryker bed/frame** a proprietary bed. Designed to allow rotation of patients to the prone or supine position. Main uses include spinal injuries and burns.

**S-T segment** ⇒ P-QRS-T complex.

**student's elbow** olecranon bursitis.

**Student's paired test** a parametric test for statistical significance. Used to test differences in mean values for two related measurements such as those obtained from the same subject. ⇒ Wilcoxon test.

**Student's t-test for independent groups** a parametric test for statistical significance. Used to test differences in mean values of two groups. ⇒ Mann–Whitney *U* test.

**stunting** *n* poor growth in height of children, leading to shorter stature for age, generally resulting in lifelong short stature. Especially associated with insufficient protein intake.

**stupor** *n* a state of marked impairment of, but not complete loss of, consciousness. The victim shows a gross lack of responsiveness, usually reacting only to noxious stimuli—**stuporous** *adj*.

**Sturge–Weber syndrome** (*syn* naevoid amentia) (W Sturge, British physician, 1850–1919; F Weber, British physician, 1863–1962) a genetically determined congenital ectodermosis, i.e. a capillary haemangioma above the eye may be accompanied by similar changes in vessels inside the skull giving rise to epilepsy and other cerebral manifestations.

**St Vitus' dance** ⇒ chorea.

**stye** *n* (*syn* external hordeolum) an abscess in the follicle of an eyelash.

**styloid** *adj* long and pointed; resembling a pen or stylus.

**styloid process** a projection of the temporal bone, or those on the radius and ulna.

**styptic** *n* an astringent applied to arrest bleeding.

**subacute** *adj* neither acute nor chronic. Often the stage between the acute and chronic phases of disease.

**subacute bacterial endocarditis** ⇒ infective endocarditis.

**subacute combined degeneration of the spinal cord** a complication of untreated pernicious anaemia (PA) that affects the posterior and lateral columns of the spinal cord.

**subacute sclerosing panencephalitis (SSPE)** a rare late complication of measles with progressive and fatal loss of neurological and cognitive function due to inflammation and destruction of brain tissue.

**subarachnoid haemorrhage (SAH)** the loss of blood from a vessel in the brain which leaks into the subarachnoid space. This is typically due to an intracerebral aneurysm or arteriovenous malformation and can be fatal. Blood is present in the cerebrospinal fluid (CSF).

**subarachnoid space** the space beneath the arachnoid membrane, between it and the pia mater. It contains cerebrospinal fluid.

**subcarinal** *adj* below a carina, usually referring to the carina tracheae.

**subclavian** *adj* beneath the clavicle.

**subclavian artery** one of two arteries with branches that supply blood to the neck, spinal cord, brain and upper limbs. The right subclavian artery branches from the brachiocephalic artery and the left subclavian artery branches directly from the aortic arch. ⇒ Appendix 1, Figure 9.

**subclavian steal syndrome** an occlusion of the subclavian artery (proximal to the vertebral artery) causes a reversal of blood flow in the vertebral artery on the same side from the basilar artery to the subclavian artery past the blockage. It can deprive areas of the brain of blood.

**subclavian vein** one of two veins that carry venous blood from the neck and upper arms to the brachiocephalic veins. ⇒ Appendix 1, Figure 10.

**subclinical** *adj* insufficient to cause the classical identifiable disease.

**subconjunctival** *adj* deep to the conjunctiva—**subconjunctivally** *adv*.

**subconscious** *adj, n* that part of the mind outside the range of consciousness and full awareness, but still able to affect conscious mental or physical reactions.

**subcostal** *adj* beneath the rib.

**subcutaneous** *adj* beneath the skin—**subcutaneously** *adv. subcutaneous oedema* is demonstrable by the 'pitting' produced by pressure of the finger. *subcutaneous tissue* ⇒ Appendix 1, Figure 12.

**subdural** *adj* beneath the dura mater; between the dura and arachnoid membranes.

**subdural haematoma (SDH)** the accumulation of blood beneath the dura lining the skull that can occur after head trauma. It develops slowly and may present as a space-occupying lesion with vomiting, papilloedema, fluctuating level of consciousness, weakness, usually hemiplegia on the opposite side to the clot. Finally there is a rise in blood pressure and a fall in pulse rate.

**subendocardial** *adj* immediately beneath the endocardium.

**subgingival** *adj* below the gingiva.

**subglossal** *adj* ⇒ sublingual.

**subhepatic** *adj* beneath the liver.

**subinvolution** *n* failure of the gravid uterus to return to its normal size within a normal time after childbirth. ⇒ involution.

**subjective** *adj* internal; personal; arising from the senses and not perceptible to others. ⇒ objective *opp*.

**sublimate** *n* a solid deposit resulting from the condensation of a vapour.

**sublimation** *n* a mental defence mechanism whereby undesirable basic instinctive drives are unconsciously redirected to, and expressed through, personally approved and socially accepted behaviour, such as aggression redirected to sporting activity.

**subliminal** *adj* inadequate for perceptible response. Below the threshold of consciousness. ⇒ liminal.

**sublingual** *adj* beneath the tongue. A route used for the administration of medicines, such as glyceryl trinitrate, which are subject to first-pass metabolism/effect in the liver. *sublingual glands* ⇒ salivary glands.

**subluxation** *n* incomplete dislocation of a joint.

**submandibular** *adj* below the mandible. *submandibular glands* ⇒ salivary glands.

**submaxillary** *adj* below the maxilla.

**submucosa** *n* the layer of connective tissue beneath a mucous membrane—**submucous, submucosal** *adj*.

**submucosal plexus** Meissner's plexus. A plexus of autonomic (sympathetic and parasympathetic) nerves that innervate the mucosal lining of the gastrointestinal tract.

**submucous** *adj* beneath a mucous membrane. *submucous resection (SMR)* (of the nasal septum) surgical correction of a deviated nasal septum.

**suboccipital** *adj* beneath the occiput; in the nape of the neck.

**subperiosteal** *adj* beneath the periosteum of bone.

**subphrenic** *adj* beneath the diaphragm. *subphrenic abscess* presence of pus under the diaphragm.

**subpoena** *n* a court order requiring a person to appear as a witness or to bring documents to court.

**substance misuse** the misuse of alcohol, tobacco, drugs and other substances that include solvents to the point when health and/or social functioning is adversely affected.

**substance P** a peptide neurotransmitter found in nerve cells and some endocrine cells in the gastrointestinal tract. It is a very powerful vasodilator, increases gastrointestinal smooth muscle contraction and is involved in pain transmission.

**substrate** *n* chemical upon which a specific enzyme is active.

**subsultus** *n* muscular tremor. *subsultus tendinum* twitching of tendons and muscles, particularly around the wrist, in severe fever, such as typhoid.

**subtalar joint** the complex joint between the talus and the calcaneus.

**subthalamus** an area below the thalamus containing many important nuclei.

**subungual** *adj* under a nail, such as a haematoma. ⊙DVD *subungual exostosis* a small outgrowth of bone under the nail plate near to, or immediately distal to, the free edge. *subungual heloma* (corn) the development of a corn or keratinized lesion under the nail plate.

**succedaneous tooth** a permanent tooth with a predecessor in the primary dentition (e.g. incisors).

**succussion** *n* **1.** splashing sound produced by fluid in a hollow cavity when the patient moves, e.g. liquid content of dilated stomach in pyloric stenosis. **2.** a term in homeopathy describing the vigorous shaking of natural diluted substances.

**sucrase** *n* intestinal enzyme that converts sucrose to glucose and fructose.

**sucrose** *n* a disaccharide that is hydrolysed into glucose and fructose during digestion. It occurs naturally in sugar and is added to many manufactured foods.

**suction** *n* aspiration of fluid or gas, such as clearing the airway or wound drainage.

**S**

**sudamina** *n* sweat rash.

**Sudan blindness** ⇒ onchocerciasis.

**sudden adult/arrhythmia death syndrome (SADS)** ⇒ long Q-T syndrome.

**sudden unexpected death in infancy (SUDI)** (*syn* cot death, sudden infant death syndrome [SIDS]) the unexpected sudden death of an infant, usually occurring overnight while sleeping in a cot, but may occur in other situations and under other circumstances. A common mode of death in infants between the ages of 1 month and 1 year, usually in the first 8 months of life, neither clinical nor postmortem findings being adequate to account for death. Risk factors include sleeping in the prone position, overheating, respiratory illness and infection, maternal smoking during pregnancy and being in an environment where people smoke. Parents/carers are recommended: (a) to put babies to sleep on their backs; (b) to place the baby at the foot of the cot to prevent him or her wriggling under the bedclothes; (c) to ensure that the baby's head does not become covered; (d) that for the first 6 months the baby sleeps in a cot in the parents' room; (e) not to have the baby in the parents' bed if one of the parents is very tired, is a smoker, or has consumed alcohol, medicines or drugs that may cause drowsiness; (f) not to overheat the room; (g) not to smoke in the same room; and (h) to seek advice from a health professional if the baby seems unwell.

**Sudeck's atrophy** (P Sudeck, German surgeon, 1866–1945) ⇒ complex regional pain syndrome.

**SUDI** *abbr* sudden unexpected death in infancy.

**sudor** *n* sweat—**sudoriferous** *adj*.

**sudorific** *adj, n* (*syn* diaphoretic) describes an agent which induces sweating.

**suffocation** *n* cessation of breathing caused by an airway obstruction.

**suggestibility** *n* abnormal vulnerability to suggestion. May be increased in individuals who have dependence on others such as those in hospital and people with a learning disability.

**suggestion** *n* the implanting in a person's mind of an idea which he or she accepts fully. In psychology suggestion may be used as a therapeutic measure during hypnosis.

**suicide** *n* intentional taking of one's own life. Usually related to depression and hopelessness. Attitudes to suicide are culturally determined, and stigma may be present in some communities. ⇒ deliberate self-harm, parasuicide.

**sulcus** *n* a furrow or groove, particularly those separating the gyri (convolutions) of the cerebral cortex—**sulci** *pl*.

**sulphaemoglobin** *n* (*syn* sulphmethaemoglobin) a sulphide oxidation product of haemoglobin, produced in vivo by certain drugs. It cannot transport oxygen or carbon dioxide and, not being reversible in the body, is an indirect poison.

**sulphaemoglobinaemia** *n* a condition of circulating sulphaemoglobin in the blood.

**sulphate** *n* salt of sulphuric acid, e.g. magnesium sulphate.

**sulphonamides** *npl* a group of bacteriostatic antibacterial agents, e.g. sulfadiazine. ⇒ Appendix 5.

**sulphones** *npl* a group of synthetic antileprotic drugs, e.g. dapsone. ⇒ Appendix 5.

**sulphonylureas** *npl* a group of oral hypoglycaemic drugs, e.g. glipizide. ⇒ Appendix 5.

**sulphur** *n* an insoluble yellow powder. Used in topical preparations and baths for acne and other skin disorders.

**sulphuric acid** inorganic acid. Highly corrosive.

**sunstroke** *n* ⇒ heatstroke.

**supercilium** *n* the eyebrow—**superciliary** *adj*.

**superego** *n* one of the three main aspects of the personality (the others being the ego and id); part of the mind concerned with moral sanctions, inhibitions and self criticism; it functions at a partly conscious, but mostly unconscious level. Roughly equates to the 'conscience'. ⇒ ego, id.

**superfecundation** *n* the fertilization of two oocytes, released during the same menstrual cycle, by spermatozoa from sexual intercourse with different partners.

**superfetation** *n* the presence of two fetuses resulting from oocytes released during different menstrual cycles.

**superficial** *adj* near the surface such as the superficial veins of the leg. *superficial bursitis* an adventitious bursa found superficial to the insertion of the Achilles tendon. It is a common condition and mainly affects adolescent females.

**superinfection** *n* infection that follows the elimination of the normal flora by antibiotic usage. This permits other micro-organisms, such as *Clostridium difficile*, to thrive in the intestine without competition from micro-

**S**

organisms of the normal flora. ⇒ pseudomembranous colitis, *Pseudomonas*.

**superior** *adj* in anatomy, the upper of two parts—**superiorly** *adj*.

**supernumerary** *adj* in excess of the normal number; additional. *supernumerary digits* ⇒ polydactyly.

**superovulation** *n* the production of many more oocytes than normal, usually as a result of gonadotrophin administration during assisted conception techniques. ⇒ ovarian hyperstimulation syndrome.

**superoxide** *n* $O_2^-$. ⇒ free radical, reactive oxygen species.

**superoxide dismutases** a group of enzymes that have metal ion cofactors such as copper, zinc and manganese. They clear harmful superoxide radicals from the body. ⇒ free radical, reactive oxygen species.

**supinate** *vt* turn or lay face or palm upward. ⇒ pronate *opp*—**supination** *n*.

**supinator** *n* that which supinates, usually applied to a muscle. For example, the *supinator*, a deep muscle of the forearm. Its origin is on the lateral epicondyle of the humerus and the proximal ulna; it inserts on to the proximal radius. Assists in forearm supination. ⇒ pronator *opp*.

**supine** *adj* **1.** lying on the back with face upwards. **2.** of the hand with palm upwards. ⇒ prone *opp*.

**supine hypotensive syndrome** affects pregnant women during the late second and third trimesters. When lying supine the gravid uterus compresses the inferior vena cava and reduces venous return to the heart, thereby reducing cardiac output and hence blood pressure.

**suppository** *n* medicament in a base that melts at body temperature. Administered rectally.

**suppression** *n* **1.** in psychology, a mental defence mechanism, whereby people voluntarily force difficult or painful thoughts out of the mind; it can precipitate mental health problems. **2.** cessation of a secretion (e.g. urine) or a normal process (e.g. menstruation).

**suppressor T cell** T lymphocytes which slow or stop the activity of other T cells and B cells once the antigen is dealt with. ⇒ CD8 cells, cytotoxic T cell.

**suppuration** *n* the formation of pus—**suppurative** *adj*, **suppurate** *vi*.

**supraclavicular** *adj* above the clavicle.

**supracondylar** *adj* above a condyle.

**supracondylar fracture** one affecting the lower end of the femur or humerus. The latter may interfere with the blood supply to the forearm. ⇒ Volkmann's ischaemic contracture.

**supraorbital** *adj* above the orbits. *supraorbital ridge* the ridge covered by the eyebrows.

**suprapubic** *adj* above the pubis.

**suprapubic catheter** catheter inserted into the urinary bladder through the abdominal wall.

**suprarenal** *adj* above the kidney. ⇒ adrenal.

**suprasternal** *adj* above the sternum.

**supraventricular** *adj* above the ventricles.

**supraventricular tachycardia (SVT)** any tachycardia originating from a focus in atrial tissue. The heart rate is greater than 100 beats/min and may be as fast as 280 beats/min. ⇒ Wolff–Parkinson–White syndrome.

**surfactant** *n* a mixture of phospholipids secreted by type II pneumocytes. It reduces surface tension in the alveoli, allows lung inflation and prevents alveolar collapse between breaths. ⇒ neonatal respiratory distress syndrome, pneumocytes.

**surgeon** *n* a qualified doctor who specializes in surgery.

**surgery** *n* that branch of medicine which treats diseases, deformities and injuries, wholly or in part, by manual or operative procedures.

**surgical** *adj* pertaining to surgery.

**surgical dressings** ⇒ wound dressings.

**surgical emphysema** air in the subcutaneous tissue planes following the trauma of surgery or injury.

**surrogate** *n* a substitute for an object or person. *surrogate motherhood* where a woman agrees to have a child for an infertile couple. Surrogacy is allowed in the UK, but women may only receive reasonable financial expenses. There are, however, many informal arrangements for surrogacy.

**survey** *n* a data collection method. Includes: interview, postal, telephone, or via the internet.

**susceptibility** *n* the opposite of resistance. Includes a state of reduced capacity to deal with infection.

**suspensory ligaments** supporting or suspending such as that supporting the lens. ⇒ Appendix 1, Figure 15.

**suture** *n, v* **1.** the junction of cranial bones. **2.** in surgery, a stitch or series of stitches used to appose the edges of a surgical or traumatic wound (Figure S.11). Also describes the placement of such stitches. ⇒ ligature.

**S$\bar{v}O_2$** *abbr* mixed venous oxygen saturation.

**SV** *abbr* stroke volume.

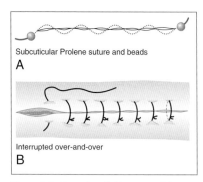

Subcuticular Prolene suture and beads

**A**

Interrupted over-and-over

**B**

**Figure S.11** Examples of skin sutures: (A) continuous subcuticular Prolene and beads; (B) interrupted over-and-over *(reproduced from Pudner 2000 with permission).*

**SVR** *abbr* systemic vascular resistance.

**SVT** *abbr* supraventricular tachycardia.

**swab** *n* **1.** a small piece of cotton wool or gauze. **2.** a small piece of sterile cotton wool, or similar material, on the end of a shaft of plastic, wire or wood, inside a protecting tube. It is used to collect material for microbiological examination.

**swallowing** *n* deglutition. Part voluntary and part involuntary activity with three stages: oral (buccal), pharyngeal and oesophageal. ⇒ dysphagia.

**sweat** *n* the secretion from the sweat (sudoriferous) glands. Contains water, electrolytes (mainly sodium and chloride) and waste. Sweat production is primarily concerned with temperature regulation but has a small excretory role.

**sweat gland** two types of skin gland that produce sweat. ⇒ apocrine sweat gland, eccrine, Appendix 1, Figure 12.

**sweat test** used to measure the amount of sodium and chloride in sweat, to confirm a diagnosis of cystic fibrosis. The drug pilocarpine is introduced into the skin by iontophoresis to induce sweating. The sweat is collected and tested.

**sycosis barbae** (*syn* barber's itch) a pustular folliculitis of the beard area in men.

**sycosis nuchae** a folliculitis at the nape of the neck which leads to keloid thickening (acne keloid).

**Sydenham's chorea** (T Sydenham, British physician, 1624–1689) ⇒ chorea.

**symbiosis** *n* a relationship between two or more organisms in which the participants are of mutual aid and benefit to one another. ⇒ antibiosis *opp*—**symbiotic** *adj*.

**symblepharon** *n* adhesion of the lid to the eyeball.

**symmelia** *n* a congenital anomaly in which the lower limbs are fused.

**sympathectomy** *n* surgical excision of part of the sympathetic nervous system.

**sympathetic nervous system** part of the peripheral nervous system (PNS), it describes a division of the autonomic nervous system (ANS). It is composed of a chain of ganglia on either side of the vertebral column and nerve fibres having thoracolumbar outflow. It opposes the parasympathetic nervous system and is usually involved with body stimulation. Its action is augmented by adrenaline (epinephrine) and noradrenaline (norepinephrine).

**sympatholytic** *n* an antagonist. A drug which impedes or opposes the effects of the sympathetic nervous system. ⇒ alpha (α)-adrenoceptor antagonists, beta (β)-adrenoceptor antagonists.

**sympathomimetic** *adj* an agonist. Producing effects similar to those produced by stimulation of the sympathetic nerves. ⇒ alpha (α)-adrenoceptor agonists, beta (β)-adrenoceptor agonists.

**symphysiotomy** *n* an operation to separate the symphysis pubis and enlarge the pelvis to facilitate delivery. Rarely undertaken.

**symphysis** *n* a fibrocartilaginous union of bones such as the symphysis pubis—**symphyseal** *adj*.

**symphysis pubis dysfunction** previously known as diastasis symphysis pubis. A painful condition occurring during late pregnancy, in labour or following delivery. It is caused by the abnormal relaxation of the ligaments associated with the pubic joint. The relaxation is due to high levels of pregnancy hormones such as relaxin.

**sympodia** *n* a congenital anomaly in which the legs are fused and the feet are missing.

**symptom** *n* a subjective phenomenon or manifestation of disease—**symptomatic** *adj*.

**symptom complex** a group of symptoms which, occurring together, typify a particular disease or syndrome.

**symptomatology** *n* **1.** the branch of medicine concerned with symptoms. **2.** the combined symptoms typical of a particular disease.

S

**Synacthen test** ⇒ tetracosactide (Synacthen) test.

**synaesthesia** *n* the occurrence of a secondary sensation accompanying another sensation, such as a particular sound producing a visual sensation.

**synapse** *n* the gap between the axon of one neuron and the dendrites of another, or the gap between the axon and a gland or muscle. Most operate chemically but a few are electrical. The synapse permits the passage of an impulse across the gap. This is achieved chemically by the release of calcium ions and a neurotransmitter such as acetylcholine.

**synapsis** *n* during meiosis, the pairing of homologous chromosomes.

**synarthrosis** *n* an immovable fibrous joint, such as the skull sutures.

**synbiotics** *npl* supplements containing both prebiotics and probiotics.

**synchondrosis** *n* a type of amphiarthrosis or cartilaginous joint formed by the epiphyseal plate before ossification.

**synchronized intermittent mandatory ventilation (SIMV)** mode of positive-pressure ventilation in which the timing of the breaths is varied according to the patient's own respiratory effort.

**synchysis scintillans** cholesterol crystals in the vitreous body (humour) of the eye, often following vitreous haemorrhage.

**syncope** *n* (*syn* faint) literally, sudden loss of strength. Caused by reduced cerebral circulation often following a fright, when vasodilation is responsible. May be symptomatic of cardiac arrhythmia, e.g. heart block.

**syncytium** *n* a mass of tissue with several nuclei. Boundaries between individual cells are absent or poorly defined.

**syndactyly, syndactylism, syndactylia** *n* (*syn* webbed toes, zygodactyly) a term applied to a total or partial fusion of adjacent digits. It is very common, usually bilateral and often familial. Multiple syndactyly occurs in hands and feet associated with other anomalies, as in Apert's syndrome, an autosomal dominant disorder—acrocephalosyndactyly. Treatment is not required for webbing of the toes—**syndactylous** *adj*.

**syndesmophyte** *n* abnormal bony growth between vertebrae, such as in ankylosing spondylitis.

**syndesmosis** *n* a type of fibrous joint in which an interosseous ligament connects two bones, e.g. tibiofibular joint.

**syndrome** *n* a group of symptoms and/or signs which, occurring together, produce a pattern or symptom complex, typical of a particular disease.

**syndrome of inappropriate ADH secretion (SIADH)** syndrome in which excessive antidiuretic hormone leads to water retention and low serum sodium.

**syndrome X** ⇒ metabolic syndrome.

**synechia** *n* abnormal union of structures, especially adhesion of the iris to the cornea in front, or the lens capsule behind—**synechiae** *pl*.

**synergism, synergy** *n* the harmonious working together of two agents, such as drugs, micro-organisms, muscles, etc.—**synergistic** *adj*.

**synergist** *n* an agent co-operating with another.

**synergistic action** that brought about by the co-operation of two or more muscles, neither of which could bring about the action alone.

**synkinesis** *n* the ability to carry out precision movements.

**synostosis** *n* union between bones occurring by ossification.

**synovectomy** *n* excision of synovial membrane.

**synovial fluid** the fluid secreted by the membrane lining a freely movable joint cavity.

**synovial joint** diarthrosis or freely movable joint. (Figure S.12). One of the three main classes of joint.

**synovial membrane** ⇒ membrane.

**synovioma** *n* a tumour of synovial membrane—benign or malignant.

**synovitis** *n* inflammation of a synovial membrane.

**synthesis** *n* the process of compiling complex substances from less complex ones by chemical reactions—**synthetic** *adj*.

**syphilide** *n* a syphilitic skin lesion.

**syphilis** *n* a sexually transmitted infection caused by the spirochaete *Treponema pallidum* (ssp. *pallidum*). It may be congenital or acquired. *acquired syphilis* is contracted during sexual intercourse with an infected person. There are two main stages: (a) early, characterized by a primary lesion (chancre) at the site of entry into the body that heals within about 1 month, and may be followed by a generalized illness (secondary syphilis) characterized by a skin rash, fever, generalized lymph node enlargement, mucosal ulcers (snail track); (b) late (occurring many years after the infection) with skin or visceral lesions

**S**

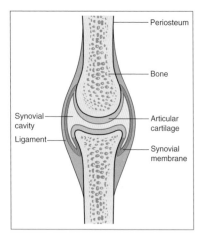

**Figure S.12** Typical synovial joint *(reproduced from Waugh & Grant 2006 with permission).*

(gumma), neurosyphilis (tabes dorsalis and general paralysis of the insane) or cardiovascular syphilis (including aneurysm formation in the ascending aorta). In many individuals there may be no clinical signs of syphilis (latent syphilis), the diagnosis being made on the basis of positive serological tests for *T. pallidum. congenital syphilis* the spirochaete is transmitted from mother to fetus via the placenta. The affected infant may exhibit characteristic features that include a generalized rash, generalized lymphadenopathy and hepatitis.

**syringe** *n* a device for injecting, instilling or withdrawing fluids. Consists of a cylindrical barrel to one end of which a hollow needle is attached, and a close-fitting plunger.

**syringe driver** medical device for the continuous delivery of drugs intravenously or subcutaneously. Commonly used in palliative care to control symptoms, including pain.

**syringomyelia** *n* an uncommon, progressive disease of the spinal cord of unknown cause, beginning mainly in early adult life. Cavitation and surrounding fibrous tissue reaction, in the upper spinal cord, interfere with sensation of pain and temperature, and sometimes with the motor pathways. There is painless injury, particularly of the hands. Touch sensation is typically intact in the early stages. ⇒ Charcot's joint.

**syringomyelocele** *n* the most severe form of meningeal hernia (spina bifida). The central canal is dilated and the thinned-out posterior part of the spinal cord is in the hernia.

**syrinx** *n* a cyst-like cavity in the spinal cord.

**systematic desensitization** a technique that utilizes classical conditioning to treat anxiety disorders and phobias. ⇒ conditioning, desensitization.

**systematic review** a systematic approach to literature reviews of both published and unpublished material that lessens bias and random errors.

**Système International d'Unités (SI) (International System of Units)** system of measurement used for scientific, technical and medical purposes. There are seven base units: ampere, candela, kelvin, kilogram, metre, mole and second, and various derived units, e.g. pascal, becquerel, etc. ⇒ Appendix 2.

**system for identifying motivated abilities (SIMA)** a self-explanatory term. The tests are especially useful in diagnosing the level of mental deterioration.

**systemic circulation** oxygenated blood leaves the left ventricle and, after flowing throughout the body, returns deoxygenated to the right atrium.

**systemic inflammatory response syndrome (SIRS)** generalized inflammatory response, which may be triggered by a range of processes (e.g. poor perfusion). Features include: abnormal temperature, altered white cell count, increased respiratory rate and increased heart rate. SIRS and multiple-organ dysfunction syndrome frequently occur together in critically ill patients.

**systemic lupus erythematosus (SLE)** a connective tissue disease where autoantibodies cause effects in many parts of the body, e.g. sun-exposed skin, lungs, heart and blood vessels, kidneys and joints. The aetiology is multifactorial. There may be skin changes with a typically butterfly-shaped facial rash, ⊙DVD alopecia, pyrexia, pleurisy, pericarditis, alveolitis, arthritis and renal damage. ⇒ connective tissue diseases.

**systemic sclerosis** a multisystem connective tissue disease. The most characteristic features are scleroderma (thickening of the skin) and Raynaud's phenomenon. Most internal organs are affected.

**systemic vascular resistance (SVR)** the resistance against which the left ventricle must pump blood into the systemic circulation. It is influenced by the degree of vasoconstriction in the peripheral arterioles, i.e. peripheral resistance.

**systole** *n* the contraction phase of the cardiac cycle, as opposed to diastole——**systolic** *adj*.

**systolic blood pressure** the maximum blood pressure measured during the cardiac contraction phase of the cardiac cycle, i.e. when blood is ejected from the heart into the aorta and the systemic arteries.

**systolic murmur** a cardiac murmur occurring between the first and second heart sounds due to valvular disease, e.g. mitral systolic murmur.

S

# T

**T₃** *abbr* triiodothyronine.

**T₄** *abbr* thyroxine.

**tabes** *n* wasting away—**tabetic** *adj*. *tabes dorsalis* a variety of neurosyphilis characterized by a staggering gait and 'lightning' limb pains. ⇒ Charcot's joint, locomotor ataxia.

**tabetic gait** ⇒ gait.

**tablet** *n* a solid form of a drug. It may be designed to be swallowed whole, or chewed, or dissolved in water, or absorbed from the buccal cavity, or sublingually. It may be a slow-release preparation, or enteric-coated to ensure that absorption occurs in the small intestine.

**taboo** *n* a behaviour forbidden by individual societies, such as incest or cannibalism.

**taboparesis** *n* a form of neurosyphilis in which there are clinical features of both brain and spinal cord involvement.

**tache noir** the black lesion that forms at the bite site in tick-borne boutonneuse fever.

**tachycardia** *n* excessively rapid action of the heart at rest (in excess of 100 beats/min in adults). *paroxysmal tachycardia* a temporary but sudden marked increase in frequency of heart beats, because the conducting stimulus is originating in an abnormal focus.

**tachyphagia** *n* eating very rapidly.

**tachyphasia** *n* extreme rapidity of speech. It can be a feature of some mental health disorders.

**tachyphylaxis** *n* the decreasing effectiveness of some drugs during long-term administration.

**tachypnoea** *n* abnormal frequency of respiration (in excess of 20 respirations per minute in adults at rest)—**tachypnoeic** *adj*.

**tactile** *adj* relating to the sense of touch.

**taenia** *n* a flat strip. *taenia coli* three bands of longitudinal muscle of the colon: because they are shorter than the colon, they produce haustrations or puckering.

*Taenia* *n* a genus of flat, parasitic worms; cestodes or tapeworms. *Taenia saginata* larvae present in infested, undercooked beef. In the human (the definitive host) intestinal lumen they develop into the adult tapeworm, which attaches itself by its four suckers to the wall of the intestine. *Taenia solium* has hooklets as well as suckers. The larvae are ingested in infested, undercooked pork; humans can also be the intermediate host for this worm by ingesting eggs, which develop into larvae in the stomach and pass via the intestinal wall

to reach organs where they develop into cysts. In the brain these may cause seizures. ⇒ cysticercosis, cysticercus, *Echinococcus*.

**taeniacide** *n* an agent that destroys tapeworms—**taeniacidal** *adj*.

**taeniafuge** *n* an agent that causes the expulsion of a tapeworm.

**Takayasu's disease** (M Takayasu, Japanese ophthalmologist, 1860–1938) ⇒ pulseless disease.

**talipes** *n* any of a number of deformities of the foot and ankle. For example, *talipes calcaneovalgus* a condition usually caused by intrauterine posture, the foot having been fixed in an upturned position with the sole against the uterine wall. Improvement and usually complete recovery occur with active movement after birth. *talipes equinovarus* the heel is drawn up, the foot inverted and the hindfoot adducted—in the equinovarus position.

**talus** *n* the astragalus. A tarsal bone situated between the tibia proximally and the calcaneus distally, thus directly bearing the weight of the body. It is the second largest bone of the ankle and articulates with the malleoli of the tibia and fibula at the ankle, with the calcaneus at the subtalar joint and with the navicular bone.

**tampon** *n* a plug used in the nose, vagina or other orifice to absorb blood or secretions. *tampon shock syndrome* ⇒ toxic shock syndrome.

**tamponade** *n* **1.** insertion of a tampon to apply pressure to a structure in order to control haemorrhage. **2.** the abnormal compression of an organ, such as the heart, caused by the accumulation of blood or other fluid. ⇒ cardiac tamponade.

**tannins** *npl* substances present in some plants. They bind to divalent metal ions such as zinc, ferrous iron, calcium, etc., present in foods, thus reducing the bioavailability of these ions for absorption from the food. Can lead to a deficiency of certain nutrients (e.g. iron) if intake is marginal, such as can occur with a strict vegetarian diet.

**tantalum (Ta)** *n* a metal used for various prostheses, including plates for repairing defects in the skull.

**tapeworm** *n* cestodes. They include *Taenia saginata* (beef tapeworm), *Taenia solium* (pork tapeworm) and *Diphyllobothrium latum* (fish tapeworm). Dogs and cats are the definitive host for the tapeworm *Dipylidium caninum*, which may cause human disease. ⇒ *Diphyllobothrium, Taenia*.

**tapôtement** *n* (*syn* tapping) massage manipulations in which the hands strike, or percuss, the body alternately and rhythmically; used to eliminate secretions, as in postural drainage, and in an invigorating massage. It may involve: beating with loosely clenched fists, clapping using clapped hands and producing a deep-toned sound, hacking using the ulnar (little-finger-side) borders of the hands and fingers, and pounding with the ulnar sides of loosely clenched fists.

**tapping** *n* **1.** ⇒ aspiration. **2.** ⇒ tapôtement.

**tardive dyskinesia** abnormal movements. Repeated involuntary movements of the face, tongue, trunk and limbs. Associated with the long-term use of typical antipsychotic (neuroleptic) drugs, particularly the phenothiazines, e.g. fluphenazine.

**target cell** **1.** a leptocyte. A red blood cell that has a dark centre surrounded by a paler ring. It can occur in various blood disorders, such as haemoglobinopathies, iron-deficiency anaemia, or in liver disease, or following splenectomy. **2.** a general term applied to cells that have a specific receptor that is targeted by specific T cells, antibodies, hormones, other chemicals, etc.

**target zone** (*syn* training zone) the use of heart rate ranges to indicate the intensity of effort required during exercise programmes.

**tarsal** **1.** *adj* relating to the seven bones of the ankle or tarsus. **2.** *adj* relating to the fibrous tissue of the eyelids (tarsus), or the tarsal glands. **3.** *n* one of the seven bones of the ankle or tarsus.

**tarsal coalition (peroneal spastic flat foot)** an anomaly in which adjacent tarsal bones are fused together. Fusion may be bony or cartilaginous. The most common occurs between the calcaneus and the navicular with union across the mid-tarsal joint. Talocalcaneal coalition also occurs.

**tarsalgia** *n* pain in the foot.

**tarsal gland** also called meibomian glands. Modified sebaceous glands of the eyelid. ⇒ meibomian glands.

**tarsometatarsal** *adj* relating to the tarsal and metatarsal region.

**tarsoplasty** *n* blepharoplasty. Plastic surgery of the eyelid.

**tarsorrhaphy** *n* suturing of the eyelids together to protect the cornea.

**tarsus** *n* **1.** the seven bones of the ankle. They are the talus, calcaneus, navicular, cuboid and three cuneiform bones (⇒ Appendix 1, Figure 2). **2.** the dense connective tissue found in each eyelid, contributing to its form and support—**tarsal** *adj*.

**tartar** *n* ⇒ calculus.

**task** *n* an autonomous, purposeful, component part of an activity.

**taste** *n* gustation. A chemical sense closely linked with olfaction (smell). *taste buds* sensory receptors found on the tongue, epiglottis and pharynx.

**taurine** *n* substance derived from the amino acid cysteine; it has a role in the conjugation of bile salts.

**taurocholic acid** one of the bile acids.

**taxis** *n* **1.** movement towards or away from a stimulus. **2.** manual manipulation for restoring a structure to its normal position, such as a hernia.

**taxonomy** *n* a classification system for naming organisms.

**Tay–Sachs disease** (*syn* gangliosidosis) (W Tay, British ophthalmologist, 1843–1927; B Sachs, American neurologist/psychiatrist, 1858–1944) an inherited lipid storage disease in which $GM_2$ ganglioside (carbohydrate-rich sphingolipid) accumulates within the nervous system. It is due to a deficiency of the enzyme β-N-acetylhexosaminidase and results in mental deterioration, blindness and death. The gene responsible is most commonly carried by individuals of Ashkenazi Jewish origins.

**TB** *abbr* tuberculosis.

**TBI** *abbr* ⇒ total body irradiation.

**TBSA** *abbr* total burn surface area.

**TCA** *abbr* tricyclic antidepressants.

**T cell** ⇒ lymphocyte.

**T-cell receptor (TCR)** receptor situated on the surface of T cells. They recognize specific antigens presented to them by antigen-presenting cells (APCs).

**TCR** *abbr* T-cell receptor.

**TCRE** *abbr* transcervical resection of endometrium.

**T-cytotoxic (killer) cell** ⇒ cytotoxic T cell.

**T-delayed hypersensitivity cell** ⇒ delayed hypersensitivity T cell.

**tears** *npl* the secretion produced by the lacrimal gland. Tears contain the bactericidal enzyme lysozyme.

**technetium (Tc)** *n* a radioactive element. The isotope $^{99m}$Tc derived from molybdenum is used in radioisotope (radionuclide) imaging (scans).

**TEDs** *acron* **t**hrombo**e**mbolic **d**eterrents.

**teeth** *npl* the 20 teeth of first or primary dentition (deciduous, milk teeth) erupt between the age of 5/6 months and 2½ years (Figure T.1A). The second dentition (permanent, adult teeth) of 32 teeth starts to replace the deciduous teeth at

471

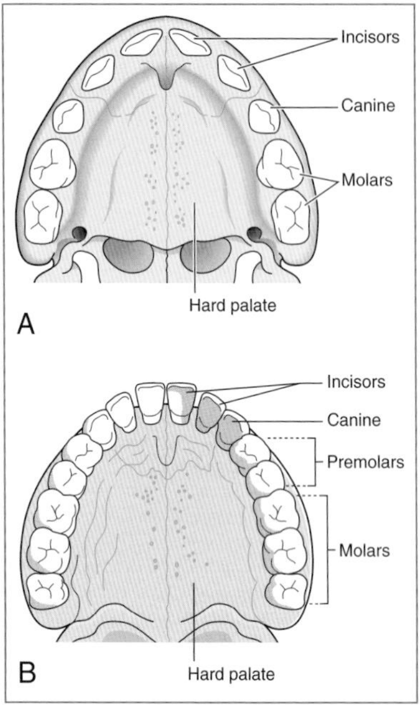

**Figure T.1** (A) First dentition; (B) second dentition *(reproduced from Waugh & Grant 2006 with permission).*

about 6 years of age. The process is nearly complete by 12 years of age; the third molars or 'wisdom' teeth, if they erupt, will do so during the late teens and early 20s (Figure T.1B).

**teething** *n* lay term for the discomfort during the eruption of the primary dentition in babies.

**tegument** *n* the skin or covering of the body.

**teichopsia** *n* also called scintillating scotoma. The appearance of shimmering zigzag lines that move across the visual field. Occurs during the aura of some types of migraine.

**telangiectasis** *n* dilatation of small blood vessels.

**telemedicine** *n* the use of electronic technologies, such as telephone and the internet, for consultations and diagnosis, monitoring patients with chronic diseases, for health professionals to seek advice from an expert and for patients to seek advice, etc. ⇒ telemetry.

**telemetry** *n* the electronic transmission of data, including clinical measurement, between distant sites. May be used for cardiac monitoring.

**telencephalon** *n* one of the secondary enlargements during embryonic development of the brain. It becomes the cerebrum and the basal nuclei.

**teletherapy** *n* treatment with a radiation source that is distant from the patient such as cobalt-60 or X-rays—**teletherapeutic** *adj.* **teletherapeutically** *adv.*

**telocentric** *adj* describes a chromosome that has the centromere at one end.

**telogen** *n* the resting stage in the hair growth cycle prior to shedding. ⇒ anagen, catogen.

**telomeres** *npl* protective regions of DNA at the ends of chromosomes that become shorter with age. Normally they stop chromosomal damage during cell division, but with increasing age the telomeres no longer function properly. Eventually results in genetic damage and cell death. ⇒ apoptosis.

**telophase** *n* the last stage of nuclear division in mitosis (see Figure M.6, p. 308) and in both divisions of meiosis (see Figure M.3, p. 296.). The set of chromosomes at each pole of the cell uncoil, the nuclear membrane reforms, the nucleoli reform and the mitotic spindle disappears. If the cell is to divide, the cleavage furrow develops further until two cells are produced by cytokinesis. ⇒ anaphase, metaphase, prophase.

**temperament** *n* the usual mental attitude of the person.

**temple** *n* that part of the head situated between the outer angle of the eye and the top of the pinna.

**temporal** *adj* relating to the temple.

**temporal arteritis** also known as giant cell arteritis. Occurs in older people and mainly affects the external carotid artery and its branches, e.g. the temporal artery supplying the scalp. Blindness can ensue if there is thrombosis of the ophthalmic vessels. Early treatment with corticosteroids is effective.

**temporal artery** a branch of the external carotid. It has three branches that supply blood to the skin and muscles of the temporal, frontal and parietal scalp.

**temporal bones** one on each side of the skull below the parietal bone, containing the cavity of the middle ear.

**temporalis** *n* a fan-shaped muscle of the head. Its origin is on the zygomatic arch and it inserts on to the mandible. Important in mastication as it closes the jaw.

**temporal lobe** lateral lobe of the cerebrum, beneath the temporal bone. It is concerned with audition and olfaction and also contains some association areas for learning and memory.

**temporal lobe epilepsy** ⇒ epilepsy.

**temporomandibular** *adj* relating to the temporal region or bone, and the lower jaw. *temporomandibular joint* (TMJ) a synovial joint (modified hinge or bicondylar joint) between the temporal bone and mandible.

**temporomandibular joint (TMJ) pain dysfunction syndrome** pain in the region of the temporomandibular joint, frequently caused by malocclusion of the teeth, resulting in malposition of the condylar heads in the joint and abnormal muscle activity, and by bruxism.

**TEN** *acron* **t**oxic **e**pidermal **n**ecrolysis.

**tenaculum** *n* **1.** an instrument for grasping and holding tissue. **2.** band of tissue that secures a body part in place. ⇒ retinaculum.

**Tenckhoff catheter** (H Tenckhoff, American nephrologist, 20th century) a commonly used peritoneal dialysis catheter.

**tendinitis** *n* inflammation of a tendon.

**tendon** *n* a band of white, fibrous connective tissue that joins muscle to bone—**tendinous** *adj*.

**tendon organ** ⇒ Golgi tendon organ.

**tendonosis** *n* degenerative changes in tendons.

**tenesmus** *n* painful, ineffectual straining to empty the bowel or bladder.

**tennis elbow** lateral epicondylitis. ⇒ epicondylitis.

**Tenon's capsule** (J Tenon, French pathologist/surgeon, 1724–1816) the fascia around the eyeball in the socket.

**tenoplasty** *n* a reconstructive operation on a tendon—**tenoplastic** *adj*.

**tenorrhaphy** *n* the suturing of a tendon.

**tenosynovitis** *n* also called tendosynovitis. Inflammation of the thin synovial lining of a tendon sheath, as distinct from its outer fibrous sheath. It may be caused by mechanical irritation or by bacterial infection.

**tenotomy** *n* division of a tendon.

**TENS** *acron* **t**ranscutaneous **e**lectrical **n**erve **s**timulation.

**tensile force** force applied along the fibres of a tissue. Excessive tensile forces cause a tearing of the tissues as they are stretched beyond their normal length.

**tensor tympani** a tiny muscle of the middle ear. It contracts reflexly (sound attenuation reflex), with another muscle the stapedius, to protect the ear from very loud sounds by reducing conduction. ⇒ stapedius.

**tentorium cerebelli** a fold of dura mater between the cerebellum and cerebrum.

Damage during birth may result in intracranial bleeding.

**TEPP** *abbr* tetraethyl pyrophosphate.

**teratogen** *n* anything capable of disrupting embryonic/fetal growth and producing malformation. Classified as drugs, poisons, radiations, physical agents such as electroconvulsive therapy, infections, e.g. rubella and Rhesus and thyroid antibodies—**teratogenic, teratogenetic** *adj*, **teratogenicity, teratogenesis** *n*.

**teratogenesis** *n* the processes by which teratogens, such as drugs, produce physical malformations, particularly during organogenesis in embryonic development.

**teratology** *n* the scientific study of teratogens and their mode of action—**teratological** *adj*, **teratologist** *n*, **teratologically** *adv*.

**teratoma** *n* commonly a tumour of the testis or ovary. It is of embryonic origin and usually malignant. Some testicular tumours have both seminoma and teratoma components. The cure rate for germ cell tumours has increased 10-fold with the use of platinum-based chemotherapy—**teratomata** *pl*, **teratomatous** *adj*.

**teres** *adj*, *n* rounded and smooth. *ligamentum teres* a ligament that secures the femur in the acetabulum, or the fibrous remnant of the fetal umbilical vein within the falciform ligament of the liver. *teres major* and *teres minor* two muscles of the shoulder.

**term** *n* **1.** normal gestation period, a pregnancy of 40 weeks' gestation. **2.** a specific period of time, e.g. a fixed-term contract.

**terminal hair** coarse pigmented hair of the scalp and eyebrows. During puberty it replaces the vellus hair found around the external genitalia and axillae in both sexes, and forms the facial and body hair in males. ⇒ lanugo, vellus hair.

**termination of pregnancy (TOP)** ⇒ abortion.

**termination or stop codon** the three-nucleotide sequence in mRNA that signals the end of a sequence of amino acids in a polypeptide chain. There are three stop codons: UAG, UGA and UAA (A, adenine, G, guanine, U, uracil).

**tertian** *adj* recurring every 48 hours, such as the fever in some types of malaria.

**tertiary** *adj* third in order.

**tertiary care** highly specialized health care services accessed through indirect referral via secondary care. Usually deals with uncommon or rare conditions. The specialized hospital care is provided by a regional or national centre, e.g. spinal injuries, certain cancers.

**T**

**tertiary prevention** ⇒ disease prevention.

**testicle** *n* ⇒ testis—**testicular** *adj*.

**testicular artery** one of two arteries that branch from the abdominal aorta to supply blood to the testes.

**testicular cancer** relatively rare cancers, but the most common cancer in young men under 35 years of age. Early detection is vital, as the cancer is highly curable if detected at an early stage; all men should be encouraged to examine their testes on a regular basis. Presentation is usually with a lump or painless swelling in one testis, or a dull ache or heavy feeling in the lower abdomen, anal or scrotal area. The treatment modalities, which can be used alone or in combination, include orchidectomy, chemotherapy or radiotherapy.

**testicular self-examination (TSE)** regular examination undertaken by men to detect cancers or other abnormalities.

**testis** *n* a male gonad. One of the two glandular structures contained in the scrotum of the male (⇒ Appendix 1, Figure 16); they produce spermatozoa and the male sex hormones. ⇒ spermatogenesis. *undescended testis* the testis remains within the bony pelvis or inguinal canal. ⇒ cryptorchism—**testes** *pl*.

**testosterone** *n* the major androgen, an anabolic steroid hormone produced by the testes. It is responsible for the development of the male secondary sexual characteristics and reproductive functioning.

**test-tube baby** one produced by in vitro fertilization.

**tetanus** *n* **1.** (*syn* lockjaw) disease caused by the bacterium *Clostridium tetani*, an anaerobic spore-forming micro-organism present in the intestine of domestic animals and humans, commonly found in soil, dust and manure. It produces a powerful exotoxin that affects the motor nerves, causing muscle spasms, rigidity and convulsions. Active immunization with tetanus toxoid (TT) is available as part of routine programmes, as regular booster doses and when risk is increased. Tetanus immunoglobulin is available for passive immunization. ⇒ opisthotonos, risus sardonicus, trismus—**tetanic** *adj*. **2.** in the contraction of muscle, the summation that increases the force of contraction by increasing the frequency of stimulation to the maximum to produce a sustained contraction.

**tetany** *n* condition of muscular hyperexcitability in which mild stimuli produce cramps and muscle spasms in the hands and feet (carpopedal spasm). It is due to a reduction in ionized calcium levels in the blood, for example as a result of alkalosis from hyperventilation or alkali ingestion, or hypocalcaemia associated with hypoparathyroidism. ⇒ Chvostek's sign, Trousseau's sign.

**tetracosactide (Synacthen) test** a test of adrenocortical function. Adrenocortical insufficiency is indicated if the plasma cortisol concentration fails to rise following an intramuscular injection of tetracosactide (an adrenocorticotrophic hormone analogue).

**tetracyclines** *npl* a group of broad-spectrum antibiotics, e.g. doxycycline. Problems associated with the tetracyclines include superinfection with gastrointestinal disturbances, bacterial resistance and vitamin B deficiency. They are also deposited in teeth and bone and should not be prescribed for pregnant or lactating women, or for children, because they can lead to discoloration of the second dentition and bone abnormalities. ⇒ Appendix 5.

**tetradactylous** *adj* having four digits on each limb.

**tetraethyl pyrophosphate (TEPP)** organophosphorous compound used as a commercial insecticide. Toxicity results from its powerful and irreversible anticholinesterase action.

**tetralogy of Fallot** ⇒ Fallot's tetralogy.

**tetraplegia** *n* (*syn* quadriplegia) paralysis of all four limbs—**tetraplegic** *adj*.

**tetrodotoxin** *n* the toxin present in the puffer fish.

**TFR** *abbr* total fertility rate.

**TGF** *abbr* transforming growth factor.

**thalamencephalon** *n* the area of the brain containing the thalamus, epithalamus and subthalamus.

**thalamic syndrome** damage to the thalamus, usually caused by a stroke, leading to intractable pain and increased sensitivity affecting the contralateral side of the body.

**thalamotomy** *n* usually operative (stereotaxic) destruction of a portion of thalamus. Can be done for intractable pain.

**thalamus** *n* a collection of grey matter at the base of the cerebrum. Sensory impulses from the whole body pass through the thalamus en route to the cerebral cortex—**thalami** *pl*, **thalamic** *adj*. ⇒ limbic system.

**thalassaemia** *n* a group of inherited haemoglobinopathies in which mutation or deletion of one or more globin genes results in an imbalance in the production of α- and β-globin molecules. Because it affects the deformability of the red cell, this imbalance leads to increased red cell breakdown and a failure of

T

bone marrow red cell precursors to produce fully mature erythrocytes. This in turn leads to anaemia, the severity of which depends on the nature of the genetic defect. *beta-thalassaemia* results most often from genetic mutations in the β-globin genes. If both copies of the gene are affected (patient is homozygous for a mutation), a severe, transfusion-dependent anaemia, with jaundice and hepatosplenomegaly may result (beta-thalassaemia major). By contrast, in the carrier (heterozygous) state where only one copy of the gene is mutated, there is often only a mild asymptomatic anaemia. The situation with *alpha-thalassaemia* is more complex as there are four α-globin genes, and the severity of alpha-thalassaemia varies from asymptomatic, if only one gene is affected, to usually fatal in utero if four genes are affected (hydrops fetalis). Persons with three affected genes have so-called haemoglobin H disease and are often transfusion-dependent.

**thallium (Tl)** *n* a metallic element. Many thallium compounds are highly toxic.

**thallium-201 myocardial perfusion scintigraphy scan** the radioisotope (radionuclide) thallium-201 ($^{201}$Tl) is administered intravenously to study myocardial perfusion. Useful in identifying myocardial ischaemia in the diagnosis of coronary artery disease when it can be combined with an exercise stress test; or a resting scan in the localization of a myocardial infarction.

**thanatology** *n* the scientific study of death, including its cause and diagnosis.

**theca** *n* an enveloping sheath, especially of a tendon, or the dura mater—**thecal** *adj*.

**thelarche** *n* the commencement of female breast development; normally starts very early in puberty.

**T-helper cell** ⇒ helper T cells.

**thenar** *adj* relating to the palm (hand) and the sole (foot). *thenar eminence* the palmar eminence below the thumb.

**therapeutic abortion** ⇒ abortion.

**therapeutic index** an indicator of the difference between the therapeutic dose of a drug and a dose that causes toxicity. It can vary between individuals.

**therapeutic play** play that is structured and initiated by adults. It can be used for distraction, creating normality, helping children to express their fears and wishes, giving information, assessing developmental stages, etc. ⇒ normative play.

**therapeutics** *n* the branch of medicine concerned with the treatment of disease states—**therapeutic** *adj*, **therapeutically** *adv*.

**therapy** *n* treatment of a range of psychological or physical conditions. ⇒ occupational therapy, physiotherapy, speech and language therapy.

**thermal** *adj* pertaining to heat.

**thermal strain** the physiological and psychological reaction to environmental thermal stress.

**thermal stress** the build-up of environmental conditions that stress the thermoregulatory structures.

**thermic effect of food** ⇒ diet-induced thermogenesis.

**thermistor** *n* a device used to detect very small changes in temperature.

**thermoalgesia** *n* pain caused by high temperature.

**thermoanaesthesia** *n* also known as thermoanalgesia. The inability to perceive the sensations of cold or heat.

**thermoduric** *adj* describes bacteria that are not destroyed by pasteurization.

**thermogenesis** *n* the production of heat by the body. It might be for maintaining temperature, or in response to food intake or drugs—**thermogenetic** *adj*. ⇒ brown adipose tissue (brown fat), diet-induced thermogenesis.

**thermography** *n* an investigation that detects minute temperature differences over different body areas by use of an infrared thermograph that is sensitive to radiant heat. The uses include the study of blood flow and detection of cancers, such as breast cancer.

**thermolabile** *adj* capable of being easily changed or destroyed by heat.

**thermolysis** *n* heat-induced chemical dissociation. Dissipation of body heat—**thermolytic** *adj*.

**thermometer** *n* an instrument for measuring temperature—**thermometric** *adj*. ⇒ clinical thermometer.

**thermophiles** *npl* bacteria that grow best at temperatures above 55°C and can tolerate temperatures up to 80°C—**thermophilic** *adj*.

**thermoreceptor** *n* a specialized nerve ending that responds to heat and cold.

**thermoregulation** *n* the homeostatic mechanisms that maintain core body temperature within a normal range.

**T**

**thermostable** *adj* unaffected by heat. Remaining unaltered at a high temperature, which is usually specified—**thermostability** *n*.

**thermotherapy** *n* heat treatment, such as diathermy, warm compresses, electric pads, warm baths, etc.

**thiamin(e)** *n* a member of the vitamin B complex. It is concerned in carbohydrate, fat and alcohol metabolism. Deficiency causes beriberi, mental confusion or cardiomyopathy. ⇒ Appendix 4, Korsakoff's psychosis/syndrome, Wernicke's encephalopathy.

**thiazide diuretics** a group of diuretics, e.g. bendroflumethiazide (bendrofluazide), that act on the first part of the distal tubule of the nephron. They reduce sodium and chloride reabsorption, which increases the amount of water, sodium and chloride excreted. ⇒ Appendix 5.

**thiazolidinediones** *npl* a group of antidiabetic drugs (oral hypoglycaemics), e.g. rosiglitazone, which reduce blood glucose. ⇒ Appendix 5.

**Thiersch skin graft** (K Thiersch, German surgeon, 1822–1895) ⇒ skin graft.

**third-degree tear** ⇒ perineal tear.

**Thomas' splint** (H Thomas, British orthopaedic surgeon, 1834–1899) splint used to immobilize fractures of the leg during transportation, and for use with various types of traction (Figure T.2).

**thoracentesis** *n* aspiration of the pleural cavity.

**thoracic** *adj* pertaining to the thorax. *thoracic aorta* that portion of the descending aorta within the thorax. ⇒ Appendix 1, Figure 9. *thoracic nerves* 12 pairs of spinal nerves that do not form a plexus. They innervate the ribs, intercostal muscles and the overlying skin. In addition the 7th to the 12th spinal nerves supply the skin and muscles of the anterior and posterior abdominal wall. ⇒ Appendix 1, Figure 11.

**thoracic cage** framework of bones (ribs, sternum and vertebrae) which protects the thoracic structures and provides muscle attachments.

**thoracic cavity** the chest. Cavity above the diaphragm containing the lungs, heart, great vessels and oesophagus.

**thoracic duct** the main channel commencing in the abdomen (cisterna chyli) that conveys lymph (chyle) from the legs, abdomen, left side of the chest and head and the left arm to the left subclavian vein.

**thoracic inlet syndrome** (*syn* cervical rib) a supernumerary rib in the cervical region, which may present no symptoms or it may press on nerves of the brachial plexus.

**thoracic vertebrae** 12 bones of the vertebral column. They have facets on their transverse processes and bodies for articulation with the ribs. ⇒ Appendix 1, Figure 3.

**thoracoplasty** *n* an operation on the thorax in which the ribs are resected to allow the chest wall to collapse and the lung to rest; previously used in the treatment of tuberculosis. Since the advent of antituberculous drugs it is extremely rare.

**thoracoscope** *n* an instrument which can be inserted into the pleural cavity through a small incision in the chest wall, to permit inspection of the pleural surfaces and division of adhesions by electric diathermy—**thoracoscopic** *adj*, **thoracoscopy** *n*.

**thoracotomy** *n* surgical exposure of the thoracic cavity.

**thorax** *n* the chest cavity—**thoracic** *adj*.

**threadworm (pinworm)** *n* Enterobius vermicularis. Tiny thread-like nematode worm that infests the intestine. ⇒ enterobiasis.

**threatened abortion** ⇒ miscarriage.

**threonine** *n* an essential (indispensable) amino acid.

**threshold** *n* the level at which a stimulus produces an effect or response. ⇒ pain threshold.

**thrill** *n* vibration as perceived by the sense of touch.

**thrombectomy** *n* surgical removal of a thrombus from within a blood vessel.

**thrombin** *n* the active enzyme formed from prothrombin. Thrombin is formed during both the extrinsic and intrinsic coagulation pathways; it converts fibrinogen to fibrin. ⇒ coagulation, prothrombin, thromboplastin.

**thromboangiitis** *n* clot formation within an inflamed vessel. *thromboangiitis obliterans* ⇒ Buerger's disease.

**thromboarteritis** *n* inflammation of an artery with clot formation.

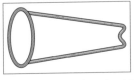

**Figure T.2** Thomas' splint (*reproduced from Brooker 2006A with permission*).

**thromboasthenia** *n* also called thrombasthenia. A decrease in platelet function. A rare inherited haemorrhagic disorder in which the platelets do not function normally in haemostasis.

**thrombocyte** *n* (*syn* platelet) functions in the coagulation of blood. ⇒ blood, platelet.

**thrombocythaemia** *n* a condition in which there is an increase in circulating blood platelets, which can encourage clotting within blood vessels. ⇒ myeloproliferative disorders, thrombocytosis.

**thrombocytopenia** *n* a reduction in the number of platelets in the blood, which can result in spontaneous bruising and prolonged bleeding after injury—**thrombocytopenic** *adj.* ⇒ idiopathic thrombocytopenic purpura (ITP).

**thrombocytosis** *n* an increase in the number of platelets in the blood. It may arise in reaction to infection, bleeding, inflammation or malignancy or may indicate the presence of a bone marrow disorder.

**thromboembolic** *adj* describes the phenomenon whereby a thrombus or clot detaches itself and is carried to another part of the body in the blood stream to block a blood vessel there. ⇒ deep-vein thrombosis, pulmonary embolus.

**thromboembolic deterrents (TEDs)** ⇒ antiembolism hosiery/stockings.

**thromboendarterectomy** *n* removal of a thrombus and atheromatous plaques from an artery.

**thromboendarteritis** *n* inflammation of the inner lining of an artery with clot formation.

**thrombogenic** *adj* capable of clotting blood—**thrombogenesis, thrombogenicity** *n,* **thrombogenically** *adv.*

**thrombokinase** *n* ⇒ thromboplastin.

**thrombolytic** *adj* pertaining to disintegration of a blood clot—**thrombolysis** *n.*

**thrombolytic therapy** the use of fibrinolytic drugs, such as alteplase, reteplase, tenecteplase and streptokinase, to dissolve preformed intravascular fibrin occlusions in acute myocardial infarction, acute arterial thrombosis, deep-vein thrombosis, pulmonary embolus and central retinal venous and arterial thrombosis.

**thrombophilia** *n* an inherited or acquired tendency to develop venous thrombosis. ⇒ factor V Leiden.

**thrombophlebitis** *n* inflammation of the wall of a vein with secondary thrombosis within the involved segment—**thrombophlebitic** *adj. thrombophlebitis migrans* recurrent episodes of thrombophlebitis affecting short lengths of superficial veins: deep-vein throm-bosis is uncommon and pulmonary embolism is rare.

**thromboplastin** *n* (*syn* thrombokinase) a substance released from damaged tissue to start the extrinsic coagulation pathway. *intrinsic thromboplastin* produced by the interaction of several factors during coagulation. It is more active than *tissue thromboplastin* (factor III) of blood coagulation, which interacts with other factors in the formation of a fibrin clot. ⇒ activated partial thromboplastin time (APTT).

**thrombopoiesis** *n* the formation of platelets from megakaryocytes in the bone marrow. The process is stimulated by cytokines, such as thrombopoietin.

**thrombosis** *n* the unwanted, intravascular formation of a blood clot—**thromboses** *pl,* **thrombotic** *adj.* ⇒ coronary thrombosis, deep-vein thrombosis.

**thromboxanes** *npl* regulatory lipids derived from arachidonic acid (fatty acid). They are released from platelets and cause vasospasm and platelet aggregation during platelet plug formation. ⇒ haemostasis.

**thrombus** *n* an intravascular blood clot—**thrombi** *pl.*

**thrush** *n* ⇒ candidiasis.

**thymectomy** *n* surgical excision of the thymus gland.

**thymic aplasia** absence of the thymus gland. ⇒ DiGeorge's syndrome.

**thymine** *n* a nitrogenous base derived from pyrimidines. With other bases, one or more phosphate groups and a sugar, it is part of the nucleic acid DNA. ⇒ deoxyribonucleic acid.

**thymocytes** *npl* cells found in the dense lymphoid tissue of the thymus gland—**thymocytic** *adj.*

**thymoma** *n* a tumour arising in the thymus—**thymomata** *pl.*

**thymopoietin** *n* peptide hormone secreted by the thymus gland.

**thymosin** *n* peptide hormone secreted by the thymus gland.

**thymus** *n* a lymphoid gland lying behind the sternum and extending upward as far as the thyroid gland. It is well developed in infancy and attains maximum size during puberty; thereafter the lymphatic tissue is replaced by fatty tissue. It produces thymic hormones (thymosins and thymopoietin) that ensure the proper development of T lymphocytes. The autoimmune condition myasthenia gravis results from pathology of the thymus gland—**thymic** *adj.*

**thyrocalcitonin** *n* ⇒ calcitonin.

**thyroglobulin** *n* a colloid stored in the thyroid follicles used for the production of thyroxine, one of the thyroid hormones.

**thyroglossal** *adj* pertaining to the thyroid gland and the tongue. *thyroglossal cyst* a retention cyst caused by blockage of the thyroglossal duct: it appears on one or other side of the neck. *thyroglossal duct* the embryonic passage from the thyroid gland to the back of the tongue. In this area thyroglossal cyst or fistula can occur.

**thyrohyoid** *n* a muscle of the throat involved in the co-ordinated events of swallowing. Its origin is on the thyroid cartilage and it inserts on to the hyoid bone.

**thyroid** *adj* pertaining to the thyroid gland.

**thyroid acropachy** periosteal hypertrophy of the digits that occurs rarely in some thyroid diseases.

**thyroid antibody test** the presence and severity of autoimmune thyroid disease are diagnosed by the levels of thyroid-stimulating immunoglobulins in the blood.

**thyroid cartilage** the main cartilage of the larynx; it has two halves, which fuse in the midline. ⇒ Appendix 1, Figure 6.

**thyroid crisis** also known as hyperthyroid crisis or thyroid storm. A very rare complication of hyperthyroidism caused by a sudden release of thyroid hormones into the blood. It is associated with infection or may occur following thyroidectomy in a patient insufficiently prepared with antithyroid drugs, or undergoing treatment with radioactive iodine. It is a life-threatening medical emergency characterized by pyrexia, tachycardia, atrial fibrillation, restlessness, confusion, agitation and possibly altered consciousness.

**thyroid gland** a two-lobed endocrine gland, either side of the trachea (Figure T.3). It secretes three hormones: triiodothyronine ($T_3$) and thyroxine ($T_4$) under pituitary control, which stimulate metabolism; and calcitonin from the follicular cells, which helps to regulate calcium and phosphate homeostasis. ⇒ hyperthyroidism, hypothyroidism.

**thyroid-stimulating hormone (TSH)** also called thyrotrophin. Pituitary hormone that stimulates the secretion of the thyroid hormones thyroxine and triiodothyronine.

**thyroid-stimulating hormone assay** radioimmunoassay of the level of thyroid-stimulating hormone in the serum. Used in the diagnosis of hypothyroidism.

**thyroidectomy** *n* surgical removal of part or all of the thyroid gland.

**thyroiditis** *n* inflammation of the thyroid gland; can occur postpartum, following viral

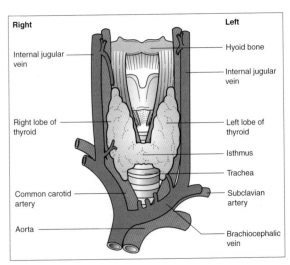

**Figure T.3** Thyroid gland *(reproduced from Watson 2000 with permission).*

infection (De Quervain's), or due to autoimmune diseases. ⇒ Hashimoto's disease, Riedel's thyroiditis.

**thyrotoxicosis** *n* ⇒ hyperthyroidism.

**thyrotrophic** *adj* (describes) any substance that stimulates the thyroid gland, e.g. thyrotrophin (thyroid-stimulating hormone [TSH]) secreted by the anterior pituitary gland.

**thyrotrophin-releasing hormone (TRH)** a hypothalamic peptide which stimulates the release of thyroid-stimulating hormone by cells in the anterior pituitary gland.

**thyroxine (T₄)** *n* the principal hormone of the thyroid gland, it contains four atoms of iodine. It is essential for metabolism and development. Used in the treatment of hypothyroidism. ⇒ triiodothyronine.

**TIA** *abbr* transient ischaemic attack.

**tibia** *n* the shin bone; the larger of the two bones in the lower part of the leg; it articulates with the femur, fibula and talus. ⇒ Appendix 1, Figures 2 and 3.

**tibial** *adj* relating to the tibia. *tibial arteries* anterior and posterior tibial arteries formed by the division of the popliteal artery, supply blood to the lower leg. *tibial nerve* a branch of the sciatic nerve, it innervates the skin and muscles of the posterior part of the leg and the sole of the foot and toes. *tibial veins* anterior and posterior tibial veins form the popliteal vein ⇒ Appendix 1, Figures 9, 10 and 11.

**tibiofibular** *adj* pertaining to the tibia and the fibula. *proximal tibiofibular joint* (also called anterior or superior tibiofibular joint) a joint between the lateral condyle of the tibia and the head of the fibula. *distal tibiofibular joint* (also called inferior tibiofibular joint) a fibrous joint between the distal ends of the tibia and fibula.

**tic** *n* purposeless involuntary, spasmodic muscular movements and twitchings, due partly to habit, but may be associated with a psychological factor.

**tic douloureux** ⇒ trigeminal neuralgia.

**tick** *n* a blood-sucking parasite, larger than a mite. Some of them are involved in the transmission of relapsing fever, typhus, etc.

**tidal volume/air (TV)** the volume of air that passes in and out of the lungs in normal breathing.

**Tietze syndrome** (A Tietze, German surgeon, 1864–1927) costochondritis. A self-limiting condition of unknown aetiology. There is no specific treatment. Differential diagnosis is myocardial infarction.

**tight junction** a junction between cells where the cell membranes are tightly bound together. It limits or prevents the movement of molecules between cells. ⇒ gap junction.

**tilt table** a standing device that can be used for patients who are unable to stand, such as those with paraplegia or quadriplegia. It can be used to position patients at any angle between horizontal and vertical.

**tincture** *n* a drug or other substance prepared in an alcoholic solution.

**tinea** *n* (*syn* ringworm) a fungal infection of the skin, hair or nails caused by a variety of dermatophytes: *Trichophyton*, *Epidermophyton* and *Microsporum*. Usually named for the area of the body affected, i.e. *tinea barbae*, the beard area; *tinea capitis*, the head; *tinea corporis* (circinata), the body; *tinea cruris* (dhobie itch), the groin; *tinea pedis*, the foot (athlete's foot); *tinea unguium*, the nails.

**Tinel's sign** (J Tinel, French neurologist, 1879–1952) a test of nerve regeneration. Tapping the area over the nerve causes tingling distal to the injury. It can also be used as a diagnostic sign in carpal tunnel syndrome.

**tinnitus** *n* an abnormal perception of buzzing, thumping or ringing sounds in the ears.

**TIPSS** *abbr* transjugular intrahepatic portasystemic stent shunting.

**tissue** *n* a collection of cells or fibres of similar function, forming a structure, often in a background stroma.

**tissue culture** cells or tissues grown in vitro and maintained artificially.

**tissue plasminogen activator (t-PA)** an endopeptidase enzyme that activates plasminogens. Produced naturally by endothelial cells lining blood vessels and other cells. Needed for fibrinolysis, the last stage of haemostasis, in which the fibrin clot is dissolved by plasmin when healing is complete. Also produced by recombinant DNA technology for use in thrombolytic therapy. *urinary plasminogen* ⇒ urokinase.

**tissue respiration** ⇒ respiration.

**tissue typing** a number of tests used to determine the degree of histocompatibility between the tissue of the donor and prospective recipient. ⇒ human leucocyte antigen, major histocompatibility complex.

**tissue viability** primarily the management of wounds, but also involves the prevention of tissue damage, protecting vulnerable skin and maintaining the health of tissue.

**T**

**titration** *n* volumetric analysis using standard solutions to determine the concentration of a substance in solution.

**titre** *n* a standard of concentration per volume, as determined by titration. Unit of measure used to assess antibody concentration in serum.

**titubation** *n* abnormal head and trunk movements when sitting, and unsteady stumbling gait.

**TIVA** *abbr* total intravenous anaesthesia.

**TLC** *abbr* total lung capacity.

**TLS** *abbr* tumour lysis syndrome.

**T lymphocyte (T cell)** ⇒ lymphocyte.

**TMJ** *abbr* temporomandibular joint.

**TNF** *abbr* tumour necrosis factor.

**TNM classification** *abbr* tumour, node (lymph) and metastasis. ⇒ staging.

**tobacco amblyopia** toxic amblyopia.

**tocography** *n* process of recording uterine contractions using a tocograph or a parturiometer. ⇒ cardiotocography.

**tocolytics** *npl* a group of drugs that relax uterine muscle. They have a restricted role in the inhibition of preterm labour. ⇒ beta (β)-adrenoceptor agonists. ⇒ Appendix 5.

**tocopherols** *npl* group of chemicals with vitamin E activity which includes the important α-tocopherols. They are widely distributed in many foods and function as important antioxidants in biological membranes.

**tocotrienols** *npl* a group of chemicals that have vitamin E activity. They have similar biological action to tocopherols but are less potent.

**Todd's paralysis** (R Todd, British physician, 1809–1860) the short-lived paralysis that can follow some types of epileptic seizure.

**togaviruses** *npl* a family of RNA viruses, they include the rubella virus and several spread by insects, such as those causing yellow fever, dengue and encephalitis.

**tokophobia** *n* morbid fear of childbirth.

**tolerable upper intake level** the maximum intake of a nutrient through foods with added nutrients or nutritional supplements that is not likely to pose the risk of being harmful to health.

**tolerance** *n* ability to endure the application or administration of a substance, usually a drug. ⇒ drug tolerance. *exercise tolerance* exercise undertaken without marked dyspnoea or pain. American Heart Association's classification of functional capacity: class I—no symptoms with ordinary effort; class II—slight disability with ordinary effort (usually subdivided into class IIa—able to carry on with normal housework under difficulty—and class IIb—cannot manage shopping or bedmaking except very slowly); class III—marked disability with ordinary effort which precludes any attempt at housework; and class IV—symptoms at rest or heart failure.

**tomography** *n* a technique of using X-rays to create an image of a specific, thin layer through the body (rather than the whole body)—**tomographic** *adj*, **tomogram** *n*, **tomograph** *n*, **tomographically** *adv*.

**tone** *n* a quality of sound, or the normal, healthy state of tension.

**tongue** *n* the mobile muscular organ situated in the mouth; it is concerned with mastication, swallowing, taste and speech. ⇒ strawberry tongue.

**tongue tie** ankyloglossia. A congenital condition in which the tongue is fixed to the floor of the mouth.

**tonic 1.** *adj* used to describe a state of continuous muscular contraction, as opposed to intermittent contraction. **2.** *n* a lay term for a medicinal product that increases general well-being.

**tonicity** *n* **1.** the normal tone or tension present in muscle. **2.** describes the effective osmotic pressure of a solution. ⇒ hyperosmolarity, hypo-osmolarity.

**tonic pupil** ⇒ Adie's pupil.

**tonofibril** *n* bundles of very fine tonofilaments present in epithelial cells. They are part of the supportive cytoskeleton of cells and are involved in intercellular contact and adhesion by converging at the desmosomes.

**tonography** *n* continuous measurement of blood, or intraocular, pressure. *carotid compression tonography* normally occlusion of one common carotid artery causes an ipsilateral fall of intraocular pressure. Used as a screening test for carotid insufficiency.

**tonometer** *n* an instrument for measuring intraocular pressure. ⇒ applanation, Goldmann tonometer.

**tonometry** *n* the measurement of pressure or tension. Usually applied to intraocular pressure (IOP).

**tonsillectomy** *n* surgical removal of the palatine tonsils.

**tonsillectomy position** the three-quarters prone position to prevent inhalation (aspiration) pneumonia and asphyxiation.

**tonsillitis** *n* inflammation of the tonsils. It is often caused by *Streptococcus pyogenes*. There is a severe sore throat, dysphagia, pyrexia, earache and enlarged lymph nodes.

**tonsilloliths** *npl* concretions arising in the body of the tonsil.

**tonsillopharyngeal** *adj* relating to the tonsils and pharynx.

**tonsils** *npl* small aggregations of lymphoid tissue located around the pharynx. Forming part of body defences, they contain macrophages and are a site for lymphocyte proliferation. There are *lingual tonsils* under the tongue, *nasopharyngeal tonsils* located on the posterior wall of the nasopharynx (called adenoids when enlarged) and the *palatine tonsils* found in the oropharynx, one on each side in the fauces between the palatine arch—**tonsillar** *adj*. ⇒ Waldeyer's ring.

**tonus** *n* muscle tone. The normal condition of partial muscle contraction controlled by reflexes.

**tooth** *n* hard calcified structures in the mouth used for masticating food. Composed largely of dentine with enamel covering the crown and cementum covering the root surface. The pulp occupies the cavity at the core of the crown (pulp chamber) and the channel running along the length of the root (root canal) (Figure T.4A)—**teeth** *pl*. There are four basic types: incisor, canine, premolar, molar (Figure T.4B). ⇒ canine, Hutchinson's teeth, incisor tooth, molar tooth, premolar tooth, teeth, wisdom tooth.

**tooth buds** the embryonic teeth. The deciduous teeth by 6 weeks' gestation and those of the permanent teeth by week 10.

**tooth drifting** the migration of teeth from their normal position in the dental arches.

**TOP** *abbr* termination of pregnancy.

**tophus** *n* a small, hard concretion forming on the ear lobe, on the joints of the phalanges, etc. in gout—**tophi** *pl*.

**topical** *adj* describes the local application of drugs to skin and mucous membrane—**topically** *adv*.

**topography** *n* a description of the regions of the body—**topographical** *adj*, **topographically** *adv*.

**torpor** *n* **1.** decreased response to a stimulus. **2.** physical or mental inactivity.

**torsion** *n* twisting, for example *torsion of the testis* twisting of the structures supporting the testis. The blood supply is disrupted and can result in testicular infarction.

**torticollis** *n* (*syn* wryneck) a painless contraction of one sternocleidomastoid muscle. The head is slightly flexed and drawn towards the contracted side, with the face rotated over the other shoulder.

**torulosis** *n* ⇒ cryptococcosis.

**total-body irradiation (TBI)** a treatment used in the treatment of some cancers, e.g. haemopoietic tissue. Usually carried out before a haemopoietic stem cell transplantation.

**total burn surface area (TBSA)** a formula for predicting outcomes after a burn injury: 100 − (age + TBSA) = percentage chance of surviving. ⇒ Lund and Browder's charts, rule of nines.

**total fertility rate (TFR)** a fertility rate expressed as the average number of children per woman. ⇒ fertility rate.

**total intravenous anaesthesia (TIVA)** general anaesthetic produced with intravenous drugs only and no gases.

**total lung capacity (TLC)** the volume of air in the lungs after the greatest inspiratory effort.

**total parenteral nutrition (TPN)** ⇒ parenteral nutrition.

**total quality management (TQM)** a whole-organization approach to quality where all employees are expected to take responsibility for quality. It aims to ensure quality at every interface and improve effectiveness and flexibility throughout the organization.

**Tourette's syndrome** also known as Gilles de la Tourette syndrome. A disorder characterized by involuntary grimaces, tics, arm movements and shouting, and the use of obscene language (coprolalia) and rude gestures.

**tourniquet** *n* an apparatus for the compression of the blood vessels of a limb. Designed for compression of a main artery to control bleeding. It is also often used to obstruct the venous return from a limb and so facilitate the withdrawal of blood from a vein. Tourniquets vary from a simple rubber band to a pneumatic cuff.

**Townsend index** composite index of deprivation in the population. Sum of the standardized values of the percentages of households without cars, households not owner-occupied, overcrowded and unemployed in an electoral ward. The components (socioeconomic variables) are drawn from census information. ⇒ Jarman.

**toxaemia** *n* a generalized poisoning of the body by the products of bacteria or damaged tissue—**toxaemic** *adj*.

**toxic** *adj* poisonous, caused by a poison.

**toxic epidermal/epidermolytic necrolysis (TEN)** also known as Lyell's syndrome or non-staphylococcal scalded-skin syndrome. A condition that usually occurs in adults in

**T**

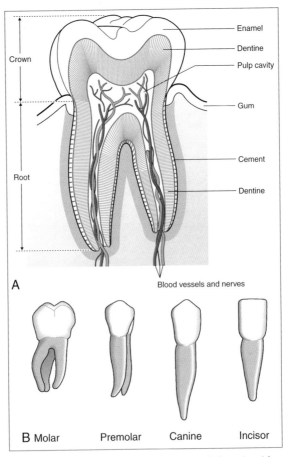

**Figure T.4** (A) Structure of a tooth. (B) Shapes of permanent teeth *(reproduced from Waugh & Grant 2006 with permission).*

response to an adverse drug reaction. There is erythema and hyperpigmentation, the formation of bullae and scaling, which gives the appearance of scalded skin. ⇒ staphylococcal scalded-skin syndrome. ⊙DVD

**toxic shock syndrome (TSS)** (*syn* tampon shock syndrome) a potential but rare complication of tampon use which also occurs in non-menstruating women and men. It is caused by the toxins of the bacterium *Staphylococcus aureus* found at various sites, including the perineal area in healthy people. Bacterial contamination of the tampon occurs and the bacteria multiply within the vagina. The bacterial toxins enter the blood stream and cause pyrexia, headache, vomiting and diarrhoea, rash, and sometimes life-threatening hypovolaemic shock.

**toxicity** *n* the quality or degree of being poisonous.

**toxicology** *n* the science dealing with poisons, their mechanisms of action and antidotes to them—**toxicological** *adj.* **toxicologically** *adv.*

**toxin** *n* a poison, for example bacterial toxin that damages or kills cells, or a chemical. ⇒ endotoxin, exotoxin.

**Toxocara** *n* genus of nematode roundworm of the dog and cat, e.g. *Toxocara canis, T. cati.* Humans can be infested. ⇒ toxocariasis.

**toxocariasis** *n* also known as visceral larva migrans. Infestation with *Toxocara*. Infestation occurs by eating with hands contaminated from contact with affected animals, especially puppies. The ova can exist for several months in soil contaminated by infected faeces from dogs or cats. Because the worms cannot develop properly in humans (incorrect host) the larvae move through the body before dying. This can lead to problems in the skin, liver and the eye: rashes, skin irritation, fever, hepatomegaly and possible blindness.

**toxoid** *n* a toxin altered in such a way that it has lost its poisonous properties but retained its antigenic properties. *toxoid antitoxin* a mixture of toxoid and homologous antitoxin in floccule form, used as a vaccine, e.g. in immunization against diphtheria.

**Toxoplasma** *n* a genus of protozoon, e.g. *Toxoplasma gondii*. It is an intracellular parasite and the definitive host is the domestic cat: other felines and rodents are the intermediate host. It can cause serious infections in humans and other mammals, e.g. sheep. ⇒ toxoplasmosis.

**toxoplasmosis** *n* infection with *Toxoplasma gondii*. Infected animals contaminate the environment with faeces containing cysts. Human infection occurs through environmental contact, such as gardening, playing and cleaning cat litter trays, by contacting infected animals or by eating undercooked meat. Most infections are symptomless or may cause a mild non-specific illness with tiredness and myalgia. However, it can be more serious with pyrexia and lymphadenopathy, with complications that include myocarditis. There is serious disease in immunocompromised individuals, e.g. acquired immunodeficiency syndrome (AIDS) patients, who develop encephalitis and eye involvement. It is possible to be infected from a donated organ during transplant surgery. Primary toxoplasmosis during pregnancy can lead to the disease being passed to the fetus via the placenta. This is extremely serious and can lead to stillbirth or an infant with problems such as microcephaly or hydrocephaly,

convulsions, or liver damage, thrombocytopenia and purpura or eye involvement. Infants who survive may have a learning disability and develop encephalitis, liver cirrhosis and blindness.

**t-PA** *abbr* tissue plasminogen activator.

**TPHA** *abbr Treponema pallidum* haemagglutination assay.

**TPN** *abbr* total parenteral nutrition.

**TQM** *abbr* total quality management.

**trabeculae** *npl* the septa or fibrous bands projecting into the interior of an organ, e.g. the spleen—**trabecula** *sing*, **trabecular** *adj.*

**trabeculectomy** *n* operation used in glaucoma to reduce intraocular pressure by creating a drainage channel from the anterior chamber of the eye to the subconjunctival space.

**trabeculoplasty** *n* various laser-assisted procedures used in glaucoma to reduce intraocular pressure. It involves the modification of the trabecular meshwork in order to improve drainage of aqueous fluid.

**trabeculotomy** *n* operation for congenital glaucoma. Creation of a channel from the scleral venous sinus (canal of Schlemm) into the anterior chamber.

**trace elements** elements that are present in very small amounts in the tissues and known to be essential for normal metabolism. For example: chromium (Cr) appears to be involved with insulin activity; cobalt (Co), utilized as vitamin $B_{12}$; copper (Cu), needed for many enzymes, e.g. superoxide dismutase, cytochrome oxidase and the production of neuropeptides and amines, e.g. enkephalins, catecholamines; fluorine (F), a constituent of bone and teeth such as calcium fluorapatite; iodine (I), a constituent of the thyroid hormones thyroxine ($T_4$) and triiodothyronine ($T_3$); manganese (Mn), a component of many enzymes, e.g. superoxide dismutase, and involved in the activation of other enzymes, e.g. kinases; molybdenum (Mo), needed for enzymes involved in the metabolism of DNA; selenium (Se), needed for the enzyme glutathione peroxidase.

**tracer** *n* a substance or instrument used to gain information. Radioactive tracers are used in the diagnosis of some cancers, e.g. brain, and thyroid disease.

**trachea** *n* (*syn* windpipe) the fibrocartilaginous tube lined with ciliated mucosa passing from the larynx to the bronchi (⇒ Appendix 1, Figure 6). It is about 115 mm long and 25 mm wide—**tracheal** *adj.*

**tracheitis** *n* inflammation of the trachea; most commonly the result of a viral infection such as the common cold.

**trachelorrhaphy** *n* operative repair of a uterine cervical laceration.

**tracheobronchial** *adj* pertaining to the trachea and the bronchi.

**tracheobronchitis** *n* inflammation of the trachea and bronchi. ⇒ bronchitis.

**tracheo-oesophageal** *adj* pertaining to the trachea and the oesophagus.

**tracheo-oesophageal fistula** a congenital defect that often occurs in conjunction with oesophageal atresia. The fistula usually connects the distal oesophagus to the trachea.

**tracheostomy** *n* surgical opening between the front of the neck and the trachea to create an artificial airway. It is kept open with a tracheostomy tube (Figure T.5). A tracheostomy may be short- or long-term. It may be performed for a variety of reasons, including: to bypass an obstruction in the upper airway; for long-term mechanical ventilation; to facilitate tracheobronchial suction when sputum is retained; to prevent the aspiration of secretions; following head and neck surgery; and in situations where laryngeal reflexes are absent, such as after brain injury or stroke—**tracheostome** *n*.

**tracheotomy** *n* vertical slit in the anterior wall of the trachea at the level of the third and fourth cartilaginous rings. Undertaken to access the airway below an obstruction caused by swelling or a foreign body. It may be performed as an emergency both in hospital and in the community.

**trachoma** *n* an eye disease caused by infection with *Chlamydia trachomatis*, which is transmitted by flies. It is common in communities with sparse water and therefore poor facial hygiene. It is characterized by a chronic, scarring, follicular conjunctivitis which may lead to corneal scarring and blindness. Infection occurs through contact, during birth, when a baby may become infected from vaginal secretions, or from unhygienic use of personal articles. Also called trachoma inclusion conjunctivitis (TRIC)—**trachomatous** *adj*.

**traction** *n* a drawing or pulling on the patient's body to overcome muscle spasm and to reduce or prevent deformity. A steady pulling exerted on some part (limb or head) by means of weights, pulleys and cords in conjunction with a variety of splints or frames. *skeletal traction* applied on a bone by means of a wire or pin passed through the lower fragment. *skin traction or extension* involves the application of weights to foam or extension plaster attached

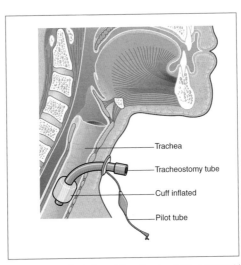

**Figure T.5** Cuffed tracheostomy tube *(adapted from Brooker & Nicol 2003 with permission)*.

to the skin. ⇒ beam, Braun's frame, Bryant's gallows traction, hoop traction, halopelvic traction, Kirschner wire, Steinmann's pin, Thomas' splint.

**tractotomy** n incision of a nerve tract. Surgical relief of intractable pain, using stereotactic measures.

**tragus** n the projection in front of the external auditory meatus/canal—**tragi** pl.

**traife** n items of food that do not comply with the dietary laws of Judaism. ⇒ kosher.

**trait** n an individual physical or mental characteristic which is inherited or develops.

**training** n in sports medicine describes a deliberate scheme or programme to assist learning and/or improve fitness. The four principles of training are: specificity, individual differences, overload and reversibility. Training programmes will vary depending on the nature of the sport or activity being trained for and the goals to be achieved.

**TRAM flap** acron **t**ransverse **r**ectus **a**bdominis **m**yocutaneous flap.

**trance** n a term used for hypnotic sleep and for certain self-induced hysterical stuporous states.

**tranquillizers** npl drugs that relieve anxiety or deal with psychotic symptoms without excessive sedation. ⇒ anxiolytics, antipsychotic drugs (neuroleptics). ⇒ Appendix 5.

**transabdominal** adj through the abdomen—**transabdominally** adv.

**transactional analysis** a form of psychotherapy based on the theory that interrelationships between people can be analysed in terms of transactions with each other as representing 'child', 'adult' and 'parent'. The aim is to give the adult ego decision-making power over the child and parent egos.

**transaminases** npl ⇒ aminotransferases.

**transamniotic** adj through the amniotic membrane and fluid, such as a transamniotic transfusion of the fetus for haemolytic disease.

**transcervical resection of endometrium (TCRE)** a hysteroscopic procedure of removing the endometrium in cases of menorrhagia.

**trans configuration** means on the opposite side. In chemistry, describes an isomerism in which the two substituent groups are on the opposite side of a carbon-carbon double bond. ⇒ cis configuration, trans fatty acids.

**transcription** n first stage in protein synthesis where genetic information is transferred from DNA to mRNA. ⇒ translation.

**transcutaneous** adj through the skin, for example monitoring, e.g. oxygen saturation by pulse oximetry, or drug absorption.

**transcutaneous electrical nerve stimulation (TENS)** a method of non-invasive pain control using pads placed either side of the spine to apply a mild electric current from a battery-operated device, which can be controlled by the patient for pain relief. Used with good effect by women during labour, and in the control of chronic pain symptoms.

**transdermal** adj through the skin. A drug administration system using patches, creams and gels. Thus drugs delivered in this way, e.g. hormone replacement, avoid first-pass metabolism/first-pass effect in the liver.

**transducer** n device that converts one form of energy into another to facilitate its electrical transmission.

**transduction** n the process by which genetic material (DNA) is transferred from one bacterium to another by a bacteriophage (a parasitic virus of bacteria).

**transection** n the cutting across or mechanical severance of a structure.

**trans fatty acids** npl stereoisomers of cis fatty acids formed during food processing, such as those produced by the hydrogenation of oils during the manufacture of margarine and other fats. They appear to have the same adverse effects on health as saturated fats, thus food manufacturers are reducing or eliminating them from foods.

**transfer RNA (tRNA)** ⇒ ribonucleic acid.

**transferable skills** particular skills—academic, problem solving, interpersonal, practical, etc.—that can be transferred to new or different situations.

**transferase** n an enzyme that catalyses the transfer of chemical radicals or groups between molecules, such as aminotransferases.

**transference** n in psychotherapy or psychoanalysis, the unconscious transfer of a client's emotions regarding a significant person, usually a person from childhood such as a dominant parent, to the therapist. countertransference the unconscious or conscious emotional reaction of therapist to client.

**transferrin** n a plasma protein that has a high affinity for ferric iron. It binds the iron and transports it around the body in the blood.

**transformation** n the process by which genetic material (DNA) is transferred from one bacterium to another through the cell wall.

**transformation zone** ⇒ squamocolumnar junction.

**transforming growth factor (TGF)** a cytokine produced by some T cells.

485

**transfrontal** *adj* through the frontal bone; an approach used for hypophysectomy.

**transfusion** *n* the introduction of fluid into the tissue or into a blood vessel. *blood transfusion* the intravenous replacement of lost or destroyed blood by compatible citrated human blood. Also used for severe anaemia with deficient blood production. Fresh blood from a donor or stored blood from a blood bank may be used. It can be given whole, or as plasma-depleted blood (packed-cell transfusion). If incompatible blood is given, severe reaction follows. ⇒ blood groups. *intrauterine transfusion* can be used from about 20 weeks' gestation for a fetus endangered by Rhesus incompatibility. Red cells may be administered by intraperitoneal transfusion, but increasingly intravascular transfusion is possible with the development of more advanced ultrasound equipment. One or more transfusions may be needed. This enables the induction of labour to be postponed until a time more favourable to fetal survival.

**transient flora** the micro-organisms that are present on a host for a short period. They colonize the superficial layers of the skin and health care workers acquire them during contact with patients, contaminated equipment or the environment.

**transient ischaemic attack (TIA)** a brief loss of neurological function as a result of a disturbance of blood supply that lasts for minutes to hours. Depending on the site involved there may be visual and speech disturbances, numbness, dizziness and weakness.

**transillumination** *n* the transmission of light through the sinuses for diagnostic purposes.

**transitional cell carcinoma** a malignant tumour of the transitional epithelium of the urinary tract (urothelium) present in the urethra, bladder, ureters and the renal pelvis.

**transjugular intrahepatic portasystemic stent shunting (TIPSS)** a stent placed between the hepatic portal vein and the hepatic vein in the liver to reduce hepatic portal pressure by providing a shunt between the hepatic portal and systemic circulations. Performed to prevent further bleeding from oesophageal varices.

**translation** *n* the second stage of protein synthesis in which tRNA and rRNA translate the base sequences required to make a new polypeptide. ⇒ transcription.

**translocation** *n* transfer of a chromosomal segment to a different site on the same chromosome (shift) or to a different chromosome. Can be a cause of several congenital abnormalities.

**translucent** *adj* in between transparent and opaque.

**translumbar** *adj* through the lumbar region. Route used for injecting contrast medium into the aorta prior to aortography.

**transmethylation** *n* a process in which methyl groups are donated by amino acids and transferred to other compounds.

**transmigration** *n* ⇒ diapedesis.

**transmural** *adj* through the wall, e.g. of an organ, etc. For example, a transmural myocardial infarction that extends from the epicardium to the endocardium—**transmurally** *adv*.

**transmyocardial revascularization** a laser technique used to increase the blood supply to the myocardium and reduce anginal pain by creating a series of tiny channels from the subepicardial surface to the endothelium. It may be a treatment option for patients with severe angina in whom angioplasty or coronary artery bypass surgery is not appropriate.

**transnasal** *adj* through the nose—**transnasally** *adv*.

**transoesophageal echocardiography** ⇒ echocardiography.

**transonic** *adj* allowing the passage of ultrasound.

**transperitoneal** *adj* across or through the peritoneal cavity. ⇒ dialysis, laparoscopy.

**transplacental** *adj* through the placenta, such as the exchange of substances between maternal and fetal blood—**transplacentally** *adv*.

**transplant** *n* customarily refers to the surgical operation of grafting an organ which has been removed from a person who has been declared brain-dead, or from a living relative. If the recipient's malfunctioning organ is removed and the transplant is placed in its bed, this is referred to as an *orthotopic transplant* (e.g. liver and heart). If the transplanted organ is not placed in its normal anatomical site the term *heterotopic transplant* (e.g. a kidney) is used—**transplantation** *n*, **transplant** *vt*. **transplantation** *n* ⇒ graft.

**transposition** *n* **1.** the movement of genetic material from one chromosome to another. Associated with various congenital abnormalities. **2.** an embryonic developmental abnormality in which a structure is located on the right side of the body when it is normally on the left or vice versa. *transposition of the great vessels* a congenital anomaly in which the pulmonary artery arises from the left ventricle and the aorta from the right ventricle.

**transpulmonary pressure** the difference between intrapleural pressure and alveolar pressure.

**transrectal** *adj* through the rectum.

**transrectal ultrasonography (TRUS)** method used to perform an ultrasound examination of the prostate gland—**transrectally** *adv*.

**trans-sexualism** *n* a condition in which individuals feel intensely uncomfortable with their biological gender and wish to live as the opposite sex. They may cross-dress, but some will eventually have hormonal modification and surgery. Extensive counselling is required before any medical or surgical treatment is undertaken.

**trans-sphenoidal** *adj* through the sphenoid bone; an approach used for hypophysectomy.

**transthoracic** *adj* across or through the chest, as in transthoracic needle biopsy of a lung mass, or transthoracic echocardiography. ⇒ echocardiography.

**transudate** *n* a fluid that has passed out of the cells into a body cavity (e.g. ascitic fluid in the peritoneal cavity); it contains few cells and only small amounts of protein. ⇒ exudate.

**transudation** *n* the movement of fluid through a membrane or cell boundary.

**transurethral** *adj* through the urethra.

**transurethral resection of prostate (TUR, TURP)** the procedure whereby prostatic tissue is resected from within the urethra using electric cautery. ⇒ prostatectomy, resectoscope.

**transurethral vaporization of the prostate (TUVP)** a minimally invasive technique used to reduce the effects of benign prostatic enlargement. An electric current vaporizes the prostate gland using an electrode passed through a resectoscope.

**transvaginal** *adj* through the vagina—**transvaginally** *adv*.

**transvaginal ultrasound** ultrasound examination of the pelvic structures using a vaginal probe. It produces higher-resolution images than the use of a transabdominal probe. Used in assisted conception techniques, in early pregnancy and to examine the uterus and ovaries.

**transventricular** *adj* through a ventricle. Term used mainly in cardiac surgery—**transventricularly** *adv*.

**transverse colon** the part of the colon between the right colonic (hepatic) flexure and the left colonic (splenic) flexure. ⇒ Appendix 1, Figure 18B.

**transverse plane** a horizontal plane that divides the body into superior and inferior parts. Also called the horizontal plane (Figure T.6).

**transverse rectus abdominis myocutaneous (TRAM ) flap** a flap from the abdominal wall muscle, which is used in breast reconstruction following mastectomy.

**transvesical** *adj* through the urinary bladder—**transvesically** *adv*.

**transvestism** *n* cross-dressing in clothes of the opposite gender.

**trapezium** *n* one of the carpal bones of the wrist. It articulates with other carpal bones, scaphoid and trapezoid, and the first and second metacarpal bones.

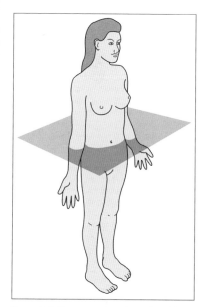

**Figure T.6** Transverse plane *(reproduced from Hinchliff et al. 1996 with permission).*

**trapezius** *n* large muscle of the neck and thorax. ⇒ Appendix 1, Figures 4 and 5.

**trapezoid** *n* one of the carpal bones of the wrist. It articulates with the scaphoid bone, and the second metacarpal bone.

**trauma** *n* bodily injury—**traumatic** *adj.* ⇒ Abbreviated Injury Scale, advanced trauma life support, post-traumatic stress disorder.

**traumatologist** *n* a doctor or nurse who specializes in traumatology.

**traumatology** *n* the branch of medicine dealing with injury—**traumatological** *adj,* **traumatologically** *adv.*

**Treacher Collins syndrome** (E Treacher Collins, British ophthalmologist, 1862–1932) a form of mandibulofacial dysostosis inherited as an autosomal dominant trait. It is characterized by slanting eyes, microtia, poorly developed facial bones and micrognathia.

**treatment** *n* methods of curing, minimizing or controlling the effects, or preventing a disease, disorder or injury. *conservative treatment* using drugs, rest, exercise or diet rather than surgery or other drastic means. *curative treatment* measures aimed at complete cure. *palliative treatment* the measures taken to control symptoms such as pain, without hope of cure. *prophylactic treatment* measures taken to prevent disease, such as taking antibiotics after exposure to an infectious disease, or immunization. *radical treatment* measures aimed at complete cure, which may for example involve extensive surgery, radiotherapy and drugs.

**Trematoda** *n* a class of parasitic flukes which include many human pathogens of the blood, hepatobiliary system, the lungs and the intestine, such as the *Schistosoma* of schistosomiasis.

**tremor** *n* rhythmic movement disorder that can affect any part of the body, typically the hands, and which can be seen in Parkinson's disease. *intention tremor* a type of tremor that becomes manifest as the hand approaches the target, typically seen in disease of the cerebellum.

**trench foot** (*syn* immersion foot) occurs in frostbite or other conditions of exposure when local blood supply is impaired and secondary bacterial infection is present.

**Trendelenburg's position** (F Trendelenburg, German surgeon, 1844–1924) lying on an operating or examination table, with the head lower than the pelvis and the legs raised. It is used for varicose vein surgery and pelvic surgery.

**Trendelenburg's sign** (F Trendelenburg) a test of the stability of the hip, and particularly of the ability of the hip abductors (gluteus medius and minimus) to steady the pelvis upon the femur. Normally, when one leg is raised from the ground the pelvis tilts upwards on that side, through the hip abductors of the standing limb. If the abductors are inefficient (e.g. in poliomyelitis, severe coxa vara and developmental dysplasia of the hip), they are unable to sustain the pelvis against the body weight and it tilts downwards instead of rising.

**trephine** *n* an instrument with sawlike edges for removing a circular piece of tissue, such as the cornea or skull.

**Treponema** *n* a genus of slender spiral-shaped bacteria that are actively motile. Best visualized with dark-ground illumination. Cultivated in the laboratory with great difficulty. *Treponema carateum* causes pinta; *T. pallidum* causes syphilis; *T. pertenue* causes yaws.

**Treponema pallidum haemagglutination assay (TPHA)** *n* a specific serological test for syphilis and other treponemal diseases.

**treponematosis** *n* any treponemal diseases.

**treponemicide** *n* lethal to *Treponema*—**treponemicidal** *adj.*

**trespass against the person** a general term that covers any interference with the person's bodily integrity and liberty, it includes assault and battery. ⇒ assault, battery.

**Trexler isolator** a flexible-film, negative-pressure, bed isolator for dangerous infections such as viral haemorrhagic disease.

**TRH** *abbr* thyrotrophin-releasing hormone.

**triacylglycerol** *n* triglyceride.

**triad** *n* a group of three. *portal triad (tract)* a branch of the hepatic artery, a branch of the hepatic portal vein and a small bile duct.

**triage** *n* a system of priority classification of casualties in any emergency situation.

**Triatoma** *n* a genus of blood-sucking bugs of the family Reduviidae. They act as vectors for the protozoon *Trypanosoma cruzi* which causes Chagas' disease, a form of trypanosomiasis, present in South America.

**TRIC** *abbr* trachoma inclusion conjunctivitis. ⇒ trachoma.

**triceps brachii** *n* the three-headed (long, lateral and medial heads) muscle on the back of the upper arm. Its three origins are one on the scapula and two on the humerus and it inserts by a long single tendon on to the olecranon process of the ulna. It contracts to extend the forearm and adduct the arm. ⇒ Appendix 1, Figures 4 and 5.

**trichiasis** *n* abnormal ingrowing eyelashes.

*Trichinella* *n* a genus of parasitic nematode worms, e.g. *Trichinella spiralis*, a parasite of pigs and rats that causes human disease. ⇒ trichinosis.

**trichinosis** *n* also called trichiniasis. Caused by eating undercooked pork infected with *Trichinella spiralis* (the trichina worm). The female worms in the small intestine produce larvae which invade the body and, in particular, form cysts in skeletal muscles; usually causes diarrhoea, nausea, colicky pain, fever, facial oedema, muscle pains and stiffness.

**trichobezoar** *n* a mass of hair present in the stomach. Individuals may swallow their own hair, or animal hair. ⇒ bezoar.

**trichoglossia** *n* 'hairy tongue', associated with fungal infection.

**trichology** *n* the study of hair and the scalp, and related diseases.

**trichomonacide** *n* an agent that is lethal to the protozoa belonging to the genus *Trichomonas*.

*Trichomonas* *n* a genus of motile protozoan parasites; e.g. *Trichomonas vaginalis* causes vaginitis in females and urethral infection in males. The organism is easily recognized by wet microscope preparations of the discharge. ⇒ trichomoniasis.

**trichomoniasis** *n* inflammation of the vagina (urethra in males) caused by the protozoan *Trichomonas vaginalis*.

**trichomycosis** *n* fungal disease affecting the hair.

*Trichophyton* *n* a genus of fungi affecting the skin and nails. ⇒ dermatophytes, tinea.

**trichophytosis** *n* infection with a species of the fungus *Trichophyton*, e.g. ringworm of the hair or skin.

*Trichosporon* *n* a genus of fungi. ⇒ piedra.

**trichotillomania** *n* an impulsive disorder in which individuals pull out their hair. It may be a feature of some learning disabilities.

**trichromatic** *adj* pertaining to normal colour vision; having cones with the three visual pigments that respond to bright light of green, blue or red wavelength.

**trichuriasis** *n* infestation with *Trichuris trichiura*. Infestation occurs from ingesting contaminated soil or food. Usually produces few symptoms but heavy infestation may cause blood-stained diarrhoea, abdominal pain and sometimes anaemia if blood loss is severe.

*Trichuris* *n* a genus of nematode worms. *Trichuris trichiura* (whipworm) common in hot, humid regions. ⇒ trichuriasis.

**tricuspid** *adj* having three cusps. *tricuspid valve* the right atrioventricular valve of the heart.

**tricyclic antidepressants (TCA)** a group of antidepressant drugs, e.g. amitriptyline. They act by inhibiting the uptake of the neurotransmitters serotonin (5-hydroxytryptamine) and noradrenaline (norepinephrine). ⇒ Appendix 5.

**tridactyly** *n* a congenital absence of digits. There are only three on a hand or foot.

**trigeminal** *adj* triple; separating into three sections, e.g. the trigeminal nerve, the fifth cranial nerve, which has three branches, ophthalmic, maxillary and mandibular.

**trigeminal neuralgia** also known as tic douloureux. Spasms of sudden, excruciating pain in the distribution of the trigeminal nerve. Although the pain may soon pass, it can be repeated rapidly over several hours. The location of pain depends on the branch of the nerve involved, but it may be the forehead, around the eye; the nose, upper lip and cheek; or the lower lip and jaw. Various activities can trigger an attack and include touching or moving the face and mouth, such as during eating and talking, or cold air blowing on the face. It usually affects people aged over 50 years and more women are affected than men.

**trigeminy** *n* a group of three. Often applied to abnormal heart rhythms in which the arrhythmia occurs in groups of three, such as two ectopic beats followed by a normal beat.

**trigger finger** a condition in which the finger can be actively bent but cannot be straightened without help; usually due to tenosynovitis of the flexor tendon sheath resulting in thickening or nodules which prevent free gliding.

**trigger point** a hypersensitive fibrous band of tissue.

**triglyceride** *n* triacylglycerol or neutral fat. A lipid with three fatty acids and a glycerol molecule. Forms the fat deposits of the body within the cytoplasm of the adipocytes (fat cells) in adipose tissue and is the major source of stored energy.

**trigone** *n* a triangular area, especially applied to the bladder base, bounded by the two ureteral openings at the back and the urethral opening at the front—**trigonal** *adj*.

**trigonocephaly** *n* a congenital malformation that results in a skull with a sharp angulation

**T**

present on the forehead; there is defective closure of the suture between the two parts of the frontal bone.

**triiodothyronine (T₃)** *n* a thyroid hormone that is involved in the regulation of growth, development and in maintaining the body's metabolic processes. It contains three iodine atoms and is more active than thyroxine from which it is formed.

**trimester** *n* a period of 3 months. Applied especially to the first, second and third trimesters of pregnancy.

**triose** *n* a monosaccharide containing three carbon atoms, such as glyceraldehyde.

**triple response** the triple response of Lewis. A three-part response to skin injury: redness caused by vasodilation of arterioles and venules; increased capillary permeability caused by the release of inflammatory chemicals results in a wheal as fluid leaks from the capillaries into the tissues; and lastly a more generalized flare occurs when adjacent arterioles dilate, which is initiated by a local axon reflex.

**triple test** blood test offered to some pregnant women at 15–18 weeks' gestation. It measures three markers—alphafetoprotein (AFP), unconjugated oestriol and total human chorionic gonadotrophin (hCG)—in maternal serum and is used in conjunction with maternal age to predict the estimated risk of conditions such as Down's syndrome and neural tube defects. Further diagnostic tests are offered if the results indicate that the risk is high, e.g. typically 1 in 250 for Down's syndrome. ⇒ amniocentesis, chorionic villus sampling, nuchal thickness scanning.

**triple vaccine** contains diphtheria, tetanus and pertussis antigens (DTaP). Offered as part of a routine immunization programme.

**triplet** *n* **1.** one of three infants resulting from a single pregnancy. **2.** the three sequential bases in a molecule of deoxyribonucleic acid or ribonucleic acid, which code for a specific amino acid in the synthesis of a polypeptide chain. ⇒ codon.

**triploid** *adj* possessing three chromosomal sets (3n). ⇒ diploid, genome, haploid, polyploidy.

**triquetral** *n* one of the proximal carpal bones of the wrist. It is situated between the pisiform and lunate bones.

**trismus** *n* spasm in the muscles of mastication such as that occurring in tetanus.

**trisomy** *n* a type of aneuploidy. The presence of three chromosomes where normally they

would be paired. Results in an increase in the chromosome number by one (single trisomy), e.g. to 47 in humans. For example, *trisomy* 13 ⇒ Patau's syndrome. *trisomy* 18 ⇒ Edward's syndrome. *trisomy* 21 ⇒ Down's syndrome. ⇒ aneuploidy, monosomy, polyploidy.

**trocar** *n* a pointed rod which fits inside a cannula.

**trochanters** *npl* two processes, the larger one (greater *trochanter*) on the outer, the other (lesser *trochanter*) on the inner side of the femur between the neck and shaft; they provide attachment for muscles—**trochanteric** *adj*.

**trochlea** *n* any part which is like a pulley in structure or function—**trochlear** *adj*.

**trochlear nerves** the fourth pair of cranial nerves. They innervate the extraocular/extrinsic muscle that moves the eyeball in an outwards and downward direction.

**trochoid joint** a pivot joint.

**Troisier's sign** (C Troisier, French pathologist, 1844–1919) ⇒ signal node.

**Trombiculidae** *n* a family of mites that include harvest mites. They act as vectors for diseases, including scrub typhus.

**trophic** *adj* pertaining to nutrition.

**trophoblast** *n* cells covering the embedding ovum and concerned with the nutrition of the ovum, invasion of the endometrium and secretion of human chorionic gonadotrophin (hCG)—**trophoblastic** *adj*.

**tropia** *n* manifest strabismus. May be used as a suffix.

**tropical sprue** chronic malabsorption of unknown aetiology occurring in residents or visitors to tropical regions.

**tropomyosin** *n* one of the proteins located in the thin filaments of a muscle myofibril.

**troponin** *n* one of the proteins present in a muscle myofibril. ⇒ cardiac enzymes.

**Trousseau's sign** (A Trousseau, French physician, 1801–1867) a test for latent tetany. Spasm of the forearm muscle is observed within 3–4 minutes of inflating a cuff on the upper arm to a pressure above the systolic blood pressure. ⇒ carpopedal spasm, Chvostek's sign.

**truncal ataxia** unco-ordinated movements of the postural muscles of the trunk.

**truncus** *n* main part of an anatomical structure, such as a vessel, from which smaller branches arise.

**truncus arteriosus** an early embryonic structure that opens from both primitive ventricles;

it will become the pulmonary artery and the aorta.

**TRUS** *abbr* transrectal ultrasonography.

**trypanocide** *n* a drug that kills trypanosomes.

***Trypanosoma*** *n* a genus of parasitic protozoa. Their life cycle alternates between blood-sucking arthropods and vertebrate hosts. A limited number of species are pathogenic to humans. ⇒ trypanosomiasis.

**trypanosomiasis** *n* disease caused by infection with *Trypanosoma*. In Africa these include: *Trypanosoma rhodesiense* or *T. brucei gambiense*. Both are transmitted by the bite of infected tsetse flies. The disease caused by *T. brucei gambiense* is usually chronic. Central nervous system involvement causes headache, confusion, insomnia, daytime sleepiness and eventually coma and death. ⇒ sleeping sickness. Infection with *T. rhodesiense* is more acute, with myocarditis, hepatitis, pleural effusion and central nervous system involvement that leads to coma, tremors and death. In South America, trypanosomiasis is also known as Chagas' disease. It is caused by *T. cruzi* transmitted by bugs. ⇒ *Triatoma*.

**trypsin** *n* active proteolytic enzyme. ⇒ trypsinogen.

**trypsinogen** *n* inactive precursor of trypsin secreted by the pancreas. It is activated by enterokinase (enteropeptidase) in the intestine.

**tryptophan** *n* one of the essential (indispensable) amino acids necessary for growth. It is a precursor of serotonin. Nicotinamide is synthesized from tryptophan.

**TSE** *abbr* testicular self-examination.

**tsetse fly** a fly of the genus *Glossina*, the vector of *Trypanosoma* in Africa. The *Trypanosoma* are transferred to new hosts, including humans, in the salivary juices when the fly bites for a blood meal.

**TSH** *abbr* thyroid-stimulating hormone.

**TSS** *abbr* toxic shock syndrome.

**T-suppressor cell** ⇒ suppressor T cell.

**Tsutsugamushi disease** scrub typhus. ⇒ rickettsial fevers, typhus.

**TTTS** *abbr* twin-to-twin transfusion syndrome.

**tubal** *adj* pertaining to a tube. *tubal abortion* ⇒ miscarriage.

**tubal ligation** tying of both uterine (fallopian) tubes as a means of sterilization.

**tubal pregnancy** ⇒ ectopic pregnancy.

**tubercle** *n* **1.** a small rounded prominence, usually on bone. Often used interchangeably with tuberosity. **2.** the specific lesion produced by *Mycobacterium tuberculosis*.

**tuberculide, tuberculid** *n* a small lump. Metastatic manifestation of tuberculosis, producing a skin lesion, e.g. papulonecrotic tuberculide, rosacea-like tuberculide.

**tuberculin** *n* a sterile extract of tuberculoprotein. Utilized in skin testing for tuberculosis or in some cases before administration of bacille Calmette–Guérin (BCG) immunization. ⇒ Heaf test, Mantoux test.

**tuberculoid** *adj* resembling tuberculosis. One of the two types of leprosy.

**tuberculoma** *n* a caseous tubercle, usually large, its size suggesting a tumour.

**tuberculosis (TB)** *n* chronic granulomatous infection caused by *Mycobacterium tuberculosis* (human type). Immunization with bacille Calmette–Guérin (BCG) is used to protect vulnerable individuals. ⇒ BCG. Tuberculosis (TB) causes systemic effects such as pyrexia, night sweats, anorexia and weight loss, plus site-dependent signs and symptoms, e.g. cough and purulent sputum in lung disease (pulmonary TB), haematuria in renal TB and infertility if the uterine tubes are affected. A diagnosis of pulmonary TB is made on clinical signs, chest X-ray, biopsy, skin tests (e.g. Heaf, Mantoux) and the presence of acid-fast bacilli in cultures of sputum or gastric washings. However, treatment is started ahead of culture results if clinical signs and histology are indicative of TB. In the UK treatment is with a combination of antituberculosis drugs in two distinct phases, initial and continuation. Four drugs are used in the initial phase: rifampicin, ethambutol, isoniazid and pyrazinamide, for a period of 2 months. Rifampicin and isoniazid are used during the continuation phase for another 4 months. The incidence, especially of multidrug-resistant tuberculosis (MDR-TB), is increasing in Asia, Africa and Eastern Europe, in association with poverty and homelessness, and in those who are immunocompromised. Bovine tuberculosis (caused by *Mycobacterium bovis*) is endemic in cattle and transmitted to humans when they drink infected milk. Pasteurization of milk and monitoring of dairy herds are the mainstays of disease control. *M. avium intracellulare (MAI)* is an atypical mycobacterium, which may infect severely immunocompromised individuals (such as those with advanced acquired immunodeficiency syndrome [AIDS]). *miliary tuberculosis* is so called because of the appearance of many small areas resembling millet seeds on the chest X-ray. There is widespread disease with dissemination of tubercle bacilli in

**T**

the blood. It can affect bone, spleen, liver and the meninges. *primary tuberculosis* occurs during childhood and there is lung involvement, fever and skin rash. *postprimary tuberculosis* the most common form of pulmonary TB but other sites may be affected—**tubercular, tuberculous** *adj*.

**tuberosity** *n* a bony prominence, such as that of the humerus. Often used interchangeably with tubercle.

**tuberous sclerosis** (*syn* epiloia) also known as Bourneville's disease. An inherited autosomal dominant disorder characterized by cognitive defects, skin lesions and epilepsy. There may also be gum hyperplasia, changes in the basal nuclei, tumour formation and retinal changes.

**tubo-ovarian** *adj* pertaining to or involving both uterine tube and ovary, e.g. tubo-ovarian abscess.

**tubule** *n* a small tube. *collecting tubule* straight tube in the kidney medulla conveying urine to the renal pelvis. *convoluted tubule* coiled tube in the kidney cortex. *renal tubule* part of a nephron. *seminiferous tubule* coiled tube in the testis.

**tularaemia** *n* (*syn* deer-fly fever, rabbit fever, tick fever) an infection of mammals, including wild rabbits, domestic cats and dogs, and birds caused by the Gram-negative bacterium *Francisella tularensis*; it occurs in the northern hemisphere and is transmitted by bites from ticks and flies. Humans acquire the infection either from ticks or from handling infected animal carcasses, such as rabbits. Skin ulceration at the inoculation site is followed by painful lymphadenopathy and fever with constitutional upset. It can be acquired by the inhalation of infected material that leads to pulmonary tularaemia and pneumonia. An infrequent presentation is conjunctivitis with ulceration. Rarely it causes septicaemia. Treatment is with an aminoglycoside antimicrobial drug, gentamicin or streptomycin—**tularaemic** *adj*.

**tumescence** *n* a state of swelling; turgidity. Usually due to oedema, or the collection of blood in the part.

**tumor** *n* swelling; usually used in the context of being one of the five classical signs and symptoms of inflammation, the others being calor, dolor, loss of function and rubor.

**tumour** *n* a swelling. A mass of abnormal tissue which resembles the normal tissues in structure, but which fulfils no useful function and which grows at the expense of the body. Benign, simple or innocent tumours are encapsulated, do not infiltrate adjacent tissue or cause metastases and are unlikely to recur if removed—**tumorous** *adj*. *malignant tumour* not encapsulated, infiltrates adjacent tissue and causes metastases. ⇒ cancer.

**tumour-infiltrating lymphocyte** lymphocytes found in solid cancers; when cultured in interleukin-2 they exhibit specific activity against the cancer from which they originated.

**tumour lysis syndrome (TLS)** may occur following intensive chemotherapy treatment for some haematological malignancies. As cancer cells are destroyed there is release of cellular breakdown products. This results in metabolic problems (e.g. hyperkalaemia, hypocalcaemia, hyperuricaemia, hyperphosphataemia) that may cause renal failure and possibly circulatory and respiratory failure.

**tumour marker** chemical detected in the serum that may be associated with a specific cancer or sometimes non-malignant diseases. They include: alphafetoprotein (AFP), cancer cell surface antigen 125 (CA-125), carcinoembryonic antigen (CEA), human chorionic gonadotrophin (hCG), pancreatic oncofetal antigen (POA) and prostate-specific antigen (PSA). They may be used for monitoring disease progress and efficacy of treatment, but are of limited use for population screening.

**tumour necrosis factor (TNF)** a cytokine that is toxic to cancer cells and activates other leucocytes. It causes profound metabolic effects that include inflammatory responses, pyrexia and weight loss leading to cachexia.

**tumour-specific antigen** an antigen produced by specific cancer cells, but that is not present on non-cancerous cells in the tissue from which the cancer was derived.

**tunica** *n* a lining membrane; a coat. *tunica adventitia* the outer fibrous coat of an artery, arteriole or vein. *tunica albuginea* the inner fibrous tissue covering of the testis; it is beneath the tunica vaginalis. It dips down into the glandular substance of the testis to form septa that divide the substance of the testis into many wedge-shaped lobules. *tunica intima* the smooth endothelial (squamous epithelium) lining of an artery, arteriole or vein. *tunica media* the middle smooth muscle and elastic tissue coat of an artery and arteriole; the tunica media of veins is thinner with less muscle and elastic tissue. *tunica vaginalis* the outer, double membrane covering the testis; it is derived from the pelvic and abdominal peritoneum during embryonic development when the testes are within the abdomen. *tunica vasculosa* a network of connective tissue and capillaries within the testis.

**tunnel vision** the loss of the peripheral part of the visual field. It may be indicative of primary open-angle glaucoma (POAG). The onset of POAG is insidious and, because central vision remains intact, patients may fail to discern the peripheral loss of vision. Occasionally patients suffer more bumps and scrapes because of visual field loss, which they erroneously attribute to ageing.

**TUR/TURP** *abbr* transurethral resection of prostate.

**turbid** *adj* cloudy, not clear. Normal urine containing mucus may be turbid. However, urine may be cloudy because it contains abnormal substances, e.g. protein, or pus and white blood cells if a urinary tract infection is present.

**turbinate** *adj* shaped like an inverted cone.

**turbinate bone** also known as nasal concha. One of three bones on either side forming the lateral nasal walls.

**turbinectomy** *n* removal of a nasal turbinate bone.

**turf toe** a colloquial expression used in sports medicine to describe the sprain and subsequent inflammation of the first metatarsophalangeal joint.

**turgid** *adj* swollen; firmly distended, as with blood by congestion—**turgescence** *n*, **turgidity** *n*.

**turgor** *n* indicates the elasticity and resilience of the skin; these are influenced by the amount of fluid in the cells and the interstitial spaces. Skin turgor decreases with age, but it can be useful as part of a holistic assessment of the state of hydration. Skin turgor is assessed by lifting a fold of skin, usually on the back of the hand. On release, it should quickly return to its original position. During normal ageing the skin loses elasticity and takes longer to return to its original position in older people. Reduced turgor may be an early sign of dehydration. Conversely the presence of oedema will increase turgor: the skin is tight and shiny and cannot be lifted.

**Turner's syndrome** (H Turner, American endocrinologist, 1892–1970) a chromosomal abnormality affecting around 1 in 2500/3000 females who have a single sex chromosome, the X, and thus they have one less chromosome than normal. The karyotype is usually XO with a total of only 45 chromosomes, but there may be mosaic forms (e.g. XO/XX). The condition is characterized by multiple abnormalities, which include webbed neck, low-set ears, abnormal facial structure, short stature, cubitus valgus, shield chest, aortic coarctation and other cardiovascular abnormalities. There may be some degree of learning disability and spatial processing defects are common. There is infantile genital development and underdeveloped breasts; the ovaries are almost completely devoid of germ cells and there is failure of pubertal development. Affected women are at risk of poor bone mineral density, hypertension and type 2 diabetes.

**tussis** *n* a cough.

**TUVP** *abbr* transurethral vaporization of the prostate.

**TV** *abbr* tidal volume/air.

**twins** *npl* one of two infants resulting from a single pregnancy. ⇒ binovular, conjoined twins, dichorionic twins, monoamniotic twins, monochorionic twins, monozygotic, uniovular.

**twin-to-twin transfusion syndrome (TTTS)** ⇒ fetofetal transfusion syndrome.

**tylosis** *n* ⇒ keratosis.

**tympanic** *adj* pertaining to the tympanum.

**tympanic cavity** the cavity of the middle ear, containing the three ossicles.

**tympanic light reflex** a reflection of light shining on the tympanic membrane. Normally this is seen as a cone of bright light in the anteroinferior segment of the tympanic membrane.

**tympanic membrane** the eardrum. It separates the outer ear from the middle ear and transmits sound vibrations to the ossicles. Most of the tympanic membrane comprises three layers—an epithelial lining continuous with the external auditory meatus/canal, a fibrous layer which provides strength and the ability to vibrate, and a mucosal layer that is continuous with that of the middle ear. The three layers are present in the lower four-fifths of the tympanic membrane, known as the pars tensa. The fibrous layer is absent in the upper tympanic membrane, known as the pars flaccida.

**tympanic thermometer** accurate core body temperature recorded by means of an electronic probe introduced into the external auditory meatus/canal.

**tympanites, tympanism** *n* (*syn* meteorism) abdominal distension due to accumulation of gas in the intestine.

**tympanoplasty** *n* reconstructive operation on the middle ear designed to improve hearing or prevent otorrhoea in ears damaged by chronic suppurative otitis media—**tympano-plastic** adj.

**tympanum** n the cavity of the middle ear.

**type I error (α error)** in research, rejecting a null hypothesis that is true.

**type II error (β error)** in research, not rejecting a null hypothesis that is false.

**typhlitis** n inflammation of the caecum.

**typhoid fever** an infectious enteric fever usually spread by contamination of food, milk or water supplies with *Salmonella typhi*, either directly by sewage, indirectly by flies or by poor personal hygiene. Symptomless carriers harbouring the micro-organism in the gallbladder and excreting it in faeces are the main source of outbreaks of disease in the UK. The average incubation period is 10–14 days. A progressive febrile illness with a 'stepladder' rise in temperature marks the onset of the disease, which develops as the micro-organism invades lymphoid tissue, including the spleen and that of the small intestine (Peyer's patches), to produce profuse diarrhoeal (pea soup) stools which may become frankly haemorrhagic due to bowel ulceration. The bowel can perforate. Patients may have a slow pulse, headache, drowsiness, delirium and a cough. A rose-coloured rash may appear on the upper abdomen and back at the end of the first week. Ultimate recovery usually begins at the end of the third week. Immunization is available for travellers to regions where sanitation is poor and the infection is endemic, and for laboratory staff, but it is not a substitute for meticulous personal hygiene measures. ⇒ paratyphoid.

**typhoid vaccine** a capsular polysaccharide vaccine for intramuscular administration and a live attenuated vaccine for oral administration.

**typhus** n a group of acute infectious diseases. The presentation varies between types but generally includes sudden onset of high fever, a skin eruption (maculopapular or petechial, depending on type), lymphadenopathy, severe headache, weakness, cough, bronchitis and limb pains. In severe infections there may be pneumonia, haemorrhage, renal failure and heart failure. It is a disease of war, famine or catastrophe, being spread by lice, ticks, mites or fleas. It is only sporadic in the UK. ⇒ rickettsial fevers.

**tyramine** n a monoamine derived from the amino acid tyrosine that is present in several foodstuffs and beverages, especially mature cheese, red wine, ripe fruit, broad beans, fermented foods, e.g. tofu and soy sauce, meat and yeast extracts. It has a similar effect in the body to adrenaline (epinephrine) and causes an increase in systemic blood pressure. It is normally metabolized by the enzyme monoamine oxidase in the wall of the intestine and in the liver; consequently patients taking drugs in the monoamine oxidase inhibitor (MAOI) group, such as some antidepressants, should not eat foods containing tyramine such as cheese, otherwise a dangerously high blood pressure may result.

**tyrosinaemia** n an aminoacidopathy resulting from abnormal metabolism of tyrosine and the build-up of toxic metabolites caused by a specific enzyme deficiency; there are several types: **1.** neonatal tyrosinaemia, in which there is a transitory inability to metabolize tyrosine, especially in preterm infants. It results in increased levels in the blood and increased excretion of tyrosine and its metabolites in the urine (aminoaciduria). **2.** type I tyrosinaemia is inherited as an autosomal recessive trait. It is due to a deficiency of the enzyme fumarylacetoacetate hydrolase. This is the most severe type and leads to liver and kidney damage. It may be acute, with symptoms occurring soon after birth. The infant fails to thrive, there is a cabbage-like odour, diarrhoea and vomiting, jaundice, liver damage, liver failure and death without a successful liver transplant. The chronic form occurs later during childhood and is characterized by delays in achieving developmental milestones, renal tubular malfunction, chronic liver disease and polyneuropathy. **3.** type II tyrosinaemia is inherited as an autosomal recessive trait in which the enzyme tyrosine aminotransferase is deficient. There are hyperkeratotic lesions on the palms and soles and affected individuals have photophobia, excessive tearing and eye pain. A learning disability is often present. **4.** type III tyrosinaemia, an autosomal dominant condition which occurs much less commonly, is caused by the lack of the enzyme 4-hydroxyphenylpyruvate dioxygenase. Affected individuals have a learning disability and experience seizures and intermittent problems with co-ordination and balance.

**tyrosine** n a conditionally essential (indispensable) amino acid required for growth. Combines with iodine to form the hormone thyroxine. If phenylalanine intake is restricted, as in phenylketonuria (PKU), the diet needs to be supplemented with tyrosine.

**tyrosinosis** n abnormal metabolism of tyrosine. Usually known as tyrosinaemia.

# U

**ubiquinone** *n* formerly known as coenzyme Q. A quinone derivative that acts as an electron carrier in the mitochondrial respiratory chain (electron transport chain).

**ulcer** *n* destruction of either mucous membrane or skin from whatever cause, producing a crater or indentation. An inflammatory reaction occurs and if it penetrates a blood vessel bleeding ensues. If the ulcer is in the lining of a hollow organ it can perforate through the wall. ⇒ arterial ulcer, leg ulcer, peptic ulcer, pressure ulcer, venous ulcer.

**ulcerative** *adj* pertaining to or of the nature of an ulcer.

**ulcerative colitis** superficial inflammatory condition affecting the colon. It always involves the rectum and spreads continuously for a variable distance. It is characterized by diarrhoea containing blood, passage of mucus and pus, pain, loss of weight and anaemia. Complications include severe inflammation, perforation of the bowel, haemorrhage, fistulae, fluid and electrolyte imbalance, toxic dilatation (megacolon) and colorectal cancer. Systemic complications include liver disease, iritis, arthralgia, mouth ulcers, gallstones, etc. ⇒ colitis, inflammatory bowel disease.

**ulcerative gingivitis** ⇒ acute necrotizing ulcerative gingivitis, necrotizing ulcerative periodontitis.

**ulcerogenic** *adj* capable of producing an ulcer.

**Ullrich syndrome** (O Ullrich, German paediatrician, 1894–1957) ⇒ Noonan's syndrome.

**ulna** *n* the inner bone of the forearm. It articulates with the humerus at the elbow, the carpals at the wrist and with the radius at the proximal and distal radioulnar joints. ⇒ Appendix 1, Figure 2.

**ulnar** *adj* pertaining to the ulna. *ulnar artery* the artery running down the medial aspect of the forearm that carries blood to muscles of the forearm and wrist. It crosses the wrist to become the superior palmar arch of the hand. *ulnar nerve* a branch of the brachial plexus, it innervates the muscles on the medial aspect of the forearm and those of the palm, and some of the skin of the digits. ⇒ cubital tunnel external compression syndrome. *ulnar vein* one of the deep veins of the forearm. ⇒ Appendix 1, Figures 9 to 11.

**ultradian** *adj* pertaining to a biological rhythm that has a cycle of less than 24 hours. ⇒ circadian.

**ultrafiltration** *n* filtration under pressure, e.g. in haemofiltration, where the blood is filtered under pressure.

**ultrasonic** *adj* relating to mechanical vibrations of very high frequency.

**ultrasonography (sonography)** *n* formation of a visible image from the use of ultrasound. A controlled beam of sound is directed into the relevant part of the body. The reflected ultrasound is used to build up an electronic image of the various structures of the body (Figure U.1). ⇒ transrectal ultrasonography, ultrasound. Routinely offered during pregnancy to monitor progress and detect fetal and placental abnormalities. *diagnostic ultrasonography* information is derived from echoes which occur when a controlled beam of sound energy crosses the boundary between adjacent tissues of differing physical properties. *real-time ultrasonography* an ultrasound imaging technique involving rapid pulsing to enable continuous viewing of movement to be obtained, rather than stationary images—**ultrasonograph** *n*, **ultrasonographically** *adv*.

**ultrasound** *n* sound waves with a frequency of over 20 000 Hz, not audible to the human ear.

**ultraviolet (UV) rays** short-wavelength electromagnetic rays outside the visible spectrum.

**umbilical cord** the cord connecting the fetus to the placenta. It contains a vein and two arteries and a gelatinous embryonic connective tissue called Wharton's jelly (Figure U.2).

**umbilical cord blood stem cells** stem cells harvested from blood taken from the umbilical cord or the placenta soon after birth. The stem cells, which will only produce blood cells, are stored and subsequently used in haemopoietic stem cell transplantation for a variety of conditions, including some types of leukaemia.

**umbilical hernia** ⇒ hernia.

**umbilicated** *adj* having a central depression.

**umbilicus, omphalus** *n* (*syn* navel) the abdominal scar left by the separation of the remnant of umbilical cord after birth—**umbilical** *adj*.

**unciform bone** ⇒ hamate.

**uncinate** *adj* hook-shaped, or having hooks. *uncinate epilepsy* a variant of temporal lobe epilepsy involving the uncinate area in which the person experiences olfactory and gustatory hallucinations.

**unconscious** *adj* **1.** unresponsive to stimuli. **2.** that part of the mind comprising the instincts, feelings, emotions and experiences of which the person is not normally aware.

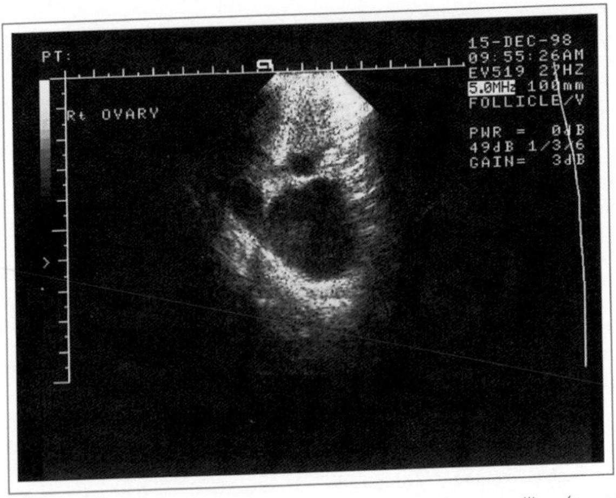

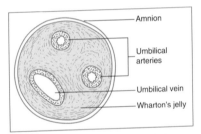

**Figure U.1** Ultrasound image showing a right-sided 6-cm cyst ovarian swelling *(reproduced from Gangar 2001 with permission).*

**Figure U.2** Umbilical cord (cross-section) *(reproduced from Fraser & Cooper 2003 with permission).*

Although such feelings are not easily recalled they may influence behaviour.

**unconsciousness** *n* state of being unconscious; insensible. ⇒ Glasgow Coma Scale.

**underclass** *n* a group who are deprived, disenfranchised and marginalized in society, such as rough sleepers.

**underwater seal** a type of drainage whereby a tube exiting from the chest is placed under water (the seal) to prevent air entering the chest. The underwater seal drain may be used to remove air, blood or other fluids from the pleural cavity. ⇒ haemothorax, pneumothorax.

**undine** *n* a small glass flask with a spout that produces a fine stream of liquid; used for irrigating the eye.

**undulant fever** brucellosis.

**unexplained underperformance syndrome (UUPS)** also known as overtraining syndrome, sports fatigue syndrome, staleness, etc. In sports medicine, a decline in performance lasting for more than 2 weeks despite sufficient recovery.

**ungual** *adj* pertaining to the fingernails and toenails.

**unguentum** *n* ointment.

**unguis** *n* a nail.

**unicellular** *adj* consisting of only one cell, such as a bacterium.

**unilateral** *adj* relating to or on one side only— **unilaterally** *adv*.

**unilateral neglect** also called spatial neglect. It is recognized by a person's failure to respond, integrate or use stimuli from one side of the body or the surroundings. May occur after brain injury when it affects the side contralateral to the brain injury.

**uniocular** *adj* pertaining to, or affecting, one eye.

**union** *n* healing; restoration of continuity, as in the healing of a fractured bone.

**uniovular** *adj* (*syn* monovular) pertaining to one ovum, as uniovular twins (identical, same-sex). ⇒ binovular *opp.*

**unipara** *n* a woman who has borne only one child. ⇒ primipara—**uniparous** *adj*.

**unipolar** *adj* having a single pole. Also describes a neuron that has a single process.

**unipolar disorder** a disorder of mood that is characterized by repeated episodes of depression. ⇒ bipolar affective disorder, depression.

**unit cost** an average cost for a specific activity, for example a surgical procedure, an investigative procedure, or a home visit. It is calculated by dividing the total cost of the service by the number of outputs.

**univariate statistics** descriptive statistics that analyse one variable, such as frequency distributions.

**universal precautions** the routine infection control precautions taken during contact, or the possibility of contact, with blood and body fluids, such as wearing gloves or using eye protection. The aim is to prevent the transmission of blood-borne viruses such as hepatitis B and C. These infection control activities are now part of standard precautions. ⇒ infection, standard precautions.

**unstable lie** in obstetrics, the lie of a fetus that changes between longitudinal, oblique or transverse after 36 weeks' gestation. Causes include placenta praevia, contracted pelvis, polyhydramnios.

**upper respiratory tract infection (URTI)** the upper respiratory tract is the commonest site of infection in all age groups. The infections include rhinitis (usually viral), sinusitis, tonsillitis, adenoiditis, pharyngitis, otitis media and croup (laryngitis), often involving the tonsils and cervical lymph nodes. Such infections seldom require hospital treatment, but epiglottitis can be rapidly fatal.

**UPPP** *abbr* uvulopalatopharyngoplasty.

**urachus** *n* the stem-like structure connecting the bladder with the umbilicus in the fetus; after birth it becomes a fibrous cord situated between the apex of the bladder and the umbilicus, known as the median umbilical ligament—**urachal** *adj*.

**uracil** *n* nitrogenous base derived from pyrimidines. With other bases, one or more phosphate groups and a sugar, it is part of the nucleic acid RNA. ⇒ ribonucleic acid.

**uraemia** *n* azotaemia. A syndrome in which endogenous waste products, including urea and other nitrogenous substances, accumulate in the blood, accompanied by disturbance of electrolytes and acid–base balance. It is caused by severely impaired renal function or renal failure, which may be due to renal disease, or to conditions such as systemic inflammatory response syndrome. It leads to a number of symptoms, particularly nausea, vomiting, headache, lethargy, altered taste, hiccups, anorexia, pruritus, visual problems, cardiac arrhythmias, altered consciousness and seizures. Renal replacement therapy such as haemodialysis may be required—**uraemic** *adj*.

**urataemia** *n* the presence of urates in the blood.

**urate** *n* any salt of uric acid.

**uraturia** *n* the excretion of urates in the urine.

**urea** *n* the main nitrogenous end-product of protein metabolism; produced in the liver, it is excreted in the urine.

**urea breath test** a non-invasive diagnostic test for the presence of *Helicobacter pylori* in the stomach.

**urea cycle** the biochemical reactions occurring in the liver in which the ammonia derived from the metabolism of amino acids is detoxified through conversion to urea by the addition of carbon and oxygen from carbon dioxide.

*Ureaplasma urealyticum* *n* a bacterium of the genus *Ureaplasma*. Commonly found in the genitourinary system of women and men where it may be asymptomatic. One of the micro-organisms responsible for non-gonococcal urethritis.

**urease** *n* bacterial enzyme that splits urea.

**ureter** *n* the tube passing from each kidney to the bladder for the conveyance of urine (⇒ Appendix 1, Figures 19 and 20); its average length in an adult is 25–30 cm. It comprises an outer fibrous layer, a middle layer of smooth muscle, which contracts to produce the peristaltic movements by which urine passes down the tube, and a mucosal lining called urothelium—**ureteric, ureteral** *adj*.

**ureterectomy** *n* excision of a ureter.

**ureteritis** *n* inflammation of a ureter.

**ureterocele** *n* prolapse of the distal portion of the ureter into the bladder. It may obstruct the flow of urine and lead to ureteral dilatation and hydronephrosis.

**ureterocolic** *adj* pertaining to the ureter and colon, usually indicating anastomosis of the two structures.

**ureteroileal** *adj* pertaining to the ureters and ileum as in the anastomosis necessary in ileal conduit.

**ureterolith** *n* a calculus in the ureter.

**ureterolithotomy** *n* surgical removal of a stone from a ureter.

**ureterolysis** *n* surgical technique of freeing encased ureters.

**U**

**ureteroneocystostomy** *n* reimplantation of the ureters; usually as treatment for vesicoureteric reflux. Also known as ureterocystoneostomy, ureterocystostomy, ureterovesicostomy. ⇒ Leadbetter–Politano operation.

**ureteronephrectomy** *n* surgical excision of the ureter and kidney. Also called nephroureterectomy.

**ureteroplasty** *n* a plastic operation on the ureter, such as that to relieve a stricture.

**ureteroscope** *n* a fibreoptic endoscope that can be used to examine the ureters and renal pelvis, and to remove stones. ⇒ nephroscope.

**ureteroscopy** *n* endoscopic visualization of the ureters.

**ureterosigmoidostomy** *n* operation to implant a ureter into the sigmoid colon.

**ureterostomy** *n* the formation of a permanent fistula through which the ureter discharges urine. ⇒ cutaneous, ileal conduit.

**ureterotomy** *n* surgical incision into a ureter.

**ureterovaginal** *adj* pertaining to the ureter and vagina.

**ureterovesical** *adj* pertaining to the ureter and urinary bladder.

**urethra** *n* the passage that drains urine from the bladder to the outside at the external urinary meatus; in the vestibule in females and the glans penis in males (⇒ Appendix 1, Figure 19). The female urethra is straight and approximately 4–5 cm in length. The male urethra, which has several curves and is surrounded by the prostate gland, is around 20–25 cm in length. Additionally the male urethra transports semen during ejaculation. The urethra has two muscular sphincters: an internal and external sphincter. The urethral muscle layer is formed from smooth muscle with elastic tissue at its junction with the bladder; this forms an internal muscular sphincter under the control of autonomic nerves. Further down the urethra it changes to skeletal muscle, which forms the external sphincter and is under voluntary control once continence is achieved during childhood. In addition there is a submucosal layer and a mucosal lining, which is continuous with the urothelium of the bladder in the upper part but changes to stratified squamous epithelium in the lower part—**urethral** *adj*.

**urethral caruncle** *n* prolapse of urethral mucosa at the external urinary meatus in women. It is prone to bleeding.

**urethral dilatation** the use of instruments to dilate the urethra narrowed by stricture.

**urethral syndrome** symptoms of urinary infection, although the urine is sterile when withdrawn by catheter.

**urethritis** *n* inflammation of the urethra from any cause, but usually caused by a bacterial or viral infection. Commonly part of infection affecting the bladder or the kidneys. It is characterized by dysuria and with some infections (e.g. gonorrhoea) a purulent discharge. *nonspecific urethritis* ⇒ non-gonococcal urethritis.

**urethrocele** *n* prolapse of the urethra, usually into the anterior vaginal wall.

**urethrography** *n* radiological examination of the urethra. Can be an inclusion with cystography, either retrograde (ascending) or during micturition—**urethrographic** *adj*, **urethrogram** *n*, **urethrograph** *n*, **urethrographically** *adv*.

**urethrometry** *n* measurement of the urethral lumen using a urethrometer—**urethrometric** *adj*, **urethrometrically** *adv*.

**urethroplasty** *n* any reconstructive operation on the urethra.

**urethrorrhaphy** *n* repair of the urethra, such as after an injury.

**urethrorrhoea** *n* abnormal discharge from the urethra; mucus or pus.

**urethroscope** *n* an instrument designed to allow visualization of the interior of the urethra—**urethroscopic** *adj*, **urethroscopy** *n*, **urethroscopically** *adv*.

**urethrostomy** *n* a surgical procedure in which the urethra is opened in the perineum in men.

**urethrotomy** *n* incision into the urethra; usually part of an operation for urethral stricture.

**urethrotrigonitis** *n* inflammation of the urethra and the trigone area of the urinary bladder between the ureteric openings and the urethra. ⇒ trigone.

**urgency** *n* the feeling of an immediate need to pass urine; it can lead to urge incontinence. It may be associated with a high intake of caffeine-containing drinks, diuretic drugs, detrusor muscle instability, urinary tract infection or bladder outflow obstruction, e.g. benign prostatic enlargement.

**uric acid** substance formed during purine metabolism, which is present in nucleic acids and some foods and beverages. Uric acid is excreted in the urine and may give rise to kidney stones. High levels of uric acid in the blood may be due to faulty excretion of uric acid or excessive cell breakdown, or associated with high purine intake. ⇒ gout.

**uricosuria** *n* ⇒ hyperuricuria.

**uricosuric agents** drugs that enhance renal excretion of uric acid, e.g. allopurinol. ⇒ Appendix 5.

**uridrosis** *n* excess of urea in the sweat; it may be deposited on the skin as fine white crystals (sometimes referred to as urea snow or frost).

**urinalysis** *n* physical, chemical or microbiological examination of the urine. Routine ward or clinic-based urinalysis involves checking the colour, clarity and odour of urine and testing with reagent strips for pH, specific gravity, protein, blood, glucose, ketones, urobilinogen and bilirubin. Some reagent strips also test for the presence of nitrites and white blood cells, which may be indicative of bacteriuria and urinary tract infection. Microbiological examination is used to detect infection, blood cells, crystals or casts.

**urinary** *adj* pertaining to urine.

**urinary bladder** a muscular distensible bag situated in the pelvis (⇒ Appendix 1, Figures 16 and 19). The bladder has an outer connective tissue layer, a middle smooth muscle layer known as the detrusor muscle and a mucosal lining of transitional epithelium (urothelium), which has folds known as rugae that allow the bladder to distend as it fills with urine. It receives urine from the kidneys via two ureters and stores it until micturition occurs.

**urinary plasminogen activator** ⇒ urokinase.

**urinary system** comprises two kidneys, two ureters, one urinary bladder and one urethra. The kidneys produce urine of variable content; the ureters convey the urine to the bladder, which stores it until there is sufficient volume to elicit reflex emptying or the desire to pass urine, and it is then conveyed to the exterior by the urethra. ⇒ Appendix 1, Figures 19 and 20.

**urinary tract infection (UTI)** includes urethritis, cystitis, pyelonephritis. A common health care-associated infection. It occurs most frequently in the presence of an indwelling catheter. It is most commonly caused by a Gram-negative bacterium, such as *Escherichia coli*, suggesting that self-infection via the periurethral route is a common pathway. ⇒ bacteriuria.

**urination** *n* ⇒ micturition.

**urine** *n* the clear straw-coloured fluid excreted by the kidneys. Urine contains water, nitrogenous waste and electrolytes. Normally adults produce about 1500 mL every 24 h, but this depends on fluid intake, activity and age. Usually slightly acidic (pH 6.0), but varies between 4.5 and 8.0. Specific gravity is usually within the range 1005–1030.

**uriniferous tubule** ⇒ renal tubule.

**urinogenital** *n* ⇒ urogenital.

**urinometer** *n* an instrument for estimating the specific gravity of urine.

**urobilin** *n* a brownish pigment excreted in the faeces. Formed by the oxidation of urobilinogen.

**urobilinogen** *n* (*syn* stercobilinogen) a pigment formed from bilirubin in the intestine by bacterial action. It may be reabsorbed into the circulation and converted back to bilirubin in the liver and re-excreted in the bile or urine.

**urobilinuria** *n* the presence of increased amounts of urobilin in the urine. Evidence of increased production of bilirubin in the liver, e.g. after haemolysis.

**urocele** *n* a swelling in the scrotum caused by extravasated urine.

**urochezia** *n* the passage of urine in faeces.

**urodynamics** *n* the method used to study bladder function. ⇒ cystometry.

**urogenital** *adj* (*syn* urinogenital) pertaining to the urinary and the genital organs.

**urography** *n* radiographic visualization of the renal pelvis and ureter by injection of a contrast medium. The medium may be injected into the blood stream whence it is excreted by the kidney (intravenous urography) or it may be injected directly into the renal pelvis or ureter by way of a fine catheter introduced through a cystoscope (retrograde or ascending urography)—**urographic** *adj*, **urogram** *n*, **urographically** *adv*. intravenous urography (IVU), also called intravenous pyelography, although other structures are demonstrated. The demonstration of the urinary tract following an intravenous injection of an opaque medium.

**urokinase** *n* an endopeptidase enzyme that activates plasminogens. Produced naturally by the kidney and excreted in the urine. It is used therapeutically in vitreous haemorrhage (eye), to clear intravenous catheters, thrombosed arteriovenous shunts and other thromboembolic conditions.

**urolith** *n* a stone or calculus that forms in the urinary tract.

**urologist** *n* a medically qualified person who specializes in disorders of the female urinary tract and the male genitourinary tract.

**urology** *n* that branch of biomedical science which deals with disorders of the female urinary tract and the male genitourinary tract—**urological** *adj*, **urologically** *adv*.

**U**

**uropathy** *n* disease in any part of the urinary system.

**uroporphyrin** *n* a naturally occurring porphyrin excreted in the urine in small amounts. The excretion of excessive amounts is indicative of porphyria.

**urostomy** *n* the collective term for cutaneous ureterostomy, ileal conduit, ureterosigmoidostomy.

**URTI** *abbr* upper respiratory tract infection.

**urticaria** *n* (*syn* nettlerash, hives) skin eruption characterized by multiple circumscribed, smooth, raised, pinkish, itchy weals, developing very suddenly, usually lasting a few days and leaving no visible trace. ⊙ DVD The cause is unknown in most cases. ⇒ angioedema. *factitial urticaria* ⇒ dermographia.

**uterine** *adj* pertaining to the uterus.

**uterine arterial embolization** ⇒ embolization.

**uterine inertia** lack of contraction of parturient uterus. Weak or poorly co-ordinated contractions during labour. Can lead to prolonged labour, or haemorrhage from the placental site.

**uterine supports** muscles of the pelvic floor, the peritoneum and various ligaments; pubocervical, round, transverse cervical (Mackenrodt's or cardinal) and the uterosacral ligaments that hold the uterus in the correct anteverted and anteflexed position.

**uterine tubes** (*syn* fallopian tubes, oviducts) two tubes that extend laterally from the upper part of the uterus to open into the peritoneal cavity. Each measures 10 cm in length, but the diameter varies greatly along the length. The tube is divided into several parts: a funnel-like infundibulum ending in the finger-like projections known as fimbriae, which help to waft the oocyte from the ovary into the tube; a dilated ampulla where fertilization usually occurs; an isthmus; and an interstitial part within the uterine wall which is extremely narrow (⇒ Appendix 1, Figure 17). The wall of a tube has three layers: it is covered with and supported by part of the broad ligament known as the mesosalpinx, a middle layer of smooth muscle, which contracts to produce the peristaltic movements that assist in moving the oocyte towards the uterus, and a highly specialized, ciliated mucosal lining containing secreting cells with microvilli. Rhythmic ciliary movements move the oocyte into the uterus and the secretions help to maintain the oocyte and spermatozoa in good condition.

**uteroplacental** *adj* pertaining to the uterus and placenta.

**uterorectal** *adj* pertaining to the uterus and rectum.

**uterosacral** *adj* pertaining to the uterus and sacrum.

**uterosalpingography** *n* (*syn* hysterosalpingography) radiological examination of the uterus and uterine tubes involving retrograde introduction of an opaque medium during fluoroscopy. Used to investigate patency of uterine (fallopian) tubes. Being superseded by ultrasound examination.

**uterovaginal** *adj* pertaining to the uterus and the vagina.

**uterovesical** *adj* pertaining to the uterus and the urinary bladder.

**uterus** *n* the womb (⇒ Appendix 1, Figure 17); a hollow muscular organ into which the ovum is received through the uterine (fallopian) tubes and where it is retained during development, and from which the fetus is expelled through the vagina. The uterus is divided into the fundus (top), corpus (body) and the cervix (neck). The corpus and the cervix are divided by a narrow isthmus. The wall of the uterus has three layers—an outer layer of peritoneum known as the perimetrium, the myometrium, a middle layer of interlocking smooth muscle fibres, which form a 'living ligature' by compressing blood vessels to prevent bleeding after childbirth, and the mucosal lining, the highly vascular endometrium that contains many glands. The endometrium has two layers, the permanent stratum basalis and the stratum functionalis, which is shed each month during menstruation. ⇒ bicornuate—**uteri** *pl.* **uterine** *adj*.

**uterus didelphys** a double uterus. ⇒ bicornuate.

**UTI** *abbr* urinary tract infection.

**utilitarianism** *n* ethical theory that holds that an action should always produce more benefits than harm. It aims to provide the greatest good for the majority of individuals. ⇒ deontological.

**utricle** *n* a little sac or pocket. A fluid-filled sac in the membranous labyrinth of the inner ear. Part of the vestibular apparatus; contains the hair cells and otoliths that are concerned with static equilibrium. ⇒ saccule.

**UUPS** *abbr* unexplained underperformance syndrome.

**UV** *abbr* ultraviolet.

**uvea** *n* the uveal tract. The pigmented middle coat of the eye, comprising the iris, ciliary body and choroid—**uveal** *adj*.

**uveitis** *n* inflammation of the uvea of the eye.

**uvula** *n* the central tag hanging down from the free edge of the soft palate.

**uvulectomy** *n* excision of the uvula. Also known as staphylectomy.

**uvulitis** *n* inflammation of the uvula.

**uvulopalatopharyngoplasty (UPPP)** *n* also known as palatopharyngoplasty, uvulopalatoplasty. An operation on the soft palate and pharyngeal tissue for relief of excessive snoring and obstructive sleep apnoea (hypopnoea) syndrome.

U

**V**

**vaccination** *n* originally described the process of inoculating persons with discharge from cowpox to protect them from smallpox. Now applied to the inoculation of any antigenic material for the purpose of producing active artificial immunity.

**vaccines** *npl* suspensions or products of infectious agents, e.g. attenuated or killed micro-organisms, used chiefly for producing active immunity. ⇒ BCG, Hib vaccine, human papillomavirus, immunization, MMR, Sabin, Salk, triple vaccine, typhoid vaccine.

**vaccinia** *n* a pox virus causing disease in cattle. Used when it is necessary to provide immunity against smallpox such as in laboratory staff.

**vacuole** *n* a small cavity or space within the cytoplasm of a cell. Some types contain water, whereas others are part of the Golgi apparatus where they contain and condense cellular secretions prior to discharging them at the cell surface.

**vacuum extractor 1.** a device used to assist delivery of the fetus. ⇒ Ventouse extraction. **2.** an aspiration device used as a method of terminating a pregnancy.

**VADAS** *abbr* voice-activated domestic appliance system.

**vagal** *adj* pertaining to the vagus nerve.

**vagina** *n* literally, a sheath; the musculomembranous passage extending from the cervix uteri to the vulva; it runs backwards at an angle of 45°. The anterior wall is about 7 cm in length and is close to the urethra and bladder, and the posterior wall, which is longer, at 9 cm, is in front of the rectum and the rectovaginal pouch. Normally the vaginal walls are in apposition, but the presence of rugae (folds) allows the vagina to distend in order to facilitate coitus and childbirth. The projection of the cervix into the vagina forms four fornices (deep folds or gutters). The hymen, a perforated membrane, partially occludes the distal opening of the vagina. The vagina has an outer layer of fibrous tissue, a layer of smooth muscle, a loose areolar layer and the stratified squamous epithelial lining, which affords some protection against the trauma of childbirth. In addition, during a woman's reproductive years the vagina is acidic (pH 4.5) due to the production of lactic acid by bacteria of the *Lactobacillus* spp., which form part of the normal flora. The lactic acid produced helps protect the vagina from many pathogenic organisms. (⇒ Appendix 1, Figure 17)—**vaginal** *adj*.

**vaginismus** *n* painful muscular spasm of the vaginal walls occurring when the external genitalia are touched, such as during medical examination or sexual contact. It results in dyspareunia or painful coitus, or indeed preventing coitus in extreme cases.

**vaginitis** *n* inflammation of the vagina. It is caused by a variety of micro-organisms that include: *Chlamydia trachomatis*, *Trichomonas vaginalis*, *Gardnerella vaginalis*, *Neisseria gonorrhoeae* and yeasts, particularly *Candida albicans*. There is discharge, intense pruritus, vulval excoriation and soreness and sometimes dysuria. *atrophic vaginitis* is characterized by thinning of the vaginal mucosa and reduced acid secretions associated with the postmenopausal decrease in oestrogen secretion, which make the vagina more prone to infection. Infection with *C. albicans* is particularly common in older women. Atrophic changes affecting the vaginal mucosa may cause inflammation, dryness, itching and dyspareunia, even when infection is not present. Any associated postmenopausal bleeding must be fully investigated.

**vaginoplasty** *n* also called colpoplasty. A plastic surgical procedure undertaken on the vagina.

**vaginosis** *n* vaginal infection caused by a proliferation of commensal micro-organisms such as *Gardnerella vaginalis*.

**vagolytic** *adj*, *n* that which neutralizes the effect of a stimulated vagus nerve.

**vagotomy** *n* surgical division of the branches of the vagus nerves that innervate the stomach; done in conjunction with gastroenterostomy in the treatment of peptic ulcer, or with pyloroplasty.

**vagus nerve** the 10th cranial nerve, composed of both motor and sensory fibres, with a wide distribution in the neck, thorax and abdomen, sending important parasympathetic branches to the heart, lungs, stomach, etc.—**vagi** *pl*, **vagal** *adj*.

**valgus, valga, valgum** *adj* exhibiting angulation away from the midline of the body, e.g. hallux valgus.

**validity (external)** *n* a term that indicates the degree to which research findings can be generalized to other populations and in other settings.

**validity (internal)** *n* in research, a term that indicates the extent to which a method or test measures what it intends to measure.

**valine** *n* an essential (indispensable) amino acid.

**Valsalva manoeuvre** (A Valsalva, Italian anatomist, 1666–1723) the maximum intrathoracic pressure achieved by forced expiration against a closed glottis; occurs in such activities as lifting heavy objects, changing position and during defecation: the glottis narrows simultaneously with contraction of the abdominal muscles.

**value for money (VFM)** a means of obtaining the best quality of service within the resource allocation. It involves economy, efficiency and effectiveness.

**values** *npl* the individual and personal view of the worth of an idea or specific behaviour. Principles of living which are refined from life experiences that guide behaviour. *value systems* an accepted set of values, conduct and way of behaving in a particular social group. ⇒ beliefs, secular beliefs.

**valve** *n* a fold of membrane in a passage or tube normally permitting the flow of contents in one direction only. For example, the atrioventricular valves of the heart—**valvular** *adj*.

**valvoplasty** *n* a plastic operation on a valve, usually reserved for the heart; to be distinguished from valve replacement or valvotomy—**valvoplastic** *adj*.

**valvotomy, valvulotomy** *n* incision of a stenotic valve, by custom referring to the heart, to restore normal function.

**valvulitis** *n* inflammation of a valve, particularly in the heart.

**valvulotomy** *n* ⇒ valvotomy.

**vancomycin-resistant enterococci (VRE)** also known as glycopeptide-resistant enterococci (GRE). Enterococci such as *Enterococcus faecium* that have developed resistance to vancomycin (a glycopeptide antibiotic). ⇒ *Enterococcus*.

**vancomycin-resistant *Staphylococcus aureus* (VRSA)** strains of meticillin (methicillin)-resistant *Staphylococcus aureus* that have developed full resistance to the antibiotic vancomycin. Although the strain is sensitive to some older antibiotics and some newer drugs, this development further restricts the choice of antibiotic treatment for serious infections caused by *S. aureus*.

**van den Bergh's test** (A van den Bergh, Dutch physician, 1869–1943) estimation of serum bilirubin. Direct positive reaction (conjugated) occurs in obstructive and hepatic jaundice. Indirect positive reaction (unconjugated) occurs in haemolytic jaundice.

**vanillylmandelic acid (VMA)** a metabolite of adrenaline (epinephrine) which is excreted in the urine. The level in a 24-hour urine collection is used to assess adrenal medulla function and in the diagnosis of adrenal tumours.

**vanishing-twin syndrome** a situation in which one fetus in a twin pregnancy is reabsorbed, usually during the first trimester.

**vaporizer** *n* a device that produces a vapour containing small droplets of a drug in liquid form for inhalation. ⇒ nebulizer.

**Vaquez–Osler disease** *n* (L Vaquez, French physician, 1860–1936; W Osler, Canadian physician, 1849–1919) primary proliferative polycythaemia. ⇒ polycythaemia.

**variable** *n* a research term that describes any factor or circumstance that is part of the study. *confounding variable* one that affects the conditions of the independent variables unequally. *dependent variable* one that depends on the experimental conditions. *independent variable* the variable conditions of an experimental situation, e.g. control or experimental. *random variable* background factors such as environmental conditions that may affect any conditions of the independent variables equally.

**variance** *n* a mathematical term used in statistics. The distribution range of a set of results around the mean. ⇒ standard deviation.

**varicella** *n* ⇒ chickenpox—**varicelliform** *adj*.

**varicella-zoster immunoglobulin (VZIG)** polyclonal immunoglobulin (largely IgG) from donors exposed to varicella-zoster. Contains high concentrations of specific antibody, and used to convey passive immunity to varicella.

**varicella-zoster virus (VZV)** herpesvirus causing chickenpox (varicella) and shingles (herpes zoster).

**varices** *npl* dilated, tortuous (or varicose) veins. ⇒ oesophageal varices, varicose veins—**varix** *sing*.

**varicocele** *n* varicosity of the veins of the pampiniform plexus in the spermatic cord.

**varicose ulcer** (*syn* gravitational ulcer) ⇒ venous ulcer.

**varicose veins** dilated veins, the valves of which become incompetent so that blood flow may be reversed (Figure V.1). Most commonly found in the lower limbs where they can result in a gravitational ulcer; in the rectum, when the term 'rectal varices' (haemorrhoids) is used; and in the lower oesophagus, when they are called oesophageal varices.

**varicotomy** *n* an incision into a varix.

**variola** *n* ⇒ smallpox.

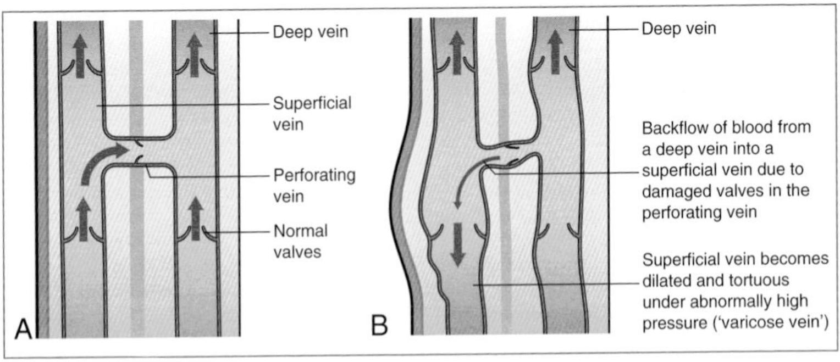

**Figure V.1** Formation of varicose veins: (A) normal veins and valves; (B) valve damage and backflow (*reproduced from Bale & Jones 1997 with permission*).

**varioloid** *n* attack of smallpox modified by previous vaccination.

**varix** *n* ⇒ varices.

**varus, vara, varum** *adj* displaying displacement or angulation towards the midline of the body, e.g. coxa vara.

**VAS** *abbr* visual analogue scale.

**vas** *n* a vessel—**vasa** *pl.*

**vasa praevia** a situation in which the umbilical blood vessels run through the membranes before inserting into the placenta (a velamentous insertion). If the placenta is sited low down in the uterus the blood vessels may be across the internal os, ahead of the presenting part. In this situation there is a high risk of damage to the vessels when the membranes rupture, resulting in fetal exsanguination.

**vasa vasorum** the minute nutrient vessels of the artery and vein walls.

**vascular** *adj* supplied with vessels, especially referring to blood vessels.

**vascularization** *n* the acquisition of a blood supply; the process of becoming vascular.

**vasculitis** *n* (*syn* angiitis) inflammation of blood vessels. May be part of a systemic disease.

**vasculotoxic** *adj* any substance or agent that causes harmful changes in blood vessels.

**vas deferens** duct carrying spermatozoa from the epididymis. ⇒ deferent duct.

**vasectomy** *n* surgical excision of all or part of the deferent duct (vas deferens), usually for male sterilization.

**vasoactive** *adj* having an effect on the diameter of blood vessels, causing vasoconstriction or vasodilation.

**vasoactive intestinal peptide (VIP)** a regulatory peptide hormone/neurotransmitter present in the hypothalamus, other areas of the brain, the intestine and pancreas. It acts to relax smooth muscle in the intestine, increases the amount of water and electrolytes in pancreatic and intestinal juices, stimulates the release of pancreatic hormones and inhibits gastric acid secretion and motility. ⇒ VIPoma.

**vasoconstriction** *n* any narrowing of the lumen of a blood vessel. Also the first stage of the four overlapping stages of haemostasis. ⇒ coagulation, fibrinolysis, platelet plug.

**vasoconstrictor** *n* any agent causing vasoconstriction.

**vasodilation** *n* widening of the lumen of a blood vessel.

**vasodilator** *n* any agent causing vasodilation.

**vasoepididymostomy** *n* anastomosis of the vas deferens to the epididymis.

**vasography** *n* radiographic demonstration of the deferent duct (vas deferens) after the introduction of contrast medium.

**vasomotor** *adj* relating to nerves and muscles that control blood vessel lumen size.

**vasomotor centre (VMC)** a centre, located in the cardiovascular centre in the medulla oblongata. Concerned with controlling lumen size of peripheral arterioles and peripheral resistance and heart rate as part of the regulation of arterial blood pressure. It operates through autonomic sympathetic nerve activity in response to baroreceptor signals. The degree of VMC activity depends on the amount of inhibition by the baroreceptors, the pressure receptors located in the carotid sinus and aortic arch.

**vasomotor symptoms** symptoms caused by vasomotor instability experienced by many women during the climacteric; typically hot flushes (flashes) and excess sweating, including night sweats.

**vasopressin** *n* antidiuretic hormone. The substance produced in the hypothalamus and stored in the posterior lobe of the pituitary gland. ⇒ antidiuretic hormone.

**vasopressor** *n* a drug which increases blood pressure, usually by constricting arterioles but not always.

**vasospasm** *n* constricting spasm of blood vessel walls—**vasospastic** *adj*.

**vasovagal** *adj* pertaining to the effects of the vagus nerve upon the vascular system.

**vasovagal reflex** stimulation of the vagus nerve that results in a rapid fall in blood pressure and heart rate. Frequently associated with the transient loss of consciousness (vasovagal syncope) caused by insufficient blood reaching the brain, pallor, nausea and sweating. May be caused by stimulation of the soft palate (gag reflex), Valsalva manoeuvre, pain or emotional episodes.

**vasovasostomy** *n* a surgical procedure to restore the patency of the deferent ducts (vas deferens), which aims to re-establish fertility; the reversal of a previous vasectomy.

**vastus** *n* one of three muscles of the fourpart quadriceps femoris muscle. *vastus intermedius* on the anterior aspect of the thigh beneath the rectus femoris muscle. *vastus lateralis* on the lateral aspect of the thigh. *vastus medialis* on the inferior medial aspect of the thigh. All three extend the knee—**vasti** *pl*.

**VBI** *abbr* vertebrobasilar insufficiency.

**VC** *abbr* vital capacity.

**vector** *n* a carrier of disease, e.g. ticks, fleas, mites, lice, mosquitoes, sandflies.

**vegan** *n* a person who excludes all animal flesh and products from the diet, so does not eat meat, fish, eggs or dairy produce. Protein is provided by nuts, grains and pulses. With careful food choices and combinations the diet can be nutritionally adequate but may be deficient in iron and vitamin $B_{12}$.

**vegetarian** *n* ⇒ lacto-ovovegetarian, lactovegetarian.

**vegetations** *npl* growths or accretions composed of fibrin and platelets occurring on the edge of the cardiac valves in infective endocarditis.

**vegetative** *adj* relating to the non-sporing stage of a bacterium.

**vehicle** *n* a substance with which a drug is mixed for administration, such as sterile water.

**vein** *n* a vessel conveying blood from the capillaries and venules back to the heart in the pulmonary and systemic circulations. It has the same basic three coats as an artery, but with some differences, including an inner coat which is modified to form valves in some veins to aid venous return to the heart—**venous** *adj*. ⇒ tunica.

**vellus hair** short downy hair found on most hair-bearing parts of the body in children and in women, except that on the scalp and the axillae and external genitalia. ⇒ lanugo, terminal hair.

**vena cava** one of two large veins emptying into the right atrium of the heart. The superior vena cava drains venous blood from the head, neck and upper limbs, and the inferior vena cava drains venous blood from structures below the diaphragm—**venae cavae** *pl*, **vena caval** *adj*. ⇒ Appendix 1, Figures 8 and 10.

**veneer** *n* in dentistry, a thin restoration that covers the surface of a tooth; usually made from composite resin or porcelain.

**venepuncture** *n* also called venipuncture. The insertion of a needle into a vein.

**venereal** *adj* pertaining to or caused by sexual intercourse. *venereal disease* ⇒ sexually transmitted infection.

**Venereal Disease Research Laboratory (VDRL) test** a non-specific serological test for syphilis.

**venereology** *n* the study and treatment of sexually transmitted infections.

**venesection** *n* (*syn* phlebotomy) a clinical procedure whereby blood is removed via venepuncture. It is used in the treatment of iron overload, e.g. haemochromatosis, and occasionally acutely for congestive heart failure.

**venography** *n* (*syn* phlebography) radiological examination of the venous system involving injection of a contrast medium. Mostly replaced by ultrasound—**venographic** *adj*, **venogram** *n*, **venograph** *n*, **venographically** *adv*.

**venom** *n* a poisonous fluid produced by some snakes, spiders and scorpions.

**venotomy** *n* incision of a vein. ⇒ venesection.

**venous** *adj* pertaining to the veins.

**venous sinus** any one of the sinuses or channels that convey venous blood from the dura

**V**

mater, or the coronary sinus which conveys venous blood from the myocardium. ⇒ coronary sinus, dural sinuses, sagittal sinuses.

**venous ulcer** (*syn* gravitational ulcer) ulcer with a venous aetiology. They usually occur close to the ankle or between ankle and knee (Figure V.2). There is often brown staining to the skin and dermatitis. Ulcers are large and shallow with large amounts of exudate. They frequently occur in people who have a history of deep-vein thrombosis or varicose veins. They are chronic wounds and can be difficult to treat effectively. ⇒ ankle–brachial pressure index (ABPI), compression therapy, larval therapy. ⊙DVD

**ventilation** *n* the supply of fresh air. Also used to describe the mechanical process of breathing. ⇒ pulmonary ventilation.

**ventilation–perfusion (V/Q) ratio** the ratio between gases in the alveoli (alveolar ventilation) and blood flow in the pulmonary capillaries (pulmonary perfusion). Homeostatic autoregulatory mechanisms normally control the ratio to ensure that gas exchange is as efficient as possible. For example, mechanisms operate to compensate for adopting an upright posture. However, differences between the apex and the base of the lung are not fully compensated by the autoregulatory mechanisms; even in healthy lungs there will be areas of lung where ventilated alveoli are not perfused and areas where poorly ventilated alveoli are perfused, which results in less efficient gas exchange. Where a substantial mismatch occurs, gas exchange is impaired and leads to the development of hypoxia and possibly hypercapnia. The mismatch may be due to alveolar underventilation (e.g. with chronic obstructive pulmonary disease) or poor blood flow in the pulmonary capillaries (e.g. after pulmonary embolus and infarction).

**ventilation–perfusion scanning** an imaging technique used in nuclear medicine to investigate lung ventilation and perfusion, such as after pulmonary embolus. The investigation has two parts; a radioactive gas (e.g. krypton [Kr-81m], xenon [Xe-133] ) is inhaled to investigate ventilation and radioactive albumin is administered intravenously to demonstrate perfusion.

**ventilator** *n* specialized equipment for mechanically inflating a patient's lungs. Used to support or replace the patient's own breathing. Known colloquially as a 'life support machine'.

**Ventouse extraction** use of the vacuum extractor in obstetrics to facilitate the delivery of the fetus.

**ventral** *adj* pertaining to the abdomen or the anterior surface of the body—**ventrally** *adv*.

**ventricle** *n* a small belly-like cavity—**ventricular** *adj*. *ventricle of the brain* four cavities filled

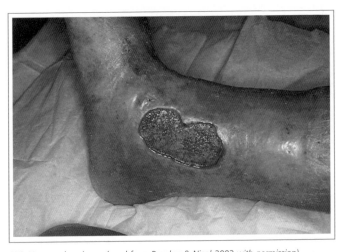

**Figure V.2** Venous ulcer *(reproduced from Brooker & Nicol 2003 with permission).*

with cerebrospinal fluid within the brain. *ventricle of the heart* the two lower muscular pumping chambers of the heart. ⇒ Appendix 1, Figure 8.

**ventricular fibrillation (VF)** a serious, life-threatening cardiac arrhythmia where unco-ordinated ventricular activity, which is characterized by fast quivering rather than contraction, fails to produce any output of blood into the circulation. Thus the person will have neither a pulse nor a blood pressure. VF occurs when abnormal foci in the ventricles fire in a completely chaotic manner. The electrocardiograph shows rapid fibrillation (Figure V.3). VF becomes a fatal arrhythmia in the absence of initial basic life support, successful defibrillation and advanced life support. A common cause of sudden death following myocardial infarction. ⇒ automated external defibrillator (AED), cardiac arrest. ⊙DVD

**ventricular septal defect (VSD)** *n* a hole or holes in the interventricular septum. Most commonly due to a congenital defect, but can also follow a myocardial infarction. VSD is the commonest congenital heart defect and accounts for 30% of defects, and can be associated with maternal rubella infection during pregnancy or Down's syndrome; it is also a feature of complex congenital heart defects, such as Fallot's tetralogy. The defect results in a left-to-right shunt of blood in the heart with a murmur, and sometimes cardiac failure in infants aged 4 to 6 weeks. Small defects may close spontaneously, but where surgical repair is indicated it is increasingly performed using percutaneous minimally invasive techniques. VSD can result in ventricular overload and hypertrophy, changes to pulmonary vascular resistance and pulmonary hypertension that lead eventually to shunt reversal and Eisenmenger's syndrome.

**ventricular tachycardia (VT)** a very serious ventricular arrhythmia characterized by a rapid ventricular rate of 140–200 beats/min. It may lead to cardiac arrest—ventricular fibrillation or pulseless ventricular tachycardia.

**ventriculitis** *n* inflammation of a ventricle. Usually refers to that affecting the cerebral ventricles in conjunction with encephalitis.

**ventriculoatrial shunt** *n* an artificial communication between the cerebral ventricles and the right atrium of the heart. Accomplished by the use of a plastic tube, which contains a pressure–flow regulator. Used to drain excess cerebrospinal fluid in hydrocephalus.

**ventriculoatriostomy** *n* ⇒ ventriculoatrial shunt.

**ventriculocysternostomy** *n* ventriculocisternal shunt. An artificial communication between the cerebral ventricles and the cisterna magna. Previously used as a drainage procedure for hydrocephalus.

**ventriculography** *n* **1.** radiographic demonstration of the cardiac ventricles following the insertion of contrast medium, or an imaging technique using a radioisotope (radionuclide). **2.** an obsolete radiographic examination of the cerebral ventricles, now replaced by computed tomography (CT) and magnetic resonance imaging (MRI) scanning.

**ventriculoperitoneal shunt** *n* an artificial communication between the cerebral ventricles and the peritoneal cavity. Accomplished by the use of a plastic tube, which contains a non-return valve. A commonly used technique for draining excess cerebrospinal fluid in hydrocephalus.

**ventriculopleural shunt** *n* an artificial communication between the cerebral ventricles and the pleural cavity. Accomplished by the use of a plastic tube, which contains a pressure-flow regulator. Used to drain excess cerebrospinal fluid in hydrocephalus.

**V**

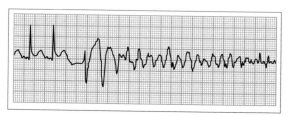

**Figure V.3** Ventricular fibrillation *(reproduced from Boon et al. 2006 with permission).*

**ventriculoscopy** *n* direct visualization of the cerebral ventricles using an endoscope.

**ventriculostomy** *n* an artificial opening into a ventricle. Usually refers to a drainage operation for hydrocephalus.

**ventriculovenous shunt** *n* an artificial communication between the cerebral ventricles and the internal jugular vein. Accomplished by the use of a plastic tube, which contains a pressure–flow regulator. Used to drain excess cerebrospinal fluid in hydrocephalus.

**ventrosuspension** *n* fixation of a displaced uterus to the anterior abdominal wall.

**Venturi effect** (G Venturi, Italian physicist, 1746–1822) a principle of gas behaviour used for the mixing and delivery of gases, such as oxygen masks. ⇒ Venturi mask.

**Venturi mask** an oxygen therapy mask designed to direct atmospheric air to mix it with a given flow of prescribed oxygen. A variety of masks are available that allow the administration of oxygen at different concentrations.

**venule** *n* a small vein that connects the capillary bed to larger veins.

**VEP** *abbr* visual-evoked potentials.

**verbigeration** *n* the stereotyped repetition of words and phrases; a feature of some types of schizophrenia.

**Veress needle** a sharp needle with a blunt-ended trocar which has a lateral hole; it is used for a pneumoperitoneum. When the trocar projects from the needle, the gut is pushed safely away from the needle point.

**vermicide** *n* an agent which kills intestinal worms—**vermicidal** *adj*.

**vermiform** *adj* wormlike. *vermiform appendix* the vestigial, hollow, wormlike structure attached to the caecum.

**vermifuge** *n* an agent that expels intestinal worms.

**vermis** *n* **1.** a worm. **2.** the narrow worm-like structure situated between the two hemispheres of the cerebellum.

**vernix caseosa** the fatty substance which covers and protects the skin of the fetus from maceration caused by amniotic fluid and friction. It is present from 18 weeks' gestation, but increases during the last trimester.

**verocytotoxin** *n* powerful enterotoxin produced by enterohaemorrhagic *Escherichia coli* such as *E. coli* O157. It can cause haemolytic–uraemic syndrome. ⇒ haemolytic–uraemic syndrome.

**verruca** *n* ⇒ wart, condyloma—**verrucae** *pl*, **verrucous, verrucose** *adj*.

**version** *n* turning—applied to the manoeuvre to alter the position of the fetus in utero. *cephalic version* turning the fetus so that the head presents. *external cephalic version (ECV)* the conversion of a breech to a cephalic presentation by manipulation through the abdominal wall. The technique is safer with the use of ultrasound and tachographic monitoring. *internal version* is turning the fetus by one hand in the uterus, and the other on the woman's abdomen. *podalic version* turning the fetus to a breech presentation. This version may be external or internal.

**vertebra** *n* one of the irregular bones making up the spinal column—**vertebrae** *pl*, **vertebral** *adj*.

**vertebral arch (neural arch)** *n* the arch formed by the pedicles and laminae at the posterior part of a vertebra; encloses the vertebral canal or foramen.

**vertebral artery** *n* one of two arteries. They contribute to the circulus arteriosus (circle of Willis) that supplies blood to the brain. The two vertebral arteries branch from the subclavian arteries, run upwards through foramina in the cervical vertebrae and pass into the skull through the foramen magnum to form the basilar artery.

**vertebral canal (neural canal)** also called vertebral foramen. The cavity within the vertebral column that houses and protects the spinal cord.

**vertebral column** (*syn* spinal column) made up of 33/34 vertebrae, articulating with the skull above and the pelvic girdle below. There are 24 individual bones—7 cervical, 12 thoracic, 5 lumbar—and 9 or 10 fused bones—5 sacral and 4 or 5 coccygeal. The vertebrae are so shaped that they enclose a cavity (vertebral or neural canal) which houses the spinal cord.

**vertebrobasilar insufficiency (VBI)** a poorly understood condition in which there is thought to be transient disturbances in the blood flow to the brainstem.

**vertex** *n* the top of the head.

**vertical transmission** transmission of disease from mother to fetus, via the placenta, during delivery or via breast milk, e.g. human immunodeficiency virus (HIV).

**vertigo** *n* giddiness, dizziness—**vertiginous** *adj*.

**very-low-density lipoprotein (VLDL)** ⇒ lipoprotein.

**vesical** *adj* pertaining to the urinary bladder.

**vesicant** *n* a drug or other substance that causes blistering of the skin.

**V**

**vesicle** *n* **1.** a small bladder, cell or hollow structure. **2.** a fluid-filled skin blister less than 5 mm in diameter—**vesicular** *adj*. **vesiculation** *n*.

**vesicocolic** *adj* pertaining to the urinary bladder and the colon. *vesicocolic fistula* an abnormal communication between the urinary bladder and the colon, for example with diverticular disease. ⇒ pneumaturia.

**vesicostomy** *n* ⇒ cystostomy.

**vesicoureteric** *adj* pertaining to the urinary bladder and ureter.

**vesicoureteric reflux (VUR)** retrograde passage of urine up the ureters following a rise of pressure within the bladder during voiding. It can lead to reflux nephropathy (chronic pyelonephritis). ⇒ reflux nephropathy.

**vesicovaginal** *adj* pertaining to the urinary bladder and vagina. *vesicovaginal fistula* an abnormal communication between the bladder and the vagina. Causes include advanced cancer of the cervix, radiotherapy and damage during labour.

**vesiculitis** *n* inflammation of a vesicle, particularly the seminal vesicles.

**vesiculography** *n* radiographic demonstration of the seminal vesicles following the introduction of contrast medium.

**vesiculopapular** *adj* pertaining to or exhibiting both vesicles and papules.

**vesiculopustular** *adj* pertaining to or exhibiting both vesicles and pustules.

**vessel** *n* a tube, duct or canal, holding or conveying fluid, especially blood and lymph.

**vestibular apparatus** the structures of the inner ear concerned with position sense and balance—the saccule and utricle of the vestibule and the semicircular canals.

**vestibular glands** four mucus-secreting glands that open into the vestibule of the female external genitalia. The greater vestibular glands (Bartholin's glands) and the lesser vestibular or paraurethral glands (Skene's glands).

**vestibule** *n* **1.** the middle part of the inner ear, lying between the semicircular canals and the cochlea. **2.** the triangular area between the labia minora. **3.** the area of the mouth between the lips and the gums/teeth—**vestibular** *adj*.

**vestibulocochlear** *adj* relating to the vestibule and the cochlea.

**vestibulocochlear nerve** auditory nerve. The eighth pair of cranial nerves. There are two branches: the vestibular, which transmits impulses from the vestibular apparatus of the ear to the cerebellum, and the cochlear, which transmits impulses from the cochlea in the ear to the auditory cortex situated in the temporal lobe of the cerebrum.

**vestibulo-ocular reflex** compensatory eye movement stimulated by head movement to stabilize gaze in space.

**vestigial** *adj* pertaining to a rudimentary structure, a remnant of something formerly present.

**VF** *abbr* ventricular fibrillation.

**VFM** *abbr* value for money.

**viable** *adj* capable of living a separate existence—**viability** *n*.

**vibration** *n* a form of massage manipulation. A fine tremor transmitted through the hands and finger tips to body cavities in order to move fluids and gases.

**vibration syndrome** (*syn* Raynaud's phenomenon) ⇒ hand–arm vibration syndrome.

**vibration—whole body** arises from use of equipment in which the worker is supported by the vibrating machinery, e.g. a vehicle seat or ship's deck. The cardiovascular system is affected, with an increase in heart rate and interference with circulation; musculoskeletal problems are common, particularly involving the spine. Fatigue and poor concentration are also thought to be significant.

***Vibrio*** *n* a genus of curved, motile microorganisms. *Vibrio cholerae* causes cholera.

**vibrissae** *npl* the coarse hairs growing within the nasal cavity.

**vicarious** *adj* substituting the function of one organ for another. *vicarious liability* describes the liability of the employer for the wrongful acts of an employee committed during the course of employment.

**videokymography** *n* recording vibrations, such as those of the vocal folds of the larynx, using a high-speed camera.

**villus** *n* a microscopic finger-like projection; found on the mucosal surface of the small intestine, or on the outside of the chorion of the embryonic sac. Those on the intestinal mucosa increase the surface area available for the absorption of water and nutrients. The villus contains blood vessels and a central lymphatic lacteal for absorption—**villi** *pl*. **villous** *adj*.

**vinca alkaloids** a group of cytotoxic drugs extracted from the periwinkle plant, e.g. vincristine. They prevent mitosis and cell division by inhibiting microtubule formation. ⇒ cytotoxic. ⇒ Appendix 5.

**Vincent's angina** (*syn* ulcerative gingivitis) (H Vincent, French physician, 1862–1950) outdated term for acute necrotizing ulcerative gingivitis.

**VIP** *abbr* vasoactive intestinal peptide.

**VIPoma** *n* a rare tumour that secretes vasoactive intestinal peptide. Usually occurs in the pancreas where it is often malignant, but it does occur elsewhere. They cause diarrhoea, hypokalaemia (reduced potassium level in the blood) and hypochlorhydria (reduced gastric acid).

**viraemia** *n* the presence of viruses in the blood—**viraemic** *adj*.

**viral haemorrhagic fevers** fevers occurring mainly in tropical areas; they are often transmitted by mosquitoes or ticks; they may have a petechial skin rash. They include: chikungunya, Ebola, dengue, Lassa fever, Marburg disease, Rift Valley fever and yellow fever.

**viral hepatitis** ⇒ hepatitis.

**Virchow's node** (R Virchow, German pathologist, 1821–1902) ⇒ signal node.

**Virchow's triad** (R Virchow) three factors that predispose to the formation of deep-vein thrombosis—slowing of blood flow (venous stasis), abnormal or inappropriate coagulation processes, or damage to veins. ⇒ deep-vein thrombosis.

**virement** *n* financial term meaning to move money from one expenditure category to another.

**viricidal** *adj* lethal to a virus—**viricide** *n*.

**virilism** *n* the appearance of secondary male characteristics in the female. It may be caused by abnormal adrenal secretion of androgenic substances, or by drugs.

**virologist** *n* an expert in viruses and viral diseases.

**virology** *n* the study of viruses and the diseases caused by them—**virological** *adj*.

**virtue ethics** an ethical approach that focuses on and encourages the intellectual and moral characteristics that allow individuals and groups to analyse ethical dilemmas and make sound ethical judgements.

**virulence** *n* infectiousness; the disease-producing power of a micro-organism and its power to overcome host resistance—**virulent** *adj*.

**viruses** *npl* a diverse group of micro-organisms which are only visible using electron microscopy. They contain either DNA or RNA, and can only replicate within the host cell. Viruses infect humans, animals, plants and other micro-organisms (bacteriophages). Diseases caused by viruses in humans include: colds, influenza, measles, rabies, hepatitis, chickenpox, poliomyelitis, dengue and acquired immunodeficiency syndrome (AIDS). Some viruses are associated with cancer of the cervix, Burkitt's lymphoma and some types of leukaemia. ⇒ Epstein–Barr virus, human T-cell lymphotropic virus, human papillomavirus.

**viscera** *n* the internal organs—**viscus** *sing*, **visceral** *adj*.

**viscid** *adj* thick, sticky and glutinous, may be used to describe sputum, mucus, etc.

**visual** *adj* pertaining to vision.

**visual acuity** the sharpness of vision; the ability to see the difference between two points of light. A measure of the ability of the eye to resolve detail. ⇒ Snellen test type chart.

**visual analogue scale (VAS)** a self-reporting scale for pain. Uses a 10-cm horizontal line with indicators of pain severity such as 'pain-free/no pain' at one end right up to 'worst pain possible' at the other end (Figure V.4A). Patients are asked to indicate the point on the scale that best describes their current pain. It can be modified by adding numbers (a verbal numerical rating scale), for example 0 = no pain and 10 = worst possible pain. These can be more reliable in measuring pain (Figure V.4B).

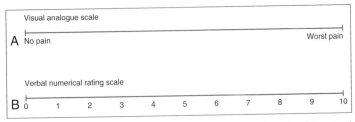

**Figure V.4** (A) Visual analogue scale. (B) Verbal numerical rating scale *(reproduced from Brooker & Waugh 2007 with permission).*

**visual-evoked potentials (VEP)** during electroencephalography a flashing light is used to stimulate the retina and changes to evoked cortical potentials are recorded over the occipital cortex. Used to diagnose problems with the optic nerve and the visual pathways; especially useful in the diagnosis of demyelinating diseases such as multiple sclerosis, which have early optic nerve damage.

**visual field** also called field of vision. The area in which objects can be seen without moving the eye. In binocular vision, the overlap of the fields of both eyes across the nose allows perception of depth (stereoscopic vision).

**visual impairment** some degree of low vision, sight impairment or blindness. Common causes worldwide include: macular degeneration, diabetic and other retinopathies, glaucoma, cataracts, vitamin A deficiency, infections (e.g. trachoma) and trauma.

**visual purple** rhodopsin. ⇒ opsins, rhodopsin.

**vital capacity (VC)** the amount of air expelled from the lungs after a maximal inspiratory effort. ⇒ forced vital capacity.

**vital centre** specialized nerve cells usually located in the brainstem or the hypothalamus that control vital autonomic functions that include heart rate, respiration, blood pressure, etc. For example, the cardiac centre, respiratory centres and vasomotor centre.

**vital signs** those signs that indicate life. Usually refers to the measurement of temperature, pulse and respiration. Within the context of basic monitoring of the condition of patients, it is usual also to record blood pressure.

**vitallium** *n* an alloy used in the manufacture of nails, plates, etc., used in orthopaedic and other surgical procedures.

**vitalograph** *n* apparatus for measuring the forced vital capacity.

**vital signs monitor** apparatus that automatically records and displays physiological measurements such as blood pressure and electrocardiogram (ECG).

**vitamin A** (*syn* retinol) a fat-soluble anti-infective substance present in all animal fats. In its provitamin form, β-carotene, it is present in carrots, cabbage, lettuce, tomatoes and other fruits and vegetables: in the body it is converted into retinol. It is essential for healthy skin and mucous membranes: it aids night vision. Deficiency can result in stunted growth, night blindness and xerophthalmia and it is an important cause of blindness in certain parts of the world, e.g. India.

**vitamin B** any one of a group of water-soluble vitamins—the vitamin B complex, all chemically related and often occurring in the same foods. ⇒ biotin, cobalamins, folate, nicotinic acid, pantothenic acid, pyridoxine, riboflavin, thiamin.

**vitamin B₁** thiamin diphosphate or thiamin pyrophosphate. It occurs in wheatgerm, wheat products, yeast extracts, meat and fortified breakfast cereals. Functions as a coenzyme in carbohydrate metabolism. Deficiency results in beri-beri and Wernicke–Korsakoff syndrome. ⇒ Korsakoff's syndrome, Wernicke's encephalopathy.

**vitamin B₂** riboflavin. Occurs in most foods: the best sources are milk, milk products, offal and fortified breakfast cereals. It functions as part of the coenzymes flavin mononucleotide (FMN) and flavin adenine dinucleotide (FAD), the electron carrier/transfer molecules involved in the oxidation of fuel molecules in the mitochondria. ⇒ oxidative phosphorylation. Deficiency symptoms are angular stomatitis, cheilosis and anaemia.

**vitamin B₃** niacin, nicotinic acid, nicotinamide. Occurs in meat, fish, pulses, wholegrains, fortified breakfast cereals, etc. It functions as part of the coenzymes nicotinamide adenine dinucleotide (NAD) and nicotinamide adenine dinucleotide phosphate (NADP), the electron carriers in the oxidation of fuel molecules and the synthesis of molecules that include fatty acids. Deficiency leads to pellagra.

**vitamin B₅** pantothenic acid. It is widespread in foods, e.g. eggs, liver, pulses, cereals, vegetables, etc., and deficiency is rare. It functions in the metabolism of protein, carbohydrate and fat.

**vitamin B₆** pyridoxine. Occurs in unprocessed cereal foods, vegetables, meat and eggs. It functions as a coenzyme in protein metabolism. Deficiency symptoms include general weakness, peripheral neuropathy, dermatitis, glossitis and impaired immunity.

**vitamin B₁₂** cobalamins. Occurs in meat, eggs, milk and cheese. It functions as a coenzyme in protein metabolism. Deficiency may develop in vegans and symptoms include megaloblastic anaemia and neurological dysfunction. ⇒ pernicious anaemia.

**vitamin C** ascorbic acid. A water-soluble antioxidant vitamin, which is present in fruits (e.g. citrus, blackcurrants) and vegetables (e.g. potato, green leafy vegetables). It is destroyed by cooking in the presence of air and by plant

**V**

enzymes released when chopping, cutting or grating food; it is also lost during storage. Deficiency leads to scurvy, sore gums and mouth, poor wound healing, etc. ⇒ ascorbic acid.

**vitamin D** a fat-soluble vitamin needed for the absorption of calcium and the calcification of the skeleton. It occurs in two forms—cholecalciferol (vitamin $D_3$) formed by the action of ultraviolet radiation on 7-dehydrocholesterol, which occurs naturally in the skin, and ergocalciferol (vitamin $D_2$, calciferol), formed by the action of ultraviolet radiation on ergosterol, which occurs naturally in plants. Occurs in oily fish, eggs and fortified margarine. Deficiency leads to rickets and osteomalacia.

**vitamin E** a group of chemically related compounds known as tocopherols and tocotrienols. It is an intracellular fat-soluble antioxidant and maintains the stability of polyunsaturated fatty acids and other fat-like substances. It is thought that deficiency results in muscle degeneration, a haemolytic blood disease, and is associated with the ageing process. *vitamin E deficiency syndrome* occurs in small infants, less than 2 kg and under 35 weeks' gestation. Diagnosis at between 6 and 11 weeks reveals low haemoglobin and reticulocytosis; there is good response to vitamin E, including a rise in haemoglobin and loss of oedema. The condition is aggravated by giving iron. Deficiency in older children results in cerebellar ataxia and is associated with abetalipoproteinaemia.

**vitamin K** occurs in three forms—phylloquinone, menaquinones and menadione. Phylloquinone occurs in green vegetables and menaquinones are produced by bacteria in the gastrointestinal tract. It is required for the synthesis of several clotting factors. Deficiency leads to reduced blood clotting.

**vitaminoids** *npl* compounds that display vitamin-like activity. For example choline, flavonoids, inositol and essential fatty acids.

**vitamins** *npl* organic substance or group of substances that have specific biochemical functions in the body. They are either fat-soluble—vitamins A, D, E and K—or water-soluble—vitamin B complex and vitamin C. They are essential for normal metabolism and are provided by the diet. Some vitamins can also be synthesized in the body, e.g. vitamin D. Their absence causes deficiency diseases.

**vitiligo** *n* a skin disease of probable autoimmune origin characterized by areas of complete loss of pigment, often on the face and hands.

**vitrectomy** *n* surgical removal of the vitreous body (humour) from the vitreous chamber.

**vitreous** *adj* resembling glass.

**vitreous body (humour)** the clear, jelly-like substance contained by a membrane within the vitreous chamber. It is formed during embryonic life within a closed system and it lasts for life. ⇒ Appendix 1, Figure 15.

**vitreous chamber** the posterior cavity inside the eyeball and behind the lens; contains the vitreous body.

**vitreous detachment** detachment from the posterior retina can occur as the vitreous body liquefies during normal ageing. It is also associated with diabetes mellitus. Vitreous detachment can cause tears in the retina and possible retinal detachment.

**vitritis** *n* inflammation within the vitreous body.

**VLDL** *abbr* very-low-density lipoprotein.

**VMA** *abbr* vanillylmandelic acid.

**VMC** *abbr* vasomotor centre.

**$V_{max}$** *abbr* the maximum velocity of an enzyme-catalysed reaction in which the substrate concentration is not limiting.

**$VO_2$** *abbr* oxygen consumption/uptake.

**$VO_{2max}$** *abbr* maximum oxygen consumption/uptake.

**vocal folds (cords)** the vocal folds (true vocal cords) are two membranous folds stretched anteroposteriorly across the larynx. The ventricular folds (or false vocal cords) are situated lateral to the vocal folds. Sound is produced by vibration of the vocal folds as air from the lungs passes between them. Their length varies, which is why men, with longer vocal cords, have deeper voices than women. An opening (the glottis) between the true vocal cords allows air movement through the larynx.

**vocational assessment** the objective evaluation of a person's ability to perform a specific job consistently and competently. This may include the identification of the need for training or the provision of compensatory techniques.

**voice-activated domestic appliance system (VADAS)** a microprocessor and voice input system that allows people with severe physical impairments to control their environment and live as independently as possible.

**volatile** *adj* evaporating rapidly. *volatile anaesthetic agent* drug in the form of a liquid which when vaporized induces general anaesthesia.

**volition** *n* the will to act—**volitional** *adj*. ⇒ conation.

**Volkmann's ischaemic contracture** (R von Volkmann, German surgeon, 1830–1889) a flexion deformity of the wrist and fingers from fixed contracture of the flexor muscles in the forearm. The cause is ischaemia of the muscles by injury or obstruction to the brachial artery, near the elbow, for example, caused by a supracondylar fracture of the humerus.

**volt (V)** *n* the derived SI unit (International System of Units) for electromotive force (also known as potential difference or electrical potential). ⇒ Appendix 2.

**voluntary** *adj* under the control of the will; free and unrestricted, as opposed to reflex or involuntary.

**voluntary muscle** ⇒ skeletal muscle.

**voluntary patient** informal patient. A person with a mental health problem who is an inpatient on a voluntary basis, i.e. not detained there under any provision of mental health legislation.

**voluntary sector** the organizations controlled and run by volunteers, e.g. Samaritans, MIND. Many have charitable status, some receive grants from government, and some employ professionals and other paid staff to facilitate their work.

**volvulus** *n* torsion of a loop of intestine, so as to occlude the lumen, causing intestinal obstruction.

**vomer** *n* bone forming part of the nasal septum.

**vomit** *n* **1.** *v* ejection of the stomach contents through the mouth and sometimes the nose; sickness. **2.** *n* the material vomited, the vomitus.

**vomiting** *n* reflex expulsion of stomach contents through the mouth, often accompanied by feelings of nausea. It may occur effortlessly, be accompanied by abdominal pain, or be projectile, such as with pyloric stenosis. The vomiting reflex is initiated and co-ordinated by two centres in the medulla of the brain—the vomiting (emetic) centre and the chemoreceptor trigger zone (CTZ).

**vomiting (emetic) centre** a centre in the medulla oblongata that has overall control of vomiting. It responds to various stimuli such as those from the gastrointestinal organs. ⇒ chemical trigger zone.

**vomiting of pregnancy** ⇒ hyperemesis.

**vomitus** *n* vomited matter.

**von Recklinghausen's disease** (*syn* Recklinghausen's disease) (F von Recklinghausen,

German pathologist, 1833–1910) describes two conditions: (a) osteitis fibrosa cystica—the result of hyperparathyroidism leading to decalcification of bones and formation of cysts; (b) multiple neurofibromatosis—the tumours can be felt beneath the skin along the course of nerves. There may be pigmented spots (café au lait) on the skin and neurofibroma in the endocrine glands and the gastrointestinal tract.

**von Willebrand's disease** (E von Willebrand, Finnish physician, 1870–1949) an inherited bleeding disease due to deficiencies relating to the von Willebrand factor in plasma. The inheritance is autosomal dominant, affecting both sexes. Essentially a disorder of the primary haemostatic mechanism with abnormal platelet–endothelial cell interaction. In rare, severe cases von Willebrand's disease results in a clotting defect resembling haemophilia.

**V/Q** *abbr* ventilation–perfusion.

**VRE** *abbr* vancomycin-resistant enterococci.

**VRSA** *abbr* vancomycin-resistant *Staphylococcus aureus.*

**VSD** *abbr* ventricular septal defect.

**VT** *abbr* ventricular tachycardia.

**vulva** *n* the external genitalia of the female—**vulval** *adj.*

**vulvectomy** *n* excision of the vulva.

**vulvitis** *n* inflammation of the vulva.

**vulvodynia** *n* chronic painful vulval discomfort such as burning, rawness and stinging. Previously regarded by many as a psychogenic condition, vulvodynia is an organic disease that presents with surface changes or as an aberration of sensory function in which surface changes may be absent.

**vulvovaginal** *adj* pertaining to the vulva and the vagina.

**vulvovaginitis** *n* inflammation of the vulva and vagina.

**vulvovaginoplasty** *n* operation for congenital absence of the vagina, or acquired disabling stenosis—**vulvovaginoplastic** *adj.*

**VUR** *abbr* vesicoureteric reflux.

**VZIG** *abbr* varicella-zoster (hyperimmune) immunoglobulin.

**VZV** *abbr* varicella-zoster virus.

V

# W

**Waardenburg's syndrome** (P Waardenburg, Dutch ophthalmologist, 1886–1979) a syndrome inherited as an autosomal dominant trait. There are facial abnormalities, multicolour irises (heterochromia), a striking white forelock and white eyelashes, and sometimes hearing impairment. **2.** also known as Klein–Waardenburg syndrome. Inherited as an autosomal dominant trait. Problems include cranial and facial abnormalities, cleft palate, short digits, congenital heart defects and glaucoma.

**WAGR syndrome** **W**ilms' tumour–**a**nhidria–**g**enitourinary abnormalities–learning disability (mental **r**etardation), caused by a deletion affecting chromosome number 11.

**waist:hip ratio** a way of assessing the distribution of fatty tissue: whether it is mainly subcutaneous or intra-abdominal. A waist-to-hip ratio of 0.95 or above for men and 0.85 or above for women increases the risk of cardiovascular disease and diabetes mellitus.

**Waldeyer's ring** (H Waldeyer, German anatomist, 1836–1921) a lymphoid tissue circle surrounding the pharynx; the lingual, palatine and pharyngeal tonsils. ⇒ tonsils.

**walking aids** walking sticks, crutches, tripods and various types of metal frame that allow people to regain or retain independence for walking.

**Wallace's rule of nines** ⇒ rule of nines.

**wallerian degeneration** (A Waller, British physician/physiologist, 1816–1870) degeneration in a nerve fibre that is separated from its nerve cell body.

**warm-up** *n* techniques used to increase local muscle and core body temperature prior to vigorous exercise. Can be either active or passive and may be specific to the sport or exercise about to be performed.

**wart** *n* verruca. *common warts* are due to human papillomavirus (HPV) and usually occur on the hands or feet. *seborrhoeic warts* (*syn* basal cell papilloma) the brown, greasy warts seen in older people, commonly on the chest or back. ⊙DVD *plane warts* flat small papules commonly seen on the face or hands in children.

**Wassermann reaction** (A von Wassermann, German bacteriologist, 1866–1925) an early complement fixation test on blood or cerebrospinal fluid for syphilis. Now obsolete.

**waterbrash** *n* ⇒ pyrosis.

**Waterhouse–Friderichsen syndrome** (R Waterhouse, British physician, 1873–1958; C Friderichsen, Danish paediatrician, 1886–1979) shock with widespread skin haemorrhages occurring in meningitis, especially meningococcal. There is bleeding into the adrenal glands.

**water-soluble vitamins** those of the B-group and vitamin C. ⇒ fat-soluble vitamins.

**watt (W)** *n* derived SI unit (International System of Units) for electrical power. ⇒ Appendix 2.

**WBC** *abbr* white blood cell (leucocyte). ⇒ blood.

**weal** *n* a superficial swelling, characteristic of urticaria, nettle stings, etc.

**Weber–Christian disease** (F Weber, British physician, 1863–1962; H Christian, American physician, 1876–1951) ⇒ panniculitis.

**Weber's test** a tuning fork (512 Hz) test for the interpretation of asymmetric deafness. ⇒ Rinne's test.

**Wechsler Intelligence Scales** (D Wechsler, American psychologist, 1896–1981) a set of standardized tests for measuring the IQ of children and adults.

**Wegener's granulomatosis** (F Wegener, German pathologist, 1907–1990) a rare anti-neutrophil cytoplasmic antibody (ANCA)-associated vasculitis affecting small vessels. It is characterized by epistaxis, nasal discharge, haemoptysis, sinusitis, deafness, visual problems caused by inflammation behind the eye and sometimes glomerulonephritis.

**Weil–Felix test** (E Weil, Austrian bacteriologist, 1879–1922; A Felix, Polish bacteriologist, 1887–1956) a non-specific agglutination reaction used in the diagnosis of rickettsial disease, e.g. typhus.

**Weil's disease** (A Weil, German physician, 1848–1916) serious bacterial disease caused by infection with spirochaetes of the genus *Leptospira* such as *L. icterohaemorrhagica*. Transmission is via the infected urine of rats and other animals. ⇒ leptospirosis.

**wen** *n* ⇒ sebaceous cyst.

**Wenckebach heart block/phenomenon** (K Wenckebach, Dutch/Austrian physician, 1864–1940). ⇒ Mobitz I heart block.

**Werdnig–Hoffmann disease** (G Werdnig, Austrian neurologist, 1844–1919; J Hoffmann, German neurologist, 1857–1919) a type of spinal muscular atrophy inherited as an autosomal recessive trait. Death occurs from respiratory complications/failure during early childhood.

**Wermer's syndrome** (P Wermer, American physician, 1898–1975) a type of multiple endocrine neoplasia (MEN) in which the inheritance is usually autosomal dominant. It is characterized by the presence of a pituitary adenoma causing excessive anterior-lobe hormone secretion which, in turn, causes overstimulation of the thyroid and adrenal glands, parathyroid tumours or hyperplasia leading to overactivity, and tumours of the pancreatic islet cells, insulinomas and gastrinomas. ⇒ Sipple's syndrome, Zollinger–Ellison syndrome.

**Wernicke's area** (K Wernicke, Polish/German neurologist, 1848–1905) a sensory speech area located in the temporal lobe of the brain. In right-handed people it is dominant in the left cerebral hemisphere and vice versa.

**Wernicke's encephalopathy** (K Wernicke) a level of impaired consciousness and thinking due to thiamin(e) deficiency and which is therefore commonly seen in long-term alcohol misuse.

**Wertheim's hysterectomy** (E Wertheim, Austrian gynaecologist, 1864–1920) a radical and extensive abdominal operation performed for cancer of the cervix, where the uterus, cervix, upper vagina, uterine (fallopian) tubes, ovaries and regional lymph nodes are removed.

**Western blot** also known as immunoblotting, a process of identifying antigens in a mixture using specific antibodies. The antigens are separated using an electrophoretic technique, transferred to a sheet of nitrocellulose, and then identified by radio- or enzyme-labelled antibodies.

**West Nile fever** a sporadic disease caused by a virus of the genus *Flavivirus*. It is found in wild birds and transmitted to humans from a bite by an infected *Culex* mosquito. There have been reports of infection after a blood transfusion. The infection may be asymptomatic, or present with fever, headache, a rash, lymphadenopathy and vague muscle aches and pains. Rarely there is encephalitis or meningoencephalitis (inflammation of the brain and spinal cord). Deaths have occurred, especially in older adults and immunocompromised individuals.

**WFP** *abbr* World Food Programme.

**Wharton's jelly** (T Wharton, English anatomist, 1614–1673) embryonic connective tissue contained in the umbilical cord.

**wheezing** *n* a whistling or rasping breathing sound. Associated with the bronchospasm of asthma and other conditions.

**whiplash injury** damage to the structures of the cervical region (ligaments, muscles or cervical vertebrae) caused by sudden, jerking back and forth movements of the head and neck. It is particularly associated with road traffic accidents in which there is sudden deceleration or acceleration, such as a vehicle being struck from behind.

**Whipple's disease** (G Whipple, American pathologist, 1878–1976) a rare condition with steatorrhoea, malabsorption, weight loss, anaemia and joint pain.

**Whipple's operation** (A Whipple, American surgeon, 1881–1963) radical operation sometimes performed for cancer of the head of pancreas. It involves partial pancreatectomy, and excision of the pylorus, duodenum and bile duct with a gastrojejunostomy, choledochojejunostomy and pancreaticojejunostomy (Figure W.1).

**Whipple's triad** (A Whipple) three essential features of an insulinoma: spontaneous attacks of severe hypoglycaemia; symptoms including sweating and dizziness associated with the hypoglycaemia; and symptoms are reversed by the administration of glucose.

**whipworm** *n Trichuris trichiura*. ⇒ trichuriasis.

**white blood cell** ⇒ leucocyte.

**white finger** ⇒ hand–arm vibration syndrome (HAVS), Raynaud's phenomenon.

**white leg** thrombophlebitis occurring in women after childbirth. ⇒ phlegmasia alba dolens.

**white matter** white nerve tissue of the central nervous system, the myelinated fibres. ⇒ grey matter.

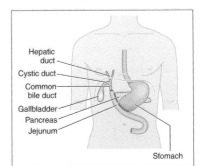

**Figure W.1** Whipple's operation *(reproduced from Brooker & Nicol 2003 with permission).*

W

**white muscle** a term used to describe muscle consisting mainly of fast-twitch fibres. It is white because there is very little myoglobin and a less abundant blood supply than in red muscle.

**white noise** sounds of different frequency within a specific band, all having equal intensity. Used in noise generators worn to mask the distressing symptoms of tinnitus.

**whitlow** *n* acute paronychia or purulent infection of the finger pulp. ⇒ paronychia.

**WHO** *abbr* World Health Organization.

**wholefoods** *npl* unrefined foods, those subjected to the minimum amount of processing. The food has no additions and nothing has been taken out. For example, wholemeal flour made by grinding the entire cereal grain.

**whooping cough** ⇒ pertussis.

**Widal reaction/test** (G Widal, French physician, 1862–1929) an agglutination reaction for typhoid fever.

**Wilcoxon test** a statistical test used as a non-parametric alternative to Student's paired test.

**Williams' syndrome** (J Williams, New Zealand and cardiologist, 20th century) rare genetic disorder usually caused by a deletion affecting chromosome number 7. It is characterized by a learning disability, distinctive elfin facial features, short stature, cardiac problems (e.g. aortic stenosis), episodes of hypercalcaemia and an excessively friendly, outgoing personality.

**Wilms' tumour** (M Wilms, German surgeon, 1867–1918) the commonest abdominal tumour of childhood, and one that usually affects the kidneys. Usually diagnosed during the pre-school period. Prognosis is uncertain and depends on the stage of the tumour and child's age at onset of diagnosis and treatment. ⇒ nephroblastoma.

**Wilson's disease** (S Wilson, British neurologist, 1878–1937) rare inherited hepaticolenticular degeneration. Due to disturbance of copper metabolism with copper deposition in various organs, such as the liver and basal nuclei (ganglia). Associated with dementia, tremor, chorea, cirrhosis, hepatic portal hypertension and liver failure. Treatment is with penicillamine, which binds the copper. Relatives with the disease should have prophylactic penicillamine, even if they have no symptoms. ⇒ Kayser–Fleischer ring.

**windchill** *n* the heat loss from the body caused by exposure to cool air currents. It is directly related to wind speed.

**windpipe** *n* ⇒ trachea.

**wisdom tooth** lay term for the molar tooth placed eighth from the midline in the secondary dentition. The last teeth to erupt, usually during late teens or early twenties.

**wobble board** a device used by physiotherapists and others during rehabilitation in order to improve proprioception and balance (Figure W.2).

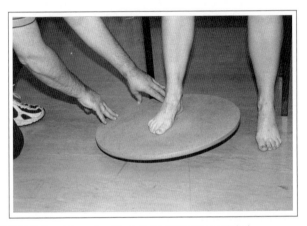

**Figure W.2** Wobble board *(reproduced from Porter 2005 with permission).*

**Wolfe graft** ⇒ skin graft.

**wolffian body** (K Wolff, German anatomist/embryologist, 1733–1794) ⇒ mesonephros.

**wolffian duct** (K Wolff) ⇒ mesonephric duct.

**Wolff–Parkinson–White (WPW) syndrome** (L Wolff, American cardiologist, 1898–1972; J Parkinson, British cardiologist, 1885–1976; P White, American cardiologist, 1886–1973) an arrhythmia resulting from an abnormal conduction pathway between the atria and ventricles. Usually results in a supraventricular tachycardia.

**Wolfram syndrome** (D Wolfram, American physician, 20th century) also called DIDMOAD syndrome—diabetes insipidus, diabetes mellitus, optic atrophy and deafness. A rare syndrome inherited as an autosomal recessive trait.

**womb** *n* the uterus.

**Wood's light** (R Wood, American physicist, 1868–1955) special ultraviolet light used for the detection of fungal diseases such as ringworm. The infected hair or skin becomes fluorescent under the light.

**Wood's manoeuvre** an invasive manoeuvre that can be used in shoulder dystocia.

**woolsorter's disease** the pulmonary form of anthrax, haemorrhagic bronchopneumonia. ⇒ anthrax.

**word blindness** ⇒ alexia.

**work** *n* productive, purposeful engagement in physical and cognitive activities by individuals in order to support themselves and their dependants, and make a useful contribution to society.

**work-related upper limb disorder (WRULD)** occurs as a result of prolonged persistent repetitive overuse of the upper limb with maintenance of static postures. It is common in keyboard workers, production workers and telephonists. The soft tissues in the shoulders, arms, wrists and hands are affected, leading to various diagnoses, e.g. tendinitis, tenosynovitis, carpal tunnel syndrome and tennis elbow. It can be prevented by adequate ergonomic-based risk assessment of the workplace.

**World Food Programme (WFP)** international food aid donated by countries with a surplus; organized and implemented by the United Nations.

**World Health Organization (WHO)** health organization that co-ordinates health activity and promotes public health worldwide. Established through a declaration during the United Nations Conference on International Organization held in San Francisco in 1945. A number of disparate health organizations were joined together under the aegis of the United Nations with a headquarters in Geneva, Switzerland.

**wormian bone** *n* (O Worm, Danish anatomist, 1588–1654) any of the tiny bones located within the sutures (fibrous joints) between the skull bones.

**worms** *npl* cestode, helminth, nematodes, *Taenia, Trematoda.*

**wound** *n* most commonly used when referring to injury to the skin or underlying tissues or organs by a blow, cut, missile or stab. It also includes injury to the skin caused by chemicals, cold, friction, heat, pressure and radiation. Wounds may be acute, e.g. surgical incision, or chronic, such as venous leg ulcers and pressure ulcers. Surgical wounds are usually classified according to the risk of wound infection, as being: (a) clean—non-traumatic wounds, such as during planned surgery using aseptic technique, which neither involves opening an organ nor has septic focus, e.g. excision of a breast lump; (b) clean contaminated—non-traumatic wounds, such as planned elective surgery, which involves opening an organ but without significant spillage of its contents, e.g. cholecystectomy, or with only a negligible breach in aseptic technique; (c) contaminated—traumatic wounds that are from a relatively clean source, such as a clean kitchen knife, or significant spillage of contents from an open organ, or when aseptic technique is seriously breached, or when acute non-purulent infection is present, e.g. removal of an inflamed appendix; and (d) dirty—traumatic wounds from a dirty source, such as a puncture wound from a garden fork, or a delay in treating a wound, or when there is acute bacterial contamination or release of pus, e.g. surgery following trauma sustained in a road traffic accident or where an organ such as the bowel is perforated and peritonitis is present. ⇒ incised wound, laceration, penetrating wound, puncture, tissue viability.

**wound drains** most commonly used in surgical wounds. They may be inserted as treatment, e.g. to drain pus, or prophylactically, e.g. to prevent haematoma formation. Drains may be attached to a vacuum system or suction apparatus, producing a closed system of wound suction.

**wound dressings** a variety of proprietary materials applied to surgical or medical wounds, e.g. leg ulcers. Modern dressings

**W**

should be permeable to water vapour and gases but not to bacteria or liquids, thus retaining serous exudate. They do not adhere to the wound surface and can be removed without damage to new tissue.

**wound healing** there are four stages/phases in normal wound healing: haemostasis, inflammation, proliferation and maturation, which may take many months. Wound healing may be delayed by local factors, e.g. mechanical stress, inadequate blood supply, or by general factors that include: malnutrition, ageing, drugs such as corticosteroids, etc. ⇒ angiogenesis, débridement, epithelialization, granulation, moist wound healing. Wound healing may be by *primary (or first) intention* in a clean wound with the edges in apposition. There is minimal scarring and deformity; *secondary (or second) intention* when the wound edges are not in apposition and there is loss of tissue the gap must be filled by granulation tissue before epithelialization can take place; or by *third intention* when a wound is left open until local factors such as infection have been treated before the wound edges are brought together.

**WPW** *abbr* Wolff–Parkinson–White syndrome.

**wrinkle** *n* furrow or skin crease, increase in number with ageing.

**wrist** *n* the carpus formed by eight carpal bones. *wrist joint* the condyloid joint between the distal radius and three of the proximal carpals, the scaphoid, lunate and triquetral. ⇒ carpus (⇒ Appendix 1, Figure 2).

**wrist drop** paralysis of the extensor muscles of the hand which are needed to raise the wrist result in the wrist being flexed. It is due to damage to the radial nerve, such as compression caused by sleeping with the arm in an abnormal position over the back of a chair.

**WRULD** *abbr* work-related upper limb disorder.

**wryneck** *n* ⇒ torticollis.

**Wuchereria** *n* (O Wucherer, German physician, 1820–1873) a genus of parasitic filarial worms, such as *Wuchereria bancrofti* that causes elephantiasis. They are found in subtropical and tropical regions that are warm and humid. ⇒ elephantiasis, *Filaria*, filariasis.

**W**

# X

**xanthaemia** *n* ⇒ carotenaemia, carotinaemia.

**xanthelasma** *n* a variety of xanthomas. *xanthelasma palpebrarum* small yellowish plaques on the eyelids.

**xanthine** *n* an intermediate product formed during the breakdown of nucleic acids to uric acid. It is excreted in the urine.

**xanthinuria** *n* **1.** the excretion of excessive amounts of xanthine in the urine. **2.** a rare inherited disorder of purine metabolism in which the enzyme xanthine oxidase is lacking, resulting in excessive urinary xanthine and hypoxanthine instead of uric acid. It is inherited as an autosomal recessive trait and may cause the formation of renal calculi.

**xanthochromia** *n* yellow discoloration of the cerebrospinal fluid due to the presence of breakdown products of haemoglobin, such as after subarachnoid haemorrhage.

**xanthogranulomatous pyelonephritis** a granulomatous reaction within the kidney, usually secondary to chronic infection and stone disease.

**xanthoma** *n* nodules showing a yellow discoloration—**xanthomata** *pl*.

**xanthomatosis** *n* yellow discoloration present in many tissues, such as that occurring in various inherited disorders of fat metabolism.

**xanthophylls** *npl* yellow-orange derivatives of carotene.

**xanthopsia** *n* a disorder of vision in which all objects are seen as yellow.

**X chromosome** sex chromosome that is paired in genetic females. Present in every oocyte and in half of spermatozoa. It is larger than the Y chromosome and carries many major genes. ⇒ sex-linked, Y chromosome.

**xenobiotic** *adj* relating to substances, such as drugs, that are foreign to the body.

**xenograft** *n* (*syn* heterograft) a graft between individuals of two different species.

**xenon (Xe)** *n* a rare inert gas. *xenon-133* ($^{133}$Xe) radioactive isotope used in ventilation–perfusion scanning of the lungs.

**xenotransplantation** *n* ⇒ xenograft.

*Xenopsylla* *n* a genus of fleas. *Xenopsylla cheopis* is the rat flea that transmits diseases, including bubonic plague.

**xeroderma, xerodermia** *n* dryness of the skin. ⇒ ichthyosis. *xeroderma pigmentosum* (*syn* Kaposi's disease) a rare inherited skin condition where there is severe photosensitivity to ultraviolet radiation. It is characterized by the formation of freckles, keratoses, telangiectases and malignant skin tumours. Those affected must avoid exposure to ultraviolet radiation.

**xerophthalmia** *n* dryness and ulceration of the cornea which may lead to blindness. Can be associated with lack of vitamin A.

**xerosis** *n* dryness. *xerosis conjunctivae* ⇒ Bitot's spots.

**xerostomia** *n* dry mouth.

**xiphoid process** also called ensiform process, xiphoid, xiphisternum. The sword-shaped cartilage at the lower end of the sternum.

**X-linked agammaglobulinaemia (XLA)** a primary (inherited) immunodeficiency affecting boys. A gene mutation results in absent B cells and hence absent immunoglobulin production.

**X-linked hyper-IgM syndrome (XHIM)** a primary (inherited) immunodeficiency affecting boys. There is defective antibody production, particularly very high immunoglobulin M (IgM) levels, and impaired cellular immunity.

**X-linked lymphoproliferative syndrome (XLP)** Duncan disease/syndrome. A rare X-linked immunodeficiency disorder. Affected individuals have abnormal immune responses to the Epstein–Barr virus (EBV). There is lymphoproliferation, B-cell lymphomas, severe infectious mononucleosis with hepatitis, or hypogammaglobulinaemia.

**XO** the anomaly in which cells have a single sex chromosome. All those with XO are female and have Turner's syndrome. Although the karyotype is usually XO with only 45 chromosomes, there may be mosaic forms.

**X-rays** *npl* short-wavelength, penetrating rays of electromagnetic spectrum, produced by electrical equipment. The word is popularly used to mean radiographs.

**XX** sex chromosomes of normal females.

**XXY syndrome** Klinefelter's syndrome.

**XY** sex chromosomes of normal males.

**xylose** *n* a five-carbon sugar (a pentose) present in plant material.

**xylose absorption test** a test for malabsorption. Xylose is given orally and its urinary excretion is measured. Less than 16% excretion indicates malabsorption.

**XYY syndrome** males with an extra Y chromosome, thus having 47 chromosomes in total. Occasionally there are two extra Y chromosomes (XYYY). The extra Y chromosome may be associated with tallness, learning disability and behavioural problems. However, it does occur in normal men.

X

**Y**

**YAG** *abbr* yttrium aluminium garnet. A crystal used in certain lasers (YAG laser).

**yawning** *n* an involuntary action whereby the person takes a deep breath in through an open mouth and exhales slowly. Often occurs with stretching and moving the upper body. It is associated with boredom, tiredness and drowsiness.

**yaws** *n* a contact disease of children, particularly in Africa, characterized by crops of infectious skin lesions, and later, periostitis. Caused by *Treponema pallidum* (ssp. *pertenue*). ⇒ bejel, pinta.

**Y chromosome** the sex chromosome found singly in the genetic male. Present in half of spermatozoa and none of the oocytes. It is shorter than the X chromosome and has fewer major genes, but carries the genes that stimulate the development of male characteristics.

**yeast** *n* a unicellular fungus, some of which are opportunistic human pathogens, e.g. *Candida albicans*, *Cryptococcus neoformans*, *Malassezia furfur*. For example, candidiasis or cryptococcosis can be particular problems for immunocompromised individuals.

**yellow card reporting** in the UK a system for reporting suspected adverse drug reactions (ADRs). This includes prescription medicines, over-the-counter drugs and herbal remedies. It is administered by the Medicines and Healthcare products Regulatory Agency (MHRA) and the Commission on Human Medicines (CHM). All health professionals (both prescribers and non-prescribers) and patients or their families are encouraged to report ADRs. Online reporting, using an electronic yellow card accessed on the MHRA website, is encouraged, but yellow cards are available from various sources, including from the MHRA, regional offices, in the *British National Formulary* or as a download from the MHRA.

**yellow fever** an acute haemorrhagic febrile illness of tropical areas, caused by a group B arbovirus and spread by a mosquito (*Aedes aegypti*). There is fever, headache, nausea and vomiting, gastrointestinal bleeding, jaundice, petechial haemorrhages, backache and oliguria or anuria. Management is supportive; there is no specific treatment. Immunization is available for those travelling to areas where yellow fever is endemic.

**yellow spot** *n* ⇒ macula lutea.

***Yersinia*** *n* (A Yersin, French bacteriologist, 1862–1943) a genus of Gram-negative bacilli of the family Enterobacteriaceae. For example, the species *Yersinia pestis*, the cause of plague; and *Yersinia enterocolitica* is a cause of gastroenteritis and mesenteric lymphadenitis.

**yin and yang** the philosophy of complementary therapies, such as acupuncture and shiatsu. They describe a dynamic, symbiotic relationship between active and passive energy forces believed to be present in the universe (true Qi) and the human body (Qi). Keeping equilibrium between the two aspects is important in maintaining health and well-being.

**yoga** *n* complementary therapy that utilizes breathing techniques, postures and exercises to relax, reduce stress and generally enhance well-being.

**yolk** *n* nutrient of the ovum. *yolk sac* early embryonic structure, it provides nutrients until the early placenta takes over, and is a site for very early blood cell formation. The blood formed from yolk sac mesoderm provides the embryo with blood until the liver commences haemopoiesis around week 5. Part of the yolk sac is eventually incorporated into the embryo to form the lining epithelium of the gut tube.

**Young's syndrome** a rare condition in which there is obstructive azoospermia, and primary ciliary dyskinesia that leads to rhinosinusitis, recurrent respiratory tract infection and bronchiectasis.

**Y-plasty** in plastic surgery, the use of a Y-shaped incision to relieve scar tissue or contractures.

**yttrium 90 ($^{90}$Y)** a substance emitting beta particles with a half-life of 64 h. Implantations of $^{90}$Y in bone wax are left in the pituitary fossa after hypophysectomy for breast cancer. Also used in a number of interstitial cancer treatments.

**Y**

## Z

**Zavanelli manoeuvre** an invasive manipulation for shoulder dystocia when all other manoeuvres have been unsuccessful. It is performed by an obstetrician; the fetal head is returned to the vagina, in order to facilitate delivery of a live infant by caesarean section.

**zeitgeber** *n* 'time-givers'. The external cues that act as signals to influence the circadian rhythms. They may be natural events that fluctuate, such as the light–dark cycle, or be socially constructed, e.g. work shift times, set meal times, alarm clocks, etc.

**Ziehl–Neelsen stain (ZN)** (F Ziehl, German bacteriologist, 1857–1926; F Neelsen, German pathologist, 1854–1894) a microbiological staining technique used in the identification of acid-fast bacilli, e.g. *Mycobacterium tuberculosis*.

**Zieve's syndrome** (L Zieve, American physician, b. 1915) a syndrome associated with an excessive intake of alcohol. It is characterized by mild anaemia, high levels of cholesterol and triglyceride in the blood, hepatosplenomegaly and a fatty liver.

**ZIFT** *abbr* zygote intrafallopian tube transfer.

**Zimmer frame** a four-point walking aid used in rehabilitation and to enhance independence in people with enduring mobility problems.

**zinc (Zn)** *n* a metallic element needed by the body in small amounts for certain enzyme reactions, insulin storage, cell multiplication and wound healing. Phytates in the diet can reduce absorption.

**zinc oxide** a widely used mild astringent, present in calamine lotion and cream and several other dermatological applications.

**zinc sulphate** used as a supplement in zinc deficiency, such as that caused by deficient intake, malabsorption or loss of zinc (e.g. with extensive burns).

**Z-line** the point of insertion of thin filaments of a myofibril. The region between two Z-lines constitutes one sarcomere (the smallest contractile unit of skeletal muscle).

**ZN** *abbr* Ziehl–Neelsen stain.

**Zollinger–Ellison syndrome** (R Zollinger, American surgeon, 1903–1992; E Ellison, American physician, 1918–1970) gastrin-secreting tumour (gastrinoma) of the pancreatic islets resulting in hypersecretion of gastric acid, fulminating ulceration of the oesophagus, stomach and duodenum and jejunum. Diagnosed by high basal gastric acid secretion and elevated fasting serum gastrin levels. ⇒ multiple endocrine neoplasia, Wermer's syndrome.

**zona** *n* a zone; a girdle; a term applied to shingles. *zona fasciculata* middle layer of the adrenal cortex, secretes glucocorticoid hormones. *zona glomerulosa* outer layer of the adrenal cortex, secretes mineralocorticoid hormones. *zona pellucida* membrane around the oocyte. *zona reticularis* inner layer of the adrenal cortex, secretes some glucocorticoids and sex hormones (androgens and oestrogens).

**zones** *npl* a term used in reflexology. The suggestion is that inborn Qi energy flows through different zones (reflexes) that end in the feet or hands.

**zonula** *n* also called zonule. A small zone, belt or girdle.

**zonula ciliaris** *n* also called the zonule of Zinn (J Zinn, German anatomist/botanist, 1727–1759). A suspensory ligament attaching the periphery of the lens of the eye to the ciliary body.

**zonulolysis** *n* enzymic breakdown of the zonula ciliaris of the eye. Previously used prior to intracapsular lens extraction.

**zoonosis** *n* disease in humans transmitted from animals, e.g. anthrax, brucellosis, leptospirosis, rabies—**zoonoses** *pl*.

**zoophilia** *n* **1.** an abnormal and excessive liking for animals. **2.** a psychosexual disorder in which an individual derives sexual gratification from close contact with animals (e.g. fondling/stroking), sexual activity with animals or fantasy involving animals.

**zoophobia** *n* an excessive and irrational fear of animals, such as mice, rats, snakes, dogs, etc.

**zoster** *n* herpes zoster. ⇒ herpes zoster, shingles.

**Z-plasty** in plastic surgery, the use of a Z-shaped incision to relieve scar tissue or contractures.

**Z-track** a technique used during intramuscular injection of substances that can irritate or stain the tissues if tracking and leakage occur, for example preparations of iron (Figure Z.1).

**zwitterions** *npl* molecules that contain both negatively and positively charged regions, such as amino acids in neutral solutions.

**zygomatic (zygoma) bones** also called malar bones. The two bones of the cheek. They form the prominent part of the cheek and contribute to the orbit. They join with the zygomatic processes of the temporal bone to form the zygomatic arch, and to the maxilla.

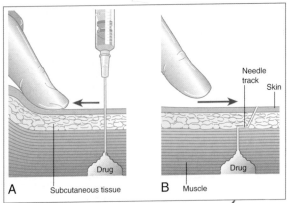

**Figure Z.1** Z-track intramuscular injection technique *(reproduced from Downie et al. 2003).*

**zygote** *n* the fertilized ovum. The diploid cell derived from the fusion after fertilization of the female and male pronuclei, each of which has the haploid, chromosome complement.

**zygote intrafallopian tube transfer (ZIFT)** a technique used in assisted conception whereby the fertilized conceptus is transferred laparoscopically into the uterine (fallopian) tube.

**zymogen** *n* a proenzyme. An inactive precursor of a proteolytic enzyme, e.g. a clotting factor, or the precursor of proteolytic enzymes produced by the stomach and pancreas. May be activated by another enzyme.

Z

# Appendices

## Appendix 1

## Illustrations of major body systems

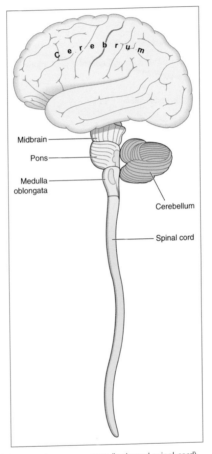

**Figure 1** The parts of the central nervous system (brain and spinal cord).

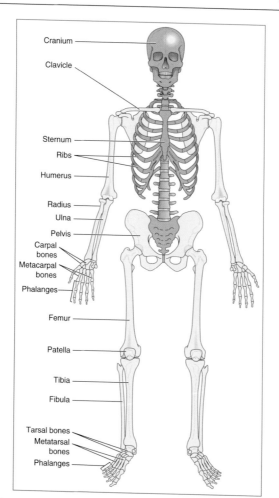

**Figure 2** Skeleton—anterior view (axial skeleton, gold, appendicular skeleton, brown).

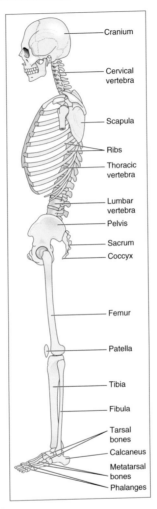

**Figure 3** Skeleton—lateral view.

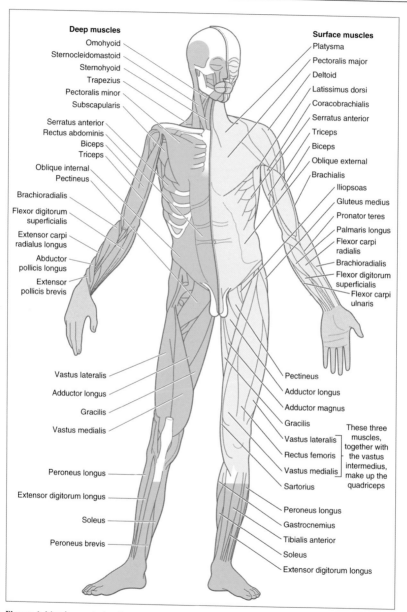

**Deep muscles**

- Omohyoid
- Sternocleidomastoid
- Sternohyoid
- Trapezius
- Pectoralis minor
- Subscapularis
- Serratus anterior
- Rectus abdominis
- Biceps
- Triceps
- Oblique internal
- Pectineus
- Brachioradialis
- Flexor digitorum superficialis
- Extensor carpi radialus longus
- Abductor pollicis longus
- Extensor pollicis brevis
- Vastus lateralis
- Adductor longus
- Gracilis
- Vastus medialis
- Peroneus longus
- Extensor digitorum longus
- Soleus
- Peroneus brevis

**Surface muscles**

- Platysma
- Pectoralis major
- Deltoid
- Latissimus dorsi
- Coracobrachialis
- Serratus anterior
- Triceps
- Biceps
- Oblique external
- Brachialis
- Iliopsoas
- Gluteus medius
- Pronator teres
- Palmaris longus
- Flexor carpi radialis
- Brachioradialis
- Flexor digitorum superficialis
- Flexor carpi ulnaris
- Pectineus
- Adductor longus
- Adductor magnus
- Gracilis
- Vastus lateralis
- Rectus femoris
- Vastus medialis
- Sartorius
- Peroneus longus
- Gastrocnemius
- Tibialis anterior
- Soleus
- Extensor digitorum longus

These three muscles, together with the vastus intermedius, make up the quadriceps

**Figure 4** Muscles—anterior view.

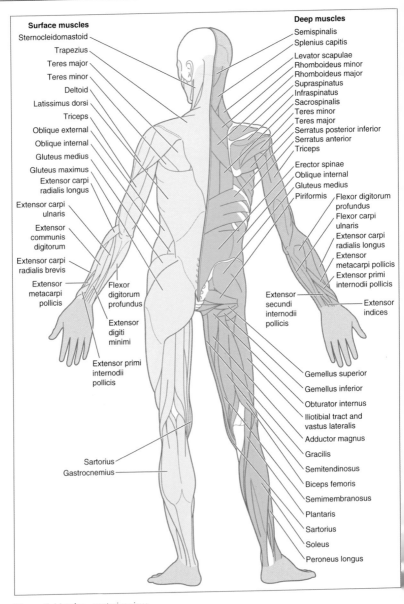

**Figure 5** Muscles—posterior view.

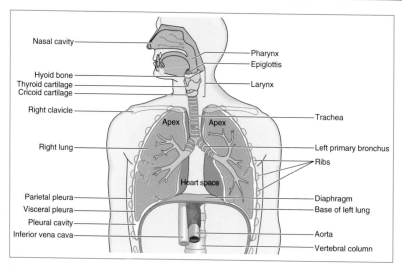

**Figure 6** Respiratory system and related structures.

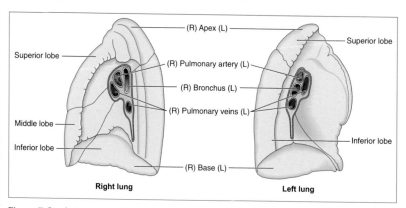

**Figure 7** Respiratory system—lungs showing lobes and vessels and airways of each hilum (medial views).

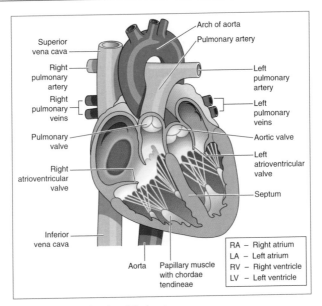

**Figure 8** Circulatory system—interior of the heart.

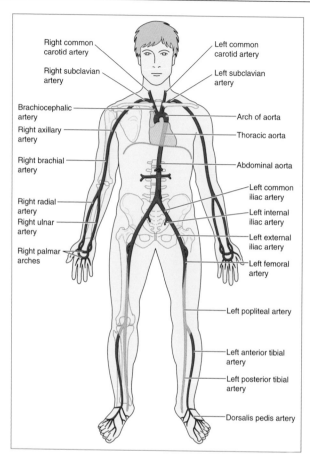

**Figure 9** Circulatory system—arteries (aorta and main arteries of the limbs).

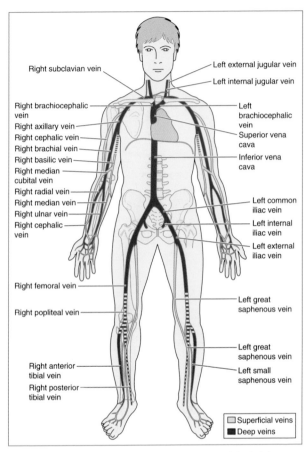

**Figure 10** Circulatory system—veins (venae cavae and main veins of the limbs).

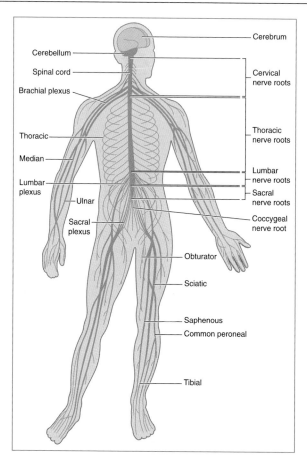

**Figure 11** Nervous system.

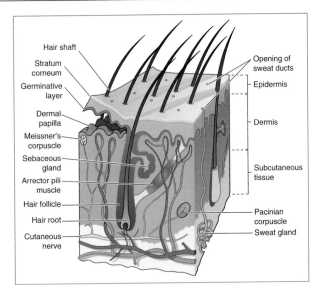

**Figure 12** Skin.

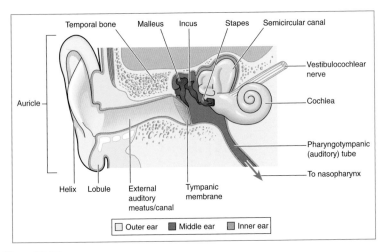

**Figure 13** Ear.

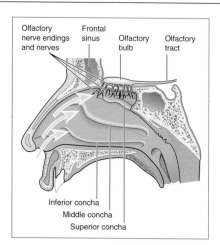

**Figure 14** Nose—olfactory structures.

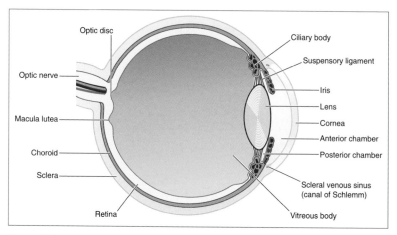

**Figure 15** Eye.

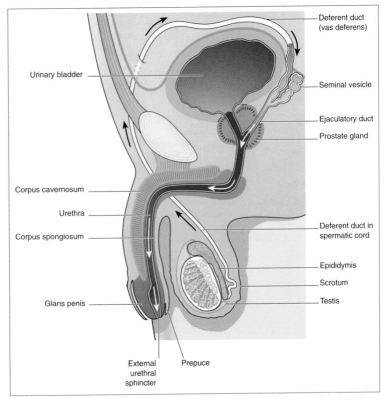

**Figure 16** Male reproductive system (showing route taken by spermatozoa during ejaculation).

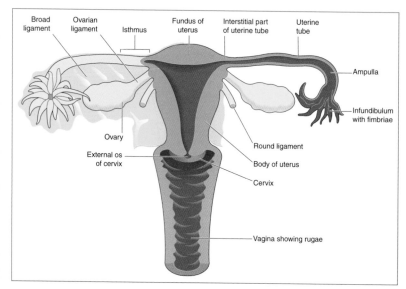

**Figure 17** Female reproductive system.

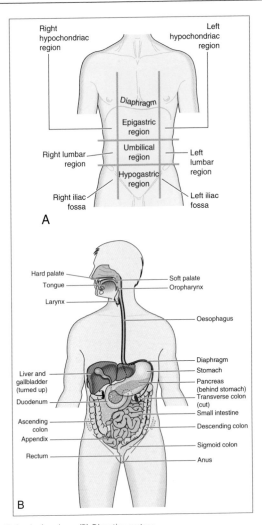

**Figure 18** (A) Abdominal regions. (B) Digestive system.

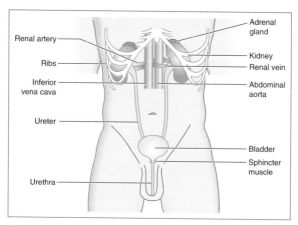

**Figure 19** Urinary system.

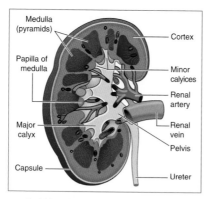

**Figure 20** Urinary system—the kidney (longitudinal section).

## Acknowledgements

Figures 1, 2, 3, 6, 7, 8, 9, 10, 12, 13, 14, 15, 16, 17, 18 (A and B) and 20 are reproduced with permission from Waugh A, Grant A (2006) *Ross and Wilson Anatomy and Physiology in Health and Illness*, 10th edn, Churchill Livingstone, Edinburgh.

## Appendix 2

## SI units and the metric system

### Système International (SI) Units

At an international convention in 1960, the General Conference of Weights and Measures agreed to promulgate an International System of Units, frequently described as SI or Système International. This is merely the name for the current version of the metric system, first introduced in France at the end of the 18th century.

In any system of measurement, the magnitude of some physical quantities must be arbitrarily selected and declared to have unit value. These magnitudes form a set of standards and are called *base units*. All other units are *derived units*.

The SI measurement system is used for medical, scientific and technical purposes in most countries and comprises seven base units with several derived units. Each unit has its own symbol and is expressed as a decimal multiple or submultiple of the base unit by use of the appropriate prefix; for example, millimetre is one thousandth of a metre.

### Base units

| Name of SI unit | Symbol for SI unit | Quantity |
| --- | --- | --- |
| metre | m | length |
| kilogram | kg | mass |
| second | s | time |
| mole | mol | amount of substance |
| ampere | A | electric current |
| kelvin | °K | thermodynamic temperature |
| candela | cd | luminous intensity |

### Derived units
Derived units are obtained by dividing or multiplying any two or more of the seven base units.

| Name of SI unit | Symbol for SI unit | Quantity |
| --- | --- | --- |
| joule | J | work, energy, quantity of heat |
| pascal | Pa | pressure |
| newton | N | force |
| watt | W | power |
| volt | V | electrical potential, potential difference, electromotive force |
| hertz | Hz | frequency |
| becquerel | Bq | radioactivity |
| gray | Gy | adsorbed dose of radiation |
| sievert | Sv | dose equivalent |

## Decimal multiples and submultiples

The metric system uses multiples of 10 to express number.

Multiples and submultiples of the base unit are expressed as decimals and the following prefixes (see below):

The most widely used prefixes are kilo, milli and micro:

$$0.000\ 001\ g\ =10^{-6}g\ =1\ \text{microgram (microgram is used in full for drug prescriptions to avoid dose errors)}$$

Multiples and submultiples of units

| Multiplication factor | | Prefix | Symbol |
|---|---|---|---|
| 1 000 000 000 000 | $10^{12}$ | tera | T |
| 1 000 000 000 | $10^{9}$ | giga | G |
| 1 000 000 | $10^{6}$ | mega | M |
| 1 000 | $10^{3}$ | kilo | k |
| 100 | $10^{2}$ | hecto | h |
| 10 | $10^{1}$ | deca | da |
| 0.1 | $10^{-1}$ | deci | d |
| 0.01 | $10^{-2}$ | centi | c |
| 0.001 | $10^{-3}$ | milli | m |
| 0.000 001 | $10^{-6}$ | micro | μ |
| 0.000 000 001 | $10^{-9}$ | nano | n |
| 0.000 000 000 001 | $10^{-12}$ | pico | p |
| 0.000 000 000 000 001 | $10^{-15}$ | femto | f |
| 0.000 000 000 000 000 001 | $10^{-18}$ | atto | a |

## Rules for using units

1. The symbol for a unit is unaltered in the plural and should not be followed by a full stop except at the end of the sentence:

   5 cm *not* 5 cm. or 5 cms.

2. The decimal sign between digits is indicated by a full stop positioned near the line. No commas are used to divide large numbers into groups of three, but a half-space (whole space in typing) is left after every third digit. If the numerical value of the number is less than 1 unit, a zero should precede the decimal sign:

   0.123 456 *not* .123,456

3. The SI symbol for 'day' (i.e. 24 hours) is 'd', but urine and faecal excretion of substances should preferably be expressed as 'per 24 hours':

   g/24 h

4. 'Squared' and 'cubed' are expressed as numerical powers and not by abbreviation:

   square centimetre is $cm^2$ *not* sq cm.

## Commonly used measurements

1. The SI base unit for temperature is the kelvin; however, temperature is expressed as degrees Celsius (°C).

   1°Celsius = 1°Centigrade

2. The calorie is replaced by the joule:

   1 calorie = 4.2 J

   1 kilocalorie (dietetic 'large' Calorie) = 4.2 kilojoules

   The energy of food or individual requirements for energy are measured in kilojoules (kJ), but in practice the kilocalorie (kcal) is still in common use.

3. The SI base unit for amount of substance is the mole (mol). The concentration of many substances is expressed in moles per litre (mol/L) or millimoles per litre (mmol/L), which replaces milliequivalents per litre (mEq/L). Some exceptions exist and include: haemoglobin, expressed in grams per litre (g/L) or grams per decilitre (g/dL), and plasma proteins, expressed in g/L. Enzyme activity is expressed in International Units (IU, U or iu).

4. The SI unit of pressure is the pascal (Pa), and the kilopascal (kPa) replaces millimetres of mercury pressure (mmHg) for blood pressure and blood gases.

    1 mmHg = 133.32 Pa
    1 kPa = 7.5006 mmHg

    However, blood pressure is still widely measured in mmHg pressure and cerebrospinal fluid in millimetres of water (mmH$_2$O). Central venous pressure may be measured in centimetres of water (cmH$_2$O) using manual systems with a water manometer, and in either mmHg or cmH$_2$O using a pressure transducer.

5. Volume is calculated by multiplying length, width and depth. The SI unit for length, the metre (m), is not appropriate, as a cubic metre is not practical for most purposes. The volume of a 10-cm cube; the litre (L), is used instead. The millilitre (mL) is commonly used in clinical practice.

## Weights and measures

### Linear measure

| | |
|---|---|
| 1 kilometre (km) | = 1000 metres (m) |
| 1 metre (m) | = 100 centimetres (cm) or 1000 millimetres (mm) |
| 1 centimetre (cm) | = 10 millimetres (mm) |
| 1 millimetre (mm) | = 1000 micrometres (μm) |
| 1 micrometre (μm) | = 1000 nanometres (nm) |

Conversions

| Metric | Imperial |
|---|---|
| 1 metre (m) | = 39.370 inches (in) |
| 1 centimetre (cm) | = 0.3937 inches (in) |
| 30.48 centimetres (cm) | = 1 foot (ft) |
| 2.54 centimetres (cm) | = 1 inch (in) |

### Volume

| | |
|---|---|
| 1 litre (L) | = 1000 millilitres (mL) |
| 1 millilitre (mL) | = 1000 microlitres (μL) |

Conversions

| Metric | Imperial |
|---|---|
| 1 litre (L) | = 1.76 pints (pt) |
| 568.25 millilitres (mL) | = 1 pint (pt) |
| 28.4 millilitres (mL) | = 1 fluid ounce (fl oz) |

### Weight (mass)

| | |
|---|---|
| 1 kilogram (kg) | = 1000 grams (g) |
| 1 gram (g) | = 1000 milligrams (mg) |
| 1 milligram (mg) | = 1000 micrograms (μg) |
| 1 microgram (μg) | = 1000 nanograms (ng) |

N.B.: In order to avoid any confusion with milligram (mg), the word microgram should be written in full on prescriptions.

Conversions

| Metric | Imperial |
|---|---|
| 1 kilogram (kg) | 2.204 pounds (lb) |
| 1 gram (g) | 0.0353 ounce (oz) |
| 453.59 grams (g) | 1 pound (lb) |
| 28.34 grams (g) | 1 ounce (oz) |

**Temperature**

$$°\text{Fahrenheit} = \left(\frac{9}{5} \times x°\text{C}\right) + 32$$

$$°\text{Centigrade} = \frac{5}{9} \times (x°\text{F} - 32)$$

where $x$ is the temperature to be converted.

## Conversion scales for certain chemical pathology tests and units of measurement

Chemical Pathology Blood Plasma

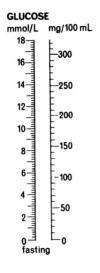

**GLUCOSE**
mmol/L    mg/100 mL

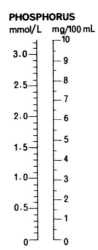

**PHOSPHORUS**
mmol/L    mg/100 mL

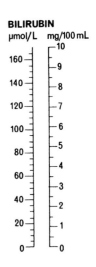

**BILIRUBIN**
µmol/L    mg/100 mL

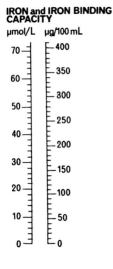

**IRON and IRON BINDING CAPACITY**
µmol/L    µg/100 mL

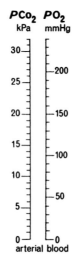

$P\text{Co}_2$   $P\text{O}_2$
kPa    mmHg

arterial blood

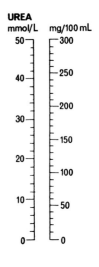

**UREA**
mmol/L    mg/100 mL

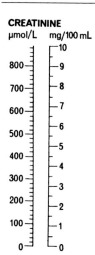

**CREATININE**

μmol/L    mg/100 mL

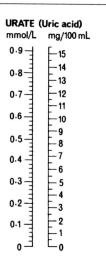

**URATE (Uric acid)**

mmol/L    mg/100 mL

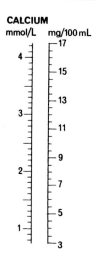

**CALCIUM**

mmol/L    mg/100 mL

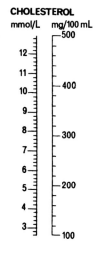

**CHOLESTEROL**

mmol/L    mg/100 mL

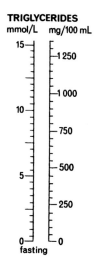

**TRIGLYCERIDES**

mmol/L    mg/100 mL

fasting

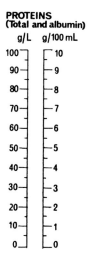

**PROTEINS**
**(Total and albumin)**

g/L    g/100 mL

**PBI**

nmol/L    µg/100 mL

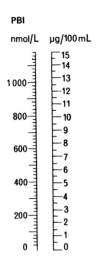

**CORTISOL**

nmol/L    µg/100 mL

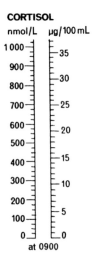

at 0900

**Urine OESTRIOL ('Oestrogens')**

µmol/24 h    mg/24 h

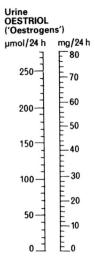

General measurements

**HEIGHT**

cm    inches

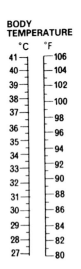

**BODY TEMPERATURE**

°C    °F

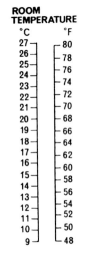

**ROOM TEMPERATURE**

°C    °F

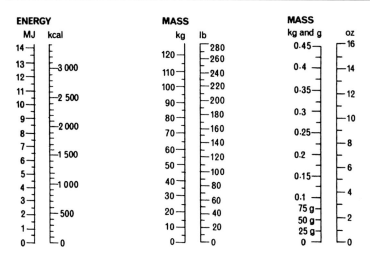

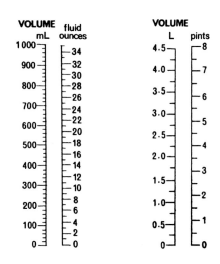

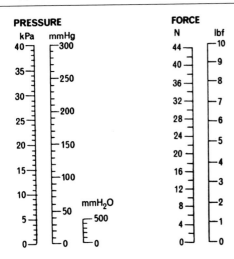

**PRESSURE**

**FORCE**

**Acknowledgement**

Conversion scales are taken from Goodsell D (1975) Coming to terms with SI metric. *Nursing Mirror* 141: 55–59 and are reproduced by kind permission of the author and *Nursing Mirror*.

# Normal values

The values below represent an 'average' reference range, in adults, for blood, cerebrospinal fluid, faeces and urine, and should only be used as a guide. Reference ranges vary between laboratories and readers should consult their own laboratory for those used locally. Reference ranges for some hormones in venous blood are provided on the DVD. ⊙ DVD

## Blood—biochemistry (venous serum or plasma unless otherwise stated)

| Test | Reference range |
| --- | --- |
| Acid phosphatase | 0.1–0.6 U/L |
| Alanine aminotransferase (ALT) | 10–40 U/L |
| Albumin | 35–50 g/L |
| Alkali phosphatase | 40–125 U/L |
| $\alpha_1$-antitrypsin | 1.1–2.1 g/L |
| Amylase | 25–125 U/L |
| Aspartate aminotransferase (AST) | 10–45 U/L |
| Base excess | −2 to +2 |
| Bicarbonate (arterial blood analysis) | 22–28 mmol/L |
| Bilirubin—total | 2–17 μmol/L |
| Caeruloplasmin | 150–600 mg/L |
| Calcium | 2.1–2.6 mmol/L |
| Chloride | 97–106 mmol/L |
| Cholesterol (total) | Less than 5.2 mmol/L: ideal 5.2–6.5 mmol/L: mild increase 6.5–7.8 mmol/L: moderate increase greater than 7.8 mmol/L: severe increase |
| High-density lipoprotein (HDL) cholesterol | Greater than 1.0 mmol/L |
| $PaCO_2$ (arterial blood analysis) | 4.6–6.0 kPa |
| Copper | 13–24 μmol/L |
| C-reactive protein | <5 mg/L |
| Creatine kinase (total) | |
| Female | 30–135 U/L |
| Male | 55–170 U/L |
| Creatine kinase MB isoenzyme | <6% of total creatine kinase |
| Creatinine | 60–120 μmol/L |
| Ferritin | |
| Female | 7–280 μg/L premenopausal 4–233 μg/L postmenopausal |
| Male | 17–300 μg/L |

*Continued*

**Blood**—biochemistry (venous serum or plasma unless otherwise stated)—
Continued

| Test | Reference range |
|------|-----------------|
| Gamma-glutamyl transferase (GGT) | 5–55 U/L |
| Glucose (venous blood, fasting) | 3.6–5.8 mmol/L |
| Glycosylated (glycated) haemoglobin (HbA$_{1c}$) | 4–6% |
| Hydrogen ion concentration (arterial blood analysis) | 35–44 nmol/L |
| Immunoglobulins | |
|   IgA | 0.8–4 g/L |
|   IgG | 5.5–16 g/L |
|   IgM | 0.4–2.9 g/L |
| Iron | |
|   Female | 10–28 μmol/L |
|   Male | 14–32 μmol/L |
| Iron-binding capacity total (TIBC) | 45–80 μmol/L |
| Lactate (arterial blood) | 0.6–1.7 mmol/L |
| Lactate dehydrogenase (total) | 230–460 U/L |
| Lead | <1.0 μmol/L |
| Magnesium | 0.75–1.0 mmol/L |
| Osmolality | 275–295 mOsm/kg |
| Osmolarity | 275–295 mOsm/L |
| Oxygen saturation | >97% |
| PaO$_2$ (arterial blood analysis) | 10.0–13.3 kPa |
| pH (arterial blood analysis) | 7.35–7.45 |
| Phosphate (fasting) | 0.8–1.4 mmol/L |
| Potassium (plasma) | 3.3–4.7 mmol/L |
| Potassium (serum) | 3.6–5.0 mmol/L |
| Protein (total) | 60–80 g/L |
| Sodium | 135–143 mmol/L |
| Transferrin | 2.0–4.0 g/L |
| Triglycerides (fasting) | 0.5–1.7 mmol/L |
| Urates | |
|   Female | 0.12–0.36 mmol/L |
|   Male | 0.12–0.42 mmol/L |
| Urea | 2.5–6.5 mmol/L |
| Vitamin A | 0.5–2.01 μmol/L |
| Vitamin D | |
|   25-hydroxy | 15–100 nmol/L depending on season |
|   1,25-dihydroxy | 20–120 nmol/L |
| Zinc | 11–22 μmol/L |

## Blood—haematology

| | |
|---|---|
| Activated partial thromboplastin time (APTT) | 20–35 s |
| Bleeding time (Ivy) | 2–8 min |
| Erythrocyte sedimentation rate (ESR) (adult) | |
|     Female | 0–15 mm/h |
|     Male | 0–10 mm/h |
| | N.B.: Older people may have higher values |
| Fibrinogen | 1.5–4.0 g/L |
| Folate (serum) | 2.0–13.5 µg/L |
| Folate (red blood cell) | 95–570 µg/L |
| Haematocrit *see* packed cell volume | |
| Haemoglobin | |
|     Female | 115–165 g/L (11.5–16.5 g/dL) |
|     Male | 130–180 g/L (13–18 g/dL) |
| Haptoglobins | 0.3–2.0 g/L |
| Mean cell haemoglobin (MCH) | 27–32 pg |
| Mean cell haemoglobin concentration (MCHC) | 30–35 g/dL |
| Mean cell volume (MCV) | 78–94 fL |
| Packed cell volume (PCV) (haematocrit) | |
|     Female | 0.37–0.47 (37–47%) |
|     Male | 0.40–0.54 (40–54%) |
| Platelets | $150–400 \times 10^9$/L |
| Prothrombin time | 11–14 s |
| Red cell count | |
|     Female | $3.8–5.3 \times 10^{12}$/L |
|     Male | $4.5–6.5 \times 10^{12}$/L |
| Reticulocytes (adults) | $25–85 \times 10^9$/L |
| White blood cells | |
| Total | $4.0–11.0 \times 10^9$/L |
| Differential | |
|     Neutrophils | $2.0–7.5 \times 10^9$/L |
|     Eosinophils | $0.04–0.4 \times 10^9$/L |
|     Basophils | $0.01–0.10 \times 10^9$/L |
|     Lymphocytes | $1.5–4.0 \times 10^9$/L |
|     Monocytes | $0.2–0.8 \times 10^9$/L |

## Cerebrospinal fluid

| | |
|---|---|
| Pressure (adult) | 50–200 mm water |
| Cells | $<5 \times 10^6$/L all mononuclear |
| Glucose | 2.5–4.0 mmol/L |
| Protein | 150–450 mg/L |
| Immunoglobulin G (IgG) index | <0.6 |

## Faeces

| | |
|---|---|
| Fat content (daily output on normal diet) | <7 g/24 h |
| Fat (as stearic acid) | 11–18 mmol/24 h |

## Urine

| | |
|---|---|
| Albumin/creatinine ratio (ACR) (used to detect microalbuminuria) | <3.5 mg albumin/mmol creatinine |
| Albumin excretion rate (AER) (used to detect microalbuminuria) | <20 µg albumin/min |
| Calcium (depends on diet) | up to 12 mmol/24 h (normal diet) |
| Copper | 0.2–0.6 µmol/24 h |
| Cortisol (24-h urine collection) | 25–250 nmol/24 h |
| Creatinine | 10–20 mmol/24 h |
| 5-Hydroxyindole-3-acetic acid (5HIAA) | 10–60 µmol/24 h |
| Metadrenaline | 0.3–1.7 µmol/24 h |
| Magnesium | 3.3–5.0 mmol/24 h |
| Normetadrenaline | 0.4–3.4 µmol/24 h |
| Oxalate | 0.04–0.49 mmol/24 h |
| Phosphate | 15–50 mmol/24 h |
| pH | 4–8 |
| Potassium (depends on dietary intake) | 25–100 mmol/24 h |
| Protein (total) | < 0.3 g/L |
| Sodium (depends on dietary intake) | 100–200 mmol/24 h |
| Urate | 1.2–3.0 mmol/24 h |
| Urea | 170–500 mmol/24 h |

## Nutrients

The maintenance of health requires the correct intake of nutrients for the production of energy and the molecules needed for cell growth and repair. These nutrients are the energy-yielding macronutrients—carbohydrate (including non-starch polysaccharide), protein and fat—and the micronutrients—vitamins (water-soluble and fat-soluble) and minerals (including trace elements).

### Further reading

Barker H 2002 Nutrition/Dietetics for Healthcare, 10th edn. Edinburgh: Churchill Livingstone
Geissler C, Powers H 2005 Human Nutrition, 11th edn. Edinburgh: Churchill Livingstone

### Reference

Department of Health 1991 Report on Health and Social Subjects 41. Dietary Reference Values for Food Eergy and Nutrients for the United Kingdom. London: HMSO

## Macronutrients

| Nutrient and energy value | Recommended nutritional intake (RNI: Department of Health 1991) | Sources | Action/functions | Deficiency | Excess | Special points |
|---|---|---|---|---|---|---|
| **Carbohydrate** 1 g yields 16 kJ (3.75 kcal) | A minimum of 47% of total daily energy intake should be provided by carbohydrate. This should include no more than 10% as non-milk extrinsic sugars. The RNI for non-starch polysaccharide is 18 g/day | Rice, pasta, noodles, chapatti, bread, breakfast cereals, sugar, yam, plantain and potato | Provides energy for metabolic processes | Weight loss, ketosis | Obesity, hypertriglyceridaemia | Diets high in carbohydrate tend to be low in fat |
| **Protein** 1 g yields 17 kJ (4 kcal) | Female 45 g/day Male 55 g/day | Meat, fish, eggs, nuts, pulses, dairy products, tofu, and quorn | A component of all body tissues; energy source in some situations | Retarded growth; weight loss and muscle wasting, poor wound healing; impaired immune system; fat deposition in the liver | Possible link with loss of minerals from bone and age-related deterioration in renal function | Protein content of western diets usually higher than the RNI |
| **Fat** 1 g yields 37 kJ (9 kcal) | Should not exceed 33% of total daily energy intake and of this, no more than 10% should be saturated fatty acids | Pastry, cakes, biscuits, chocolate and crisps, cooking oils, ghee, margarine, fried foods, full-fat dairy products, meat, oily fish, seeds, nuts | Source of energy, energy storage, absorption of fat-soluble vitamins, synthesis of steroid hormones, integrity of nerve and cell membranes, insulation | Weight loss; deficiency of essential fatty acids can lead to neurological damage | Obesity; increased risk of many conditions, including cardiovascular disease and some cancers | The normal development of the nervous system depends on two essential fatty acids— linoleic acid and alpha-linolenic acid |

# Micronutrients: Vitamins—water-soluble

| Vitamin | Recommended nutritional intake (RNI: Department of Health 1991) | Sources | Action/functions | Deficiency | Excess | Special points |
|---|---|---|---|---|---|---|
| **Vitamin B group** | | | | | | |
| $B_1$ Thiamin(e) | 0.4 mg/ 1000 kcal | Fortified breakfast cereals, yeast extract, vegetables, fruit, wholegrain cereals, milk, liver, eggs, pork | Coenzyme for carbohydrate metabolism | Beri-beri; neuritis; mental confusion; fatigue; poor growth in children. Wernicke–Korsakoff syndrome occurring with alcohol misuse | Headache, insomnia, irritability, contact dermatitis | Requirement related to the amount of carbohydrate intake |
| $B_2$ Riboflavin | Female: 1.1 mg/day Male: 1.3 mg/day | Milk, milk products, offal, yeast extract, fortified breakfast cereals | Coenzyme for the metabolism of carbohydrate, fat and protein | Fissures at corner of mouth; tongue inflammation; corneal vascularization | Large quantities are not absorbed thus preventing toxicity | Destroyed by sunlight |
| $B_3$ Niacin (nicotinic acid and nicotinamide) | 6.6 mg/ 1000 kcal as nicotinic acid equivalents | Meat, fish, yeast extract, pulses, wholegrains, fortified breakfast cereals | Energy metabolism, as part of coenzymes NAD and NADP involved in oxidation and reduction reactions | Pellagra—dermatitis, diarrhoea and dementia | Liver damage, skin irritation | Also synthesized from the amino acid tryptophan |
| $B_5$ Pantothenic acid | None set | Widespread in food, e.g. liver, eggs, yeast, vegetables, pulses, cereals | Protein, fat, carbohydrate and alcohol metabolism | Vomiting, insomnia | Not reported | |

*Continued*

## Micronutrients: Vitamins—water-soluble—Continued

| Vitamin | Recommended nutritional intake (RNI: Department of Health 1991) | Sources | Action/functions | Deficiency | Excess | Special points |
|---|---|---|---|---|---|---|
| B₆ Pyridoxine | Female: 1.2 mg/day Male: 1.4 mg/day | Meat, fish, eggs, some vegetables, wholegrains | Amino acid metabolism. Needed for haemoglobin production | Rare: metabolic abnormalities and convulsions | Peripheral nerve damage | Requirement is related to protein intake |
| Biotin | None set | Widely distributed in many foods, e.g. offal, egg yolk, legumes, etc. Can be synthesized by intestinal bacteria | Essential in fat metabolism | Rare: dermatitis, hair loss, fatigue and anorexia. May be seen in patients having long-term total parenteral nutrition and where large quantities of raw egg are eaten | None known | |
| B₁₂ Cobalamins | 15 µg/g of protein | Animal products, meat, eggs, fish, dairy products, yeast extract | Essential for red blood cell formation and nerve myelination. Needed for folate use | Megaloblastic anaemia. Irreversible spinal cord damage | Not reported | Requires the intrinsic factor produced by the stomach for absorption; only found in foods of animal origin; therefore, strict vegetarians and vegans require a dietary supplement |

| | | | | | |
|---|---|---|---|---|---|
| Folates (folic acid) | 200 µg/day | Green leafy vegetables, bread, fortified breakfast cereals, yeast extract, liver | Red blood cell production, DNA synthesis | Megaloblastic anaemia; growth retardation | Can mask the megaloblastic anaemia of $B_{12}$ deficiency | Supplement recommended prior to conception and during first 3 months of pregnancy to reduce the incidence of neural tube defects |
| **Vitamin C (ascorbic acid)** | 40 mg/day | Citrus fruits, kiwi fruit, blackcurrants; green peppers, green leafy vegetables; potato; strawberries; tomatoes. Content decreases with storage | Collagen synthesis, formation of bones, connective tissue, teeth. Iron absorption for red blood cell production. Acts as an antioxidant | Sore mouth and gums; capillary bleeding; scurvy; delayed wound healing, scar breakdown | Diarrhoea; oxalate stones in kidneys | Destroyed by cooking in the presence of air and by plant enzymes released when cutting and grating raw food |

## Micronutrients: Vitamins—fat-soluble

| Vitamin | Recommended nutritional intake (RNI: Department of Health 1991) | Sources | Action/functions | Deficiency | Excess | Special points |
|---|---|---|---|---|---|---|
| **Vitamin A**—retinol | Female: 600 µg/day Male: 700 µg/day | As retinol in liver, kidney, oily fish, egg yolk, full-fat dairy produce. As the provitamin carotenes in green, yellow, orange and red fruit and vegetables, e.g. broccoli, carrots, apricots, mangoes, sweet potatoes and tomatoes | Visual pigments in retina, aids night vision. Normal growth and development of tissues; essential for healthy skin and mucosae. Acts as an antioxidant | Poor growth; rough, dry skin and mucosae; xerophthalmia and eventual blindness; increased risk of infection; poor night vision | High doses are teratogenic | Synthesized in the body from carotenes present in the diet |
| **Vitamin D**—cholecalciferol and ergosterol | 10 µg/day for the house-bound | Oily fish, egg yolk, butter, fortified margarine; action of ultraviolet rays (sunlight) on the provitamin (7-dehydrocholesterol) in the skin | Calcium and phosphorus homeostasis | Rickets (children); osteomalacia (adults) | Rare: weight loss and diarrhoea | Produced in the body by the action of sunlight on a provitamin in the skin; deficiency develops in those who are not exposed to sun, for example, the house-bound |

| | | | | |
|---|---|---|---|---|
| **Vitamin E**—tocopherols and tocotrienes | None set | Wheat germ, vegetable oils, nuts, seeds, egg yolk, cereals, dark green vegetables | An antioxidant. Protects against cell membrane damage | Haemolytic anaemia, can develop in premature infants and malabsorption syndrome | Breast pain, muscle weakness, gastrointestinal disorders | Requirement is increased with increased intake of polyunsaturated fatty acids |
| **Vitamin K**—phylloquinones and menaquinones | None set | Green leafy vegetables, fruit and dairy products | Needed for the production of prothrombin and other coagulation factors | Impaired clotting; liver damage | Not yet observed from naturally occurring vitamin | Synthesized by intestinal bacteria so deficiency unusual; can occur in newborns (haemorrhagic disease of the newborn) and those on anticoagulant therapy |

## Micronutrients: Minerals

| Mineral and chemical symbol | Recommended nutritional intake (RNI: Department of Health 1991) | Sources | Action/functions | Deficiency | Excess | Special points |
|---|---|---|---|---|---|---|
| **Calcium—Ca** | 700 mg/day | Milk and milk products, green leafy vegetables, soya beans, white bread, hard water | Strengthening the skeleton and teeth; blood coagulation; normal neuromuscular function | Osteomalacia; rickets; tetany. Reduced bone density, osteoporosis | Calcium deposits in soft tissue, hypercalcaemia | Absorption helped by vitamin D and parathyroid hormone |
| **Iodine—I** | 140 µg/day | Seafood; iodized salt; milk and milk products, meat and eggs | Production of the thyroid hormones: thyroxine and triiodothyronine | Goitre; retarded growth; impaired brain development; congenital abnormalities | Goitre and hyperthyroidism | Some vegetables contain goitrogens that inhibit iodine absorption |
| **Iron—Fe** | Female: 14.8 mg/day Male: 8.7 mg/day | Liver, kidney, red meat, egg yolk, wholegrains, pulses, dark green vegetables, dried fruit, treacle, cocoa, molasses | Component of haemoglobin, myoglobin and many enzymes | Iron-deficiency anaemia. Poor growth; impaired intellectual development | Liver damage | Absorption is aided by vitamin C and inhibited by phytates and tannins |
| **Magnesium— Mg** | Female: 270 mg/day Male: 300 mg/day | Cereals, milk, nuts, seeds, and green vegetables | Cofactor for many enzymes essential for carbohydrate and protein metabolism; important role in calcium homeostasis and skeletal development. Neuromuscular function | Unlikely, mainly in cases of chronic malabsorption and chronic renal failure when it will accompany hypocalcaemia | Unlikely from dietary sources | Absorption inhibited by phytate |

| | | | | | |
|---|---|---|---|---|---|
| **Potassium—K** | 3500 mg/day | Major intracellular electrolyte; influences muscle contraction and nerve excitability. Regulation of acid–base balance | Muscular weakness; depression; confusion; arrhythmias; cardiac arrest | Hyperkalaemia, cardiac arrest | Kidney controls secretion and absorption; deficiency is rare due to poor dietary intake but can occur following prolonged use of diuretics and purgatives |
| **Sodium—Na** | 1600 mg/day | Major extracellular electrolyte; important for regulating water balance. Regulation of acid–base balance | Weakness; cramp; faintness | Oedema, hypertension | Lost through fever, sweat and diarrhoea |
| **Zinc—Zn** | Female: 7.0 mg/day Male: 9.5 mg/day | Cofactor needed for many enzymes. Structural role in some proteins; wound healing; functioning of immune system; sexual and physical development | Fatigue; retarded growth and sexual maturity | Nausea, vomiting, fever, or anaemia with chronic excess | Present in all tissues |

Plus other minerals, such as chloride, and trace elements (needed in minute quantities) that include: copper; chromium; fluoride; phosphorus as phosphates; manganese; molybdenum and selenium.

# Drugs—the law, measurement and drug groups in common use
Revised by Jennifer Kelly

## Drugs and the law

The main Acts governing the use of medicines in the UK are the Medicines Act 1968, the Misuse of Drugs Act 1971, the Medicinal Products: Prescription by Nurses Act 1992 and the Health and Social Care Act 2001.

At the time of writing there are proposals to extend the prescribing of controlled drugs by independent nurse prescribers, and under patient group directions. Readers are advised to check new legislation that may affect practice.

### The Medicines Act 1968

Under this Act, medicines are divided into three groups:

1. Prescription-only medicines (POM)—includes most of the potent drugs in common use, from antibiotics to hypnotics. These are drugs that may only be supplied or administered to a patient on the instructions of an appropriate practitioner.
2. Pharmacy-only medicines (P)—drugs supplied under the control and supervision of a registered pharmacist without the need for a prescription.
3. General sales list (GSL) medicines—includes commonly used drugs such as aspirin and paracetamol, available through many retail outlets.

These distinctions of POM, P and GSL medicines do not apply to hospitals where it is accepted practice that medicines are supplied only on prescription.

### The Misuse of Drugs Act 1971

This Act imposes controls on those drugs liable to cause dependency and harm when misused, e.g. for recreational purposes. It grades drugs into three classes based on their potential harmfulness:

1. Class A—e.g. cocaine, diamorphine, methylenedioxymethamfetamine (ecstasy), morphine, injectable class B drugs (the 2005 Drugs Act gives the police increased powers to test for class A drugs)
2. Class B—e.g. oral amfetamines, barbiturates, codeine
3. Class C—e.g. most benzodiazepines, cannabis, cannabis resin, buprenorphine, zolpidem, androgenic and anabolic steroids. In the UK debate continues on reclassifying cannabis to Class B.

The Act categorizes these drugs into five separate schedules according to different levels of control over production, supply, possession, prescribing and record-keeping. The current level of control is defined by the Misuse of Drugs Regulations 2001 (see table below). Health care practitioners should be familiar with regulations governing Schedule 2 and 3 drugs, which are frequently referred to as 'controlled drugs' (CDs); although all five schedules are technically controlled drugs.

| Schedule | Examples |
| --- | --- |
| 1 | Drugs that have no medicinal use, e.g. cannabis and hallucinogens such as lysergide (LSD). Possession and supply are only permitted with Home Office authority |
| 2 | Addictive drugs including: amfetamine, cocaine, diamorphine (heroin), morphine, pethidine, secobarbital. Their prescription, safe custody (except secobarbital) must fulfil the full controlled drug requirements, which includes maintaining registers |
| 3 | These include barbiturates (except secobarbital), buprenorphine, phentermine and temazepam. All schedule 3 drugs, except temazepam, are subject to special prescription requirements, but not to safe custody requirements with some exceptions (e.g. buprenorphine). CD registers are not required |
| 4 | These are subject neither to controlled drug prescription rules nor to safe custody requirements. Part I includes benzodiazepines (except temazepam) and zolpidem, in which some controls exist. Part II includes androgenic and anabolic steroids, clenbuterol, chorionic gonadotrophin (hCG), somatropin |
| 5 | These medicines, such as some cough mixtures and kaolin and morphine, contain only small amounts of the CD and so are exempt from most CD regulations except the keeping of invoices for 2 years |

Amendments in 2006 to the Misuse of Drugs Regulations 2001 mean that prescriptions involving CDs can now be computer-generated, except for the signature. A computer-generated prescription must include:

- Patient's name and address
- Dose and dosage form, e.g. tablets, capsules
- Total quantity to be supplied written in words and figures
- Prescriber's signature in ink and the date

In hospital CDs must be:

- Stored in a double-locked cupboard attached to the wall and reserved for CDs alone, with the key being kept and carried by the nurse in charge
- Obtained by a prescription signed by a medical officer. Alternatively, ward stocks of CDs in frequent use can be ordered in special CDs order books. Each order must be signed by the nurse in charge
- Recorded in a special book every time a dose is given. The record must state the date, patient's name, time administered and dosage. This record is signed by the nurse giving the drug and another person who has checked the source of the drug as well as the dosage against the prescription
- Checked regularly to ensure that the contents of the CDs cupboard match the record books. Any discrepancies require full investigation, which may involve the police.

As a result of the Shipman Inquiry legislation is being introduced to tighten controls over the management of CDs and to ensure there is an audit trail to monitor their movement from prescriber through dispenser to patient. For example, people collecting CDs need to provide proof of identity.

Until recently, only registered medical practitioners and dentists could prescribe preparations containing CDs, with a special licence being required from the Home Office to prescribe CDs for the treatment of addiction. However, the Misuse of Drugs (Amendment) (no. 3) Regulations 2003 allow specialist nurses to prescribe diazepam, lorazepam, midazolam, codeine phosphate, dihydrocodeine, and co-phenotrope for minor ailments and in some specific situations. Furthermore nurses will also be able to prescribe the following drugs under a patient group direction:

- Diamorphine, but only for the treatment of cardiac pain by specialist nurses in accident and emergency and coronary care units in hospitals
- All drugs listed in Schedule 4 (except anabolic steroids) and Schedule 5 of the 2001 regulations.

## Medicinal Products: Prescription by Nurses Act 1992 and Health and Social Care Act 2001

These two Acts contain the primary legislation to allow nurse prescribing and its subsequent extension to 'non-medical prescribing'. Initially nurses and health visitors working in the community who had completed an appropriate educational programme were able to prescribe from a limited formulary. This formulary was expanded in 2002 and nurses in secondary care were enabled to take on a prescribing role. In May 2006 amendments to the legislation enabled nurses, midwives and pharmacists to prescribe, in theory, any drug in the *British National Formulary*, with the exception of unlicensed drugs and most CDs. These prescribers are referred to as independent prescribers as they take responsibility for the clinical assessment of the patient, establishing a diagnosis and the clinical management required, as well as taking responsibility for prescribing where necessary. However, the Commission on Human Medicines (formerly Committee on Safety of Medicines and the Medicines Commission) advise that these independent prescribers should *only* prescribe medicines for an identified list of medical conditions (www.bnf.org.uk).

As well as independent prescribers, supplementary or dependent prescribing was introduced in 2003, allowing first-level registered nurses, registered midwives and pharmacists, who have undertaken appropriate training, to implement an agreed patient-specific clinical management plan once the patient has been clinically assessed by an independent prescriber (a doctor or dentist). The clinical management plan specifies the range and circumstances within which the supplementary prescriber can vary the dosage, frequency and formulation of the medicines identified and contains relevant warnings about known sensitivities of the patient to particular medicines and includes arrangements for notification of adverse drug reactions. Other health care professionals, including optometrists, physiotherapists, podiatrists and radiographers, are now also able to become supplementary prescribers.

Although, not considered a form of 'prescribing', patient group directions allow a variety of health professionals, including nurses, physiotherapists, paramedics and radiographers to supply or administer a named medicine in an identified clinical situation.

### Further reading and information sources

*British National Formulary* and *British National Formulary for Children* revised twice yearly (March and September) by the British Medical Association and the Royal Pharmaceutical Society of Great Britain. Available online at www.bnf.org.uk.

Department of Health: www.dh.gov.uk.

Medicines and Health Products Regulatory Agency (MHRA): www.mhra.gov.uk.

National Prescribing Centre: www.npc.co.uk.

### Drug measurement

The International System of Units (SI) is used for drug doses and concentrations and for patient data (including weight and body surface area), drug levels in the body and other measurements (see Appendix 2).

### Weight

Grams (g) and milligrams (mg) are the units most often encountered in drug dosages. Doses of less than 1 g should be expressed in milligrams, e.g. 250 mg rather than 0.25 g. Similarly, doses less than 1 mg should be expressed in micrograms, e.g. 200 micrograms, rather than 0.2 mg. Whenever drugs are prescribed in microgram dosages, the units should be written in full, e.g. digoxin 250 micrograms, as the use of the contracted terms μg or mcg may in practice be mistaken for mg and, as this dose is 1000 times greater, disastrous consequences may follow.

Drug dosages are often described in terms of unit dose per kg of body weight, i.e. mg/kg, microgram/kg, etc. This method of dosage is frequently used for children and allows dosages to be tailored to the individual patient's size.

## Volume

Litres (L rather than 'l', which can be misread as 'one') and millilitres (mL) account for almost all measurements expressed in unit volume for the prescription and administration of drugs.

## Concentration

When expressing concentration of dosages of a medicine in liquid form, several methods are available:

- Unit weight per unit volume—describes the unit of weight of a drug contained in unit volume, e.g. 1 mg in 1 mL, 40 mg in 2 mL. For example, pethidine injection 100 mg in 2 mL; chloral hydrate mixture 500 mg in 5 mL.
- Percentage (weight in volume)—describes the weight of a drug, expressed in grams (g), which is contained in 100 mL of solution, e.g. calcium gluconate injection 10% which contains 10 g in each 100 mL of solution, or 1 g in each 10 mL, or 100 mg (0.1 g) in each 1 mL.
- Percentage (weight in weight)—describes the weight of a drug, expressed in grams (g), which is contained in 100 g of a solid or semisolid medicament, such as ointments and creams, e.g. fusidic acid ointment 2%, which contains 2 g of fusidic acid in each 100 g of ointment.
- Volume containing '1 part'—a few liquids and, to a lesser extent, gases, particularly those containing drugs in very low concentrations, are often described as containing 1 part per 'x' units of volume. For liquids, 'parts' are equivalent to grams and volume to millimetres, e.g. adrenaline injection 1 in 1000, which contains 1 g in 1000 mL or expressed as a percentage (w/v)—0.1%.
- Molar concentration—only very occasionally are drugs in liquid form expressed in molar concentration. The mole is the molecular weight of a drug expressed in grams and a one molar (1 M) solution contains this weight dissolved in each litre. More often the millimole (mmol) is used to describe a medicinal product, e.g. potassium chloride solution 15 mmol in 10 mL indicates a solution containing the molecular weight of potassium chloride in milligrams $\times$ 15 dissolved in 10 mL of solution.

## Body height and surface area

Drug doses may be expressed in terms of microgram, milligram or gram per unit of body surface area. This is frequently the case where precise dosages tailored to individual patients' needs are required. Typical examples may be seen in cytotoxic chemotherapy or in drugs given to children. Body surface area is expressed as square metres or $m^2$ and drug dosages as units per square metre or units/$m^2$, e.g. cytarabine injection 100 mg/$m^2$.

## Formulae for calculation of drug doses and drip rates

Oral drugs (solids, liquids)

$$\text{Amount required} = \frac{\text{Strength required} \times \text{Volume of stock strength}}{\text{Stock strength}}$$

Parenteral drugs

(a) Solutions (intramuscular (IM), intravenous (IV) injections)

$$\text{Volume required} = \frac{\text{Strength required} \times \text{Volume of stock strength}}{\text{Stock strength}}$$

(b) Powders

It is essential to follow the manufacturer's directions for dilution, then use the appropriate formula.

(c) IV Infusions

$$\text{Rate(drops/min)} = \frac{\text{Volume of solution(mL)} \times \text{Number of drops/mL}}{\text{Time(min)}}$$

Macrodrip (20 drops/mL)—clear fluids

$$\text{Rate(drops/min)} = \frac{\text{Volume of solution(mL)} \times 20}{\text{Time(min)}}$$

Macrodrip (15 drops/mL)—blood

$$\text{Rate(drops/min)} = \frac{\text{Volume of solution(mL)} \times 15}{\text{Time(min)}}$$

(d) Infusion pumps

$$\text{Rate(mL/h)} = \frac{\text{Volume(mL)}}{\text{Time(h)}}$$

(e) IV infusions with drugs

$$\text{Rate(mL/h)} = \frac{\text{Amount of drug required(mg/h)} \times \text{Volume of solution(mL)}}{\text{Total amount of drug(mg)}}$$

N.B.: After selecting the appropriate formula, ensure that all strengths are in the same units, otherwise convert.

1% solution contains 1 g of solute dissolved in 100 mL of solution.

1:1000 means 1 g in 1000 mL of solution, therefore 1 g in 1000 mL is equivalent to 1 mg in 1 mL.

Other useful formulae

Children's dose (Clarke's body weight rule)

$$\text{Child's dose} = \frac{\text{Adult dose} \times \text{Weight of child(kg)}}{\text{Average adult weight(70 kg)}}$$

N.B.: Young children may require higher doses per kg than adults because of their higher metabolic rates. In obesity calculation by body weight can result in higher than necessary doses, so doses should be calculated from ideal weight, related to age and height.

Children's dose (Clarke's body surface area rule)

$$\text{Child's dose} = \frac{\text{Adult dose} \times \text{Surface area of child(m}^2)}{\text{Surface area of adult(1.8 m}^2)}$$

## Acknowledgement

The measurement section was adapted from Henney CR *et al.* 1995 Drugs in Nursing Practice, 5th edn. Edinburgh: Churchill Livingstone, with permission; and the formulae from Havard M 1994 A Nursing Guide to Drugs, 4th edn. Edinburgh: Churchill Livingstone, with permission.

## Drug groups in common use

| Drug groups and subgroups | Examples | Main indications |
|---|---|---|
| **Acetylcholinesterase-inhibiting drugs** | Donepezil, galantamine, rivastigmine | Alzheimer's disease. dementia associated with Parkinson's disease |
| **Alpha₁-adrenoceptor antagonists (alpha blockers)** | Doxazosin, prazosin | Benign prostatic enlargement, hypertension |
| **Anabolic steroids** | Nandrolone, stanozolol | Aplastic anaemia, pruritus in palliative care |
| **Analgesics** | | |
| 1. Non-opioids (see also non-steroidal anti-inflammatory drugs) | 1. Aspirin, paracetamol | 1. Mild to moderate pain, e.g. simple headache and pyrexia |
| 2. Opioids | 2. Diamorphine, morphine, dihydrocodeine, fentanyl, tramadol, etc. | 2. Moderate to severe pain, e.g. postoperative, palliative care |
| 3. Used for neuropathic pain | 3. Amitriptyline, carbamazepine, gabapentin | 3. Trigeminal neuralgia, complex regional pain syndrome |
| **Antacids** | Aluminium hydroxide, magnesium trisilicate, simeticone, alginate | Dyspepsia, gastro-oesophageal reflux disease |
| **Anthelmintics** | | |
| 1. Benzimidazoles | 1. Mebendazole, tiabendazole | 1. Intestinal nematodes, e.g. threadworm, roundworm, whipworm, hookworm |
| 2. Filaricides | 2. Ivermectin | 2. Tissue nematodes, e.g. onchocerciasis. Also cutaneous larva migrans, strongyloidiasis |
| 3. Taenicides | 3. Praziquantel | 3. Tapeworm. Also schistosomiasis (bilharziasis) |
| **Antiandrogens** | 1. Cyproterone acetate | 1. Male hypersexuality, prostate cancer, acne and hirsutism in women |
| | 2. Dutasteride, finasteride (5α-reductase inhibitors) | 2. Benign prostatic enlargement |
| **Antiarrhythmics** | | |
| 1. Supraventricular arrhythmias | 1. Verapamil, adenosine | 1. Supraventricular tachycardia |
| 2. Ventricular arrhythmias | 2. Lidocaine (lignocaine) | 2. Ventricular tachycardia |
| 3. Both supraventricular and ventricular arrhythmias | 3. Amiodarone, disopyramide | 3. Atrial fibrillation and flutter, ventricular tachycardia |

*Continued*

## Drug groups in common use—Continued

| Drug groups and subgroups | Examples | Main indications |
|---|---|---|
| **Antibacterials (antibiotics), antiprotozoals** | | |
| 1. Aminoglycosides | 1. Gentamicin, netilmicin | 1. Life-threatening Gram-negative infections, e.g. septicaemia, acute pyelonephritis, etc. |
| 2. Antituberculosis | 2. Initial phase—ethambutol, isoniazid, pyrazinamide, rifampicin (in combination) | 2. Tuberculosis |
| 3. Carbapenems | 3. Meropenem | 3. Aerobic and anaerobic Gram-positive and Gram-negative bacteria |
| 4. Cephalosporins | 4. Cefadroxil, cefuroxime, ceftazidime | 4. Meningitis, pneumonia, septicaemia |
| 5. Fluoroquinolones | 5. Ciprofloxacin | 5. Gram-positive and -negative infections, e.g. *Escherichia coli*, *Pseudomonas*, *Salmonella*, *Campylobacter* |
| 6. Glycopeptides | 6. Vancomycin, teicoplanin | 6. Gram-positive cocci infections, e.g. meticillin-resistant *Staphylococcus aureus* (MRSA), septicaemia, endocarditis |
| 7. Macrolides | 7. Erythromycin, clarithromycin | 7. Gram-positive infections in penicillin-sensitive patients, *Mycoplasma* pneumonia, legionnaires' disease |
| 8. 5-Nitroimidazoles | 8. Metronidazole | 8. Anaerobic infections and protozoal infections with *Trichomonas vaginalis* |
| 9. Oxazolidones | 9. Linezolid | 9. Gram-positive infections including those caused by MRSA and vancomycin-resistant enterococci (VRE) |
| 10. Penicillins | 10. (a) Broad-spectrum, e.g. ampicillin | 10. (a) Gram-positive infections, e.g. bronchitis, gonorrhoea, otitis media |
| | 10. (b) Beta-lactamase-resistant, e.g. flucloxacillin | 10. (b) Staphylococcal cellulitis, pneumonia, etc. |
| 11. Streptogramin | 11. Quinupristin and dalfopristin (as a combination) | 11. Gram-positive infections that have not responded to other drugs |
| 12. Sulphonamides and trimethoprim | 12. Co-trimoxazole | 12. Urinary tract infection, *Pneumocystis jirovecii* (formerly *P. carinii*) pneumonia, toxoplasmosis, etc. |
| 13. Tetracyclines | 13. Tetracycline, doxycycline | 13. Chlamydial infections, rickettsia, Lyme disease |

**Anticoagulants**

1. Coumarins
   1. Warfarin
      1. Deep-vein thrombosis, pulmonary embolus and patients with mechanical prosthetic heart valves

2. Heparin
   2. Standard and low-molecular-weight heparin
      2. Treatment and prophylaxis of deep-vein thrombosis and pulmonary embolus

**Antidepressants**

1. Monoamine oxidase inhibitors (MAOI)
   1. Phenelzine
      1. Depressive illness, severe phobias

2. Selective serotonin reuptake inhibitors (SSRI)
   2. Citalopram, fluoxetine
      2. Depressive illness, obsessive-compulsive disorder and panic disorders

3. Tricyclic antidepressants (TCA)
   3. Amitriptyline
      3. Depressive illness; neuropathic pain, bedwetting in children

**Antidiabetic drugs (oral hypoglycaemics)**

1. Alpha-glucosidase inhibitors
   1. Acarbose
      1. Type 2 diabetes

2. Biguanides
   2. Metformin
      2. Type 2 diabetes

3. Glitazones (thiazolidinediones)
   3. Pioglitazone, rosiglitazone
      3. Type 2 diabetes

4. Prandial glucose regulators
   4. Repaglinide
      4. Type 2 diabetes

5. Sulphonylureas
   5. Glipizide, tolbutamide
      5. Type 2 diabetes

**Antidiarrhoeals**

Codeine phosphate, loperamide (antimotility drugs)

Adjuncts to rehydration in acute diarrhoea

**Antiemetics**

Nausea and vomiting:

1. Cannabinoids
   1. Nabilone
      1. Caused by cytotoxic chemotherapy

2. Drugs that act centrally on the chemoreceptor trigger zone
   2. Domperidone
      2. Caused by cytotoxic chemotherapy

3. D2-receptor antagonists: phenothiazines
   3. Prochlorperazine
      Metoclopramide acts in a similar way to the phenothiazines but also directly affects the gastrointestinal tract
      3. Caused by gastrointestinal disorders, radiation and chemotherapy

4. H1-receptor antagonists (antihistamines)
   4. Cinnarizine, cyclizine
      4. Caused by motion sickness, vestibular disorders

5. 5-HT3-receptor antagonists
   5. Dolasetron, ondansetron
      5. Caused by chemotherapy, radiation and postoperatively

6. Muscarinic (acetylcholine) receptor antagonists
   6. Hyoscine hydrobromide
      6. Caused by motion sickness

*Continued*

## Drug groups in common use—Continued

| Drug groups and subgroups | Examples | Main indications |
|---|---|---|
| 7. Neurokinin 1 receptor antagonist | 7. Aprepitant | 7. Used with other drugs to prevent nausea and vomiting associated with cisplatin-based chemotherapy |
| **Antiepileptic (anticonvulsant)** | Carbamazepine, gabapentin, phenytoin | Seizure control |
| **Antifibrinolytics and haemostatics** | Tranexamic acid, aprotinin | Prevention of bleeding, menorrhagia |
| **Antifungal** | | |
| 1. Imidazoles | 1. Clotrimazole, miconazole | 1. Topical candidiasis |
| 2. Polyenes | 2. (a) Amphotericin | 2. (a) Systemic aspergillosis, candidiasis, cryptococcosis |
| | 2. (b) Nystatin | 2. (b) Topical candidiasis |
| 3. Triazoles | 3. Fluconazole | 3. Systemic candidiasis, cryptococcal meningitis in acquired immunodeficiency syndrome (AIDS) patients |
| 4. Others | 4. Griseofulvin, terbinafine | 4. Dermatophytosis, e.g. scalp ringworm |
| **Antihistamines** | Chlorphenamine, cetirizine, loratadine | Hayfever; emergency treatment of anaphylactic reactions |
| **Antihypertensives** | | |
| 1. Angiotensin-converting enzyme (ACE) inhibitor | 1. Captopril, ramipril | 1. Hypertension; also heart failure, left ventricular dysfunction, diabetic nephropathy |
| 2. Angiotensin II receptor antagonists | 2. Candesartan, losartan | 2. Hypertension; also in heart failure, diabetic nephropathy |
| 3. Beta-adrenoreceptor antagonists (beta-blockers) | 3. Propranolol (non-selective) Atenolol (selective for $\beta_1$ receptors) | 3. Hypertension; also angina, myocardial infarction, arrhythmias, heart failure, hyperthyroidism, anxiety |
| 4. Calcium channel blockers | 4. Verapamil, nifedipine, diltiazem | 4. Hypertension; also angina, arrhythmias |
| 5. Centrally acting | 5. Clonidine, methyldopa | 5. Hypertension; migraine |
| 6. Vasodilators | 6. Hydralazine | 6. Hypertension; also heart failure |
| **Antileprotics** | Dapsone, rifampicin, clofazimine | Leprosy |
| **Antimalarials** | Chloroquine, mefloquine, primaquine, proguanil, quinine | Malaria—chemoprophylaxis and treatment |
| **Antimigraine 5-HT$_1$ agonists** | Sumatriptan | Migraine—treatment |

**Antiobesity**
1. Lipase inhibitor
2. Appetite suppressant (centrally acting)

    1. Orlistat
    2. Sibutramine

    1. Adjunct in obesity—weight loss
    2. Adjunct in obesity—weight loss

**Antioestrogens**
1. Negative-feedback inhibitor
2. Oestrogen receptor antagonist
3. Aromatase inhibitors

    1. Clomifene
    2. Tamoxifen
    3. Anastrozole, letrozole

    1. Anovulatory infertility
    2. Breast cancer; female infertility
    3. Metastatic breast cancer

**Antiparkinson**
1. Dopaminergics

    1 (a) Amantadine
    1 (b) Catechol-O-methyltransferase inhibitors, e.g. entacapone
    1 (c) Dopamine receptor agonists, e.g. bromocriptine, pergolide, rotigotine
    1 (d) Levodopa, e.g. co-beneldopa (levodopa plus benserazide)
    1 (e) Monoamine-oxidase-B inhibitor, selegiline

    1. Parkinsonism

2. Antimuscarinics

    2. Orphenadrine

    2. Parkinsonism, drug-induced extrapyramidal effects

**Antiplatelet drugs**

Aspirin, clopidogrel, dipyridamole, tirofiban

Prophylaxis of thrombotic cerebrovascular and cardiovascular disease

**Antipsychotics (neuroleptics)**
1. Typical (phenothiazines)

    1. Fluphenazine, chlorpromazine

    1. Disturbed individuals, e.g. agitated depression. Short-term treatment of severe anxiety. Long-term management of schizophrenia

2. Atypical

    2. Clozapine, risperidone

    2. As above

**Antirheumatics (see disease-modifying antirheumatic drugs [DMARD])**

**Antispasmodics**

Dicycloverine, mebeverine, peppermint oil

Gastrointestinal smooth muscle spasm, irritable bowel syndrome

**Antithyroid**

Carbimazole

Hyperthyroidism

**Antivirals**
1. Nucleoside reverse transcriptase inhibitors
2. Protease inhibitors

    1. Zidovudine
    2. Ritonavir

    1. Human immunodeficiency virus (HIV) infection
    2. Progressive or advanced HIV infection

*Continued*

## Drug groups in common use—Continued

| Drug groups and subgroups | Examples | Main indications |
|---|---|---|
| 3. Non-nucleoside reverse transcriptase inhibitors | 3. Efavirenz | 3. HIV infection |
| 4. Nucleic acid synthesis inhibitors | 4. Aciclovir | 4. Herpes simplex, varicella-zoster |
| **Anxiolytics** Benzodiazepines | Diazepam, temazepam | Short-term for anxiety and insomnia, status epilepticus, alcohol withdrawal (acute), etc. |
| **Bisphosphonates** | Alendronic acid, disodium etidronate | Osteoporosis, Paget's disease, hypercalcaemia of cancer |
| **Bronchodilators** | | |
| 1. Beta$_2$-adrenoceptor agonists | 1. Salbutamol, salmeterol | 1. Asthma, chronic obstructive pulmonary disease |
| 2. Muscarinic antagonists | 2. Ipratropium, tiotropium | 2. Asthma, chronic obstructive pulmonary disease |
| 3. Xanthines | 3. Aminophylline, theophylline | 3. Asthma, chronic obstructive pulmonary disease |
| **Cardiac glycosides** | Digoxin (positive inotropic) | Supraventicular tachycardia |
| **Central nervous system stimulants** | Atomoxetine, dexamfetamine methylphenidate, modafinil | Attention deficit hyperactivity disorder (ADHD): narcolepsy; sleepiness due to obstructive sleep apnoea syndrome |
| **Chelating agents** | (a) Desferrioxamine | (a) Poisoning with iron salts, treatment for iron overload |
| | (b) Penicillamine | (b) Copper deposition in Wilson's disease |
| **Contraceptives** | | |
| 1. Combined contraceptive (an oestrogen and a progestogen in various formulations) | 1 (a) Oral—ethinylestradiol + a progestogen, e.g. norethisterone or levonorgestrel | 1. Contraception, menstrual problems |
| | 1 (b) Transdermal patch—ethinylestradiol + norelgestromin | |
| 2. Progestogen-only | 2 (a) Parenteral—long-acting medroxyprogesterone acetate administered by intramuscular injection | 2 (a), (b), (c) Contraception |
| | 2 (b) Intrauterine device—levonorgestrel | |
| | 2 (c) Oral daily (continuous)—desogestrel, levonorgestrel, norethisterone | 2 (b) also used for primary menorrhagia |
| 3. Emergency contraception—hormonal | 3. Levonorgestrel | 3. Emergency contraception used within 72 hours of unprotected intercourse |
| **Corticosteroids (see glucocorticoids and mineralocorticoids)** | | |
| **Cromoglicate** | Sodium cromoglicate (cromoglycate) | Asthma prophylaxis, food allergy, allergic rhinitis and conjunctivitis |

**Cytotoxic agents**

| | |
|---|---|
| 1. Alkylating agent | 1. Chlorambucil, cyclophosphamide, mephalan | 1. Chronic lymphocytic leukaemia, Hodgkin's disease, ovarian cancer, etc. |
| 2. Antimetabolite | 2. Fluorouracil, methotrexate | 2. Acute lymphoblastic leukaemia, non-Hodgkin's lymphoma, solid tumours, etc. |
| 3. Cytotoxic antibiotics including the anthracyclines | 3. Bleomycin, doxorubicin | 3. Acute leukaemia, lymphomas, solid tumours |
| 4. Vinca alkaloids and etoposide | 4. Vincristine, etoposide | 4. Acute leukaemias, lymphomas, solid tumours (lung, breast, testicular) |

**5–9. Selection of other anticancer drugs**

| | |
|---|---|
| 5. Monoclonal antibodies (see also separate entry for monoclonal antibodies) | 5. Alemtuzumab, rituximab, trastuzumab | 5. Chronic lymphocytic leukaemia, non-Hodgkin's lymphoma, HER2-positive breast cancers |
| 6. Platinum compounds | 6. Carboplatin, cisplatin | 6. Solid tumours (ovarian, lung, testicular, bladder, cervical) |
| 7. Protein kinase inhibitors | 7. Dasatinib, erlotinib, etc. | 7. Various leukaemias, some metastatic lung cancer |
| 8. Taxanes | 8. Docetaxel, paclitaxel | 8. Solid tumours (ovarian, breast, lung) |
| 9. Topoisomerase I inhibitors | 9. Irinotecan, topotecan | 9. Colorectal cancer (metastatic), ovarian cancer (metastatic) |

| | | |
|---|---|---|
| **Decongestant** | Pseudoephedrine | Nasal congestion |
| **Dementia drugs (see acetylcholinesterase-inhibiting drugs)** | | |
| **Disease-modifying antirheumatic drugs (DMARD)** | Gold, penicillamine, chloroquine, sulfasalazine | Suppression of juvenile and rheumatoid arthritis |

**Diuretics**

| | | |
|---|---|---|
| 1. Aldosterone antagonists | 1. Spironolactone | 1. Oedema, primary hyperaldosteronism |
| 2. Carbonic anhydrase inhibitors | 2. Acetazolamide | 2. Glaucoma |
| 3. Loop diuretic | 3. Furosemide (frusemide) | 3. Oedema, heart failure |
| 4. Osmotic diuretic | 4. Mannitol | 4. Cerebral oedema, glaucoma |

*Continued*

## Drug groups in common use—Continued

| Drug groups and subgroups | Examples | Main indications |
|---|---|---|
| 5. Potassium-sparing | 5. Amiloride, triamterene | 5. Oedema, conservation of potassium |
| 6. Thiazide | 6. Bendroflumethiazide (bendrofluazide) | 6. Heart failure, oedema, hypertension |
| **Fibrinolytic drugs** | Streptokinase, alteplase, reteplase | Deep-vein thrombosis, pulmonary embolus, acute myocardial infarction, arterial thromboembolism, etc. |
| **Glucocorticoids (corticosteroids)** | Beclometasone, cortisone, dexamethasone, hydrocortisone, prednisolone | Replacement, acute transplant rejection, asthma, dermatitis, inflammatory bowel disease, malignant disease, rheumatoid arthritis |
| **H₂-receptor antagonists (see ulcer-healing drugs)** | | |
| **HMG-CoA reductase inhibitors (see lipid regulators)** | | |
| **5-HT₁ agonists (see antimigraine)** | | |
| **Hypnotics** | Zaleplon | Insomnia (short-term only) |
| **Immunosuppressants (see also glucocorticoids)** | Azathioprine, ciclosporin, sirolimus, basiliximab | Organ transplantation, autoimmune and chronic inflammatory diseases |
| **Inotropic sympathomimetics** | Dobutamine, dopamine | Cardiogenic shock after cardiac surgery or infarction |
| **Insulin** | Short-acting—soluble insulin, insulin analogues (e.g. insulin lispro); intermediate, long-acting—insulin zinc suspension, protamine zinc suspension, biphasic isophane insulin, analogues (e.g. insulin glargine) | Type 1 and 2 diabetes mellitus |
| **Laxatives (aperients)** | | |
| 1. Bulk-forming laxatives | 1. Ispaghula, methylcellulose | 1. Constipation |
| 2. Faecal softeners | 2. Arachis oil (enema) | 2. Constipation |
| 3. Osmotic laxative | 3. Lactulose, phosphate and sodium citrate (enema) | 3. Constipation |
| 4. Stimulant | 4. Senna, bisacodyl (oral and suppositories), glycerol (suppositories), sodium picosulfate (oral) | 4. Constipation |
| 5. Bowel cleansing | 5. Sodium picosulfate (oral) | 5. Prior to examination, barium enema or bowel surgery |
| **Lipid regulators** | | |
| 1. Anion exchange resins | 1. Colestyramine | 1. Hypercholesterolaemia, hyperlipidaemia; also pruritus associated with biliary obstruction and diarrhoea |

| | |
|---|---|
| 2. Fibrates | 2. Ciprofibrate, gemfibrozil | 2. Hyperlipidaemia, prevention of coronary events in patients with coronary heart disease (CHD) |
| 3. Statins (HMG-CoA reductase inhibitors) | 3. Pravastatin, simvastatin | 3. Hypercholesterolaemia, hyperlipidaemia, prevention of coronary events in patients with CHD |
| **Mineralocorticoids** | Fludrocortisone | Adrenocortical insufficiency |
| **Miotics** | Pilocarpine | Glaucoma |
| **Monoclonal antibodies** | Infliximab | Inflammatory bowel disease, ankylosing spondylitis, rheumatoid arthritis |
| **Mucolytics** | Dornase alpha (inhaled) | Cystic fibrosis |
| **Mydriatics** | Tropicamide | Pupil dilatation for ophthalmic examination |
| **Myometrial relaxants (tocolytics)** | Atosiban, terbutaline sulphate | Uncomplicated premature labour |
| **Neuroleptics (see antipsychotics)** | | |
| **Nitrates** | Glyceryl trinitrate, isosorbide dinitrate | Angina, left ventricular failure |
| **Non-steroidal anti-inflammatory drugs (NSAIDs)** | Diclofenac, ibuprofen, indometacin, naproxen | Pain relief, dental pain, dysmenorrhoea, antipyretic, reduction of inflammation and stiffness in arthritis |
| **Oestrogens** | Oestradiol, oesterone | Hormone replacement therapy (with progesterone for women with an intact uterus) |
| **Opioids (see analgesics)** | | |
| **Oxytocics** | Oxytocin | Induction of labour, prevention and treatment of postpartum haemorrhage |
| **Potassium channel activator** | Nicorandil | Angina |
| **Progestogens** | Medroxyprogesterone, progesterone | Dysmenorrhoea, with hormone replacement therapy, infertility, premenstrual syndrome, postnatal depression |
| **Prostaglandins** | Gemeprost, mifepristone | Induction of labour, termination of pregnancy |
| **Proton pump inhibitors (see ulcer-healing drugs)** | | |
| **Retinoids** | Acitretin, isotretinoin | Severe psoriasis, acne |

*Continued*

575

## Drug groups in common use—Continued

| Drug groups and subgroups | Examples | Main indications |
|---|---|---|
| **Selective (o)estrogen receptor modulators (SERMS)** | Raloxifene | Prevention and treatment of postmenopausal osteoporosis |
| **Skeletal muscle relaxants** | Baclofen, dantrolene, diazepam | Chronic muscle spasm, e.g. multiple sclerosis; malignant hyperthermia |
| **Stimulants (see central nervous system stimulants)** | | |
| **Thyroid hormones** | Thyroxine (levothyroxine) | Hypothyroidism |
| **Tocolytics (see myometrial relaxants)** | | |
| **Tranquillizers (see antipsychotics, anxiolytics)** | | |
| **Ulcer-healing drugs** | | |
| 1. $H_2$-receptor antagonists | 1. Cimetidine, ranitidine | 1. Peptic ulceration, gastro-oesophageal reflux disease |
| 2. Proton pump inhibitors | 2. Omeprazole, lansoprazole | 2. Peptic ulceration, eradication of *Helicobacter pylori*, gastro-oesophageal reflux disease, Zollinger–Ellison syndrome |
| **Uricosuric** | Probenecid | Prevention of gout |
| **Vasoconstrictor sympathomimetics** | Phenylephrine | Acute hypotension |

Readers should be aware that some drugs used as examples for a particular drug group may also have other uses; for example, acetazolamide, a carbonic anhydrase inhibitor, is occasionally used as a second-line antiepileptic drug.

# Appendix 6

## Abbreviations—medical terms and related organizations

| | |
|---|---|
| AA | Alcoholics Anonymous |
| AAA | abdominal aortic aneurysm |
| AABR | automated auditory brainstem response |
| AAMI | age-associated memory impairment |
| ABGs | arterial blood gases |
| ABPI | ankle–brachial pressure index |
| ACBT | active cycle of breathing technique |
| ACE | angiotensin-converting enzyme |
| ACh | acetylcholine |
| ACTH | adrenocorticotrophic hormone |
| ADD | attention deficit disorder |
| ADH | antidiuretic hormone |
| ADHD | attention deficit hyperactivity disorder |
| ADI | acceptable daily intake |
| ADLs | activities of daily living |
| ADP | adenosine diphosphate |
| ADRs | adverse drug reactions |
| AED | automated external defibrillator |
| AFB | acid-fast bacilli |
| AFP | alphafetoprotein |
| AHF/G | antihaemophilic factor/globulin |
| AHI | apnoea hypopnoea index |
| AICD | automatic implantable cardioverter defibrillator |
| AID | artificial insemination using donor semen |
| AIDS | acquired immune deficiency syndrome |
| AIH | artificial insemination using husband's (partner's) semen |
| AIS | abbreviated injury scale |
| ALA | alpha ($\alpha$)-linolenic acid |
| ALD | adrenoleucodystrophy |
| ALG | antilymphocyte globulin |
| ALL | acute lymphoblastic leukaemia |
| ALS | **1.** advanced life support **2.** amyotrophic lateral sclerosis |
| ALT | alanine aminotransferase |
| AMA | antimitochondrial antibody |
| AMD | age-related macular degeneration |
| AMED | Allied and Complementary Medicine Database |
| AMI | acute myocardial infarction |
| AML | acute myeloblastic leukaemia |
| AMP | adenosine monophosphate |
| ANA | antinuclear antibody |
| ANCA | antineutrophil cytoplasmic antibody |
| ANOVA | analysis of variance |
| ANP | atrial natriuretic peptide |
| ANS | autonomic nervous system |
| ANUG | acute necrotizing ulcerative gingivitis |
| AP | anaesthesia practitioner |
| APC | antigen-presenting cell |
| APD | **1.** auditory processing disorder **2.** automated peritoneal dialysis |
| APH | antepartum haemorrhage |
| APKD | adult polycystic kidney disease |

| APTT | activated partial thromboplastin time |
| ARC | AIDS-related complex |
| ARDS | acute/adult respiratory distress syndrome |
| ARF | **1.** acute renal failure **2.** acute respiratory failure |
| ARM | artificial rupture of membranes |
| AROM | active range of motion |
| ASD | atrial septal defect |
| ASO | antistreptolysin O |
| ASOM | acute suppurative otitis media |
| AST | aspartate aminotransferase |
| ASW | approved social worker |
| ATLS | advanced trauma life support |
| ATN | acute tubular necrosis |
| ATP | adenosine triphosphate |
| AVP | arginine vasopressin |

| BACUP | British Association of Cancer United Patients |
| BAL | bronchial alveolar lavage |
| BAOT/COT | British Association/College of Occupational Therapists |
| BBA | born before arrival |
| BBB | **1.** blood–brain barrier **2.** bundle branch block |
| BBV | blood-borne virus |
| BCC | basal cell carcinoma |
| BCG | bacille Calmette–Guérin |
| BDA | **1.** British Dental Association **2.** British Dietetic Association |
| BDD | body dysmorphic disorder |
| BEI | bioelectrical impedance |
| BID | brought in dead |
| BIH | benign intracranial hypertension |
| BIPAP | biphasic positive airways pressure |
| BLS | basic life support |
| BM | bowel movement |
| BMA | British Medical Association |
| BMD | bone mineral density |
| BME | benign myalgic encephalomyelitis |
| BMI | body mass index |
| BMR | basal metabolic rate |
| BMT | bone marrow transplant |
| BNF | *British National Formulary* |
| BOS | bronchiolitis obliterans syndrome |
| BP | **1.** blood pressure **2.** British Pharmacopoeia |
| BPD | bronchopulmonary dysplasia |
| BPE | benign prostatic enlargement |
| BPH | benign prostatic hyperplasia |
| bpm | beats per minute |
| BPPV | benign paroxysmal positional vertigo |
| Bq | becquerel |
| BRM | biological response modifier |
| BRSC | British Red Cross Society |
| BSA | body surface area |
| BSE | **1.** bovine spongiform encephalopathy **2.** breast self-examination |
| BSL | British sign language |
| BST | bovine somatotrophin |
| BUN | blood urea nitrogen |

| | |
|---|---|
| BV | biological value |
| Bx | biopsy |
| BXO | balanitis xerotica obliterans |

| | |
|---|---|
| CA-125 | cancer cell surface antigen 125 |
| CABG | coronary artery bypass graft |
| CAD | coronary artery disease |
| CAH | congenital adrenal hyperplasia |
| CAL | computer-assisted learning |
| CAM | **1.** cell adhesion molecule **2.** complementary and alternative medicine |
| cAMP | cyclic adenosine monophosphate |
| CAPD | continuous ambulatory peritoneal dialysis |
| CAPE | Clifton Assessment Procedures for the Elderly |
| C&S | culture and sensitivity |
| CAT | computed axial tomography |
| CBA | cost–benefit analysis |
| CBF | cerebral blood flow |
| CCF | congestive cardiac failure |
| CCK | cholecystokinin |
| CCPNS | cell cycle phase non-specific |
| CCPS | cell cycle phase-specific |
| CCU | coronary care unit |
| CD | controlled drug |
| Cd | candela |
| CDC | Centers for Disease Control and Prevention |
| CDH | congenital dislocation of the hip |
| CEA | **1.** carcinoembryonic antigen **2.** cost-effectiveness analysis |
| CEHR | Commission for Equality and Human Rights |
| CF | cystic fibrosis |
| CFM | cerebral function monitor |
| CFS/ME | chronic fatigue syndrome/myalgic encephalomyelitis |
| CFT | complement fixation test |
| CFTR | cystic fibrosis transmembrane regulator |
| CGM | continuous glucose monitoring |
| CHART | continuous hyperfractionated accelerated radiotherapy |
| CHD | coronary heart disease |
| CHF | congestive heart failure |
| CHI | creatinine height index |
| CHM | Commission on Human Medicines |
| CHO | carbohydrate |
| CHRE | Council for Healthcare Regulatory Excellence |
| CI | cardiac index |
| CIN | cervical intraepithelial neoplasia |
| CINAHL | Cumulative Index to Nursing and Allied Health Literature |
| CIS | carcinoma in situ |
| CJD | Creutzfeldt–Jakob disease |
| CLL | chronic lymphocytic leukaemia |
| CLO | columnar-lined oesophagus |
| CML | chronic myeloid leukaemia |
| CMO | Chief Medical Officer |
| CMV | **1.** controlled mandatory ventilation **2.** cytomegalovirus |
| CNO | Chief Nursing Officer |
| CNS | **1.** central nervous system **2.** clinical nurse specialist |
| CO | cardiac output |

| COC | combined oral contraceptive |
| COMA | Committee on Medical Aspects of Food Policy |
| COPD | chronic obstructive pulmonary disease |
| COSHH | Control of Substances Hazardous to Health |
| COT | College of Occupational Therapists |
| CPAP | continuous positive airways pressure |
| CPD | continuing professional development |
| CPK | creatine kinase/phosphokinase |
| CPM | continuous passive motion |
| CPN | community psychiatric nurse |
| CPP | cerebral perfusion pressure |
| CPR | cardiopulmonary resuscitation |
| CREST | calcinosis, Raynaud's phenomenon, (o)esophageal dysfunction, sclerodactyly and telangiectasis |
| CRF | chronic renal failure |
| CRH | corticotrophin-releasing hormone |
| CRP | C-reactive protein (test) |
| CRPS | complex regional pain syndrome |
| CS | caesarean section |
| CSF | **1.** cerebrospinal fluid **2.** colony-stimulating factor |
| CSII | continuous subcutaneous insulin infusion |
| CSM | Committee on Safety of Medicines ⇒ CHM |
| CSOM | chronic suppurative otitis media |
| CSP | Chartered Society of Physiotherapy |
| CSSD | central sterile supplies department |
| CSSU | central sterile supply unit |
| CT | **1.** cerebral tumour **2.** computed tomography **3.** coronary thrombosis |
| CTG | cardiotocography |
| CTZ | chemoreceptor trigger zone |
| CUA | cost–utility analysis |
| CV | curriculum vitae |
| CVA | cerebrovascular accident |
| CVD | cardiovascular disease |
| CVID | common variable immunodeficiency |
| CVP | central venous pressure |
| CVS | **1.** cardiovascular system **2.** chorionic villus sampling |
| CVVH | continuous veno-venous haemofiltration |
| CVVHD | continuous veno-venous haemodiafiltration |
| CXR | chest X-ray |

| DADL | domestic activities of daily living |
| D and C | dilatation and curettage |
| D and E | dilatation and evacuation |
| DAS | disease activity score |
| Db | decibel |
| DC | direct current |
| DCIS | ductal carcinoma in situ |
| DCR | dacryocystorhinostomy |
| DDH | developmental dysplasia of the hip |
| DEF | decayed, extracted, filled |
| DEXA | dual-energy X-ray absorptiometry |
| DHA | docosahexaenoic acid |
| DHEA | dehydroepiandrosterone |
| DIC | disseminated intravascular coagulation |
| DIDMOAD | diabetes insipidus, diabetes mellitus, optic atrophy and deafness |

| | |
|---|---|
| DMARD | disease-modifying antirheumatic drug |
| DMD | Duchenne muscular dystrophy |
| DMF | decayed, missing, filled |
| DMS | Director of Medical Services |
| DNA | deoxyribonucleic acid |
| DNAR | do not attempt resuscitation |
| DNase | deoxyribonuclease |
| DNR | do not resuscitate |
| $DO_2$ | oxygen delivery |
| DOA | dead on arrival |
| DOB | date of birth |
| DOMS | delayed-onset muscle soreness |
| 2,3-DPG | 2,3-diphosphoglycerate |
| DR | digital radiography |
| DRVs | dietary reference values |
| DSA | digital subtraction angiography |
| DSH | deliberate self-harm |
| DSM | *Diagnostic and Statistical Manual of Mental Disorder* |
| DT | delirium tremens |
| DUB | dysfunctional uterine bleeding |
| DVT | deep-vein thrombosis |

| | |
|---|---|
| EAR | estimated average requirement |
| EBM | **1.** evidence-based medicine **2.** expressed breast milk |
| EBP | evidence-based practice |
| EBV | Epstein–Barr virus |
| ECF | extracellular fluid |
| ECG | electrocardiogram |
| ECM | extracellular matrix |
| ECMO | extracorporeal membrane oxygenation |
| ECoG | electrocochleography |
| ECT | electroconvulsive therapy |
| ECV | external cephalic version |
| ED | erectile dysfunction |
| EDD | expected date of delivery |
| EDRF | endothelium-derived relaxing factor |
| EDTA | ethylene diamine tetra-acetic acid |
| EDV | end-diastolic volume |
| EEG | electroencephalogram |
| EFAs | essential fatty acids |
| EFSA | European Food Safety Authority |
| EHEC | enterohaemorrhagic *Escherichia coli* |
| EIA | exercise-induced asthma |
| EIEC | enteroinvasive *Escherichia coli* |
| ELISA | enzyme-linked immunosorbent assay |
| EMD | electromechanical dissociation |
| EMEA | European Medicines Agency |
| EMF | electromotive force |
| EMG | electromyography |
| EMLA | eutectic mixture of local anaesthetics |
| EMRSA | epidemic meticillin-resistant *Staphylococcus aureus* |
| ENT | ear, nose and throat |
| EOG | electro-oculogram |
| EPA | eicosapentaenoic acid |
| EPEC | enteropathic *Escherichia coli* |

| EPO | erythropoietin |
|---|---|
| EPOC | excess postexercise oxygen consumption |
| ER | endoplasmic reticulum |
| ERCP | endoscopic retrograde cholangiopancreatography |
| ERG | **1.** electroretinogram **2.** epidermal growth factor |
| ERPC | evacuation of retained products of conception |
| ESP | **1.** extended-scope physiotherapy practitioner **2.** extrasensory perception |
| ESR | erythrocyte sedimentation rate |
| ESRD/F | end-stage renal disease/failure |
| ESWL | extracorporeal shock-wave lithotripsy |
| ESV | end-systolic volume |
| $ETCO_2$ | end-tidal carbon dioxide |
| ETEC | enterotoxigenic *Escherichia coli* |
| EUA | examination under anaesthetic |

| FAD | flavin adenine dinucleotide |
|---|---|
| FAS | fetal alcohol syndrome |
| FBS | **1.** fasting blood sugar **2.** fetal blood sampling |
| FBC | full blood count |
| FESS | functional endoscopic sinus surgery |
| FEV | forced expiratory volume |
| FHS | Family Health Services |
| FIM | Functional Independence Measure |
| $FiO_2$ | fractional inspired oxygen concentration |
| FMN | flavin mononucleotide |
| FOB | faecal occult blood |
| FPA | Family Planning Association |
| FRC | functional residual capacity |
| FSA | Food Standards Agency |
| FSH | follicle-stimulating hormone |
| FTA-Abs | fluorescent treponemal antibody absorbed test |
| FVC | forced vital capacity |

| GABA | gamma-aminobutyric acid |
|---|---|
| GAS | general adaptation syndrome |
| GBM | glomerular basement membrane |
| GBS | Guillain–Barré syndrome |
| GCS | Glasgow Coma Scale |
| G-CSF | granulocyte colony-stimulating factor |
| GDC | General Dental Council |
| GDS | geriatric depression scale |
| GFR | glomerular filtration rate |
| GGT | gamma-glutamyltransferase |
| GH | growth hormone |
| GHRH | growth hormone-releasing hormone |
| GHRIH | growth hormone release-inhibiting hormone |
| GI | gastrointestinal |
| GIFT | gamete intrafallopian transfer |
| GIP | gastric inhibitory peptide |
| GLA | gamma ($\gamma$)-linolenic acid |
| GMC | General Medical Council |
| GM-CSF | granulocyte–macrophage colony-stimulating factor |
| GMS | general medical services |
| GnRH | gonadotrophin-releasing hormone |
| GORD | gastro-oesophageal reflux disease |

| GP | general practitioner |
| G6PD | glucose-6-phosphate dehydrogenase |
| GPI | general paralysis of the insane |
| GSL | general sales list |
| GU | genitourinary |
| GUM | genitourinary medicine |
| GVHD | graft-versus-host disease |
| Gy | gray |

| HAI | hospital-acquired infection |
| HAV | hepatitis A virus |
| HAVS | hand–arm vibration syndrome |
| Hb | haemoglobin |
| HBIG | hepatitis B immunoglobulin |
| HBV | hepatitis B virus |
| HCA | health care assistant |
| HCAI | health care-associated infection |
| hCG | human chorionic gonadotrophin |
| HCV | hepatitis C virus |
| HDL | high-density lipoprotein |
| HDU | high-dependency unit |
| HELLP | haemolysis, elevated liver enzymes and low platelets |
| HER2 | human epidermal growth factor receptor-2 |
| HFEA | Human Fertilization and Embryology Authority |
| HHNK | hyperglycaemic hyperosmolar non-ketotic (coma) |
| 5-HIAA | 5-hydroxyindoleacetic acid |
| Hib | *Haemophilus influenzae* type B |
| HIV | human immunodeficiency virus |
| HLA | human leucocyte antigen |
| HONK | hyperosmolar non-ketotic (coma) |
| HPA | Health Protection Agency |
| HPC | Health Professions Council |
| HPL | human placental lactogen |
| HPV | human papillomavirus |
| $HR_{max}$ | maximum heart rate |
| HRT | hormone replacement therapy |
| HSC | Health and Safety Commission |
| HSCT | haemopoietic stem cell transplantation |
| HSDU | hospital sterilization and disinfection unit |
| HSE | Health and Safety Executive |
| HSSU | hospital sterile supply unit |
| HSV | herpes simplex virus |
| 5-HT | 5-hydroxytryptamine |
| HTLV | human T-cell lymphotropic virus |
| HUS | haemolytic–uraemic syndrome |
| HV | health visitor |

| IABP | intra-aortic balloon pump |
| IADL | instrumental activities of daily living |
| IBD | inflammatory bowel disease |
| IBS | irritable bowel syndrome |
| IBW | ideal body weight |
| IC | inspiratory capacity |
| ICD | *International Classification of Diseases* |
| ICE | ice, compress and elevation |

| | |
|---|---|
| ICF | **1.** *International Classification of Functioning, Disability and Health* **2.** intracellular fluid |
| ICP | **1.** integrated care pathway **2.** intracranial pressure |
| ICSH | interstitial cell-stimulating hormone |
| ICSI | intracytoplasmic sperm injection |
| ICU | intensive care unit |
| IDDM | insulin-dependent diabetes mellitus |
| IE | infective endocarditis |
| IFG | impaired fasting glucose/glycaemia |
| IFN | interferon |
| Ig | immunoglobulin |
| IGF | insulin-like growth factors |
| IGT | impaired glucose tolerance |
| IHD | ischaemic heart disease |
| IL | interleukin |
| IMRT | intensity-modulated radiotherapy |
| IOP | intraocular pressure |
| $IP_3$ | inostitol triphosphate |
| IPE | interprofessional education |
| IPPV | intermittent positive-pressure ventilation |
| IQ | intelligence quotient |
| ISC | intermittent self-catheterization |
| ITP | idiopathic thrombocytopenic purpura |
| ITU | intensive therapy unit |
| IUCD | intrauterine contraceptive device |
| IUD | intrauterine device |
| IUGR | intrauterine growth restriction/retardation |
| IUI | intrauterine insemination |
| IV | intravenous |
| IVC | inferior vena cava |
| IVF | in vitro fertilization |
| IVI | intravenous infusion |
| IVIG | intravenous immunoglobulin |
| IVU/IVP | intravenous urogram/pyelogram |
| | |
| J | joule |
| JCA | juvenile chronic arthritis |
| JGA | juxtaglomerular apparatus |
| JVP | jugular venous pressure |
| | |
| kJ | kilojoule |
| KP | keratic precipitates |
| KUB | kidney, ureter and bladder |
| | |
| LAK cells | lymphokine-activated killer cells |
| LASER | light amplification by stimulated emission of radiation |
| LASIK | laser in situ keratomileusis |
| LAUP | laser-assisted uvulopalatoplasty |
| LAVH | laporoscopic-assisted vaginal hysterectomy |
| LBC | liquid-based cytology |
| LBW | low birth weight |
| $LD_{50}$ | lethal dose in 50% |
| LDH | lactate dehydrogenase |
| LDL | low-density lipoprotein |
| LE | lupus erythematosus |

| | |
|---|---|
| LFTs | liver function tests |
| LGVCFT | lymphogranuloma venereum complement fixation test |
| LH | luteinizing hormone |
| LMA | laryngeal mask airway |
| LMP | last menstrual period |
| LOA | left occipitoanterior |
| LOC | level of consciousness |
| LOP | left occipitoposterior |
| LP | lumbar puncture |
| LRNI | lower reference nutrient intake |
| LRTI | lower respiratory tract infection |
| LS | lecithin–sphingomyelin ratio |
| LSD | lysergic acid diethylamide |
| LTM | long-term memory |
| LTOT | long-term oxygen therapy |
| LUTS | lower urinary tract symptoms |
| LVAD | left ventricular assist device |
| LVF | left ventricular failure |

| | |
|---|---|
| MAb | monoclonal antibody |
| MAC | 1. mid-arm circumference 2. *Mycobacterium avium* complex |
| MAG3 | mercaptoacetyltriglycine |
| MAI | *Mycobacterium avium intracellulare* |
| MALT | mucosa-associated lymphoid tissue |
| MAOI | monoamine oxidase inhibitor |
| MAP | mean arterial pressure |
| MAST | military antishock trousers |
| MBC | maximal breathing capacity |
| MCA | Medicines Control Agency ⇒ MHRA |
| MCADD | medium-chain acyl-CoA dehydrogenase deficiency |
| MCH | mean cell haemoglobin |
| MCHC | mean cell haemoglobin concentration |
| MCP | multiple cosmetic phlebectomy |
| MCU | micturating cystourethrogram |
| MCV | mean cell volume |
| MDA | Medical Devices Agency ⇒ MHRA |
| MDM | mental defence mechanism |
| MDR-TB | multidrug-resistant tuberculosis |
| MDT | multidisciplinary team |
| ME | myalgic encephalomyelitis |
| MEDLARS | medical literature analysis retrieval system |
| MELAS | mitochondrial encephalopathy lactic acidosis and stroke-like episodes |
| MEN | multiple endocrine neoplasia |
| MEP | maximum expiratory pressure |
| MESA | microsurgical epididymal sperm aspiration |
| MESH/MeSH | Medical Subject Headings |
| METS | metabolic equivalents |
| mg | milligram |
| MHC | major histocompatibility complex |
| MHRA | Medicines and Healthcare products Regulatory Agency |
| MIP | maximum inspiratory pressure |
| MIS | minimally invasive surgery |
| mL | millilitre |
| MLC | multileaf collimation |
| MLNS | mucocutaneous lymph node syndrome |

| MLSO | Medical Laboratory Scientific Officer |
| mm | millimetre |
| mmHg | millimetres of mercury |
| mmol | millimole |
| MMR | measles, mumps and rubella (vaccine) |
| MMSE | Mini Mental State Examination |
| MND | motor neuron disease |
| MO | Medical Officer |
| MODS | multiple-organ dysfunction syndrome |
| MODY | maturity-onset diabetes of the young |
| MOH | Medical Officer of Health |
| mol | mole |
| MRC | Medical Research Council |
| MRI | magnetic resonance imaging |
| mRNA | messenger ribonucleic acid |
| MRSA | meticillin (methicillin)-resistant *Staphylococcus aureus* |
| MS | **1.** multiple sclerosis **2.** musculoskeletal system |
| MSA | multiple systems atrophy |
| MSH | melanocyte-stimulating hormones |
| MSP | Munchausen syndrome by proxy |
| MSU/MSSU | midstream specimen of urine |
| MSW | medical social worker |
| MUAC | mid-upper-arm circumference |

| N | Newton |
| NACNE | National Advisory Committee on Nutrition Education |
| NAD | nicotinamide adenine dinucleotide |
| NADP | nicotinamide adenine dinucleotide phosphate |
| NAI | non-accidental injury |
| NAMCW | National Association for Maternal and Child Welfare |
| NAWCH | National Association for the Welfare of Children in Hospital |
| NBM | nil (nothing) by mouth |
| NCVQ | National Council for Vocational Qualifications |
| NEC | necrotizing enterocolitis |
| ng | nanogram |
| NG | nasogastric |
| NGF | nerve growth factor |
| NGU | non-gonococcal urethritis |
| NHL | non-Hodgkin's lymphoma |
| NHS | National Health Service |
| NHSLA | NHS Litigation Authority |
| NICE | National Institute for Health and Clinical Excellence |
| NICU | Neonatal Intensive Care Unit |
| NIDDM | non-insulin-dependent diabetes mellitus |
| NIPPV | non-invasive positive-pressure ventilation |
| NK | natural killer cells |
| NLH | National Library for Health |
| NLP | neurolinguistic programming |
| nm | nanometre |
| NMC | Nursing and Midwifery Council |
| NMR | nuclear magnetic resonance |
| NNU | neonatal unit |
| NPF | *Nurse Prescribers' Formulary* |
| NPN | non-protein nitrogen |
| NPSA | National Patient Safety Agency |

| NRDS | neonatal respiratory distress syndrome |
| NREM | non-rapid eye movement (sleep) |
| NSAIDs | non-steroidal anti-inflammatory drugs |
| NSCLC | non-small cell lung carcinoma |
| NSFs | National Service Frameworks |
| NSP | non-starch polysaccharide |
| NSU | non-specific urethritis |
| NTD | neural tube defect |
| NVQ | National Vocational Qualification |

| OAE | otoacoustic emission |
| OBLA | onset of blood lactate accumulation |
| OBS | organic brain syndrome |
| OCD | obsessive compulsive disorder |
| ODA | operating department assistant |
| ODD | oppositional defiant disorder |
| ODP | operating department practitioner |
| OGD | oesophagogastroduodenoscopy |
| ORS | oral rehydration solution |
| ORT | oral rehydration therapy |
| OSAS | obstructive sleep apnoea (hypopnoea) syndrome |
| OSAHS | obstructive sleep apnoea hypopnoea syndrome |
| OT | occupational therapy/therapist |
| OTC | over-the-counter (medicines) |

| Pa | pascal |
| PA | pernicious anaemia |
| $PaCO_2$ | partial pressure of carbon dioxide in arterial blood |
| $PACO_2$ | partial pressure of carbon dioxide in alveolar air |
| PACS | picture archiving communication system |
| PADL | personal activities of daily living |
| PAFC | pulmonary artery flotation catheter |
| PAL | physical activity level |
| PALS | **1.** paediatric advanced life support **2.** Patient Advocacy Liaison Service |
| PAO | peak acid output |
| $PaO_2$ | partial pressure of oxygen in arterial blood |
| $PAO_2$ | partial pressure of oxygen in alveolar air |
| PAOP | pulmonary artery occlusion pressure |
| Pap | Papanicolaou smear test |
| PAR | physical activity ratio |
| PARNUTS | foods for particular nutritional purposes |
| PAWP | pulmonary artery wedge pressure |
| PBD | peak bone density |
| PBM | peak bone mass |
| PBMC | peripheral blood mononuclear cells |
| PCAG | primary closed-angle glaucoma |
| PCA(S) | patient-controlled analgesia (system) |
| PCEA | patient-controlled epidural analgesia |
| PCI | percutaneous coronary intervention |
| PCM | protein–calorie malnutrition |
| $PCO_2$ | partial pressure of carbon dioxide |
| PCOS | polycystic ovary syndrome |
| PCP | pneumocystis pneumonia |
| PCR | polymerase chain reaction |
| PCT | Primary Care Trust |

| PCV | packed cell volume |
| PCWP | pulmonary capillary wedge pressure |
| PDA | patent ductus arteriosus |
| PDP | personal development plan |
| PDGF | platelet-derived growth factor |
| PDT | photodynamic therapy |
| PE | pulmonary embolus |
| PEA | pulseless electrical activity |
| PEEP | positive end-expiratory pressure |
| PEFR | peak expiratory flow rate |
| PEG | percutaneous endoscopic gastrostomy |
| PEM | protein–energy malnutrition |
| PERRLA | pupils equal, round, react to light, accommodation |
| PESA | percutaneous epididymal sperm aspiration |
| PET | positron emission tomography |
| PFI | private finance initiative |
| PGD | preimplantation genetic diagnosis |
| PGDRS | psychogeriatric dependency rating scale |
| PGH | preimplantation genetic haplotyping |
| pH | hydrogen ion concentration |
| Ph | Philadelphia chromosome |
| PHC | primary health care |
| PI | performance indicator |
| PICC | peripherally inserted central catheter |
| PICU | Paediatric Intensive Care Unit |
| PID | **1.** pelvic inflammatory disease **2.** prolapsed intervertebral disc |
| PKU | phenylketonuria |
| PMB | postmenopausal bleeding |
| PMI | point of maximum impulse |
| PMS | premenstrual syndrome |
| PND | paroxysmal nocturnal dyspnoea |
| PNF | proprioceptive neuromuscular facilitation |
| PNI | psychoneuroimmunology |
| PNS | peripheral nervous system |
| $PO_2$ | partial pressure of oxygen |
| POA | pancreatic oncofetal antigen |
| POAG | primary open-angle glaucoma |
| POM | prescription-only medicine |
| POMC | pro-opiomelanocortin |
| POMR | problem-oriented medical record |
| PONV | postoperative nausea and vomiting |
| POP | **1.** plaster of Paris **2.** progestogen-only pill |
| PPE | personal protective equipment |
| PPLO | pleuropneumonia-like organism |
| PPS | pelvic pain syndrome |
| PPV | positive-pressure ventilation |
| PR | **1.** per rectum **2.** peripheral resistance |
| PRL | prolactin |
| PRP | panretinal photocoagulation |
| PSA | prostate-specific antigen |
| PT | **1.** physiotherapist **2.** prothrombin |
| PTA | percutaneous transluminal angioplasty |
| PTC | percutaneous transhepatic cholangiography |
| PTCA | percutaneous transluminal coronary angioplasty |

| | |
|---|---|
| PTH | parathyroid hormone |
| PTSD | post-traumatic stress disorder |
| PUFA | polyunsaturated fatty acid |
| PUJ | pelviureteric junction |
| PUO | pyrexia of unknown origin |
| PUVA | psoralen plus ultraviolet light A |
| PV | per vagina |
| PVD | peripheral vascular disease |
| PVL | Panton–Valentine leukocidin |
| PVR | pulmonary vascular resistance |
| PVS | persistent vegetative state |

| | |
|---|---|
| QALYs | quality-adjusted life years |

| | |
|---|---|
| RADAR | Royal Association for Disability and Rehabilitation |
| RADC | Royal Army Dental Corps |
| RAMC | Royal Army Medical Corps |
| RAS | reticular activating system |
| RAST | radioallergosorbent test |
| RBC | red blood cell |
| RCT | randomized controlled trial |
| RDA | recommended daily allowance |
| RDI | recommended daily intake |
| RDS | respiratory distress syndrome |
| REF | renal erythropoietic factor |
| REM | rapid eye movement (sleep) |
| RES | reticuloendothelial system |
| RF | rheumatoid factor |
| Rh | Rhesus |
| RHD | rheumatic heart disease |
| RICE | rest, ice, compress, elevation |
| RIHSA | radioiodinated human serum albumin |
| rINN | recommended International Non-proprietary Name |
| RIP | raised intracranial pressure |
| RMO | resident medical officer |
| RNA | ribonucleic acid |
| RNI | reference nutrient intake |
| RNIB | Royal National Institute of the Blind |
| RNID | Royal National Institute for the Deaf and hard of hearing people |
| RO | reality orientation |
| ROA | right occipitoanterior |
| ROM | **1.** range of motion **2.** resisted range of movement |
| ROP | right occipitoposterior |
| ROS | reactive oxygen species |
| RPR | rapid plasma reagin test |
| rRNA | ribosomal ribonucleic acid |
| RSI | repetitive strain injury |
| RSV | respiratory syncytial virus |
| RTA | **1.** renal tubular acidosis **2.** road traffic accident |
| RVF | right ventricular failure |

| | |
|---|---|
| SACN | Scientific Advisory Committee on Nutrition |
| SAD | seasonal affective disorder |
| SADS | sudden adult/arrhythmia death syndrome |

| SAH | subarachnoid haemorrhage |
|---|---|
| SAID | specific adaptation to imposed demands |
| SANDS | Stillbirth and Neonatal Death Society |
| StAAA | St Andrew's Ambulance Association |
| StJAA | St John Ambulance Association |
| StJAB | St John Ambulance Brigade |
| $SaO_2$ | arterial oxygen saturation |
| SARA | sexually acquired reactive arthritis |
| SARS | severe acute respiratory syndrome |
| SBLA syndrome | sarcoma, breast, leukaemia and adrenal gland syndrome |
| SBS | short-bowel syndrome |
| SCAT | sheep cell agglutination test |
| SCBU | special care baby unit |
| SCC | 1. spinal cord compression 2. squamous cell carcinoma |
| SCID | severe combined immunodeficiency |
| SCJ | squamocolumnar junction |
| SD | standard deviation |
| SDA | specific dynamic action |
| SDH | subdural haematoma |
| SE | standard error |
| SERMs | selective (o)estrogen receptor modulators |
| SFD | small for dates |
| SFS | Social Functioning Scale |
| SGA | small for gestational age |
| SGOT | serum glutamic oxaloacetic transaminase (aspartate aminotransferase) |
| SGPT | serum glutamic pyruvic transaminase (alanine aminotransferase) |
| SHO | senior house officer |
| SI units | Système International d'Unités |
| SIADH | syndrome of inappropriate antidiuretic hormone |
| SIB | self-injurious behaviour |
| SIDS | sudden infant death syndrome |
| SIMA | system for identifying motivated abilities |
| SIMV | synchronized intermittent mandatory ventilation |
| SIRS | systemic inflammatory response syndrome |
| SLE | systemic lupus erythematosus |
| SLT | speech and language therapist/therapy |
| SMA | spinal muscular atrophy |
| SMART (goals) | specific measurable achievable realistic time oriented |
| SMBG | self-monitoring blood glucose |
| SMBR | standardized morbidity ratio |
| SMR | 1. standardized mortality ratio 2. submucous resection |
| SNB | sentinel node biopsy |
| SNP | single-nucleotide polymorphism |
| SOB | shortness of breath |
| SOAP | subjective objective assessment plan |
| SPECT | single-photon emission computed tomography |
| SPMSQ | Short Portable Mental State Questionnaire |
| SPOD | sexual problems of the disabled |
| SPSS | Statistical Package for Social Sciences |
| SSPE | subacute sclerosing panencephalitis |
| SSRIs | selective serotonin reuptake inhibitors |
| SSSS | staphylococcal scalded-skin syndrome |
| STD | sexually transmitted disease |
| STI | sexually transmitted infection |
| STM | short-term memory |

| | |
|---|---|
| SUDI | sudden unexpected death in infancy |
| Sv | sievert |
| SV | stroke volume |
| SVQs | Scottish Vocational Qualifications |
| SVR | systemic vascular resistance |
| SVT | supraventricular tachycardia |

| | |
|---|---|
| $T_3$ | triiodothyronine |
| $T_4$ | thyroxine |
| $t_{1/2}$ | half-life |
| TB | tuberculosis (tubercle bacillus) |
| TBI | total body irradiation |
| TBSA | total burn surface area |
| TCA | tricyclic antidepressant |
| TCR | T-cell receptor |
| TCRE | transcervical resection of endometrium |
| TED | thromboembolic deterrents |
| TEN | toxic epidermal necrolysis |
| TENS | transcutaneous electrical nerve stimulation |
| TEPP | tetraethyl pyrophosphate |
| TFR | total fertility rate |
| TGF | transforming growth factor |
| TIA | transient ischaemic attack |
| TIBC | total iron-binding capacity |
| TIPSS | transjugular intrahepatic portasystemic stent shunting |
| TIVA | total intravenous anaesthesia |
| TLC | total lung capacity |
| TLS | tumour lysis syndrome |
| TMJ | temporomandibular joint |
| TNF | tumour necrosis factor |
| TNM | tumour, node (lymph), metastasis |
| TOP | termination of pregnancy |
| tPA | tissue plasminogen activator |
| TPHA | *Treponema pallidum* haemagglutination assay |
| TPN | total parenteral nutrition |
| TPR | temperature, pulse, respiration |
| TQM | total quality management |
| TRH | thyrotrophin-releasing hormone |
| TRIC | trachoma inclusion conjunctivitis |
| tRNA | transfer ribonucleic acid |
| TRUS | transrectal ultrasonography |
| TSE | testicular self-examination |
| TSF | triceps skinfold thickness |
| TSH | thyroid-stimulating hormone |
| TSS | toxic shock syndrome |
| TT | tetanus toxoid |
| TTTS | twin-to-twin transfusion syndrome |
| TUR/TURP | transurethral resection of the prostate |
| TUVP | transurethral vaporization of the prostate |
| TV | tidal volume |

| | |
|---|---|
| UPPP | uvulopalatopharyngoplasty |
| URTI | upper respiratory tract infection |
| USS | ultrasound scan |
| UTI | urinary tract infection |

| | |
|---|---|
| UUPS | unexplained underperformance syndrome |
| UV | ultraviolet |

| | |
|---|---|
| v | volt |
| VADAS | voice-activated domestic appliance system |
| VAS | visual analogue scale |
| VBI | vertebrobasilar insufficiency |
| VC | vital capacity |
| VDRL | venereal disease research laboratory (test) |
| VEP | visual-evoked potentials |
| VF | ventricular fibrillation |
| VFM | value for money |
| VIP | vasoactive intestinal peptide |
| VLDL | very-low-density lipoprotein |
| VMA | vanillylmandelic acid |
| VMC | vasomotor centre |
| $VO_2$ | oxygen consumption |
| $VO_{2max}$ | maximum oxygen consumption/uptake |
| $V/Q$ | ventilation–perfusion ratio |
| VRE | vancomycin-resistant enterococci |
| VRSA | vancomycin-resistant *Staphylococcus aureus* |
| VSD | ventricular septal defect |
| VSO | Voluntary Service Overseas |
| VT | ventricular tachycardia |
| VUR | vesicoureteric reflux |
| VZIG | varicella-zoster (hyperimmune) immunoglobulin |
| VZV | varicella-zoster virus |

| | |
|---|---|
| W | watt |
| WBC | white blood cell |
| WFP | World Food Programme |
| WHO | World Health Organization |
| WPW | Wolff–Parkinson–White (syndrome) |
| WRULD | work-related upper limb disorder |

| | |
|---|---|
| XLA | X-linked agammaglobulinaemia |
| XHIM | X-linked hyper-IgM syndrome |

| | |
|---|---|
| YAG | yttrium aluminium garnet |

| | |
|---|---|
| ZIFT | zygote intrafallopian tube transfer |
| ZN | Ziehl–Neelsen (stain) |

# Appendix 7

## Useful websites

Action for Sick Children http://www.actionforsickchildren.org/
Action on Smoking and Health (ASH) http://www.ash.org.uk/
Age Concern England http://www.ace.org.uk/
Alcoholics Anonymous http://www.alcoholics-anonymous.org.uk/
Alzheimer's Society http://www.alzheimers.org.uk/
Arthritis Care http://www.arthritiscare.org.uk/
Asthma UK http://www.asthma.org.uk/
BACUP (British Association of Cancer United Patients and their Families and Friends)
    http://www.cancerbacup.org.uk
Bandolier—evidence-based thinking about healthcare http://www.jr2.ox.ac.uk/Bandolier/
Breast Cancer Care http://www.breastcancercare.org.uk/
British Allergy Foundation http://www.allergyfoundation.com
British Association/College of Occupational Therapists http://www.cot.org.uk/
British Deaf Association http://www.bda.org.uk/
British Heart Foundation http://www.bhf.org.uk/
British Liver Trust http://www.britishlivertrust.org.uk/
*British National Formulary* http://www.bnf.org.uk/
British Organ Donor Society http://www.argonet.co.uk/body
British Pregnancy Advisory Service (BPAS) http://www.bpas.org/
British Red Cross Society (BRCS) http://www.redcross.org.uk/
British Society of Hearing Therapists http://www.hearingtherapy.org/
Cancer Research UK http://www.cancerresearchuk.org/
Cardiomyopathy Association http://www.cardiomyopathy.org/
Carers UK http://www.carersonline.org.uk/
Centre for Reviews and Dissemination (York) http://www.york.ac.uk/inst/crd
Chartered Society of Physiotherapy http://www.csp.org.uk/
Cochrane Library http://www.cochrane.co.uk/
Coeliac Society http://www.coeliac.co.uk/
Commission for Equality and Human Rights http://www.cehr.org.uk/
Council for Healthcare Regulatory Excellence http://www.crhp.org.uk/
Cruse http://www.crusebereavementcare.org.uk/
Department of Health http://www.dh.gov.uk/
Diabetes UK http://www.diabetes.org.uk/
Disabled Living Foundation http://www.dlf.org.uk/
Eating Disorders Association http://www.b-eat.co.uk/
Epilepsy Action http://www.epilepsy.org.uk/
Equal Opportunities Commission http://www.eoc.org.uk
General Medical Council http://www.gmc-uk.org/
Guide Dogs for the Blind Association http://www.gdba.org.uk/
Guillain–Barré Syndrome Society http://www.gbs.org.uk/
Haemophilia Society http://www.haemophilia.org.uk/
Headway—brain injury association http://www.headway.org.uk/
Health and Safety Executive http://www.hse.gov.uk
Health Professions Council http://www.hpc-uk.org/
Health Protection Agency http://www.hpa.org.uk/
Healthcare Commission http://www.healthcarecommission.org.uk/
Help the Aged http://www.helptheaged.org.uk/

Ileostomy and Internal Pouch Support Group http://www.ileostomypouch.demon.co.uk/
Institute of Complementary Medicine http://www.icmedicine.co.uk/
International Glaucoma Association (IGA) http://www.iga.org.uk
King's Fund http://www.kingsfund.org.uk/
Leukaemia Care Society http://www.leukaemiacare.org.uk/
Leukaemia Society http://www.leukaemiasociety.org.uk/
Macmillan Cancer Support http://www.macmillan.org.uk/
Marie Curie Cancer Care http://www.mariecurie.org.uk/
Medicines and Healthcare products Regulatory Agency http://www.mhra.gov.uk/
Mencap http://www.mencap.org.uk/
Meningitis Research Foundation http://www.meningitis.org.uk/
Migraine Action Association http://www.migraine.org.uk/
MIND—National Association for Mental Health http://www.mind.org.uk/
Multiple Sclerosis Society http://www.mssociety.org.uk/
Muscular Dystrophy Campaign (MDC) http://www.muscular-dystrophy.org/
National Aids Trust http://www.nat.org.uk/
National Childbirth Trust (NCT) http://www.nctpregnancyandbabycare.com/
National Institute for Health and Clinical Excellence (NICE) http://www.nice.org.uk/
National Institute of Medical Herbalists http://www.nimh.org.uk/
National Library for Health http://www.library.nhs.uk/
National Osteoporosis Society http://www.nos.org.uk/
National Society for the Prevention of Cruelty to Children (NSPCC) http://www.nspcc.org.uk/
NHS Centre for Reviews and Dissemination (York) http://www.york.ac.uk/inst/crd
Parkinson's Disease Society http://www.parkinsons.org.uk/
Royal Association for Disability and Rehabilitation (RADAR) http://www.radar.org.uk/
Royal National Institute for the Deaf and hard of hearing people (RNID) http://www.rnid.org.uk/
Royal National Institute of the Blind (RNIB) http://www.rnib.org.uk/
Royal Society for the Prevention of Accidents (RoSPA) http://www.rospa.co.uk/
Royal Society of Medicine http://www.rsm.ac.uk/
Samaritans http://www.samaritans.org.uk/
Scoliosis Association (UK) http://www.sauk.org.uk/
Scottish Executive http://www.scotland.gov.uk/
Scottish Intercollegiate Guidelines Network (SIGN) http://www.sign.ac.uk/
Sickle Cell Society http://www.sicklecellsociety.org/
Society and College of Radiographers http://www.sor.org/
Society of Chiropodists and Podiatrists http://www.scpod.org/
St Andrew's Ambulance Association http://www.firstaid.org.uk/
St John Ambulance Association and Brigade http://www.sja.org.uk/
Stillbirth and Neonatal Death Society (SANDS) http://www.uk-sands.org/
Stroke Association http://www.stroke.org.uk/
Terrence Higgins Trust http://www.tht.org.uk/
UK National Poisons Information Services http://www.npis.org/NPIS/uknpis.htm
UK Thalassaemia Society http://www.ukts.org/
VSO (Voluntary Service Overseas) http://www.vso.org.uk/
World Health Organization http://www.who.org

## Appendix 8

### Chemical symbols and formulae

| | | | |
|---|---|---|---|
| Aluminium | Al | Mercury | Hg |
| Ammonia | $NH_3$ | Molybdenum | Mo |
| Ammonium | $NH_4$ | Nickel | Ni |
| Barium | Ba | Nitrate | $NO_3$ |
| Bicarbonate (hydrogen carbonate) | $HCO_3$ | Nitric acid | $HNO_3$ |
| Cadmium | Cd | Nitrogen | N |
| Caesium | Cs | Oxygen | O |
| Calcium | Ca | Phosphate | $PO_4$ |
| Carbon | C | Phosphorus | P |
| Carbonic acid | $H_2CO_3$ | Potassium | K |
| Carbon dioxide | $CO_2$ | Potassium chloride | KCl |
| Chlorine | Cl | Radium | Ra |
| Chromium | Cr | Selenium | Se |
| Cobalt | Co | Silicon | Si |
| Copper | Cu | Silver | Ag |
| Fluorine | F | Sodium | Na |
| Gold | Au | Sodium bicarbonate | $NaHCO_3$ |
| Helium | He | Sodium chloride | NaCl |
| Hydrochloric acid | HCl | Sodium hydroxide | NaOH |
| Hydrogen | H | Strontium | Sr |
| Hydrogen phosphate | $HPO_4$ | Sulphate | $SO_4$ |
| Hydroxide | OH | Sulphur | S |
| Iodine | I | Sulphuric acid | $H_2SO_4$ |
| Iridium | Ir | Technetium | Tc |
| Iron | Fe | Thallium | Tl |
| Lead | Pb | Vanadium | V |
| Lithium | Li | Water | $H_2O$ |
| Magnesium | Mg | Xenon | Xe |
| Magnesium sulphate | $MgSO_4$ | Yttrium | Y |
| Manganese | Mn | Zinc | Zn |

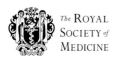

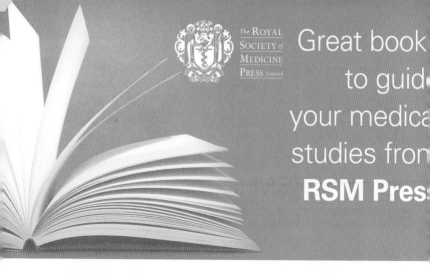
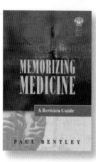
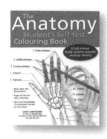

## ELSEVIER DVD-ROM LICENCE AGREEMENT

PLEASE READ THE FOLLOWING AGREEMENT CAREFULLY BEFORE USING THIS PRODUCT. THIS PRODUCT IS LICENSED UNDER THE TERMS CONTAINED IN THIS LICENCE AGREEMENT ('Agreement'). BY USING THIS PRODUCT, YOU, AN INDIVIDUAL OR ENTITY INCLUDING EMPLOYEES, AGENTS AND REPRESENTATIVES ('You' or 'Your'), ACKNOWLEDGE THAT YOU HAVE READ THIS AGREEMENT, THAT YOU UNDERSTAND IT, AND THAT YOU AGREE TO BE BOUND BY THE TERMS AND CONDITIONS OF THIS AGREEMENT. ELSEVIER LIMITED ('Elsevier') EXPRESSLY DOES NOT AGREE TO LICENSE THIS PRODUCT TO YOU UNLESS YOU ASSENT TO THIS AGREEMENT. IF YOU DO NOT AGREE WITH ANY OF THE FOLLOWING TERMS, YOU MAY, WITHIN THIRTY (30) DAYS AFTER YOUR RECEIPT OF THIS PRODUCT RETURN THE UNUSED PRODUCT AND ALL ACCOMPANYING DOCUMENTATION TO ELSEVIER FOR A FULL REFUND.

**DEFINITIONS** As used in this Agreement, these terms shall have the following meanings:

'Proprietary Material' means the valuable and proprietary information content of this Product including without limitation all indexes and graphic materials and software used to access, index, search and retrieve the information content from this Product developed or licensed by Elsevier and/or its affiliates, suppliers and licensors.

'Product' means the copy of the Proprietary Material and any other material delivered on DVD-ROM and any other human-readable or machine-readable materials enclosed with this Agreement, including without limitation documentation relating to the same.

**OWNERSHIP** This Product has been supplied by and is proprietary to Elsevier and/or its affiliates, suppliers and licensors. The copyright in the Product belongs to Elsevier and/or its affiliates, suppliers and licensors and is protected by the copyright, trademark, trade secret and other intellectual property laws of the United Kingdom and international treaty provisions, including without limitation the Universal Copyright Convention and the Berne Copyright Convention. You have no ownership rights in this Product. Except as expressly set forth herein, no part of this Product, including without limitation the Proprietary Material, may be modified, copied or distributed in hardcopy or machine-readable form without prior written consent from Elsevier. All rights not expressly granted to You herein are expressly reserved. Any other use of this Product by any person or entity is strictly prohibited and a violation of this Agreement.

**SCOPE OF RIGHTS LICENSED (PERMITTED USES)** Elsevier is granting to You a limited, non-exclusive, non-transferable licence to use this Product in accordance with the terms of this Agreement. You may use or provide access to this Product on a single computer or terminal physically located at Your premises and in a secure network or move this Product to and use it on another single computer or terminal at the same location for personal use only, but under no circumstances may You use or provide access to any part or parts of this Product on more than one computer or terminal simultaneously.

You shall not (a) copy, download, or otherwise reproduce the Product or any part(s) thereof in any medium, including, without limitation, online transmissions, local area networks, wide area networks, intranets, extranets and the Internet, or in any way, in whole or in part, except for printing out or downloading nonsubstantial portions of the text and images in the Product for Your own personal use; (b) alter, modify, or adapt the Product or any part(s) thereof, including but not limited to decompiling, disassembling, reverse engineering, or creating derivative works, without the prior written approval of Elsevier; (c) sell, license or otherwise distribute to third parties the Product or any part(s) thereof; or (d) alter, remove, obscure or obstruct the display of any copyright, trademark or other proprietary notice on or in the Product or on any printout or download of portions of the Proprietary Materials.

**RESTRICTIONS ON TRANSFER** This Licence is personal to You, and neither Your rights hereunder nor the tangible embodiments of this Product, including without limitation the Proprietary Material, may be sold, assigned, transferred or sublicensed to any other person, including without limitation by operation of law, without the prior written consent of Elsevier. Any purported sale, assignment, transfer or sublicense without the prior written consent of Elsevier will be void and will automatically terminate the Licence granted hereunder.

**TERM** This Agreement will remain in effect until terminated pursuant to the terms of this Agreement. You may terminate this Agreement at any time by removing from Your system and destroying the Product and any copies of the Proprietary Material. Unauthorized copying of the Product, including without limitation, the Proprietary Material and documentation, or otherwise failing to comply with the terms and conditions of this Agreement shall result in automatic termination of this licence and will make available to Elsevier legal remedies. Upon termination of this Agreement, the licence granted herein will terminate and You must immediately destroy the Product and all copies of the Product and of the Proprietary Material, together with any and all accompanying documentation. All provisions relating to proprietary rights shall survive termination of this Agreement.

**LIMITED WARRANTY AND LIMITATION OF LIABILITY** Elsevier warrants that the software embodied in this Product will perform in substantial compliance with the documentation supplied in this Product, unless the performance problems are the result of hardware failure or improper use. If You report a significant defect in performance in writing to Elsevier within ninety (90) calendar days of your having purchased the Product, and Elsevier is not able to correct same within sixty (60) days after its receipt of Your notification, You may return this Product, including all copies and documentation, to Elsevier and Elsevier will refund Your money. In order to apply for a refund on your purchased Product, please contact the return address on the invoice to obtain the refund request form ('Refund Request Form'), and either fax or mail your signed request and your proof of purchase to the address indicated on the Refund Request Form. Incomplete forms will not be processed. Defined terms in the Refund Request Form shall have the same meaning as in this Agreement.

YOU UNDERSTAND THAT, EXCEPT FOR THE LIMITED WARRANTY RECITED ABOVE, ELSEVIER, ITS AFFILIATES, LICENSORS, THIRD PARTY SUPPLIERS AND AGENTS (TOGETHER 'THE SUPPLIERS') MAKE NO REPRESENTATIONS OR WARRANTIES, WITH RESPECT TO THE PRODUCT, INCLUDING, WITHOUT LIMITATION THE PROPRIETARY MATERIAL. ALL OTHER REPRESENTATIONS, WARRANTIES, CONDITIONS OR OTHER TERMS, WHETHER EXPRESS OR IMPLIED BY STATUTE OR COMMON LAW, ARE HEREBY EXCLUDED TO THE FULLEST EXTENT PERMITTED BY LAW.

IN PARTICULAR BUT WITHOUT LIMITATION TO THE FOREGOING NONE OF THE SUPPLIERS MAKE ANY REPRESENTIONS OR WARRANTIES (WHETHER EXPRESS OR IMPLIED) REGARDING THE PERFORMANCE OF YOUR PAD, NETWORK OR COMPUTER SYSTEM WHEN USED IN CONJUNCTION WITH THE PRODUCT, NOR THAT THE PRODUCT WILL MEET YOUR REQUIREMENTS OR THAT ITS OPERATION WILL BE UNINTERRUPTED OR ERROR-FREE.

EXCEPT IN RESPECT OF DEATH OR PERSONAL INJURY CAUSED BY THE SUPPLIERS' NEGLIGENCE AND TO THE FULLEST EXTENT PERMITTED BY LAW, IN NO EVENT (AND REGARDLESS OF WHETHER SUCH DAMAGES ARE FORESEEABLE AND OF WHETHER SUCH

LIABILITY IS BASED IN TORT, CONTRACT OR OTHERWISE) WILL ANY OF THE SUPPLIERS BE LIABLE TO YOU FOR ANY DAMAGES (INCLUDING, WITHOUT LIMITATION, ANY LOST PROFITS, LOST SAVINGS OR OTHER SPECIAL, INDIRECT, INCIDENTAL OR CONSEQUENTIAL DAMAGES ARISING OUT OF OR RESULTING FROM: (I) YOUR USE OF, OR INABILITY TO USE, THE PRODUCT; (II) DATA LOSS OR CORRUPTION; AND/OR (III) ERRORS OR OMISSIONS IN THE PROPRIETARY MATERIAL.

IF THE FOREGOING LIMITATION IS HELD TO BE UNENFORCEABLE, OUR MAXIMUM LIABILITY TO YOU IN RESPECT THEREOF SHALL NOT EXCEED THE AMOUNT OF THE LICENCE FEE PAID BY YOU FOR THE PRODUCT. THE REMEDIES AVAILABLE TO YOU AGAINST ELSEVIER AND THE LICENSORS OF MATERIALS INCLUDED IN THE PRODUCT ARE EXCLUSIVE.

If the information provided in the Product contains medical or health sciences information, it is intended for professional use within the medical field. Information about medical treatment or drug dosages is intended strictly for professional use, and because of rapid advances in the medical sciences, independent verification of diagnosis and drug dosages should be made.

The provisions of this Agreement shall be severable, and in the event that any provision of this Agreement is found to be legally unenforceable, such unenforceability shall not prevent the enforcement or any other provision of this Agreement.

**GOVERNING LAW** This Agreement shall be governed by the laws of England and Wales. In any dispute arising out of this Agreement, you and Elsevier each consent to the exclusive personal jurisdiction and venue in the courts of England and Wales.